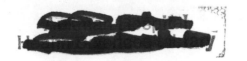

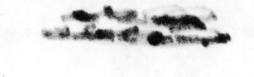

DIFFERENTIAL DIAGNOSIS
OF ACUTE PAIN
BY
BODY
REGION

DIFFERENTIAL DIAGNOSIS
OF ACUTE PAIN
BY
BODY
REGION

Stanley L. Wiener, M.D.

Professor of Medicine
Formerly, Chief, Section of General Internal Medicine
The University of Illinois
College of Medicine at Chicago
Chicago, Illinois

McGRAW-HILL, INC.
Health Professions Division

New York   St. Louis   San Francisco   Auckland   Bogotá   Caracas
Lisbon   London   Madrid   Mexico   Milan   Montreal   New Delhi
Paris   San Juan   Singapore   Sydney   Tokyo   Toronto

14156

2 3 4 5 6 7 8 9   DOWDOW   9 8 7 6 5 4 3

INTERNATIONAL EDITION ISBN 0-07-112996-0

ISBN 0-07-070177-6

This book was set in Times Roman by Waldman Graphics, Inc.
The editors were J. Dereck Jeffers and Lester A. Sheinis; the
production supervisor was Clare Stanley; the text designer was
Judy Allan / The Designing Woman Concepts; the front matter
and cover designer was Edward R. Schultheis; the internal art
designer was Shiere Melin; the indexer was Irving Conde Tullar.
R. R. Donnelley & Sons Company was printer and binder.

Library of Congress Cataloging-in-Publication Data

Wiener, Stanley L.
    Differential diagnosis of acute pain : by body region /
Stanley L. Wiener.
        p.   cm.
    Includes bibliographical references and index.
    ISBN 0-07-070177-6
    1. Pain—Diagnosis. 2. Diagnosis, Differential. I. Title.
    [DNLM: 1. Acute Disease. 2. Diagnosis, Differential.
3. Pain— diagnosis.   WB 176 W647d]
RB127.W53   1993
616′.0472—dc20
DNLM/DLC
for Library of Congress   92-49473
                                                       CIP

To my father, Irving I. Wiener (1902–1991),
whose honesty, integrity, kindness, and concern for the less fortunate
have been a major influence in my life.

CONTENTS

PREFACE

This book is designed and written to make the differential diagnosis of acute pain in any region easier, faster, and more thorough. Acute pain is defined as pain that is severe, unremitting, of recent or abrupt onset, associated with other severe and worrisome symptoms, and resistant to simple medication and other measures. This is not another volume on pain management designed to deal with the less than 1 percent of patients who suffer from severe, difficult to control, chronic pain.

The diagnosis of the cause of regional or generalized pain is a fundamental and high-frequency problem in clinical medicine. The National Ambulatory Care Survey (NAMCS) in 1975 determined that 9 of the top 15 new problem encounters with patients were for pain in a specific region. For example, sore throat, lower extremity, abdominal, and upper extremity pain were the top 4 reasons for a visit to a physician.

Clinical studies at the University of Illinois College of Medicine Walk-In Clinic during the mid-1980s confirmed the NAMCS data. Fifty-eight percent of 3427 patients' chief complaints involved pain in a specific location. The top 6 chief complaints were pain in the abdomen, low back, chest, lower extremity, head, and upper extremity, accounting for 78 percent of the patients with the 10 most frequent complaints.

At Illinois Masonic Hospital, a major Chicago community hospital, 36 percent of admission chief complaints on the Medical Service (575 admissions) were a regional or generalized pain. Pain in the chest, abdomen, extremities, or low back constituted 4 of the top 5 reasons for admission to the Medical Service.

One of the major difficulties with the diagnosis of regional or generalized pain and other symptoms of disease is that the possible causes fall into many specialties and subspecialties. The diagnostic lists in this text cross all clinical subspecialty and specialty boundaries. The probability that the cause of a regional or generalized pain is not listed is very low and difficult to estimate, but it is probably less than 1 percent.

The book is "user friendly." A "rogues' gallery" of shaded pain diagrams of different body regions appears in the front. The reader can match the patient's pain location to one or more diagrams that contain the patient's pain site within their shaded area. The chapter number under the selected diagram will direct the reader to the appropriate chapter that discusses pain in that location. In cases where the chapter title matches the patient's complaint (e.g., Chapter 2), use of the diagrams is unnecessary.

Each chapter begins with a Diagnostic List of the causes of pain in the region covered by that chapter. The Summary provides the reader with a brief account of each of the disorders

listed, and a concise discussion of the clinical, laboratory, imaging, and response to therapy differences between them.

A Table of Incidence is included to inform the reader about the relative frequency of the diseases on the Diagnostic List. It provides only an approximate estimate of what is common, uncommon, or rare. The frequency or prior probability of a cause of a specific regional pain may vary with age, sex, race, ethnic origin, family history, risk factors, climate, season, geographic region, and other variables. The Table of Incidence is derived from the clinical experience of the author and subspecialists at the University of Illinois College of Medicine at Chicago, incidence data available in the medical literature, and the size of reported series of specific diagnostic entities published by major medical centers.

The Description of Listed Diseases section discusses each disorder on the Diagnostic List and provides a careful and detailed description of the clinical characteristics of the regional pain associated with that disorder, as well as a discussion of the common examination, laboratory, and imaging findings associated with that disease. When appropriate, the effects of a specific therapy on the listed disorder are also used for diagnosis. Criteria for establishing specific diagnoses have been provided when they were available in the literature and developed by a major subspecialty organization (e.g., American Rheumatism Association).

Because painful diseases may masquerade as other diseases, many chapters have sections on diseases that mimic high-frequency disorders.

This is the first time that acute pain as a symptom of disease has been covered in great detail for the entire human body in a single volume. Diagnostic lists cover the entire body (e.g., generalized pain), large regions (e.g., generalized abdominal pain, upper and lower arm pain), smaller regions (e.g., the wrist and hand, the foot), and small areas within a region (e.g., forefoot, midfoot, and hindfoot pain). The reason for the explicit treatment of acute pain in such detail in this volume is that the book is patterned after the way patients with pain frequently present.

General textbooks in internal medicine, surgery, and obstetrics and gynecology are of greatest value once a diagnosis is established. This book begins with a symptom (e.g., pain in a specific region) and helps the physician establish a specific diagnosis. Further reading in excellent textbooks, like *Harrison's Principles of Internal Medicine* or Schwartz's *Principles of Surgery*, will provide supplementary information on pathophysiology, therapy, and prophylaxis, and the management of the diagnosed disease.

Primary care physicians in internal medicine and family practice, emergency physicians, medical and surgical residents, and medical students should find this book helpful because they encounter many patients every day with pain as a symptom of disease. Subspecialists will also benefit because they may be unfamiliar with the other causes of pain in a specific region that fall outside their area of expertise. For example, an orthopedic surgeon may be unfamiliar with some of the rheumatologic, infectious, neurologic, vascular, and hematologic diseases that can cause knee or leg pain and masquerade as an orthopedic problem. This book will facilitate rapid acquisition of information for the subspecialist who wishes to expand his or her knowledge of the causes of pain and methods of diagnosis.

ACKNOWLEDGMENTS

Many of the detailed descriptions of the pain associated with a specific disease were recorded by the author and other faculty members (e.g., Mark Kushner, M.D., and Reza Kiani, M.D.) during interviews with patients with a confirmed diagnosis. I express my appreciation for the cooperation of these people.

I also wish to express my gratitude to the following past and present University of Illinois College of Medicine faculty for lectures, conferences, personal discussions, or reprints of their articles and other publications that they provided me with during the writing of this book: Lloyd M. Nyhus, M.D., Professor of Surgery (abdominal pain); Richard L. Nelson, M.D., Associate Professor of Surgery (anorectal pain); Bruce Brundage, M.D., Professor of Medicine and Chief of the Section of Cardiology (chest pain of cardiac origin); Melvin Lopata, M.D., Professor of Medicine and Chief, Section of Pulmonary Medicine (chest pain of pulmonary origin); Paul K. Schlesinger, M.D., Associate Professor of Clinical Medicine and Gastroenterology (esophageal chest pain); Edward Applebaum, M.D., Professor of Otolaryngology, and Barry Wenig, M.D., Director of Head and Neck Surgery (otolaryngology) (facial, nose, ear, throat, and neck pain); Bernardo Duarte, M.D., Clinical Assistant Professor of Surgery (neck pain); John Spellacy, M.D., Professor and Head of the Department of Obstetrics and Gynecology (pelvic, perineal, and labial pain); Morton Goldberg, M.D., Professor and Head of the Department of Ophthalmology, and Jacob Wilensky, M.D., Professor of Ophthalmology (eye pain); Cathy Helgason, M.D., Assistant Professor of Neurology (half body, neuropathic limb pain, headache); Lawrence M. Solomon, M.D., Professor and Head of Dermatology (generalized and localized skin pain); John Skosey, M.D., Professor of Medicine and Chief of the Section of Rheumatology (generalized and localized joint pain); Andrew Wilbur, M.D., Assistant Professor of Radiology (CT radiology); Martin Lazarus, M.D., Assistant Professor of Radiology (bone radiology and MRI); Riad Barmada, M.D., Professor and Head of Orthopedics (low back, hip pain); David L. Spencer, M.D., Associate Professor of Orthopedics (back and buttock pain); Alon Winnie, M.D., Professor of Anesthesiology, Director, Pain Control Center (psychogenic pain, reflex sympathetic dystrophy, and other causes of limb pain); Mabel Koshy, M.D., Professor of Medicine (sickle cell pain crisis); Roohollah Sharifi, M.D., Professor of Clinical Surgery and Urology (perineal, suprapubic, and prostate-related pain); Jose A.L. Arruda, M.D., Professor of Medicine and Chief of the Section of Nephrology (flank and renal pain); and James J. Schuler, M.D., Associate Professor and Chief, Division of Vascular Surgery (vascular limb pain).

In addition, I wish to thank Richard Corzatt, M.D. (Orthopedics), formerly a Chicago White Sox physician (back and limb pain).

I wish to thank Shiere Melin for her excellent line drawings and Sheila (Rosner) Heusmann for photocopying thousands of articles, aiding me in preparing reprint files, and for rapid, accurate, and meticulous manuscript preparation. I wish to thank copy editors Howard Runyon and Pamela Ann Lloyd, and editors J. Dereck Jeffers (editor-in-chief) and Lester A. Sheinis at McGraw-Hill for their efficient help and support.

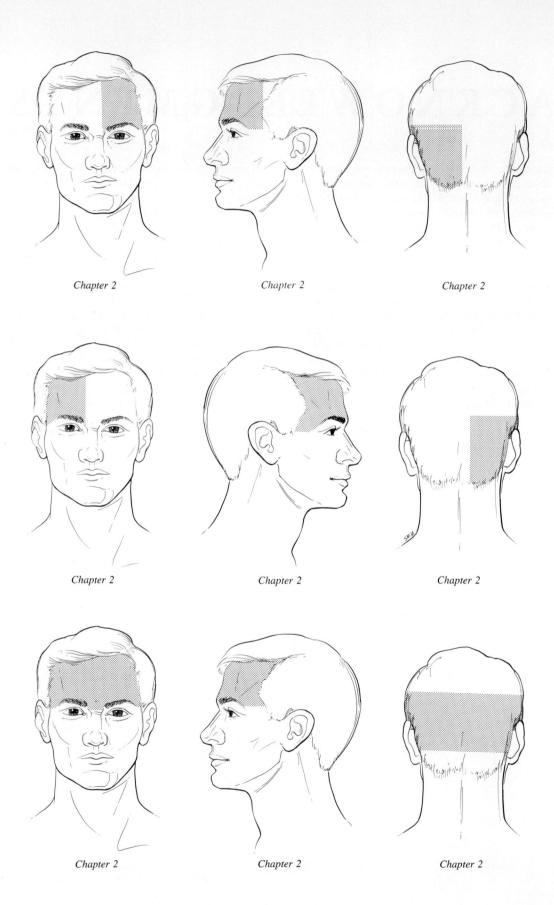

Chapter 2

Chapter 2

Chapter 2

Chapter 2

Chapter 2

Chapter 2

Chapter 2

Chapter 2

Chapter 2

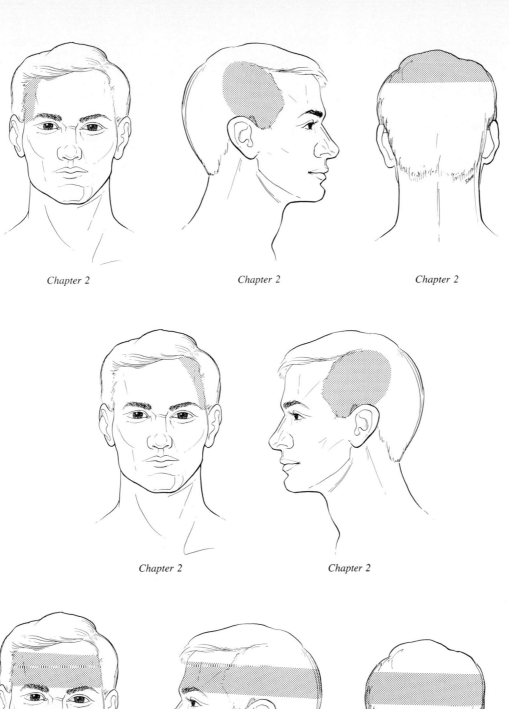

Chapter 2   *Chapter 2*   *Chapter 2*

Chapter 2   *Chapter 2*

Chapter 2   *Chapter 2*   *Chapter 2*

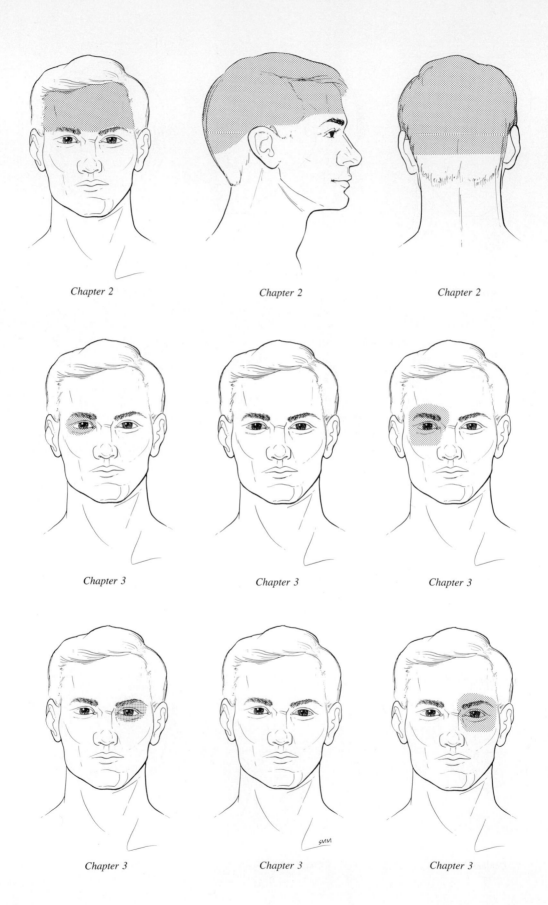

Chapter 2   *Chapter 2*   *Chapter 2*

Chapter 3   *Chapter 3*   *Chapter 3*

Chapter 3   *Chapter 3*   *Chapter 3*

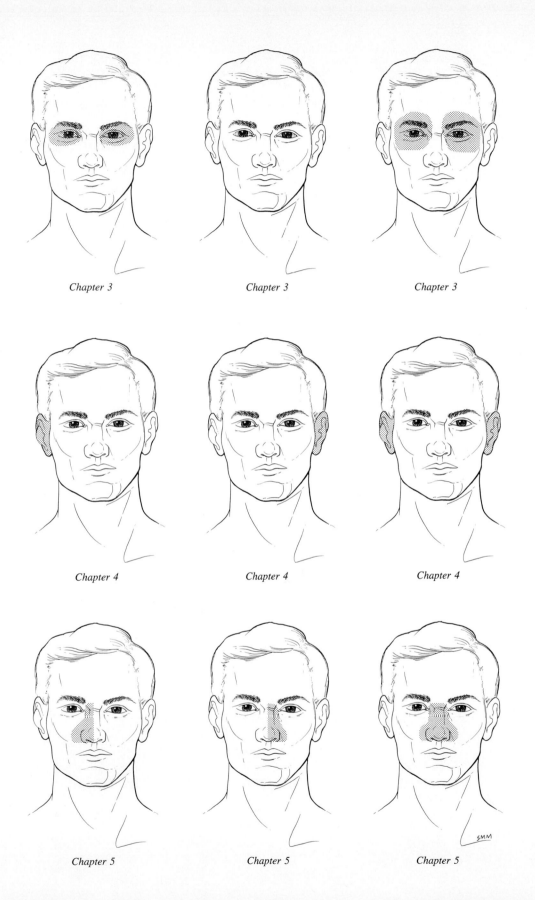

Chapter 3 Chapter 3 Chapter 3

Chapter 4 Chapter 4 Chapter 4

Chapter 5 Chapter 5 Chapter 5

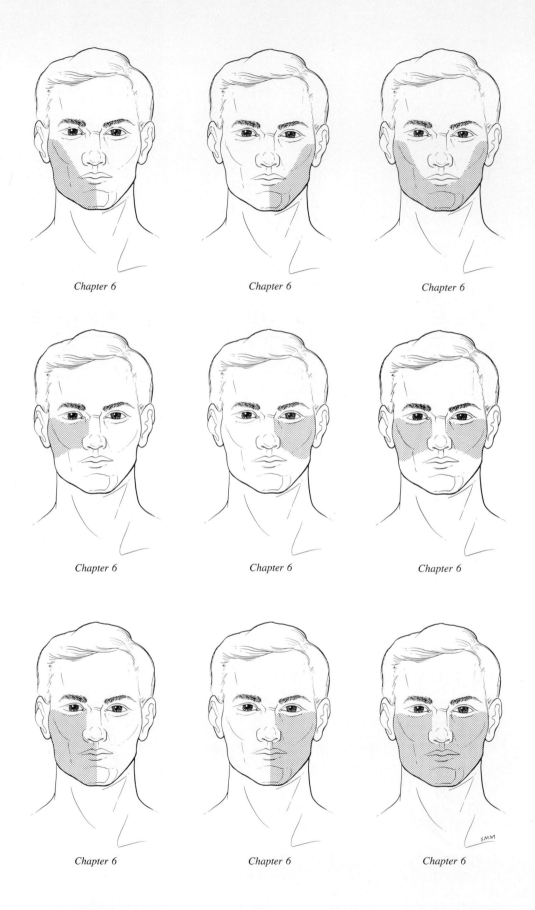

Chapter 6

Chapter 6

Chapter 6

Chapter 6

Chapter 6

Chapter 6

Chapter 6

Chapter 6

Chapter 6

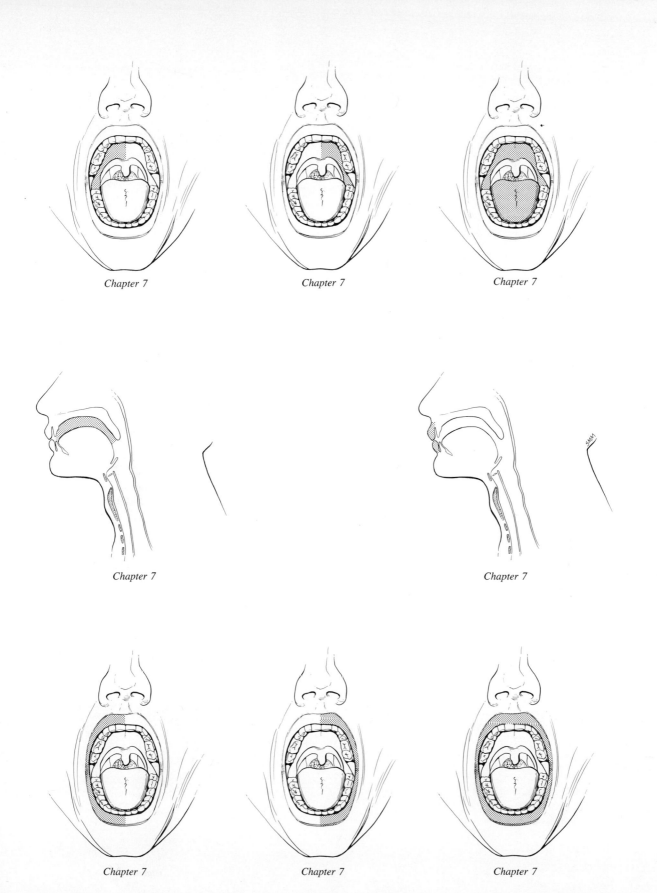

Chapter 7

Chapter 7

Chapter 7

Chapter 7

Chapter 7

Chapter 7

Chapter 7

Chapter 7

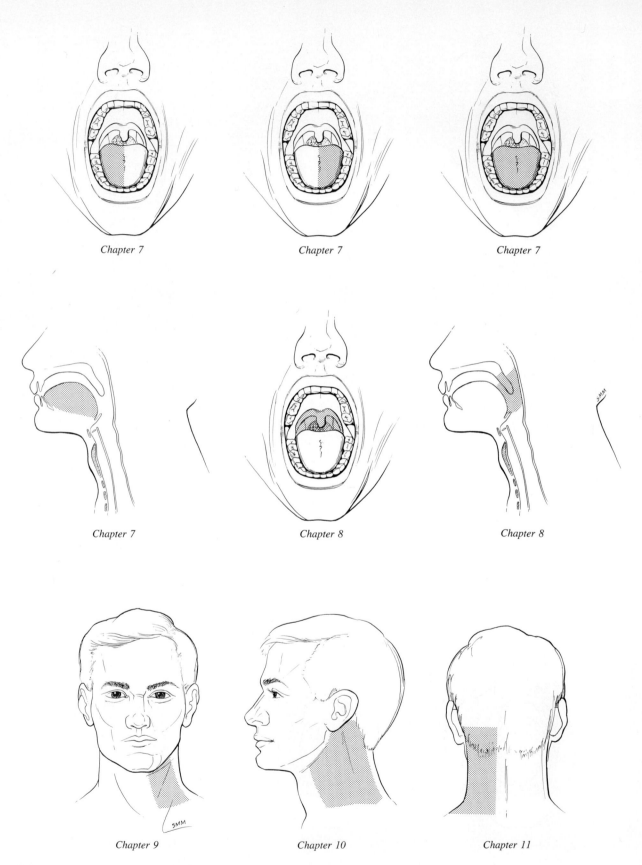

Chapter 7

Chapter 7

Chapter 7

Chapter 7

Chapter 8

Chapter 8

Chapter 9

Chapter 10

Chapter 11

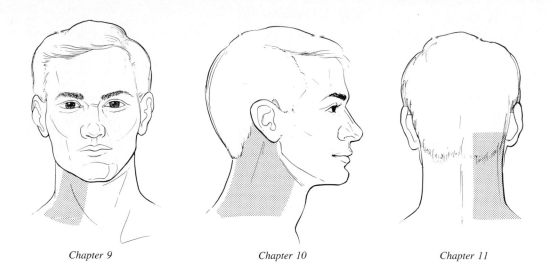

Chapter 9   *Chapter 10*   *Chapter 11*

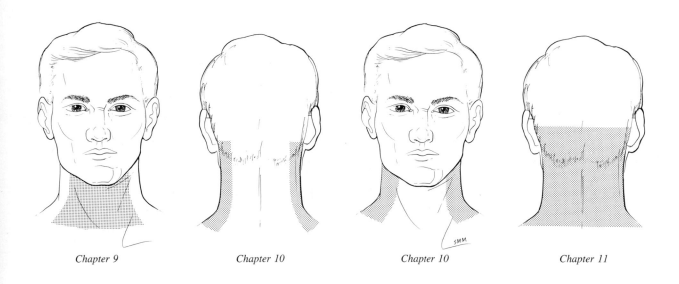

Chapter 9   *Chapter 10*   *Chapter 10*   *Chapter 11*

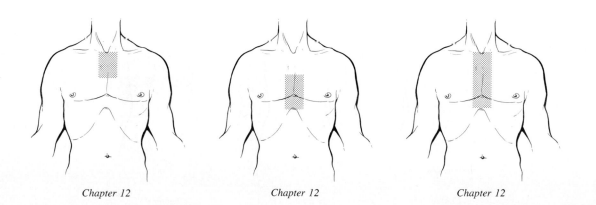

Chapter 12   *Chapter 12*   *Chapter 12*

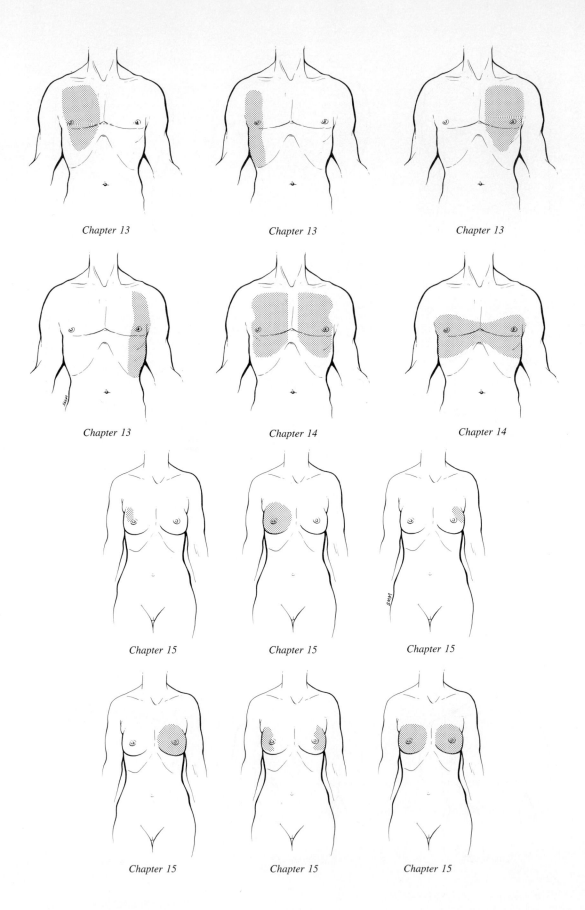

Chapter 13

Chapter 13

Chapter 13

Chapter 13

Chapter 14

Chapter 14

Chapter 15

Chapter 15

Chapter 15

Chapter 15

Chapter 15

Chapter 15

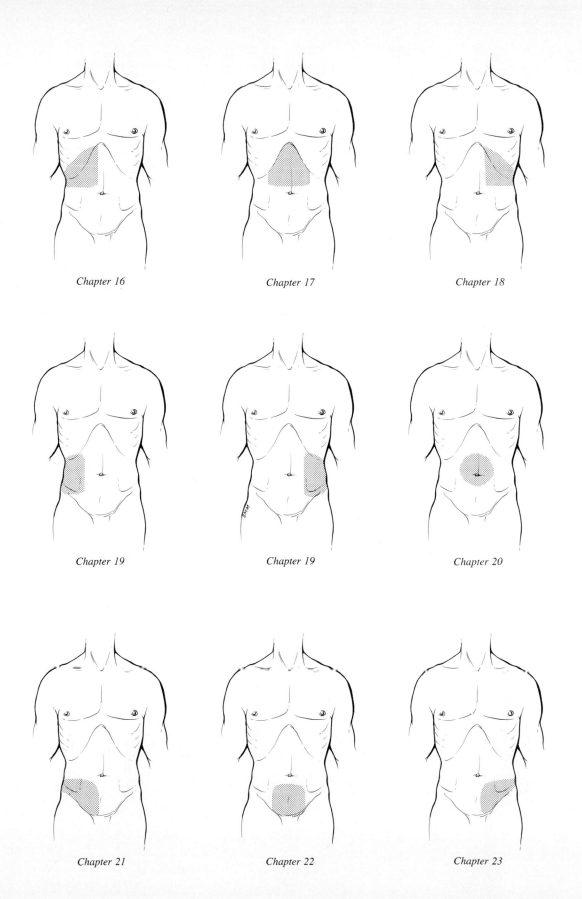

Chapter 16

Chapter 17

Chapter 18

Chapter 19

Chapter 19

Chapter 20

Chapter 21

Chapter 22

Chapter 23

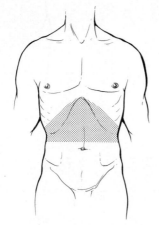

Chapter 24

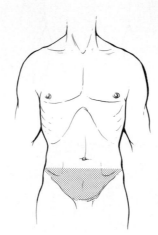

Chapter 25

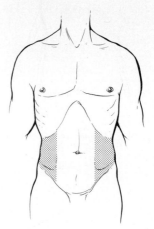

Chapter 26

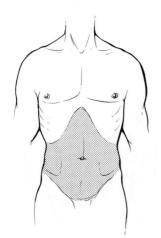

Chapter 27

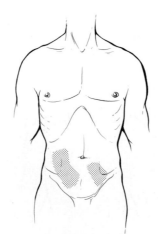

Chapter 28

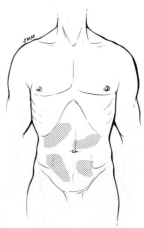

Chapter 28

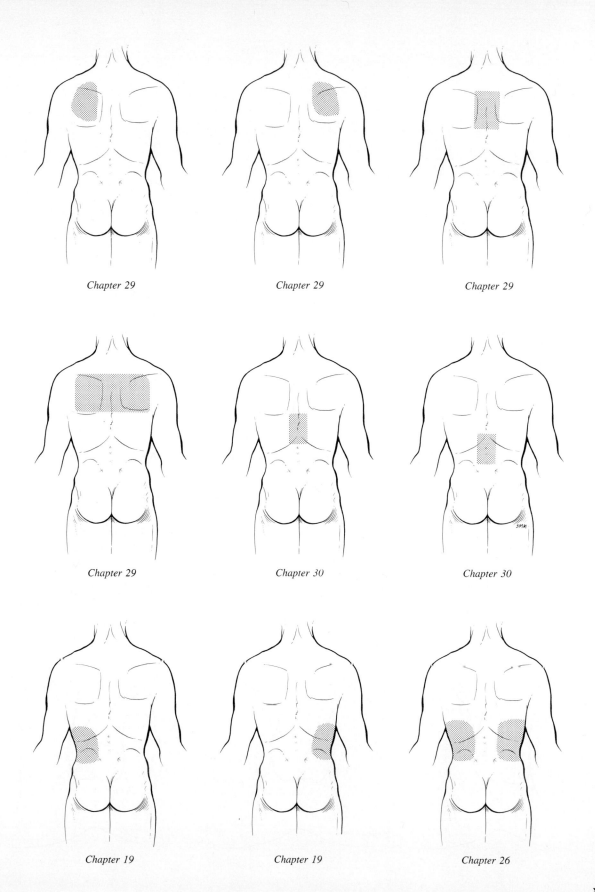

Chapter 29

Chapter 29

Chapter 29

Chapter 29

Chapter 30

Chapter 30

Chapter 19

Chapter 19

Chapter 26

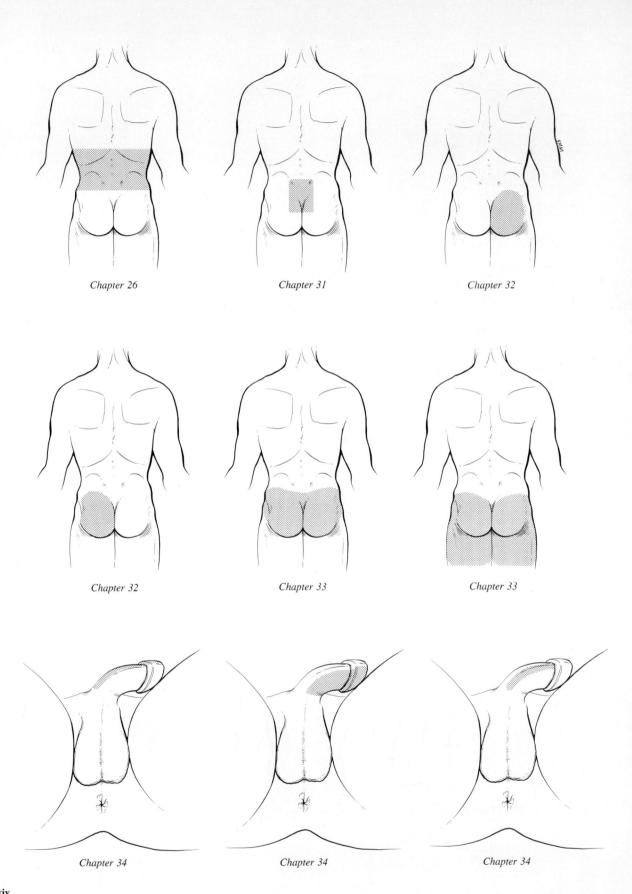

Chapter 26

Chapter 31

Chapter 32

Chapter 32

Chapter 33

Chapter 33

Chapter 34

Chapter 34

Chapter 34

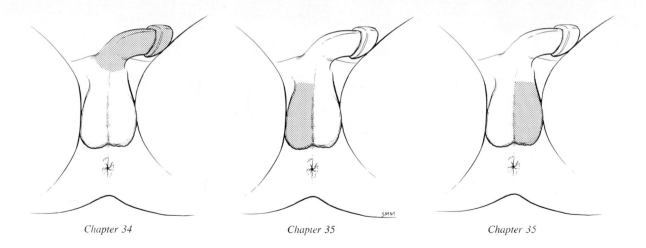

Chapter 34

Chapter 35

Chapter 35

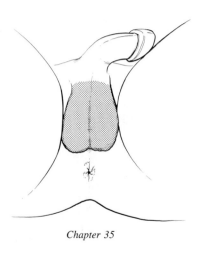

Chapter 35

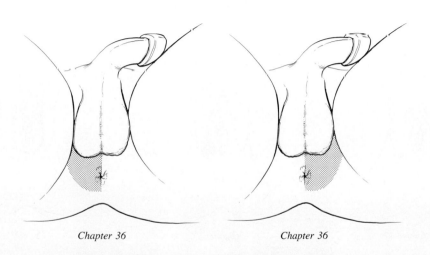

Chapter 36

Chapter 36

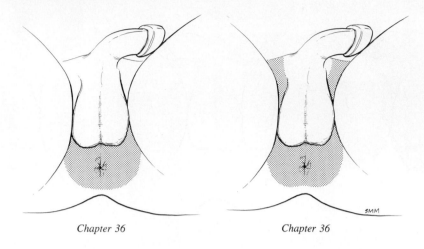

Chapter 36   *Chapter 36*

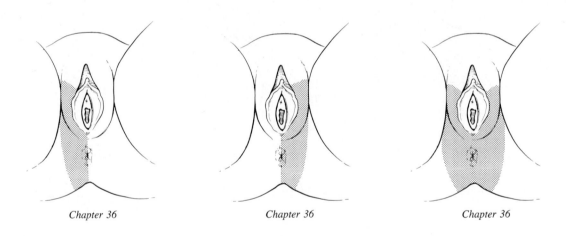

Chapter 36   *Chapter 36*   *Chapter 36*

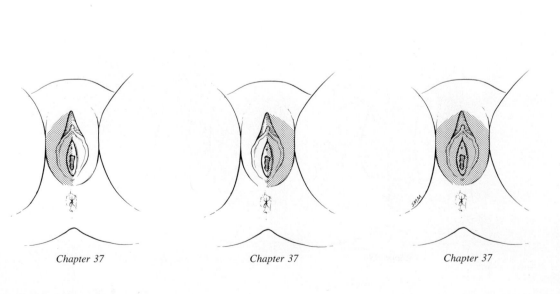

Chapter 37   *Chapter 37*   *Chapter 37*

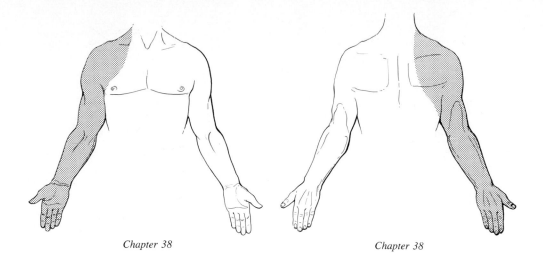

Chapter 38

Chapter 38

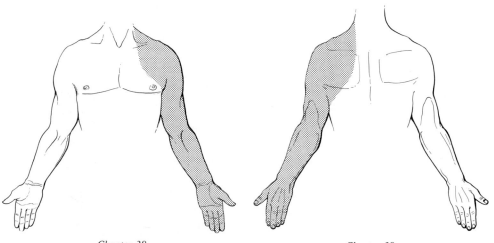

Chapter 38

Chapter 38

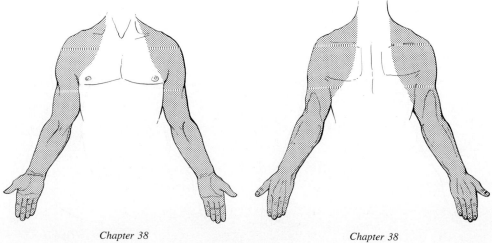

Chapter 38

Chapter 38

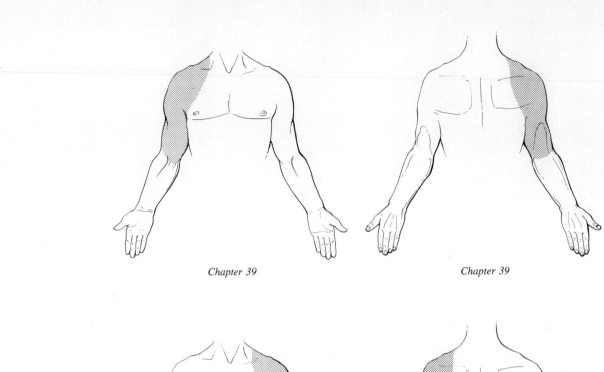

Chapter 39

Chapter 39

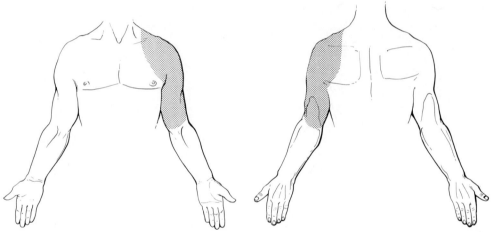

Chapter 39

Chapter 39

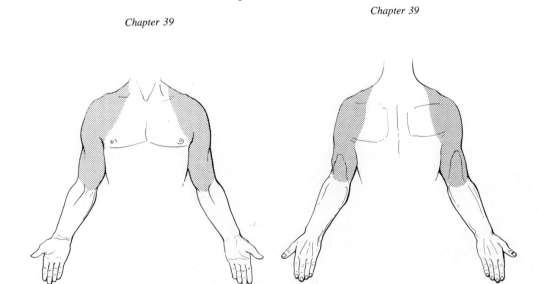

Chapter 39

Chapter 39

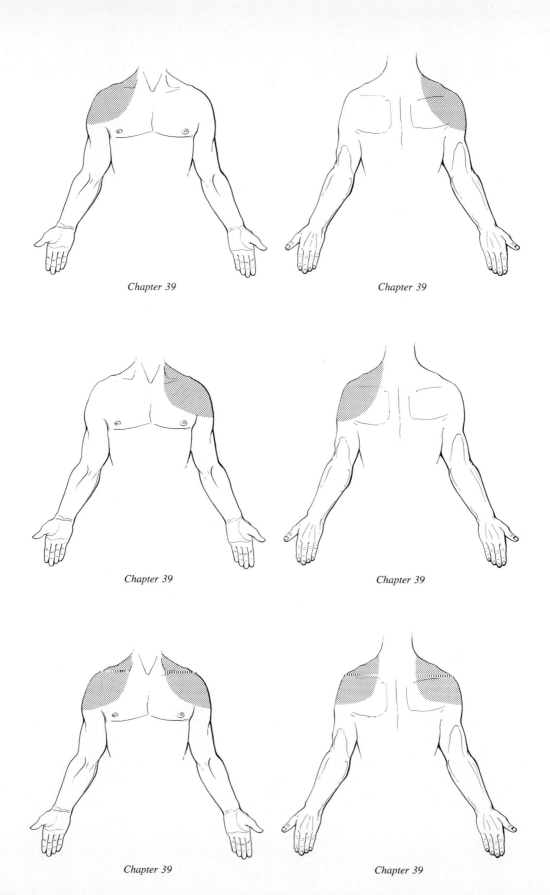

Chapter 39

Chapter 39

Chapter 39

Chapter 39

Chapter 39

Chapter 39

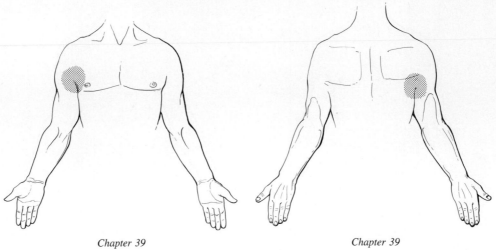

Chapter 39   *Chapter 39*

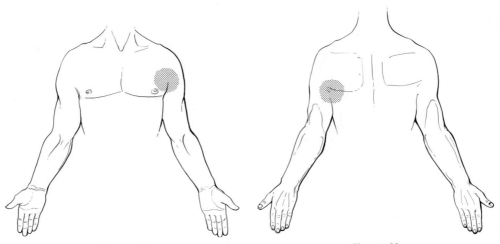

Chapter 39   *Chapter 39*

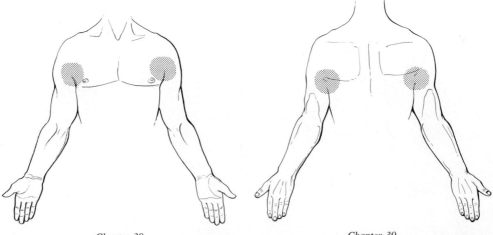

Chapter 39   *Chapter 39*

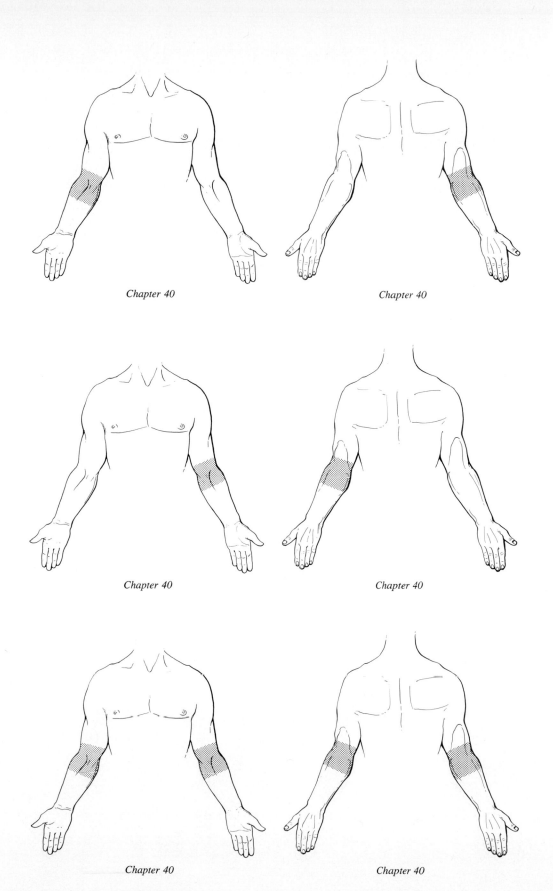

Chapter 40 *Chapter 40*

Chapter 40 *Chapter 40*

Chapter 40 *Chapter 40*

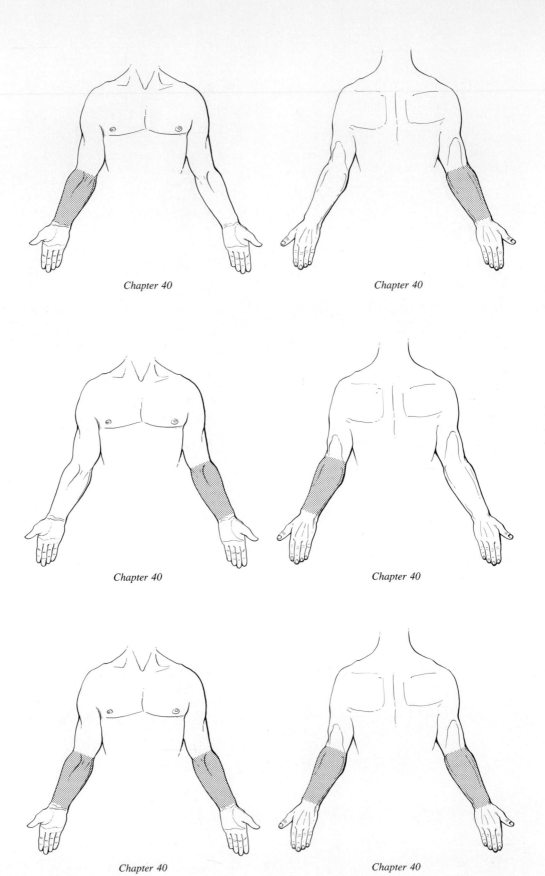

Chapter 40

Chapter 40

Chapter 40

Chapter 40

Chapter 40

Chapter 40

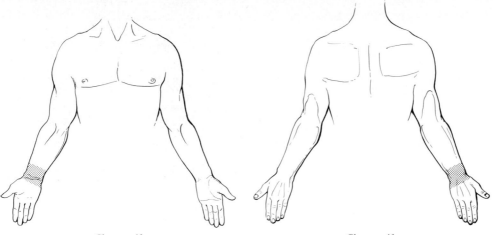

Chapter 41

Chapter 41

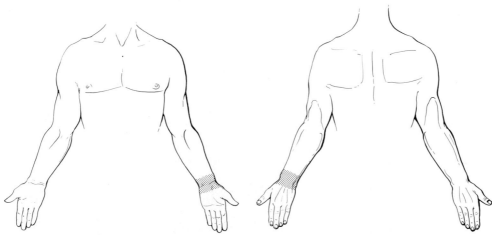

Chapter 41

Chapter 41

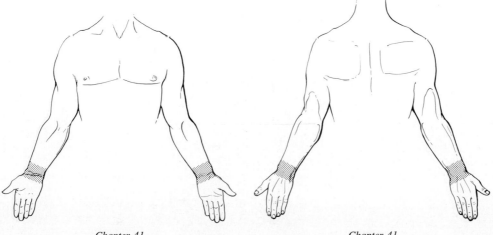

Chapter 41

Chapter 41

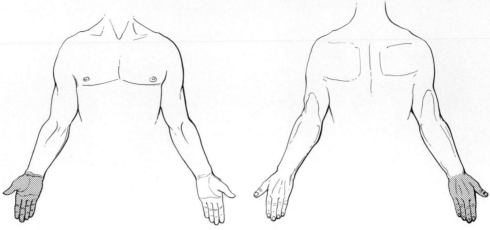

Chapter 41   *Chapter 41*

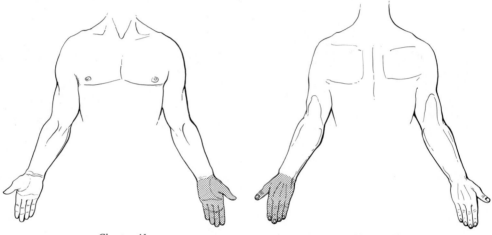

Chapter 41   *Chapter 41*

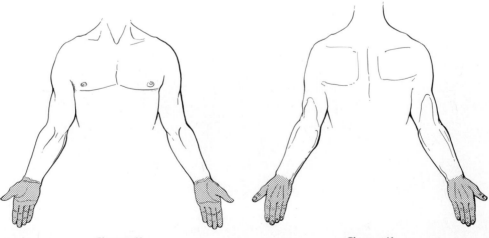

Chapter 41   *Chapter 41*

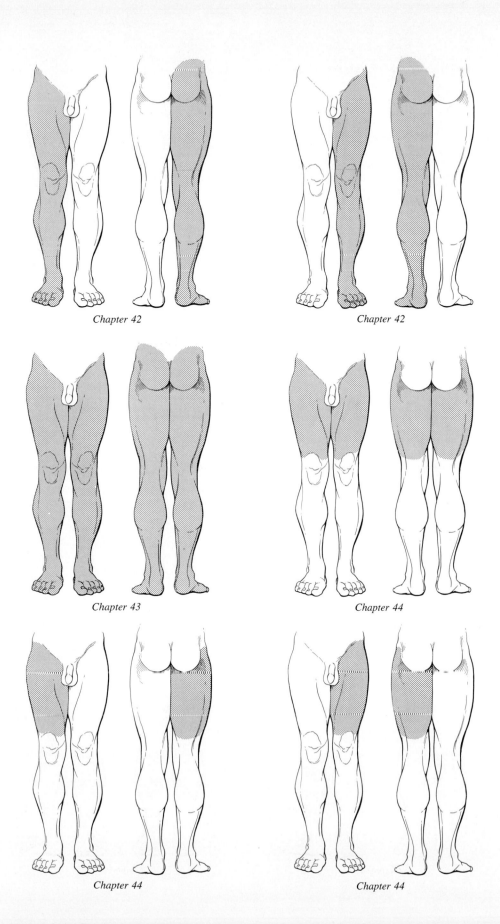

Chapter 42

Chapter 42

Chapter 43

Chapter 44

Chapter 44

Chapter 44

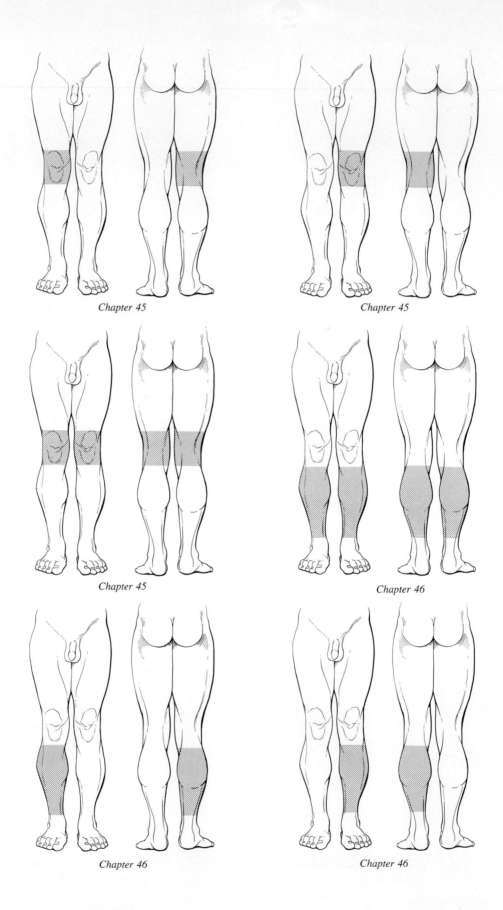

Chapter 45

Chapter 45

Chapter 45

Chapter 46

Chapter 46

Chapter 46

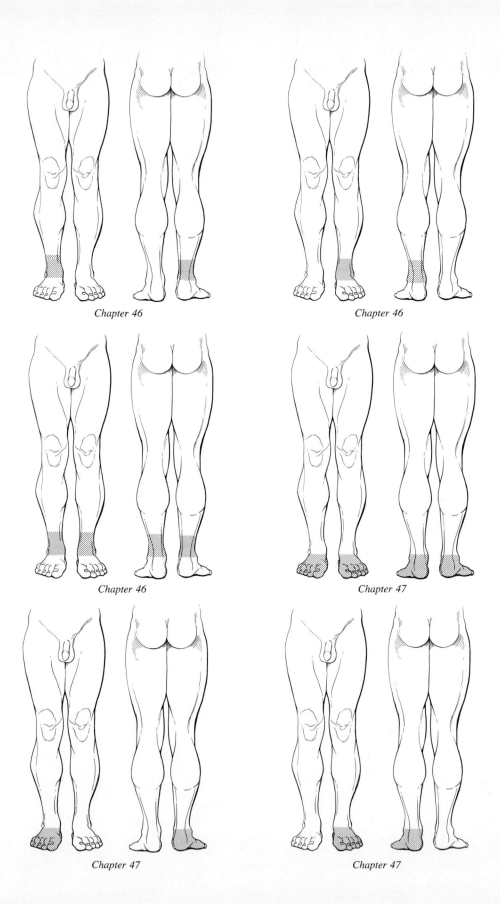

Chapter 46

Chapter 46

Chapter 46

Chapter 47

Chapter 47

Chapter 47

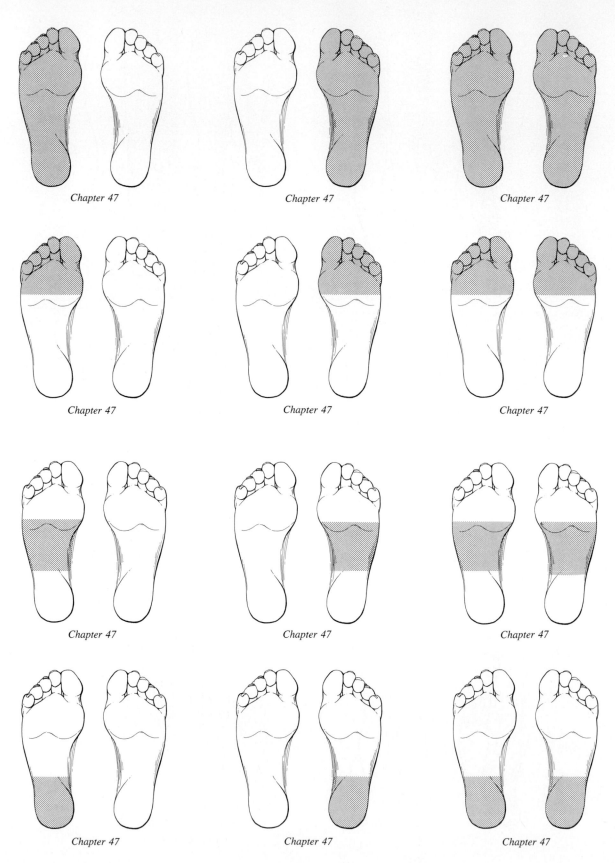

Chapter 47

Chapter 47

Chapter 47

Chapter 47

Chapter 47

Chapter 47

Chapter 47

Chapter 47

Chapter 47

Chapter 47

Chapter 47

Chapter 47

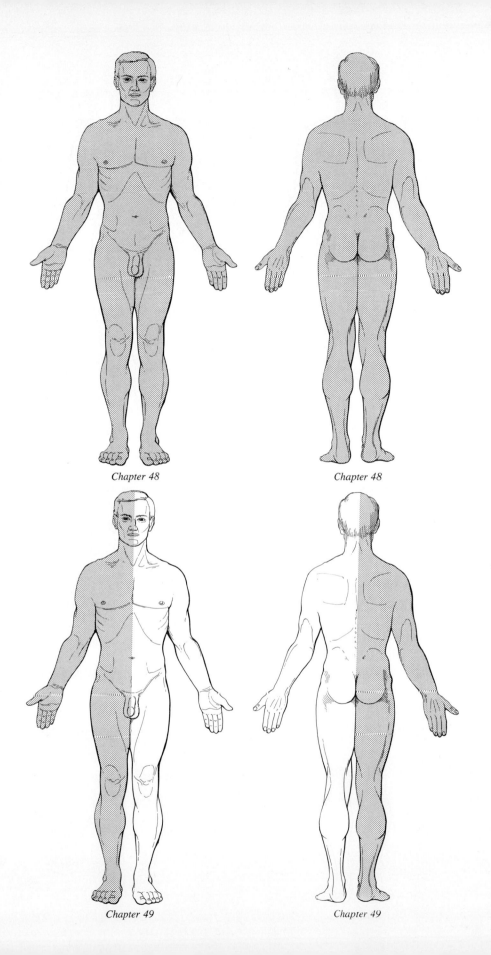

Chapter 48

Chapter 48

Chapter 49

Chapter 49

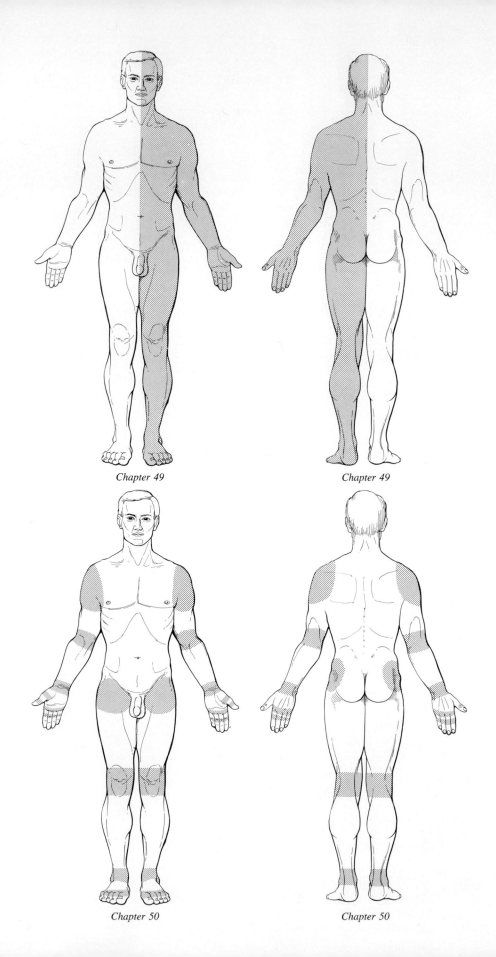

Chapter 49

Chapter 49

Chapter 50

Chapter 50

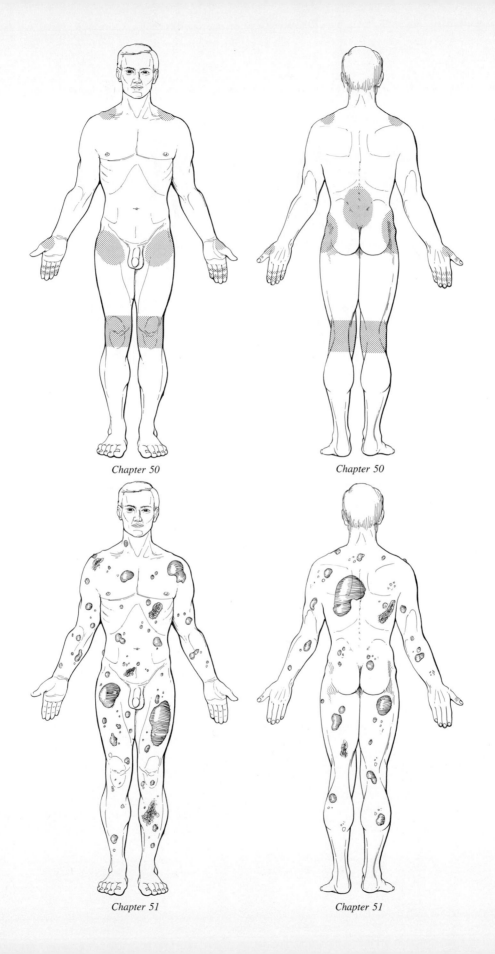

Chapter 50

Chapter 50

Chapter 51

Chapter 51

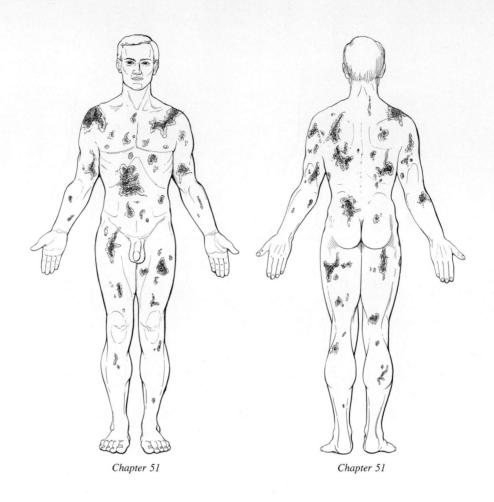

Chapter 51 *Chapter 51*

DIFFERENTIAL DIAGNOSIS OF ACUTE PAIN BY BODY REGION

CHAPTER 1

Organization and Use of This Book

☐ INTRODUCTION

Pain is one of the most common symptoms experienced by patients; some type of pain accounts for a major portion of symptom-provoked visits to physicians' offices and emergency rooms. This book is a comprehensive text designed to aid in the differential diagnosis of acute pain. The pain area diagrams have been selected to represent the most frequent pain patterns that a physician will encounter.

The diagnostic lists in each chapter contain the common and uncommon causes of pain in the region represented by that chapter; and most of the rare disorders capable of causing similar pain.

☐ ORGANIZATION OF THIS BOOK

This book is organized by body region. The patient's description of pain location is matched to one or more shaded body diagrams. The chapter referenced beneath each shaded diagram lists and describes the disorders that can cause pain in the shaded region. The pain patterns selected for discussion in individual chapters are those that occur most frequently in clinical practice.

Diseases that cause pain at two or more sites are listed and described in chapters dealing with each of those sites.

Further differentiation of the cause of a patient's pain requires matching other clinical descriptors obtained in the history, physical signs, and abnormal laboratory and/or imaging findings to those associated with the disorders listed in the chapter.

☐ ACUTE PAIN AND ITS CHARACTERISTICS

Acute pain is pain that precipitates a visit to (or a desire to visit) a physician, in the office or emergency room, within minutes, hours, or a few days after onset. It causes the patient to seek care with minimal delay because of one or more of the following characteristics:

1. It is new and never experienced before, in terms of location and pain quality (e.g., central squeezing chest pain experienced for the first time by a previously asymptomatic middle-aged man), and is anxiety-provoking.

2. The pain may be so severe and disabling that relief is sought (e.g., the excruciating pain of renal colic, subarachnoid hemorrhage, or dissecting aneurysm). Simple measures available to the patient (e.g., rest, heat, mild analgesics, or change of position) are ineffective.

3. The pain is continuous or recurs so many times during the first day or two that relief is sought as soon as possible (e.g., unstable angina or renal colic).

4. The site of the pain may cause alarm (e.g., the front of the chest, the eye, the entire abdomen).

5. The associated symptoms may be alarming and they may drive the patient to seek care (e.g., head pain associated with a high fever and a seizure; central chest pain associated with severe weakness, generalized pallor and sweating; generalized abdominal pain associated with distension and bloody diarrhea).

6. The setting may be alarming (e.g., a patient with chest pain whose family members have all died of heart attacks before age 50).

This description may be contrasted with that of chronic pain, which has the following characteristics:

1. It has been experienced before and has remitted spontaneously, or after simple measures or medical care.
2. It is usually mild to moderate in intensity, and not so severe as to be disabling.
3. Usually it is of limited duration and is improved by simple measures or by medical or surgical care. It often tends to recur one or more times before definitive therapy is sought. Constant pain may be of such low intensity that it does not provoke a physician visit.
4. The pain site does not cause alarm (e.g., an elbow, a knee, or the lower back) because it is a common site for pain in the general population.
5. There are no alarming associated symptoms.
6. The pain may be ameliorated or controlled by simple measures (e.g., angina controlled by avoiding stair-climbing, or headaches controlled by not drinking red wine).
7. The setting is not alarming.

☐ CHAPTER PLAN AND CONTENT EACH CHAPTER HAS THE FOLLOWING PARTS:

1. DIAGNOSTIC LIST

This is a list of the disorders that can cause pain in the topographic anatomic region covered by the chapter. It is very complete and is designed as a checklist to jog the reader's memory, since a diagnosis will be missed if it is not considered.

2. SUMMARY

This section presents further information about the listed diseases, with special attention given to the points of *difference*—in pain character, associated symptoms and signs, and laboratory, endoscopic, and imaging data—that help differentiate one disease from another. In some cases the response to specific therapy is also described (where it is helpful in differentiating one disorder from another).

3. TABLE OF DISEASE INCIDENCE

This table divides the disorders on the diagnostic list into three categories (common, uncommon, and rare). The incidence ranges given are only estimates, since accurate data are not available for all diseases listed.

Common disorders are those seen every day, or several times a week, in our clinics and wards. The medical literature contains papers describing large groups of patients with these disorders, collected over a 1- or 2-year interval.

Uncommon disorders are those seen once every 2 or 3 months in our clinics and wards. The medical literature contains papers reporting on small groups of patients, collected over a 5- to 10-year period or longer.

Rare disorders are those that are seen once or twice a year or less. The medical literature usually contains only case reports, and a reported series seldom contains more than five patients.

The above classification is only semiquantitative and is based on clinical experience, detailed surveys of 3000 outpatient visits and 2000 medical admissions at our institution, and a review of the medical literature from 1966 to the present. It does not specify frequency estimates for specific age, sex, and demographic groups.

4. DESCRIPTION OF LISTED DISEASES

The major portion of each chapter is dedicated to a detailed description of the pain produced by each disorder on the diagnostic list. A description is given of the pain's quality; severity; setting of onset; provoking, exacerbating, and ameliorating circumstances; response to specific therapy; and associated complaints. Physical signs, laboratory abnormalities, and endoscopic and imaging abnormalities that contribute to confirmation of the diagnosis (and to differentiation from other entities) are included for each disease. Careful characterization of pain in a specific region is helpful in limiting the number of entities to be considered in the differential diagnosis. Specific physical signs, and imaging and laboratory results, are also helpful in differentiating disorders with pains that have similar characteristics. Pain is characterized by the following parameters:

A. Location and Radiation Pain location is defined by the shaded areas in the line drawings associated with each chapter. However, subtle differences within a shaded area may support one diagnosis over another. For example, in patients with central chest pain, a parasternal location is more likely to indicate costochondritis than ischemic pain. Pain radiation and referral may be helpful. Anterolateral chest pain associated with ipsilateral shoulder pain indicates an inflammatory diaphragmatic process, while central chest pain and associated left lateral neck and trapezius ridge pain are characteristic of acute pericarditis.

B. Chronology Acute pain may be persistent for hours (e.g., acute myocardial infarction, acute biliary colic), or recurrent with symptom-free intervals of minutes or hours (e.g., acute coronary insufficiency, intestinal colic). The presence of an acute persistent or recurrent pain pattern in association with a specific disorder is described when it has diagnostic usefulness.

C. Quality of the Pain Patients' descriptions of the quality of pain may aid in differentiating one cause of pain from another.

In the chest, pressurelike or squeezing central pain suggests ischemia or esophageal spasm; stabbing or sticking pain, pleuritis; a dull parasternal ache, costochondritis; lancinating or stabbing pain radiating around the hemithorax from the back, intercostal neuritis; and tearing or ripping central chest pain, aortic dissection. In the abdomen, gnawing or aching, poorly localized epigastric pain suggests ulcer disease, while a constant aching or burning right lower abdominal pain occurs with acute appendicitis. Aching and sharp, stabbing transient lower abdominal pains occur in patients with gastroenteritis and are related to gaseous distension and spasm. Dull aching midline abdominal pain may be due to ischemia, while periumbilical colic with pain-free intervals suggests an early phase of intestinal obstruction.

D. Severity of the Pain This may be quantitated by its effect on the patient's ability to function, and the requirement for analgesics. *Mild* pain allows the patient to carry on all activities without need for analgesics. *Moderate* pain interferes with concentration and work efficiency, and requires the use of oral analgesics. (Some examples of moderate pain are a streptococcal tonsillitis, recent lumbosacral strain, a myofascial syndrome involving the neck muscles, and a constant toothache.) *Severe* pain interferes with the patient's ability to work, but is not completely incapacitating. Narcotic injections may be required. Examples include the bone pain of metastatic cancer, the joint pain of gonococcal arthritis, and the low back and leg pain of a herniated disc. *Very severe or excruciating* pain occurs with renal, biliary, or intestinal colic; aortic dissection; and acute myocardial infarction. The patient is completely incapacitated, and narcotic injections are required but may not always be effective.

E. Setting in Which the Pain Occurs This parameter refers to the immediate events preceding the onset of pain and/or the patient's prior medical, social, work, and family history.

Pain in the chest occurring during unaccustomed exertion suggests ischemic heart disease, while sharp chest pain occurring during heavy lifting suggests a musculoskeletal disorder. Sudden stabbing chest pain occurring in a patient while inhaling cocaine, using a Valsalva maneuver, suggests a diagnosis of pneumothorax.

Risk factors can also provide a profile that may aid in establishing a diagnosis. An obese, diabetic, hypertensive smoker who develops severe substernal chest pain is likely to have coronary ischemic pain. A similar pain in a psychiatric patient who has recurrent panic attacks with diaphoresis, dyspnea, inner trembling and lightheadedness, and fear of impending death is less likely to be ischemic. Crampy abdominal pain, especially in a person whose history shows risk factors for infection with human immunodeficiency virus (HIV), may represent HIV infection with cryptosporidiosis. New-onset lower abdominal crampy abdominal pain in a middle-aged man whose father and brother died of colon cancer should be evaluated carefully to rule out a large-bowel malignancy. Risk factors are useful insofar as they may support a diagnosis, but their absence does not exclude a diagnosis. For example, one may see acute myocardial infarction or iliofemoral vein thrombosis in patients without known risk factors for those disorders.

F. Precipitating and Exacerbating Circumstances The ability to provoke or intensify a pain by a specific action provides valuable information as to its cause. Although such maneuvers are not completely specific, they may reduce the number of disorders on the final differential list. For example, left chest pain, intensified by a deep breath, may be caused by pericarditis, pleuritis, or a chest wall disorder; but not by myocardial infarction, esophageal spasm, or aortic dissection.

Central chest pain provoked by exertion may be caused by myocardial ischemia, reflux esophagitis, or costochondritis. Central chest pain that is intensified by lying down may be due to pericarditis or a mediastinal tumor. Lying on the side of the chest with a fractured rib may intensify the pain, while the same position—with its splinting effect—may alleviate the pain of pleuritis. Ingestion of orange or tomato juice, or a diet cola, may intensify the pain of reflux esophagitis, but has no effect on chest wall or ischemic pain.

G. Alleviating Circumstances and the Effects of Therapy Pain in the chest, brought on by exertion and relieved by rest, suggests ischemic pain, although similar rest-associated relief may occur with chest wall pain. The pain of pericarditis and mediastinal and spinal cord tumors may be alleviated by sitting up. Sublingual nitroglycerin may relieve the central chest pain of ischemic heart disease or an esophageal motility disorder. Prednisone may dramatically relieve the chest pain of idiopathic pericarditis and the headache of temporal arteritis. Calcium channel–blocking drugs may relieve the rest pain of Prinzmetal's angina. Antibiotic therapy may relieve the lower abdominal pain of pelvic infection and the pleuritic pain of acute pneumonia. H_2 blockers and antacids may relieve the epigastric pain of duodenal ulcer.

H. Associated Symptoms Associated complaints are helpful in attributing a pain to a specific organ dysfunction. Pleuritic pain associated with cough, hemoptysis, and dyspnea occurs with lung disorders, such as pneumonia and pulmonary embolism.

Dull epigastric pain associated with melena or hematemesis is associated with gastric or duodenal ulcer disease or a gastric neoplasm.

Right upper abdominal aching pain associated with dark urine and jaundice directs attention to the liver, the common bile duct, and the head of the pancreas. Chest pain associated with palpitations and dyspnea directs attention to the heart; similar pain associated with odynophagia, pyrosis, and dysphagia is likely to have an esophageal origin.

I. Physical Examination Findings   Specific individual findings or clusters of findings are useful in differential diagnosis. In a patient with central chest pain, a pericardial friction rub suggests myocardial infarction or idiopathic pericarditis; a Hamman's sign, mediastinal emphysema or Boerhaave's syndrome; a new-onset diastolic aortic murmur, aortic dissection; and an S_3 gallop, acute myocardial infarction or myopericarditis.

Certain clusters of findings may have particular meanings. Fever, right upper abdominal tenderness, guarding, and jaundice together suggest gallbladder disease; a butterfly facial rash, symmetrical arthritis of the hands and knees, and a pleural friction rub suggest systemic lupus erythematosus; distended neck veins, muffled heart sounds, and a paradoxical pulse occur with pericarditis and an effusion; and decreased breath sounds over a hemithorax, distended neck veins, and contralateral deviation of the trachea occur with a tension pneumothorax.

J. Laboratory and Imaging Studies   Some disorders may present with indistinguishable clusters of historical and physical findings (e.g., cecal diverticulitis, mesenteric adenitis, and acute appendicitis). Ultrasound and CT scanning may differentiate these disorders preoperatively. Crohn's disease of the colon, ulcerative colitis, and ischemic colitis may present similar clinical findings, and may be differentiated by colonoscopy and/or barium enema. Boerhaave's syndrome and aortic dissection may cause similar clinical and plain radiographic findings (i.e., widened mediastinum), but can be differentiated by a contrast CT study of the mediastinum. In a patient with acute upper abdominal pain and tenderness, elevated serum amylase and lipase values support a diagnosis of pancreatitis; free air under the diaphragm is usually due to a perforated ulcer. Specific laboratory, imaging, and endoscopic findings, useful in differentiating one disorder from another, are included in the entries on individual diseases.

☐ ILLUSTRATIONS

Line drawings of the body are presented in panels at the beginning of the book (i.e., head, face, neck, chest, abdomen, back and buttocks, perineum and genitalia, upper extremity, lower extremity, and the entire body).

A chapter is referenced beneath each shaded drawing. This chapter will list and describe diseases causing acute pain in the area shaded. Matching the patient's pain location to one or more drawings (e.g., the patient's pain may correspond to a shaded area or fall slightly within or outside the area) will refer the physician to one or more appropriate chapters. These will list and describe the disorders that are possible causes of the patient's pain. Further differentiation of the cause will depend on matching other descriptors of the patient's pain (associated symptoms, pain quality, severity, setting of onset, alleviating and exacerbating events); physical signs; laboratory and imaging findings; to those of the listed disorders.

☐ MODULAR DESIGN

Each chapter is a complete module and contains descriptions of the listed disorders. In a few cases not all the disorders causing a particular pathophysiologic problem are discussed in detail but are listed in the text or a table (e.g., the many causes of intestinal obstruction). Some disorders appear on lists related to several anatomic areas. (For example, myocardial infarction may appear in the substernal, jaw, and interscapular pain chapters; dental pain may appear in the mouth and ear chapters.)

☐ USE OF THIS BOOK

To determine the cause of a specific pain:

1. Carefully define the location and characteristics of your patient's pain and positive physical findings.
2. Locate the shaded line drawing that includes the site of the patient's pain (i.e., provides the best match to the patient's description of pain location).
3. Decide that the pain is acute using the descriptions of acute and chronic pain provided in this chapter.
4. Consult the appropriate chapter designated under the pain diagram.
5. Read the Diagnostic List and the Summary. Consult the Description of Listed Diseases and review those disorders that seem most likely, as well as the descriptions of diseases that are unfamiliar.
6. If the diagnosis is still uncertain and requires more information to differentiate between competing possibilities, recheck the patient for specific physical signs; and order laboratory tests, special procedures, and imaging studies to confirm or exclude positively the disorders on the now-shortened list of possible diagnoses.
7. Consider a therapeutic trial if the results of tests are likely to be delayed for weeks (e.g., cultures for tuberculosis); or if the completed tests and imaging studies are negative or indeterminate, but the clinical findings suggest a specific treatable disorder.

PART ONE

Acute Head Pain

Acute Head Pain

☐ DIAGNOSTIC LIST

1. Posttraumatic headache
   A. Scalp injury and superficial neuropathy
   B. Migraine-like
   C. Muscle contraction-like
   D. Cluster-like
   E. Migraine-muscle contraction
   F. Cervical injury–related headache
      1. Posttraumatic dysautonomic cephalgia
      2. Posttraumatic occipital neuralgia
      3. Posttraumatic basilar artery migraine
      4. Traumatic dissection of the internal carotid artery
      5. Blunt trauma to the spine, ligaments, and muscles
   G. Post-head injury syndrome (postconcussion syndrome)
   H. Headache caused by structural intracranial injury
      1. Acute subdural hematoma
      2. Acute epidural hematoma
      3. Cerebral contusion
      4. Intracerebral hematoma
      5. Epidural hematoma in the posterior fossa

2. Spontaneous subarachnoid hemorrhage
   A. Aneurysm
      1. Minor leak and sentinel headache
      2. Thunderclap headache due to aneurysm without bleeding
      3. Aneurysmal rupture and onset headache
      4. Thunderclap headache without aneurysm or hemorrhage
   B. Arteriovenous malformation
   C. Spinal subarachnoid hemorrhage

3. Intracranial infection
   A. Acute bacterial meningitis
   B. Unusual forms of bacterial meningitis
      1. Lyme disease and meningitis
      2. *Listeria monocytogenes* meningitis
      3. *Mycobacterium tuberculosis* meningitis
      4. Anaerobic bacterial meningitis
      5. Mixed bacterial meningitis

C. Mimics of acute bacterial
meningitis
   1. Amebic
      meningoencephalitis
   2. Viral meningitis
   3. Meningitis secondary to
      intracranial tumors and
      cysts
   4. Drug-related meningitis
   5. Collagen vascular disease
      and aseptic meningitis
   6. Behçet's disease and
      aseptic meningitis
   7. Mollaret's meningitis
   8. Fungal meningitis
   9. Brain abscess with
      parameningeal reaction
   10. AIDS and contrast-
       enhancing brain lesions
   11. Subdural empyema
   12. Cranial epidural abscess
   13. Pituitary apoplexy
   14. Pituitary abscess
4. Cerebrovascular disease and
   headache
   A. Intraparenchymal hemorrhage
      1. Putaminal hemorrhage
      2. Thalamic hemorrhage
      3. Lobar cerebral hemorrhage
      4. Midbrain hemorrhage
      5. Cerebellar hemorrhage
   B. Ischemic stroke
   C. Transient ischemic attack
   D. Hypertensive encephalopathy
   E. Intracranial venous thrombosis
   F. Cervical artery dissection
      1. Carotid artery dissection
      2. Vertebral artery dissection
5. Brain tumor and acute headache
   A. Paroxysmal headache
   B. Uncal and cerebellar
      herniation
   C. Hemorrhage into a tumor
   D. Subarachnoid hemorrhage
   E. Acute meningitis
   F. Acute stroke
6. Encephalitis
   A. Herpes simplex
   B. Arthropod-borne
      1. Eastern equine
      2. Western equine

      3. St. Louis
      4. California and La Crosse
7. Systemic infections with headache
   and/or meningismus
   A. Rickettsial diseases
      1. Rocky Mountain spotted
         fever
      2. Q fever
      3. Typhus
   B. Spirochetal diseases
      1. Lyme disease
      2. Leptospirosis
      3. Meningovascular syphilis
   C. Pneumonias and meningismus
      1. *Chlamydia psittaci*
      2. *Mycoplasma pneumoniae*
      3. *Histoplasma capsulatum*
   D. Typhoid fever
   E. Pyelonephritis
   F. Primary HIV infection
8. Provoked vascular headaches
   A. Exertional
      1. Acute-effort migraine
      2. Low-intensity
         exercise–induced headache
      3. Minimal-effort headache
   B. Sexual activity
   C. Cough and straining
   D. Hunger
   E. Food and beverage
   F. Drug
   G. Decompression
   H. Altitude and hypoxia
   I. Hypercapnia
   J. Menstruation
   K. Carbon monoxide
   L. Hypoglycemia
   M. Pheochromocytoma
9. Temporal arteritis
10. Acute sinusitis
11. Acute occipital neuralgia
12. Multiple sclerosis
13. Eclampsia
14. Cerebrospinal fluid hypotension
   A. Post–lumbar puncture
      headache
   B. Acute postural headache with
      infectious disease
   C. Spontaneous intracranial
      hypotension

☐ SUMMARY

Posttraumatic headache may occur in several forms. Local *scalp pain and paresthesias* are associated with tenderness at the impact site. Finger pressure may intensify the pain and provoke paresthesias. Other posttraumatic head pains take the form of classic or common *migraine, muscle contraction,* or *cluster* headaches, or a *mixed type,* with muscle contraction and migraine elements.

A *neck injury* to the carotid region may cause attacks of severe unilateral headache associated with ipsilateral mydriasis and facial sweating. As the pain resolves, a *Horner's syndrome* may appear (*posttraumatic dysautonomic cephalgia*). *Occipital neuralgia,* with unilateral posterior neck and head pain, and paresthesias and/or hypesthesia of the scalp may follow sleeping on a hard-edged surface or severe hyperextension and rotation of the neck. *Basilar artery migraine* may be provoked by a whiplash-type injury. Attacks of occipital headache, vertigo, ataxia, dysarthria, four-limb paresthesias, loss of vision, and coma may occur. *Dissection of a carotid artery* may follow a neck injury. Frontal, orbital, and/or temporal pain occur on the side of neck injury. A Horner's syndrome may be associated with the headache, and focal neurologic signs may develop. These usually begin minutes or hours after the injury and may include hemiparesis, hemisensory loss, dysphasia, diplopia, and amaurosis fugax. Flexion or hyperextension injuries may cause *spine or soft tissue damage* in the posterior upper neck and occiput. This results in aching neck and occipital pain, which is intensified by neck movement.

A *post–head injury syndrome* consisting of headache, lightheadedness, vertigo, gait abnormalities, defects in memory and concentration, and personality change has been observed. *Acute subdural hematoma* may cause headache, persistent loss of consciousness, or unconscious alternating with periods of lucidity. Focal neurologic symptoms and signs, such as hemiparesis, posturing, and a fixed dilated pupil, also may occur. Head pain, coma, or unconsciousness alternating with lucidity, ipsilateral pupillary dilatation and hemiparesis, decerebrate posturing, and sometimes papilledema may be caused by an *acute epidural hematoma* resulting from a temporal bone fracture. A *cerebral contusion* may mimic the symptoms of an intracranial hematoma. These disorders can be differentiated by a CT scan or MRI. An *intracerebral hematoma* may cause a similar headache, change in mental status, and focal signs. CT or MRI can easily visualize the hematoma. An *epidural hematoma in the posterior fossa* results from a blow to the back of the head. Occipital and neck pain, meningismus, and limb and gait ataxia occur. CT scan or MRI can detect the epidural hematoma.

A *minor leak from a cerebral aneurysm* may occur hours or days prior to rupture. Such headaches are severe, generalized or localized, and abrupt in onset and have been called *thunderclap headaches.* In only a minority of cases are they associated with photophobia, neck stiffness, or a change in the level of consciousness. In up to 50 percent of cases with *hemorrhage,* the headaches are severe enough to initiate a visit to a physician. Since a CT scan will detect a minor leak in only 44 percent, lumbar puncture is required to rule out minor bleeding. Up to 80 percent of patients investigated for thunderclap headaches will show no evidence of subarachnoid hemorrhage, and these patients probably have a severe form of migraine. An unusual case of thunderclap headache associated with a nonbleeding aneurysm has been reported.

Rupture of an aneurysm causes an explosive severe headache that may be associated with transient loss of consciousness, photophobia, meningismus, and mental confusion or a decrement in the level of consciousness. The diagnosis can be confirmed by a CT scan (85–95 percent sensitive if done within 72 h), and the aneurysm can be imaged by cerebral angiography. *AV malformations* usually cause a more gradual onset of generalized headache, neck stiffness, and photophobia. There may be a history of seizures and of one or more subarachnoid hemorrhages. The diagnosis can be confirmed by a contrast-enhanced CT scan or cerebral angiogram. *Spinal subarachnoid bleeding* begins suddenly, with stabbing midline neck or back pain; generalized headache; meningismus; and chest, abdominal, rectal, or sciatic pain, depending on the level of the bleeding lesion in the spinal canal.

Acute bacterial meningitis begins with a severe generalized headache, fever, chills, vomiting, prostration, and meningismus. The headache is not of the thunderclap variety, and it develops gradually over several hours. Fever and chills are prominent, and the CSF contains an increased number of cells with a polymorphonuclear leukocyte predominance, an elevated protein level, and a low glucose level. Gram's stain and/or bacterial culture is usually positive.

Meningitis with a polymorphonuclear leukocyte predominance and a low or normal glucose may be caused by *Streptococcus pneumoniae; Neisseria meningitidis; Haemophilus influenzae,* and other, less common, microorganisms. *Lyme disease* may present with a rash (erythema chronicum migrans), systemic symptoms, aseptic meningitis, and a cranial and/or peripheral radiculoneuritis. *Listeria monocytogenes* causes a bacterial meningitis in patients with leukemia or lymphoma, or immunosuppressed by corticosteroids. *Mycobacterium tuberculosis* may present with headache, fever, and meningismus of gradual onset over a 1- to 4-week period in association with a CSF that may show a polymorphonuclear leukocyte predominance and a low glucose level in up to 22 percent of cases. *Anaerobic meningitis* is associated with sinusitis or otitis media in adults. *Mixed bacterial meningitis* may be caused by gram-positive cocci, gram-negative aerobes, and anaerobes. This polymicrobial infection is associated with fistulous connections between the airway, colon, rectum, or skin and the subarachnoid space.

A polymorphonuclear cell exudate in the CSF is associated with a negative Gram's stain and culture in a patient who has another disorder that mimics the clinical and laboratory abnormalities of bacterial meningitis. *Naegleria (amebic)* infection causes a CSF polymorphonuclear predominance and a clinical picture indistinguishable from bacterial meningitis. Amebas may be identified by their motility in a cell-counting chamber. *Viral meningitis* causes milder meningismus, fever, and headache. If a polymorphonuclear leukocyte predominance is present, a second lumbar puncture, 12 h later, will usually show a shift to a lymphocyte predominance. Necrosis of a *brain tumor* or emptying of an epidermoid *cyst* can cause an acute chemical meningitis that mimics the clinical and CSF findings of bacterial meningitis. The correct diagnosis can be established by imaging the tumor by a contrast-enhanced CT scan or MRI.

Some drugs, such as sulfamethoxazole, ibuprofen, or sulindac, may provoke a *drug-related meningitis,* especially in women with systemic lupus erythematosus or *mixed connective tissue disease.* Disorders of unknown cause such as collagen vascular diseases and Behçet's disease may cause aseptic meningitis.

Mollaret's meningitis is a recurrent disorder. Cultures and Gram's-stain smears are negative. Large "endothelial" or mononuclear cells may constitute 75 percent of the cells present on day 1. It is necessary to exclude other causes of meningeal inflammation before making a diagnosis of Mollaret's meningitis. Coccidiodal meningitis may present with fever meningismus, nausea, and vomiting. Cases occur in the endemic area or in recent visitors to that area. CSF findings may mimic an acute bacterial meningitis. Cultures of CSF may be falsely negative, but CSF complement fixing antibodies to *C. immitis* are present in up to 95 percent of cases.

Brain abscess is associated with headache; focal neurological signs; and, in some cases, nuchal pain and stiffness. The CSF may show a polymorphonuclear predominance and a normal or low glucose level, but cultures are usually negative. The diagnosis can be established by CT or MRI. AIDS patients with headache should be evaluated for cerebral toxoplasmosis, *M. tuberculosis,* a *Candida* abscess, or a B-cell lymphoma.

Subdural empyema arises in an infected sinus or middle ear. Headache, drowsiness, fever, periorbital and/or frontal area swelling, seizures, and focal neurologic signs occur. Nuchal rigidity is present in almost all cases. The diagnosis of a subdural or *epidural empyema* can be made by CT scan.

Pituitary apoplexy causes a severe bilateral frontal headache, drowsiness, diplopia, and visual loss. Pituitary tumor necrosis may cause a chemical meningitis or result in a subarachnoid hemorrhage. A CT or MRI scan will demonstrate the tumor.

Pituitary abscess mimics the symptoms and signs of pituitary apoplexy. An aseptic or bacterial meningitis may occur.

Headache (48–67 percent of cases) and focal neurologic signs often accompany a *parenchymal brain hemorrhage.* The location of the hemorrhage can be established by a CT study. *Ischemic strokes* and *transient ischemic attacks* (TIAs) are also associated with headache in up to 25 percent of cases.

Hypertensive encephalopathy presents with a markedly elevated blood pressure (systolic ≥230 mmHg, diastolic ≥130 mmHg), a severe generalized headache, a change in mental status (e.g., confusion, somnolence, or agitation), visual blurring, and seizures. The fundoscopic examination reveals a grade III or IV hypertensive retinopathy. Symptoms and signs resolve with effective antihypertensive therapy.

Venous sinus thrombosis may result from a contiguous otitis media or sinusitis, or from altered blood coagulability. This disorder presents with headache, vomiting, visual blurring, and diplopia in association with signs of increased intracranial pressure (e.g., papilledema). Focal neurologic signs may occur, and some patients with an underlying otitis media or sinusitis may develop fever, chills, and other manifestations of sepsis. The diagnosis can be established by MRI or jugular venography. *Carotid artery dissection* may cause ipsilateral neck pain, frontal headache, a partial Horner's syndrome, and an audible bruit associated with focal neurologic signs. *Vertebral artery dissection* causes posterior neck and occipital pain and a lateral medullary or basilar artery syndrome.

Brain tumors may present acutely as a paroxysmal headache that begins within seconds. Vomiting; neck pain; loss of consciousness; and episodes of mental confusion, diplopia, vertigo, and ataxia may be associated with the headache. Colloid cysts of the third ventricle and posterior fossa tumors may cause paroxysmal head pain. Sudden increases in intracranial pressure may be the cause of such headaches. Herniation of the uncus of the temporal lobe produces an ipsilateral dilated pupil, hemiparesis, and a decreased level of consciousness. *Cerebellar tonsillar herniation* causes neck pain and stiffness, a head tilt, unconsciousness, and cerebellar fits. *Hemorrhage into a tumor* may cause a strokelike syndrome. Tumor necrosis can lead to an acute meningitis or to a *subarachnoid hemorrhage. Herpes simplex encephalitis* may present acutely with headache, seizures, confusion, meningismus, and limb paresis. The CSF shows an elevated protein level and a lymphocytic predominance. A CT scan may show a mass effect and hypodense lesions in the temporal lobe. EEG and radionuclide brain scans confirm involvement of one or both temporal lobes. Biopsy reveals a necrotizing encephalitis, and herpes simplex virus can be grown from biopsied brain tissue.

Arthropod-borne encephalitis occurs in epidemics in the summer and early fall. Most cases are subclinical, but some patients develop aseptic meningitis and a mild to severe encephalitis.

Some *systemic infections* are known to cause very severe headache, and meningismus. These infections include *rickettsial diseases* (e.g., *Rocky Mountain spotted fever*, *Q fever*, and *typhus*) and *spirochetal diseases* (e.g., *Lyme disease*, *leptospirosis*, and *meningovascular syphilis*). Some forms of *pulmonary infection* (e.g., *psittacccis*, *mycoplasma*, and *histoplasmosis*) are associated with headache and meningismus. Similarly, these symptoms may occur in *typhoid fever* and in some cases of *pyelonephritis*, leading to lumbar puncture to exclude meningitis. Aseptic meningitis is part of the *acute human immunodeficiency virus (HIV) syndrome.* This disorder presents with fever, sore throat, headache, photophobia, a diffuse macular rash in 50 percent of cases, and generalized lymphadenopathy.

Provoked headaches are *vascular*, or *muscle contraction* headaches named for the provoking stimulus or setting in which they occur. These include *exertional*, *sexual activity* or coital, *cough*, *hunger*, *food-induced,* ice cream, and *drug-*

TABLE OF DISEASE INCIDENCE

INCIDENCE PER 100,000 (APPROXIMATE)

Common (>100)

Posttraumatic headache: scalp injury and superficial neuropathy, migraine-like, muscle contraction–like, migraine-muscle contraction–like

Cervical injury: blunt trauma to posterior or anterior neck involving ligaments and muscles

Post–head injury syndrome (postconcussion syndrome)

Intraparenchymal hemorrhage

Ischemic stroke

Transient ischemic attack

Provoked headaches: exertional, sexual activity, cough and straining, hunger-related, food and beverage, drug-related, altitude and hypoxia, hypercapnia, menstruation

Acute sinusitis

Uncommon (>5–100)

Intracranial trauma: cerebral contusion, intracerebral hematoma

Minor leak due to aneurysm

Subarachnoid hemorrhage due to aneurysm

Thunderclap headache without subarachnoid hemorrhage or aneurysm

Acute bacterial meningitis

Viral meningitis

Behcet's disease

Temporal arteritis

Brain abscess with parameningeal reaction

Hypertensive encephalopathy

AIDS and CT-enhancing brain lesions

Systemic infections with meningismus: rickettsial diseases (Rocky Mountain spotted fever, Q fever); spirochetial diseases (Lyme, leptospirosis); *Mycoplasma pneumoniae*, *Chlamydia psittaci*, pulmonary histoplasmosis

Typhoid fever

Pyelonephritis

Primary HIV infection

Provoked headaches: hypoglycemia, decompression sickness, carbon monoxide

Brain tumor with paroxysmal headache, hemorrhage into the tumor, acute stroke syndrome

Temporal arteritis

Eclampsia

Rare (>0–5)

Posttraumatic headache: cluster-like

Cervical injury–related headache: dysautonomic cephalgia, occipital neuralgia, basilar artery migraine, dissection of internal carotid artery

Intracranial trauma: acute subdural hematoma, acute epidural hematoma, posterior fossa epidural hematoma

Thunderclap headache with aneurysm but without bleeding

Subarachnoid hemorrhage due to AV malformation or spinal lesion

Lyme disease meningitis

Listeria meningitis

Tuberculous meningitis

Anaerobic bacterial meningitis

Mixed bacterial meningitis

Amebic meningoencephalitis

Tumor-related meningitis

Drug-related meningitis

Collagen vascular disease meningitis

Mollaret's meningitis

Fungal meningitis

Cranial subdural empyema

Cranial epidural abscess

Pituitary apoplexy

Pituitary abscess

Intracranial venous thrombosis

Carotid artery dissection

Vertebral artery dissection

Brain tumor with uncal or cerebellar herniation, subarachnoid hemorrhage, acute meningitis

Herpes simplex encephalitis

Arthropod-borne encephalitis

Systemic infections with meningismus: typhus, meningovascular syphilis

Pheochromocytoma

Acute occipital neuralgia

Multiple sclerosis

Cerebrospinal fluid hypotension

Acute postural headache with infectious disease

---

induced headaches. *Decompression* during sports diving or flying and sudden arrival in a *high-altitude* mountainous area may result in the acute onset of headache. *Hypercapnia* resulting from pulmonary disease, *menstruation*, *CO poisoning*, *hypoglycemia*, and *pheochromocytoma* may be associated with severe headaches.

Temporal arteritis causes headaches and tenderness of the scalp in patients over age 55. The head pain is usually localized to one or both temples. Jaw claudication, visual loss, and an elevated sedimentation rate are variably present components. Temporal artery biopsy and/or a dramatic improvement within 48 h of starting prednisone therapy confirms the diagnosis.

Acute sinusitis causes pharyngeal and nasal discharge of purulent and/or blood-streaked mucus, fever, localized or generalized head and face pain, nasal stuffiness, and sinus tenderness. Plain sinus radiographs or CT studies of the sinuses will confirm the diagnosis. Fiberoptic rhinoscopy is also useful and will identify purulent material coming from a sinus orifice. There is a therapeutic response to antibiotic therapy. *Acute occipital neuralgia* causes occipital pain, scalp paresthesias, and hypesthesia. It may be caused by trauma, scalp compression, osteoarthritis, cerebellar herniation, gout, and infections.

Multiple sclerosis may present with a diffuse throbbing headache and remitting neurologic abnormalities such as optic neuritis, cerebellar dysfunction with vertigo and ataxia, and lower extremity weakness and numbness. *Eclampsia* occurs in a setting of pregnancy and labor and causes a severe headache, edema, hypertension, proteinuria, and seizures. The seizures can be controlled by intravenous magnesium sulfate.

Cerebrospinal fluid hypotension may cause a postural headache that is provoked or exacerbated by standing and relieved by lying down. This type of headache usually follows lumbar puncture but may occur spontaneously. A similar type of head-ache may occur in patients with fever and systemic infection, but the mechanism of this form of postural cephalgia is unknown.

☐ DESCRIPTION OF LISTED DISEASES

1. POSTTRAUMATIC HEADACHE

Mild or severe head injuries may be associated with a posttraumatic headache. Loss of consciousness is not a prerequisite for the development of this disabling complaint. Several different types of headache may occur.

A. Scalp Injury and Superficial Neuropathy Superficial scalp injury–related headache is maximal in the region injured by the impact. Well-localized tenderness is present. The head pain expands outward from the site of injury and is often continuous. Percussion or pressure over the injured site may provoke sharp, stabbing pain and paresthesias. It may be uncomfortable to lie on the affected area or even to wear a hat. Paresthesias and/or hypesthesia are often present in and around the area of injury. Local injection of lidocaine into the painful site may relieve the pain. Use of indomethacin for 5 to 7 days may lead to complete or partial resolution of the head pain.

B. Migraine-Like Posttraumatic migraine-like headache may begin at impact or within hours or days of the injury. The pain may be aching, throbbing, or both. The headache may be localized to one frontotemporal or occipital area, but it is often bilateral. It may be constantly present or intermittent. Exertion, bending, rapid head movements, coughing, sneezing, and mental activity may provoke more intense pain. Retro-orbital and facial pain may be associated. Local scalp tenderness is commonly present in the painful area. This disorder may behave much like a migraine headache; and nausea, vomiting, scintillating scotoma, and photophobia may be present. The pain may respond to treatment with ergotamine, and administration of a beta-adrenergic blocker may prevent recurrent episodes.

C. Muscle Contraction–Like Some patients develop a muscle contraction–type headache, subjectively perceived as a pressure or tight band around the head or a more localized occipital or bitemporal ache. Local scalp sensitivity may be present. These headaches are usually intermittent, lasting several hours, or they may be continuous for days or weeks. Nausea and light-headedness may

accompany the pain. A suboccipital and nuchal distribution of the pain may be associated with a whiplash-type neck injury.

A muscle contraction-type headache is the most common variety of posttraumatic headache. It may respond to the use of simple analgesics or require the use of tricyclic antidepressants.

D. Cluster-Like Cluster-type headaches have also been described in the postinjury period but are relatively rare. Several attacks of excruciating unilateral, frontotemporal, and orbital pain lasting 30 to 120 min occur each day. These episodes are associated with redness and tearing of the ipsilateral eye, stuffiness of the nose, and rhinorrhea. Recurrent attacks may occur each day for weeks or months and then cease, only to recur months or years later. Cluster headaches may be provoked by alcohol, emotional stress, fatigue, bright lights, rainy weather, and sleep. Up to 16 percent of patients with cluster headaches have a history of head injury. Nitroglycerin or histamine may also provoke an attack of headache. Administration of ergotamine or inhalation of O_2 will shorten the period of headache. Prednisone therapy may decrease the frequency and severity of attacks.

E. Migraine-Muscle Contraction Combinations of migraine and muscle contraction headaches may also occur after head trauma, as they do spontaneously.

F. Cervical Injury–Related Headaches

1. Posttraumatic Dysautonomic Cephalgia Injury to the anterior neck may damage sympathetic neurons. After a latent period of several weeks, a severe unilateral headache associated with mydriasis and hyperhidrosis on the painful side may occur. This headache may have an aching or throbbing quality, and it may persist for hours to days. As the pain subsides, the patient develops ipsilateral miosis and ptosis (Horner's syndrome). Several such attacks may occur each month, and they may be prevented by propranolol or other beta blocking drugs.

2. Posttraumatic Occipital Neuralgia Unilateral neck and occipital pain follows a hyperextension whip-lash-type injury of the neck. Eye and face discomfort may occur on the same side. The pain is intensified by head movements. Some patients describe an exploding feeling in the head and neck at the instant of injury. Pressure over the suboccipital region may cause local pain. Upper posterior neck and scalp hypesthesia is present on the affected side. This disorder may be caused by injury to the C2 ganglion and nerve root by compression between the lamina of the axis and atlas during extreme neck hyperextension and rotation. Surgical ablation of the C2 nerve root may be required.

3. Posttraumatic Basilar Artery Migraine Basilar artery migraine, with unilateral throbbing occipital head pain, may follow a cervical whiplash injury. Vertigo, ataxia, dysarthria, limb paresthesias, bilateral loss of vision, and coma may occur in association with the head pain.

4. Traumatic Dissection of the Internal Carotid Artery Hyperextension and rotation, or forced flexion of the neck may stretch or compress the internal carotid artery, leading to dissection. These effects on the neck commonly occur in motor vehicle accidents but can result from direct blows, falls, manipulative chiropractic therapy, or attempted suicide by hanging. Neck pain and tenderness may occur but are relatively uncommon. Ipsilateral headache (frontotemporal and orbital) is associated with an oculosympathetic paralysis and/or focal neurologic signs of a transient or persistent nature. Bruits may be audible in 39 percent of cases and may be the only sign of abnormality. The neurologic findings may include contralateral hemiparesis and hemisensory loss, dysphasia, amaurosis fugax, and diplopia. Focal neurologic signs may also occur without unilateral headache. The time interval between injury and the onset of symptoms of cerebral ischemia was within 3 weeks in 71 percent of cases in one reported series, but a delay of up to 14 years has been recorded. Bilateral headache may be seen with bilateral dissection. The diagnosis can be confirmed by carotid angiography.

5. Blunt Trauma to the Spine, Ligaments, and Muscles Blunt trauma to the neck may injure posterior neck muscles, ligaments, facet joints, discs, and vertebral bodies, producing neck and occipital pain on one or both sides. Plain cervical spine, CT with contrast, or MRI may be required to identify these disorders. Posttraumatic myofascial syndromes involving one or more of the posterolateral neck muscles may also account for cases of posterior neck and occipital pain. Identification and injection of trigger points in these muscles will provide relief.

G. Post–Head Trauma Syndrome A post–head injury syndrome may follow severe, as well as seemingly trivial, head injuries. This syndrome may include headache, lightheadedness, unsteadiness of gait, vertigo, irritability, nausea, decrease in the ability to concentrate, ease of fatigue, a memory disorder, a flat affect, and other personality changes. When this collection of symptoms follows a brief trauma-related loss of consciousness, this disorder has been called the postconcussion syndrome.

MRI may detect subtle brain injury not imaged by a CT scan. MRI may detect small brain contusions that may lead to encephalomalacia, small subdural or epidural hematomas, cerebral edema, and demyelinating white matter injuries. Some authorities believe that difficult-to-

demonstrate trauma-related injuries such as these have an etiologic role in the post–head trauma syndrome.

H. Headache Associated with Structural Intracranial Injury Headache alone or associated with other symptoms and signs occurring after trauma may be an important clue to significant intracranial injury.

A depressed or a decreasing level of consciousness, focal neurologic signs, a penetrating head injury, or a depressed skull fracture mandates a CT scan and neurosurgical consultation.

A progressively severe headache, a change in the level of consciousness, a seizure, vomiting, amnesia, serious facial injury, a basilar skull fracture, intoxication, or an unreliable history are strong, but not absolute, indications for obtaining a CT study.

1. Acute Subdural Hematoma Up to 29 percent of patients with this disorder never lose consciousness, while an additional 42 percent have periods of lucidity and unconsciousness. Headache is an important symptom in those alert enough to complain. Other findings include hemiparesis (20 percent), hemiplegia (18 percent), decerebrate posturing (35 percent), decorticate posturing (6 percent), and a dilated ($\geq$6 mm) fixed pupil ipsilateral to the hematoma (31 percent). Papilledema may occur in up to 37 percent and a nerve VI palsy in 3 percent. Pupillary dilatation contralateral to the hematoma may occur in 9 to 44 percent, and a hemiparesis ipsilateral to the subdural collection in 15 to 39 percent. Contralateral hemiparesis may also occur. A CT scan with contrast or MRI will demonstrate the subdural hematoma and associated lesions, such as a cerebral contusion or hemorrhage, subarachnoid bleeding, or an associated epidural hematoma. Evacuation of the hematoma by a craniotomy approach will relieve the headache, improve the level of consciousness, and reverse neurologic signs. Delay in proceeding to surgery, deep coma on presentation, or associated parenchymal injuries result in an operative mortality of 40 to 65 percent.

2. Acute Epidural Hematoma Injury to the middle meningeal artery (50 percent of cases) or veins (33 percent), injury to the diploic veins or dural sinuses (10 percent), or laceration of a carotid artery before it enters the intracranial dura can cause an epidural hematoma. Up to 50 percent of epidural hematomas occur in the temporal region with extension to other sites. Up to 68 percent of patients with epidural bleeding have no other intracranial injury. Lucid patients may complain of head pain and tenderness at the site of temporal bone fracture, but a more generalized constant headache may occur. The course of these patients may be: (1) no loss of consciousness (9–25 percent); (2) unconscious throughout (14–56 percent); (3) unconscious-lucid-unconscious (11–67 percent); (4) unconscious-lucid (0–26 percent); or (5) lucid-unconscious (0–21 percent). The initial unconscious period is caused by a concussion, while the expanding hematoma produces the second episode of unconsciousness. Lucidity may be only relative. On careful testing, these ''clear'' periods may be associated with an abnormal mental status examination. Pupillary dilatation and fixation, hemiparesis, and decerebrate or decorticate posturing are associated. Early in the course, papilledema may be absent, but retinal hemorrhages may be present. A CT scan will image the hematoma and fracture; and surgical evacuation, with control of the bleeding vessel, will produce a survival rate of 85 percent.

3. Cerebral Contusion   This is the commonest intracranial lesion following head injury. In a contused region, the brain is necrotic, edematous, and hemorrhagic. The frontal and temporal lobes are most commonly affected, and ''coup'' and ''contre-coup'' lesions may occur. There may be an initial loss of consciousness after injury due to concussion, followed by recovery of mental clarity. Localized or diffuse headache, a decreased level of consciousness, and focal motor and/or speech deficits occur. Diffuse cerebral edema may result in an increase in intracranial pressure, with papilledema and retinal hemorrhages. The diagnosis of hemorrhagic contusion can be made by a CT scan, while MRI is more sensitive for detection of nonhemorrhagic lesions. Surgical resection of a large contusion may be required to prevent dangerous increases in intracranial pressure. Delayed bleeding into a contusion or CT ''normal brain'' can occur and is signaled by a deterioration in the level of consciousness and new neurologic symptoms and signs. New bleeding can be confirmed by repeating the CT scan.

4. Intracerebral Hematoma   This manifestation of head injury is difficult to distinguish clinically from an acute subdural or epidural hematoma. Unconsciousness followed by lucidity and then unconsciousness, lucidity followed by unconsciousness, unconsciousness or lucidity throughout, or unconsciousness and then lucidity are the clinical patterns observed. Focal motor signs, loss of speech, dilated pupils, and signs of increased intracranial pressure may also occur. A CT scan without contrast will establish the diagnosis.

Large hematomas may require operative evacuation because of the danger of herniation secondary to increased intracranial pressure.

5. Epidural Hematoma in the Posterior Fossa   This disorder occurs after a blow to the back of the head. Skull x-rays show an occipital fracture in 67 to 100 percent of cases. Bleeding occurs from the wall of a transverse or sigmoid venous sinus at or adjacent to the fracture site. Occipital and posterior neck pain and nuchal rigidity may be associated with gait and extremity ataxia, but cerebellar signs may be absent in rapidly progressive cases. Hemiparesis occurs frequently and is usually due to a coincident supratentorial lesion. This disorder may be diagnosed by a CT scan directed at delineating posterior fossa structures or by MRI.

2. SPONTANEOUS SUBARACHNOID HEMORRHAGE

A. Aneurysm

1. Minor Leak and Sentinel Headache   A warning or sentinel headache may occur in 30 to 60 percent of patients who subsequently have a major subarachnoid hemorrhage. The headache produced by a minor leak has been described as abrupt in onset and extremely severe (thunderclap headache). The pain may be constant, throbbing, or both. The location may reflect the site of the bleeding aneurysm. Anterior communicating aneurysms cause bifrontal, bioccipital headache or hemicranial, periorbital, and hemifacial pain, while internal carotid and posterior communicating aneurysms are more likely to cause a hemicranial, hemifacial, and/or periorbital headache. The headache may continue for several hours or as long as 14 days. It may never cease and may be followed by a massive rupture and more pain. In one reported series, rupture followed minor leak within 24 h in 26 percent, and in 2 to 30 days in the remaining patients, providing ample time for intervention if the diagnosis is considered. Only 50 percent of patients with minor leak consult a physician, and approximately half of these will be correctly diagnosed. Associated symptoms of a minor leak include nausea (18 percent); vomiting (18 percent), and neck pain (18 percent); confusion, ataxia, and third nerve palsy occur in less than 3 percent of cases. The diagnosis of a minor subarachnoid hemorrhage may be confirmed by CT scan in only 44 percent. Lumbar puncture has a sensitivity approaching 100 percent, and should be performed in such cases if the CT scan is normal. Lumbar puncture will reveal red blood cells and/or xanthochromia. Differentiation of a minor leak hemorrhage from a traumatic tap is facilitated by a decrease in the red blood cell count from collection tube 1 to 3, the absence of xanthochromia, and a negative D-dimer assay for fibrin breakdown products (<200 mcg/liter) in patients without true hemorrhage. Discovery of a minor leak requires immediate arteriography and surgical intervention before a major rupture occurs.

2. Thunderclap Headache Due to Aneurysm without Bleeding   A case of recurrent occipital and bitemporal thunderclap headache of 12- to 16-h duration associated with a normal spinal fluid and an unruptured internal carotid aneurysm with associated vasospasm has been reported. This case suggests that occasionally a patient may have a warning headache without evidence of bleeding.

3. Aneurysmal Rupture and Onset Headache Major rupture is signaled by an onset headache. The headache begins abruptly and is severe to excruciating. Qualitative descriptions by patients include ''bursting,'' ''crushing,'' ''struck by a hammer,'' and ''something popped or snapped in my head.'' Quantitative assessments of severity include ''tremendous,'' ''awful,'' ''excruciating,'' and ''intolerable.'' Up to 8 percent may note a mild headache at onset, and 1.5 percent may never have a severe headache. The sensitivity of severe headache as a symptom of subarachnoid bleeding is given as 98 to 100 percent in some series, and 59 to 71 percent in others. The lower range of sensitivity reported may reflect inclusion of obtunded patients who were unable to give an accurate history.

The headache is generalized in 70 percent, and lateralized in 30 percent. Unilateral headaches are usually frontal or frontoparietal, are associated with carotid-posterior communicating and middle cerebral artery aneurysms, and are ipsilateral to the bleeding lesion. Retro-orbital and orbital pain is seen in carotid and posterior communicating aneurysms. Generalized headache is more common with rupture of anterior communicating aneurysms. The headache onset may be associated with a transient or persistent loss of consciousness. Nausea and vomiting may occur during the first few hours, and neck stiffness and pain develop over the first 24 h. Photophobia and the tendency to keep the eyelids closed begins during the first day after onset. Mental obtundation, confusion, and evidence of motor weakness and dysphasia may appear within the first few hours.

A small percentage of patients may also have lumbar or thoracic backache and unilateral or bilateral leg pain. Difficulty in straightening the legs may be reported, due to hamstring muscle tightness. A positive Kernig sign may be present.

Physical examination may reveal hypertension (32 percent), fever (5 percent), focal neurologic findings (10 percent), confusion and lethargy, seizures (7 percent), nuchal rigidity (70 to 95 percent), photophobia, and subhyaloid and preretinal hemorrhages (5 percent). A CT scan performed within 72 h of onset has a sensitivity of 91 to 96 percent for the detection of subarachnoid hemorrhage. CT performed at 72 h may have a sensitivity below 80 percent. Lumbar puncture may be associated with uncal herniation and neurologic deterioration. Patients with this complication have had subdural or parenchymal hemorrhages present on CT scans done immediately after a lumbar puncture. The presence of midline shift or an intracranial hematoma are contraindications to lumbar puncture. Lumbar

puncture should be performed on patients with suspected subarachnoid hemorrhage and a negative CT scan. The CT scan is less sensitive after 72 h, and some patients seen after a delay of more than 3 days may go undiagnosed without a lumbar puncture. A normal CT scan, the absence of CSF red blood cells, xanthochromia (measured spectrophotometrically at 415–460 nm), and/or a negative D-dimer assay excludes subarachnoid hemorrhage. CSF xanthochromia is present in 100 percent of patients between 12 h and 2 weeks and in 70 percent for 3 weeks. The sensitivity of a CT scan for detection of subarachnoid bleeding is only 30 to 50 percent at 1 week and 30 percent at 2 weeks. Spinal fluid obtained within the first 12 h after the onset of a thunderclap headache will contain many red blood cells, but the cell lysis required to produce free CSF oxyhemoglobin and bilirubin, the pigments causing xanthochromia, may not yet have occurred, accounting for an absence of xanthochromia in such samples.

An uncommon subset of patients have a thunderclap headache, a normal CT scan, and blood-containing CSF without xanthochromia. These patients have a good prognosis. In three cases, angiograms were negative. The most likely explanation for the blood-stained fluid is a traumatic tap in a patient with a nonhemorrhagic thunderclap headache.

Cerebral angiography will usually demonstrate the aneurysm and vasospasm of adjacent vessels. Rarely, aneurysmal rupture will occur in the absence of a demonstrable aneurysm (false-negative study) on the initial angiogram. Clinical confirmation of acute subarachnoid hemorrhage and a CT scan showing a septum pellucidum hematoma or blood in the cistern of the lamina terminalis and the anterior interhemispheric fissure is suggestive of rupture of an anterior communicating aneurysm. The additional presence of angiographically demonstrable arterial spasm without a visible aneurysm is supportive of the diagnosis of aneurysmal rupture. Patients with such findings have been surgically explored, and the suspected aneurysm has been found and clipped, excluding it from the circulation.

Common misdiagnoses in patients with subarachnoid bleeding include systemic febrile illness, migraine, a hypertensive crisis, cervical disc disease or arthritis, aseptic meningitis, brain tumor, and sinusitis. An initial incorrect diagnosis occurs in 23 to 25 percent of cases with aneurysmal rupture.

Cerebral angiography is usually highly sensitive for the demonstration of an aneurysm in the cerebral circulation. Associated vasospasm may aid in determining which aneurysm has ruptured in the 22 percent of cases with multiple aneurysms. Clipping of the bleeding aneurysm excludes it from the circulation and is definitive therapy. Use of nimodipine intravenously in the perioperative period reduces the frequency of ischemic complications and the mortality rate.

4. Thunderclap Headache without Aneurysm or Hemorrhage Up to 80 percent of patients with the explosive or abrupt onset of a severe or excruciating headache have a negative CT scan and lumbar puncture. Such patients mimic subarachnoid hemorrhage clinically but show no evidence of bleeding and do not usually develop meningismus. The etiology of these headaches is unknown, and their course is benign. They may represent severe attacks of common migraine or other type of vascular headache. A small number may eventually prove to have expanding aneurysms that have not yet leaked, but demonstration requires angiography.

B. Arteriovenous Malformation This congenital malformation may present with the abrupt onset of headache, due to subarachnoid hemorrhage, nuchal pain, and stiffness (50–67 percent of cases). Focal or grand mal seizures may be the initial manifestation of this disorder in up to 50 percent of cases.

Recurrent migraine-like headaches may occur in 8 to 10 percent of cases. A vascular steal syndrome can cause progressive hemiparesis and dementia. The latter may also occur secondary to normal pressure hydrocephalus resulting from repeated episodes of subarachnoid hemorrhage. The diagnosis can be confirmed by a CT scan with contrast. The malformation can also be imaged and its extent and blood supply defined by angiography.

Surgical excision of the malformation is feasible if it is located in the frontal, occipital, or temporal pole of the brain.

Microsurgical techniques have lowered the morbidity and mortality associated with resection of arteriovenous malformations. Bleeding from an AV malformation accounts for up to 10 percent of episodes of spontaneous subarachnoid hemorrhage.

C. Spinal Subarachnoid Hemorrhage Spinal subarachnoid hemorrhage results from spontaneous bleeding from an AV malformation, because of anticoagulant therapy, from a blood dyscrasia, or from an ependymoma. Severe midline neck or back pain, and tenderness at the level of rupture occur abruptly (like the ''strike of the dagger''). Radicular involvement may result in acute anterior chest pain (upper thoracic spine lesion), abdominal pain (lower thoracic or lumbar lesion), or rectal pain (cauda equina lesion). Headache, stiff neck, and fever may follow, in association with spine pain and tenderness. Subarachnoid hemorrhage, sciatica, and headache constitute what has been called the Fincher syndrome.

MRI or a CT-enhanced myelogram will demonstrate a spinal cord tumor, AV malformation, or spinal subarachnoid hematoma secondary to bleeding in a patient on anticoagulant therapy.

A spinal subarachnoid hematoma may produce back pain of abrupt onset, meningismus with headache, sciatica or abdominal pain, bilateral or unilateral leg weakness, patchy lower extremity sensory loss or a sensory level, and impairment of sphincter function. A spinal subarachnoid hematoma can also result from bleeding from an arteriovenous malformation, from a tumor, or from vasculitis associated with a collagen vascular disease. Only 1 percent of subarachnoid hemorrhages are of spinal origin. It is of interest that the presence of blood of spinal cord level origin may result in papilledema, retinal hemorrhages, and mental confusion in a small number of patients. Prompt spinal cord decompression will relieve motor, sensory, and sphincter symptoms.

Head injury is the commonest cause of subarachnoid bleeding. Spontaneous subarachnoid hemorrhage is caused by aneurysm (90 percent of cases), AV malformation (8 percent), and a heterogeneous group of rare disorders (1–2 percent) that are listed in Table 2-1.

3. INTRACRANIAL INFECTION

A. Acute Bacterial Meningitis In older children and adults, this disorder usually presents acutely, with a generalized headache and sometimes bilateral retro-orbital pain, chills, fever, nausea, and vomiting. A painful stiff neck is usually present or develops within hours. Confusion, lethargy, combativeness, and irritability may occur. Severe myalgias and generalized limb weakness and stiffness may develop. Reports of fulminant meningitis occurring in the absence of meningeal signs suggest that the presence of fever, headache, and a change in mental alertness or a gait disturbance warrant CT study and/or lumbar puncture.

Table 2-1
CAUSES OF ACUTE SPONTANEOUS SUBARACHNOID HEMORRHAGE

	Relative Frequency (%)
Aneurysm	90
Arteriovenous malformation	8
Developmental disorders	
Sturge-Weber disease	
Osler-Weber-Rendu syndrome	
Ehlers-Danlos syndrome	
Pseudoxanthoma elasticum	
Infectious disorders	
Myocotic aneurysm	
Brain abscess	
Meningitis	
Herpes encephalitis	
Syphilitic meningoencephalitis	
Brain neoplasms	
Blood dyscrasias and coagulopathies	
Vasculitis	
Hypertensive encephalopathy	
Rupture of an atherosclerotic artery	
Spinal subarachnoid hemorrhage	1

A subset of patients with bacterial meningitis may develop meningeal signs gradually over a period of 1 to 7 days. Fever, headache, and flexion-extension and/or rotational neck pain and stiffness may occur. The slower time course of symptom development in these patients may sometimes be due to partial treatment with oral antibiotics.

Examination reveals pain and nuchal stiffness on attempted flexion, but in early cases Kernig's sign and Brudzinski's sign may be absent. Lethargy, confusion, episodes of screaming, combativeness, garbled speech, or an ataxic gait may occur in some patients. Meningococcal disease may be associated with a diffuse erythematous maculopapular or petechial rash. Focal neurologic signs such as hemiparesis, facial weakness, quadriparesis, dysphasia, paresis of extraocular muscles, hearing loss, visual blurring, and coma may occur in a small percentage of cases during the first 96 h.

N. meningitidis infection occurs as a sporadic illness or as a community epidemic in urban areas and in new military recruits. *S. pneumoniae* meningitis is a nonepidemic disease, and it is associated with acute otitis and/or mastoiditis, pneumonia, sinusitis, a prior skull fracture (recent or past), splenectomy, and immunoglobulin deficiency. *H. influenzae* meningitis does not occur over age 5 unless an anatomic or immunologic problem is present.

Meningeal infection by gram-negative bacteria may follow trauma or neurosurgery and is associated with diabetes mellitus (*Klebsiella*), cirrhosis, neoplastic disease, alcoholism, and urinary tract infections.

The more gradual development of headache and the early prominence of fever, rigors, and chills separate bacterial meningitis from an acute subarachnoid hemorrhage.

The CSF reveals an elevation of the total leukocyte count with a range of 10 to more than 20,000 cells/mm^3. The predominant cell (>50 percent of the cells counted) is the polymorphonuclear leukocyte. In patients with bacterial meningitis and a cell count below 1000/mm^3, as many as 32 percent may have CSF lymphocytosis (60–70 percent lymphocytes); and/or the total cell count may be normal (1 percent of cases). Since a CSF Gram's stain will identify bacteria in 80 percent of cases, only 6.4 percent of the total number of cases would be misclassified as nonbacterial after a cell count and Gram's stain. Newer methods of antigen detection are 95 percent sensitive and can make a specific diagnosis in patients with culture-negative CSF resulting from prior antibiotic therapy. These include latex agglutination (LA) and counterimmunoelectrophoresis (CIE) tests. The sensitivity of the latter is 50 to 90 percent with meningococcal disease and 50 to 100 percent with *S. pneumoniae* meningitis. Measurement of CSF lactate reveals levels of more than 35 mg/dl in 90 to 95 percent of cases of bacterial meningitis. Measurement of CSF glucose has proved to be insensitive (sensitivity = 50 percent) and nonspecific for the diagnosis of bacterial infection. CSF protein levels are frequently elevated, but such increases are nonspecific, occurring in many types of central nervous system disorders. Cultures will provide specific identification of the cause of meningitis and are 20 percent more sensitive than are Gram's stains.

Meningitis due to *S. pneumoniae* and *N. meningitidis* will respond to 20 to 24 million units of intravenous penicillin per day, while gram-negative meningitis may be treated with a third-generation cephalosporin or aztreonam.

The clinical syndrome of fever; frontal, orbital, and/or generalized headache; meningismus; and altered mental status may occur in other forms of meningitis produced by unusual bacteria or resulting from etiologies other than bacterial infection. These disorders may be confused with pneumococcal, meningococcal, or gram-negative meningeal infections, since they may have a similar clinical presentation and a CSF that contains an increased leukocyte count with a polymorphonuclear leukocyte predominance and a CSF glucose level below 40 mg/dl or 0.4 of the blood glucose. Unusual infectious causes of acute meningitis and mimics of acute bacterial meningitis are discussed below.

B. Unusual Forms of Bacterial Meningitis

1. Lyme Disease   Three to 32 days (median = 7 days) after a tick bite (macule or small papule), a characteristic skin rash (erythema chronicum migrans) appears at the bite site. It is an expanding, annular, flat or elevated erythematous ringlike lesion, with the bite at its center. The inner area is a paler pink or normal skin color, and may be indurated. Up to 86 percent of patients may develop this rash. Smaller secondary annular lesions may occur within a few days in up to 50 percent of patients. Systemic symptoms such as fever, chills, headache, photophobia, neck discomfort and stiffness, malaise, fatigue, diffuse myalgias and arthralgias, and dysesthesias in the limbs may occur in some cases (stage 1). Lumbar puncture during stage 1 is usually normal, but *Borrelia burgdorferi* antigen has been detected in such fluid. Within 4 to 10 weeks after the appearance of the rash, a severe frontal, occipital, bitemporal, posterior neck, or generalized headache occurs, accompanied by fever, nausea, vomiting, photophobia, and pain on eye motion (stage 2). Mild stiffness of the neck may be demonstrable on physical examination, but other meningeal signs are usually absent. The total cell count ranges from 15 to 700/mm^3, with 5 to 100 percent lymphocytes; and the CSF glucose level varies from 33 to 61 mg/dl. Most patients have a lymphocytic pleocytosis, but others have presented with a 95 percent neutrophilic predominance. CSF sugar values are usually in the normal range, and cultures and Gram's stain are negative. Meningitis may present in association with a mild encephalitis (difficulty concentrating, insomnia, memory difficulties, irritability, and emotional lability); an inflammatory neuritis of multiple cranial nerves (unilateral or bilateral facial paresis, abducens paresis, or only subjective diplopia); and sometimes a peripheral neuritis. The latter may take the form of a sensory radiculopathy, with pain, paresthesias, and skin hyperesthesia or hypesthesia; a motor radiculoneuritis, with weakness and atrophy; mononeuritis multiplex; or a brachial plexitis. The extremity radiculoneuritis is usually sensory and motor. One or more of these neurologic syndromes may be present in stage 2 Lyme disease. Serologic confirmation can be obtained by measuring the CSF IgM and IgG index for *B. burgdorferi* and by measuring the serum IgM and IgG antibody titers to the same organism. Patients with stage 2 disease are usually positive on the ELISA for IgG antibody to *B. burgdorferi*. Meningeal and other neurologic symptoms respond to a regimen of 20 million units of intravenous penicillin a day for 10 days.

2. Listeria Monocytogenes *Meningitis*   Headache, fever, and meningismus may be associated with a CSF neutrophilic predominance and a low CSF glucose level. The majority of patients with *Listeria* meningitis have acute or chronic leukemia, a lymphoma, or a collagen vascular disease under therapy with corticosteroids. Patients immunosuppressed because of renal transplantation are also at risk. The organism may be grown from the blood or CSF and is often initially mistaken for a streptococcus or diphtheroid.

Listeria may also cause cerebritis without meningitis. Such patients may have fever, headache, and focal neurologic signs. Progression to brain abscess may occur, and this can be demonstrated by detection of contrast-enhancing lesions on CT scan. Brain abscess is rare but may cause hemiparesis, aphasia, homonymous hemianopia, and a neutrophilic CSF with negative cultures. *Listeria* may also cause a rhombencephalitis with prominent signs of brain stem dysfunction (diplopia, dysarthria, dysphagia, facial dysesthesias, and/or paresis) due to involvement of cranial nerves V, VI, VII, VIII, IX, and X; fever; headache; and vomiting. Lumbar puncture may reveal a lymphocytic predominance and negative CSF cultures (parameningeal reaction). The diagnosis can sometimes be made from positive blood cultures. Parenteral therapy with ampicillin and gentamicin is effective against this organism.

3. Mycobacterium tuberculosis   The onset is more gradual than in patients with rapidly progressive bacterial meningitis, but 45 percent of patients have symptoms for only 5 to 14 days prior to admission. Up to 65 percent complain of headache, fever, nausea, and drowsiness. Up to 55 percent may have a depressed level of consciousness with stupor or coma. Nuchal rigidity occurs in 55 percent; papilledema in 6 percent; and abnormalities of cranial nerves II, III, IV, VI, and VII in 6 to 13 percent. The CSF glucose level may be low in 55 to 60 percent, the cell count may be less than 500/mm^3 in 95 percent, and a polymorphonuclear predominance may occur in 22 percent of cases, mimicking acute bacterial meningitis. The Gram's stain and routine bacterial cultures are negative. A Ziehl-Neelsen stain of CSF may be positive in 2 to 87 percent of cases, depending on how much effort is taken to find the organism. Culture for *M. tuberculosis* is the gold standard, but false-negative cultures may occur in 13 percent. A large volume of CSF (10–15 ml) should be centrifuged and the sediment cultured on Lowenstein-Jensen medium to enhance the likelihood of a positive result. Some cases have only been proved at postmortem.

An ELISA method for the detection of *M. tuberculosis* antigen in spinal fluid has been developed for rapid diagnosis. Its sensitivity is only 52 percent, but its specificity is 96 percent.

The tuberculin skin test may be falsely negative in 15 to 30 percent, the chest radiograph negative in 42 percent, the sedimentation rate normal in 35 percent, and the white blood count less than 10,000 cells/mm^3 in 68 percent of cases.

Treatment with isoniazid, rifampin, and pyrazinamide leads to resolution with a mortality rate of 12 to 22 percent.

4. *Anaerobic Bacteria*   These organisms may rarely cause acute meningitis. Most reported cases of *Bacteroides fragilis* meningitis have occurred in premature infants or in older patients with otitis media. Anaerobic bacteria are only rarely reported as a cause of meningitis. The clinical and CSF picture is typical of bacterial meningitis, but such organisms may be missed if the fluid is not cultured for anaerobes. Suspicion of anaerobic infection should be raised if the Gram's stain is positive and routine aerobic cultures are negative. In a surveillance study covering 1977–1981, 18,642 cases of meningitis occurred, with only 5 cases caused by obligate anaerobes, but the type and number of anaerobic cultures performed was not reported.

5. *Mixed Bacterial Meningitis*   Patients present with fever greater than 100°F (100 percent of cases), headache (100 percent), mental status changes (78 percent), and nuchal rigidity (88 percent), with 80 percent of total CSF cell counts greater than 949 cells/mm^3 (mean, 6261 leukocytes/mm^3) and a neutrophilic predominance of greater than 80 percent in 60 percent of cases. The CSF glucose is less than 40 mg/dl in 67 percent. In one study, Gram's stains were positive in 67 percent, but only half of these patients demonstrated more than a single organism. Positive CSF cultures grew two or more organisms, including enteric aerobic and anaerobic bacteria, orapharyngeal flora, and *Staphylococcus aureus*. Risk factors for mixed bacterial meningitis include a fistula connecting the upper airway, skin, or bowel to the subarachnoid space; a ventricular shunt; infection at a contiguous site (e.g., otitis media or sinusitis); recent neurosurgery; and malignancy (e.g., rectal cancer with fistula to meninges). In patients with one or more of these risk factors, mixed bacterial infection should be suspected; aerobic and anaerobic cultures obtained; and therapy for gram-positive, gram-negative, and anaerobic organisms started, pending the outcome of cultures.

C. Mimics of Acute Bacterial Meningitis

1. Amebic Meningoencephalitis *Naegleria fowleri* is an amcboflagellate. The trophozoites are 10 to 15 μm in diameter and have a large, centrally located nucleus with a prominent karyosome. These organisms enter the nasopharynx after head submersion during freshwater swimming, invade the nasal mucosae and the cribriform plate, and then multiply in the meninges and olfactory bulbs. The illness characteristically begins approximately 1 week after swimming in a freshwater lake in the southeastern United States, although European cases have followed bathing in a chlorinated swimming pool. The clinical picture includes fever, severe frontal headache, nausea, vomiting, and meningismus. Unusual tastes and smells are a clue to the presence of the organism in the olfactory bulbs. The CSF contains a large number of neutrophils and a low glucose level. Amebas with a characteristic slow motility are usually visible in a wet mount of cerebrospinal fluid. Amebas can also be detected in dry CSF samples with a direct fluorescent antibody stain and can be cultured on salt-free agar seeded with *Escherichia coli*. Parenteral and intrathecal amphotericin may lead to cure, but the mortality with optimum therapy is high. Acanthamoeba infections of the meninges are very rare, and they usually cause a mononuclear predominance in the CSF.

2. Aseptic (Viral) Meningitis Patients have mild to severe headache; fever; nuchal stiffness; and, uncommonly, evidence of a slight change in the level of consciousness. The CSF taken during the first 12 h of illness may show a predominance of polymorphonuclear leukocytes. If a second tap is performed 12 or more hours after the first, almost all cases of viral meningitis will demonstrate a lymphocytic predominance in the CSF. The spinal fluid sugar has been reported to be depressed in some partients with aseptic meningitis produced by mumps (10 percent in the range of 20–50 mg/dl), herpes simplex virus, and lymphocytic choriomeningitis virus.

3. Meningitis Secondary to Intracranial Tumors and Cysts Aseptic chemical meningitis due to necrotic tumor or cyst contents may mimic bacterial meningitis, since it can produce a fever, generalized headache,

meningismus, vomiting and lethargy, an elevated CSF cell count, a polymorphonuclear predominance, and a low CSF glucose level. A single or multiple episodes of acute meningitis may occur before the correct diagnosis is made. The CSF Gram's stain and cultures are negative. CSF examination for keratin and cholesterol crystals may aid in the diagnosis of an epidermoid cyst.

Lesions producing this form of chemical meningitis include intracranial or spinal epidermoid tumors or cysts; dermoid cysts of the posterior fossa; glioblastoma multiforme; craniopharyngiomas; pituitary adenomas; and spinal teratomas. These can be detected by a CT scan or MRI of the brain and spinal cord. Removal of the tumor or cyst prevents recurrence. Some cystic lesions may be difficult to image at the time of the meningitis episode, since they may have emptied their contents into the CSF and decreased in size. Scans done 3 to 6 months after recovery may image these cysts, since they may have enlarged by then.

4. Drug-Related Meningitis Fever, headache, neck ache, vomiting, and a decreased level of consciousness associated with a neutrophilic predominance in the CSF and low or normal glucose levels may be associated with hypersensitivity to drugs such as ibuprofen, sulindac, tolmetin, trimethoprim-sulfamethoxasole, and azathioprine. Other drugs that have been associated with aseptic meningitis include penicillin, isoniazid, phenazopyridine, and sulfonamides.

Drug-induced meningitis may be associated with facial swelling, urticaria, pruritus, conjunctivitis, and the rapid cessation of symptoms of meningitis after discontinuation of the offending drug.

Drug-induced meningitis is more common in women and in patients with systemic lupus erythematosus, mixed connective tissue disease, and Sjogren's syndrome.

5. Collagen Vascular Disorders and Aseptic Meningitis (Systemic Lupus Erythematosus and Mixed Connective Tissue Disease) In one series, aseptic meningitis occurred in 2 to 4.5 percent of SLE cases over an 11-year period. A clinical picture of fever, headache, meningismus, and CSF findings of a neutrophilic predominance and a depressed glucose level may mimic bacterial meningitis. Other symptoms and signs of lupus are usually present, and CSF Gram's stain and bacterial cultures are negative. Prednisone may suppress all symptoms and signs. The ANA test and LE preparation are usually positive.

There is a single case report of mixed connective tissue disease in association with aseptic meningitis without a provoking drug. This patient had fever, headache, meningismus, a lymphocytic pleocytosis, and a normal CSF glucose level.

6. Behçet's Disease Recurrent aphthous stomatitis occurs with two or more of the following: recurrent aphthous genital ulcers, uveitis, meningoencephalitis, arthritis or arthralgia, and skin nodules or pustules. Headache, fever, and meningismus are usually associated with an elevated CSF cell count, lymphocytic predominance, and normal glucose levels. These findings are sometimes confused with bacterial meningitis, since up to 32 percent of patients with bacterial meningitis and total CSF cell counts less then 1000/mm^3 may show a lymphocytic predominance. CSF Gram's stain and cultures are required to exclude bacterial meningitis.

An associated encephalitis may cause focal or multifocal corticospinal tract disease with limb weakness, cerebellar ataxia, pseudobulbar palsy, and diplopia secondary to oculomotor nerve lesions. Other findings associated with Behçet's disease include superficial thrombophlebitis, ulcerative enterocolitis, epididymitis, erythema nodosum, and a peculiar tendency of the skin to form papules at sites of an aseptic needle stick.

Meningeal and encephalitic manifestations can be suppressed by chlorambucil.

7. Mollaret's Meningitis   This is a recurrent disorder that may go undiagnosed for years. The clinical picture includes fever, generalized headache, shoulder and arm pain, meningismus, and lethargy. The cell count is usually less than 3000/mm^3, and a lymphocytic predominance is usual, but polymorphonuclear neutrophils may exceed 50 percent of the cell number in some episodes. Large CSF ''Mollaret cells'' demonstrable by a Papanicolaou smear may constitute 60 to 70 percent of the cells present during the first 24 h of illness. Similar cells may occur in herpes simplex meningitis. The CSF glucose level is usually normal. Colchicine may decrease the severity and frequency of attacks. Some cases originally thought to be Mollaret's meningitis have been found to be caused by central nervous system tumors or cysts.

The presence of a tumor, an infection, or an immunologic disorder should be excluded before a diagnosis of an idiopathic disorder such as Mollaret's meningitis is accepted.

8. Fungal Meningitis (Coccidioidal Meningitis)   An acute form may occur, with fever, headache, meningismus, nausea, and vomiting. Most cases occur in the endemic area (e.g., southwestern United States) or in recent visitors to that region. Lumbar puncture may reveal a total cell count greater than 1000/mm^3, a predominance of polymorphonuclear neutrophils, a low CSF glucose level, and sometimes the presence of CSF eosinophils. Complement-fixing antibodies to *Coccidioides immitis* may be present in the serum and CSF. Cultures of CSF are positive in only 20 to 40 percent of cases.

A persistent serum CF titer of 1:32 or more suggests disseminated coccidioidomycosis, and any spinal fluid CF titer (present in up to 95 percent of cases of meningitis) is diagnostic of coccidioidal meningitis. CSF titers range from 1:1 to greater than 1:32. Therapy with amphotericin B or fluconazole is effective, but relapse after treatment is common.

9. Brain Abscess   Patients who develop a brain abscess usually have a history of a contiguous infection (e.g., draining ear, sinusitis, or mastoiditis); a pulmonary, cardiac, or other remote infection (e.g., pneumonia, lung abscess, bronchiectasis, endocarditis, cyanotic heart disease, or skin infection); dental disease (e.g., caries, periapical abscess, a recent root canal procedure or extraction, or periodontitis); penetrating brain trauma, or a recent neurosurgical or otolaryngolical procedure.

Symptoms include a unilateral or generalized headache (65–80 percent), a decrease in mental status (26–68 percent), fever and chills (34–52 percent), nausea and vomiting (35–50 percent), focal or generalized seizures (25–36 percent), and focal neurologic deficits. The latter include hemiparesis (9–25 percent), aphasia (9 percent), visual field defects, and cranial nerve lesions. The duration of symptoms prior to diagnosis may be as short as 1 week or as long as 6 months.

Physical examination reveals fever (60 percent); lethargy (71 percent); stupor (6 percent); coma (6 percent); hemiparesis (23 percent); monoparesis (5 percent); a visual field loss (14 percent); dysfunction of cranial nerves III, IV, VI, and VIII (29 percent); dysphasia (12 percent); papilledema (10 percent); and nuchal rigidity (49 percent).

The CSF is usually abnormal but may not be in up to 11 percent of cases. Cell counts are elevated in 80 percent, and in 42 percent there is a polymorphonuclear predominance. The glucose level is usually normal, but it may be less than 40 mg/dl in 20 percent of cases. CSF cultures may be positive in up to 10 percent of cases. CSF findings of a polymorphonuclear leukocyte predominance and a low sugar level in a patient with headache, fever, and nuchal rigidity simulates a bacterial meningitis. In some cases, bacterial meningitis does occur, secondary to abscess rupture into the subarachnoid space. In these cases, cell counts are very high and may exceed 150,000/mm^3 of CSF, and the Gram's stain is positive.

The diagnosis of brain abscess can be confirmed by a contrast-enhanced CT scan that demonstrates one or more ring-enhancing lesions surrounded by cerebral edema (57 percent), nodular enhancement (17 percent), and areas of attenuation without enhancement (13 percent). Initially negative scans may become positive within 5 to 13 days, resulting in a prevalence of ring-enhancing lesions of 77 percent by the third week of hospitalization.

Technetium 99m brain scans have a high sensitivity (100 percent). Sixty percent show spherical accumulations of radioactivity, and 20 percent doughnut-shaped collections. The technetium 99m scan is more likely than a CT scan to be positive in a patient with acute cerebritis during the first few days of illness before the lesion has progressed to abscess formation. Detection of such early lesions may allow for complete resolution with antibiotic therapy alone.

MRI has been as sensitive as contrast-enhanced CT for abscess detection. Abscesses appear hypointense with respect to brain on short TR/short TE scans and hyperintense on long TR/intermediate or long TR/long TE scans. On short TR/short TE scans, the abscess rim is hyperintense relative to white matter (white rim) or isointense. On long TR/intermediate to long TE scans, the rim was hypointense (dark rim). MRI is useful for differentiating an abscess from other lesions by allowing visualization of the morphologic features of the abscess capsule on long TR scans.

A single organism may be etiologic in 53 percent of cases, two organisms in 22 percent, and three or more in 9 percent. Aerobic organisms (38 percent of cases) such as streptococci, gram-negative enteric bacteria, *S. aureus*, and *S. pneumoniae*; anaerobes (40 percent); and microaerophilic streptococci (21 percent) have been obtained as single or multiple isolates from cultured pus. Broad-spectrum antibiotic therapy, combined with abscess drainage and/or excision, results in recovery in 90 percent of cases. Penicillin or cefotaxime (e.g., for abscesses secondary to ear infections) and anti-anaerobic antibiotics provide effective coverage for the organisms usually isolated.

10. AIDS and Contrast-Enhancing Brain Lesions
Patients with AIDS may present with headache, fever, focal neurologic abnormalities, and seizures. Toxoplasma abscesses, B-cell lymphoma, fungal abscesses, tuberculosis, and occasionally cryptococcosis may be seen as enhancing lesions on CT or as well-delineated lesions by MRI. MRI may be more sensitive for toxoplasmosis than a contrast-enhanced CT.

In a patient with a suspected abscess, a CT scan or MRI should be done initially, and if an abscess is demonstrated, a lumbar puncture should be avoided because of the danger of neurologic deterioration secondary to uncal or cerebellar herniation. A technetium 99m scan should be done if an early abscess or cerebritis is thought to be present. The presence of a ring-enhancing lesion in an AIDS patient may require biopsy for definitive diagnosis. In some centers, therapy for toxoplasmosis is given and the clinical response evaluated before resorting to brain biopsy.

11. Subdural Empyema This disorder has a predilection for adolescent males, but cases may occur at any age, and women may be affected. Most cases arise from a symptomatic or clinically silent sinusitis (70 percent), while other cases are associated with otitis media or mastoiditis (10–20 percent), skull trauma or craniotomy, osteomyelitis of the skull, or meningitis. Frontal or generalized headache (75 percent), fever (75 percent), malaise, and periorbital swelling (in cases associated with sinusitis) occur initially and are followed within 1 week by drowsiness, lethargy, or stupor (75 percent). Focal neurologic symptoms such as hemiparesis (92 percent), dysphasia (43 percent), cranial nerve lesions (21 percent), and papilledema (25 percent) are associated with an altered sensorium. Focal or generalized seizures may occur in 29 percent, and status epilepticus may develop. Fever and nuchal rigidity (100 percent) suggest the possibility of acute bacterial meningitis. The CSF shows an increased cell count in the 40 to 2000/mm^3 range and a polymorphonuclear neutrophil predominance, although lymphocytic predominance may occur in some fluids. The CSF glucose level remains normal, and cultures and Gram's stain are negative. This disorder should be considered in patients with a clinical picture of meningitis associated with seizures and focal neurologic symptoms and signs. Plain sinus films usually reveal sinus opacification in cases associated with sinusitis. Disease in the frontal (71 percent), ethmoid (57 percent), and maxillary (43 percent) sinuses occurs, and multiple sinuses are usually involved (pansinusitis in 36 percent).

A contrast-enhanced CT scan will identify a crescentic frontoparietal or a sliver-shaped parafalcine lucency, with fine irregular enhancement of the margins of the lucency, as well as evidence of sinus opacification. False-negative or inconclusive CT scans may occur in 12 to 50 percent of patients on the initial examination. If the diagnosis is suspected but unproven by CT, a cerebral angiogram may be helpful. Some diagnoses have been confirmed by repetition of the CT scan several days later or by surgical exploration. Surgical drainage of the empyema and antibiotic therapy directed at common isolates are required for eradication of this potentially lethal infection. Isolates obtained during surgical drainage have included microaerophilic streptococci (*S. milleri*), anaerobic streptococci, *S. aureus*, *S. pneumoniae*, anaerobes, and gram-negative aerobic bacteria. Single or mixed bacterial infections occur.

12. Cranial Epidural Abscess This rare disorder may present with frontal and/or generalized headache and fever, chills, and anorexia. Symptoms similar to those produced by a subdural empyema or meningitis develop. The diagnosis can be confirmed by a CT scan, but arteriography may be necessary in CT-negative cases. Organisms similar to those found in cases of subdural empyema are usually isolated. Treatment requires surgical (burr-hole) drainage and parenteral antibiotic therapy. This disorder may be associated with a fluctuant soft tissue swelling over the frontal bone (Pott's puffy tumor), frontal sinusitis, and an underlying osteomyelitis of the frontal bone.

13. Pituitary Apoplexy   Severe bilateral frontal or frontotemporal headache, nausea, and sometimes fever begin abruptly. Drowsiness and diplopia are common associated complaints. Visual acuity may be decreased in one or both eyes to the point of complete blindness, or specific field defects may occur (bitemporal hemianopia and, rarely, central or homonymous field defects). Fundoscopy may show optic atrophy or temporal pallor of the disc. Pressure on ocular motor nerves in the cavernous sinus by an enlarged pituitary gland may cause an isolated abducens or oculomotor nerve palsy or a panophthalmoplegia. This disorder occurs secondary to sterile necrosis and infarction of a pituitary neoplasm. Blood and necrotic tumor may be released into the subarachnoid space, causing a chemical meningitis, with headache, neck pain, and nuchal rigidity. This clinical picture may also suggest an acute subarachnoid hemorrhage. Lumbar puncture may reveal a xanthochromia, an elevated leukocyte count, a polymorphonuclear predominance, and negative cultures. The diagnosis can be confirmed by a CT scan that demonstrates a tumor mass, sella enlargement, and rim enhancement in the sella area. A careful history reveals evidence of amenorrhea or other menstrual abnormalities, galactorrhea, hair loss, weakness, infertility, and loss of libido. Pituitary hypofunction and/or increased prolactin levels may be present.

Successful recovery of vision requires rapid surgical intervention and the administration of corticosteroids. Patients with severely impaired vision may recover completely.

14. Pituitary Abscess (Aseptic or Infectious)   The symptoms and signs resemble those of pituitary apoplexy with headache, hypopituitarism and visual field defects, ocular motor nerve palsies, symptoms of sphenoid sinusitis, and radiologic evidence of sella erosion or enlargement. Abscess can be associated with an aseptic meningitis, as described above, or with bacterial infection. There is controversy as to whether a pituitary abscess is caused by bacterial infection or is noninfectious in origin. The associated aseptic meningitis may produce a lymphocytic pleocytosis in association with a normal glucose level in the CSF. Infection is believed to invade from the adjacent sphenoid sinuses or from a cavernous sinus thrombosis. Pituitary abscess has also been reported in association with otitis media; mastoiditis; and peritonsillar abscess. Infection is more likely in a patient with a chromophobe adenoma or a craniopharyngioma.

4. CEREBROVASCULAR DISEASE AND HEADACHE

A. Intraparenchymal Hemorrhage   Sentinel headache occurs in only 14 percent of cases. The frequency of headache is dependent on the site and size of hemorrhage. Headache was associated with 13 to 62 percent of putaminal, 46 to 68 percent of lobar, 30 percent of thalamic, 35 percent of pontine, and 48 to 80 percent of cerebellar hemorrhages in one series. Small hemorrhages (1–2 cm) may occur without an associated headache. Putaminal hemorrhage may cause a unilateral frontal headache in 67 percent of cases. A differential diagnosis of intraparenchymal hemorrhage is presented in Table 2-2 and that of acute stroke in Table 2-3.

1. Putaminal Hemorrhage   Putaminal hemorrhage may develop gradually over a period of 6 to 12 h (60 percent) or rapidly (40 percent). Contralateral hemiparesis, homonymous hemianopia, gaze palsy, contralateral neglect, and hemisensory loss occur. Right hemiparesis may be associated with aphasia. Patients with hemorrhages larger then 3 cm in diameter may lapse into a stupor or coma. Small putaminal hemorrhages may occur without headache and would be diagnosed as a thrombotic or embolic stroke without a CT scan. This procedure demonstrates the hemorrhage as a hyperdense round-to-ovoid collection in the putamen. This localization is more prevalent in hypertensives.

2. Thalamic Hemorrhage   Contralateral hemiparesis, hemisensory loss, and a homonymous hemianopia occur. Dominant-side hemorrhage causes aphasia, and

Table 2-2
CAUSES OF INTRAPARENCHYMAL HEMORRHAGE

	Relative Frequency (%)
Hypertension	30–45
Aneurysms	15–20
Arteriovenous malformation	5–15
Bleeding disorders	10–30
Thrombocytopenia	
Thrombocytosis	
Hemophilia	
Anticoagulant therapy	
Thrombolytic therapy	
Brain tumors	5–10
Cortical vein/venous sinus thrombosis	
Vasculitis	5
Collagen vascular disease	
Amphetamine-induced	
Giant cell arteritis	
Granulomatous arteritis	
Primary central nervous system angiitis	
Miscellaneous	
Amyloid angiopathy	
Cryptic arteriovenous malformations	
Moyamoya disease	

Table 2-3
THE DIFFERENTIAL DIAGNOSIS OF STROKE

	Time Course and Symptoms	Risk Factors and Associated Disorders	Unique Features
Atherothrombotic infarction	Headache in only 26% Onset in seconds, minutes, hours, or days, in a series of steps Gradual, but often incomplete, improvement over weeks or months	TIAs Coronary disease and peripheral vascular disease, hypertension, elevated cholesterol, and diabetes Age >50 Carotid bruits	Normal CSF cell counts and sugar with normal or elevated protein CT scan showing an area of focal attenuation (infarction and edema) in the subcortical region of the brain Hemiparesis and/or dysphasia may be present, but patient is alert
Cerebral embolism	Headache in only 14% Onset of completed stroke in seconds or minutes, and rapid improvement in minutes, hours, or days	No prior TIAs Sources of emboli include the heart (atrial fibrillation, mitral stenosis, prosthetic valve, myocardial infarction, ventricular aneurysm, endocarditis, mitral valve prolapse, patent foramen ovale with paradoxic embolization) Carotid stenosis Large-vessel disease at the aortic arch Evidence of recent infarction may be present in other areas of the brain and at other sites in the body	Young age Associated headache Clear CSF CT scan showing an area of focal attenuation (infarction and edema) in the subcortical region of the brain
Venous thrombosis	Headache common Abrupt or gradual onset Stroke with seizures and signs of increased intracranial pressure Gradual recovery over months	Postpartum or postoperative period Recent ear or sinus infection, meningitis, polycythemia vera, or sickle cell disease	Young age Positive MRI for venous sinus thrombosis
Cerebral hemorrhage	Onset in minutes to several hours, and stroke complete within hours Onset when awake Gradual recovery Headache common	Hypertension May be no prior warning	Positive CT scan for intraparenchymal hemorrhage Red cells and xanthocromia in CSF Hemiparesis and stupor Neck stiffness and associated headache
Aneurysmal subarachnoid hemorrhage	Sudden onset of headache in 98% and stiff neck in 90% Absence of focal signs Seizure, syncope, or transient weakness or numbness at onset Hemiparesis may follow in 7–10 days due to ischemic infarction secondary to spasm	Sentinel headache (minor leak) Coarctation of aorta Polycystic kidneys Hypertension	CT scan positive for subarachnoid hemorrhage CT scan negative for intraparenchymal hemorrhage CSF grossly bloody with xanthocromia
AV malformation hemorrhage	Sudden onset of headache, neck stiffness, and hemiparesis	History of a seizure disorder Subjective bruit Recurrent bouts of subarachnoid hemorrhage	Young age CT scan with contrast demonstrating AV malformation and subarachnoid bleeding
Arteritis	Gradual progressive course without reversal over days or weeks, with multiple sites of CNS involvement	Arteritis elsewhere, syphilis, or tuberculosis	Young age Elevated sedimentation rate Muscle or skin biopsy showing arteritis Brain and meningeal biopsies showing arteritis CT scan may be normal Cerebral angiogram may demonstrate ''beading'' of vessels

(continued on page 24)

Table 2-3 *(continued)*
THE DIFFERENTIAL DIAGNOSIS OF STROKE

Hypertensive encephalopathy	Abrupt onset with severe headache, mental confusion, seizures, and visual loss BP >220 systolic, >130 diastolic Transient hemiparesis	Uncontrolled hypertension due to acute glomerulonephritis, renal failure, essential hypertension, pheochromocytoma, monoamine oxidase therapy, and tyramine ingestion Cushing's syndrome Eclampsia Abrupt withdrawl of antihypertensive therapy Grade III or IV hypertensive retinopathy	Recovery with blood pressure reduction Negative CT scan for hemorrhage, subarachnoid bleeding, or infarction
Brain tumor with stroke-like onset	Abrupt onset with hemiparesis, dysphasia, hemianopia Headaches Papilledema Deficits may improve transiently and partially, but tend to persist and progress	Prior history of recurrent headache Intellectual deterioration and personality change	CSF pressure and protein level may be increased CT or MRI evidence of brain tumor with surrounding edema or hemorrhage into the tumor

nondominant lesions cause contralateral neglect. Extension of the hemorrhage into the subthalamus causes paralysis of vertical and lateral gaze, downward and inward deviation of the eyes, loss of the light reflex, and convergence and convergence-retraction nystagmus.

3. Lobar Cerebral Hemorrhage With *occipital lobe* hemorrhage, severe ipsilateral eye pain occurs in association with a contralateral homonymous hemianopia. A portion of the superior quadrants may be spared.

Left *temporal lobe* hemorrhage may cause left-sided headache centered near the ear and a fluent dysphasia with poor understanding and frequent paraphasias. Repetition is preserved. Logorrhea may occur. Right-sided weakness may occasionally be present. Contralateral homonymous hemianopia or inferior quadrantic defects may be present.

Frontal lobe hemorrhage may cause frontal or bifrontal headache associated with contralateral arm weakness. Leg and facial weakness are absent or mild. A mild gaze preference toward the side of the lesion is noted in some patients. Drowsiness may occur.

Parietal lobe hemorrhage may cause temporal headache accompanied by contralateral arm and leg weakness and hemisensory loss. A contralateral homonymous hemianopia may be present, and dysphasia may occur with lesions of the dominant lobe.

4. Midbrain Hemorrhage Patients may experience a unilateral supraorbital or occipital headache that may become generalized. Paralysis of vertical gaze may occur, in association with diplopia, hemiparesis or quadriparesis, ocular motor palsies, and loss of pupillary response to light. Gait and limb ataxia may occur. The

diagnosis can be established by detecting a hemorrhage in the midbrain by a CT scan or MRI.

5. Cerebellar Hemorrhage Headache, nausea, and vomiting are associated with vertigo, and gait and limb ataxia. Progression occurs over several hours. There is a loss of the ability to sit, stand, and walk. Paresis of conjugate gaze to the side of the hemorrhage occurs, with deviation of the eyes to the contralateral side. Dysarthria and dysphagia may occur. A spastic paraplegia or quadriplegia may be present.

A precise and sensitive diagnosis can be made by a CT scan. Lumbar puncture can be used in cases where CT scanning is unavailable and there is no evidence of increased intracranial pressure.

The association of severe headache and vomiting with focal neurologic deficits is helpful in differentiating intraparenchymal hemorrhage from an ischemic stroke. A CT scan or MRI will clearly differentiate a hemorrhagic from an ischemic stroke.

B. Ischemic Stroke Headache may occur at the onset of focal neurologic symptoms in 17 percent of patients with an ischemic stroke. The incidence varies with the type of stroke and is 14 percent for cerebral embolism, 26 percent in large artery occlusive disease, and 6 percent in lacunar infarction. Such headaches are usually focal, unilateral, and severe. Retro-orbital and frontal headache frequently occurs ipsilateral to the side of a carotid artery thrombosis or a middle cerebral artery embolism, but head pain has been nonlocalizing in patients with middle cerebral artery thrombosis.

Occlusion of the middle cerebral or the internal carotid artery may cause the following focal deficits: contralateral hemiparesis or hemiplegia, contralateral peripheral and cortical hemisensory loss, aphasia, a contralateral homonymous hemianopia or superior homonymous quadrantanopia, contralateral gaze paralysis, a Gerstmann syndrome (i.e., agraphia, acalculia, finger agnosia, right-left confusion), apractagnosia, anosognosia, unilateral neglect, agnosia for the left half of external space (i.e., nondominant parietal lobe lesion), dressing and constructional apraxia, and visual illusions. Carotid occlusion may also affect the area of perfusion of the anterior cerebral artery, resulting in urinary incontinence, akinetic mutism, gait apraxia, and dementia.

Not all of these findings occur with a specific episode of internal carotid or middle cerebral artery occlusion, since collateral circulation may modify the clinical picture.

C. Transient Ischemic Attack   Headache in one retro-orbital and/or frontal location (57 percent) or bilaterally (43 percent) occurs in 25 percent of patients with internal carotid TIAs. The headache is rarely the presenting symptom and usually occurs in association with other neurologic symptoms or follows spontaneous resolution of these deficits.

Neurologic symptoms arising from a carotid TIA include either ocular (amaurosis fugax) or hemispheric attacks. These do not usually occur together in the same episode. Hemispheric attacks may cause partial or complete contralateral hemiparesis and numbness of the contralateral arm and hand, face and lips, fingers and lips, fingers only, or contralateral hand and foot. Sometimes, transient confusion or aphasia may be part of the attack.

Headache occurs in 10 to 45 percent of vertebrobasilar TIAs. Pain location is usually occipital or nuchal (87 percent), and it accompanies or follows the attack. Symptoms that may occur with a posterior circulation TIA include dizziness, diplopia, facial numbness, dysarthria, hemiparesis or quadriparesis and sensory deficits on one or both sides of the body.

Less common manifestations of vertebrobasilar insufficiency include gait ataxia, a feeling of being ''cross-eyed,'' visual loss, ptosis, a dilated pupil, gaze paralysis, dysphagia, and tunnel vision. Drop attacks may occur in up to 15 percent of cases. Headaches associated with vertebrobasilar TIAs tend to be persistent, and they may be intensified by straining or stooping. A similar type of headache may accompany the neurologic symptoms associated with the subclavian steal syndrome. Claudication and weakness of the left arm, a diminished pulse in the wrist, and symptoms of basilar artery insufficiency on use of the arm constitute this syndrome.

Headache usually accompanies each recurrent episode of vertebrobasilar insufficiency.

In patients with recurrent attacks of carotid insufficiency, headache is present as a component of subsequent episodes in only one-third of the patients who experience headache during their initial attack.

D. Hypertensive Encephalopathy   A severe throbbing generalized headache occurs and is accompanied by nausea, vomiting, mental confusion, visual blurring, focal or generalized seizures, and somnolence. Transient hemiparesis, dysphasia, and homonymous hemianopia may occur. Some of the visual symptoms are due to ischemia of the visual cortex and others to hypertensive retinopathy. Many patients have retinal hemorrhages, exudates, and papilledema, but others may only show focal retinal arterial narrowing. The blood pressure usually exceeds 230 systolic and 130 diastolic. Encephalopathy may progress to stupor or coma if not promptly treated.

Hypertensive encephalopathy may occur in patients with essential hypertension, acute glomerulonephritis, chronic renal failure, eclampsia, or pheochromocytoma; after use of monoamine oxidase drugs and ingestion of tyramine-containing foods; and in Cushing's syndrome. Abrupt withdrawal of antihypertensives (e.g., clonidine) or marked bladder or gastric distension in a spinal cord–injured patient can precipitate this syndrome. The focal neurologic findings associated with hypertensive encephalopathy are usually transient but may persist. Space-occupying intracranial lesions or obstructive hydrocephalus may also cause a marked rise in intracranial and systemic blood pressure. These disorders may be associated with papilledema, but without diffuse exudates and hemorrhages in the retina.

Sodium nitroprusside or other drugs can be used to lower blood pressure in patients with hypertensive encephalopathy. Careful titration of the blood pressure into a mildly elevated or normotensive range leads to resolution of the headache, visual complaints, and focal neurologic signs and cessation of seizures. Mental status improves gradually over a period of several days.

Marked cerebral edema, and microscopic and macroscopic brain hemorrhages occur. Small areas of cerebral infarction, necrosis, and/or thrombosis of small cerebral vessels (arterioles) are part of the neuropathologic findings. Since uncal or cerebellar herniation has been found at autopsy, secondary to elevated intracranial pressure, lumbar puncture should be avoided. CT or MRI can be used to detect intracranial bleeding or ischemic infarction.

E. Intracranial Venous Thrombosis   Superior longitudinal sinus occlusion presents with an occipitofrontal headache that is intensified by head motion or sitting up. Focal or grand mal seizures may occur, as may paresis of one or both legs. Subjective numbness of one or both sides of the body, as well as a cortical sensory deficit, may occur. Homonymous hemianopia or quadrantanopia, aphasia, conjugate gaze paresis, and urinary incontinence may occur. Headache may be associated with nausea, vomiting, papilledema, and diplopia (nerve VI paresis), a group of symptoms and signs caused by elevated intracranial pressure. The thrombosis in the sinus can be visualized noninvasively by MRI or invasively with a cerebral angiogram or a jugular venogram. Lumbar puncture may reveal an elevated CSF pressure and protein concentration, but no other abnormalities.

Lateral sinus thrombosis is usually secondary to otitis media and/or mastoiditis. Severe headache, diplopia due to an abducens nerve paralysis, photophobia, visual loss, bilateral papilledema, and intraretinal hemorrhages occur. Neurologic signs may appear in a minority of patients and include facial paralysis, hemiparesis, ataxia, or an altered level of consciousness. The diagnosis can be confirmed by MRI or venography.

Aseptic forms of this disorder usually present with symptoms and signs of increased intracranial pressure and, on occasion, focal neurologic signs. There is no fever or toxicity. Aseptic thrombosis may occur with ear and sinus infections or in patients with altered coagulability of the blood. The latter group includes postpartum or postoperative patients and patients with sickle cell disease or primary or secondary polycythemia. This syndrome is indistinguishable clinically from benign intracranial hypertension, and when associated with otitis media it has been called otitic hydrocephalus.

Septic thrombophlebitis of these venous sinuses is usually secondary to ear and sinus disease, as described above. Clot propagation may extend to the lateral, transverse, and superior longitudinal sinuses and the internal jugular vein. High fever, chills, and rigors occur in association with symptoms and signs of intracranial hypertension. Propagation of a septic thrombus from a lateral sinus to the internal jugular vein may be associated with otalgia; a tender, painful mass in the upper anterior neck; nuchal stiffness; torticollis, paresis of nerves IX, X, and XI (jugular foramen syndrome); a positive Queckenstedt maneuver during lumbar puncture; and evidence of septic pulmonary and systemic embolization. Septic sinus thrombosis requires surgical intervention and antibiotics for survival. Aseptic occlusions frequently recanalize spontaneously.

Therapy for intracranial venous thrombosis includes supportive care and antiseizure medications. Heparin has been used, but no controlled trials are available proving its efficacy. Measures to control intracranial hypertension (e.g., repeated lumbar puncture, steroids, subtemporal decompression, sinus thrombectomy, or a ventriculo-peritoneal shunt) may be necessary to relieve headache and preserve vision if spontaneous recanalization does not occur.

F. Cervical Artery Dissection

1. Carotid Artery Dissection   There is an abrupt onset of unilateral frontal, fronto-orbital, or temporal head pain of an aching and/or throbbing quality. It may be associated with ipsilateral upper anterior neck pain (22 percent) and tenderness. A partial Horner's syndrome may accompany the headache. This includes ptosis, miosis, and visual blurring with preservation of facial sweating. Focal neurologic symptoms follow within minutes, hours, or days and may include a contralateral hemiparesis, a hemisensory deficit, aphasia, amaurosis fugax, and diplopia. Subjective and/or objective bruits over the carotid region may be present. Bilateral neck and head pain, associated with bilateral focal neurologic symptoms and signs, is suggestive of dissection of both carotid arteries. The diagnosis can be confirmed by carotid angiography that may demonstrate a segmental stenosis, an abrupt luminal reconstitution, an intimal flap, an aneurysm, or complete occlusion of the internal carotid artery. Spontaneous resolution of symptoms and arteriographic abnormalities occur in 85 percent of patients within a 6-month period.

2. Vertebral Artery Dissection   This disorder begins suddenly with a unilateral posterior neck and occipital pain. Vertigo, oscillopsia, and focal neurologic symptoms are other initial symptoms. Within 5 h to 14 days, ischemic symptoms and signs develop. Completed strokes occur in 75 percent of cases, and TIAs in the remainder. The most common neurologic presentation is a lateral medullary syndrome, which consists of all or a portion of the following symptoms and signs: (1) pain and numbness of the ipsilateral face; (2) limb and gait ataxia; (3) vertigo, nausea, and vomiting; (4) nystagmus, diplopia, and oscillopsia; (5) Horner's syndrome; (6) dysphagia, hoarseness, and vocal cord paralysis; (7) numbness of the ipsilateral arm, trunk, and leg; and (8) hiccups. Other focal symptoms may be superimposed, including hemiparesis, diplopia, ipsilateral facial weakness, and tinnitus (an add-on syndrome). Patients presenting with bilateral brain stem signs may have a basilar artery occlusion, secondary to a unilateral dissection or bilateral vertebral artery dissection. These patients may have quadriparesis, dysarthria, dysphagia, diplopia, visual loss, and ataxia. The diagnosis can be confirmed by vertebrobasilar angiography. Spontaneous recovery of neurologic findings and angiographic abnormalities occur in 85 percent of cases within a 6-month period.

5. BRAIN TUMOR AND ACUTE HEADACHE

Tumors of the brain may present acutely in the following ways:

A. Paroxysmal Headaches   There is an abrupt onset (within seconds) of a severe bifrontal or generalized headache. The pain is associated with vomiting, and it may persist for hours or days, or recur several times a day.

Neck pain and episodes of loss of consciousness, a decrease in level of awareness or confusion, vertigo, ataxia, diplopia, visual loss, or photophobia may also occur. Certain positions or movements of the head may provoke or intensify the pain, and others may relieve it.

Some patients with colloid cysts of the third ventricle present with paroxysmal headaches that are affected by changes of head position, but most cases have headaches unaffected by positional changes. Paroxysmal headaches may also occur with brain stem gliomas; tumors of the lateral ventricle, hemisphere, or cerebellum; craniopharyngiomas; and pinealomas. Sudden increases in intracranial pressure may be the cause of such headaches and associated vomiting, mental dysfunction, and diplopia. Colloid cysts and other tumors can be diagnosed by a CT scan or MRI.

Patients with symptomatic colloid cysts usually have dilated lateral ventricles. Even in the absence of hydrocephalus, removal of the colloid cyst may improve memory and resolve emotional abnormalities.

B. Uncal and Cerebellar Herniation Tumor alone or in association with a lumbar puncture may cause rapid herniation of the brain. A bilateral headache in the fronto-occipital region, vomiting, diplopia, and a decrease in mental awareness may represent the presence of a mass lesion and elevated intracranial pressure. Uncal herniation causes ipsilateral ptosis and mydriasis; a decrease in the level of consciousness; and, later, ophthalmoplegia and ipsilateral hemiplegia. This may progress rapidly to posturing (decerebrate or decorticate).

Cerebellar herniation is associated with posterior fossa tumors or masses, which can cause unilateral tonsillar herniation. Cerebral tumor or severe bilateral hemispheric edema may cause bilateral tonsillar herniation.

Neck pain, stiffness, and cerebellar tonsillar head tilt occur during early herniation. The neck may be stiff and Brudzinski's sign positive. Episodes of tonic extension of the neck and decerebrate posturing; unconsciousness; and disturbances of cardiac rate and rhythm, and respiratory drive occur. Tonic contractions of the limbs and body (cerebellar fits) may occur. Rapid progression (within minutes) to apnea, hypotension, dilated fixed pupils, and irreversible brain damage may occur.

Delayed tumor diagnosis, a rapid increase in size of a supratentorial or posterior fossa lesion, or a lumbar puncture can cause herniation. In the presence of a mass lesion such as a tumor, cyst, intracranial hematoma, or abscess, or generalized cerebral edema, a lumbar puncture is contraindicated because there is a possibility that it may precipitate herniation.

C. Acute Hemorrhage into a Tumor There is abrupt onset of a severe localized headache or facial pain in association with nausea and vomiting. Drowsiness, disorientation, severe confusion, or stupor may follow. Focal neurologic symptoms and signs may appear. These may be related to the location of the tumor. For example, an acoustic neurinoma with intratumoral hemorrhage may present with headache, ipsilateral facial paresis, hearing loss, and ataxia. A CT scan will demonstrate the hemorrhage and may or may not identify the underlying tumor. An angiogram will exclude an aneurysm or AV malformation and may demonstrate a tumor blush or vessel displacement. Intratumoral bleeding with an abrupt onset of headache, sweating, vomiting, and focal neurologic findings may occur with a glioma, meningioma, melanoma, choriocarcinoma, pituitary adenoma, or oligodendroglioma. Surgical removal of the tumor is required. Hemorrhage into the tumor and subarachnoid bleeding may occur simultaneously. Hemorrhage from a pituitary tumor into the subarachnoid space is an important cause of subarachnoid bleeding in patients with negative angiograms.

D. Acute Subarachnoid Hemorrhage There is a sudden onset of severe headache, vomiting, a decreased level of awareness, neck stiffness, and pain. A CT scan will demonstrate subarachnoid and intraventricular bleeding. Brain tumors account for 0.4 percent of all cases of subarachnoid bleeding. Glioblastoma multiforme, oligodendroglioma, melanoma, choriocarcinoma, pituitary adenoma, meningioma, and choroid plexus papilloma are the tumors most likely to cause a spontaneous subarachnoid hemorrhage.

E. Acute Meningitis This mimic of bacterial meningitis can be caused by the discharge of chemically irritating necrotic tumor or cyst contents into the subarachnoid space. This syndrome is described above (Section 3C3).

F. Acute Stroke Syndrome There may be an abrupt onset of focal neurologic symptoms, such as hemiparesis, hemisensory loss, homonymous hemianopia, and dysphasia. Bleeding into the tumor, a sudden increase in edema adjacent to the lesion, or tumor necrosis may precipitate a course similar to an acute stroke. Headache of an intermittent or persistent type may occur on the same side as the tumor. The tumor can be demonstrated by a CT scan or MRI. Prior symptoms of intermittent or persistent headache, vomiting, mental changes, or seizures may precede the onset of acute neurologic symptoms by weeks, months, or years. Tumor and other causes of acute stroke are compared in Table 2-3.

6. ENCEPHALITIS

A. Herpes Simplex This disorder may begin with a prodromal influenza-like illness (46 percent) or with fever (90–100 percent), bifrontal or generalized headache, and mental confusion (54 percent). Neck pain and stiffness are present in 65 percent. Changes in level of consciousness include drowsiness, disorientation, stupor, and coma. Focal signs such as limb pareses, aphasia (46 percent), and focal or grand mal seizures (61 percent) occur. Early symptoms indicating temporal lobe involvement include olfactory hallucinations or distortions of taste, anosmia, temporal lobe seizures, and bizarre behavior. The latter may lead to psychiatric referral and a delayed diagnosis.

The electroencephalogram shows periodic high-voltage sharp waves and slow-wave complexes at 2 to 3/s over the frontotemporal region on one (79 percent) or both sides. These findings are suggestive, but not specific, for herpes simplex virus encephalitis.

A CT scan may show hypodense lesions in one temporal and/or frontal lobe (58 percent). Contrast enhancement occurs in the frontal and temporal lobes on one or both sides, and a mass effect with midline shift may be present in 46 percent of cases. A radionuclide scan will localize uptake to one or both temporal lobes.

CSF examination reveals leukocyte counts of 0 to 1100/mm^3. Early in the course (first 3 days), the CSF may be normal. The differential cell count shows a lymphocytic predominance, although occasionally polymorphonuclear leukocytes may exceed lymphocytes in number. The protein concentration may range from 34 to 280 mg/dl. Red blood cell concentrations may range from 12 to 4000/mm^3, and xanthochromia may occur. The CSF glucose level is usually normal, but it may be decreased. Cerebral biopsy reveals an acute necrotizing encephalitis in 93 percent of cases, and herpes simplex virus can be isolated by culture in 73 percent and detected by immunofluorescence studies of brain in 11 percent. This disorder usually responds to a 14-day course of intravenous acyclovir. Herpes simplex virus is the most common cause of encephalitis that occurs throughout the year and the most important cause of fatal acute encephalitis. It has an average annual incidence of one case per million.

B. Arthropod-Borne Viral Encephalitis These disorders occur in epidemics beginning in the summer or autumn.

1. Eastern Equine Encephalitis This disorder occurs in the United States east of the Mississippi River, in the Atlantic and Gulf coastal regions. Outbreaks occur in the summer and fall. There may be an abrupt onset of headache, vomiting, fever, drowsiness, myoclonus, and generalized seizures. Sialorrhea and dyspnea may occur. Paresis of limbs, hyperactive reflexes, and Babinski signs may appear. Confusion, defective memory, and personality and behavioral changes frequently develop. The CSF shows a neutrophilic predominance (counts 500–2000 cells/mm^3). Red blood cells may be present; an elevated protein concentration; and a normal

glucose level. The diagnosis can be confirmed by serologic methods. A peripheral leukocytosis with a left shift is commonly present.

2. Western Equine Encephalitis This disorder occurs in the western United States from the Mississippi River to the Rocky Mountains. Equine cases precede human ones by several weeks and provide a warning of a coming epidemic. The inapparent/apparent infection ratio in adults is 1000:1.

Headache of a generalized nature, fever myalgias, and malaise are followed within 1 to 4 days by drowsiness, neck pain and stiffness, vomiting, and photophobia. Limb paresis, tremors, cranial nerve lesions, and seizures may occur. Most adults recover without sequelae. The CSF shows a polymorphonuclear leukocyte predominance with the total count less than 500/mm^3, a normal glucose level, and a moderately elevated protein level. The diagnosis can be confirmed by serologic studies using hemagglutination inhibition, neutralizing, or IgM ELISA assays.

3. St. Louis Encephalitis Epidemics occur in urban-suburban centers in the midwest, Texas, and Florida. Summer-fall epidemics are the rule, except in warm regions such as Florida. Encephalitis is the most frequent presentation in adults over age 55. Acute headache, fever, myalgias, drowsiness, and meningismus are the initial symptoms. Neurologic abnormalities include facial palsy, delirium, myoclonus, nystagmus, and ataxia. Tremors of the tongue, face, and limbs; mental confusion; and lethargy are important components of this disorder. The Guillain-Barré syndrome may be associated.

The CSF shows a polymorphonuclear leukocyte predominance and an elevated protein level. Elevated serum CPK, SGOT, and aldolase activity occur. An EEG may show amorphous delta activity and diffuse slowing in the frontal and temporal regions. Urinary frequency, urgency and retention, or incontinence may occur, in association with pyuria, hematuria and proteinuria, and an elevated creatinine level. These urinary symptoms and laboratory abnormalities are due to viral invasion of the renal system. The diagnosis can be confirmed by serologic methods.

4. California Encephalitis (California, LaCrosse, Jamestown Canyon, and Snowshoe Hare Viruses) California virus causes disease in the western United States, while LaCrosse virus is more prevalent in the midwest and the eastern United States. These viruses cause summer-fall cases, and the pattern of infection is endemic and localized to specific ''hot spots'' (community centers of viral activity). Headache, fever, meningeal signs, altered consciousness, and seizures may occur. The disorder is usually self-limited. The CSF shows a lymphocytic predominance and an elevated protein level. Serologic studies are required to establish the diagnosis. The hemagglutination inhibition test for LaCrosse viral antigen and the IgM antibody-capture ELISA are the most accurate serologic tests.

7. SYSTEMIC INFECTIONS WITH HEADACHE

Almost all infectious diseases may be associated with fever and headache. The disorders discussed below are known to present with severe headache and/or meningismus as important components of the clinical picture.

A. Rickettsial Diseases

1. Rocky Mountain Spotted Fever This disorder begins abruptly with a high fever and bilateral frontal or frontotemporal headache. A maculopapular and/or petechial rash appears 2 to 14 days after the onset. The rash occurs in 96 percent of cases, but may not become petechial in up to 46 percent. It classically begins on the distal portions of the extremities and spreads up the limb to the trunk. Biopsy of the rash may detect rickettsiae in skin capillaries, confirming the diagnosis 5 to 7 days before serologic tests become positive. Headache and abnormalities of mental status are common (42–54 percent), and lethargy occurs in 12 to 21 percent. Nuchal pain and stiffness occur in 30 percent; and focal neurologic signs, such as limb paresis, cranial nerve palsies, deafness, hemiparesis, and transverse myelitis, may develop in a small percentage of cases. The CSF may be abnormal in up to 66 percent of cases, with an elevated protein level (45–120 mg/dl), a normal glucose level, and a lymphocytic pleocytosis. Up to 6 percent may have mild hypoglycorrhachia, and 9 percent may show a neutrophilic predominance. Myalgias may be severe in up to 46 percent. Hepatosplenomegaly occurs in 12 to 50 percent, and adenopathy in 15 to 42 percent. Hyponatremia (91 percent), thrombocytopenia, and a left shift of the peripheral leukocyte count in a febrile patient with myalgias and headache should suggest the diagnosis prior to the onset of the rash. Only 56 percent of patients recall a tick bite, but most patients have dog contact or possible exposure to ticks. Serologic tests are required to confirm the diagnosis.

2. Q Fever Patients experience fever, rigors, severe frontal and retrobulbar headache, myalgias, and chest pain. The presence of a nonproductive cough and patchy segmental or lobar infiltrates is consistent with Q fever pneumonia. Hepatitis, with hepatomegaly, tenderness, and jaundice, may occur. The diagnosis can be confirmed by complement fixation or an indirect fluorescent antibody test.

3. Typhus High fever, headache, and rash occur in typhus and other rickettsial diseases.

B. Spirochetal Diseases

1. Lyme Disease Patients may present with a characteristic skin rash, fever, headache, myalgias, arthralgias, and meningismus, as discussed above (Section 3B1).

2. Leptospirosis This disorder may present with fever, conjunctival injection, nausea, vomiting, adenopathy (50 percent), myalgias and muscle tenderness (50 percent), neck pain and stiffness (35 percent), hepatosplenomegaly (15 percent), proteinuria and cylinduria, an elevated creatinine level, and evidence of abnormal liver function with clinical jaundice or bilirubinuria.

The CSF may be normal (10 percent of cases), or the cell count may be elevated to 500 cells/mm^3, with a neutrophilic or lymphocytic predominance. The CSF protein level is elevated. The patient's serum can be screened for antibodies to *Leptospira interrogans* by a macroagglutination test. Sanitation or slaughterhouse work, dairy farming, and fishing are occupations at increased risk for acquiring leptospirosis. Exposure to infected animals or their urine by washing or swimming in infected water may also result in infection. Penicillin therapy given within 3 days of onset accelerates recovery.

3. Syphilis Meningovascular syphilis with headache, meningismus, fever, and a spinal fluid lymphocytic pleocytosis with a positive CSF VDRL may occur within 1 year of primary syphilitic infection. Multiple cranial nerve abnormalities occur. In 10 percent of cases, the onset coincides with the rash of secondary syphilis.

Penicillin therapy is effective, but it may intensify fever, headache, and other symptoms during the first day of therapy due to a Jarisch-Herxheimer reaction (related to massive release of antigen).

C. Pneumonia and Meningismus Fever and severe headache, neck pain, and stiffness may occur in patients with a respiratory illness with cough and/or pleuritic or nonspecific chest pain. The headache is usually bifrontal or diffuse, and is so intense that meningitis is suspected. The respiratory infections associated with headache and meningismus include the following:

1. Chlamydia psittaci (Psittacosis) Fever, rigors, and sweats are associated with a severe headache, myalgias, a nonproductive cough, and meningismus. Lumbar puncture reveals a normal cell count in 98 percent, a normal glucose level, and a CSF protein level above 40 mg/dl in 44 percent of cases. Ninety-one percent of patients have an abnormal chest x-ray with a pulmonary infiltrate confined to one lobe (90 percent of positive films) or positive pulmonary physical findings. The diagnosis can be confirmed by serologic methods. In 80 to 90 percent of patients, there is a history of exposure to birds.

2. **Mycoplasma** *pneumoniae* Symptoms include fever, headache, and a nagging nonproductive cough, as well as meningismus (in up to 14 percent of cases) severe enough to require lumbar puncture. The CSF is usually normal. Chest radiographs show patchy, subsegmental, or segmental infiltrates.

3. **Histoplasma** *capsulatum* Acute pulmonary histoplasmosis causes fever, severe headache, cough, arthralgias, myalgias, and meningismus requiring lumbar puncture in 10 to 15 percent of symptomatic cases. The CSF is usually normal. Chest radiographs show patchy subsegmental and segmental infiltrates, scattered miliary lesions, and/or hilar adenopathy.

D. Typhoid Fever Patients may have fever, diarrhea (73 percent), abdominal pain (60 percent), headache (47 percent), cough (33 percent), vomiting (33 percent), and an abnormal mental status. Meningismus, delirium, "toxic" staring, and stupor may also occur. Physical findings may include fever, relative bradycardia, diffuse abdominal tenderness (47 percent) and distension (13 percent), splenomegaly (40 percent), rose spots, and nuchal stiffness. The diagnosis can be confirmed by stool or blood cultures and by the Widal test. An O agglutinin titer of 1:80 or more or a fourfold rise in titer supports the diagnosis. False-positive serologic results are common in endemic areas, and false-negative results may also occur. The CSF examination reveals a normal sugar and cell count.

E. Pyelonephritis Patients may have fever; chills; rigors; thoracolumbar, interscapular, and posterior neck pain; and neck stiffness associated with costovertebral and diffuse back muscle tenderness. A bifrontal or generalized headache may accompany the neck pain and stiffness. The urine contains neutrophils singly, in clumps, and in casts. Abnormal concentrations of bacteria are present in the urine. The symptoms respond to oral or intravenous antibiotics. CSF examination reveals no evidence of abnormality. In the elderly, the possibility of gram-negative meningitis, secondary to urinary tract infection, must be considered.

F. Primary HIV Infection This disorder begins 1 to 7 weeks after exposure to HIV by a needle stick, transfusion, or sexual contact. Fever, headache, photophobia, myalgias, arthralgias, and lymphadenopathy are associated with a diffuse macular rash in up to 50 percent of cases. Meningismus, with a stiff neck and a spinal fluid lymphocytic pleocytosis, may occur. Leukopenia, lymphopenia, and thrombocytopenia develop during the first 2 weeks. Encephalopathy and peripheral or cranial neuropathy, and myelopathy, may occur. Antibody to HIV appears within 6 to 12 weeks of the onset of the acute illness. HIV antigen in peripheral blood and/or positive HIV blood cultures are usually present during the acute illness.

8. PROVOKED VASCULAR HEADACHES

Vascular and/or muscle contraction headaches may be provoked by certain activities, such as exertion, cough, change in head position, and sexual activity, or by foods, beverages, hunger, drugs, occupational exposures, a low Po_2, high altitude, a high Pco_2, carbon monoxide, caffeine withdrawal, ice cream, alcohol, sun exposure, menses, trauma, arguments, or upsetting life events, or they may "appear out of the blue" in a patient living in a chronically stressful setting.

The provoking stimuli have given a name to the headache, which is usually vascular, muscle contraction, or a combination of these types. The vast majority of provoked headaches are benign and can be dismissed without further evaluation, but a small subset require CT or MR imaging and sometimes lumbar puncture, angiography, or metabolic investigation.

A. Exertional Headache Three types have been described and are arbitrarily classified by the amount and intensity of activity required to precipitate head pain.

1. Acute-Effort Migraine An acute, throbbing, unilateral headache with nausea and vomiting occurs. It may be frontal, temporal, and/or retro-orbital. Scintillating scotoma may precede the attack. The provoking activity is a high-intensity athletic effort, such as a quarter- or full-mile race. Running at high altitude may increase the incidence of this disorder.

2. Low-Intensity Exercise–Induced Headaches These headaches may occur in joggers or cyclists who are not well-conditioned. The pain may be intense, throbbing, bilateral, unilateral, occipital, or frontal. Nonthrobbing unilateral occipital pain may also occur. The pain may begin during the effort, immediately after stopping, or 1 to 24 h later.

3. Minimal-Effort Headache Some individuals develop occipital head pain with minimal exertion. Movement of the neck or changes of neck position may intensify or decrease the severity of the pain. The headache may cease with continued exertion or within 24 h. Exertional headaches may occur in a cluster for several days or weeks, and then may disappear spontaneously. Up to 30 percent of patients are exertion headache–free within 5 years, and 70 percent within 10 years. Prophylactic use of drugs such as analgesics, beta blockers, ergotamine, or indomethacin before exertion may be effective.

Up to 10 percent of patients with exertional headache may have disorders such as a Chiari malformation and basilar impression, a subdural hematoma, or a brain tumor. Careful workup should be done to exclude structural intracranial disease.

B. Sexual Activity or Coital Headache Head pain may begin in one or both occipital regions during the early buildup phase of sexual intercourse or masturbation, at the point of orgasm, or seconds to hours later. The occipital pain associated with increasing sexual excitement may be dull, aching, and nonpulsatile, and associated with neck extension and jaw clenching. Neck movement into flexion may partially relieve the pain. This type of headache may intensify at orgasm and then gradually resolve over the next 24 h.

An explosive headache may begin at any time during the heightened phase of sexual excitement or at orgasm. Such headaches mimic the thunderclap headache of a ruptured aneurysm and provoke great fear and anxiety. Nausea and vomiting may occur with benign sexual headache but are uncommon, and the pain may disappear in minutes or after several days. A residual discomfort for up to 48 h may occur in patients with nonstructural disease. It is not clinically possible to separate the "thunderclap headache" of sexual intercourse from the sentinel bleed of a leaking aneurysm. The majority of sentinel headaches do not cause vomiting, photophobia, or neck stiffness and pain. Exclusion of subarachnoid hemorrhage is necessary in patients with sexual activity–provoked headache, unless the headache disappears a few minutes after it starts. A CT scan is not always sensitive enough (sensitivity = 55 percent) to detect leakage from an aneurysm, and lumbar puncture is required. Occasionally, a "thunderclap headache" is caused by aneurysmal enlargement or distension without bleeding, and the diagnosis requires angiography. In most cases, sexual activity–provoked cephalgia workups are negative for bleeding. In one series of over 100 patients with bleeding aneurysms, only 2 percent occurred during intercourse.

A rare form of postcoital headache resembles the low CSF pressure headache of lumbar puncture. The headache is intensified by standing and relieved by lying down.

C. "Cough" Headache and Its Equivalents Sneezing, straining at stool, rapid performance of Valsalva's maneuver, laughing, stooping, or bending may provoke headaches that last minutes to hours. Only 5 percent of headaches associated with brain tumor are provoked by cough, and the vast majority of patients with this symptom have a benign vascular headache. A CT scan or MRI to exclude an intracranial mass lesion should be performed.

D. Hunger-Induced Headache Missing meals or religious fasting may provoke throbbing frontal, temporal, and/or retro-orbital headaches and/or facial pain on one

or both sides. These may not respond immediately to ingestion of food.

E. Food and Beverage–Provoked Pain Frontal, retro-orbital, and/or nasal and midfacial pain may follow minutes or hours after ingestion of certain foods and beverages. Individual migraine patients are intolerant of different foods, but a higher frequency of headache is associated with the following foods and drinks: cured meats containing sodium nitrite (e.g., "hot dog" headache, as well as bacon, ham, and salami); cheese; chocolate; onions, scallions, chives, and shallots; citrus fruits; smoked and pickled fish and meat; pork products; chicken livers; mushrooms; beef concentrate; nuts; monosodium glutamate; dark beer; and red wine. For example, nitrite headache may begin 30 min after ingestion of a cured meat and persist for 1 to 2 h. The larger the dose, the more severe and persistent the headache. Inexplicably, the same dose of nitrite given on a different day may not provoke pain.

A food diary can be kept, and specific foods relating temporally to the provocation of headache identified and eliminated from the diet. Alternatively, a limited diet may be initiated and additional foods gradually reintroduced into the patient's diet in hope of identifying headache-provoking foods.

Ice cream headaches occur in patients with a history of migraine. Placement of ice chips in the region of the hard palate or oropharynx can cause a brief head pain located in the frontal and/or retro-orbital region, vertex, or retroauricular area. In one study, 93 percent of patients with migraine developed an acute ice cream headache, compared to 31 percent of a control group.

F. Drugs Some drugs may provoke a moderate-to-severe headache by causing hypertension (e.g., epinephrine; bretylium; monoamine oxidase inhibitors accompanied by ingestion of tyramine-rich foods) or by abrupt withdrawal of antihypertensives (e.g., clonidine and beta blockers). Drugs causing vasodilatation (e.g., nitrates, dipyridamole, calcium channel blockers, caffeine, and theophylline) may also provoke pain. Rarely, drug-related headaches may be caused by increased intracranial pressure produced by anesthetics (e.g., ketamine and enflurane), antibiotics (e.g., tetracycline, ampicillin, griseofulvin, sulfamethoxazole, and metronidazole), prednisone, vitamin A, perhexilene, hydralazine, and indomethacin. Some drugs produce headaches by an unknown mechanism (e.g., digoxin, amphotericin B, allopurinol, rifampin, and primidone). Caffeine or ergotamine withdrawal may be associated with headache.

G. Decompression Sickness Bilateral throbbing head pain may be caused by decompression sickness. This disorder has been reported frequently as a result of sports diving. Neurologic findings such as scintillating scotomas, homonymous field deficits, vertigo, transient confusion, hemiparesis, and hemisensory deficits and seizures may be associated with the headache. Spinal cord involvement is signaled by low back and root pain, girdle pain, leg weakness, and loss of bladder and sphincter control. Recompression in a chamber is required to relieve headache and reverse neurologic damage.

Exposure to high altitude in a decompression chamber or in actual flight may cause type 2 decompression sickness, with joint and limb pain, headache, visual disturbances, limb weakness and paresthesias, and sometimes a change in level of consciousness. Treatment in a hyperbaric chamber resolves these symptoms.

H. Altitude and Hypoxia Altitude-related headache may begin after sudden arrival at an altitude exceeding 10,000 ft. Such headaches usually begin after hours of breathing low concentrations of oxygen and are unresponsive to O_2 therapy. Cough, straining, the supine position, head jarring, and exertion may intensify the pain. Papilledema and retinal hemorrhages may occur in patients with acute mountain sickness. Headache and other complaints, such as dyspnea and orthopnea, usually develop within 24 h and resolve after 4 to 8 days.

I. Carbon Dioxide Retention Patients with alveolar hypoventilation, secondary to chronic pulmonary disease, may develop a bilateral dull aching frontal, occipital, or generalized headache. There is a tendency for such headaches to occur at night.

The headache may be accompanied by a high-frequency tremor of the outstretched hands, myoclonic jerks, muscle twitching, and asterixis. Venous congestion, hemorrhages, and bilateral papilledema may be detected on fundoscopic examination. Drowsiness, inattentiveness, memory difficulties, indifference, and mental confusion may be intermittent or constant, and progressive to stupor or coma. Lumbar puncture often reveals an elevated CSF pressure. Blood gases reveal a Pco_2 of 75 mmHg or more and a variable amount of hypoxemia. The EEG may demonstrate slow activity bilaterally. Attacks of hypercapneic headache progressive to stupor can be precipitated by too much sedation or O_2 administration, both of which may blunt the respiratory drive. Use of mechanical ventilation, venesection to reduce the hematocrit, and diuretics may relieve the headache and reverse the abnormal mental changes and retinal abnormalities.

J. Menstruation A severe aching or throbbing unilateral or bilateral headache may occur 1 to 2 days prior to or during menses. Photophobia; nausea; vomiting; dizziness; profound weakness; and a desire to be in a quiet, dark room may accompany the attack. Such a headache may incapacitate the patient for 2 to 3 days and may require narcotics for relief. Some patients may also suffer from attacks of classical or common migraine that occur spontaneously throughout the month. Occurrence with menses may be an isolated event or may become a common monthly association. Some authors report that migraine, muscle contraction, and combined (muscle contraction and migraine) headaches may all increase in frequency and severity during the menstrual period.

K. Carbon Monoxide Bilateral aching and/or throbbing headache is associated with a carboxyhemoglobin level greater than 10 percent. Cases may present during the winter season with refractory head pain. There is often a history of use of a gas space heater or gas stove in a confined, poorly ventilated dwelling. Coinhabitants of the same living quarters may also suffer from headache and/or irritability, mild loss of intellectual ability, and personality changes. Diffuse encephalopathic abnormalities may be detected by EEG, and the diagnosis can be confirmed by measuring the carboxyhemoglobin level. Other groups at risk for this disorder include automobile mechanics and traffic officers in vehicle-congested cities, and survivors of fires. Indoor barbecueing or a faulty automobile exhaust system can also lead to CO poisoning.

L. Hypoglycemia Insulin or oral hypoglycemic overdosage, islet cell pancreatic tumors, and alcoholic or other forms of liver disease (e.g., Reye's syndrome) may cause hypoglycemia.

Diffuse sweating, an aching and/or throbbing anterior or generalized headache, profound weakness and faintness, irritability, jitteriness, impatience, and inability to concentrate occur. Some patients progress rapidly through this phase to disorientation, confusion, stupor, and unconsciousness. Symptoms begin with blood sugar levels in the 30- to 40-mg/dl range. Deep coma ensues at a blood sugar level of 10 mg/dl. At this time, the pupils may be dilated, the skin pale and cool, respirations shallow, and the pulse slow. Intravenous administration of glucose will rapidly reverse many of the symptoms of acute hypoglycemia, including headache. Deep coma and focal neurologic signs may require a longer time for recovery. Headache is a relatively infrequent complaint (<10 percent of cases) of patients with hypoglycemia.

M. Pheochromocytoma A severe throbbing bilateral, frontal, frontotemporal, or occipital headache accompanies paroxysms of hypertension in 92 percent of patients with intermittent hypertension. A similar headache occurs in 72 percent of patients with sustained hypertension who have paroxysms of increased blood pressure.

Diaphoresis occurs in 60 to 70 percent of patients and affects the upper body. Palpitations occur in 73 percent with paroxysmal hypertension and in 51 percent with sustained hypertension. Anginal chest pain occurs in 34 percent during paroxysms and in 13 percent of patients with only sustained hypertension. Epigastric pain, nausea, and vomiting are common, but the mechanism is unknown. Weight loss may occur in 25 percent with paroxysms.

Paresthesias and arm pain may occur in 0 to 11 percent of cases.

In 40 to 50 percent of cases, the blood pressure is normal between paroxysms. During an attack, the blood pressure may rise to 330/180. The duration of an attack may be minutes or hours, and the frequency may vary from 20 per day to 3 or 4 per year. Patients with sustained hypertension may have orthostatic hypotension and tachycardia. Poor control of hypertension by drugs should suggest the possibility of pheochromocytoma.

Patients with paroxysmal hypertension have normal fundi or gr I-II hypertensive retinopathy. Patients with sustained hypertension have gr III-IV retinopathy (53 percent), gr I-II retinopathy (40 percent), and normal fundi (5 percent). The retinal changes are reversible after removal of the tumor. Temperature elevation occurs in up to 66 percent of cases and may reach 105°F. Loud systolic murmurs may occur over the aortic, mitral, or pulmonic areas, and cardiomegaly can occur. Attacks of hypertension may be precipitated by alcohol, anesthesia, metoclopramide, propylthiouracil, and glucocorticoids. Daily activities, including exercise, bending, stooping, straining during urination, or sleeping, may provoke an attack. Measurement of urinary VMA and metanephrine excretion and/or plasma catecholamine concentration will confirm the diagnosis. Plasma catecholamine measurement provides the greatest accuracy. In less than 2 percent of cases, the urinary catecholamines may be in the normal range. Catecholamine metabolite excretion can be expressed per milligram of creatinine, allowing for use of the test in renal failure and without a need for a 24-h urine collection. CT scans will identify most clinically active tumors. Lesions as small as 1 cm may be imaged.

The differential diagnosis of pheochromocytoma includes two syndromes that can produce elevated plasma catecholamines and urinary VMA and metanephrine excretion.

Administration of monoamine oxidase inhibitors such as tranylcypromine, isocarboxazid, and phenelzine for the treatment of depression puts the patient at risk for a severe paroxysm of hypertension following ingestion of tyramine-rich foods or beverages (e.g., cheddar cheese, pickled herring, beer, sherry, and yeast extract). Ingestion of drugs such as amphetamines, ephedrine, imipramine, or amitriptyline by patients taking monoamine oxidase inhibitors can also cause a similar crisis.

Abrupt withdrawal of clonidine therapy may also precipitate a hypertensive paroxysm similar to that produced by a pheochromocytoma. Similar episodes may follow autonomic discharges in paraplegics.

9. TEMPORAL ARTERITIS

This disorder occurs in patients older than age 55. It may begin abruptly, causing a severe headache, and sometimes jaw claudication and visual loss within a few days, or it may develop more gradually over a period of weeks or months.

A continuous boring or aching pain occurs (90 percent) in one or both temporal areas. Lancinating pains may be superimposed, and scalp tenderness (69 percent), maximal over the temporal artery (95 percent), occurs. Hair combing, lying on the tender regions, or even the pressure of an eyeglass frame on the temple may trigger severe paroxysms of stabbing pain. Jaw weakness, fatigue, or aching pain provoked by chewing or talking (i.e., jaw claudication) occurs in 69 percent of cases. Weight loss and the polymyalgia syndrome occur in 48 to 52 percent of cases. Amaurosis fugax may occur one or more times, and, within days of the first episode, permanent partial or complete visual loss may occur in one or both eyes. Ophthalmologic symptoms are present in up to 40 percent of cases. Permanent complete visual loss occurs in 10 percent, and partial loss in an additional 10 percent. Fever occurs in 21 percent and may be associated with other systemic complaints, such as anorexia, weakness, fatigue, and malaise. The sedimentation rate is greater than 40 mm in 95 to 100 percent of cases. The diagnosis can be confirmed by a temporal artery biopsy and/or by observation of a clinical response to oral prednisone (40–60 mg/dl) within 48 h. In one series, 13.7 percent of cases had positive biopsies and responded to prednisone, and an additional 21.6% had negative biopsies but were steroid-responsive. The remainder had a negative biopsy and no response to steroids. Other studies have reported an 82 percent sensitivity for biopsy. Recent-onset headache; jaw claudication; and tenderness, thickening, or redness of a temporal artery are specific for temporal arteritis. If all three findings are present, the likelihood of the diagnosis is close to 100 percent. Patients with negative biopsies may be found to have a lymphoma (18 percent), carotid disease (15 percent), diabetes mellitus (15 percent), or connective tissue disorders such as lupus erythematosus, vasculitis, or rheumatoid arthritis.

10. ACUTE SINUSITIS

The location of face and/or head pain is related to the site(s) of sinus infection. Frontal sinusitis may cause unilateral or bilateral supraorbital and orbital pain and tenderness. Maxillary involvement causes aching pain in one or both cheeks, frontal headache, and sometimes aching of the premolars and molars of the ipsilateral upper jaw. Pain may also radiate to the temperomandibular joint area. Tenderness is usually maximal over one or both cheeks.

Sphenoid sinus infection causes unilateral head pain in the frontal, temporal, or occipital region, or in two or more of these locations. Pain may also be felt in the vertex, eye, nasal cavity, cheek, and teeth, on one or both sides. Ethmoid sinus pain occurs in the lateral nasal cavity, eye, and frontal region.

The pain of sinus infection may be dull and continuous or severe and sharp. Throbbing pain may be superimposed. Maxillary sinus pain may be intensified or provoked by lowering the head. Sinus infection causes nasal and posterior pharyngeal discharge, which is usually yellow, green, or bloody. Blood-streaked mucus may be blown from the nose. Fever, chills, myalgias, and malaise may occur but are frequently absent.

Flexible fiberoptic rhinoscopy will detect erythema of the turbinates and purulent drainage coming from a specific sinus drainage region. Plain sinus radiographs and a sinus CT scan may miss cases of sinusitis detected by clinical findings and rhinoscopy. A marked improvement in pain, fever, and nasopharyngeal exudate follows the administration of specific antibiotics, and such a response to therapy serves to support the diagnosis. If symptoms worsen or fail to improve on antibiotic therapy, surgical drainage of the involved sinus(es) may be required.

Pansinusitis may cause bilateral face pain and/or frontal, temporal, or occipital head pain with the same associated symptoms as described above.

11. ACUTE OCCIPITAL NEURALGIA

This disorder produces aching upper neck and occipital pain on one side, associated with tingling and/or crawling paresthesias and hypesthesia of the posterior scalp. The causes of acute occipital neuralgia include (1) scalp trauma from a direct blow; (2) compression neuropathy from lying with the head on a hard, angular surface or edge; (3) hyperextension injury to the ganglion and root of C2 with compression between the lamina of the axis and atlas; (4) fracture of the atlas or axis; (5) gout; (6) mastoiditis; (7) infections such as typhoid, influenza, malaria, and syphilis; (8) osteoarthritis of the facet joints of C1-C2 and C2-C3; and (9) cerebellar tonsillar herniation compressing the C1 and C2 roots caused by a posterior fossa tumor, cyst, or Chiari malformation.

12. MULTIPLE SCLEROSIS

A migraine-like vascular headache may occur in association with optic or retrobulbar neuritis, vertigo, diplopia, leg weakness, and/or hypesthesia and paresthesias of the legs and feet. These symptoms may remit in whole or in part. An acute syndrome, beginning with a severe pounding headache and associated with ataxia, vertigo, diplopia, leg weakness, and sensory loss in the limbs, may occur in up to 2 percent of cases. Up to 1 percent of patients present with a vascular headache as part of their initial episode. The CSF may show an elevated protein level, pleocytosis, an increased concentration of gamma globulin, and oligoclonal gamma globulin bands. De-

myelinating central nervous system lesions may be visualized by MRI.

13. ECLAMPSIA

This disorder may begin prior to or during labor or up to 10 days postpartem. A severe frontal headache is accompanied by visual blurring or loss; face, arm, and leg edema; hypertension; and proteinuria. Focal and grand mal seizures may occur. The CSF is usually normal. MRI of the brain may reveal multiple cortical infarctions. The electroencephalogram may show sharp wave activity and focal slowing in one or more areas consistent with seizure activity. There is a therapeutic response to intravenous magnesium sulfate.

14. CEREBROSPINAL FLUID HYPOTENSION

A. Post-Lumbar Puncture Headache   Headache begins within hours to a week after lumbar puncture. It is more common in women and younger adults. The pain is bifrontal and/or bioccipital, and is exacerbated by standing or sitting and relieved by lying down. Associated complaints may include neck, shoulder, and low back pain, nuchal rigidity simulating meningitis, nausea, and vomiting. The incidence of post–lumbar puncture headache after spinal anesthesia is reported as 1.5 to 15 percent. Most cases resolve within 14 days with supine bed rest, oral hydration, and analgesics. Isolated abducens nerve paralysis with diplopia may occur in 0.08 to 0.009 percent. Nerve VI paralysis usually occurs several days after the onset of the headache. Refractory cases of post–lumbar puncture headache have been treated successfully with one or more epidural blood patches. Persistence of headache beyond 2 to 3 weeks requires neurologic evaluation. Rarely, it is symptomatic of an intracranial mass lesion.

B. Acute Postural Headache with Infectious Disease   Acute febrile infectious diseases may cause frontal or occipital headache increased by standing and relieved by lying down. The pathyphysiology of this type of headache is unknown.

C. Spontaneous Intracranial Hypotension   Headache, neck pain and stiffness, nausea, and vomiting occur in a standing or sitting position and are relieved in the supine position. There may be a history of a fall, straining, or no identifiable cause. Rest in a supine position for several days to a week relieves symptoms, and there is no tendency for recurrence. The mechanism may be an arachnoid tear around a nerve root sleeve or other site with CSF leakage. CSF pressure is low, and 20 to 50 mononuclear cells may be present in the CSF, but cultures are negative.

HEAD PAIN REFERENCES

Abscess—Epidural/Subdural

Berenson CS, Bia FJ: Fever, frontal sinus mass, and CSF pleocytosis in a 44-year-old man. *Yale J Biol Med* 59: 613–620, 1986.

Harris LF, Haws FP, Triplett JN Jr, et al: Subdural empyema and epidural abscess: Recent experience in a community hospital. *South Med J* 80(10):1254–1258, 1987.

Hodges J, Anslow P, Gillett G: Subdural empyema: Continuing diagnostic problems in the CT scan era. *Q J Med* 59(228):387–393, 1986.

Tudor RB, Carson JP, Pulliam MW, et al: Pott's puffy tumor, frontal sinusitis, frontal bone osteomyelitis, and epidural abscess secondary to a wrestling injury. *Am J Sports Med* 9(6):390–391, 1981.

Yoshikawa TT, Quinn W: The aching head: Intracranial suppuration due to head and neck infections. *Infect Dis Clin North Am* 2(1):265–277, 1988.

Abscess—Pituitary

Berger SA, Edberg SC, David G: Infectious disease in the sella turcica. *Rev Infect Dis* 8(5):747–755, 1986.

Ford J, Torres LF, Cox T, et al: Recurrent sterile meningitis caused by a pituitary abscess. *Postgrad Med J* 62:929–931, 1986.

AIDS and Neurosyphilis

Johns DR, Tierney M, Felsenstein D: Alteration in the natural history of neurosyphilis by concurrent infection with the human immunodeficiency virus. *N Engl J Med* 316:1569–1572, 1987.

Apoplexy—Pituitary

Rusnak RA: Adrenal and pituitary emergencies. *Emerg Med Clin North Am* 7(4):903–925, 1989.

Arteritis—Temporal

Goodman BW Jr: Temoral arteritis. *Am J Med* 67(5):839–852, 1979.

Huston KA, Hunder GG, Lie JT, et al: Temporal arteritis: A 25-year epidemiologic, clinical, and pathologic study. *Ann Intern Med* 88:162–167, 1978.

Malmvall B-E, Bengtsson B-A, Alestig K, et al: The clinical pictures of giant cell arteritis. *Postgrad Med* 67(1):141–143, 146–147, 150, 1980.

Pereira M, Kaine JL: Polymyalgia rheumatica and temporal arteritis: Managing older patients. *Geriatrics* 41(6):54–55, 59–60, 63–66, 1986.

Roth AM, Milsow L, Keltner JL: The ultimate diagnoses of patients undergoing temporal artery biopsies. *Arch Ophthalmol* 102:901–903, 1984.

Simmons RJ, Cogan DG: Occult temporal arteritis. *Arch Ophthalmol* 68:38–47, 1962.

Vilaseca J, González A, Cid MC, et al: Clinical usefulness of temporal artery biopsy. *Ann Rheum Dis* 46:282–285, 1987.

Wykes WN, Cullen JF: Headache and temporal arteritis. *Scott Med J* 30.42, 1985.

Cerebral Embolism

Auerbach SH, Butler RB, Levine HL: Headache in cerebral embolic disease. *Stroke* 12(3):367–369, 1981.

Tipton BK, Robertson JT, Robertson JH: Embolism to the central nervous system from cardiac myxoma. *J Neurosurg* 47:937–940, 1977.

Cerebrovascular Aspects of Headache

Appenzeller O: Cerebrovascular aspects of headache. *Med Clin North Am* 62(3):467–480, 1978.

Headache—Review Articles

Headache Classification Committee of the International Headache Society: Classification and diagnostic criteria for headache disorders, cranial neuralgias and facial pain. *Cephalalgia* 8(suppl 7):9–92, 1988.

Hematoma—Epidural/Subdural

McDermott M, Fleming JFR, Vanderlinden RG, et al: Spontaneous arterial subdural hematoma. *Neurosurgery* 14(1):13–18, 1984.

Stone JL, Rifai MHS, Sugar O, et al: Subdural hematomas: 1. Acute subdural hematoma: Progress in definition, clinical pathology, and therapy. *Surg Neurol* 19:216–231, 1983.

Hemorrhage—Intracerebral

Fingerote RJ, Shuaib A, Brownell AKW: Spontaneous midbrain hemorrhage. *South Med J* 83(3):280–282, 1990.

Godersky JC, Biller J: Diagnosis and treatment of spontaneous intracerebral hemorrhage. *Compr Ther* 13(9):22–30, 1987.

Ropper AH, Davis KR: Lobar cerebral hemorrhages: Acute clinical syndromes in 26 cases. *Ann Neurol* 8:141–147, 1980.

Steiger HJ, Tew JM Jr: Hemorrhage and epilepsy in cryptic cerebrovascular malformations. *Arch Neurol* 41:722–724, 1984.

Hemorrhage—Parenchymal

Catapano MS, Marx JA: Central nervous system cysticercosis simulating an acute cerebellar hemorrhage. *Ann Emerg Med* 15:847–849, 1986.

Hemorrhage—Spinal/Subarachnoid

Barton CW: Subarachnoid hemorrhage presenting as acute chest pain: A variant of le coup de poignard. *Ann Emerg Med* 17(9):977–978, 1988.

Gaitzsch J, Berney J: Spinal subarachnoid hematoma of spontaneous origin and complicating anticoagulation: Report of four cases and review of the literature. *Surg Neurol* 21:534–538, 1984.

Rappaport B, Emsellem HA, Shesser R, et al: An unusual case of proctalgia. *Ann Emerg Med* 19(2):201–203, 1990.

Ueda S, Saito A, Inomori S, et al: Cavernous angioma of the cauda equina producing subarachnoid hemorrhage. *J Neurosurg* 66:134–136, 1987.

Hemorrhage—Subarachnoid/Aneurysm-Related

Adams HP Jr, Kassell NF, Torner JC, et al: CT and clinical correlations in recent aneurysmal subarachnoid hemorrhage: A preliminary report of the Cooperative Aneurysm Study. *Neurology* 33:981–988, 1983.

Adams HP, Sahs AL: Aneurysmal subarachnoid hemorrhage. *Mod Concepts Cardiovasc Dis* 50(9):49–54, 1981.

Alvord EC Jr, Thorn RB: Natural history of subarachnoid hemorrhage: Early prognosis. *Clin Neurosurg* 24:167–175, 1977.

Bartlett JR: Subarachnoid haemorrhage. *Br Med J* [Clin Res] 283(6303):1347–1348, 1981.

Bjerre P, Videbaek H, Lindholm J: Subarachnoid hemorrhage with normal cerebral angiography: A prospective study on sellar abnormalities and pituitary function. *Neurosurgery* 19(6):1012–1015, 1986.

DiLorenzo N, Guidetti G: Anterior communicating aneurysm missed at angiography: Report of two cases treated surgically. *Neurosurgery* 23(4):494–499, 1988.

Duffy GP: Lumbar puncture in spontaneous subarachnoid haemorrhage. *Br Med J* [Clin Res] 285:1163–1164, 1982.

Heros RC, Zervas NT: Subarachnoid hemorrhage. *Ann Rev Med* 34:367–375, 1983.

Hitchcock EK: Ruptured aneurysms. *Br Med J* [Clin Res] 286:1299–1301, 1983.

Hunt WE, Meagher JN, Hess RM: Intracranial aneurysm: A nine-year study. *Ohio State Med J* 62(11):1168–1171, 1966.

Lindsay KW, Teasdale GM, Knill-Jones RP: Observer variability in assessing the clinical features of subarachnoid hemorrhage. *J Neurosurg* 58:57–62, 1983.

Lindsay KW, Teasdale G, Knill-Jones RP, et al: Observer variability in grading patients with subarachnoid hemorrhage. *J Neurosurg* 56:628–633, 1982.

Locksley HB: Report on the cooperative study of intracranial aneurysms and subarachnoid hemorrhage: Section 5, part 1. Natural history of subarachnoid hemorrhage, intracranial aneurysms and arteriovenous malformations: Based on 6368 cases in the cooperative study. *J Neurosurg* 25(2):219–239, 1966; part 2. Natural history of subarachnoid hemorrhage, intracranial aneurysms and arteriovenous malformations: Based on 6368 cases in the cooperative study. *J Neurosurg* 25(2):321–368, 1966.

Öhman J, Heiskanen O: Effect of nimodipine on the outcome of patients after aneurysmal subarachnoid hemorrhage and surgery. *J Neurosurg* 69:683–686, 1988.

Seiler RW, Reulen HJ, Huber P, et al: Outcome of aneurysmal subarachnoid hemorrhage in a hospital population: A prospective study including early operation, intravenous nimodipine, and transcranial Doppler ultrasound. *Neurosurgery* 23:598–604, 1988.

Sicuteri F: Headache and meningismus evoked by lumbar puncture and subarachnoid hemorrhage: A biochemical interpretation. *Headache* 5(4):108–110, 1966.

Six EG, Clark JB, Early CB: Subarachnoid hemorrhage and intracranial aneurysms: A review of assessment and early management. *Mil Med* 148:497–501, 1983.

Sundt TM Jr, Whisnant JP: Subarachnoid hemorrhage from intracranial aneurysms. Surgical management and natural history of disease. *N Engl J Med* 299:116–122, 1978.

Welty TE, Horner TG: Pathophysiology and treatment of subarachnoid hemorrhage. *Clin Pharm* 9:35–39, 1990.

Zervas NT: Subarachnoid hemorrhage (editorial). *N Engl J Med* 299(3):147–148, 1978.

Hemorrhage—Subarachnoid/AV Malformations

Davis C, Symon L: The management of cerebral arteriovenous malformations. *Acta Neurochir* 74:4–11, 1985.

Selecki BR: Some aspects of intracranial arteriovenous malformations. *Med J Aust* 1(11):495–496, 1983.

Hemorrhage—Subarachnoid/Early Diagnosis

Adams HP Jr, Jergenson DD, Kassell NF, et al: Pitfalls in the recognition of subarachnoid hemorrhage, *JAMA* 244:794–796, 1980.

Ball MJ: Pathogenesis of the "sentinel headache" preceding berry aneurysm rupture. *Can Med Assoc J* 112:78–79, 1975.

Black P: Recognizing and treating spontaneous intracranial hemorrhage. *Drug Ther (Hosp)* 5(9):33–47, 1980.

Brust JCM: Subarachnoid hemorrhage: Early detection and diagnosis. *Hosp Pract [Off]* 17(2):73–80, 1982.

Day JW, Raskin NH: Thunderclap headache: Symptom of unruptured cerebral aneurysm. *Lancet* 2(8518):1247–1248, 1986.

Drexler ED: Severe headaches: When to worry, what to do. *Postgrad Med* 87(4):164–165, 168–170, 173–176, 178, 180, 1990.

Edmeads J: The worst headache ever: 1. Ominous causes. *Postgrad Med* 86(1):93–96, 103–104, 1989: 2. Innocuous causes. *Postgrad Med* 86(1):107–110, 1989.

Fontanarosa PB: Recognition of subarachnoid hemorrhage. *Ann Emerg Med* 18:1199–1205, 1989.

Hillman J: Should computed tomography scanning replace lumbar puncture in the diagnostic process in suspected subarachnoid hemorrhage? *Surg Neurol* 26:547–550, 1986.

Klara PM, George ED: Warning leaks and sentinel headaches associated with subarachnoid hemorrhage. *Mil Med* 147:660–662, 1982.

Knaus WA, Wagner DP, Davis DO: CT for headache: Cost/benefit for subarachnoid hemorrhage. *AJR* 136:537–542, 1981.

Lang DT, Berberian LB, Lee S, et al: Rapid differentiation of subarachnoid hemorrhage from traumatic lumbar puncture using the D-dimer assay. *Am J Clin Pathol* 93:403–405, 1990.

Leblanc R, Winfield JA: The warning leak in subarachnoid hemorrhage and the importance of its early diagnosis. *Can Med Assoc J* 131:1235–1236, 1984.

Shapiro SA: Sentinel symptoms and signs of intracranial aneurysms. *Ind Med* 83(1):20–22, 1990.

Shesser R: Headache caused by serious illness: Evaluation in an emergency setting. *Postgrad Med* 81(3):117–121, 124–125, 1987.

Shuttleworth EC, Parker JM, Wise GR, et al: Differentiation of early subarachnoid hemorrhage from traumatic lumbar puncture. *Stroke* 8(5):613–617, 1977.

Vermeulen M, Hasan D, Blijenberg BG, et al: Xanthochromia after subarachnoid haemorrhage needs no revisitation. *J Neurol Neurosurg Psychiatry* 52:826–828, 1989.

Verweij RD, Wijdicks EFM, van Gijn J: Warning headache in aneurysmal subarachnoid hemorrhage: A case-control study. *Arch Neurol* 45:1019–1020, 1988.

Hemorrhage—Subarachnoid/Tumor-Related

Goetting MG, Swanson SE: Massive hemorrhage into intracranial neurinomas. *Surg Neurol* 27:168–172, 1987.

Lee J-P, Wang AD-J: Acoustic neurinoma presenting as intratumoral bleeding. *Neurosurgery* 24:764–768, 1989.

Yonemitsu T, Niizuma H, Kodama N, et al: Acoustic neurinoma presenting as subarachnoid hemorrhage. *Surg Neurol* 20:125–130, 1983.

Herpes Simplex Encephalitis

Kennedy PGE: A retrospective analysis of forty-six cases of herpes simplex encephalitis seen in Glasgow between 1962 and 1985. *Q J Med* 68(255):533–540, 1988.

Kennedy PGE, Adams JH, Graham DI, et al: A clinico-pathological study of herpes simplex encephalitis. *Neuropathol Appl Neurobiol* 14:395–415, 1988.

Whitley RJ: Antiviral treatment of a serious herpes simplex infection: Encephalitis. *J Am Acad Dermatol* 18:209–211, 1988.

Hypertensive Encephalopathy

Barnett HJM: Cerebral ischemia and infarction, in Wyngaarden JB, Smith LH Jr (eds): *Cecil Textbook of Medicine*, 18th ed. Philadelphia, Saunders, 1988, pp 2162–2173.

Infectious Diseases and Headache

Cohen JI, Corson AP, Corey GR: Late appearance of skin rash in Rocky Mountain spotted fever. *South Med J* 76(11):1457–1458, 1983.

Denning DW: The neurological features of acute HIV infection. *Biomed Pharmacother* 42:11–14, 1988.

Downey D, Anzimlt JC, Ellis-Pegler RB: *Salmonella typhi* infection in adults is not limited to travellers returning from the tropics. *N Z Med J* 99(804):443–446, 1986.

Gaines H, von Sydow M, Pehrson PO, et al: Clinical picture of primary HIV infection presenting as a glandular-fever-like illness. *Br Med J* 297(6660):1363–1368, 1988.

Giannoulis E, Arvanitakis C, Zaphiropoulos A, et al: Disseminated strongyloidiasis with uncommon manifestations in Greece. *J Trop Med Hyg* 89:171–178, 1986.

Jevon TR, Knudson MP, Smith PA, et al: A point-source epidemic of leptospirosis: Description of cases, cause, and prevention. *Postgrad Med* 80(8):121–122, 127–129, 1986.

Kelleher RJ, Murray JAM, Welsby PD: Recurrent meningitis associated with meningioma of the mastoid cavity. *J Laryngol Otol* 108:99–100, 1989.

Kirk JL, Fine DP, Sexton J, et al: Rocky Mountain spotted fever: A clinical review based on 48 confirmed cases, 1943–1986. *Medicine* 69(1):35–45, 1990.

Lee SMK: Viscerotropic Rocky Mountain spotted fever in southeastern Texas: Report of a survivor with atypical manifestations and multiple organ failure. *South Med J* 82(5):640–642, 1989.

Mousa ARM, Elhag KM, Khogali M, et al: The nature of human brucellosis in Kuwait: Study of 379 cases. *Rev Infect Dis* 10(1):211–217, 1988.

Sawyer LA, Fishbein DB, McDade JE: Q fever: Current concepts. *Rev Infect Dis* 9(5):935–946, 1987.

Yung AP, Grayson ML: Psittacosis: A review of 135 cases. *Med J Aust* 148:228–233, 1988.

Lateral Sinus Thrombosis

Adams RD, Victor M: Cerebrovascular diseases, in *Principles of Neurology,* 4th ed. New York, McGraw-Hill, 1989, pp 618–685.

Adams RD, Victor M: Nonviral infections of the nervous system, in *Principles of Neurology,* 4th ed. New York, McGraw-Hill, 1989, pp 565–566.

Goldenberg RA: Lateral sinus thrombosis: Medical or surgical treatment? *Arch Otolaryngol* 111:56–58, 1985.

Mathews TJ: Lateral sinus pathology: 22 cases managed at Groote Schuur Hospital. *J Laryngol Otol* 102:118–120, 1988.

Lumbar Puncture

Alfery DD, Marsh ML, Shapiro HM: Post-spinal headache or intracranial tumor after obstetric anesthesia. *Anesthesiology* 51:92–94, 1979.

Mayer FA, Clark RW, Scheinin GS: Post-lumbar puncture headache as a complication of spinal anesthesia. *J Foot Surg* 26(3):242–245, 1987.

Sternbach, G: Lumbar puncture. *J Emerg Med* 2:199–203, 1985.

Meningismus

Chapel TA: The signs and symptoms of secondary syphilis. *Sex Trans Dis* 7(4):161–164, 1980.

Polk DB, Steele RW: Bacterial meningitis presenting with normal cerebrospinal fluid. *Pediatr Infect Dis J* 6:1040–1042, 1987.

Steingrub JS, Mikolich DJ, Schlaeffer F: Delirium tremens with meningismus. *Isr J Med Sci* 23:839–840, 1987.

Meningitis—Amebic

Ma P, Visvesvara GS, Martinez AJ, et al: *Naegleria* and *Acanthamoeba* infections: Review. *Rev Infect Dis* 12(3):490–514, 1990.

Meningitis—Bacterial

Callaham M: Fulminant bacterial meningitis without meningeal signs. *Ann Emerg Med* 18:90–93, 1989.

Dougherty JM, Jones J: Cerebrospinal fluid cultures and analysis. *Ann Emerg Med* 15:317–323, 1986.

Downs NJ, Hodges GR, Taylor SA: Mixed bacterial meningitis. *Rev Infect Dis* 9(4):693–704, 1987.

Gorelick PB, Biller J: Lumbar puncture: Technique, indications, and complications. *Postgrad Med* 79(8):257–261, 265–266, 268, 1986.

Salih MAM, Ahmed HS, Hofvander Y, et al: Rapid diagnosis of bacterial meningitis by an enzyme immunoassay of cerebrospinal fluid. *Epidemiol Infect* 103:301–310, 1989.

Siegman-Igra Y, Schwartz D, Alperin H, et al: Invasive pneumococcal infection in Israel: Review of 90 cases. *Scand J Infect Dis* 18:511–517, 1986.

Waltman WD II, Gray B, McDaniel LS, et al: Cross-reactive monoclonal antibodies for diagnosis of pneumococcal meningitis. *J Clin Microbiol* 26(9):1635–1640, 1988.

Williams RG, Hart CA: Rapid identification of bacterial antigen in blood cultures and cerebrospinal fluid. *J Clin Pathol* 41:691–693, 1988.

Witt DJ, Craven DE, McCabe WR: Bacterial infections in adult patients with the acquired immune deficiency syndrome (AIDS) and AIDS-related complex. *Am J Med* 82(5):900–906, 1987.

Meningitis—Bacterial/Problems and Complications

Behrman RE, Meyers BR, Mendelson MH, et al: Central nervous system infections in the elderly. *Arch Intern Med* 149:1596–1599, 1989.

Feris, J, Moledina N, Rodriguez WJ, et al: Aztreonam in the treatment of gram-negative meningitis and other gram-negative infections. *Chemotherapy* 35 (suppl 1):31–38, 1989.

Phelan M, Manson JI: Spinal cord dysfunction with quadriplegia complicating pneumococcal meningitis. *Aust Paediatr J* 23:57–59, 1987.

Powers WJ: Cerebrospinal fluid lymphocytosis in acute bacterial meningitis. *Am J Med* 79(2):216–220, 1985.

Taft TA, Chusid MJ, Sty JR: Cerebral infarction in *Hemophilus influenzae* type B meningitis. *Clin Pediatr* 25(4):177–180, 1986.

Wong VK, Hitchcock W, Mason WH: Meningococcal infections in children: A review of 100 cases. *Pediatr Infect Dis J* 8:224–227, 1989.

Meningitis—Bacterial/Uncommon Causes

Bach MC, Davis KM: *Listeria rhombencephalitis* mimicking tuberculous meningitis. *Rev Infect Dis* 9(1):130–140, 1987.

Bayne LL, Schmidley JW, Goodin DS: Acute syphilitic meningitis: Its occurrence after clinical and serologic cure of secondary syphilis with penicillin G. *Arch Neurol* 43:137–138, 1986.

Dee RR, Lorber B: Brain abscess due to *Listeria monocytogenes:* Case report and literature review. *Rev Infect Dis* 8(6)968–978, 1986.

Farber JM, Losos JZ: *Listeria monocytogenes:* A foodborne pathogen. *Can Med Assoc J* 138(5):413–418, 1988.

Feder HM Jr: *Bacteroides fragilis* meningitis. *Rev Infect Dis* 9(4):783–786, 1987.

Hira SK, Patel JS, Bhat SG, et al: Clinical manifestations of secondary syphilis. *Int J Dermatol* 26(2)103–107, 1987.

Muder RR, Yu VL, Dummer JS, et al: Infections caused by *Pseudomonas maltophilia:* Expanding clinical spectrum. *Arch Intern Med* 147:1672–1674, 1987.

Pachner AR, Steere AC: The triad of neurologic manifestations of Lyme disease: Meningitis, cranial neuritis, and radiculoneuritis. *Neurology* 35:47–53, 1985.

Pal GS, Baker JT, Humphrey PRD: Lyme disease presenting as recurrent acute meningitis. *Br Med J [Clin Res]* 295(6594):367, 1987.

Spitzer, PG, Hammer SM, Karchmer AW: Treatment of *Listeria monocytogenes* infection with trimethoprim-sulfamethoxazole: Case report and review of the literature. *Rev Infect Dis* 8(3):427–430, 1986.

Meningitis—Drug-Related

Gordon MF, Allon M, Coyle PK: Drug-induced meningitis. *Neurology* 40:163–164, 1990.

Greenberg GN: Recurrent sulindac-induced aseptic meningitis in a patient tolerant to other nonsteroidal anti-inflammatory drugs. *South Med J* 81(11):1463–1464, 1988.

Holdiness MR: Neurological manifestations and toxicities of the antituberculosis drugs: A review. *Med Toxicol* 2:33–51, 1987.

Mifsud AJ: Drug-related recurrent meningitis. *J Infect* 17(2):151–153, 1988.

Ruppert GB, Barth WF: Tolmetin-induced aseptic meningitis. *JAMA* 245:67–68, 1981.

Meningitis—Herpetic

Kaufman RH: Clinical features of herpes genitalis. *J Reprod Med* 31(supp l5):379–383, 1986.

Mertz G, Corey L: Genital herpes simplex virus infections in adults. *Urol Clin North Am* 11(1):103–119, 1984.

Meningitis—Immunologic

de la Monte S, Gupta PK, Hutchins GM: Polymorphous exudates and atypical mononuclear cells in the cerebrospinal fluid of patients with Sjögren's syndrome. *Acta Cytol* 29(4):634–637, 1985.

Harris GJ, Franson TR, Ryan LM: Recurrent aseptic meningitis as a manifestation of mixed connective tissue disease (MCTD). *Wis Med J* 86(3):31–33, 1987.

O'Duffy JD, Robertson DM, Goldstein NP: Chlorambucil in the treatment of uveitis and meningoencephalitis of Behçet's disease. *Am J Med* 76(1):75–84, 1984.

Sands ML, Ryczak M, Brown RB: Recurrent aseptic meningitis followed by transverse myelitis as a presentation of systemic lupus erythematosus. *J Rheumatol* 15:862–864, 1988.

Meningitis—Mollaret's

Kwong YL, Woo E, Fong PC, et al: Mollaret's meningitis revisited:

Report of a case with a review of the literature. *Clin Neurol Neurosurg* 90(2):163–167, 1988.

Mascia RA, Smith CW Jr: Mollaret's meningitis: An unusual disease with a characteristic presentation. *Am J Med Sci* 287(1):52–53, 1984.

Meningitis Secondary to CNS Tumor

Becker WJ, Watters GV, de Chadarevian J-P, et al: Recurrent aseptic meningitis secondary to intracranial epidermoids. *Can J Neurol Sci* 11:387–389, 1984.

Krueger DW, Larson EB: Recurrent fever of unknown origin, coma, and meningismus due to a leaking craniopharyngioma. *Am J Med* 84(3):543–545, 1988.

Starinsky R, Wald U, Michowitz SD, et al: Dermoids of the posterior fossa: Case reports and review. *Clin Pediatr* 27(12):579–582, 1988.

Otitic Headache

Gillanders DA: Gradenigo's syndrome revisited: *J Otolaryngol* 12(3):169–174, 1983.

Review Articles—Acute Headache

Diehr P, Wood RW, Barr V, et al: Acute headaches: Presenting symptoms and diagnostic rules to identify patients with tension and migraine headache. *J Chron Dis* 34:147–158, 1981.

Olenick JS, Taylor RB: Emergency evaluation and treatment of headache. *Prim Care* 13(1):97–107, 1986.

Trauma—Head

Cooper PR: Post-traumatic intracranial mass lesions, in Cooper PR (ed): *Head Injuries*. Baltimore, Williams & Wilkins, 1982, pp 185–232.

Elkind AH: Headache and facial pain associated with head injury. *Otolaryngol Clin North Am* 22(6):1251–1271, 1989.

Gennarelli TA, Thibault LE: Biomechanics of acute subdural hematoma. *J Trauma* 22(8):680–686, 1982.

Gurdjian ES, Gurdjian ES: Acute head injuries. *Surg Gynecol Obstet* 146:805–820, 1978.

Kishore PRS, Kipper MH: Craniocerebral trauma, in Lee SH, Rae KCVG (eds): *Cranial Computed Tomography*. New York, McGraw-Hill, 1983, pp 479–504.

Mokri B, Piepgras DG, Houser OW: Traumatic dissections of the extracranial internal carotid artery. *J Neurosurg* 68:189–197, 1988.

Peyster RG, Hoover ED: CT in head trauma. *J Trauma* 22(1):25–38, 1982.

Pozzato E, Gaist G, Vinci A, et al: Traumatic interhemispheric subdural hematomas. *J Trauma* 22(3):241–243, 1982.

Wallis A, Donald PJ: Frontal sinus fractures: A review of 72 cases. *Laryngoscope* 98:593–598, 1988.

Vascular Headache

Dalessio DJ: Major vascular diseases and headaches, in Dalessio DJ (ed): *Wolfe's Headache and Other Head Pain,* 5th ed. New York, Oxford University Press, 1987, pp 204–214.

Grindal AB, Toole JF: Headache and transient ischemic attacks. *Stroke* 5(5):603–606, 1974.

Jones HR Jr, Siekert RG: Neurological manifestations of infective endocarditis. *Brain* 112:1295–1315, 1989.

Louis S: A bedside test for determining the sub-types of vascular headache. *Headache* 21:87–88, 1981.

PART TWO
Acute Facial Pain

Acute Eye Pain

☐ DIAGNOSTIC LIST

1. Eyelids
   A. Hordeolum (stye)—external and internal
   B. Chalazion
   C. Sebaceous carcinoma of the lid
   D. Blepharitis
   E. Dacryoadenitis
   F. Dacryocystitis
   G. Erysipelas of the face
2. Conjunctiva, iris, cornea, sclera, and globe
   A. Foreign body in the conjunctiva or cornea
   B. Herpes zoster ophthalmicus
   C. Conjunctivitis
      1. Bacterial and viral
      2. Purulent
      3. *Chlamydia trachomatis*
      4. Epidemic keratoconjunctivitis
   D. Acute iritis and iridocyclitis
      1. Suppurative
      2. Nonsuppurative
      3. Mimics of iritis
   E. Corneal injury and foreign body
   F. Herpes simplex keratitis
   G. Acute glaucoma
   H. Episcleritis
   I. Scleritis
      1. Anterior
      2. Posterior

   J. Endophthalmitis and panophthalmitis
   K. Preseptal cellulitis
3. Orbital disease—"red eye," proptosis, and diplopia
   A. Idiopathic orbital pseudotumor
   B. Subperiosteal orbital abscess
   C. Orbital cellulitis and/or abscess
   D. Rhinocerebral mucormycosis
   E. Bacterial cavernous sinus thrombosis
   F. Thyroid ophthalmopathy—acute type
   G. Orbital hematoma
   H. Intracavernous carotid artery aneurysm
   I. Carotid cavernous sinus fistula
   J. Dural cavernous sinus shunt
   K. Pituitary apoplexy
4. Referred orbital pain
   A. Minor leak from an internal carotid or anterior communicating aneurysm
   B. Carotid artery dissection
   C. Occipital lobe and cerebellar lesions
5. Orbital pain and diplopia
   A. Supraclinoid internal carotid or posterior communicating aneurysm
   B. Diabetic or nondiabetic ischemic neuropathy

C. Ophthalmoplegic migraine
6. Ocular pain and visual loss
   A. Idiopathic optic neuritis and multiple sclerosis
   B. Devic's disease
   C. Mimics of optic neuritis
      1. Autoimmune disorders— systemic lupus erythematosus and Sjögren's syndrome
      2. Parasellar region inflammatory disorders— chronic tuberculous or fungal meningitis, and sarcoidosis
      3. Parainfectious associations
      4. Neuroretinitis
      5. Parasellar masses—cysts, tumors, and aneurysms
      6. Temporal (giant cell) arteritis
      7. Amaurosis fugax and ocular infarction
7. Infectious diseases causing bilateral ocular pain
   A. Nonspecific viral syndromes
   B. Varicella
   C. Epstein-Barr virus
   D. Lymphogranuloma venereum and cat-scratch fever
   E. Trichinosis
   G. Q fever
8. Skin disorders with acute eye involvement
   A. Toxic epidermal necrolysis
   B. Stevens-Johnson syndrome
9. Referred dental pain
10. Pain distribution (unilateral or bilateral) in acute ophthalmic disorders

☐ SUMMARY

A furuncle-like lesion on the lid margin or surface is usually due to a staphylococcal infection of the glands of the lid *(hordeolum)*. A *chalazion* presents as a mildly tender and painful skin-colored nodule caused by granulomatous inflammation of a lid gland. *Sebaceous carcinoma* is a highly malignant lesion of the eyelid. It is often indistinguishable from a chalazion, or it may present as conjunctivitis or blepharitis. A chalazion recurrent at the same site after curettage requires biopsy. Clues to the malignant nature of a chalazion-like lesion are induration, fixation to eyelid skin, recurrence after treatment, and an insidious onset.

Blepharitis causes eye and lid pain, scaling, crusting, and redness of the lid margin, with distortion and discoloration of the eyelashes. A painful conjunctivitis and/or keratitis may be associated and result in more pain, photophobia, and lacrimation. *Acute dacryoadenitis* causes upper lateral lid pain, tenderness, swelling, and sometimes redness. It is associated with viral infections and local bacterial infections of the eye. *Dacryocystitis* causes pain, swelling, and redness below the inner canthus of the eye and epiphora. *Erysipelas* causes erythematous edema, firmness, and tenderness of the skin of the face and lid(s), accompanied by fever and malaise. This disorder responds to antibiotic therapy. A *foreign body* in the eye causes pain, lacrimation, and conjunctival injection. *Herpes zoster* may cause unilateral burning and stabbing eye, cheek, and forehead pain and upper facial edema, associated with the eruption of groups of small, red-based vesicles or crusted ulcers on the lids, forehead, and nose. *Conjunctivitis* may cause conjunctival edema, hyperemia, burning ocular pain, discharge, lacrimation, and photophobia. A watery discharge, lid

follicles, and preauricular adenopathy have been associated with *viral conjunctivitis*. *Purulent unilateral conjunctivitis* in a patient with a urethral discharge is likely to be due to *Neisseria gonorrhoeae*, while a mucoid, watery, or mildly purulent discharge in the same setting may be caused by a chlamydial infection. These agents can be differentiated by stained smears and cultures.

Epidemic keratoconjunctivitis usually causes conjunctival injection, tearing, and photophobia associated with a decrease in visual acuity. A keratitis begins during the first week and may persist for months.

Acute iritis may be due to pyogenic organisms, chronic infections, or immunologic disorders. Aching and at times sharp, stabbing ocular pain is associated with circumcorneal hyperemia. The pain is intensified by focusing to read or by staring into a light and is relieved by cycloplegics. Slit lamp examination shows protein (e.g., flare) and cells in the anterior chamber. Shining a light in the unaffected eye may cause pain intensification in the involved eye. Suppurative and nonsuppurative forms occur. The former occurs in patients with sepsis, endocarditis, or penetrating trauma. Paracentesis and culture will establish the diagnosis. Nonsuppurative iritis may be idiopathic, secondary to a chronic infection such as syphilis, tuberculosis, or histoplasmosis, or it may occur as a component of a systemic disorder of unknown etiology (e.g., Behçet's disease, Reiter's syndrome). Vascular or malignant disease may affect the iris and mimic iritis.

Corneal injury causes constant aching and/or stabbing anterior eye pain that is increased by eye or lid movement. The lid may be red and swollen, and the eye red and tender to palpation. Photophobia, lacrimation, and blepharospasm are common associated findings. A drop of local anesthetic may produce immediate pain relief. Fluorescence staining will identify corneal abrasions and ulcers and direct attention to *foreign bodies*. Slit lamp examination and corneal microscopy aid in the evaluation of corneal injury.

Herpes simplex keratitis causes ocular pain and redness, photophobia, tearing, and visual blurring. Fluorescence staining shows dendritic, star-shaped, linear, or punctate corneal lesions. Cultures will isolate herpes simplex virus frequently, but the clinical presentation may be sufficient for diagnosis. *Acute glaucoma* presents with a red, painful eye and blurred vision. The cornea is edematous and hazy, and the pupil dilated and poorly responsive to light. The intraocular pressure usually exceeds 50 mmHg. There is evidence of a narrow angle, and improvement follows use of a laser to create an opening in the peripheral iris that facilitates fluid passage to the anterior chamber.

Episcleritis causes burning or stinging pain in a quadrant of the anterior portion of the eye associated with local hyperemia of the episcleral membrane. A nodular form may also occur.

Anterior scleritis causes diffuse or nodular hyperemic scleral lesions in the white portion of the eye associated with deep aching eye and/or orbital pain. Keratitis may occur, with loss of visual acuity, photophobia, lacrimation, and anterior eye pain.

Posterior scleritis causes deep, boring eye and orbital pain in one or both eyes. An associated anterior scleritis may be present, or the sclera may be white. Proptosis, ptosis, and periorbital edema may occur secondary to orbital inflammation. The pain may be intensified by ocular movement. Fundoscopic examination reveals a fundal mass and/or chorioidal folds and retinal striae. Evidence of exudative retinal detachment or cystoid macular edema may be present. Ultrasound or CT scans will show posterior global flattening and scleral thickening, and edema of the orbital fat. Scleritis may be idiopathic or associated with collagen vascular disorders or other diseases with prominent immunologic abnormalities.

Endophthalmitis presents with a painful, tender, red eye; loss of vision; a hazy or opaque cornea; hypopyon; and a history of recent lid trauma, adjacent or systemic infection, or intraocular surgery. Endogenous clostridial ophthalmitis occurs spontaneously in a setting of bowel or gallbladder-related sepsis.

Preseptal cellulitis causes mildly painful and tender erythema and edema of the lids. It is caused by bacteria that gain access to the preseptal region by trauma or by spread from an infected conjunctiva, lacrimal sac, or sinus. There may be chemosis, but proptosis, ophthalmoplegia, and visual loss do not occur.

Idiopathic orbital pseudotumor causes deep orbital pain, lid edema, chemosis, restricted ocular motility, proptosis, and diplopia. The pain may be intensified by eye movements. A CT scan may show ipsilateral infiltration of orbital fat by a streaky or homogeneous density. Early cases resolve with corticosteroid therapy.

A *subperiosteal orbital abscess* is usually secondary to an ethmoid sinusitis. Fever, preseptal cellulitis, chemosis, orbital pain, and asymmetrical proptosis occur, with limitation of ocular movement. Local tenderness may be present between the supraorbital margin and the globe. A subperiosteal abscess may be detected by a CT scan or MRI. *Orbital cellulitis* causes ipsilateral aching ocular pain and fever; preseptal cellulitis; chemosis; proptosis; and ophthalmopareses, paresthesias, and/or hypesthesia in the sensory areas of trigeminal division V_1 and sometimes V_2. Only a small percentage of cases develop cavernous sinus thrombosis. CT or MRI may detect orbital edema and infiltration, medial rectus muscle enlargement, and air fluid levels in an orbital abscess. *Rhinocerebral mucormycosis* occurs in a setting of uncontrolled diabetes, ketoacidosis, renal failure, or immunosuppression. Severe toxicity, fever, lid edema, chemosis, proptosis, and ophthalmoplegias occur. Visual loss on the affected side may be rapid. A black mucosal eschar may be observed in the nose, a sinus, or palate. Cerebral, thalamic, and brain stem lesions may result from fungal arterial occlusion or embolism. The severe orbital cellulitis produced invades the orbital apex and the optic nerve, causing visual loss or blindness. Impairment of trigeminal divisions V_1 and V_2 may also occur. CT and MRI will detect evidence of sinus, orbital, and brain disease. A small percentage of patients with mucormycosis develop cavernous sinus thrombosis and bilateral signs. *Bacterial cavernous sinus thrombosis* occurs with toxicity, high fever, ipsilateral proptosis, chemosis and lid edema, hypesthesia and paresthesias of the face, and ophthalmoplegias. Fundoscopy reveals papilledema and venous congestion. Bilateral involvement occurs within 2 to 4 days. MRI will detect a cavernous sinus clot with high sensitivity. A rare form of *thyroid ophthalmopathy* presents with orbital pain, bilateral proptosis, chemosis, and ophthalmopareses. Visual loss may occur from optic nerve compression. A CT scan shows ocular muscle enlargement and orbital edema. There is a response to prednisone and/or irradiation. An *orbital hematoma* occurs suddenly with a "pop" and then progresses to produce severe orbital pain, proptosis, and ophthalmopareses. Extensive lid edema and ecchymoses may be associated findings. A CT scan will confirm the presence of an orbital hematoma. Spontaneous cases are associated with an orbital varix. *Intracavernous carotid artery aneurysms* may present with orbital pain and ipsilateral facial pain and paresthesias, ophthalmopareses, and proptosis. A superior orbital fissure syndrome may occur in 16 percent and a cavernous sinus syndrome in 43 percent of cases. The diagnosis can be confirmed by MRI or a cerebral angiogram. A *carotid cavernous fistula* causes pulsating exophthalmos, orbital pain and chemosis with lid edema. A bruit is audible to the examiner and/or patient. Visual loss as well as ophthalmopareses, may occur. The fistula can be demonstrated by cerebral angiography. A *dural cavernous sinus shunt* can produce a similar picture and should be suspected if the cerebral angiogram is negative. These lesions can be demonstrated by an external carotid angiogram that shows early filling of the cavernous sinus. Pituitary apoplexy causes severe retro-orbital, frontal, and/or generalized head pain; diplopia (16 percent), a disturbance of consciousness (12 percent), and an abrupt partial or complete loss of vision. The cause is sudden hemorrhage into a pituitary tumor. The tumor can be detected by CT or MRI.

A *minor leak from an internal carotid or anterior communicating aneurysm* may cause an ipsilateral retro-orbital and/or frontal thunderclap headache. Confirmation of subarachnoid bleeding by CT or lumbar puncture and cerebral angiography will establish the diagnosis. *Carotid artery dissection* may cause anterior neck, retro-orbital, hemifacial, and/or hemicranial pain and sometimes an ipsilateral Horner's syndrome and/or a bruit (subjective and/or objective). These findings may be followed within several hours or days by transient or permanent cerebral deficits (e.g., hemiparesis, aphasia, and amaurosis fugax). The diagnosis can be confirmed by angiography of the carotid vessels. *Occipital lobe infarction or hemorrhage* may cause referred ipsilateral orbital pain and a macular-sparing homonymous hemianopia.

A *posterior communcating or supraclinoid carotid aneurysm* may cause severe eye pain and a third nerve palsy with a dilated, fixed pupil. *Diabetic ischemic neuropathy* may cause eye pain and oculomotor nerve paresis with pupillary sparing. *Ophthalmoplegic migraine* occurs in young patients and is transient and sometimes recurrent. There is a dilated pupil. Since up to 14 percent of patients with an aneurysm have pupillary sparing, careful evaluation of third nerve lesions without pupillary dilatation is required. Complete third nerve lesions require angiography to exclude aneurysm, and some incomplete lesions may also need this procedure.

Optic neuritis causes unilateral ocular pain intensified by motion or palpation of the globe, a loss of visual acuity and color perception, and an ipsilateral central scotoma. Loss of vision progresses to a nadir within 2 to 3 weeks and then spontaneously recovers without specific therapy. Such a course is characteristic of this disorder. Most cases are idiopathic, but 25 to 50 percent develop multiple sclerosis at a later time. A small number of patients present with bilateral optic neuritis and transverse myelitis (Devic's disease). *Mimicry of idiopathic optic neuritis* by *autoimmune diseases, chronic inflammatory disorders in the parasellar area, neuroretinitis, parasellar masses* (cysts, tumors, and aneurysms), and *temporal arteritis* may occur. Idiopathic optic neuritis may also be confused with parainfectious ocular disorders associated with HIV and mycoplasma pneumoniae infections. *Amaurosis fugax* and *ocular infarction* occur with atherosclerotic disease or *giant cell arteritis* in the elderly and with migraine or cardiogenic emboli in the young.

Orbital pain is common in *viral and rickettsial diseases,* and it occurs at the extremes of globe movement. *Varicella* may cause conjunctival ulcers and keratitis, *Epstein-Barr* may cause lacrimal gland or sac infections, and *lymphogranuloma venereum* or *cat-scratch fever* may cause conjunctivitis with preau-

TABLE OF DISEASE INCIDENCE

INCIDENCE PER 100,000 (APPROXIMATE)

Common (>100)	**Uncommon (>5–100)**	**Rare (>0–5)**
Hordoleum	Dacryoadenitis	Sebaceous carcinoma of the lid
Chalazion	Dacryocystitis	Iritis—suppurative
Blepharitis	Erysipelas of the face	Iritis mimics
Foreign body in the conjunctiva	Herpes zoster ophthalmicus	Episcleritis
Conjunctivitis—bacterial and viral	Purulent (gonococcal) conjunctivitis	Rhinocerebral mucormycosis
Epidemic keratoconjunctivitis	Chlamydial conjunctivitis	Bacterial cavernous sinus thrombosis
Corneal injury and foreign body	Iritis—nonsuppurative	Acute thyroid ophthalmopathy
Nonspecific viral diseases and ocular pain	Herpes simplex keratitis	Orbital hematoma
	Acute glaucoma	Intracavernous carotid artery aneurysm
	Scleritis	Carotid cavernous fistula
	Endophthalmitis/panophthalmitis	Dural cavernous sinus shunt
	Preseptal cellulitis	Pituitary apoplexy
	Idiopathic orbital pseudotumor	Minor leak from an aneurysm
	Subperiosteal orbital abscess	Carotid artery dissection
	Orbital cellulitis and/or abscess	Occipital lobe infarction or hematoma
	Supraclinoid or posterior communicating aneurysm and nerve III palsy	Cerebellar hemorrhage
	Diabetic ischemic neuropathy of nerve III	Ophthalmoplegic migraine
	Idiopathic optic neuritis	Devic's disease
	Optic neuritis and multiple sclerosis	Mimics of optic neuritis: autoimmune disorders, parasellar inflammatory process, parainfectious associations, neuroretinitis, parasellar masses
	Mimics of optic neuritis: temporal arteritis, amaurosis fugax and ocular infarction	Infectious diseases causing bilateral ocular pain: varicella conjunctivitis and keratitis, Epstein-Barr dacryoadenitis and dacryocystitis, lymphogranuloma venereum, keratitis, cat-scratch fever, conjunctivitis and preauricular adenopathy, trichinosis, Q fever uveitis
	Toxic epidermal necrolysis	
	Stevens-Johnson syndrome	
	Referred dental pain	

ricular adenopathy. *Trichinosis* causes orbital myositis and edema, and pain on eye movement. *Q fever* may cause anterior uveitis. *Toxic epidermal necrolysis* (TEN) causes generalized skin erythema, bullae, and skin erosions; and the conjunctiva may undergo a similar process. The *Stevens-Johnson syndrome* causes oral mucosal erosion, a severe conjunctivitis, and sometimes keratitis or corneal ulceration. A *dental abscess* or *pulpitis* may cause very severe jaw and dental pain that may extend to the ipsilateral eye.

☐ DESCRIPTION OF LISTED DISEASES

1. EYELIDS

A. Hordeolum (Stye) A painful, erythematous, tender nodule appears at the base of one or two lashes at the lid margin (external hordeolum). Pain, redness, and swelling may continue for 3 to 5 days, terminating with spontaneous drainage of purulent material. Staphylococcal infection of a lash follicle, gland of Zeis, or Moll gland is the usual cause. Meibomian gland infection (internal hordeolum) causes a localized painful red nodule deep in the lid that may drain through the conjunctival surface. Hot compresses and antibiotic drops are used for treatment and to prevent recurrence.

B. Chalazion A chalazion may be asymptomatic or painful. It presents as a skin-colored nodule at the lid margin (Zeis gland) or deep in the lid (Meibomian gland). It gradually enlarges and can be removed by a conjunctival incision and curettage. Multiple lesions of this type may be present or occur sequentially.

C. Sebaceous Carcinoma of the Lid This disorder is usually painless unless it arises in a Zeis gland at the lid margin and ulcerates early. It is nearly impossible to differentiate an early carcinoma from a chalazion without histopathologic study. Any chalazion that recurs at the same site or has an unusual consistency should be examined microscopically. Carcinomas present insidiously, are firm, and may be attached to the overlying skin. Chalazions usually present abruptly, are rubbery, and are not attached to the skin of the lid. This form of carcinoma may be overlooked until advanced. A less common clinical presentation is in the form of a chronic, persistent unilateral conjunctivitis or blepharitis due to intraepidermal growth of the tumor. The upper lid is involved 2 to 3 times more often than the lower. A full-thickness conjunctival or lid margin biopsy is required to establish a diagnosis of intraepidermal carcinoma.

D. Blepharitis Redness; crusting; and, in severe cases, painful ulceration and tenderness occur on the lid margin. Aching lid pain may occur and is intensified by blinking or touching the eyelid margin. A foreign body sensation in the eye, an associated conjunctivitis, and sometimes keratitis may occur. The latter may be signaled by photophobia and lacrimation. Chalazia and/or hordeola may complicate the course. Seborrheic dermatitis of the scalp and/or face and lid margin and staphylococcal infection are responsible for this disorder. Lashes may be lost, broken, or depigmented (poliosis) or their growth misdirected (trichiasis), leading to corneal and/or bulbar conjunctival irritation and abrasion. Hyperopic refractive errors may play a role in the causation of this disorder and should be corrected with lenses. Therapy includes control of the associated seborrheic dermatitis of the scalp with selenium sulfide; lid margin staphylococcal infection by gentle scrubbing with a cotton-tipped applicator moistened with baby shampoo; and application of an antistaphylococcal ointment to the edge of the lid.

E. Acute Dacryoadenitis Swelling, pain, redness, and tenderness occur in the lateral portion of an upper lid. This disorder may be associated with mumps, infectious mononucleosis, measles, and other systemic diseases. Invasion of the lacrimal gland duct by a bacterial infection of the lid or conjunctiva may also be responsible and respond to antibiotic therapy. A CT scan of the inflamed gland will show enlargement and molding by adjacent bone or sclera. An abscess can also be identified by a CT or ultrasound scan.

F. Dacryocystitis Aching pain, swelling, redness, and tenderness develop in the region between the inner canthus of the eye and the nose. Middle-aged women are predisposed to this disorder. Epiphora, due to duct obstruction, may precede the onset. Streptococcal species are usually responsible, but *Hemophilus influenzae, Klebsiella pneumoniae, Pseudomonas aeruginosa, Treponema pallidum, Mycobacterium tuberculosis, Chlamydia trachomatis,* or fungal species have been identified as causative in a small number of cases. Therapy involves relieving obstruction of the nasolacrimal duct and administration of antibiotics. Abscess formation requires incision and drainage.

G. Erysipelas Diffuse erythema and tenderness of the skin of the face and eyelid may occur secondary to group A streptococcal infection. Fever, malaise, and aching facial and eyelid pain occur and respond to antibiotic therapy. A similar type of bacterial infection of the lids (preseptal, or periorbital, cellulitis) is described below.

2. CONJUNCTIVA, IRIS, CORNEA, SCLERA, AND GLOBE

A. Foreign Body in the Conjunctiva of the Lid or Globe Pain begins abruptly with a sensation of something flying into the eye. This may be a speck of dust, metal, sawdust, or an insect. Eye pain that is intensified by blinking, a sensation of sand in the eye, lid edema, tearing, and photophobia may occur. Conjunctival injection may follow rubbing. Symptoms respond to removal of the foreign body, instillation of antibiotics, and patching for 24 h if a corneal abrasion has occurred.

B. Herpes Zoster Ophthalmicus Unilateral burning and/or lancinating pain in the eyelid, eye, and forehead is followed within 1 to 4 days by ipsilateral lid and facial swelling and the eruption of grouped vesicles and red-rimmed, crusted ulcers in areas of lid and facial edema. Deep, boring eye pain; a decrease in visual acuity; and photophobia signal the occurrence of keratitis and/or iridocyclitis. Conjunctival hyperemia, corneal edema, and intraepithelial infiltrates occur. A deep disciform keratitis may develop in some cases, leading to loss of visual acuity. Scleritis, hyphema, and secondary glaucoma may occur in a small number of patients. Severe forms of this disorder often occur in patients with HIV disease.

C. Conjunctivitis

1. Bacterial and Viral Viral or bacterial conjunctivitis caused diffuse conjunctival redness (81–93 percent); itching (33–38 percent); blurred vision (0–9 percent); burning discomfort (11–31 percent); a foreign body sensation (6–44 percent); pain (22–31 percent); photophobia (22–38 percent); morning lid stickiness and crusting (25–45 percent); lid edema (27–31 percent); and watery (39–50 percent), mucoid (17–19 percent), or purulent ocular discharge (25–28 percent) in one reported series. Signs in the same group of patients with conjunctivitis included palpebral follicles (33–50 percent) or papillae (0–22 percent), superficial punctate keratitis (11–13 percent), bulbar conjunctival injection (94–100 percent), preauricular nodes (6–31 percent), and conjunctival discharge (56–72 percent).

Some studies have suggested that a watery discharge; lid follicles; and tender, enlarged preauricular nodes were more likely to occur in viral or chlamydial infections and that the absence of these signs and the presence of a purulent discharge favored a diagnosis of bacterial conjunctivitis. Subsequent studies have shown a poor correlation of clinical findings with laboratory results, and in one report agreement between a clinical impression of viral or bacterial conjunctivitis and culture was present in only 35 to 47 percent of cases. Gram's and Giemsa stains of conjunctival exudate may miss 85 percent of cases with a bacterial etiology.

In a series collected in a busy inner city hospital, *Staphylococcus aureus* and *Streptococcus pneumoniae* were the most frequent causes. *H. influenzae* occurred in the pediatric age group, while *Proteus* and *Klebsiella* species were isolated in less than 10 percent of all cases. Only 3 percent were due to *N. gonorrhoeae*. The diagnosis of bacterial conjunctivitis by laboratory methods is difficult. *Staphylococcus epidermidis,* some *corynebacteria,* and streptococci may be grown from normal conjunctiva and in small amounts from infected eyes. Whether to attribute pathogenicity to such isolates is an unsettled problem.

2. Purulent Conjunctivitis Due to Neisseria gonorrhoeae Patients experience eyelid pain, swelling, redness, and conjunctival chemosis. The exudate is initially serous but soon becomes purulent. Corneal inflammation occurs, causing deep ocular pain and tenderness. This infection is usually limited to one eye and is often ipsilateral to the dominant hand of the affected male. Acute urethral gonorrhea is usually associated. A Gram's stain of the conjunctival exudate reveals gram-negative intracellular diplococci. These can be isolated as *N. gonorrhoeae* on chocolate agar or Thayer-Martin medium. There is a good response to parenteral penicillin or ceftriaxone therapy.

3. Chlamydia trachomatis An acute conjunctivitis may occur in association with urethral burning and discharge. The conjunctiva of one or both eyes may show hyperemia, lid edema, and/or chemosis. The exudate is watery or mucopurulent. Conjunctival scrapings may be positive for *C. trachomatis* by immunofluorescent antibody staining or by culture. Therapy with oral and topical tetracycline or erythromycin is effective.

4. Epidemic Keratoconjunctivitis This disorder frequently begins with a sore throat or coryza. Bilateral eyelid edema, conjunctival hyperemia, and profuse tearing occur. The eyes burn, and a foreign body sensation develops in association with photophobia. Palpebral follicles and tender preauricular adenopathy occur. During the first week, a diffuse superficial epithelial keratitis occurs, followed by the development of fluorescein-staining, slightly raised, epithelial lesions, and subepithelial granular opacities. These corneal changes give rise to a loss of visual acuity, which may impair reading and driving. Such visual loss may persist for 3 to 24 months after the conjunctivitis has resolved. The cause is a type 8 or 19 adenovirus. Up to 20 percent of cases may only have conjunctivitis. This disease may be spread person-to-person, and it has been transmitted in the offices of ophthalmologists by contaminated fingers, instruments, or tonometers.

D. Acute Iritis and Iridocyclitis

1. Suppurative There is an acute onset of deep, aching, unilateral eye pain; hyperemia of the perilimbal area; and decreased visual acuity. Slit lamp examination reveals cells and flare in the anterior chamber and cloudiness of the vitreous. Shining a light into the unaffected eye causes sharp pain in the involved eye by inducing consensual contraction of the inflamed iris. Paracentesis for culture and Gram's stain should be done, and intravenous and intraocular antibiotics started. Causes include penetrating trauma, endocarditis, and septicemia.

2. Nonsuppurative Iritis This disease frequently begins with a superficial stinging or burning eye discomfort that soon becomes a deep ache. Photophobia occurs due to ciliary spasm, and vision is impaired because of cellular and protein exudation into the anterior chamber. Sharp, stabbing eye pain, sometimes radiating straight through to the back of the head, may occur when reading (accommodation) or looking at a light (light reflex). The pupil is usually small, irregular, and poorly reactive. The cornea is usually clear, unless there is an associated keratitis. Circumcorneal and conjunctival hyperemia are present, and shining a light into the normal eye causes contralateral eye pain. Flare due to increased aqueous humor protein is observed when the anterior chamber is viewed by slit lamp. Inflammatory cell precipitates may be present on the inner surfaces of the cornea, lens, and iris. Prevention of synechiae and glaucoma is the main objective of therapy. This requires pupillary dilatation with homatropine and use of topical and sometimes systemic steroids. The cycloplegic drops put the iris at rest and usually relieve pain.

Iritis may be associated with ankylosing spondylitis; psoriatic arthritis; Reiter's syndrome; Vogt-Koyanagi-Harada disease; Behçet's syndrome; inflammatory bowel disease; sarcoidosis; and infections such as syphilis, tuberculosis, and histoplasmosis. A large percentage of cases are of unknown cause. Specific infectious agents should be treated with appropriate antimicrobial therapy.

3. Mimics of Iritis and Iridocyclitis Similar clinical findings may occur with ischemic oculopathy due to carotid stenosis, metastatic tumor, or leukemia involving the uveal tract.

E. Corneal Injury and Foreign Body Corneal trauma may cause severe unilateral eye pain and local tenderness due to an abrasion, ulceration, or perforation of the cornea. The pain is intensified by lid or eye movement. The lid may become swollen and erythematous, and the bulbar conjunctiva injected. Profuse tearing, blepharospasm, and photophobia may occur. These complaints may be dramatically relieved by a single drop of local anesthetic (proparacaine, 0.5%), and this effect has been used to differentiate a painful eye due to simple corneal injury from one caused by conjunctivitis, iritis, glaucoma, or a chronic corneal ulcer. Final pain scores are lower and changes in scores greater in the former group. Fluorescein staining of the cornea and slit lamp and corneal microscopy will confirm the clinical findings and determine the

extent and severity of the corneal injury. Instillation of antibiotic drops and patching lead to resolution of superficial ulcerations. Foreign bodies in the cornea cause similar complaints. They can be visualized directly or by slit lamp and removed. Any residual stain or ''rust ring'' should also be removed before it causes an inflammatory reaction or infection.

F. Herpes Simplex Keratitis This disorder causes eye pain secondary to blepharoconjunctivitis, uveitis, and keratitis. Tearing and photophobia accompany the pain. Corneal sensitivity may be decreased. Fluorescein staining of the cornea may reveal a dendritic, branching, superficial lesion. In some cases, the corneal lesions are punctate and diffuse, star-shaped, or linear. Conjunctival hyperemia may or may not be present. The early dendritic lesion consists of vesicles in the corneal epithelium that soon rupture, producing a superficial dendritic ulcer. Recent cold sores and vesicular lesions on the skin of the lid or the conjunctiva may be associated. Herpes simplex infection may be diagnosed by its characteristic appearance (dendritic ulcer) or by viral cultures. A DNA-DNA hybridization test using a biotinylated DNA probe to detect herpes simplex virus antigen obtained from corneal swabs is rapid and specific. Fast and accurate diagnosis allows early treatment with antiviral drugs (trifluridine or idoxuridine). This disorder may be confused with a traumatic abrasion or ulcer and treated without antiviral therapy. This is likely to occur if a geographic or large corneal epithelial staining defect is present. Herpetic ulcers are not associated with a history of trauma. A mild follicular conjunctivitis and decreased corneal sensitivity are usually present. Some cases of herpetic infection present with conjunctivitis and an area of corneal opacification without ulceration due to a disciform or stromal keratitis. Corticosteroids should not be used in patients with herpes simplex keratitis.

G. Acute Glaucoma This disorder presents abruptly with severe pain and tenderness in one eye. The ocular pain is deep and aching and may radiate to the frontotemporal region. Vision is impaired, and large haloes appear about streetlights. Nausea, vomiting, and abdominal pain may accompany the eye pain. Photophobia and blephospasm may occur. The cornea is hazy and edematous, the pupil dilated and poorly responsive to light, and the conjunctiva edematous and hyperemic with perilimbal injection. Observation of a nasal iris shadow produced by temporal illumination of the iris supports a diagnosis of narrow-angle glaucoma. Chamber depth at the angle can be estimated by use of the slit lamp or by gonioscopy.

Intraocular pressure measured with a Schiøtz tonometer usually exceeds 50 mmHg. An acute episode can be abated with 2% pilocarpine drops and acetazolamide or by creating a small opening in the peripheral iris with a laser to facilitate flow of aqueous humor to the anterior chamber. Attacks have been precipitated by the use of a long-acting mydriatic or by a prolonged period in a dark place (e.g., movie theater).

H. Episcleritis   Stinging or burning pain, vascular congestion, and tenderness occur in a quadrant of one or both globes in the region between the rectus muscle insertions and the limbus. Visual acuity is unaffected, but mild photophobia may occur. A nodular form, consisting of purplish elevations a few millimeters in diameter in an area of background hyperemia, also occurs. These nodules are located in the episcleral elastic layer and are not attached to the underlying sclera. The course is variable, with some episodes resolving spontaneously within a few days, while some cases of nodular episcleritis may persist for up to 2 months. The pain and vascular congestion respond to oral nonsteroidal anti-inflammatory drugs and/ or topical corticosteroids within a few days. The etiology is unknown, and the symptoms follow a relapsing course or occur only once. Some cases are associated with a recent viral illness, a hypersensitivity reaction, or contact with industrial solvents.

I. Scleritis   This disorder may be idiopathic or associated with collagen vascular disorders such as rheumatoid arthritis, dermatomyositis, systemic lupus erythematosus, polyarteritis nodosa, and hypersensitivity angiitis or arthritic diseases such as gout, Reiter's syndrome, psoriatic arthritis, ankylosing spondylitis, relapsing polychondritis, and Still's disease. Some cases are associated with bacterial or other infections such as herpes simplex or herpes zoster, syphilis, or tuberculosis or diseases of unknown etiology such as sarcoidosis, IgA nephropathy, Takayasu's disease, temporal arteritis, inflammatory bowel disease, Behçet's syndrome, acne rosacea, pyoderma gangrenosum, and Wegener's granulomatosis. Fungal infections, trauma, and cataract surgery have also been associated.

1. Anterior Scleritis   This disorder occurs in one or both eyes (50 percent), but since the involvement of the second eye usually occurs weeks or months later, 67 to 90 percent of cases present with symptoms related to only one eye. Bilaterality occurs within 6 years in 80 percent of cases associated with rheumatoid arthritis but in only 35 percent without that association.

Deep eye and orbital pain and diffuse or nodular regions of tender hyperemic scleral tissue are associated. The involved hyperemic region of the outer globe has a bluish-red hue. Corneal invasion is signaled by a loss of visual acuity and the onset of lacrimation and photophobia. Part of the cornea may be replaced by sclerotic tissue so that it begins to resemble the sclera (sclerosing keratitis).

In patients with rheumatoid arthritis, an anterior nodular or diffuse scleritis may occur that leads to scleral thinning and eventual perforation of the globe. This may result in uveal herniation through the defect (scleromalacia perforans) and loss of the eye secondary to infection.

2. Posterior Scleritis   Pain occurs in the eye or orbit, but it may also be referred to the frontal, temporal, or malar areas. One or both eyes (10–33 percent) may be affected. Visual acuity is usually decreased because of exudative retinal detachment, macular distortion by a scleral mass, cystoid macular edema, or optic neuritis. Some myopic patients report an improvement in their vision, while hyperopia may develop in other patients because of shortening of the diameter of the globe due to scleral thickening. Lid edema, ptosis, chemosis of the conjunctiva, decreased ocular motility, and iritis may also occur in a small number of cases.

The anterior sclera of the affected eye may be white and appear normal, or there may be dilatation of episcleral vessels in a fornix, a patchy hyperemic scleritis, or a nodular or diffuse anterior scleritis. Patients presenting with white sclera often give a history of prior episodes of mild scleral redness responsive to topical corticosteroids. Proptosis, ptosis, and periorbital edema may occur secondary to orbital inflammation resulting from extension of the periscleritis associated with this disorder.

Ocular pain may be intensified or provoked by eye movement, simulating the clinical symptomatology of optic neuritis. In some cases, diplopia may also occur because of ocular muscle weakness. Both pain and diplopia are caused by myositis of the ocular muscles.

Fundoscopic examination may reveal a circumscribed fundal mass that can mimic a tumor like a melanoma. In the case of posterior scleritis, the mass produced by the thickened sclera has the same color as the adjacent pigment epithelium and a normal choroidal vascular pattern. It is surrounded by choroidal folds or retinal striae, and a bullous retinal detachment may develop. Choroidal folds, retinal striae, and disc edema without a fundal mass may occur in patients with milder forms of diffuse inflammation. Annular ciliochoroidal detachment may occur, displacing the iris and lens forward, closing the angle, and leading to secondary glaucoma. Choroidal inflammation can result in exudative retinal detachment. The detachment may be localized to the posterior pole, or it may be bullous with shifting subretinal fluid. Cystoid macular edema may occur in a small percentage of cases.

The diagnosis of posterior scleritis can be confirmed by the use of B-scan ultrasonography, which will demonstrate posterior globe flattening, scleral thickening, and retrobulbar edema. A CT scan can demonstrate the same findings. Fluorescein angiography (FA) demonstrates multiple focal areas of retinal fluorescence that increase in size and brightness with time after injection.

In the late phase of the study, dye accumulates in the subretinal fluid. FA is helpful in differentiating posterior scleritis from a central serous chorioretinopathy, which is usually associated with only a single site of leakage. There is a good therapeutic response to retrobulbar injection of corticosteroids or oral prednisone, indomethacin, or aspirin.

J. Endophthalmitis and Panophthalmitis   Endophthalmitis involves the ocular cavities and immediately adjacent tissues. Panophthalmitis involves the sclera, choroid, retina, and Tenon's capsule. The clinical differentiation of these disorders is quantitative. Both present with severe ocular pain and tenderness, a hazy cornea, loss of vision, and hypopyon. Panophthalmitis causes lid edema and erythema and/or chemosis and exophthalmos.

Endophthalmitis may arise from penetrating trauma, intraocular surgery, or perforation of a corneal ulcer; by extension of infection from an adjacent tissue (e.g., orbital abscess); or by bacteremic spread from a distant site (e.g., endocarditis, abdominal sepsis, or meningitis).

In a series of 30 patients who developed endophthalmitis following intraocular lens implantation after cataract extraction, the presenting symptoms and their frequencies were deep, boring eye pain (73 percent); decreased visual acuity (57 percent); purulent discharge (23 percent); red eye (13 percent); and photophobia (7 percent).

Signs included lid edema (33 percent), conjunctival injection (67 percent), corneal edema/haze (67 percent), hypopyon (70 percent), and an absent red reflex (73 percent). Elevated intraocular pressure occurred in some cases. Fever was uncommon, but the leukocyte count was sometimes increased, and in rare instances a patient had a left shift. Aqueous or vitreous fluid was aspirated and cultured. The most common isolates were *Staphylococcus aureus* (31 percent) and coagulase-negative staphylococci (58 percent). Patients were treated with intravenous and topical antibiotics. Some patients received subconjunctival injections of antibiotics. Pars plana vitrectomy was frequently performed (90 percent). In the series described, an acuity of 20/70 or better was obtained in 53 percent and a poor outcome (≤20/200) in 47 percent.

Endogenous *clostridial* panophthalmitis has occurred secondary to gallbladder rupture, ischemic colitis, sigmoid diverticulitis, and adenocarcinoma of the colon. Characteristic findings are a gas bubble in the anterior chamber, rapid onset of blindness, and bloody or coffee-colored fluid in the anterior chamber. Proptosis, severe pain, and brawny lid edema are common findings. This disorder has been uniformly fatal. In one reported case, a Gram's stain of aqueous humor revealed plump grampositive bacilli with terminal spores, and the isolate was *Clostridium septicum*.

Most cases of endophthalmitis are caused by bacteria, with staphylococci, streptococci, and coliforms being the most frequent etiologic agents. Rarely, fungal infections such as mucormycosis, aspergillosis, blastomycosis, or sporotrichosis may be etiologic. Some cases result from necrosis of an intraocular tumor and are culture-negative.

K. Preseptal (Periorbital) Cellulitis   Inflammation occurs anterior to the orbital septum and is usually secondary to sinusitis, lid trauma, conjunctivitis, or dacryocystitis. There are edema, tenderness, warmth, and sometimes erythema of one or both eyelids. Chemosis and marked narrowing of the palpebral fissure may occur. Fever is more common in pediatric patients. Pain is usually mild and may be present only on attempted eyelid movement. There is no proptosis, diplopia, or limitation of extraocular movements. Full range of ocular movement without pain differentiates this disorder from orbital cellulitis. In adults, *Staphylococcus aureus* and *Streptococcus pyogenes* are the usual infectious agents, while in children under age 5, *H. influenzae* is most prevalent. Spontaneous drainage may occur from the lid surface. A Gram's stain and culture of any drainage will usually identify the causative organism. This disorder resolves after oral or intravenous therapy with a penicillinase-resistant antibiotic.

3. ORBITAL DISEASE—"RED EYE," PROPTOSIS, AND DIPLOPIA

A. Idiopathic Orbital Pseudotumor   This disorder is very similar clinically to posterior scleritis. It may present with proptosis, acute deep aching ocular pain, lid edema, ptosis, injection and chemosis of the conjunctiva, restricted ocular motility, papillitis, iritis, and retinal striae. Other fundoscopic findings, such as a scleral mass and exudative retinal detachment, are uncommon with pseudotumor. Bilateral onset may occur. B-scan ultrasonography demonstrates scleral thickening and edema in Tenon's space. A CT scan shows a diffuse orbital infiltrate and a thickened sclera. An orbital mass can usually be imaged. This disorder, like posterior scleritis, responds to corticosteroid therapy. Many authors consider posterior scleritis and orbital pseudotumor to be two forms of the same disorder. Alternative names for this disorder include acute sclerotenonitis and acute periscleritis.

B. Subperiosteal Orbital Abscess   This disorder is usually secondary to sinusitis. The abscess forms between the bony wall of the orbit and the periosteum, lining it (i.e., the periorbita). Fever and unilateral preseptal cellulitis are the earliest signs. Chemosis and asymmetrical proptosis occur, with the eye displaced away from the abscess. The globe may be directed in a lateral or downward direction. Ocular movement is limited in the direction of the abscess, and this results in diplopia in this direction of gaze. Tenderness may be present in the region between the medial orbital margin and the globe at the site of the abscess. Pus may drain through the lid, forming a fistula. Patients with an abscess may have moderately severe retro-orbital pain, and symptoms and signs may progress or fail to respond to antibiotic therapy until the involved sinus is drained and irrigated. CT scans may sometimes demonstrate the abscess, but sensitivity is limited. A subperiosteal abscess may resolve without drainage after treatment of the associated sinusitis and parenteral administration of antibiotics, but some require surgical drainage.

C. Orbital Cellulitis This complication of sinusitis presents with fever, unilateral lid edema, redness, tenderness and warmth, chemosis, and severe aching orbital pain. Axial proptosis and symmetrical limitation of eye movements are present, in contrast to the findings with a subperiosteal abscess. Pain is intensified by attempted motion of the affected eye. Hypesthesia of the upper and midface may be present secondary to involvement of trigeminal divisions V_1 and V_2 in the orbit. External ophthalmoplegia, ptosis, a dilated fixed pupil, and a decrease in visual acuity or blindness may signal formation of an orbital abscess. In the presence of an abscess, there may be evidence of papilledema, retinal venous congestion, and hemorrhage.

A CT scan may help in separating preseptal from orbital disease and will usually identify infected sinuses or an orbital abscess. Ultrasound may also identify orbital edema, a mottled appearance of the orbital fat, and edema of the extraocular muscles in patients with orbital cellulitis. Intravenous antibiotics and drainage of sinuses and/or orbital collections of pus will lead to recovery without complications (e.g., cavernous sinus thrombosis, meningitis, or brain abscess).

Sinus disease is causative in 64 to 84 percent of patients with orbital cellulitis. The most commonly involved sinuses are the ethmoid, frontal, maxillary, and sphenoid, in decreasing order of frequency. Other less frequent causes include local cellulitis of the face or eyelid, acute dacryocystitis, dental and ear infections, extradural or cerebral abscesses, panophthalmitis, penetrating trauma, Wegener's granulomatosis, rhabdomyosarcoma of the orbit, a necrotic choroidal melanoma, and iatrogenic penetration of the orbit during sinus or nasal surgery. Rarely, typhoid fever; tuberculosis; rickettsial diseases; syphilis; scarlet fever; bacterial endocarditis; and viral disorders such as herpes simplex, herpes zoster, or infectious mononucleosis may cause orbital inflammation.

Fungal infections, such as mucormycosis and aspergillosis, and parasitic infestations, such as trichinosis, echinococcosis, and cysticercosis, may involve the orbit. The most common bacterial isolates in adults are *S. aureus, S. pyogenes,* and *S. pneumoniae,* while *H. influenzae* is a frequent pathogen in children under age 5.

CT scans may fail to detect orbital involvement when it is present. CT findings include medial rectus muscle enlargement due to edema, separation of the periosteum from the lamina papyracea (i.e., evidence of a subperiosteal abscess), proptosis, orbital fat edema, and an air fluid level in an abscess cavity. In one series, the sensitivity of CT for orbital disease was only 50 percent, and subperiosteal abscesses were difficult to identify. Up to 40 percent of patients with orbital cellulitis or abscess may go undetected because of equivocal or negative clinical and CT findings.

D. Rhinocerebral Mucormycosis This highly lethal disease occurs most frequently in diabetics (80 percent). Poor control with ketoacidosis is usually present. Mucormycosis may also occur in a setting of renal failure (e.g., in renal transplant patients, renal cortical necrosis, and acute nephrotic syndrome), leukemia, Hodgkin's disease and other lymphomas, cancer chemotherapy, immunosuppression, malnutrition, chronic diarrhea, septicemia, or extensive burns.

Clinical symptoms usually begin with fever, toxicity, malaise, nasal stuffiness, and sometimes a brown or hemorrhagic nasal discharge from the involved side of the nose. Symptoms of nasal or sinus infection may be absent. Severe orbital and sometimes ipsilateral facial pain are associated with eyelid and occasionally facial edema. Lid erythema, tenderness, and chemosis may follow. Proptosis, ophthalmoplegia, ptosis, a dilated fixed pupil, and a marked decrease in visual acuity signal a severe orbital cellulitis with involvement of the orbital apex. A black eschar involving the mucosa of the nose, ethmoid sinuses, or palate may appear due to vascular infarction secondary to fungal arterial invasion. The orbital infection usually arises in an ethmoid or sphenoid sinus. It may rapidly spread to the brain through the cribriform plate, leading to frontal lobe and olfactory tract necrosis. Spread may also occur to the orbital apex and the cavernous sinus, leading to thrombosis of the ipsilateral sinus and, within days, the other sinus. The fungus may invade the intracavernous carotid artery, causing thrombosis and septic infarction of multiple sites in the ipsilateral side of the brain. Lesions due to ischemia, cerebritis, or hemorrhage may occur in any portion of the brain (i.e., hemispheres, thalamus, hypothalamus, midbrain, and pons). A CT scan will detect sinus, orbital, and cerebral disease. MRI findings have been reported for only a few cases. These have included hyperintense mucosal thickening/secretions in the ethmoid sinus, infiltration of the fat plane medial to the medial rectus muscle, edema of the medial rectus muscle, swelling of preseptal tissue, and invasion of the deep spaces of the face (i.e., infratemporal fossa and pterygomaxillary fissure). Cavernous sinus thrombosis may also be visualized by MRI and cerebral and brain stem lesions demonstrated with greater sensitivity than by CT. The diagnosis of infection by *Rhizopus, Mucor,* or *Absidia* species may be confirmed by microscopic examination of biopsied nasal or palatal tissue, or resected sinus mucosa, or orbital tissue. Large nonseptated hyphae branching at right angles identify a member of the Mucoraceae family. Members of this family have the ability to grow along the walls of blood vessels, producing vessel occlusions or emboli due to the hyphae or a necrotizing vasculitis. Control of diabetes; administration of amphotericin B; and surgical drainage and/or debridement of involved sinuses, eschars, and necrotic tissue in the orbit may result in survival. This disorder may cause bilateral cavernous sinus thrombosis and may mimic bacterial cavernous sinus thrombosis. Occurrence in a setting of severe diabetes, renal failure, or immunosuppression; a palatine, sinus, or nasal eschar; rapid loss of vision; and biopsy evidence of branching hyphae distinguish mucormycosis from bacterial infection of the cavernous sinus. Only a small percentage of patients with mucormycosis develop cavernous sinus occlusion.

E. Bacterial Cavernous Sinus Thrombosis This disorder may be preceded by a cellulitis or furuncle in the middle third of the face, a stye, a sphenoid or ethmoid sinusitis, or a dental infection involving the maxillary teeth (10 percent of cases). Rarely, it follows extension of an orbital cellulitis, otitis media, or mastoiditis. The most common isolate is *S. aureus,* but *Staphylococcus albus, S. pneumoniae, S. pyogenes,* and species of *Proteus, Pseudomonas,* or anaerobic bacteria may be causative. Rarely, bacterial infection is mimicked by invasive aspergillosis or mucormycosis, causing sinus thrombosis.

Patients present with fever, malaise, toxicity, and sometimes lethargy. There is constant orbital aching pain that may spread to the forehead and midface. The initial localizing symptoms include lid edema, which may extend to the base of the nose and frontal region, conjunctival chemosis, diplopia, and ptosis. Ophthalmoparesis or plegia is usually demonstrable, and paresthesias, hypesthesia, or hyperesthesia of the upper and midface (e.g., trigeminal division V_1 and V_2) develop in association with ptosis and a dilated and fixed pupil (cranial nerve III). Proptosis, ptosis, and chemosis are present in 90 percent of cases. Mental status changes occur in 50 percent, and meningismus occurs in 40 percent. The fundoscopic examination shows papilledema, retinal venous congestion, and hemorrhages in more than 60 percent of cases. A decrease in visual acuity occurs in 25 percent and is not as common as with mucormycosis. Seizures and hemiparesis due to cerebritis or cerebral infarction occur in less than 5 percent of cases. Progression to involve the contralateral eye usually occurs within 2 to 4 days because of spread through the intercavernous sinuses. Such patients have bilateral lid edema, proptosis, ptosis, chemosis, and ophthalmoplegia. A leukocytosis is usually present, and the CSF reveals either a mixed pleocytosis of polymorphonuclear leukocytes and mononuclear cells and a normal sugar level, or a polymorphonuclear predominance and a low CSF sugar level. Blood and CSF cultures may be positive in a small percentage of cases.

Conventional sinus films are less sensitive than a CT scan for detection of sphenoid sinusitis. A CT scan may demonstrate proptosis; bulging of the lateral walls of the cavernous sinus; irregular low-attenuation filling defects; and, rarely, air in the cavernous sinus. Unless the cavernous sinus thrombosis is secondary to spread of an orbital abscess into the cavernous sinus, the orbit appears unremarkable except for the presence of a dilated ophthalmic vein. MRI T_1- or T_2-weighted images may demonstrate hyperintense signals in the ophthalmic veins and cavernous sinus that are identifiable as thrombosed blood. The sensitivity of MRI for demonstration of cavernous sinus thrombosis has not yet been reported, but it appears to be superior to CT. A differential diagnosis of disorders presenting with a red eye, proptosis, and/or ophthalmoparesis(es) is presented in Table 3-1.

F. Thyroid Ophthalmopathy This disorder is the commonest condition affecting the orbit. It usually presents with lid retraction and mild proptosis. An unusual acute form of this disease has been reported that begins with unilateral or bilateral aching orbital pain, proptosis, a red eye with chemosis, lid edema, ptosis, and limitation of ocular movement, resulting in diplopia. Visual loss progressive to blindness may follow the onset of ophthalmopareses and is due to optic nerve compression by enlarged edematous ocular muscles. The ptosis may be due to damage to the levator palpebrae superioris. Papilledema may be present. Patients presenting in this manner may be euthyroid, hyperthyroid, or hypothyroid. Bilateral involvement with some asymmetry of severity occurs within a week of onset if the presentation is unilateral. A CT study of the orbit reveals bilateral disease with enlargement of the bellies of one or more of the ocular muscles and sparing of their tendinous insertions. An increased volume of orbital fat also may occur and, with the enlarged muscles, is responsible for the proptosis. There is a response to prednisone therapy in 66 percent, and 64 percent of the nonresponders will be benefited by orbital irradiation. This disorder is often diagnosed as orbital cellulitis and treated with antibiotics before the correct diagnosis is made.

G. Orbital Hematoma Patients experience a sudden onset of unilateral orbital pain or pressure-like discomfort, proptosis, ptosis, and diplopia due to ophthalmopareses. Nausea and vomiting may occur. Ecchymoses may appear on the lids within 24 h. With severe proptosis, lid retraction may lead to corneal drying and ulceration, and optic nerve compression can lead to visual loss. The usual cause is rupture of an orbital varix or a small branch of the ophthalmic vein, but bleeding may also occur from an orbital tumor, severe hypertension, straining during labor, or a coagulopathy. Patients with bleeding secondary to rupture of a varix may give a history of childhood exophthalmos of fluctuating severity with transient exacerba-

Table 3-1
DIFFERENTIAL DIAGNOSIS OF RED EYE, PROPTOSIS, AND/OR OPHTHALMOPARESES

	Primary Diseases	Orbital Pain	Periorbital Edema/ Chemosis	Proptosis	Eschar Nose/Palate	Trigeminal Divisions V_1 and V_2 Involvement	Superior Orbital Fissure Syndrome
Periorbital Cellulitis	Facial skin infection Sinusitis	Minimal	Present	0%	0%	None	None
Orbital Cellulitis	Sinusitis	Present 85%	Present 95%/65%	Present 89%	None, unless due to mucormycosis or aspergillosis	May occur	Rare
Rhinocerebral Mucormycosis	Ethmoid or maxillary sinusitis Diabetic ketoacidosis	Present	Present	Present	Present	Present	May occur
Bacterial Cavernous Sinus Thrombosis	Facial infection Sphenoid sinusitis Dental infection	Present	Present	Present	None	Present	May occur or similar findings
Orbital Hematoma	Orbital varix Orbital tumor Straining	Present	Mild	Present	None	None	May occur
Acute Thyroid Ophthalmopathy	Euthyroid, hyperthyroid, or hypothyroid	Present	Present	Present	None	None	None
Intracavernous Carotid Aneurysm	Hypertension Congenital aneurysm	Present	May occur	May occur	None	60%	16%
Carotid Cavernous Fistula	Trauma Aneurysm	Present	Present	Present, pulsating	None	Present	May occur or similar findings

tions related to an increase in venous pressure in the head (e.g., from straining or coughing). The diagnosis of hemorrhage can be confirmed by CT and symptoms relieved by orbital decompression if optic nerve function is threatened.

H. Intracavernous Carotid Artery Aneurysm This disorder may present acutely with unilateral boring or aching retro-orbital and eye pain and facial paresthesias and/or pain (60 percent). Ophthalmoparesis or plegia causing diplopia may occur in up to 67 percent and involve nerve III (20–40 percent), nerve IV (16–20 percent), and nerve VI (43–53 percent). A variant of the superior orbital fissure syndrome, with ocular and facial pain and diplopia, occurs in 16 percent, and a variant of the cavernous sinus syndrome may be present in 43 percent. Patients may describe the presence of a bruit on the ipsilateral side. The diagnosis can be confirmed by a CT scan or MRI, which may reveal bone erosion and/or a parasellar mass lesion. MRI may be falsely negative with small aneurysms (<1 cm) or may misdiagnose a large thrombosed aneurysm as a tumor or hematoma. Carotid angiography is

highly sensitive and specific. Giant aneurysms (>2.5 cm) occur in 16 to 73 percent, depending on the series, and may cause optic nerve or chiasmal compression, with visual loss in 20 percent, or hypopituitarism. Spontaneous rupture can cause subarachnoid hemorrhage, epistaxis, or a carotid cavernous sinus fistula.

I. Carotid Cavernous Sinus Fistula A traumatic skull fracture may be associated with an internal carotid artery tear and formation of a carotid cavernous sinus fistula. Rupture of an intracavernous aneurysm of the internal carotid artery causes most cases of spontaneous onset. Other causes of nontraumatic fistulae include collagen deficiency syndromes, carotid artery dissection, and fibromuscular dysplasia.

Unilateral pain occurs in the retro-orbital area, face, and adjacent parietotemporal area and may be associated with an objective and/or subjective orbital bruit. Rapidly progressive proptosis may occur in 1 to 3 percent. Pulsating proptosis is a common finding. Vascular injection of the conjunctiva and retina, papilledema, pulsating retinal veins, and chemosis of the conjunctiva are frequently

Superior Orbital Apex Syndrome	Visual Loss	Ophthalmo-plegia	Cerebral Infarction, Cerebritis, or Meningitis	CT or MRI Evidence of Orbital Cellulitis	Cavernous Sinus Thrombosis	Bilateral Involvement	Response to Cortico-steroids	Carotid Angiogram
None	0%	0%	0%	0%	0%	Common	None	Negative
Rare	20%	73%	2.5%	Present 50%	5% may develop cavernous sinus thrombosis	Rare	None	Negative
May occur	75%	Present	Frequent	Present	Uncommon, unless cavernous sinus thrombosis secondary to orbital cellulitis	Uncommon, unless bilateral cavernous sinus thrombosis occurs	None	May show intracavernous stenosis or occlusion
May occur or similar findings	25%	Present	Rare	Rare, unless primary disease is orbital cellulitis	Present	One side initially, and then both	None	Intracavernous stenosis or occlusion
May occur	May occur	Present	0%	None; hematoma detected	None	0%	None	Negative
May be present	May occur	Present	None	None; enlarged ocular muscles	None	One side initially, and then both	Dramatic	Negative
May occur or similar findings	20%	67%	May occur	None	Cavernous sinus thrombosis may occur	Rarely bilateral (only 28 reported cases)	None	Intracavernous carotid Aneurysm
May occur or similar findings	32%	May occur	May occur	None	Cavernous sinus thrombosis may occur	12–15% of traumatic cases	None	Carotid cavernous sinus fistula

present. Ipsilateral visual loss may occur in up to 32 percent and may progress to blindness in 5 percent. Diplopia may result from involvement of nerves III, IV, and VI in the cavernous sinus. Bleeding may occur from the fistula, leading to potentially lethal intracerebral (3 percent) or subarachnoid hemorrhage (3 percent) and epistaxis (3.1 percent). The fistula can be demonstrated by cerebral angiography, and all symptoms and signs, including visual loss and ophthalmoplegia, can be improved or eliminated by closure of the fistula.

J. Dural Cavernous Sinus Shunt Rupture of thin-walled dural vessels into the cavernous sinus with drainage anteriorly into the superior ophthalmic vein may cause unilateral ocular pain, proptosis, a red eye, ophthalmoparesis(es) with diplopia, and visual loss due to ischemia. Retinal venous congestion, papilledema, and hemorrhages may be present on the ipsilateral side. If conventional internal carotid angiography is negative, a dural cavernous sinus shunt is possible, and selective external carotid angiography should be performed. This may demonstrate early filling of the cavernous sinus or an AV malformation of the dura. Anterior drainage is often associated with

thrombosis of the cavernous sinus and/or inferior petrosal sinus. This can be demonstrated by MRI.

K. Pituitary Apoplexy This disorder is caused by sudden hemorrhage into, or hemorrhagic infarction of, a pituitary tumor. Severe retro-orbital and/or frontal or generalized head pain (63 percent) and visual loss (59 percent) may occur, abruptly. Unilateral or bilateral orbital pain may occur. Diplopia due to involvement of nerves III, IV, and VI in the adjacent cavernous sinus may occur (16 percent), and signs of ophthalmopareses or plegias may be present. Loss of visual acuity and field defects may develop. A central scotoma may be present, simulating optic neuritis. Homonymous or bitemporal hemianopias or partial field defects may also occur. A disturbance of consciousness may develop in 12 percent of cases, and there may be an associated fever and meningismus due to subarachnoid hemorrhage or to the discharge of fragments of necrotic tumor into the subarachnoid space. Severely ill patients may have nausea and vomiting and, in rare cases, proptosis or a carotid occlusion with a contralateral hemiparesis related to cavernous sinus compression by the abrupt enlargement of the pituitary tumor. Associated sexual dysfunction, gynecomastia, galactorrhea, amenorrhea, and hair loss may also provide clinical clues to the diagnosis of a pituitary tumor, and this can be confirmed by a CT scan or MRI. Decompression by removal of the tumor is required to prevent permanent visual loss and diplopia.

4. REFERRED ORBITAL PAIN

A. Minor Leak from an Aneurysm   A minor leak from an aneurysm may cause an ipsilateral thunderclap headache in the retro-orbital and frontal region. Retro-orbital and facial pain on the ipsilateral side in one series occurred in 53 percent of the patients with a leaking internal carotid or posterior communicating aneurysm. The pain was unusually severe in 50 percent of cases, and associated with nausea, vomiting, or neck pain in up to 18 percent. Symptoms such as confusion, lethargy, malaise, weakness, ataxia, or a nerve III palsy (diplopia) each appeared in only 3 percent of cases.

The diagnosis of a minor subarachnoid hemorrhage may be confirmed by a CT scan (40 percent sensitive) or lumbar puncture (95 percent sensitive during the first 3 days), and the bleeding aneurysm can be demonstrated by cerebral angiography (99 percent sensitive).

B. Carotid Artery Dissection   There is an abrupt onset of pain in one side of the face and/or head and/or a subjective bruit. Neck pain may also occur. Retro-orbital pain and facial pain are common and may be accompanied by an ipsilateral carotid bruit and a Horner's syndrome with ptosis, miosis, and preservation of facial sweating below the supraorbital ridge. Amaurosis fugax, permanent visual loss, and an abducens paralysis with diplopia may also occur. Ipsilateral scalp tenderness may be present. Transient or permanent contralateral hemiparesis and sometimes an associated dysphasia may follow the onset of face and eye pain within hours to days. Bilateral carotid dissection may occur, but it is uncommon. The diagnosis can be confirmed by carotid angiography, which may demonstrate a long, tapered, irregular carotid stenosis or occlusion; pseudoaneurysm formation; a detached intimal flap; and/or a double lumen. Follow-up within 6 months may show a high percentage of cases with resolution of all arteriographic abnormalities. Vigorous exercise, a history of hypertension, Marfan's syndrome, syphilis, fibromuscular dysplasia, and cystic medial necrosis are sometimes associated with spontaneous carotid artery dissection.

C. Occipital Lobe and Cerebellar Lesions with Referred Ocular Pain   Referred pain to the ipsilateral eye and frontal region may occur with an acute infarction or hemorrhage in the occipital lobe. A contralateral homonymous hemianopia is usually present. Vascular lesions such as posterior cerebral artery occlusion produce a homonymous hemianopia with macular sparing. Some patients with hemianopic defects may detect colored, but not achromatic, targets in the hemianopic field. Up to 20 percent of patients without pattern discrimination in the hemianopic field may be able to reach for objects accurately or view moving light in the "blind field."

Cerebellar hemorrhage may cause bifrontal headache in 18 percent of cases and ipsilateral eye pain in 7 percent. The mechanism of referral may be related to the innervation of the tentorium, posterior falx cerebri, and occipital dura by recurrent branches of the ophthalmic division of nerve V. Stimulation of the superior surface of the tentorium cerebelli results in ipsilateral eye and frontal pain, while stimulation of the inferior surface and adjacent posterior fossa dura causes only occipital pain.

5. ORBITAL PAIN AND DIPLOPIA

A. Supraclinoid Internal Carotid or Posterior Communicating Aneurysms   These may cause unilateral retro-orbital pain for as long as 2 weeks before the onset of a third cranial nerve paresis with ptosis, diplopia, and a dilated sluggish or fixed pupil. Pain may also radiate to the forehead and anterior scalp. The abducens nerve may be involved in some cases. Supraclinoid aneurysms may also compress the optic nerve or chiasm, causing a decrease in visual acuity and field defects. A cerebral angiogram will demonstrate the lesion.

B. Diabetic Ischemic Neuropathy   Diabetes may cause an acutely painful diplopia with a unilateral third nerve palsy and pupillary preservation. There is a tendency for the paresis to resolve over a period of months. This disorder has been reported in nondiabetics, but such occurrences are rare.

C. Ophthalmoplegic Migraine   Rarely, a patient with migraine (0.02 percent) may develop eye pain and headache, ptosis, diplopia, and a fixed dilated pupil. This disorder usually occurs in children and young women. Angiograms reveal no abnormalities. The ophthalmoparesis is usually transient and improves or resolves within a few days, but it may recur with subsequent episodes of headache.

A complete paralysis of the third cranial nerve should be evaluated by cerebral arteriography even in a diabetic. A partial third nerve palsy with only ptosis (levator palpabrae superioris paresis), a superior rectus paresis with diplopia on upward gaze, and pupillary sparing also require evaluation for aneurysm. Since up to 14 percent of aneurysms may cause a nerve III paresis and spare the pupil, preservation of the pupil is not an absolute sign of a benign disorder. Rarely, vasculitis may involve the third nerve and may be suggested by other findings and an elevated sedimentation rate.

6. OCULAR PAIN AND VISUAL LOSS

A. Idiopathic Optic Neuritis and Multiple Sclerosis
There is an abrupt onset of visual loss in one eye (99.5 percent of cases), with associated mild pain that increases on eye motion and with palpation of the globe. The pain usually begins with the visual loss but may precede it by days or weeks. Eye movement upward or laterally often causes maximal pain. A central scotoma is usually present in association with a loss of visual acuity and color perception.

The involved eye shows a relative afferent pupillary defect, with a decreased response to direct light stimulation and a normal consensual response. This can be demonstrated by a swinging flash light or cover test.

It is characteristic of this disorder for the visual loss and field defects to progress to a nadir of function during the first 2 weeks and then to recover spontaneously during the next 3 to 6 weeks. Such a course makes evaluation of steroid and other therapy difficult. Tumors in the orbit and parasellar region usually do not regress and allow visual improvement spontaneously, but occasional exceptions have been observed.

Intraocular involvement of the optic nerve results in papillitis associated with exudates, hemorrhages, and normal venous pulsations. Disc elevation is usually less than 2 diopters, and a central scotoma is present. Papilledema resembles papillitis on ophthalmoscopic examination, but it is associated with loss of retinal venous pulsations. In addition, it does not cause ocular pain, a central scotoma, or a severe decrease in visual acuity. If retrobulbar optic neuropathy is present, the retina and disc appear normal.

This disorder may occur as a symptom of multiple sclerosis in 25 to 50 percent of cases. Other patients have an idiopathic disorder and never progress to a full-blown demyelinating disease.

B. Devic's Disease   Bilateral optic neuritis and transverse myelitis constitute a specific demyelinating disorder that may be a variant of multiple sclerosis or a distinct entity in itself. Cerebral plaques have been detected by MRI in 60 to 70 percent of patients with optic neuritis. The optic nerve may also show demyelination by MRI.

Ocular pain on motion with visual loss may occur in iridocyclitis, acute thyrotoxic ophthalmopathy, and posterior scleritis.

C. Mimics of Idiopathic Optic Neuritis

1. Autoimmune Disorders   An autoimmune optic neuropathy responsive to steroids may occur in patients with systemic lupus erythematosus or lupus-like illnesses and in Sjögren's syndrome.

2. Parasellar Region Inflammatory Disorders   Optic nerve dysfunction can result from extension of a sphe-

noid sinusitis or involvement of the cranial nerves at the base of the brain by a chronic meningitis caused by tuberculosis, cryptococcosis, coccidioidomycosis, syphilis, carcinoma, or focal lesions related to toxoplasmosis or sarcoidosis.

3. Parainfectious Associations   These include mycoplasma pneumonia, the Guillain-Barré syndrome, and AIDS.

4. Neuroretinitis   Patients experience ocular pain, visual loss, and an exudative macular star associated with papillitis. Causes include syphilis, mumps, measles, rubella, leptospirosis, cat-scratch fever, psittacosis, herpes simplex encephalitis, and Behçet's disease.

5. Parasellar Masses—Cysts, Tumors, and Aneurysms   These include primary brain and pituitary tumors, aneurysms, metastatic tumors, lymphomas, plasmacytomas, leukemias, sphenoid sinus carcinoma, and benign lesions such as a sphenoid mucocele.

6. Temporal (Giant Cell) Arteritis   This disorder may present with an acute temporal headache and tenderness due to an inflamed, indurated temporal artery with diminished pulsations. Jaw and tongue claudication may accompany chewing and sometimes talking. Retinal artery occlusion or stenosis causes visual loss or blindness due to anterior ischemic optic neuropathy. Involvement of the short ciliary arteries may cause optic nerve ischemia with eye pain on movement, globe tenderness, and visual loss, simulating idiopathic optic neuritis. Fever and polymyalgia rheumatica may be associated. The sedimentation rate is frequently elevated (91 percent), while it is usually normal in optic neuritis. The diagnosis can be confirmed by temporal artery biopsy in 40 to 45 percent, and a probable diagnosis can be made by observing the response of headache, tenderness, and systemic symptoms to prednisone (80–100 mg/day) over a 48-h period. Bilateral ocular involvement may occur during the initial week of therapy, resulting in blindness, but this is uncommon.

7. Amaurosis Fugax and Ocular Infarction   This disorder may occur as a single episode of visual loss or obscuration associated with acute supraorbital or ocular aching and/or stabbing pain. The duration of visual loss was less than 30 min in 76 percent, and less than 1 h in 84 percent of cases. A single episode may terminate in ocular infarction, resulting in a persistent field defect, enlargement of the blind spot and/or a scotoma, and disc and/or retinal pallor with only small effects on overall visual acuity. Occasionally, patients may suffer a severe loss of visual acuity. Symptoms of transient cerebral dysfunction occurred in only 11 percent in association with amaurosis fugax. These episodes of cerebral dysfunction usually occurred independently of the attacks of amaurosis fugax, but in 33 percent they accompanied the ocular symptoms. In young adults, the etiology of amaurosis fugax and ocular infarction is unknown, but migraine appears to be the most likely cause, although cardiogenic emboli may be responsible in some cases (e.g., atrial fibrillation, mitral valve prolapse, or paradoxic embolism through a patent foramen ovale). In older patients, this disorder may be caused by common carotid or right innominate atherosclerosis at the arch level, internal carotid artery stenosis or occlusion, or giant cell arteritis. Angiography in the younger patients (<45 years of age) is usually negative, but unusual lesions, such as an isolated stenosis of the ophthalmic artery or irregularities of the cerebral arteries, have been detected in a small percentage of cases.

Optic neuritis mimics, like idiopathic orbital granuloma or the Tolosa-Hunt syndrome, may respond to high-dose corticosteroid therapy. A CT scan or MRI should be done prior to establishing a diagnosis of idiopathic optic neuritis, since mass lesions may closely mimic this disorder. Lumbar puncture with culture and cytology, a VDRL and FTA test, an ANA and ESR, and an angiotensin converting enzyme (ACE) level may help establish a specific disorder as a cause of an optic neuritis–like syndrome.

7. INFECTIOUS DISEASES AND BILATERAL OCULAR PAIN

A. Nonspecific Viral Syndromes Ocular pain may occur with eye movement in many nonspecific febrile viral infections. Associated symptoms include fever, chilliness, headache, malaise, myalgias, diaphoresis, arthralgias, anorexia, nausea, vomiting, abdominal pain or diarrhea, and/or respiratory complaints.

B. Varicella Vesicular or pustular conjunctival lesions or a keratitis may be caused by varicella.

C. Epstein-Barr Virus Patients may experience ocular pain and lid edema secondary to dacryoadenitis or dacryocystitis.

D. Lymphogranuloma Venereum (LGV) and Cat-Scratch Fever Cat-scratch fever may cause a Parinaud's syndrome with a painful conjunctivitis and preauricular adenopathy. LGV may cause a keratitis.

E. Trichinosis Patients have ocular pain on motion and bilateral lid and conjunctival edema secondary to a myositis that involves the ocular muscles. Ophthalmoparesis with diplopia may occur. This disorder begins acutely with generalized myalgias and muscle tenderness due to

Table 3-2
UNILATERAL (U) AND BILATERAL (B) INVOLVEMENT IN MAJOR PAINFUL OPHTHALMIC DISORDERS

	Initial Clinical Presentation	Fully Developed Clinical Presentation
Conjunctivitis, viral or bacterial	U or B	U or B
Iritis	U or B	U or B
Acute glaucoma	U	U
Scleritis	U or B (10–33%)	U or B (40–80%)
Acute endophthalmitis	U	U
Preseptal cellulitis	U or B	U or B
Idiopathic orbital pseudotumor	U	U or B
Subperiosteal orbital abscess	U	U
Orbital cellulitis or abscess	U	U or B if cavernous sinus thrombosis occurs
Rhinocerebral mucormycosis	U	U or B if cavernous sinus thrombosis occurs Rare/bilateral cases may occur without cavernous sinus thrombosis
Cavernous sinus thrombosis	U	B
Acute thyroid ophthalmopathy	U or B	B
Orbital hematoma	U	U
Intracavernous carotid aneurysm	U (B only 28 cases reported)	U
Carotid cavernous fistula	U or B (10–15% of traumatic cases)	U or B (10–15% of traumatic cases)
Dural cavernous sinus shunt	U	U
Pituitary apoplexy	U or B	U or B
Minor leak	U or B	U or B
Carotid artery dissection	U (B rare)	U (B rare)
Occipital lobe lesion, referred pain	U	U
Posterior communicating aneurysm and nerve III lesion	U	U
Diabetic ischemic neuropathy and nerve III lesion	U	U
Ophthalmoplegic migraine	U	U (B subsequent attacks may switch sides)
Optic neuritis	U	U (only 0.5% bilateral)
Temporal arteritis	U or B	U or B
Herpes zoster	U	U
Sebaceous carcinoma of the lid	U	U
Herpes simplex keratitis	U	U or B (<1%)
Blepharitis	U or B	U or B

myositis, fever, weakness, malaise, and headache. Small hemorrhages may be found in the nails, at the insertions of the ocular muscles on the globe, and in the retina. There is a marked peripheral eosinophilia (20–70 percent) and an elevation of serum muscle enzyme levels with a normal sedimentation rate. The diagnosis can be supported by a skin test, a serum bentonite flocculation test, or a muscle biopsy obtained during the second week of the illness.

F. Q Fever Patients may have headache and fever, cough, interstitial pneumonia, and ocular pain and photophobia due to uveitis.

8. SKIN DISORDERS WITH ACUTE EYE INVOLVEMENT

A. Toxic Epidermal Necrolysis A toxin produced by a staphylococcal phage group II infection on the skin or at a distant site may result in toxic epidermal necrolysis. It begins with diffuse skin erythema, fever, and the formation of thin-walled bullae that rapidly rupture, leaving the dermis exposed. A similar reaction occurs bilaterally in the conjunctiva, causing eye pain, redness, and exudation with adherence of the lid margins. A similar syndrome may be caused by drug allergy or viral illnesses. The Nikolsky sign is positive in erythematous areas within 24 h of onset.

B. Stevens-Johnson Syndrome Severe cases present with high fever and a generalized macular and/or papular rash with target lesions, urticarial plaques, vesicles, and bullae. Lesions may cluster over the lateral and extensor surfaces of the limbs and over lower extremity joints. The oral mucosa and lips develop bullous lesions that soon rupture. The lips and mucosa of the mouth become covered with a gray pseudomembrane and hemorrhagic crusts.

Eye pain results from severe ocular inflammation. A bilateral purulent conjunctivitis occurs and may be complicated by corneal ulceration, iridocyclitis, and panophthalmitis.

9. REFERRED DENTAL PAIN

A painful root abscess or pulpitis may cause severe aching or throbbing tooth and jaw pain that is constant or is provoked by chewing and/or cold or hot liquids. This severe pain may be referred from the upper jaw and midface to the ipsilateral eye. The eye pain is relieved by correction of the dental disorder.

10. PAIN DISTRIBUTION (UNILATERAL OR BILATERAL) IN ACUTE OPHTHALMIC DISORDERS

Painful ocular disorders may initially involve only one eye or both. Some disorders that begin on one side progress to develop similar pain and findings on the other, while some unilateral processes rarely, if ever, involve both sides. Table 3-2 summarizes these differences for many of the disorders discussed in this chapter.

EYE PAIN REFERENCES

Aneurysms and Orbital Pain

Diaz FG, Ohaegbulam S, Dujovny M, et al: Surgical alternatives in the treatment of cavernous sinus aneurysms. *J Neurosurg* 71:846–853, 1989.

Halbach VV, Hieshima GB, Higashida RT, et al: Carotid cavernous fistulae: Indications for urgent treatment. *AJR* 149:587–593, 1987.

Leblanc R: The minor leak preceding subarachnoid hemorrhage. *J Neurosurg* 66:35–39, 1987.

Linskey ME, Sekhar LN, Hirsch W Jr, et al: Aneurysms of the intracavernous carotid artery: Clinical presentation, radiographic features, and pathogenesis. *Neurosurgery* 26(1):71–79, 1990.

Little JR, Rosenfeld JV, Awad IA: Internal carotid artery occlusion for cavernous segment aneurysm. *Neurosurgery* 25(3):398–404, 1989.

Zachariades N, Papavassiliou D: Traumatic carotid-cavernous sinus fistula. *J Craniomaxillofac Surg* 16:385–388, 1988.

Cavernous Sinus Syndrome

Ben-Uri R, Palma L, Kaveh Z: Case report: Septic thrombosis of the cavernous sinus: Diagnosis with the aid of computed tomography. *Clin Radiol* 40:520–522, 1989.

Curnes JT, Creasy JL, Whaley RL, et al: Air in the cavernous sinus: A new sign of septic cavernous sinus thrombosis (letter to editor). *AJNR* 8(1):176–177, 1987.

DiNubile MJ: Septic thrombosis of the cavernous sinuses. *Arch Neurol* 45:567–572, 1988.

Hawke SHB, Mullie MA, Hoyt WF, et al: Painful oculomotor nerve palsy due to dural-cavernous sinus shunt. *Arch Neurol* 46:1252–1255, 1989.

Levine SR, Twyman RE, Gilman S: The role of anticoagulation in cavernous sinus thrombosis. *Neurology* 38:517–522, 1988.

Johnson EV, Kline LB, Julian BA, et al: Bilateral cavernous sinus thrombosis due to mucormycosis. *Arch Ophthalmol* 106:1089–1092, 1988.

Macdonald RL, Findlay JM, Tator CH: Sphenoethmoidal sinusitis complicated by cavernous sinus thrombosis and pontocerebellar infarction. *Can J Neurol Sci* 15:310–313, 1988.

Mahapatra AK: Brain abscess—an unusual complication of cavernous sinus thrombosis: A case report. *Clin Neurol Neurosurg* 90(3):241–243, 1988.

Micheli F, Schteinschnaider A, Plaghos LL, et al: Bacterial cavernous sinus aneurysm treated by detachable balloon technique. *Stroke* 20:1751–1754, 1989.

Ogundiya DA, Keith DA, Mirowski J: Cavernous sinus thrombosis and blindness as complications of an odontogenic infection: Report of a case and review of literature. *J Oral Maxillofac Surg* 47:1317–1321, 1989.

Savino PJ, Grossman RI, Schatz NJ, et al: High-field magnetic resonance imaging in the diagnosis of cavernous sinus thrombosis. *Arch Neurol* 43(10):1081–1082, 1986.

Southwick FS, Richardson EP Jr, Swartz MN: Septic thrombosis of the dural venous sinuses. *Medicine* 65(2):82–106, 1986.

Tveterås K, Kristensen S, Dommerby H: Septic cavernous and lateral sinus thrombosis: Modern diagnostic and therapeutic principles. *J Laryngol Otol* 102:877–882, 1988.

Virapongse C, Cazenave C, Quisling R, et al: The empty delta sign: Frequency and significance in 76 cases of dural sinus thrombosis. *Radiology* 162:779–785, 1987.

Cornea—Trauma

Sklar DP, Lauth JE, Johnson DR: Topical anesthesia of the eye as a diagnostic test. *Ann Emerg Med* 18:1209–1211, 1989.

Cornea—Ulcer

Martin NF, Stark WJ, Maumenee AE: Treatment of Mooren's and Mooren's-like ulcer by lamellar keratectomy: Report of six eyes and literature review. *Ophthalmic Surg* 18(8):564–569, 1987.

Dissection—Internal Carotid Artery and Orbital Pain

Kline LB, Vitek JJ, Raymon BC: Painful Horner's syndrome due to spontaneous carotid artery dissection. *Ophthalmology* 94:226–230, 1987.

Lepojärvi M, Tarkka M, Leinonen A, et al: Spontaneous dissection of the internal carotid artery. *Acta Chir Scand* 154:559–566, 1988.

Drug-Related Eye Pain

Coulter DM: Eye pain with nifedipine and disturbance of taste with captopril: A mutually controlled study showing a method of post-marketing surveillance. *Br Med J* 296(6629):1086–1088, 1988.

Johnson DW, Parkinson D, Wolpert SM, et al: Intracarotid chemotherapy with 1,3-bis-(2-chloroethyl)-1-nitrosourea (BCNU) in 5% dextrose in water in the treatment of malignant glioma. *Neurosurgery* 20(4):577–583, 1987.

Kelly SP, Walley TJ: Eye pain with nifedipine (letter to editor). *Br Med J* 296(6633):1401, 1988.

Stewart DJ, Grahovac Z, Russel NA, et al: Phase I study of intracarotid PCNU. *J Neuro-Oncol* 5:245–250, 1987.

Ectropion

Korn EL, Glotzbach RK: Carbon dioxide laser repair of medial ectropion. *Ophthalmic Surg* 19(19):653–657, 1988.

Endophthalmitis

Boisjoly HM, Jotterand VH, Bazin R, et al: Metastatic *Pseudomonas* endophthalmitis following bronchoscopy. *Can J Ophthalmol* 22(7):378–80, 1987.

Case 29-1989, Case records of the Massachusetts General Hospital. *N Engl J Med* 321(3):172–182, 1989.

Croxatto JO, Lombardi A, Malbran ES: Inflamed eye in Marfan's syndrome with posteriorly luxated lens. *Ophthalmologica* (Basel) 193:23–26, 1986.

Green MT, Font RL, Campbell JV, et al: Endogenous *Clostridium* panophthalmitis. *Ophthalmology* 94:435–438, 1987.

Weber DJ, Hoffman KL, Thoft RA, et al: Endophthalmitis following

intraocular lens implantation: Report of 30 cases and review of the literature. *Rev Infect Dis* 8(1):12–20, 1986.

Ernest Syndrome

Shankland WE II: Ernest syndrome as a consequence of stylomandibular ligament injury: A report of 68 patients. *J Prosthet Dent* 57(4):501–506, 1987.

Eyelids—Conjunctivitis

Brook I: Presence of anaerobic bacteria in conjunctivitis associated with wearing contact lenses. *Ann Ophthalmol* 20:397–399, 1988.

Enberg RN: Perennial nonallergic rhinitis: A retrospective review. *Ann Allergy* 63(6, part 1):513–516, 1989.

Fitch CP, Rapoza PA, Owens S, et al: Epidemiology and diagnosis of acute conjunctivitis at an inner-city hospital. *Ophthalmology* 96:1215–1220, 1989.

Grutzmacher RD: Ocular disease from wearing contact lenses: A potentially devastating complication. *Postgrad Med* 86(4):90–100, 1989.

Lohr JA, Austin RD, Grossman M, et al: Comparison of three topical antimicrobials for acute bacterial conjunctivitis. *Pediatr Infect Dis J* 7:626–629, 1988.

McDonnell PJ: How do general practitioners manage eye disease in the community? *Br J Ophthalmol* 72:733–736, 1988.

Prendiville KJ, Bath PE: Lateral cantholysis and eyelid necrosis secondary to *Pseudomonas aeruginosa*. *Ann Ophthalmol* 20:193–195, 1988.

Reed DB: Viral and bacterial conjunctivitis: Prevention of disastrous results. *Postgrad Med* 86(4):103–104, 107–109, 113–114, 1989.

Trimethoprim-Polymyxin B Sulphate Ophthalmic Ointment Study Group: Trimethoprim-polymyxin B sulphate ophthalmic ointment versus chloramphenicol ophthalmic ointment in the treatment of bacterial conjunctivitis: A review of four clinical studies. *J Antimicrob Chemother* 23:261–266, 1989.

Eyelids—Sebaceous Carcinoma

Kass LG, Hornblass A: Sebaceous carcinoma of the ocular adnexa. *Surv Ophthalmol* 33(6):477–490, 1989.

Eye Pain—Review Articles

Kohrman BD, Warfield CA: Eye pain: Ocular and nonocular causes. *Hosp Pract* 22(12):33–35, 38, 40–50, 1987.

Rosenblatt MA, Sakol PJ: Ocular and periocular pain. *Otolaryngol Clin North Am* 22(6):1173–1203, 1989.

Yanofsky NN: The acute painful eye. *Emerg Med Clin North Am* 6(1):21–42, 1988.

Glaucoma

Clark CV: Diabetes mellitus in primary glaucoma. *Ann Acad Med Singapore* 18(2):190–194, 1989.

Kalra L, Bone MF: The effect of nebulized bronchodilator therapy on intraocular pressures in patients with glaucoma. *Chest* 93(4):739–741, 1988.

Makabe R: Comparative studies of the width of the anterior chamber angle using echography and gonioscopy. *Klin Monatsbl Augenheilkd* 194(1):6–9, 1989.

Malukiewicz-Wisniewska G, Kaūzny J: Laser gonioplasty of the iridocorneal angle in the treatment of glaucoma. *Klin Oczna* 91(1):23–25, 1989.

Scheie HG, Albert DM: Glaucoma, in *Textbook of Ophthalmology*, 9th ed. Philadelphia, Saunders, 1977, pp 522–553.

Schiff FS: Trabeculectomy, ECCE with PC-IOL implant, and vitrectomy after malignant glaucoma. *Ophthalmic Surg* 19(4):277–278, 1988.

Striga M, Curkovic T: Treatment of narrow- or closed-angle glaucoma using combined argon and Nd-YAG laser photocoagulation. *Lijec Vjesn* 111(8):281–285, 1989.

Globe Tumors

El Baba F, Hagler WS, De La Cruz A, et al: Choroidal melanoma with pigment dispersion in vitreous and melanomalytic glaucoma. *Ophthalmology* 95:370–377, 1988.

Head Pain—Eye-Associated

Greenidge KC, Dweck M: Head pain associated with the eye, in Cooper BC, Lucente FE (eds): *Management of Facial, Head and Neck Pain*, Philadelphia, Saunders, 1989, pp 77–98.

Keratitis

Beyer CF, Arens MQ, Hill JM, et al: Penetrating keratoplasty in rabbits induces latent HSV-1 reactivation when corticosteroids are used. *Curr Eye Res* 8(12):1323–1329, 1989.

Brincker P, Gregersen E, Prause JU: *Acanthamoeba* keratitis: Clinicopathological report of 2 cases. *Acta Ophthalmol (Copenh)* 66(2):210–213, 1988.

Cashwell LF Jr, Holleman IL, Weaver RG, et al: Idiopathic true exfoliation of the lens capsule. *Ophthalmology* 96(3):348–351, 1989.

Catalano RA, Webb RM, Smith RS, et al: A modified immunoperoxidase method for rapid diagnosis of herpes simplex I keratitis. *Am J Clin Pathol* 86(1):102–104, 1986.

Chumbley LC, Thomson IM: Epidemiology of trachoma in the West Bank and Gaza Strip. *Eye* 2:463–470, 1988.

Cobo M, Foulks GN, Liesegang T, et al: Observations on the natural history of herpes zoster ophthalmicus. *Curr Eye Res* 6(1):195–199, 1987.

Collum LM, Mullaney J, Hillery M, et al: Two laboratory methods for diagnosis of herpes simplex keratitis. *Br J Ophthalmol* 71(10):742–745, 1987.

Dart JK: Predisposing factors in microbial keratitis: The significance of contact lens wear. *Br J Ophthalmol* 72(12):926–930, 1988.

Derick RJ, Kelley CG, Gersman M: Contact lens related corneal ulcers at the Ohio State University Hospitals 1983–1987. *CLAO J* 15(4):268–270, 1989.

Deutsch FH: Concurrent adenoviral and herpetic ocular infections. *Ann Ophthalmol* 21(11):432–438, 1989.

Donzis PB, Mondino BJ: Management of noninfectious corneal ulcers. *Surv Ophthalmol* 32(2):94–110, 1987.

Dugel PU, Holland GN, Brown HH, et al: *Mycobacterium fortuitum* keratitis. *Am J Ophthalmol* 105(6):661–669, 1988.

Epstein RJ, Wilson LA, Visvesvara GS, et al: Rapid diagnosis of *Acanthamoeba* keratitis from corneal scrapings using indirect fluorescent antibody staining. *Arch Ophthalmol* 104(9):1318–1321, 1986.

Fan CC, Shimomura Y, Inoue Y, et al: A case of simultaneous bilateral herpetic epithelial keratitis. *Jpn J Ophthalmol* 33(1):120–124, 1989.

Ficker LA, Kirkness CM, Rice NS, et al: The changing management and improved prognosis for corneal grafting in herpes simplex keratitis. *Ophthalmology* 96(11):1587–1596, 1989.

Friedberg DN, Stenson SM, Orenstein JM, et al: Microsporidial keratoconjunctivitis in acquired immunodeficiency syndrome. *Arch Ophthalmol* 108(4):504–508, 1990.

Gans LA: Eye lesions of epidermolysis bullosa: Clinical features, management, and prognosis. *Arch Dermatol* 124:762–764, 1988.

Gradus MS, Koenig SB, Hyndiuk RA, et al: Filter-culture technique using amoeba saline transport medium for the noninvasive diagnosis of *Acanthamoeba* keratitis. *Am J Clin Pathol* 92(5):682–685, 1989.

Hayasaka S, Watanabe M, Yamamoto Y, et al: Herpes zoster ophthalmicus complicated by hyphema and hemorrhagic glaucoma. *Ophthalmologica* (Basel) 196:185–187, 1988.

Howes DS: The red eye. *Emerg Med Clin North Am* 6(1):43–56, 1988.

Hsieh WC, Dornic DI: *Acanthamoeba* dendriform keratitis. *J Am Optom Assoc* 60(1):32–34, 1989.

Ishibashi Y, Hommura S, Matsumoto Y: Direct examination vs culture of biopsy specimens for the diagnosis of keratomycosis. *Am J Ophthalmol* 103(5):636–640, 1987.

Ishibashi Y, Kaufman HE: Corneal biopsy in the diagnosis of keratomycosis. *Am J Ophthalmol* 101(3):288–293, 1986.

Johns KJ, O'Day DM, Head WS, et al: Herpes simplex masquerade syndrome: *Acanthamoeba* keratitis. *Curr Eye Res* 6(1):207–212, 1987.

Johns KJ, Parrish CM, Seal MR, et al: *Acanthamoeba* keratitis in

Tennessee: A growing problem in patients wearing contact lenses. *J Tenn Med Assoc* 82(11):584–588, 1989.

Kent HD, Cohen EJ, Laibson PR, et al: Microbial keratitis and corneal ulceration associated with therapeutic soft contact lenses. *CLAO J* 16(1):49–52, 1990.

Laflamme MY, Poisson M, Chehade N: *Mycobacterium chelonei* keratitis following penetrating keratoplasty. *Can J Ophthalmol* 22(3):178–180, 1987.

Lee SF, Pepose JS: Sandwich enzyme immunoassay and latex agglutination test for herpes simplex virus keratitis. *J Clin Microbiol* 28(4):785–786, 1990.

Lee SF, Storch GA, Reed CA, et al: Comparative laboratory diagnosis of experimental herpes simplex keratitis. *Am J Ophthalmol* 109(1):8–12, 1990.

Lindquist TD, Sher NA, Doughman DJ: Clinical signs and medical therapy of early *Acanthamoeba* keratitis. *Arch Ophthalmol* 106(1):73–77, 1988.

MacEwen CJ, Khan ZU, Anderson E, et al: Corneal re-graft: Indications and outcome. *Ophthalmic Surg* 19(10):706–712, 1988.

Mannis MJ, Tamaru R, Roth AM, et al: *Acanthamoeba* sclerokeratitis: Determining diagnostic criteria. *Arch Ophthalmol* 104(9):1313–1317, 1986.

McClellan KA, Bernard PJ, Billson FA: Microbial investigations in keratitis at the Sydney Eye Hospital. *Aust N Z J Ophthalmol* 17(4):413–416, 1989.

Mondino BJ: Inflammatory diseases of the peripheral cornea. *Ophthalmology* 95:463–472, 1988.

Moore MB, McCulley JP: *Acanthamoeba* keratitis associated with contact lenses: Six consecutive cases of successful management. *Br J Ophthalmol* 73(4):271–275, 1989.

Moore MB, Newton C, Kaufman HE: Chronic keratitis caused by *Mycobacterium gordonae*. *Am J Ophthalmol* 102(4):516–521, 1986.

Murrah WF: Epidermic keratoconjunctivitis. *Am J Ophthalmol* 20:36–38, 1988.

Nago R, Hayashi K, Ochiai H, et al: Detection of herpes simplex virus type 1 in herpetic ocular diseases by DNA-DNA hybridization using a biotinylated DNA probe. *J Med Virol* 25:259–270, 1988.

Newton C, Moore MB, Kaufman HE: Corneal biopsy in chronic keratitis. *Arch Ophthalmol* 105(4):577–578, 1987.

O'Brien JJ, Campoli-Richards DM: Acyclovir: An updated review of its antiviral activity, pharmacokinetic properties and therapeutic efficacy. *Drugs* 37(3):233–309, 1989.

O'Day DM: Management of herpes simplex keratitis: Problems associated with epithelial disease. *Aust N Z J Ophthalmol* 15(4):263–267, 1987.

Ormerod LD, Gomez DS, Schanzlin DJ, et al: Chronic alcoholism and microbial keratitis. *Br J Ophthalmol* 72(2):155–159, 1988.

Pflugfelder SC, Flynn HW Jr, Zwickey TA, et al: Exogenous fungal endophthalmitis. *Ophthalmology* 95(1):19–30, 1988.

Portnoy SL, Insler MS, Kaufman HE: Surgical management of corneal ulceration and perforation. *Surv Ophthalmol* 34(1):47–58, 1989.

Pulido JS, Goeken JA, Nerad JA, et al: Ocular manifestations of patients with circulating antineutrophil cytoplasmic antibodies. *Arch Ophthalmol* 108(6):845–850, 1990.

Schwab IR, Abbott RL: Toxic ulcerative keratopathy: An unrecognized problem. *Ophthalmology* 96(8):1187–1193, 1989.

Sharma S, Srinivasan M, George C: *Acanthamoeba* keratitis in noncontact lens wearers. *Arch Ophthalmol* 108(5):676–678, 1990.

Shivitz IA: Bilateral simultaneous *Pseudomonas* keratitis with myopic extended-wear contact lenses. *Ann Ophthalmol* 19(6):204–206, 1987.

Silvany RE, Luckenbach MW, Moore MB: The rapid detection of *Acanthamoeba* in paraffin-embedded sections of corneal tissue with calcofluor white. *Arch Ophthalmol* 105(10):1366–1367, 1987.

Tauber J, Melamed S, Foster CS: Glaucoma in patients with ocular cicatricial pemphigoid. *Ophthalmology* 96:33–37, 1989.

Tripathi RC, Monninger RH, Tripathi BJ: Contact lens-associated

Acanthamoeba keratitis: A report from the USA. *Fortschr Ophthalmol* 86(1):67–71, 1989.

Weiss JS, Orlando F, Albert DM: The usefulness of routine alcian blue staining of corneal specimens. *Cornea* 7(2):127–132, 1988.

Wilhelmus KR: Diagnosis and management of herpes simplex stromal keratitis. *Cornea* 6(4):286–291, 1987.

Wilhelmus KR, Osato MS, Font RL, et al: Rapid diagnosis of *Acanthamoeba* keratitis using calcofluor white. *Arch Ophthalmol* 104(9):1309–1312, 1986.

Young TL, Robin JB, Holland GN, et al: Herpes simplex keratitis in patients with acquired immune deficiency syndrome. *Ophthalmology* 96(10):1476–1479, 1989.

Nasal Origin of Eye Pain

Chen M-S, Lin F-J, Tang SG, et al: Clinical significance of cranial nerve deficit in the therapy of nasopharyngeal carcinoma. *Br J Radiol* 62:739–743, 1989.

Gerbe RW, Fry TL, Fischer ND: Headache of nasal spur origin: An easily diagnosed and surgically correctable cause of facial pain. *Headache* 24:329–330, 1984.

Neuroretinitis

Margolis T, Irvine AR, Hoyt WF, et al: Acute retinal necrosis syndrome presenting with papillitis and arcuate neuroretinitis. *Ophthalmology* 95(7):937–940, 1988.

McLeish WM, Pulido JS, Holland S, et al: The ocular manifestations of syphilis in the human immunodeficiency virus type 1-infected host. *Ophthalmology* 97(2):196–203, 1990.

Weiss AH, Beck RW: Neuroretinitis in childhood. *J Pediatr Ophthalmol Strabismus* 26(4):198–203, 1989.

Ocular Injuries

Scheie HG, Albert DM: Ocular injuries, in *Textbook of Ophthalmology*, 9th ed. Philadelphia, Saunders, 1977, pp 554–576.

Ophthalmic Overview

Scheie HG, Albert DM: Ophthalmic overview: An introduction to ophthalmic diseases and their terminology, in *Textbook of Ophthalmology*, 9th ed. Philadelphia, Saunders, 1977, pp 3–44.

Ophthalmology—Medical

Scheie HG, Albert DM: Medical ophthalmology, in *Textbook of Ophthalmology*, 9th ed. Philadelphia, Saunders, 1977, pp 359–479.

Ophthalmology—Neuro-

Scheie HG, Albert DM: Neuro-ophthalmology, in *Textbook of Ophthalmology*, 9th ed. Philadelphia, Saunders, 1977, pp 480–521.

Orbit—Graves' Ophthalmopathy

Feldon SE: Graves' ophthalmopathy: Is it really thyroid disease? (editorial). *Arch Intern Med* 150:948–950, 1990.

Kahaly G, Beyer J: Immunosuppressant therapy of thyroid eye disease. *Klin Wochenschr* 66:1049–1059, 1988.

Kendall-Taylor P, Crombie AL, Stephenson AM, et al: Intravenous methylprednisolone in the treatment of Graves' ophthalmopathy. *Br Med J:* 297:1574–1578, 1988.

Khardori R, Weaver ME, Soler NG: Graves' ophthalmopathy: An unusual course. *Am J Med* 77:1121–1125, 1984.

Leone CR Jr, Piest KL, Newman RJ: Medial and lateral wall decompression for thyroid ophthalmopathy. *Am J Ophthalmol* 108:160–166, 1989.

Perrild H, Feldt-Rasmussen U, Bech K, et al: The differential diagnostic problems in unilateral euthyroid Graves' ophthalmopathy. *Acta Endocrinol (Copenh)* 106:471–476, 1984.

Perros P, Kendall-Taylor P: The pathogenesis of thyroid-associated ophthalmopathy. *J Endocrinol* 122:619–624, 1989.

Perros P, Weightman DR, Crombie AL, et al: Azathioprine in the treatment of thyroid-associated ophthalmopathy. *Acta Endocrinol (Copenh)* 122(1):8–12, 1990.

Prummel MF, Wiersinga WM, Mourits MP, et al: Effect of abnormal thyroid function on the severity of Graves' ophthalmopathy. *Arch Intern Med* 150:1098–1101, 1990.

Sanders MD, Brown P: Acute presentation of thyroid ophthalmopathy. *Trans Ophthalmol Soc U K* 105:720–722, 1986.

Sandler HM, Rubenstein JH, Fowbel BL, et al: Results of radiotherapy for thyroid ophthalmopathy. *Br J Radiat Oncology Biol Phys* 17:823–827, 1989.

Spaulding SW, Lippes H: Hyperthyroidism: Causes, clinical features, and diagnosis. *Med Clin North Am* 69(5):937–951, 1985.

Wiersinga WM, Smit T, Schuster-Uittenhoeve ALJ, et al: Therapeutic outcome of prednisone medication and of orbital irradiation in patients with Graves' ophthalmopathy. *Ophthalmologica* (Basel) 197:75–84, 1988.

Wiersinga WM, Smit T, van der Gaag R, et al: Clinical presentation of Graves' ophthalmopathy. *Ophthalmic Res* 21:73–82, 1989.

Wiersinga WM, Smit T, van der Gaag R, et al: Temporal relationship between onset of Graves' ophthalmopathy and onset of thyroidal Graves' disease. *J Endocrinol Invest* 11:615–619, 1988.

Orbit Hematoma

Jacobson DM, Itani K, Digre KB, et al: Maternal orbital hematoma associated with labor. *Am J Ophthalmol* 105(5):547–553, 1988.

Orbit—Inflammatory

Benson WE: Posterior scleritis. *Surv Ophthalmol* 32(5):297–316, 1988.

Brass LS, Amedee RG: Atypical facial pain. *J La State Med Soc* 142(1):15–18, 1990.

Curtin HD: Pseudotumor. *Radiol Clin North Am* 25(3):583–599, 1987.

Deutsch TA, Corwin HL: Lupus optic neuritis with negative serology. *Ann Ophthalmol* 20:383–384, 1988.

Garrity JA, Kennerdell JS, Johnson BL, et al: Cyclophosphamide in the treatment of orbital vasculitis. *Am J Ophthalmol* 102(1):97–103, 1986.

Glover AT, Grove AS Jr: Eosinophilic granuloma of the orbit with spontaneous healing. *Ophthalmology* 94:1008–1012, 1987.

Goadsby PJ, Lance JW: Clinicopathological correlation in a case of painful ophthalmoplegia: Tolosa-Hunt syndrome. *J Neurol Neurosurg Psychiatry* 52:1290–1293, 1989.

Gutowski WM, Mulbury PE, Hengerer AS, et al: The role of C.T. scans in managing the orbital complications of ethmoiditis. *Int J Pediatr Otorhinolaryngol* 15:117–128, 1988.

Hannerz J, Ericson K, Bergstrand G: Orbital phlebography for differentiation between multiple sclerosis and venous vasculitis in subacute blindness. *Acta Radiol* 29(5):505–507, 1988.

Hodges E, Tabbara KF: Orbital cellulitis: Review of 23 cases from Saudi Arabia. *Br J Ophthalmol* 73:205–208, 1989.

Jackson K, Baker SR: Clinical implications of orbital cellulitis. *Laryngoscope* 96(5):568–574, 1986.

Kaufman DM, Litman N, Miller MH: Sinusitis: Induced subdural empyema. *Neurology* 33:123–132, 1983.

Moloney JR, Badham NJ, McRae A: The acute orbit: Preseptal (periorbital) cellulitis, subperiosteal abscess and orbital cellulitis due to sinusitis. *J Laryngol Otol Suppl* 12:1–18, 1987.

Patchett RB, Wilson WB, Ellis PP: Ophthalmic complications with disseminated intravascular coagulation. *Br J Ophthalmol* 72:377–379, 1988.

Sergott RC: Neuro-ophthalmic evaluation of the red orbit syndrome. *Neurol Clin* 1(4):897–908, 1983.

Spires JR, Smith RJH: Bacterial infections of the orbital and periorbital soft-tissues in children. *Laryngoscope* 96(7):763–767, 1986.

Thomas DJB, Charlesworth MC, Afshar F, et al: Computerised axial tomography and magnetic resonance scanning in the Tolosa-Hunt syndrome. *Br J Ophthalmol* 72:299–302, 1988.

Wenig BL, Goldstein MN, Abramson AL: Frontal sinusitis and its intracranial complications. *Int J Pediatr Otorhinolaryngol* 5:285–302, 1984.

Wesley RE, Cooper J, Litchford DW: Orbital inflammatory pseudotumor associated with multifocal systemic neoplastic immunoincompetence. *Ann Ophthalmol* 20:150–152, 1988.

Orbit—Neoplastic Lesions

Bartley GB, Garrity JA, Waller RR, et al: Orbital exenteration at the Mayo Clinic: 1967–1986. *Ophthalmology* 96:468–474, 1989.

Boldt HC, Nerad JA: Orbital metastases from prostate carcinoma. *Arch Ophthalmol* 106:1403–1408, 1988.

Capone A Jr, Slamovits TL: Discrete metastasis of solid tumors to extraocular muscles. *Arch Ophthalmol* 108:237–243, 1990.

Gross FJ, Waxman JS, Rosenblatt MA, et al: Eosinophilic granuloma of the cavernous sinus and orbital apex in an HIV-positive patient. *Ophthalmology* 96:462–467, 1989.

Knapp AJ, Gartner S, Henkind P: Multiple myeloma and its ocular manifestations. *Surv Ophthalmol* 31:343–351, 1987.

Lyons CJ, McNab AA, Garner A, et al: Orbital malignant peripheral nerve sheath tumours. *Br J Ophthalmol* 73:731–738, 1989.

Ormerod LD, Weber AL, Rauch SD, et al: Ophthalmic manifestations of maxillary sinus mucoceles. *Ophthalmology* 94:1013–1019, 1987.

Parrish CM, O'Day DM: Brown tumor of the orbit: Case report and review of the literature. *Arch Ophthalmol* 104:1199–1202, 1986.

Reifler DM, Davison P: Histochemical analysis of breast carcinoma metastatic to the orbit. *Ophthalmology* 93:254–259, 1986.

Sarkies NJC: Optic nerve sheath meningioma: Diagnostic features and therapeutic alternatives. *Eye* 1:597–602, 1987.

Shields JA, Shields CL, Lieb WE, et al: Multiple orbital neurofibromas unassociated with von Recklinghausen's disease. *Arch Ophthalmol* 108:80–83, 1990.

Yamasaki T, Handa H, Yamashita J, et al: Intracranial and orbital cavernous angiomas: A review of 30 cases. *J Neurosurg* 64:197–208, 1986.

Orbital Varices

Phanthumchinda K, Locharernkul C, Hemachudha T: Intermittent exophthalmos. *J Med Assoc Thai* 72(6):351–354, 1989.

Parasellar Syndromes

Bitoh S, Hasegawa H, Ohtsuki H, et al: Parasellar metastases: Four autopsied cases. *Surg Neurol* 23:41–48, 1985.

Grimson BS, Thompson HS: Raeder's syndrome: A clinical review. *Surv Ophthalmol* 24(4):199–210, 1980.

Mokri B: Raeder's paratrigeminal syndrome: Original concept and subsequent deviations. *Arch Neurol* 39:395–399, 1982.

Pituitary Apoplexy

Fong LP, Fabinyi GCA: Ophthalmic manifestations of pituitary apoplexy. *Med J Aust* 142:142–143, 1985.

Petersen P, Christiansen KH, Lindholm J: Acute monocular disturbances mimicking optic neuritis in pituitary apoplexy. *Acta Neurol Scand* 78:101–103, 1988.

Rosenbaum TJ, Houser OW, Laws ER: Pituitary apoplexy producing internal carotid artery occlusion: Case report. *J Neurosurg* 47:599–604, 1977.

Tsitsopoulos P, Andrew J, Harrison MJG: Pituitary apoplexy and haemorrhage into adenomas. *Postgrad Med J* 62:623–626, 1986.

Wakai S, Fukushima T, Teramoto A, et al: Pituitary apoplexy: Its incidence and clinical significance. *J Neurosurg* 55:187–193, 1981.

Sella Region—Related Ocular Pain

Baskin DS, Wilson CB: Surgical management of craniopharyngiomas: A review of 74 cases. *J Neurosurg* 65:22–27, 1986.

Cano M, Lainez JM, Escudero J, et al: Pituitary adenoma presenting as painful intermittent third nerve palsy. *Headache* 29:451–452, 1989.

Sphenopalatine Neuralgia

Babe J: Treatment of sphenopalatine ganglion neuralgia. *An Otorrinolaringol Ibero Am* 16(5):463–474, 1989.

Onofrio BM, Campbell JK: Surgical treatment of chronic cluster headache. *Mayo Clin Proc* 61(7):537–544, 1986.

Salar G, Ori C, Iob I, et al: Percutaneous thermocoagulation for sphenopalatine ganglion neuralgia. *Acta Neurochir (Wien)* 84(1–2):24–28, 1987.

Symptomatology of Eye Diseases

Scheie HG, Albert DM: Symptomatology of eye diseases, in *Textbook of Ophthalmology*, 9th ed. Philadelphia, Saunders, 1977, pp 159–168.

Trachoma

Barnes RC: Laboratory diagnosis of human chlamydial infections. *Clin Microbiol Rev* 2(2):119–136, 1989.

Barsoum IS, Mostafa MS, Shihab AA, et al: Prevalence of trachoma in school children and ophthalmological outpatients in rural Egypt. *Am J Trop Med Hyg* 36(1):97–101, 1987.

Elbagir A, Mardh PA: Evaluation of chlamydial tests in early trachoma. *APMIS* 98(3):276–280, 1990.

Lisby SM, Nahata MC: Recognition and treatment of chlamydial infections. *Clin Pharm* 6(1):25–36, 1987.

Rahi A, Rashood A, Rahi S, et al: Immunodiagnosis of ocular chlamydial infection. *Int Ophthalmol* 12(1):65–72, 1988.

Uveitis

Appiah AP, Hirose T: Secondary causes of premacular fibrosis. *Ophthalmology* 96(3):389–392, 1989.

Baarsma GS, La Hey E, Glasius E, et al: The predictive value of serum angiotensin converting enzyme and lysozyme levels in the diagnosis of ocular sarcoidosis. *Am J Ophthalmol* 104(3):211–217, 1987.

Bienfait MF, Hoogsteden HC, Baarsma GS, et al: Diagnostic value of bronchoalveolar lavage in ocular sarcoidosis. *Acta Ophthalmol (Copenh)* 65(6):745–748, 1987.

Bopp FP, Cheney ML, Donzis PB, et al: Heerfordt syndrome: A cause of facial paralysis. *J La State Med Soc* 142(2):13–15, 1990.

Cipriani D, Landonio G, Canepari C: A case of Vogt-Koyanagi-Harada syndrome in a patient affected by Hodgkin's disease. *J Neurol* 236(5):303–304, 1989.

Corriveau C, Easterbrook M, Payne D: Lymphoma simulating uveitis (masquerade syndrome). *Can J Ophthalmol* 21(4):144–149, 1986.

Croxatto JO, Hulsbus R, Lombardi A: Unsuspected mycobacterial endophthalmitis with increased aqueous lactate dehydrogenase levels in a child. *Ann Ophthalmol* 21(6):233–237, 1989.

Dash GI, Kimmelman CP: Head and neck manifestations of sarcoidosis. *Laryngoscope* 98(1):50–53, 1988.

Dussaix E, Cerqueti PM, Pontet F, et al: New approaches to the detection of locally produced antiviral antibodies in the aqueous of patients with endogenous uveitis. *Ophthalmologica* 194(2–3):145–149, 1987.

Ficker L, Meredith TA, Wilson LA, et al: Chronic bacterial endophthalmitis. *Am J Ophthalmol* 103(6):745–748, 1987.

Goldey SH, Stern GA, Oblon DJ, et al: Immunophenotypic characterization of an unusual T-cell lymphoma presenting as anterior uveitis: A clinicopathologic case report. *Arch Ophthalmol* 107(9):1349–1353, 1989.

Graham EM: Differential diagnosis of ocular sarcoidosis. *Sarcoidosis* 3(1):34–39, 1986.

Gur S, Silverstone BZ, Zylberman R, et al: Chorioretinitis and extrapulmonary tuberculosis. *Ann Ophthalmol* 19(3):112–115, 1987.

Heidemann DG, Trese M, Murphy SF, et al: Endogenous *Listeria monocytogenes* endophthalmitis presenting as keratouveitis. *Cornea* 9(2):179–180, 1990.

Heinemann MH, Gold JM, Maisel J: Bilateral toxoplasma retinochoroiditis in a patient with acquired immune deficiency syndrome. *Retina* 6(4):224–227, 1986.

Henderly DE, Genstler AJ, Smith RE, et al: Changing patterns of uveitis. *Am J Ophthalmol* 103(2):131–136, 1987.

Hira SK, Patel JS, Bhat SG, et al: Clinical manifestations of secondary syphilis. *Int J Dermatol* 26(2):103–107, 1987.

Hoover DL, Khan JA, Giangiacomo J: Pediatric ocular sarcoidosis. *Surv Ophthalmol* 30(4):215–228, 1986.

Itami, N, Akutsu Y, Yasoshima K, et al: Acute tubulointerstitial nephritis with uveitis (letter to editor). *Arch Intern Med* 150(3):688, 1990.

Jennings T, Tessler HH: Twenty cases of sympathetic ophthalmia. *Br J Ophthalmol* 73(2):140–145, 1989.

Joos R, Veys EM, Mielants H, et al: Clinical manifestations in HLA-B27-positive patients. *Clin Exp Rheumatol* 5(suppl 1):S41–S47, 1987.

Khalil MK, Lorenzetti DW: Lens-induced inflammations. *Can J Ophthalmol* 21(3):96–102, 1986.

Khan JA, Hoover DL, Giangiacomo J, et al: Orbital and childhood sarcoidosis. *J Pediatr Ophthalmol Strabismus* 23(4):190–194, 1986.

Kijlstra A, Breebaart AC, Baarsma GS, et al: Aqueous chamber taps in toxoplasmic chorioretinitis. *Doc Ophthalmol* 64(1):53–58, 1986.

Kijlstra A, Luyendijk L, Baarsma GS, et al: Aqueous humor analysis as a diagnostic tool in toxoplasma uveitis. *Int Ophthalmol* 13(6):383–386, 1989.

Kijlstra A, Rothova A, Baarsma GS, et al: Computer registration of uveitis patients. *Doc Ophthalmol* 67(1–2):139–143, 1987.

Kirmani MH, Thomas EL, Rao NA, et al: Intraocular reticulum cell sarcoma: Diagnosis by choroidal biopsy. *Br J Ophthalmol* 71(10):748–752, 1987.

Kittiponghansa S, Prabriputaloong A, Pariyanonda S, et al: Intracameral gnathostomiasis: A cause of anterior uveitis and secondary glaucoma. *Br J Ophthalmol* 71(8):618–622, 1987.

Kunnamo I, Pelkonen P: Routine analysis of synovial fluid cells is of value in the differential diagnosis of arthritis in children. *J Rheumatol* 13(6):1076–1080, 1986.

Lappin MR, Greene CE, Winston S, et al: Clinical feline toxoplasmosis: Serologic diagnosis and therapeutic management of 15 cases. *J Vet Intern Med* 3(3):139–143, 1989.

Linssen A, Dekker-Saeys AJ, Dijkstra PF, et al: The use of HLA-B27 as a diagnostic and prognostic aid in acute anterior uveitis (AAU) in the Netherlands. *Doc Ophthalmol* 64(2):217–223, 1986.

Ljung BM, Char D, Miller TR, et al: Intraocular lymphoma: Cytologic diagnosis and the role of immunologic markers. *Acta Cytol* 32(6):840–847, 1988.

Mannis MJ, Tamaru R, Roth AM, et al: *Acanthamoeba* sclerokeratitis: Determining diagnostic criteria. *Arch Ophthalmol* 104(9):1313–1317, 1986.

McClellan KA, Coster DJ: Uveitis: A strategy for diagnosis. *Aust N Z J Ophthalmol* 15(3):227–241, 1987.

Miller P: Seronegative arthritis: Etiology and diagnosis. *Scand J Rheumatol Suppl* 66:119–127, 1987.

Morgan ED, Laszlo JD, Stumph PG: Incomplete Behçet's syndrome in the differential diagnosis of genital ulceration and postcoital bleeding: A case report. *J Reprod Med* 33(10):844–846, 1988.

Murray P: Serum autoantibodies and uveitis. *Br J Ophthalmol* 70(4):266–268, 1986.

Ohtahara A, Kotake H, Hisatome I, et al: Complete atrioventricular block with a 22-month history of ocular sarcoidosis: A case report. *Heart Lung* 16(1):66–68, 1987.

Passo MS, Rosenbaum JT: Ocular syphilis in patients with human immunodeficiency virus infection. *Am J Ophthalmol* 106(1):1–6, 1988.

Pellegrini V, Ohno S, Hirose S, et al: Subretinal neovascularisation and snow banking in a case of sarcoidosis: Case report. *Br J Ophthalmol* 70(6):474–477, 1986.

Rosenbaum JT: Characterization of uveitis associated with spondyloarthritis. *J Rheumatol* 16(6):792–796, 1989.

Rosenbaum JT: Uveitis: An internist's view. *Arch Intern Med* 149:1173–1176, 1989.

Rosenbaum JT, Bennett RM: Chronic anterior and posterior uveitis and primary Sjögren's syndrome. *Am J Ophthalmol* 104(4):346–352, 1987.

Rothova A, Meenken C, Michels RP, et al: Uveitis and diabetes mellitus. *Am J Ophthalmol* 106(1):17–20, 1988.

Rothova A, van Knapen F, Baarsma GS, et al: Serology in ocular toxoplasmosis. *Br J Ophthalmol* 70(8):615–622, 1986.

Rouwen AJ, Wijermans PW, Boen-Tan TN, et al: Intraocular non-Hodgkin's lymphoma treated with systemic and intrathecal chemotherapy and radiotherapy: A case report and review of the literature. *Graefes Arch Clin Exp Ophthalmol* 227(4):355–359, 1989.

Sabates R: Choroiditis compatible with the histopathologic diagnosis of sympathetic ophthalmia following cyclocryotherapy of neovascular glaucoma. *Ophthalmic Surg* 19(3):176–182, 1988.

Stone SP, Bendig J, Hakim J, et al: Cryptococcal meningitis presenting as uveitis. *Br J Ophthalmol* 72(3):167–170, 1988.

Sugimoto M, Nakashima H, Ando M, et al: Bronchoalveolar lavage studies in uveitis patients without radiological intrathoracic involvement of sarcoidosis. *Jpn J Med* 28(1):50–54, 1989.

Tabbut BR, Tessler HH, Williams D: Fuchs' heterochromic iridocyclitis in blacks. *Arch Ophthalmol* 106(12):1688–1690, 1988.

Trudeau M, Shepherd FA, Blackstein ME, et al: Intraocular lymphoma: Report of three cases and review of the literature. *Am J Clin Oncol* 11(2):126–130, 1988.

Veldman E, Bos PJ: Neuroretinitis in secondary syphilis. *Doc Ophthalmol* 64(1):23–29, 1986.

Wang FD, Wang LS, Liu YC, et al: Successful treatment of metastatic endophthalmitis: Case reports. *Ophthalmologica* 198(3):124–128, 1989.

Ward K, O'Connor C, Odlum C, et al: Prognostic value of bronchoalveolar lavage in sarcoidosis: The critical influence of disease presentation. *Thorax* 44(1):6–12, 1989.

Wirostko E, Johnson L, Wirostko W: Juvenile rheumatoid arthritis inflammatory eye disease: Parasitization of ocular leukocytes by mollicute-like organisms. *J Rheumatol* 16(11):1446–1453, 1989.

Wirostko E, Johnson L, Wirostko B: Sarcoidosis associated uveitis: Parasitization of vitreous leucocytes by mollicute-like organisms. *Acta Ophthalmol (Copenh)* 67(4):415–424, 1989.

Zadnik K: Cataracts, chronic uveitis, and retinal vasculitis in Behçet's disease. *Am J Optom Physiol Opt* 64(1):72–75, 1987.

Zierhut M, Kreissig I, Pickert A: Panuveitis with positive serological tests for syphilis and Lyme disease. *J Clin Neuro Ophthalmol* 9(2):71–75, 1989.

Vascular Disorders of the Eye

Dhopesh VP, Goldman WH: Eye and frontal pain in posterior lesions: A reappraisal. *Headache* 27:34, 1987.

Edmeads J: Headaches in cerebrovascular disease: A common symptom of stroke. *Postgrad Med* 81(8):191–193, 196–198, 1987.

Edwards KK, Lindsley HB, Lai C-W, et al: Takayasu arteritis presenting as retinal and vertebrobasilar ischemia. *J Rheumatol* 16:1000–1002, 1989.

Gorelick PB, Hier DB, Caplan LR, et al: Headache in acute cerebrovascular disease. *Neurology* 36:1445–1450, 1986.

Tippin J, Corbett JJ, Kerber RE, et al: Amaurosis fugax and ocular infarction in adolescents and young adults. *Ann Neurol* 26:69–77, 1989.

4 Acute Ear Pain

☐ **DIAGNOSTIC LIST**

1. Disorders of the auricle
   A. Cellulitis
   B. Trauma
   C. Sebaceous cyst
   D. Impetigo
   E. Relapsing polychondritis
   F. Cold injury
      1. Perniosis (chilblains)
      2. Frostbite
   G. Chondrodermatitis helicis
   H. Gouty tophus
   I. Varicella-zoster virus
   J. Herpes simplex virus
   K. Contact dermatitis
2. Disorders of the external and middle ear
   A. Acute otitis externa
   B. Furuncle of the external canal
   C. Malignant otitis externa
   D. Acute suppurative otitis media

   E. Bullous myringitis
   F. Aerotitis and eustachian tube insufficiency
   G. Acute mastoiditis
3. Referred pain
   A. Dental disease
   B. Tonsillitis
   C. Lingual tonsillitis
   D. Peritonsillar abscess (quinsy)
   E. Acute cervical lymphadenitis
   F. Posttonsillectomy pain
   G. Temporomandibular joint trauma
   H. Thyroiditis
      1. Acute suppurative thyroiditis
      2. Subacute thyroiditis
   I. Parotitis
      1. Acute viral parotitis
      2. Acute suppurative parotitis

☐ **SUMMARY**

Cellulitis of the auricle causes redness, swelling, pain, and tenderness of the entire auricle, including the lobule. Fever, chills, and malaise may accompany the local inflammatory response. This disorder may occur spontaneously or follow an acute or chronic external otitis, a localized skin disorder of the auricle (eczematoid dermatitis or seborrheic dermatitis), or trauma. *Trauma* may cause redness, abrasions, lacerations, chondral fractures, seromas, hematomas, and abscess forma-

tion. A *sebaceous cyst* may form a red, painful cystic mass behind the lobule. The overlying skin is red and tender. Pain and tenderness respond to excision or drainage of the cyst. *Impetigo* causes an erythematous crusting lesion on the ear and face. *Relapsing polychondritis* causes bilateral redness and tenderness of the skin overlying the auricular cartilage but spares the lobules. Ear pain is related to the erythematous swollen auricles. Similar pain, redness, and tenderness may affect the distal nose. Anterior neck pain and tenderness may be secondary to thyroid cartilage and tracheal involvement.

Cold injury of the auricles may cause *chilblains*, with reddish, cyanotic, edematous ears, fingers, and toes or *frostbite*, with redness, pain, scaling, vesicle formation, and pruritus. *Chondrodermatitis helicis* is a small, painful inflammatory nodule that forms spontaneously on the helix of one or both ears. It is more common in older men and on the right side, but bilateral lesions may occur (3–6 percent). A *gouty tophus* may simulate chondrodermatitis or a furuncle of the auricle, but the "pus" draining from it consists of chalky white urate crystals. *Varicella-zoster* virus may cause vesicles and crusted ulcers on the auricle and in the ear canal, and severe burning or aching ear pain. Facial paresis and sometimes deafness, vertigo, and tinnitus associated with ear pain and vesicular skin lesions constitute the *Ramsay Hunt syndrome*. *Herpes simplex* virus may cause auricular pain and tenderness associated with skin vesicles and crusted ulcers. Cultures may be required to differentiate this disorder from herpes zoster. *Contact dermatitis* may cause localized (e.g., from earrings in the lobule) or generalized inflammation of the auricle (e.g., shampoo or hair spray).

Acute otitis externa causes mild to severe otalgia, pain on movement of the auricle, otorrhea, and canal stenosis with partial or complete loss of hearing. The canal is red, friable, and swollen, and there is a rapid response to topical corticosteroid and polymyxin therapy.

A *furuncle of the external canal* causes localized tenderness, redness, and severe pain just within the external auditory meatus. Local pressure on the furuncle with the ear speculum provokes or intensifies the pain. *Malignant otitis externa* usually occurs in elderly diabetics and in immunosuppressed pediatric patients. Severe otalgia; otorrhea; and a swollen, tender canal are common findings. Preauricular tenderness may be present, as may temporomandibular joint pain and tenderness. Opening the mouth may provoke pain. The sedimentation rate is usually markedly elevated; the bone scan and gallium-67 scan is usually positive; and a CT scan may demonstrate bone erosion and soft tissue infiltration of the mastoid, middle ear, temporomandibular joint, and jugular bulb region. Impairment of nerve VII and sometimes nerves IX, X, XI, and XII may occur with advanced disease. There is a good therapeutic response to ciprofloxacin, rifampin, and other antipseudomonal regimens.

Acute suppurative otitis media causes ear pain in the presence of a normal canal. The tympanic membrane is reddened or yellow and bulging and has poor mobility and absent or distorted landmarks. Membrane rupture and purulent otorrhea may occur. Bullous myringitis can be diagnosed by otoscopic examination: It may be caused by mycoplasmal, viral, or bacterial infection. Otalgia, a red tympanic membrane, ear fullness, and deafness may follow descent of a pressurized aircraft. The tympanic membrane may be red and serous, or bloody fluid may be present in the middle ear. *Acute mastoiditis* causes postauricular aching, otorrhea, low-grade fever, and mastoid tenderness. Pain radiographs or a CT scan will demonstrate mastoid air cell clouding.

Referred pain to the ear simulates otic disease, but there is no abnormality of the external canal or middle ear. *Dental*

TABLE OF DISEASE INCIDENCE

INCIDENCE PER 100,000 (APPROXIMATE)

Common (>100)	Uncommon (>5–100)	Rare (>0–5)
Trauma to the auricle	Cellulitis of the auricle	Relapsing polychondritis
Sebaceous cyst	Impetigo of the auricle	Perniosis (chilblains) in United States
Frostbite	Chondrodermatitis helicis	Gouty tophus with acute inflammation
Acute external otitis	Varicella-zoster virus (Ramsay Hunt syndrome)	Herpes simplex virus infection of the auricle
Furuncle of the external canal	Contact dermatitis of the auricle	Acute suppurative thyroiditis
Dental disease	Malignant otitis externa	
Tonsillitis	Acute suppurative otitis media in adults	
Acute cervical lymphadenitis	Bullous myringitis	
Posttonsillectomy pain	Aerotitis media	
Acute viral parotitis	Acute mastoiditis	
	Lingual tonsillitis	
	Peritonsillar abscess	
	Temporomandibular joint trauma	
	Subacute thyroiditis	
	Acute suppurative parotitis	

disease (pulpitis and/or periapical abscess), *tonsillitis, lingual tonsillitis*, a *peritonsillar abscess*, or *cervical adenitis* may cause referred otalgia. Otalgia is a common *posttonsillectomy* symptom. *Temporomandibular joint injuries* may cause referred otalgia, as may *inflammatory involvement of the thyroid or parotid glands*.

☐ DESCRIPTION OF LISTED DISEASES

1. DISORDERS OF THE AURICLE

A. Cellulitis Pain, warmth, redness, tenderness, and edema of one auricle occur. The inflammatory process involves the lobule and may extend into the adjacent face, scalp, and lateral neck. Fever, chills, and malaise may occur. Cervical lymphadenitis occurs on the ipsilateral side. There may be preceding trauma, an external otitis, or a chronic eczematous dermatitis of the auricle or ear canal. There is a good response to parenteral antibiotic therapy.

B. Trauma Injury to the auricle may cause edema, redness, and ecchymosis of the auricle. A seroma or hematoma may be present, causing swelling, deformity, and fluctuance of the auricle. Infection of the seroma and/or hematoma may lead to abscess formation, with fever, chills, and malaise, and spontaneous drainage of purulent material from a fluctuant auricular mass. Seromas and/or hematomas should be aspirated to relieve pain and risk of subsequent infection. Other injuries include chondral fractures, abrasions, and lacerations.

C. Sebaceous Cyst   Local redness, tenderness, and pain may be caused by a retroauricular cystic lesion. This may become secondarily infected, resulting in redness and edema of the adjacent skin. Drainage or excision of the cyst and antibiotic therapy usually relieve the retroauricular pain and tenderness.

D. Impetigo   Local pain, redness, tenderness, crusting, and pruritus of the auricle may occur. Similar crusted lesions may occur on the side of the face and neck. Telephone use has been associated with transmission of this type of superficial streptococcal or staphylococcal infection. The right ear is most commonly affected when the telephone has been the vehicle of spread. There is a good response to the use of a local antibiotic ointment and/or oral antibiotics.

E. Relapsing Polychondritis   The initial attack of this disorder may begin with unilateral or bilateral ear pain, swelling, redness, and tenderness that spare the lobule. Bilateral involvement with an erythematous cartilaginous portion of the auricle and pale white lobule are characteristic. The distal nose may also become painful, red, and tender. Thyroid cartilage and tracheal involvement cause anterior neck pain and tenderness. Bilateral symmetrical arthralgias may occur in the hands, knees, and ankles due to a nonerosive arthritis. High-dose corticosteroid therapy or dapsone usually controls pain, tenderness, and other inflammatory signs.

F. Cold Injury

   1. Perniosis (Chilblains)   Redness or reddish-blue cyanosis and edema affect the hands, feet, auricles, and other cold-exposed areas. A burning discomfort accompanies the skin changes. These lesions occur in winter after chronic exposure to nonfreezing cold temperatures This disorder is uncommon in the United States, where central heating and warm, dry clothing are readily available. In Britain, it is estimated that in winter 10 percent of the population is affected. Small ulcerations of the fingers and toes may occur. A move to a warm, dry climate usually results in rapid resolution. Nifedipine, in doses of 60 mg/day, may prevent lesion development and speed healing.

   2. Frostbite   Stinging or burning pain occurs in both auricles on exposure to freezing cold. Within 20 to 40

min, the pain is replaced by numbness. On recovering, the pain may recur, and within 24 h the auricles may become red, edematous, and tender. Vesicle formation and peeling may follow during the next 7 days.

G. Chondrodermatitis Helicis (Winkler's Disease)   A firm, tender, and painful nodule (0.3–3 cm) appears on the auricle in the region of the helix. The pain is intermittent and may last for hours. It may be provoked by lying on the affected ear or by cold and is sometimes relieved by removal of crusts. Skin redness, ulceration, and crusting may be associated with the lesion. Middle-aged or elderly men are most commonly affected (male/female ratio is 10:1). The right ear is most commonly affected, and bilateral lesions occur in only 3 to 6 percent. Intralesional injection of a corticosteroid or excision relieves the pain and tenderness. This disorder is not associated with any systemic disease.

   Other nodular lesions that may mimic chondrodermatitis helicis include carcinomas, keratoacanthoma, and verrucae. These are usually painless, unless ulceration has occurred. Differentiation may require biopsy.

H. Gouty Tophus   Patients with a gouty tophus are usually asymptomatic. Occasionally, a tophus may enlarge and become tender, with an erythematous base simulating a furuncle. Spontaneous discharge of chalky white urate crystals may occur, mimicking drainage of a furuncle. Microscopic examination of the chalky ''pus'' will reveal a mass of urate crystals.

I. Varicella-Zoster Virus   Burning pain and/or pruritus may affect one auricle and ear canal. The onset of pain is followed within a few days by the appearance of grouped vesicles and crusted small ulcers on the skin of the auricle near the external meatus and in the ear canal. When an ipsilateral facial palsy (nerve VII) accompanies the painful eruption, this disorder is known as the Ramsay Hunt syndrome. Tinnitus, deafness, and vertigo may also be associated. An open trial of intravenous acyclovir was effective in relieving otalgia and the associated skin eruption but had only a minimal effect on hearing loss and vertigo.

J. Herpes Simplex Virus   This virus may cause grouped, painful, and tender vesicles and crusted ulcers on the skin of the auricle and side of the face. Vague otalgia and facial pain may accompany the eruption, and the local lesions may be tender. Differentiation from herpes zoster may require viral culture.

K. Contact Dermatitis   This disorder may occur on one or both sides. The auricle may become red, tender, and swollen, with weeping and crusting of the skin of the canal and pinna. Causes include soaps, hair sprays, shampoos, and perfumes. Involvement of the lobule may be caused by earrings, and of the ear canal by hearing aids and the compounds used to clean them. Removal of the causative allergen leads to relief of symptoms within 2 to 7 days.

2. DISORDERS OF THE EXTERNAL AND MIDDLE EAR

A. Acute Otitis Externa   Pain occurs in one or both ear canals, associated with drainage of cheesy white or yellowish exudate from the canal. Movement of the auricle or pressure on the tragus intensifies the pain. Fever is seldom present. The canal is usually edematous and filled with exudate. Removal of the exudate reveals an erythematous, friable canal wall that bleeds easily. The tympanic membrane may be coated with a gray-white exudate but is otherwise normal. The canal may be stenotic due to edema and may even be closed, causing hearing impairment. Cultures of the exudate usually grow *Pseudomonas aeruginosa.* There is a prompt therapeutic response to removal of exudate and instillation of polymyxin-neomycin-hydrocortisone eardrops. Rarely, spread of the infection to the auricle may occur, with pain, redness, swelling, and tenderness. This complication will usually respond to parenteral antibiotic therapy. Otitis externa usually occurs in hot and humid climates (i.e., tropical areas or summer) and is associated with water sports (swimmer's ear). Other cases may follow trauma to the canal with a hairpin or cotton swab.

B. Furuncle of the External Canal   Aching and/or throbbing pain occurs in the outer portion of one ear canal. Local tenderness may be present in the outer canal, and the pain is intensified by movement of the auricle or tragus. Local pressure with the ear speculum on the lesion reproduces or intensifies the pain. Inspection of the canal reveals a white-capped, red-based furuncle near the external meatus. Surgical or spontaneous drainage of this localized abscess provides dramatic pain relief.

C. Malignant Otitis Externa   The usual duration of symptoms before diagnosis is 3 to 8 weeks, but acute cases, with a history of only 1 week, may occur. Almost all patients have mild to severe diabetes mellitus. Elderly males are most commonly affected, but cases in children and adolescents have been recorded. This syndrome may occur rarely in patients with leukemia and granulocytopenia, children receiving chemotherapy for malignancy, and other pediatric patients with an immune deficiency state secondary to anemia and malnutrition.

Malignant otitis externa causes persistent severe to excruciating unilateral ear pain (75–100 percent of cases). The extreme severity of the pain is suggestive of the diagnosis. Severe headache in the temporal or occipital area may accompany the ear pain. Local temporomandibular joint pain and tenderness may occur, and this is intensified by opening the mouth, chewing, or talking. Purulent otorrhea occurs in 50 to 81 percent. Pressure on the tragus or

traction on the auricle intensifies the pain. The canal is edematous and red and contains exudate. Granulation tissue may be present at the juncture of the cartilaginous and bony external canal. Fever may occur. Cranial nerve dysfunction is associated and provides evidence of invasive infection. The facial nerve is most commonly affected (23–43 percent), but other neuropathies may involve nerves IX, X, and XI, causing hoarseness, dysphagia, and ipsilateral shoulder weakness (jugular foramen syndrome). Tongue weakness and dysarthria may result from nerve XII involvement in the hypoglossal canal. Treatment may sometimes reverse these cranial neuropathies.

The sedimentation rate is usually markedly elevated (Mean = 87 mm/h), with values frequently exceeding 100 mm/h. High sedimentation rates seldom occur with simple external otitis or carcinoma of the external canal.

A technetium 99m bone scan is 100 percent sensitive for malignant otitis externa, but its specificity is, unfortunately, low. Severe cases of simple external otitis may have bone scans similar to those with malignant otitis. Positive scans may also occur with temporomandibular joint disorders, fractures, and head and neck cancer. Gallium-67 scans are also highly sensitive (89–100 percent) but are also nonspecific. CT scans are useful for detection of bone erosion and soft tissue infiltration in the external canal, the region of the temporomandibular joint, the masticator space, and the hypoglossal canal. Fluid in the middle ear or mastoid air cells can also be imaged. CT is less sensitive than a radionuclide scan or MRI for the imaging of early disease.

Antibiotic therapy (oral ciprofloxacin and rifampin, intravenous cefsuloden, or intravenous piperacillin and tobramycin) will usually relieve ear pain, fever, and discharge within 1 week. Prolonged therapy beyond 8 weeks may be required to prevent relapse.

Persistent external otitis for more than 2 weeks or frequent recurrence; excruciating ear pain; evidence of cranial neuropathy; a high sedimentation rate; and a positive radionuclide bone or CT scan, or MRI support the diagnosis of malignant otitis externa.

D. Acute Suppurative Otitis Media   Constant aching pain of one or both ears is the most frequent complaint. Pressure on the tragus or traction on the auricle has no effect on the pain. Otorrhea is associated with perforation of the drum. Without an opening in the tympanic membrane, otorrhea is absent, and the external canal is normal. Signs reported to be useful in the diagnosis of otitis media include redness of the tympanic membrane, distortion of the light reflex, and disappearance of the concave contour of the tympanic membrane near the umbo. In one study, a yellow (82 percent) or red (19 percent) bulging drum (100 percent) occurred in patients with acute otitis media. Evidence of decreased tympanic membrane mobility has also been reported in children with this disorder. Air bubbles and fluid in the middle ear and hemorrhagic areas on the tympanic membrane also occur.

Acute otitis media has its peak incidences at ages 6 to 36 months and between ages 4 and 7 years, although adolescents and adults may be affected. Fever frequently may be absent in adults. Hearing loss is common, and tinnitus and vertigo may occur. There is a good response of symptoms and signs to antibiotic therapy.

E. Bullous Myringitis   Patients have pain, in one or both ears, of a constant aching quality. Otoscopic observation reveals one or more tympanic membrane bullae. The cause is a viral or mycoplasma infection, but bacterial organisms may cause similar bullous lesions. There is a response to appropriate antimicrobial therapy.

F. Aerotitis and Eustachian Tube Insufficiency   Ear pain, fullness, and unilateral or bilateral hearing loss may follow descent in a pressurized aircraft. Performance of a Valsalva maneuver one or more times or swallowing may open the eustachian tube and relieve pain, fullness, and hearing loss. Unrelieved obstruction of the eustachian tube may result in tympanic membrane redness; a serous or hemorrhagic middle ear effusion (hemotympanum); and persistent otalgia, fullness, and hearing loss. Myringotomy will relieve symptoms, and antibiotics are usually not required.

G. Acute Mastoiditis   This disorder may follow an inadequately treated acute suppurative otitis media. Dull, aching retroauricular pain; otorrhea; mastoid tenderness; and a low-grade fever are commonly present. The middle ear may contain purulent material, and the tympanic membrane may appear dull and edematous. Plain radiographs or a CT scan will demonstrate clouding of mastoid air cells and loss of bony intercellular walls. This disorder may respond to antibiotic therapy and myringotomy, but simple mastoidectomy may be required.

3. REFERRED PAIN

Otalgia, occurring without any signs of disease of the auricle, ear canal, or middle ear, is usually due to disease at another site and is not caused by otic disease.

A. Dental Disease   An acute inflammation of the dental pulp (pulpitis) or a periapical abscess can cause pressure or hot and/or cold temperature–provoked dental pain in the region of the diseased tooth, and/or ipsilateral otalgia. In some cases, ear pain without dental pain can be provoked by having the patient hold crushed ice in the ipsilateral side of the mouth. Characteristic pain is provoked in less than 2 min. In other cases, dental radiographs may provide the only clue to an obscure cause of otalgia. Such films may show caries, a restoration immediately adjacent to the dental pulp, or a periapical abscess. The ear pain is often intermittent, aching, and sometimes burning and often awak-

ens the patients 2 or 3 h after retiring, since dental pain is often intensified in the supine position. Inhalation through the mouth may intensify the pain. Extraction or root canal surgery resulting in pain relief will confirm the diagnosis.

B. Tonsillitis   An acute tonsillitis or lateral pharyngitis may cause ipsilateral or bilateral otalgia. The affected tonsil is usually red and swollen and may be covered with white or yellow-white exudate. Swallowing may or may not intensify the ear pain. There is prompt relief with antibiotic therapy.

C. Lingual Tonsillitis   This disorder may cause posterior tongue and throat pain intensified by swallowing, and unilateral or bilateral otalgia. Fever may be present. The diagnosis requires examination of the posterior tongue with a mirror.

D. Peritonsillar Abscess (Quinsy)   There is a history of a sore throat for several days that appears to be improving, but then one side becomes very painful. Odynophagia may become extreme, and the patient may sit with his or her mouth partially open, drooling saliva. The voice is muffled ("hot potato voice"), and ipsilateral otalgia occurs. Fever, chills, sweats, and cervical adenitis are present. Trismus may occur on the affected side. The tonsil bulges toward the midline and forward. The adjacent palate is red and edematous. Pus may drain spontaneously from the anterior faucial pillar. Prolonged antibiotic therapy is required to ensure control of the infection, and incision and drainage may be necessary. Tonsillectomy should be performed to prevent recurrence once the acute inflammatory edema has resolved.

E. Acute Cervical Lymphadenitis   Pharyngitis or tonsillar or dental disease may cause a unilateral or bilateral cervical adenitis with tender, enlarged nodes at the angle of the jaw. Nodes larger than 1 cm may be felt in this area, and pressure over the tender ones may reproduce the patient's otalgia. There is a prompt response to antibiotic therapy. Examination of the ear canals and tympanic membranes reveals no abnormalities.

F. Posttonsillectomy Pain   Patients may feel posttonsillectomy pain in the throat, especially on swallowing, and in one or both ears. Within a period of several weeks, this pain vanishes. Persistence after 2 months should suggest the possibility of an Eagle's syndrome caused by an elongated styloid process.

G. Temporomandibular Joint Trauma   Acute injury to the joint, associated ligaments, and muscles may cause unilateral or bilateral temporomandibular joint and ear pain. Pain may follow direct blows to the mandible or sudden acceleration or deceleration (whiplash) injuries. Associated symptoms may include head and facial pain; tinnitus; a partial loss of hearing; pain on chewing, talking, or opening the mouth; and unstable occlusal disturbances (crossbite or posterior or anterior open bite), joint crepitus, and locking. MRI and/or contrast arthrographic studies of patients with these symptoms and signs have demonstrated an internal derangement of the temporomandibular joint meniscus, retrodiscal tissue swelling, joint effusion or bleeding, condyle and condylar neck fractures, osteochondritis dissecans, avascular necrosis or musculotendinous injuries, and atrophy of masticatory muscles.

H. Thyroiditis   Pain occurs in the anterior neck in one or both paratracheal regions. It is intensified by swallowing and by direct palpation. Referral cephalad to one or both ears is common and is an important clue to the diagnosis.

1. Acute Suppurative Thyroiditis   Neck pain, local tenderness, redness, and swelling are prominent. Fever and toxicity are common, and a fluctuant abscess may become palpable, with skin erythema and pustules. Pain may radiate to the ipsilateral ear. Abscess formation usually involves one lobe. Antibiotic therapy and surgical drainage lead to recovery.

2. Subacute Thyroiditis   Patients have anterior neck and referred otalgia to one or both sides, with minimal fever and toxicity. Some patients believe they have a simple throat infection. Up to 50 percent of patients develop transient mild hyperthyroidism with palpitations, tremors, sweating, and weight loss. The thyroid scan shows a failure of radioiodine uptake during the first 6

to 8 weeks after onset, while serum levels of T_3 and T_4 are normal or elevated.

I. Parotitis

1. Acute Viral Parotitis   This infection begins with malaise, fever, ear pain, and swelling anterior to the tragus at the angle of the jaw and in the submental region. Acute mumps is the commonest cause, but parotid inflammation may occur with Coxsackie A, Epstein-Barr, influenza A, and lymphocytic choriomeningitis infections.

2. Acute Suppurative Parotitis   Patients may have acute preauricular swelling and skin redness associated with high fever, chills or rigors, sweats, and toxemia. The parotid is exquisitely tender and may rapidly become fluctuant. Preauricular and deeper ear pain may occur on the ipsilateral side. The orifice of the duct of the infected parotid gland is often red and drains purulent material. In some cases, gentle pressure on the duct is required to deliver pus from the orifice. A debilitated state, the postoperative period, use of anticholinergics or drugs with similar oral drying activity (tranquilizers and antihistamines), dehydration, sialolithiasis, diuretic therapy, oral cancer, immunosuppression, and tracheostomy are risk factors for this disorder. *Staphylococcus aureus* is the commonest infecting organism, but *Streptococcus pneumoniae*, other streptococci, and gram-negative bacilli have also been isolated. There may be a response to intravenous antibiotics alone, but in some cases surgical exploration and drainage are required.

EAR PAIN REFERENCES

Auricular Pain

Cannon CR: Bilateral chondrodermatitis helicis: Case presentation and literature review. *Am J Otol* 6(2):164–166, 1985.

Carruthers R: Chilblains (perniosis). *Aust Fam Phys* 17(11):968–969, 1988.

Dahl MV: Strategies for the management of recurrent furunculosis. *South Med J* 80(3):352–356, 1987.

Hedström SÅ: Treatment and prevention of recurrent staphylococcal furunculosis: Clinical and bacteriological follow-up. *Scand J Infect Dis* 17:55–58, 1985.

Heffner DK, Hyams VJ: Cystic chondromalacia (endochondral pseudocyst) of the auricle. *Arch Pathol Lab Med* 110:740–743, 1986.

Lazar RH, Heffner DK, Hughes GB, et al: Pseudocyst of the auricle: A review of 21 cases. *Otolaryngol Head Neck Surg* 94:360–361, 1986.

Rustin MHA, Newton JA, Smith NP, et al: The treatment of chilblains with nifedipine: The results of a pilot study, a double-blind placebo-controlled randomized study and a long-term open trial. *Br J Dermatol* 120:267–275, 1989.

Sane DC, Vidaillet HJ Jr, Burton CS: Saddle nose, red ears, and fatal airway collapse. *Chest* 91(2):268–270, 1987.

External Ear—Carcinoma

Paaske PB, Witten J, Schwer S, et al: Results in treatment of carcinoma of the external auditory canal and middle ear. *Cancer* 59:156–160, 1987.

External Ear—Malignant Otitis

Amedee RG, Mann WJ: Osteomyelitis of the skull base: An unusual manifestation. *Am J Otol* 10(5):402–404, 1989.

Benuck I, Traisman HS: Malignant external otitis in a diabetic adolescent. *J Adolesc Health Care* 7:57–59, 1986.

Giordano JA, Phillips J: Malignant external otitis: Now a medical problem. *Diabetes Care* 3:611–614, 1980.

Mendelson MH, Meyers BR, Hirschman SZ, et al: Treatment of invasive external otitis with cefsulodin. *Rev Infect Dis* 6(suppl 3):S698–S704, 1984.

Rubin J, Stoehr G, Yu VL, et al: Efficacy of oral ciprofloxacin plus rifampin for treatment of malignant external otitis. *Arch Otolaryngol Head Neck Surg* 115:1063–1069, 1989.

Rubin J, Yu VL: Malignant external otitis: Insights into pathogenesis, clinical manifestations, diagnosis, and therapy. *Am J Med* 85(3):391–398, 1988.

Lateral Sinus Thrombosis
Hawkins DB: Lateral sinus thrombosis: A sometimes unexpected diagnosis. *Laryngoscope* 95:674–677, 1985.

Otalgia
Mattucci KF, Choo YB: Otalgia, in Cooper BC, Lucente FE (eds): *Management of Facial, Head and Neck Pain.* Philadelphia, Saunders, 1989, pp 53–76.

Otalgia—Eagle's Syndrome
Correll RW, Wescott WB: Eagle's syndrome diagnosed after history of headache, dysphagia, otalgia, and limited neck movement. *J Am Dent Assoc* 104(4):491–492, 1982.

Otalgia—Geniculate Neuralgia
Sharan R, Isser DK, Narayan HP: Clinical records: Juvenile nervus intermedius otalgia. *J Laryngol Otol* 94:1069–1073, 1980.
Tralla M, Schindler RA: Twelfth nerve neurilemmoma occurring in the middle ear. *Otolaryngol Head Neck Surg* 90:662–664, 1982.
Yeh H-s, Tew JM Jr: Tic convulsif: The combination of geniculate neuralgia and hemifacial spasm relieved by vascular decompression. *Neurology* 34:682–684, 1984.

Otalgia—Neoplastic
Hahn SS, Kim J-A, Goodchild N, et al: Carcinoma of the middle ear and external auditory canal. *Int J Radiat Oncol Biol Phys* 9:1003–1007, 1983.
Harner SG, Olsen KD, Banks PM, et al: Lymphocytic lymphoma involving the middle ear. *Mayo Clin Proc* 55:645–647, 1980.
Harries MLL: Melanoma metastatic to the head and neck. *J Laryngol Otol* 102:842–844, 1988.

Otalgia—Psychogenic Pain
Dight R: Psychogenic earache: An unusual cause of otalgia. *Med J Aust* 1:76–77, 1980.
Gilbert RW, Pierse PM, Mitchell DP: Cryptic otalgia: A case of Munchausen syndrome in a pediatric patient. *J Otolaryngol* 16(4):231–233, 1987.

Otalgia—Referred Pain
Clark JL: Otalgia: Identifying the source. *Postgrad Med* 70(4):99–103, 1981.
Gooder P: Follicular carcinoma in a lingual thyroid. *J Laryngol Otol* 94:437–439, 1980.
Jackler RK, Brackmann DE: Xanthoma of the temporal bone and skull base. *Am J Otol* 8(2):111–115, 1987.
Kreisberg MK, Turner J: Dental causes of referred otalgia. *Ear Nose Throat J* 66(10):398–408, 1987.
Robertson MS, Hornibrook J: The presenting symptoms of head and neck cancer. *N Z Med J* 95(708):337–341, 1982.
Thaller SR, DeSilva A: Otalgia with a normal ear. *Am Fam Physician* 36(4):129–136, 1987.
Wazen JJ: Referred otalgia. *Otolaryngol Clin North Am* 22(6):1205–1215, 1989.
Wilder WH, Harner SG, Banks PM: Lymphoma of the nose and paranasal sinuses. *Arch Otolaryngol* 109:310–312, 1983.

Otalgia—Review Articles
Black B: Otalgia. *Aust Fam Physician* 16(3):292–296, 1987,
Johnson IT, Rood SR, Newman RK: Abnormalities in and around the ear: Congenital, traumatic, inflammatory, and neoplastic. *Postgrad Med* 72(4):123–125, 128–130, 1982.

Olsen KD: The many causes of otalgia: Infection, trauma, cancer. *Postgrad Med* 80(6):50–52, 55–56, 61–63, 1986.

Otalgia—Wegener's Granulomatosis
Halsted LA, Karmody CS, Wolff SM: Presentation of Wegener's granulomatosis in young patients. *Otolaryngol Head Neck Surg* 94:368–371, 1986.

Otitis Media
Bluestone CD: Surgical management of otitis media. *Pediatr Infect Dis* 3(4):392–396, 1984.
Bluestone CD: Treatment of otitis media with effusion. *Scand J Infect Dis Suppl* 39:26–33, 1983.
Ginsburg CM: Otitis media. *Pediatrics* 74(suppl):948–949, 1984.
Schwartz RH, Stool SE, Rodriguez WJ, et al: Acute otitis media: Toward a more precise definition. *Clin Pediatr* 20(9):549–554, 1981.
Walike JW: Management of acute ear infections. *Otolaryngol Clin North Am* 12(2):439–445, 1979.

Otitis Media and Externa
Klein JO: Otitis externa, otitis media, mastoiditis, in Mandell GL, Douglas RG Jr, Bennett JE (eds): *Principles and Practice of Infectious Diseases,* 3d ed. New York, Churchill Livingstone, 1990, pp 505–510.
Kohan D, Rothstein SG, Cohen NL: Otologic disease in patients with acquired immunodeficiency syndrome. *Ann Otol Rhinol Laryngol* 97:636–640, 1988.

Petrous Apicitis
Chole RA, Donald PJ: Petrous apicitis: Clinical considerations. *Ann Otol Rhinol Laryngol* 92:544–551, 1983.

Ramsay Hunt Syndrome
Inamura H, Aoyagi M, Tojima H, et al: Effects of acyclovir in Ramsay Hunt syndrome. *Acta Otolaryngol Suppl (Stockh)* 446:111–113, 1988.

Relapsing Polychondritis
Batsakis JG, Manning JT: Relapsing polychondritis. *Ann Otol Rhinol Laryngol* 98:83–84, 1989.
Cohen PR, Rapini RP: Relapsing polychondritis. *Int J Derm* 25:280–285, 1986.
Isaak BL, Liesegang TJ, Michet CJ Jr: Ocular and systemic findings in relapsing polychondritis. *Ophthalmology* 93:681–689, 1986.
Kitridou RC, Wittman A-L, Quismorio FP Jr: Chondritis in systemic lupus erythematosus: Clinical and immunopathologic studies. *Clin Exp Rheum* 5:349–353, 1987.
Michet CJ, McKenna CH, Luthra HS, et al: Relapsing polychondritis: Survival and predictive role of early disease manifestations. *Ann Intern Med* 104:74–78, 1986.
Schlapbach P, Gerber NJ, Ramser P, et al: Relapsing polychondritis mimicking rheumatoid arthritis. *Ann Rheum Dis* 47:1021–1026, 1988.
Stern JR: Pathologic quiz case 1. *Arch Otolaryngol Head Neck Surg* 112:674–676, 1986.
Stiles MC, Khan JA: Photo essay: Relapsing polychondritis. *Arch Ophthalmol* 107:277, 1989.
Trepel RJ, Lipnick RN, D'Angelo L: Relapsing polychondritis in an adolescent. *J Adolesc Health Care* 10:557–560, 1989.
White JW Jr: Relapsing polychondritis. *South Med J* 78(4):448–451, 1985.

Acute Nasal Pain

☐ **SUMMARY**

Folliculitis presents with pain, redness, and tenderness, that involve the mucosa just within the margin of the nostril. The area involved is at the base of one or more nasal hairs. The *furuncle* may develop within the vestibule and result in redness, warmth, edema, and aching or throbbing pain in the tip and lateral portion of one side of the nose. This lesion soon forms a yellow head and spontaneously drains pus, relieving the pain, redness, and swelling. *Fissures and small crusted ulcers* occur in the lower vestibule or near the base of the septum (i.e., ulcers). These respond to removal of crusts and application of antibiotic ointment. *Herpes simplex virus* causes pain, tenderness, and the eruption of grouped red-based vesi-

cles and tiny ulcers on the skin of the upper lip at the margin of a naris. Extension into the nose may occur. *Nasal trauma* may cause a *fracture,* with nasal bridge tenderness and sometimes bony crepitus. An asymmetrical deformity or depression of the nasal bridge may be observed if posttraumatic edema is not severe. A *nasal septal hematoma* may obstruct the nasal cavity and appear as a widened, thickened, and indentable septum. *Cartilage fracture* causes septal deviation, pain, and tenderness. *Relapsing polychondritis* causes red, painful, tender auricles with pale white lobules; nasal tip redness, pain, and tenderness; nonerosive arthritis; anterior neck pain and tenderness; and hoarseness. A biopsy of an involved auricle or nasal cartilage shows evidence of necrotizing chondritis with an inflammatory cell infiltrate.

TABLE OF DISEASE INCIDENCE

INCIDENCE PER 100,000 (APPROXIMATE)

Common (>100)	Uncommon (>5–100)	Rare (>0–5)
Folliculitis	Herpes zoster of V_1 or V_2	Relapsing polychondritis
Furunculosis	Rhinopharyngitis due to *M. pneumoniae*	
Fissures and small ulcers	Ethmoid sinusitis	
Herpex simplex virus	Nasal septum abscess	
Nasal trauma	Trigeminal neuralgia of V_1 and/or V_2	
Rhinopharyngitis-associated external nasal pain	Intranasal foreign body	
Rhinopharyngitis due to viruses, group A streptococci, and bacterial superinfection		

Herpes zoster of the ophthalmic division of the trigeminal nerve causes unilateral supraorbital and eye and lateral nasal aching or burning pain, accompanied by an eruption of grouped vesicles and crusted ulcers on the forehead, lids, and nose. Eyelid swelling, conjunctivitis, and corneal involvement (i.e., keratitis) may occur. During a cold, the external nose may become red, swollen, and tender from sneezing, wiping, and blowing. This resolves as the cold improves. *Rhinopharyngitis* may also cause deep posterior nasal pain and soreness made more intense with each sneeze. Clear mucoid rhinorrhea, nasal stuffiness, and obstruction occur, but fever and cough are uncommon. *Group A streptococcal nasopharyngitis* can mimic a viral cold, as can *Mycoplasma pneumoniae infection*. Patients with cold symptoms for 7 to 10 days who suddenly develop a yellow-green nasal and/or postnasal discharge probably have *bacterial superinfection. Ethmoid sinusitis* may follow a cold or start spontaneously. There is pain behind the bridge of the nose and in the medial orbit on one or both sides. Referred pain to the parietal region and vertex may also occur. Purulent nasal and postnasal discharge occur. The diagnosis can be confirmed by a CT study of the paranasal sinuses, and symptoms respond to antibiotic therapy. *Unusual fungi and bacteria* may cause sinus infections in patients with a defect in host defenses (e.g., diabetes, leukopenia, and AIDS).

A *nasal septal abscess* causes local pain and bilateral nasal obstruction. It may follow trauma (e.g., a nasal septal hematoma). Unusual causes include sinusitis, furunculosis of the vestibule, and nasal or dental surgery. *Trigeminal neuralgia* may cause sharp jabs of cutting or burning cheek and intranasal pain (i.e., "like a red hot poker") lasting seconds. A facial trigger point may provoke attacks, but sensorimotor abnormalities of the face cannot be detected on neurologic examination. Attacks cease in up to 60 percent of cases with carbamazepine therapy. *Nasal foreign bodies* cause pain and purulent discharge. The diagnosis can be confirmed by examination of the nasal cavity. Relief follows removal of the foreign body.

☐ DESCRIPTION OF LISTED DISEASES

1. External Nose

A. Folliculitis Local pain, tenderness, redness, and crusting occur at the base of one or more hairs in the nasal vestibule near the mucocutaneous junction of a naris. Pain and tenderness resolve spontaneously without drainage, but recurrence is common. Local treatment with antibiotic ointment may prevent recurrent episodes. One or both nares may be involved.

B. Furunculosis Pain and tenderness occur just within the nasal vestibule, associated with redness, tenderness, and swelling of the skin of the tip and side of the nose and sometimes the adjacent face. There is a severe ache and/or throbbing pain. Fever is seldom present. Within 2 to 4 days, the swelling localizes, and a white or yellow head forms on this intranasal nodule. Spontaneous drainage is facilitated by the use of local warm soaks and oral antibiotics. With drainage of pus, pain, tenderness, and redness resolve over the next few days. Recurrence at variable intervals is common, and skin furuncles at other sites may follow. Use of an antistaphylococcal nasal antibiotic and avoidance of nose picking may prevent future attacks.

C. Fissures and Small Crusted Ulcers These crusted small lesions of the nasal vestibule occur at the mucocutaneous junction of the nostril. There may be mild local pain and tenderness just within the margin of the nasal opening. Local cauterization of the fissure and use of an antibiotic ointment lead to healing. Small, painful, crusted ulcers may appear at the base of the anterior portion of the nasal septum. These may heal after gentle removal of the surface crust and daily application of an antibiotic ointment (e.g., bacitracin-neomycin).

D. Herpes Simplex Virus Small grouped vesicles and crusted ulcers appear on a tender erythematous base on the skin of the upper lip just below the nasal vestibule, often extending upward into a naris. There may be mild pain or only tenderness. Spontaneous healing occurs within 14 days, but recurrences at the same site or on the philtrum of the upper lip may follow.

E. Nasal Trauma

1. Nasal Septal Hematoma Deviation, bulging, or widening of the septum may occur. There may be nasal obstruction, but the mucosa of the septum does not appear blue. If a hematoma is present, it can be indented by a cotton-tipped applicator. The hematoma may be unilateral (one side indents) or bilateral (both sides indent).

Hematomas require drainage because persistence can lead to cartilage destruction from pressure or a nasal septal abscess.

2. Nasal Bone Fractures   Patients have epistaxis and pain over the bridge of the nose. Local tenderness and sometimes bony crepitus are present. Deformity with nasal asymmetry may be observed, as may edema and ecchymoses. Lateral nasal fractures result from a "right cross" punch. The entire bridge of the nose is shifted to the contralateral side. Severe swelling appears after 2 to 5 h. Radiographs of the nose may miss fractures. Fractures are usually transverse and run perpendicular to the longitudinal axis of the nose, while longitudinal lines on the nasal bones are usually caused by nutrient blood vessels. Nasal bone fractures may be associated with fractures of other facial bones (Le Fort–type fractures 1–3).

3. Septal fractures   A septal deviation that obstructs one nasal cavity may be caused by a septal fracture.

F. Relapsing Polychondritis   An initial attack may present with painful, violaceous, red cartilaginous auricles, and pale white auricular lobules. The pinnae are warm, swollen, and tender. The tip and lateral lower portion of the external nose may become red, painful, and tender due to nasal chondritis. Red eyes may reflect an associated conjunctivitis, iritis, scleritis, or uveitis. Costochondritis with chest pain and a mono-, pauci-, or polyarticular asymmetrical, nonerosive, nondeforming arthritis may also occur. Hoarseness, anterior neck pain, and tenderness reflect involvement of the thyroid and tracheal cartilages. Cough, dyspnea, stridor, or hemoptysis may accompany inflammatory airway changes. Cartilage biopsy from an auricle or the nose reveals a necrotizing chondritis with an inflammatory cell infiltrate.

G. Herpes Zoster of the Trigeminal Nerve   A constant aching or burning pain may precede the onset of an eruption of grouped, small, red-based vesicles on the skin of the forehead, eyelids, and side of the nose. The pain is felt in the area of the rash. The vesicles soon rupture and become covered with a reddish-brown crust. The affected side of the face and eyelids may be erythematous and swollen, and the eye red, painful, and tender. Vesicles on the side and tip of the nose are often associated with corneal lesions (e.g., keratitis and ulcers). Involvement of divisions V_1 or V_2 can cause nasal pain and vesicular lesions in their corresponding dermatomal areas. Acyclovir taken orally may benefit severe cases.

H. Rhinopharyngitis-Associated External Nasal Pain
After 2 to 3 days of sneezing, blowing, and wiping, the skin of the nose becomes red, swollen, painful, and tender. This subsides as the cold improves.

2. Internal Nose and Paranasal Sinuses

A. Rhinopharyngitis   Patients present with a scratchy, painful upper throat and aching discomfort deep within the nasal cavity. The nose and throat pain may be intensified by sneezing. Rhinorrhea with a clear mucoid discharge, paroxysms of sneezing, nasal stuffiness or obstruction, and a nasal intonation of speech may be associated. Mild aching in the forehead and over one or both cheeks may occur. The conjunctivae may be mildly injected. Fever is usually absent, but malaise, fatigue, and generalized aching discomfort may accompany the nasopharyngeal symptoms.

1. Viruses   Over 200 viruses are capable of causing this type of illness. Infections occur year-round but are most frequent in the winter. Most adults suffer one to three such infections each year. The nasal smear does not demonstrate eosinophilia. Rhinoviruses and coronaviruses are the commonest responsible agents. These infections may exacerbate asthma and chronic bronchitis and may be complicated by sinusitis or otitis media.

2. Group A Streptococci   Group A streptococcal infection in adults may mimic a rhinovirus cold. It may present with clear, watery mucoid rhinorrhea; nasal stuffiness or obstruction; and deep unilateral or bilateral nasal pain, intensified by nose-blowing. A mild to moderate sore throat, intensified by swallowing, may be present. The upper anterior cervical nodes may be enlarged and tender. Fever is frequently absent. Throat culture or a streptococcus screen is positive for group A streptococci. Penicillin or erythromycin therapy results in relief within 36 h.

3. Bacterial Superinfection   Bacterial nasopharyngitis and sinusitis may complicate a viral cold. Signs of a bacterial component include a purulent nasal or postnasal discharge and tender, enlarged upper cervical nodes. This usually occurs 7 to 10 days after the onset of the cold. Antibiotic therapy directed at *Hemophilus influenzae, Streptococcus pneumoniae, Staphylococcus aureus,* and *Streptococcus pyogenes* usually leads to prompt resolution of symptoms.

4. M. pneumoniae   Patients may present with a cold-like syndrome. Multiple cases within a family group are commonly present. There may be a response to erythromycin therapy.

B. Ethmoid Sinusitis

1. Bacterial   Symptoms may begin spontaneously or follow an episode of the common cold. Fever occurs in less than 50 percent of adults. There is aching discomfort over the bridge of the nose and in the medial portion of one or both orbits. Cheek pain may accompany antral infection. Referral of ethmoid sinus pain to the vertex and/or parietal region may also occur. A purulent and/or bloody nasal and postnasal discharge may be present. Early-morning sore throat, throat clearing to remove postnasal discharge, hoarseness, and a complicating bronchitis with a productive cough may develop. In one study, quantitative cultures were obtained by direct needle aspiration (from the maxillary sinus), and 50 percent of isolates were *S. pneumoniae* or unencapsulated *H. influenzae*. Other isolates were *S. pyogenes, Branhamella catarrhalis,* other gram-negative bacteria and anaerobes (present in up to 10 percent of cases when correct anaerobic culture techniques were used). Bacterial counts greater than 10^3/ml correlated with sinus fluid leukocytosis (>5000 leukocytes/ml). Bacteria were almost always cultured in high concentrations from purulent sinus fluid. Rarely, *Actinomyces* or *Nocardia* species cause sinus infection.

Unusual organisms may cause sinus infections in patients with underlying disorders. These pathogens, common associated disorders, and risk factors for sinus infection are discussed below.

2. Rare Causes of Sinusitis   *Aspergillus* species may cause an invasive and fulminant form of sinusitis in patients with leukopenia (i.e., from aplastic anemia and acute leukemia), neutrophil dysfunction syndromes, or alcoholism. Prolonged antibiotic and corticosteroid use is also a risk factor for invasive aspergillosis. Cases may also occur in patients immunosuppressed for organ transplantation.

Mucormycosis of the sinuses, orbit, and brain may occur in patients with diabetic ketoacidosis, leukopenia, or immunosuppression.

Candida albicans may cause noninvasive sinusitis in diabetics and patients on prolonged antibiotic therapy.

Pseudomonas aeruginosa and *S. aureus* may cause sinus and bronchial infection in patients with cystic fibrosis or the immotile cilia syndrome.

Polymicrobial sinus infections with *Serratia, Pseudomonas, Escherichia coli,* and other aerobic gram-negative bacteria occur in immunosuppressed patients and those whose nasal airway has been invaded and damaged by nasopharyngeal or nasotracheal tubes or nasal packing.

Legionella pneumophila, Acanthamoeba castellani, H. influenzae, S. pneumoniae, and a fungous *Pseudallescheria boydii* have been isolated from sinus infections in AIDS patients.

C. Abscess of the Nasal Septum   This disorder usually follows a traumatic septal hematoma. Secondary infection of this hematoma with *S. aureus* or *H. influenzae* (in children) causes local nasal pain, marked bilateral obstruction, and fever. Examination reveals a cherry-red bilateral swelling of the septum that is fluctuant and tender. Drainage of this lesion discharges pus, relieves symptoms, and preserves the nasal septum and the external shape of the nose. Delayed diagnosis can lead to septal cartilage destruction and a saddle nose deformity with septal perforation. Patients with a nasal septal abscess may develop osteomyelitis of adjacent bones, orbital cellulitis and abscess, cavernous sinus thrombosis, or an intracranial abscess and/or meningitis.

Less common causes of nasal septal abscess include nasal surgery, furunculosis of the nasal vestibule, dental extraction, and influenza. Several cases of non-trauma-associated septal abscess have been reported in association with ethmoid and isolated sphenoid sinusitis. The latter disorder may be difficult to diagnose, since false-negative sinus radiographs (15 percent) may occur. Computed tomography is a sensitive method of demonstrating sphenoid and ethmoid sinus disease. In patients with septal abscess and sphenoid sinusitis, symptoms may not resolve until the sphenoid sinus, as well as the abscess, is drained.

D. Trigeminal Neuralgia   Sharp, stabbing, or burning unilateral pain radiating up the nose and/or across the cheek is typical. These jabs last only a few seconds to a minute. Pains may appear in a cluster lasting for several minutes and then remit, or trains of jabbing pain may continue for hours. A trigger point that initiates a typical jab of pain when touched or stimulated by talking or eating may be present on the skin of the nose, cheek, or lip. There are no motor or sensory abnormalities in the region innervated by the ophthalmic and maxillary divisions of nerve V. There is a response of the pain to phenytoin or carbamazepine or to stereotactic thermocoagulation of the trigeminal roots. This disorder has been called tic douloureux because patients characteristically wince in response to the severe intensity of the pain.

E. Intranasal Foreign Bodies

1. Animate   Animate foreign bodies cause bilateral purulent nasal discharge and nasal pain. The onset of symptoms occurs within 3 days of nasal invasion by the causative parasite. Temperature may be elevated, and examination of the nasal cavity may reveal mucosal, or bony, and cartilaginous destruction.

Animate foreign bodies occur in a setting of poverty; in warm tropical regions of the United States; and in patients with severe diabetes, syphilis, or a chronic debilitating disease. Infestations include fly maggots, larvae, screw worms, black carpet beetles, and ascaris worms.

2. Inanimate   Compared to animate foreign bodies, inanimate items are less likely to cause pain. Children and psychotic or retarded adults are most likely to present with this problem. Unilateral mucoid, serosanguinous, or purulent discharge and nasal obstruction may occur. Erythema, superficial necrosis, and ulceration occur on the mucosa adjacent to the foreign body. Examples of inanimate foreign bodies that may be found along the floor of the nose below the inferior turbinate or anterior to the middle turbinate include erasers, paper, pebbles, marbles, peas, and beans.

NASAL PAIN REFERENCES

Atrophic Rhinitis
Dudley JP: Atrophic rhinitis: Antibiotic treatment. *Am J Otolaryngol* 8(6):387–390, 1987.

Cavernous Sinus Syndromes
Bosley TM, Schatz NJ: Clinical diagnosis of cavernous sinus syndromes. *Neurol Clin* 1(4):929–953, 1983.

Idiopathic Midline Destructive Disease
Costa J, Delacrétaz F: The midline granuloma syndrome. *Pathol Annu* 21(part 1):159–171, 1986.

Harrison DFN: Midline destructive granuloma: Fact or fiction. *Laryngoscope* 97(9):1049–1053, 1987.

Tsokos M, Fauci AS, Costa J: Idiopathic midline destructive disease (IMDD): A subgroup of patients with the "midline granuloma" syndrome. *Am J Clin Pathol* 77(2):162–168, 1982.

Lethal Midline Granuloma—Cocaine
Becker GD, Hill S: Midline granuloma due to illicit cocaine use. *Arch Otolaryngol Head Neck Surg* 114:90–91, 1988.

Lethal Midline Granuloma—Lymphoma
Chott A, Rappersberger K, Schlossarek W, et al: Peripheral T cell lymphoma presenting primarily as lethal midline granuloma. *Hum Pathol* 19(9):1093–1101, 1988.

Fu Y-S, Perzin KH: Nonepithelial tumors of the nasal cavity, paranasal sinuses and nasopharynx: A clinicopathologic study: 10. Malignant lymphomas. *Cancer* 43:611–621, 1979.

Laeng RH, Gerber H, Mueller J: Malignant histiocytosis (histiocytic sarcoma): A (the?) major cause of the "midline granuloma syndrome." *Acta Otolaryngol (Stockh)* 101:135–145, 1986.

Laeng RH, Gerber HA, Schaffner T, et al: Heterogeneous malignant non Hodgkin's lymphomas as a causative disorder in lethal midline granuloma. *Virchows Arch [A]* 415:265–273, 1989.

Lippman SM, Grogan TM, Spier CM, et al: Lethal midline granuloma with a novel T-cell phenotype as found in peripheral T-cell lymphoma. *Cancer* 59:936–939, 1987.

Maeda H, Aozasa K, Tsujimura T, et al: Malignant lymphomas and related conditions involving nasal cavity and paranasal sinuses: A clinicopathologic study of forty-two cases with emphasis on prognostic factors. *Eur J Surg Oncol* 14:9–15, 1988.

Platt JC, Tomich CE, Campbell S: Malignant lymphoma presenting as a midline lethal granuloma. *J Oral Maxillofac Surg* 47:511–513, 1989.

Polico C, Corti L, Rigon A, et al: Steward's midline granuloma: A case report. *Tumori* 72:447–449, 1986.

Ratech H, Burke JS, Blayney DW, et al: A clinicopathologic study of malignant lymphomas of the nose, paranasal sinuses, and hard palate, including cases of lethal midline granuloma. *Cancer* 64:2525–2531, 1989.

Yamanaka N, Kataura A, Sambe S, et al: Midfacial T cell lymphoma: Characterization by monoclonal antibodies. *Ann Otol Rhinol Laryngol* 94:207–211, 1985.

Lethal Midline Granuloma—Lymphomatoid Granulomatosis
Atichartakarn V, Nitiyanant P, Kraiphibul P, et al: Lethal midline granuloma and lymphoproliferative disorders. *J Med Assoc Thai* 72(5):243–249, 1989.

DeRemee RA, Weiland LH, McDonald TJ: Polymorphic reticulosis, lymphomatoid granulomatosis: Two diseases or one? *Mayo Clin Proc* 53:634–640, 1978.

Gaulard P, Henni T, Marolleau J-P, et al: Lethal midline granuloma (polymorphic reticulosis) and lymphomatoid granulomatosis: Evidence for a monoclonal T-cell lymphoproliferative disorder. *Cancer* 62:705–710, 1988.

Liebow AA, Carrington CRB, Friedman PJ: Lymphomatoid granulomatosis. *Hum Pathol* 3:457–558, 1972.

McDonald TJ, DeRemee RA, Harrison EG Jr, et al: The protean clinical features of polymorphic reticulosis (lethal midline granuloma). *Laryngoscope* 86:936–945, 1976.

Whittaker S, Foroni L, Luzzatto L, et al: Lymphomatoid granulomatosis: Evidence of a clonal T-cell origin and an association with lethal midline granuloma. *Q J Med* 68(256):645–655, 1988.

Lethal Midline Granuloma—Midline Malignant Reticulosis
Yamamura T, Asada H, Mike N, et al: Immunohistochemical and ultrastructural studies on disseminated skin lesions of midline malignant reticulosis. *Cancer* 58:1281–1285, 1986.

Lethal Midline Granuloma—Reviews
Aozasa K, Ohsawa M, Tajima K, et al: Nation-wide study of lethal mid-line granuloma in Japan: Frequencies of Wegener's granulomatosis, polymorphic reticulosis, malignant lymphoma and other related conditions. *Int J Cancer* 44:63–66, 1989.

Batsakis JG: Midfacial necrotizing diseases. *Ann Otol Rhinol Laryngol* 91:541–542, 1982.

Batsakis JG, Luna MA: Midfacial necrotizing lesions. *Sem Diagn Pathol* 4:90–116, 1987.

Fauci AS, Johnson RE, Wolff SM: Radiation therapy of midline granuloma. *Ann Intern Med* 84:140–147, 1976.

Galli M, Formenti A, Pettenati C, et al: Immunological features of nonhealing midline granuloma. *ORL J Otorhinolaryngol Relat Spec* 48:256–260, 1986.

O'Connor JC, Robinson RA: Review of diseases presenting as "midline granuloma." *Acta Otolaryngol Suppl (Stockh)* 439:1–16, 1987.

Pickens JP, Modica L: Current concepts of the lethal midline granuloma syndrome. *Otolaryngol Head Neck Surg* 100(6):623–630, 1989.

Ruey-Bin C, Nagase M, Nakajima T, et al: Treatment of "idiopathic midline destructive disease" by irradiation: A case report. *J Cranio-Max-Fac Surg* 16:375–378, 1988.

Lethal Midline Granuloma—Wegener's Granulomatosis
Andrassy K, Rasmussen N: Treatment of granulomatous disorders of the nose and paranasal sinuses. *Rhinology* 27(4):221–230, 1989.

Drake-Lee AB, Milford CA: A review of the role of radiology in nonhealing granulomas of the nose and nasal sinuses. *Rhinology* 27(4):231–236, 1989.

Milford CA, Drake-Lee AB, Lloyd GAS: Radiology of the paranasal sinuses in nonhealing granulomas of the nose. *Clin Otolaryngol* 11:199–204, 1986.

Lupus Pernio

Spiteri MA, Matthey F, Gordon T, et al: Lupus pernio: A clinico-radiological study of thirty-five cases. *Br J Dermatol* 112:315–322, 1985.

Mucormycosis

Perry AP, Abedi S: Diagnosis and management of rhino-orbitocerebral mucormycosis (phycomycosis): A report of 16 personally observed cases. *Ophthalmol* 90:1096–1104, 1983.

Nasal Pain—Review

Kennedy DW, Loury MC: Nasal and sinus pain: Current diagnosis and treatment. *Sem Neurol* 8(4):303–314, 1988.

Nasal/Paranasal Sinus Diseases—Malignant

Anand VK: Malignant diseases of the nose and paranasal sinuses, in Lee KJ (ed): *Textbook of Otolaryngology and Head and Neck Surgery*. New York, Elsevier, 1989, pp 304–312.

Nasal Septal Abscess

Close DM, Guinness MDG: Abscess of the nasal septum after trauma. *Med J Aust* 142:472–474, 1985.

Collins MP: Abscess of the nasal septum complicating isolated acute sphenoiditis. *J Laryngol Otol* 99:715–719, 1985.

Kryger H, Dommerby H: Haematoma and abscess of the nasal septum. *Clin Otolaryngol* 12:125–129, 1987.

Matsuba HM, Thawley SE: Nasal septal abscess: Unusual causes, complications, treatment, and sequelae. *Am Plast Surg* 16(2):161–166, 1986.

Pirsig W: Historical notes and actual observations on the nasal septal abscess especially in children. *Int J Pediatr Otorhinolaryngol* 8:43–54, 1984.

Nasal Septal Perforation

Deutsch HL, Millard DR Jr: A new cocaine abuse complex: Involvement of nose, septum, palate and pharynx. *Arch Otolaryngol Head Neck Surg* 115:235–237, 1989.

Eviatar A, Myssiorek D: Repair of nasal septal perforations with tragal cartilage and perichondrium grafts. *Otolaryngol Head Neck Surg* 100:300–302, 1989.

Lee HS, Goh CL: Occupational dermatosis among chrome platers. *Contact Dermatitis* 18:89–93, 1988.

Lindberg E, Hedenstierna G: Chrome plating: Symptoms, findings in the upper airways, and effects on lung function. *Arch Environ Health* 38(6):367–374, 1983.

Nasal Tumors

Echeverria-Zumarraga M, Kaiser C, Gavilan C: Nasal septal carcinoma: Initial symptoms of nasal septal perforation. *J Laryngol Otol* 102:834–835, 1988.

Hanna GS, Akosa AB, Ali MH: Vascular leiomyoma of the inferior turbinate: Report of a case and review of the literature. *J Laryngol Otol* 102:1159–1160, 1988.

Hills P: Malignant melanoma of the nasal cavity. *Radiography* 54(615):111–112, 1988.

Nasopharyngeal Carcinoma

Fedder M, Gonzalez MF: Nasopharyngeal carcinoma: Brief review. *Am J Med* 79:365–369, 1985.

Rhinologic Causes of Facial Pain

Kimmelman CP: Rhinologic causes of facial pain, in Cooper BC, Lucente FE (eds): *Management of Facial, Head and Neck Pain*. Philadelphia, Saunders, 1989, pp 99–114.

Sinus Disease—Infection

Berg O, Carenfelt C: Analysis of symptoms and clinical signs in the maxillary sinus empyema. *Acta Otolaryngol (Stockh)* 105:343–349, 1988.

Friedman WH, Slavin RG: Diagnosis and medical and surgical treatment of sinusitis in adults. *Clin Rev Allergy* 2:409–428, 1984.

Goodwin WJ Jr: Orbital complications of ethmoiditis. *Otolaryngol Clin North Am* 18(1):139–147, 1985.

Harrington PC: Complications of sinusitis. *Ear Nose Throat J* 63:58–71, 1984.

Jannert M, Andréasson L, Ivarsson A: Studies on the maxillary ostial function in cases with maxillary pain, intrasinusal cysts and chronic sinusitis. *Acta Otolaryngol (Stockh)* 97:325–334, 1984.

Kern EB: Suppurative (bacterial) sinusitis. *Postgrad Med* 81(4):194–198, 203–210, 1987.

Levine HL: The office diagnosis of nasal and sinus disorders using rigid nasal endoscopy. *Otolaryngol Head Neck Surg* 102:370–373, 1990.

Mulbury PE: Medical management of sinusitis. *Ear Nose Throat J* 63:35–42, 1984.

Ramsey PG, Weymuller EA: Complications of bacterial infection of the ears, paranasal sinuses, and oropharynx in adults. *Emerg Med Clin North Am* 3(1):143–160, 1985.

Rasmussen P, Laursen J, Simonsen P, et al: Chronic facial pain following diseases affecting the maxillary antrum: The influence of peripheral impulses from the maxillary air sinus is not significant in their maintenance. *Acta Neurochir (Wien)* 82:39–42, 1986.

Rihani A: Maxillary sinusitis as a differential diagnosis in temporo-mandibular joint pain-dysfunction syndrome. *J Prosthet Dent* 53(1):97–100, 1985.

Robinson KE: Roentgenographic manifestations of benign paranasal disease. *Ear Nose Throat J* 63:26–34, 1984.

Stammberger H, Wolf G: Headaches and sinus disease: The endoscopic approach. *Ann Otol Rhinol Laryngol* 134(suppl):3–23, 1988.

Urquhart AC, Fung G, McIntosh WA: Isolated sphenoiditis: A diagnostic problem. *J Laryngol Otol* 103:526–527, 1989.

Sinus Disease—Neoplastic

Rice DH: Benign and malignant tumors of the ethmoid sinus. *Otolaryngol Clin North Am* 18(1):113–124, 1985.

Trigeminal Trophic Syndrome

Arasi R, McKay M, Grist WJ: Trigeminal trophic syndrome. *Laryngoscope* 98(12):1330–1333, 1988.

Tumors

Hills P: Malignant melanoma of the nasal cavity. *Radiography* 54(615):111–112, 1988.

Holmes DK, Panje WR: Intranasal granuloma faciale. *Am J Otolaryngol* 4:184–186, 1983.

Potter AJ Jr, Khatib G, Peppard SB: Intranasal glomus tumor. *Arch Otolaryngol* 110:755–756, 1984.

VanDellen RG, McDonald TJ: Nasopharyngeal masses mimicking "allergic" nasal symptoms. *Mayo Clin Proc* 63:69–71, 1988.

6

Acute Lower and Midfacial Pain

☐ DIAGNOSTIC LIST

1. Traumatic fractures
   A. Mandible
      1. Condyle
      2. Body
   B. Maxilla
   C. Zygomatic bone
   D. Orbit
2. Pathologic fracture due to metastatic or primary tumor or osteomyelitis
3. Temporomandibular joint (TMJ) pain
   A. Acute pseudogout and gout
   B. Lyme disease
   C. TMJ pain/dysfunction (myofascial pain/dysfunction) syndrome
4. Maxillary sinusitis
   A. Acute suppurative sinusitis (empyema)
   B. Barotrauma

5. Herpes zoster (maxillary or mandibular division of nerve V)
6. Referred jaw and face pain
   A. Myocardial infarction and coronary insufficiency
   B. Dissecting aneurysm
7. Parotitis
   A. Acute viral parotitis (mumps and other viruses)
   B. Acute suppurative parotitis
   C. Sialolithiasis
   D. Iodism (chronic iodide intoxication)
8. Lateral pharyngeal space infection
9. Masticator space infection
10. Idiopathic trigeminal neuralgia (tic douloureux)
    A. Microvascular compression
    B. Multiple sclerosis

☐ SUMMARY

Fracture of the mandible usually occurs in fist fights, from assaults with blunt objects, and from motor vehicle accidents, gunshot wounds, and falls. A mandibular fracture presents with severe pain, swelling, tenderness, and crepitus adjacent to the fracture site. The pain is intensified by jaw motion during chewing, biting, swallowing, or talking. Malocclusion may occur. Ramus or angle fractures may cause trismus. Panoramic radiographs of the jaw will demonstrate the site and extent of a mandibular fracture. Fracture through a *condyle* or *condylar neck* causes pain, swelling, and tenderness of the involved

temporomandibular joint (TMJ), an occlusal disturbance, and trismus. *Body fractures* cause local pain, tenderness, and swelling. *Midfacial fractures* have been classified by Le Fort into three basic types; these are discussed below. *Zygomatic bone fractures* cause maxillary pain, tenderness, and dimpling of the cheek. *Orbital fractures* cause local pain in the orbit and maxillary area, and may cause diplopia, enophthalmus, and visual loss. Facial fractures can be clearly demonstrated by a CT scan. *Pathologic fracture of the mandible* secondary to tumor or osteomyelitis may cause local pain, tenderness, and swelling that begins spontaneously or after a minor injury.

TMJ pain, swelling, and tenderness may be secondary to an

acute uric acid (*gout*)–induced or calcium pyrophosphate dihydrate (*pseudogout*)–induced arthritis. Pseudogout patients tend to be older than gout patients and usually have chondrocalcinosis of the knees. Both groups respond to colchicine therapy or nonsteroidal anti-inflammatory drugs. *Lyme disease* has caused an acute myofascial-type syndrome. Masseter, temporalis, and/or pterygoid muscle pain and tenderness, with malocclusion and TMJ tenderness, may arise as a primary myofascial syndrome with active muscle trigger point(s), or may be secondary to a deep space infection, a TMJ internal derangement, or acute TMJ arthritis. MRI of the TMJ region can detect a deep space infection, internal derangement, and/or inflammation of the TMJ.

Maxillary sinusitis causes ipsilateral cheek pain that may be referred to the adjacent maxillary teeth, simulating a dental disorder. Nasal stuffiness, a purulent or bloody nasal and/or postnasal discharge, sore throat, cough, and hoarseness may occur. Fever may be low-grade or absent. Examination reveals hyperemia and pus in the middle meatus on the affected side. Maxillary tenderness to light percussion is usually present. Sinus radiographs may show opacification or mucosal thickening exceeding 8 mm and/or an air-fluid level.

Barotrauma resulting from flying or sea diving can cause maxillary sinus pain and tenderness. Sinus damage results from high negative or positive sinus pressures relative to ambient pressure. These pressure differences result in exudation of fluid into the sinuses, and submucosal hemorrhages. The maxillary sinuses are less often affected than the frontal and ethmoidal sinuses.

Herpes zoster may cause acute, unilateral, burning mandibular or maxillary pain, and a vesicular eruption in the painful zone. Considerable facial edema may accompany the rash.

Jaw, neck, and chest pain suggests cardiac ischemia associated with acute infarction or coronary insufficiency. The pain may improve with thrombolytic therapy. A tearing chest, neck, jaw, and back pain, associated with a widened mediastinum and, in up to 50 percent of cases, a new aortic insufficiency murmur, suggests a dissecting aneurysm of the aorta. A thoracic CT scan, with contrast, or an aortogram will confirm the diagnosis.

Mumps parotitis causes marked unilateral—and sometimes bilateral—parotid aching pain, fever, and swelling, which distorts the lower face and upper neck. The pain and swelling may continue for 5 to 10 days, and resolve spontaneously. The orifice of Stensen's duct may be red, but the saliva exiting from it is clear and watery in appearance.

Acute suppuration of the parotid causes a high fever, marked leukocytosis, and unilateral or bilateral fluctuant swelling of the parotid gland(s). Pus can be expressed from Stensen's duct in 75 percent of cases. This is a disorder of elderly debilitated patients. It is associated with dehydration, use of anticholinergic drugs, antibiotics, and poor oral hygiene. Up to 40 percent of cases may occur in the postoperative period. There is a good response to antibiotics and surgical drainage of the parotid.

Sialolithiasis may cause intermittent unilateral parotid pain and swelling. Ingestion of food and citrus juices intensifies the pain and swelling. Symptoms resolve with removal of a salivary duct stone. In some cases the parotid swelling persists between meals, until duct patency is restored.

Ingestion of *iodides* may induce a chronic intoxication with coryza-like complaints and bilateral painful swelling of the parotid glands ("iodide mumps"). Symptoms resolve after iodides are discontinued.

A *lateral pharyngeal space infection* causes fever, chills, rigors, trismus, pain, and swelling at the angle of the jaw, in the ear, and in the preauricular area. The space abscess can be imaged by a CT scan or MRI of the face and head. A confirmed lateral pharyngeal space infection requires drainage and parenteral antibiotic therapy.

A *peritonsillar abscess* may cause a persistent sore throat, fever, odynophagia, a muffled voice, and drooling. The tonsil may be displaced medially. Antibiotic therapy and drainage of the abscess relieves all symptoms. If trismus develops, invasion of the lateral pharyngeal space is likely.

An *infection in the masticator space* usually arises from a

TABLE OF DISEASE INCIDENCE

INCIDENCE PER 100,000 (APPROXIMATE)

Common (>100)	Uncommon (>5–100)	Rare (>0–5)
Traumatic fracture of the mandible, maxilla, zygomatic bone, or orbit	TMJ pain/dysfunction (myofascial pain/dysfunction)	TMJ pain: gout and pseudogout
Maxillary sinusitis (suppurative)	Maxillary sinus injury due to barotrauma	TMJ pain: Lyme disease
Viral parotitis (mumps and other viruses)	Herpes zoster (maxillary or mandibular divisions of nerve V)	Pathologic fracture of the mandible due to tumor or osteomyelitis
Suppurative parotitis	Referred pain and myocardial infarction or coronary insufficiency	Referred pain from a dissecting aneurysm
Sialolithiasis	Suppurative parotitis	Iodism (iodide mumps)
	Lateral pharyngeal space infection	Trigeminal neuralgia due to multiple sclerosis
	Masticator space infection	
	Idiopathic trigeminal neuralgia	
	Trigeminal neuralgia due to microvascular compression	

third-molar periapical abscess. Marked pain, swelling, and tenderness occur over the posterior portion of the mandible. Trismus occurs; but medial displacement of the lateral pharyngeal wall, rigors, and severe toxicity do not. Drainage and antibiotic therapy usually lead to resolution.

Typical *trigeminal neuralgia (tic douloureux)* causes severe lancinating jaw and/or midfacial pain. Lower or midfacial trigger areas, when stimulated, provoke jabs of pain. There are no demonstrable neurologic abnormalities. Up to 80 percent of cases resistant to medical therapy appear to be caused by microvascular compression of the sensory roots of the trigeminal nerve.

Acute tic douloureux may be the initial manifestation of *multiple sclerosis*. In 87 percent of cases where the two disorders are associated, the symptoms and signs of multiple sclerosis precede those of tic douloureux. Patients with multiple sclerosis appear to have typical tic douloureux, but they tend to be younger, have bilateral symptoms more frequently, and experience a high failure rate when treated with carbamazepine, because their tolerance for the drug is poor.

☐ DESCRIPTION OF LISTED DISEASES

1. TRAUMATIC FRACTURES

A. Mandible In one inner city series, fistfights (47 percent), assaults with blunt objects (18 percent), motor vehicle accidents (10 percent), gunshot wounds (10 percent), and falls (9 percent) accounted for 94 percent of the mandibular fractures seen. Single fractures occurred in 53 percent, double fractures in 41 percent, and triple fractures in 4 percent. The body (30 percent), angle (21 percent), condyles (18 percent), and parasymphyseal area (14 percent) were the most common sites of fracture. Associated injuries included facial bone fractures (22 percent), intracranial injuries (10 percent), and cervical spine fracture/dislocations (4 percent). A mandibular fracture results in localized pain, swelling, tenderness, and sometimes crepitus. Soft tissue edema and skin ecchymoses occur near the fracture site. Pain is intensified by chewing, swallowing, and talking. The upper and lower teeth may fail to come together properly. Fracture of a ramus or angle of the mandible may cause trismus. Abnormal mobility and a palpable abrupt step-off from one portion of the mandible to another may be present. Fractures of the mandible can usually be confirmed by a panoramic radiograph of the jaw.

1. Condyle Sharp pain, tenderness, and swelling occur over the TMJ region. Trismus may occur. The pain may radiate to the ear, face, head, and neck, and an occlusal disturbance is commonly present. The diagnosis can be confirmed by plain radiographs, a panoramic mandibular radiograph, a CT scan or MRI.

2. Body If the fracture is angled forward and downward, it is considered to be "favorable," since the muscle groups attached to the respective fragments impact them against each other, so that they tend to remain in good alignment. "Unfavorable" body fractures begin anteriorly and are angled posteriorly and downward. The attached muscle groups tend to pull the fragments apart. Mandibular fractures may be repaired by intermaxillary fixation, open reduction/internal fixation, or use of external stabilizing devices.

B. Maxilla Bilateral midface fractures have been classified into three types: Le Fort I fractures are horizontal fractures through the lower maxillae. The fractured segment includes the teeth of the upper jaw, the hard palate, the pterygoid plates, and the lower wall of the maxillary sinus. The alveolar ridge and palate are separated from the midface, producing a "floating upper jaw." This mobility can be demonstrated by grasping the anterior teeth of the upper jaw and initiating a push-pull movement. An anterior open bite is usually present. An intraoral hematoma may be present in the buccal sulcus in the area of the zygomatico-alveolar buttress. A midpalatal ecchymotic line may be present.

Le Fort II fractures extend across the mid-upper face and involve the nasal bones, the frontal processes of the maxillae, and the inferior rims of the orbits. They extend across the zygomatico-maxillary sutures. They involve the maxillary sinuses and pterygoid processes. Massive edema of the lips, midface, and eyes, and scattered ecchymoses may obscure an underlying "dishface" deformity of the midface. Diplopia and widening of the inner canthi of the eyes may occur. Malocclusion, with an anterior open bite, may be present.

Le Fort III fractures present with generalized facial edema and ecchymoses, lacerations, and hypesthesia of the upper lip. The fracture crosses the orbit, nose, pterygoid processes, and zygomatic arches. Craniofacial disjunction may occur, with mobility of the upper face on the cranial vault. A cranial fossa fracture may occur, with spinal fluid rhinorrhea.

C. Zygomatic Bone Pain, tenderness, and swelling occur over the cheek; there may be a dimpling or a dent in the cheek. Pain may occur on jaw motion if the coronoid process of the mandible is compressed by the fracture. There may be downward and lateral deformity of the outer canthus of the ipsilateral eye. A lower-lid deformity may occur, with widening of the palpebral fissure, and epiphora may be present. Enophthalmos, epistaxis, and subconjunctival bleeding may occur. Paresthesias and numbness may involve the upper lip. These fractures can be clearly visualized by a CT scan of the face.

D. Orbit Orbital and cheek pain, diplopia, enophthalmos, and visual loss may occur. Diplopia on vertical gaze results from muscle entrapment in the fracture. Enophthalmos results from loss of orbital fat into the maxillary sinus or expansion of the orbital space. Orbital edema and hemorrhage may also contribute to diplopia. Deformity and tenderness of the orbital margins may be present. Eyelid edema, ecchymoses, and subconjunctival bleeding occur. The pupil of the ipsilateral eye sits at a lower level than its opposite. Orbital fractures can be imaged by a CT scan.

2. PATHOLOGIC FRACTURES

Pathologic fracture of the mandible secondary to a metastatic (breast, lung, or colorectal carcinoma) or primary tumor is very rare. A neoplasm may present with persistent local aching pain and tenderness, swelling, malocclusion, loosening of teeth, trismus, and hypesthesia and paresthesias of the lips and lower face. The diagnosis of neoplasm can be made by plain radiographs and by a CT scan or MRI.

Chronic osteomyelitis, with local mandibular pain, swelling, tenderness, and draining sinus, may become acutely painful if a pathologic fracture of the mandible occurs. The diagnosis can be confirmed by a panoramic radiograph of the mandible.

3. TEMPOROMANDIBULAR JOINT (TMJ) PAIN

A. Acute Pseudogout and Gout In both disorders pain may begin abruptly in the TMJ, the ear, and the side of the face. There may be increased pain with chewing, and mild trismus may be present. The TMJ is tender and swollen. In patients with pseudogout radiographs of the TMJ may reveal a narrowed joint space with calcification; knee radiographs may show chondrocalcinosis; and polarized light microscopy of aspirated TMJ fluid may demonstrate calcium pyrophosphate dihydrate crystals. There is a good therapeutic response to nonsteroidal anti-inflammatory drugs or colchicine. Pain and dysfunction resolve without therapy in 1 to 2 weeks. Gout has been reported to cause an acute arthritis of the TMJ, but this is very rare. Uric acid crystals are present in the aspirated TMJ fluid. Other forms of arthritis affecting this joint rarely present as an acute arthritis (i.e., rheumatoid arthritis, systemic lupus erythematosus, ankylosing spondylitis, and osteoarthritis).

B. Lyme Disease A case report of Lyme disease mimicking a TMJ pain/dysfunction syndrome has been published. Meningismus and TMJ pain and tenderness were associated. No TMJ arthropathy occurred.

C. TMJ Pain/Dysfunction (Myofascial Pain Dysfunction) Syndrome Acute pain in the masseter and temporalis muscle areas on one side may occur. These muscles may be tender and firm, because of spasm. Attempts to open the jaw or chew may cause severe preauricular and jaw pain. There may be malocclusion and joint locking. This disorder may arise from a trigger point in one or more of the muscles of mastication, or may result from an internal derangement of the TMJ. Exclusion of an underlying deep space infection causing a secondary myofascial syndrome is essential for management; this can be accomplished with a CT scan or MRI of the upper neck, face, and head. Acute arthritis of the TMJ, or a displaced or torn meniscus, may cause joint pain and a secondary myofascial pain/dysfunction syndrome. MRI or contrast arthrography can detect an internal derangement or inflammatory disorder of the TMJ.

4. MAXILLARY SINUSITIS

A. Acute Suppurative Sinusitis Aching pain occurs over the cheek (37 percent of cases) and sometimes in the adjacent teeth. TMJ and ear pain are often associated. A unilateral predominance of cheek pain usually occurs, even when bilateral disease is present. There is a purulent, yellow-green, and often blood-streaked nasal and postnasal discharge. Early in the course, bloody mucoid discharge may occur. The maxillary pain may be intensified by lowering the head (i.e., as in bending over), and this may cause the pain to "pulse." Coughing and sneezing may also increase the pain. Clenching seems to ameliorate the dental ache. With infection of only one maxillary sinus, the purulent discharge is ipsilateral to the pain. Severe cacosmia occurs in 8 percent of cases and has a high predictive value for suppurative disease. Fever may or may not be present. Generalized malaise and frontal headache may also occur.

Signs include pus in the middle meatus on the affected side (41 percent of cases) and purulent ostial discharge (4 percent). Sinus percussion tenderness occurs in 43 percent. The presence of 3 or 4 of the following has a sensitivity of 81 percent and a specificity of 88 percent for the diagnosis of suppurative sinusitis: (1) purulent rhinorrhea with unilateral predominance; (2) cheek pain with unilateral predominance; (3) bilateral purulent rhinorrhea; and (4) pus in the nasal cavity. In addition, an elevated sedimentation rate increases the sensitivity beyond 81 percent.

An occipitomental, or Waters', view provides excellent radiographic imaging of the maxillary sinus. The occipitofrontal, or Caldwell, view demonstrates the frontal and ethmoid sinuses. Mucosal thickening of 6 to 8 mm or greater, opacification, or air-fluid levels have a high predictive value for purulent sinusitis. Less mucosal thickening has a low specificity (i.e., 48 to 74 percent). Sinus CT studies provide excellent imaging of all the sinuses, the adjacent orbits, and nasal cavities. The most commonly involved organisms include *Haemophilus influenzae, Streptococcus pneumoniae, Streptococcus pyogenes, Staphylococcus aureus,* and anaerobes. There is a good response to antibiotic therapy (e.g., cefaclor, cefuroxime, or amoxacillin–clavulinic acid).

Predisposing causes for the development of acute suppurative sinusitis include viral respiratory infection; sleeping in a dry, overheated environment; barotrauma; periapical dental abscess; allergy; nasal foreign bodies; polyps; underwater swimming; ostial obstruction by a septal spur or the septum; immotile cilia syndrome; and Kartagener's syndrome (bronchiectasis, sinusitis, and situs inversus). Systemic disorders that may predispose to sinusitis include diabetes mellitus, blood dyscrasias, steroid use, and antitumor chemotherapy.

B. Barotrauma   Aviation and deep-sea diving can cause painful sinus and/or ear injuries. In one series of barotrauma cases related to diving, pain occurred in the frontal region in 68 percent of cases; in the ethmoid region (bridge and side of nose) in 16 percent; and in the maxillary area in only 8 percent. Squeeze-type injuries occur on descent from altitude or from the sea surface to depth. Sinus ostial obstruction occurs at altitude or on the sea surface, and results in a sinus pressure that is lower than the ambient pressure at ground level or below the sea. This causes negative-pressure barotrauma. Pain and epistaxis or drainage of a watery, bloody discharge are the main complaints. A sinus may become partially or completely opacified by transudation of fluid and/or a submucous hematoma. Some patients with squeeze-related transudation may become symptomatic only on ascent, when ambient pressure is decreased and sinus gases cannot expand because of the contained fluid. Reverse squeeze occurs when a sinus becomes obstructed at takeoff or at a depth (in diving). With ascent, the ambient pressure decreases and a positive overpressure occurs in the sinus, leading to ischemia, mucosal injury, and bleeding. Pain and epistaxis also occur with this type of injury. Sinus radiographs may be normal (stage I), or may show mucosal thickening (stage II) or sinus opacification (stage III). Most cases of barotrauma will clear with use of decongestants and time. Surgical intervention is seldom required. Rare cases of facial hypesthesia, or even facial palsy, may occur because of barotrauma.

5. HERPES ZOSTER (MAXILLARY OR MANDIBULAR DIVISION OF NERVE V)

Burning or stinging pain may occur in the cheek, lower eyelid, and side of the nose (division II), or in the lower jaw (division III) on one side. Within 2 to 3 days, edema and redness of the skin develop in the painful area, and an eruption of small grouped vesicles on an erythematous base appears. These rupture, leaving small superficial ulcers covered with a red-brown hemorrhagic crust. In most cases the initial pain disappears within the first week, but in some the pain may persist for months. Acyclovir therapy has been used, but its efficacy has not been proved in controlled studies.

6. REFERRED PAIN

A. Myocardial Infarction and Coronary Insufficiency
Severe unilateral or bilateral lower jaw, dental, and neck pain may occur in the presence or absence of anterior crushing chest pain. Pain and/or numbness and paresthesias may radiate into one or both arms. Pallor, sweating, weakness, nausea, vomiting, and anxiety are common associated symptoms. Physical examination may reveal a gallop rhythm and/or distant heart sounds and frequent premature contractions. The ECG and serum isozyme levels will confirm a diagnosis of infarction. Similar pain may occur in patients with coronary insufficiency due to a partially obstructing intracoronary thrombus. The pain of complete or partial coronary obstruction may respond to thrombolytic therapy and/or direct angioplasty.

B. Dissecting Aneurysm   Pain begins suddenly in the midanterior chest and radiates to the neck, the jaws and lower face, the back, and the abdomen, in rapid succession. It is usually excruciating and has been described by some patients as having a tearing or ripping quality. Severe anxiety, sweating, nausea, and vomiting occur; patients may writhe in bed, unable to find a comfortable position. Examination may reveal a new aortic diastolic murmur (50 percent of cases), tachycardia, a gallop rhythm, and a loss or diminution of one or more peripheral pulses. A chest radiograph will show widening of the aortic shadow. Aortography or a CT scan with contrast will confirm the diagnosis of dissecting aneurysm of the aorta.

7. PAROTITIS

A. Acute Viral Parotitis   Mumps may begin with low-grade fever, malaise, and myalgias. A diffuse swelling develops at the angle of the jaw, preauricular region, and submandibular region on one side. This edema is accompanied by severe aching discomfort that is intensified by attempts to eat and drink. The skin over the swollen area is warm and taut, but not erythematous, and there is marked tenderness. The angle of the jaw is obscured and the examiner's fingers cannot separate the swelling from the mandible. Submaxillary swelling may occur during the next 2 days, and contralateral parotitis may also develop. Fever is usually low-grade, but temperature elevations to 103°F may occur. The serum amylase level may be markedly elevated. The pain and swelling continue for 3 to 10 days, and then gradually subside without sequelae. Analgesics and cold compresses may be required to control pain during the first week. Complications include epigastric pain and tenderness due to pancreatitis, testicular pain due to orchiitis, and headache and neck stiffness secondary to aseptic meningitis. Mumps virus is the usual cause; but Coxsackieviruses A and B, Epstein-Barr virus, influenza A, lymphocytic choriomeningitis, and parainfluenza virus may also cause acute parotitis that mimics mumps virus infection. Infection by these viruses explains second attacks of mumps occurring in some patients.

B. Acute Suppurative Parotitis   There is an abrupt onset of high fever, chills and/or rigors, and swelling of one or both (17 percent of cases) parotid glands. The overlying skin may be warm and erythematous, and the gland is firm, indurated, and tender. Pus can be expressed from Stensen's duct in 75 percent of cases. A marked polymorphonuclear leukocytosis may be present, with counts above 40,000 cells per mm³ (mean, 33,000 per mm³), as well as an elevated serum amylase level. The causative organism(s) can be obtained by needle aspiration of the gland. Aspirates should be cultured for aerobic and anaerobic bacteria, fungi, and mycobacteria. Surgical incision and drainage may be required to identify the causative organism(s).

Acute suppurative parotitis is a disease of the elderly, chronically ill, and debilitated patient. It is usually associated with xerostomia secondary to dehydration from failure to drink, overuse of diuretics, or administration of therapeutic agents with anticholinergic activity. Antibiotic therapy and poor oral hygiene also predispose patients to acute suppurative parotitis. This disorder may occur in the postoperative period (30 to 40 percent of cases in a recent series). Other factors that may increase a patient's risk for suppurative parotitis include malignancy, other foci of infection, and tracheostomy.

The most common isolates include *Staphylococcus aureus*, *Streptococcus pyogenes*, and α-hemolytic streptococci. Rare isolates include *Streptococcus pneumoniae*, *Haemophilus influenzae*, *Pseudomonas aeruginosa*, *Escherichia coli*, *Actinobacillus* species, anaerobes, mycobacteria, and *Candida* species. Parenteral antimicrobial therapy and sometimes incision and drainage are required for recovery.

C. Sialolithiasis   Aching, dull pain and parotid swelling occur on one side during meals. Citrus fruits may provoke this response more easily than other foods. The gland may decrease in size between meals, or the swelling and pain may persist. A salivary duct stone can be detected by palpation of the parotid duct or by radiography and removed, with relief of symptoms.

D. Iodism (Chronic Intoxication)   Initial symptoms consist of an abnormal metallic taste and a burning discomfort in the mouth and throat. The teeth and gums may be painful and tender. Coryza-like complaints, sneezing, headache, and eyelid edema occur. A productive cough, related to the stimulatory effect of iodide on bronchial secretion, occurs. Bilateral parotid and submaxillary gland pain, swelling, and tenderness develop, simulating mumps. Acneiform skin lesions may be present. All complaints resolve after discontinuation of the responsible iodide-containing medication.

8. LATERAL PHARYNGEAL SPACE INFECTION

Infection in the lateral pharyngeal space may arise from the lateral pharynx, tonsils (peritonsillar abscess), teeth, parotid gland, submandibular space, retropharyngeal space, or adjacent lymph nodes.

The styloid process divides the lateral pharyngeal space into an anterior, or prestyloid, compartment and a posterior, or neurovascular, compartment. Anterior compartment infection causes swelling and pain at the angle of the jaw and pain in the preauricular area, ear, and adjacent neck. Rotation of the head to the contralateral side intensifies the pain. Swallowing may be painful and impaired, and difficulty in opening the jaw (trismus) may be encountered. Fever, chills, and rigors are common associated findings. Severe cases may develop dyspnea and other symptoms of airway obstruction. Signs include toxicity and tenderness, induration, and edema at the angle of the mandible and above it. Trismus and medial bulging of the lateral pharyngeal wall may also occur. Lateral space infection can be confirmed by a CT scan or ultrasonography of the face and neck.

Posterior compartment infection may occur by extension from the anterior compartment or from another adjacent space. Severe toxicity, airway obstruction (due to laryngeal and epiglottic edema), and parotid space swelling may occur. Complications of posterior compartment infection include septic thrombophlebitis of the internal jugular vein. This may result in the appearance of a painful, tender mass in the upper anterior neck below the angle of the jaw; septic pulmonary emboli; phlebitis of adjacent veins and intracranial venous sinuses; and brain and metastatic abscesses. Infection of the common carotid artery and its branches may lead to aneurysm formation and rupture. "Herald bleeds" from the nose, mouth, or ear may be the first symptom of impending fatal rupture. Hemorrhage from the carotid may follow as long as 1 to 2 weeks after an adequate surgical drainage of the lateral pharyngeal space. Carotid infection may also be manifested by massive hemorrhage into the airway and shock, or by the formation of a neck hematoma. Lateral space infections require drainage and parenteral antibiotic therapy. Impending carotid rupture requires surgical intervention.

Peritonsillar abscess causes a persistent sore throat, fever, odynophagia, a muffled "hot potato" voice, and drooling. The tonsil is displaced medially, anteriorly, and inferiorly. Uncomplicated cases do not have severe toxicity, parotid swelling, or trismus. Development of these findings indicates spread of the infection to the lateral pharyngeal space. This can be confirmed by a CT study of the upper neck and face. Lateral space infections are an important complication of peritonsillar infection.

9. MASTICATOR SPACE INFECTION

This space contains the mandible and the muscles of mastication. Infection arises from a third molar (e.g., periapical abscess). Pain, swelling, and tenderness occur over the posterior portion of the mandible on the affected side. Trismus is usually present, while medial displacement of the lateral pharyngeal wall, rigors, and severe toxicity are not. Drainage and antibiotic therapy usually lead to resolution.

10. IDIOPATHIC TRIGEMINAL NEURALGIA (TIC DOULOUREUX)

Sharp, stabbing pain in the mandibular or maxillary area of the face, or both, may occur. The pain is described as lancinating and severe; patients wince and contort their faces as the pain is experienced (i.e., tic). Each jab lasts only seconds, but a train of pains may occur in sequence. There are trigger areas on the lower or midface or in the oral cavity. These may be stimulated by touching, chewing, talking, or shaving; by exposure to cold air; or by the eating of pungent fruit. Stimulation of a trigger area provokes a sharp shooting pain. There is no evidence of facial hypesthesia or motor impairment.

A. Microvascular Compression Idiopathic cases resistant to medical therapy may be due, in large part, to microvascular compression of the trigeminal nerve by the superior cerebellar artery (30 to 80 percent of medically resistant cases). Idiopathic trigeminal neuralgia occurs in persons past age 50, with most cases in the 60 to 85 age group.

B. Multiple Sclerosis Multiple sclerosis may present acutely with typical tic douloureux. Patients with this disease are younger, tend to have bilateral disease, and have difficulty tolerating carbamazepine or phenytoin therapy. While 13 percent of patients with multiple sclerosis and tic douloureux have no other findings of multiple sclerosis at onset, the remaining 87 percent have other symptoms and signs of demyelination (i.e., leg paresis, voice changes, optic neuritis, diplopia).

LOWER AND MIDFACIAL PAIN REFERENCES

Atypical Facial Pain

Baile WF Jr, Myers D: Psychological and behavioral dynamics in chronic atypical facial pain. *Anesth Prog* 33(5):252–257, 1986.

Brass LS, Amedee RG: Atypical facial pain. *J La State Med Soc* 142(1):15–18, 1990.

Drummond PD: Vascular changes in atypical facial pain. *Headache* 28:121–123, 1988.

Eriksson MBE, Sjölund BH, Sundbärg G: Pain relief from peripheral conditioning stimulation in patients with chronic facial pain. *J Neurosurg* 61:149–155, 1984.

Feinmann C, Harris M: The diagnosis and management of psychogenic facial pain disorders (editorial). *Clin Otolaryngol* 9:199–201, 1984.

Feinmann C, Harris M: Psychogenic facial pain: 1. The clinical presentation. *Br Dent J* 156:165–168, 1984; 2. Management and prognosis. *Br Dent J* 156:205–208, 1984.

Feinmann C, Harris M, Cawley R: Psychogenic facial pain: Presentation and treatment. *Br Med J* 288:436–438, 1984.

Gale EN: Psychophysiological treatment of facial pain syndromes. *N Y State Dent J* 51(5):273–275, 1985.

Goss AN, Speculand B, Hallet E: Diagnosis of temporomandibular joint pain in patients seen at a pain clinic. *J Oral Maxillofac Surg* 43:110–114, 1985.

Harness DM, Rome HP: Psychological and behavioral aspects of chronic facial pain. *Otolaryngol Clin North Am* 22(6):1073–1094, 1989.

Keller JT, Van Loveren H: Pathophysiology of the pain of trigeminal neuralgia and atypical facial pain: A neuroanatomical perspective. *Clin Neurosurg* 32:275–293, 1985.

Lam RW, Remick RA: The lateralization of atypical facial pain. *Can J Psychiatry* 33(2):100–102, 1988.

Lazorthes Y, Armengaud JP, Da Motta M: Chronic stimulation of the Gasserion ganglion for treatment of atypical facial neuralgia. *PACE* 10(2):257–265, 1987.

Malinow KL, Grace EG: Facial pain and monosymptomatic hypochondriasis. *J Oral Maxillofac Surg* 42:330–332, 1984.

Martins IP, Ferro JM: Atypical facial pain, ectasia of the basilar artery, and baclofen: A case report. *Headache* 29:581–583, 1989.

Mastrocola R, Gross A, Hall RE: Atypical facial pain of psychogenic origin. *Gen Dent* 35(3):207–209, 1987.

Mock D, Frydman W, Gordon AS: Atypical facial pain: A retrospective study. *Oral Surg Oral Med Oral Pathol* 59:472–474, 1985.

Ramani V: Brainstem auditory evoked potentials in atypical facial neuralgia. *J Oral Maxillofac Surg* 43:35–37, 1985.

Reik L Jr: Atypical facial pain: A reappraisal. *Headache* 25:30–32, 1985.

Carotodynia
Murray TJ: Carotidynia: A cause of neck and face pain. *Can Med Assoc J* 120:441–443, 1979.
Raskin NH, Prusiner S: Carotidynia. *Neurology* 27:43–46, 1977.

Cervical Lymphadenitis
Dossett JH, Weitekamp M: Cervical lymphadenitis, in Schlossberg D (ed): *Infections of the Head and Neck*. New York, Springer-Verlag, 1987, pp 161–167.

Cluster Headache
Eversole LR, Stone CE: Vasogenic facial pain (cluster headache). *Int J Oral Maxillofac Surg* 16:25–35, 1987.
Gerbe RW, Fry TL, Fischer ND: Headache of nasal spur origin: An easily diagnosed and surgically correctable cause of facial pain. *Headache* 24:329–330, 1984.
Joubert J: Cluster headache in black patients: A report of 7 cases. *S Afr Med J* 73:552–554, 1988.
Kudrow L: Cluster headache: New concepts. *Neurol Clin* 1(2):369–383, 1983.
McKenna JP: Cluster headaches. *Am Fam Physician* 37(4):173–178, 1988.
Onofrio BM, Campbell JK: Surgical treatment of chronic cluster headache. *Mayo Clin Proc* 61:537–544, 1986.
Tegeler CH, Bell RD: Vascular headache. *Otolaryngol Clin North Am* 20(1):65–82, 1987.

Craniomandibular Disorders
Cooper BC: Craniomandibular disorders, in Cooper BC, Lucente FE (eds): *Management of Facial, Head and Neck Pain*. Philadelphia, Saunders, 1989, pp 153–254.

Deep Neck Infections
Echevarria J: Deep neck infections, in Schlossberg D (ed): *Infections of the Head and Neck*. New York, Springer-Verlag, 1987, pp 168–184.

Eagle's Syndrome
Dolan EA, Mullen JB, Papayoanou J: Styloid-stylohyoid syndrome in the differential diagnosis of atypical facial pain. *Surg Neurol* 21:291–294, 1984.
Hampf G, Aalberg V, Tasanen A, et al: A holistic approach to sylalgia. *Int J Oral Maxillofac Surg* 15:549–552, 1986.

Facial Pain—Referred
Schnetler J, Hopper C: Intracranial tumours presenting with facial pain. *Br Dent J* 166:80–83, 1989.

Facial Pain—Review Articles
Chow AW: Infections of the oral cavity, head, and neck, in Mandell GL, Douglas RG Jr, Bennett JE (eds): *Principles and Practice of Infectious Diseases*, 3d ed. New York, Churchill Livingstone, 1990, pp 516–529.
Crews DA, Warfield CA: Facial pain. *Hosp Pract [Off]* 20(4):171–172, 175, 179, 1985.
Drinnan AJ: Differential diagnosis of orofacial pain. *Dent Clin North Am* 22(1):73–87, 1978.
Drinnan AJ: Differential diagnosis of orofacial pain. *Dent Clin North Am* 31(4):627–643, 1987.
Mandel S: Facial pain: Why does my face hurt, doctor? *Postgrad Med* 87(1):77–80, 1990.
Sessle BJ: Neural mechanisms of oral and facial pain. *Otolaryngol Clin North Am* 22(6):1059–1072, 1989.
Zilkha KJ: Facial pain. *Br J Hosp Med* 21(2):112–114, 1979.

Facial Pain—Secondary to an Underlying Lesion
Bindoff LA, Hesseltine D: Unilateral facial pain in patients with lung cancer: A referred pain via the vagus? *Lancet* 1(8589)812–815, 1988.
Broderick JP, Auger RG, DeSanto LW: Facial paralysis and occult parotid cancer. *Arch Otolaryngol Head Neck Surg* 114:195–197, 1988.

Crosher RF, Blackburn CW, Dinsdale RCW: Blue rubber-bleb naevus syndrome. *Br J Oral Maxillofac Surg* 26:160–164, 1988.
Dixon JA: Spontaneous external carotid artery occlusion. *J Laryngol Otol* 103:710–712, 1989.
Jones MT, Lawson RAM: Unilateral facial pain as a rare presentation of bronchial carcinoma. *Br J Clin Pract* 41(11):1025–1026, 1987.
Katusic SK, Beard CM, Wiederholt WC, et al: Incidence, clinical features, and prognosis in Bell's palsy, Rochester, Minnesota, 1968–1982. *Ann Neurol* 20:622–627, 1986.
Ruff T, Lenis A, Diaz JA: Atypical facial pain and orbital cancer. *Arch Otolaryngol* 111:338–339, 1985.
Watt TLP: Unilateral facial pain in patients with lung cancer (editorial). *Lancet* 1(8595):1168–1169, 1988.
Whittet HB, Quiney RE: Dehiscence of the infraorbital nerve as a new cause of facial pain. *Br Med J [Clin Res]* 296(6614):18–19, 1988.

Facial Trauma
Bell RM, Page GV, Bynoe RP, et al: Post-traumatic sinusitis. *J Trauma* 28(7):923–930, 1988.
Busuito MJ, Smith DJ Jr, Robson MC: Mandibular fractures in an urban trauma center. *J Trauma* 26(9):826–829, 1986.
Gruss JS: Complex craniomaxillofacial trauma: Evolving concepts in management, a trauma unit's experience—1989 Fraser B. Gurd lecture. *J Trauma* 30(4):377–383, 1990.
Mayer JS, Wainwright DJ, Yeakley JW, et al: The role of three-dimensional computed tomography in the management of maxillofacial trauma. *J Trauma* 28(7):1043–1053, 1988.
Reath DB, Kirby J, Lynch M, et al: Patterns of maxillofacial injuries in restrained and unrestrained motor vehicle crash victims. *J Trauma* 29(6):806–810, 1989.
Scherer M, Sullivan WG, Smith DJ Jr, et al: An analysis of 1,423 facial fractures in 788 patients at an urban trauma center. *J Trauma* 29(3):388–390, 1989.

Mandibular Infarction
Hammersley N: Mandibular infarction occurring during a sickle cell crisis. *Br J Oral Maxillofac Surg* 22:103–114, 1984.

Maxilla/Mandible Osteomyelitis
Calhoun KH, Shapiro RD, Stiernberg CM, et al: Osteomyelitis of the mandible. *Arch Otolaryngol Head Neck Surg* 114:1157–1162, 1988.
Felsberg GJ, Gore RL, Schweitzer ME, et al: Sclerosing osteomyelitis of Garrè (periostitis ossificans). *Oral Surg Oral Med Oral Pathol* 70:117–120, 1990.
Gill Y, Scully C: Orofacial odontogenic infections: Review of microbiology and current treatment. *Oral Surg Oral Med Oral Pathol* 70:155–158, 1990.
Kashima I, Tajima K, Nishimura K, et al: Diagnostic imaging of diseases affecting the mandible with the use of computed panoramic radiography. *Oral Surg Oral Med Oral Pathol* 70:110–116, 1990.
Schneider LC, Mesa ML: Differences between florid osseous dysplasia and chronic diffuse sclerosing osteomyelitis. *Oral Surg Oral Med Oral Pathol* 70:308–312, 1990.
Shannon MT, Sclaroff A, Colm SJ: Invasive aspergillosis of the maxilla in an immunocompromised patient. *Oral Surg Oral Med Oral Pathol* 70:425–427, 1990.
van Merkesteyn JPR, Groot RH, Bras J, et al: Diffuse sclerosing osteomyelitis of the mandible: A new concept of its etiology. *Oral Surg Oral Med Oral Pathol* 70:414–419, 1990.

Maxilla/Mandible Tumors
Borghelli RF, Barros RE, Zampieri J: Ewing sarcoma of the mandible: Report of case. *Oral Surg* 36:473–475, 1978.
Chuchurru JA, Luberti R, Cornicelli JC, et al: Myxoma of the mandible with unusual radiographic appearance. *J Oral Maxillofac Surg* 43:987–990, 1985.
Chuong R, Kagan LB: Diagnosis and treatment of jaw tumors in children. *J Oral Maxillofac Surg* 43(5):323–332, 1985.
Cook HE: Chondrosarcoma arising from the zygomatic arch. *J Oral Maxillofac Surg* 44:67–69, 1986.
Corio RL, Goldblatt LI, Edwards PA, et al: Ameloblastic carcinoma:

A clinicopathologic study and assessment of eight cases. *Oral Surg Oral Med Oral Pathol* 64:570–576, 1987.

Eisenberg E, Leiblich S, Glogoff M: Facial swelling in an adolescent female. *J Oral Maxillofac Surg* 47:843–848, 1989.

Garrington GE, Scofield HH, Cornyn J, et al: Osteosarcoma of the jaws: Analysis of 56 cases. *Cancer* 20:377–391, 1967.

Lindqvist C, Teppo L, Sane J, et al: Osteosarcoma of the mandible: Analysis of nine cases. *J Oral Maxillofac Surg* 44:759–764, 1986.

Moran WJ: Tumors and cysts of the maxilla and mandible, in Lee KJ (ed): *Textbook of Otolaryngology and Head and Neck Surgery*. New York, Elsevier, 1989, pp 415–432.

Morris MR, Clark SK, Porter BA, et al: Chondrosarcoma of the temporomandibular joint: Case report. *Head Neck Surg* 10:113–117, 1987.

Nortjé CJ, Farman AG, Grotepass FW, et al: Chondrosarcoma of the mandibular condyle: Report of a case with special reference to radiographic features. *Br J Oral Surg* 14:101–111, 1976.

Okuyama T, Suzuki H, Umehara I, et al: Diagnosis of aneurysmal bone cyst of the mandible: A report of two cases with emphasis on scintigraphic approaches. *Clin Nucl Med* 10:786–790, 1985.

Orden A, Laskin DM, Lew D: Chronic preauricular swelling. *J Oral Maxillofac Surg* 47:390–397, 1989.

Schwartz ML, Baredes S, Mignogna FV: Metastatic disease to the mandible. *Laryngoscope* 98(3):270–273, 1988.

Sturrock BD, Marks RB, Gross BD, et al: Giant cell tumor of the mandible. *J Oral Maxillofac Surg* 42:262–267, 1984.

Midfacial Pain

Eng CT, Vasconez LO: Facial pain due to perineural invasion by basal cell carcinoma. *Ann Plastic Surg* 12(4):374–377, 1984.

Haidar Z: Facial pain of uncommon origin. *Oral Surg Oral Med Oral Pathol* 63(6):748–749, 1987.

Midfacial Pain—Multiple Cranial Neuropathy

Juncos JL, Beal MF: Idiopathic cranial polyneuropathy: A fifteen-year experience. *Brain* 110:197–211, 1987.

Myofascial Pain Mimics

Lloyd JM, Mitchell RG: Myasthenia gravis as a cause of facial pain. *Oral Surg Oral Med Oral Pathol* 66:45–46, 1988.

Roistacher S, Tanenbaum D: Myofascial pain associated with oropharyngeal cancer. *Oral Surg Oral Med Oral Pathol* 61:459–462, 1986.

Nasopharyngeal Carcinoma

Milton CM: A retrospective study of nasopharyngeal carcinoma presenting over a 10-year period. *ORL J Otorhinolaryngol Relat Spec* 47:169–173, 1985.

Neurological Causes

Kessler JT: Neurological causes of head and face pain, in Cooper BC, Lucente FE (eds): *Management of Facial, Head and Neck Pain*. Philadelphia, Saunders, 1989, pp 23–51.

Orbital Pain

Carter JE: Ophthalmic and neuro-ophthalmic aspects of headache and head pain. *Neurol Clin* 1(2):415–443, 1983.

Johnson LN, Krohel GB, Yeon EB, et al: Sinus tumors invading the orbit. *Ophthalmology* 91:209–217, 1984.

Ryan RE Jr, Kern EB: Rhinologic causes of facial pain and headache. *Headache* 18:44–50, 1978.

Parotid Disease

Boles R: Parotid neoplasms: Surgical treatment and complications. *Otolaryngol Clin North Am* 10(2)413–420, 1977.

Grace EG, North AF: Temporomandibular joint dysfunction and orofacial pain caused by parotid gland malignancy: Report of case. *J Am Dent Assoc* 116:348–350, 1988.

Lam KH, Wei WI, Lau WF: Tumours of the parotid: The value of clinical assessment. *Aust N Z J Surg* 56:325–329, 1986.

Laudadio P, Caliceti U, Tito P, et al: Mucoepidermoid tumour of the parotid gland: A very difficult prognostic evaluation. *Clin Otolaryngol* 12:177–182, 1987.

Partridge M, Langdon JD, Borthwick-Clarke A, et al: Diagnostic techniques for parotid disease. *Br J Oral Maxillofac Surg* 24:311–322, 1986.

Perry RS: Recognition and management of acute suppurative parotitis. *Clin Pharm* 4:566–571, 1985.

Regezi JA, Batsakis JG: Histogenesis of salivary gland neoplasms. *Otolaryngol Clin North Am* 10(2):297–307, 1977.

Shaha A, Thelmo W, Jaffe BM: Is parotid lymphadenopathy a new disease or part of AIDS? *Am J Surg* 156(4):297–300, 1988.

Shemen LJ, Huvos AG, Spiro RH: Squamous cell carcinoma of salivary gland origin. *Head Neck Surg* 9:235–240, 1987.

Travis LW, Hecht DW: Acute and chronic inflammatory diseases of the salivary glands: Diagnosis and management. *Otolaryngol Clin North Am* 10(2):329–338, 1977.

Work WP: Parapharyngeal space and salivary gland neoplasms. *Otolaryngol Clin North Am* 10(2):421–426, 1977.

Wyatt MG, Coleman N, Eveson JW, et al: Management of high grade parotid carcinomas. *Br J Surg* 76:1275–1277, 1989.

Raeder's Syndrome

Kashihara K, Ito H, Yamamoto S, et al: Raeder's syndrome associated with intracranial internal carotid artery aneurysm. *Neurosurgery* 20(1):49–51, 1987.

Reflex Sympathetic Dystrophy—Face

Jaeger B, Singer E, Kroening R: Reflex sympathetic dystrophy of the face: Report of two cases and a review of the literature. *Arch Neurol* 43:693–695, 1986.

Sinus Pain

Chakeres DW: Computed tomography of the ethmoid sinuses. *Otolaryngol Clin North Am* 18(1):29–42, 1985.

Friedman WH, Rosenblum BN: Paranasal sinus etiology of headaches and facial pain. *Otolaryngol Clin North Am* 22(6):1217–1228, 1989.

Friedman WH, Slavin RG: Diagnosis and medical and surgical treatment of sinusitis in adults. *Clin Rev Allergy* 2:409–428, 1984.

Garges LM: Maxillary sinus barotrauma: Case report and review. *Aviat Space Environ Med* 56:796–802, 1985.

Joseph DJ, Renner G: Head pain from diseases of the ear, nose, and throat. *Neurol Clin* 1(2):399–414, 1983.

Kern EB: Suppurative (bacterial) sinusitis. *Postgrad Med* 81(4):194–198, 203–210, 1987.

Sphenopalatine Neuralgia

Cepero R, Miller RH, Bressler KL: Long-term results of sphenopalatine ganglioneurectomy for facial pain. *Am J Otolaryngol* 3:171–174, 1987.

Temporomandibular Joint Internal Derangements

Kaplan PA, Reiskin AB, Tu HK: Temporomandibular joint arthrography following surgical treatment of internal derangements. *Radiology* 163:217–220, 1987.

Walker RV, Kalamchi S: A surgical technique for management of internal derangement of the temporomandibular joint. *J Oral Maxillofac Surg* 45:299–305, 1987.

Temporomandibular Joint Pain—Dysfunction

Ash MM: Current concepts in the aetiology, diagnosis and treatment of TMJ and muscle dysfunction. *J Oral Rehabil* 13:1–20, 1986.

Bell WE: Temporomandibular joint pains, in *Orofacial Pains: Classification, Diagnosis, Management*, 4th ed. Chicago, Year Book Medical, 1989, pp 285–331.

Bezuur JN, Habets LMH, Lopez VJ, et al: The recognition of craniomandibular disorders: A comparison between clinical and radiographic findings in eighty-nine subjects. *J Oral Rehabil* 15:215–221, 1988.

Burgess JA, Sommers EE, Truelove EL, et al: Short-term effect of two therapeutic methods on myofascial pain and dysfunction of the masticatory system. *J Prosthet Dent* 60(5):606–610, 1988.

Bush FM: Tinnitus and otalgia in temporomandibular disorders. *J Prosthet Dent* 58(4):495–498, 1987.

Heikinheimo K, Salmi K, Myllärniemi S, et al: Symptoms of craniomandibular disorder in a sample of Finnish adolescents at the ages of 12 and 15 years. *Eur J Orthod* 11:325–331, 1989.

Hijzen TH, Slangen JL: Myofascial pain-dysfunction: Subjective signs and symptoms. *J Prosthet Dent* 54(5):705–711, 1985.

Hodges J: Managing temporomandibular joint syndrome. *Laryngoscope* 100(1):60–66, 1990.

Lipton JA, Marbach JJ: Predictors of treatment outcome in patients with myofascial pain-dysfunction syndrome and organic temporomandibular joint disorders. *J Prosthet Dent* 51(3):387–393, 1984.

Okeson JP: Diagnosis of temporomandibular disorders, in *Fundamentals of Occlusion and Temporomandibular Disorders*. St. Louis, Mosby, 1985, pp 238–260.

Okeson JP: History and examination for temporomandibular disorders, in *Fundamentals of Occlusion and Temporomandibular Disorders*. St. Louis, Mosby, 1985, pp 185–237.

Rihani A: Maxillary sinusitis as a differential diagnosis in temporomandibular joint pain-dysfunction syndrome. *J Prosthet Dent* 53(1):97–100, 1985.

Schellhas KP, Wilkes CH, Baker CC: Facial pain, headache, and temporomandibular joint inflammation. *Headache* 29:228–231, 1989.

Wänman A, Agerberg G: Mandibular dysfunction in adolescents. *Acta Odontol Scand* 44:47–54, 1986.

Yusuf H, Rothwell PS: Temporomandibular joint pain-dysfunction in patients suffering from atypical facial pain. *Br Dent J* 161:208–212, 1986.

Temporomandibular Joint Pain—Dysfunction Mimics

Ellman MH, Krieger MI, Brown N: Pseudogout mimicking synovial chondromatosis. *J Bone Jt Surg* 57-A(6):863–865, 1975.

Ettala-Ylitalo U-M, Syrjänen S, Halonen P: Functional disturbances of the masticatory system related to temporomandibular joint involvement by rheumatoid arthritis. *J Oral Rehabil* 14:415–427, 1987.

Good AE, Upton LG: Acute temporomandibular arthritis in a patient with bruxism and calcium pyrophosphate deposition disease. *Arthritis Rheum* 25(3):353–355, 1982.

Hutton CW, Doherty M, Dieppe PA: Acute pseudogout of the temporomandibular joint: A report of three cases and review of the literature. *Br J Rheumatol* 26:51–52, 1987.

Kleinman HZ, Ewbank RL: Gout of the temporomandibular joint: Report of three cases. *Oral Surg Oral Med Oral Pathol* 27(2):281–282, 1969.

Lader E: Lyme disease misdiagnosed as TMJ syndrome. *N Y State Dent J* 55(9):46, 48, 50, 52, 1989.

Marciani RD, Haley JV, Roth GI: Facial pain complaints in the elderly. *J Oral Maxillofac Surg* 43:173–176, 1985.

Merrill RG, Yih WY, Langan MJ: A histologic evaluation of the accuracy of TMJ diagnostic arthroscopy. *Oral Surg Oral Med Oral Pathol* 70:393–398, 1990.

Pritzker KPH, Phillips H, Luk SC, et al: Pseudotumor of temporomandibular joint: Destructive calcium pyrophosphate dihydrate arthropathy. *J Rheumatol* 3:70–81, 1976.

Quinn JH: Arthroscopic and histologic evidence of chondromalacia in the temporomandibular joint. *Oral Surg Oral Med Oral Pathol* 70(3):387–392, 1990.

Schellhas KP: Temporomandibular joint injuries. *Radiology* 173:211–216, 1989.

Schellhas KP, Wilkes CH, El Deeb M, et al: Permanent proplast temporomandibular joint implants: MR imaging of destructive complications. *AJR* 151:731–735, 1988.

Schellhas KP, Wilkes CH, Fritts HM, et al: MR of osteochondritis dissecans and avascular necrosis of the mandibular condyle. *AJR* 152:551–560, 1989.

Temporomandibular Joint Pain—Dysfunction—Malignant and Infectious Mimics

Cohen SG, Quinn PD: Facial trismus and myofascial pain associated with infections and malignant disease. *Oral Surg Oral Med Oral Pathol* 65:538–544, 1988.

Trigeminal Neuralgia—Idiopathic

Brown, JA, Pruel MC: Percutaneous trigeminal ganglion compression for trigeminal neuralgia: Experience in 22 patients and review of the literature. *J Neurosurg* 70:900–904, 1989.

Frank RA: Cranial neuralgias. *Neurol Clin* 1(2):501–509, 1983.

Jannetta PJ, Bissonette DJ: Management of the failed patient with trigeminal neuralgia. *Clin Neurosurg* 32:334–347, 1985.

Lunsford LD, Apfelbaum RI: Choice of surgical therapeutic modalities for treatment of trigeminal neuralgia: Microvascular decompression, percutaneous retrogasserian thermal, or glycerol rhizotomy. *Clin Neurosurg* 32:319–333, 1985.

Lunsford LD, Bennett MH: Percutaneous retrogasserian glycerol rhizotomy for tic douloureux: 1. Technique and results in 112 patients. *Neurosurgery* 14(4):424–430, 1984.

Rappaport ZH, Gomori JM: Recurrent trigeminal cistern glycerol injections for tic douloureux. *Acta Neurochir (Wien)* 90:31–34, 1988.

Roberts AM, Person P, Chandran NB, et al: Further observations on dental parameters of trigeminal and atypical facial neuralgias. *Oral Surg Oral Med Oral Pathol* 58:121–129, 1984.

Spaziante R, Cappabianca P, Peca C, et al: Percutaneous retrogasserian glycerol rhizolysis: Observations and results in about 50 cases. *J Neurosurg Sci* 31:121–128, 1987.

Trigeminal Neuralgia—Microvascular

Dahle L, von Essen C, Kourtopoulos H, et al: Microvascular decompression for trigeminal neuralgia. *Acta Neurochir (Wien)* 99:109–112, 1989.

Klun B, Prestor B: Microvascular relations of the trigeminal nerve: An anatomical study. *Neurosurg* 19(4):535–539, 1986.

Lye RH: Basilar artery ectasia: An unusual cause of trigeminal neuralgia. *J Neurol Neurosurg Psychiatry* 49:22–28, 1986.

Trigeminal Neuralgia—Secondary

Beck DW, Menezes AH: Lesions in Meckel's cave: Variable presentation and pathology. *J Neurosurg* 67:684–689, 1987.

Belal A Jr: Retrolabyrinthine surgery: Anatomy and pathology. *Am J Otol* 7(1):29–33, 1986.

Bitoh S, Hasegawa H, Ohtsuke H, et al: Parasellar metastases: Four autopsied cases. *Surg Neurol* 23:41–48, 1985.

Brisman R: Trigeminal neuralgia and multiple sclerosis. *Arch Neurol* 44:379–381, 1987.

Bullitt E, Tew JM, Boyd J: Intracranial tumors in patients with facial pain. *J Neurosurg* 64:865–871, 1986.

Dieckmann G, Veras G, Sogabe K: Retrogasserian glycerol injection or percutaneous stimulation in the treatment of typical and atypical trigeminal pain. *Neurol Res* 9(1):48–49, 1987.

Harrington HJ, Mayman CI: Carotid body tumor associated with partial Horner's syndrome and facial pain ("Raeder's syndrome"). *Arch Neurol* 40:564–566, 1983.

Linderoth B, Håkanson S: Paroxysmal facial pain in disseminated sclerosis treated by retrogasserian glycerol injection. *Acta Neurol Scand* 80:341–346, 1989.

McCormick PC, Bello JA, Post KD: Trigeminal schwannoma: Surgical series of 14 cases with review of the literature. *J Neurosurg* 69:850–860, 1988.

Nager GT: Neurinomas of the trigeminal nerve. *Am J Otolaryngol* 5:301–333, 1984.

Perkin GD, Illingworth RD: The association of hemifacial spasm and facial pain. *J Neurol Neurosurg Psychiatry* 52:663–665, 1989.

Tsubaki S-I, Fukushima T, Tamagawa T, et al: Parapontine trigeminal cryptic angiomas presenting as trigeminal neuralgia. *J Neurosurg* 71:368–374, 1989.

Vassilakis D, Phylaktakis M, Selviaridis P, et al: Symptomatic trigeminal neuralgia. *J Neurosurg Sci* 32:117–120, 1988.

Yasui T, Hakuba A, Kim SH, et al: Trigeminal neurinomas: Operative approach in eight cases. *J Neurosurg* 71:506–511, 1989.

Trigeminal Sensory Neuropathy

Lecky BRF, Hughes RAC, Murray NMF: Trigeminal sensory neuropathy: A study of 22 cases. *Brain* 110:1463–1485, 1987.

Acute Mouth, Tongue, and Lip Pain

☐ DIAGNOSTIC LIST

MOUTH PAIN
1. Dental pain
   A. Acute pulpitis or pulpal abscess
   B. Periapical abscess and dental ulcer
   C. Pericoronitis
   D. Acute complications of dental therapy
      1. Post-endodontic surgery pain
      2. Dry socket
      3. "High bite" pain after dental restoration
      4. Toothbrush-related gingival erosion and tooth injury
   E. Acute necrotizing ulcerative gingivitis (ANUG)
2. Mimics of dental disease
   A. Acute maxillary sinusitis
   B. Acute myocardial infarction
   C. Ernest syndrome
   D. Trigeminal neuralgia
   E. Sphenopalatine ganglion neuralgia
3. Acute (primary) herpetic gingivostomatitis
4. Stevens-Johnson syndrome
5. Toxic epidermal necrolysis (TEN)
6. Acute oral ulcers
   A. Trauma
   B. Burns
   C. Viral infections
      1. Varicella-zoster virus
      2. Epstein-Barr virus
      3. Hand-foot-and-mouth disease
      4. Herpangina (Coxsackievirus group A)
   D. Gonococcal stomatitis
   E. Aphthous ulcers
   F. Syphilis
      1. Primary syphilis
      2. Secondary syphilis
7. Stomatitis
   A. Contact stomatitis (stomatitis venenata)
   B. Irritant stomatitis
   C. Oral drug reactions (stomatitis medicamentosa)
      1. Allergic stomatitis
      2. Lichenoid drug reactions
      3. Pemphigus-like drug reactions
      4. Lupus erythematosus–like drug reactions
      5. Cytotoxic drug reactions
         A. Mucositis
         B. Mucositis and agranulocytic ulceration
8. Systemic disease and oral lesions
   A. Leukemia
      1. Leukemic gingivitis
      2. Oral candidiasis
      3. Dental disease
      4. Ecthyma gangrenosum (*Pseudomonas* species)
      5. Ulceronecrotic lesions of unknown cause
      6. Acute necrotizing ulcerative gingivitis

7. Herpes simplex virus infection
8. Varicella-zoster virus infection
9. Cytotoxic drug reactions
B. Acquired immunodeficiency syndrome (AIDS)
   1. Candidiasis
   2. Ulcerative lesions
      A. Herpes simplex virus (HSV) (labial and intraoral)
      B. Cytomegalovirus
      C. Idiopathic prednisone-responsive oral aphthae
      D. Herpes zoster
      E. Periodontal disease and acute necrotizing ulcerative gingivitis
      F. Necrotizing stomatitis
   3. Neoplastic disorders
      A. Kaposi's sarcoma
      B. Lymphoma
   4. Hairy leukoplakia
C. Diabetes mellitus
D. Uremia
TONGUE PAIN
9. Glossitis and/or glossodynia
   A. Candidiasis
   B. Gonococcal glossitis and ulceration
   C. *Trichomonas vaginalis* glossitis
   D. Staphylococcal glossitis
   E. *Pseudomonas* infection (ecthyma gangrenosum)

F. Gram-negative bacterial ulceration
G. Stevens-Johnson syndrome
H. Acute necrotizing ulcerative gingivitis
I. *Chlamydia trachomatis* glossitis and ulceration
J. Tularemia
K. Herpes simplex virus ulceration
L. Cytomegalovirus infection
M. Syphilis
   1. Primary syphilis
   2. Secondary syphilis
N. Tongue bites and burns
O. Contact allergy
P. Toxic epidermal necrolysis
Q. Aphthous ulcers
R. Allergic glossitis
S. Coxsackievirus or enterovirus infection
LIP PAIN
10. Acute cheilitis
   A. Actinic cheilitis
   B. Isotretinoin therapy
   C. Allergic cheilitis
   D. Herpes simplex virus infection
   E. Impetigo
   F. Factitious cheilitis
   G. Stevens-Johnson syndrome and toxic epidermal necrolysis
   H. Angular cheilitis from *Staphylococcus aureus* or *Candida* species
   I. Chapping from exposure to cold and/or wind

☐ SUMMARY

Acute pulpitis begins with brief attacks of cold-induced tooth and/or jaw pain. Soon, hot stimuli, bite pressure, and percussion of the affected tooth induce pain. Continuous prolonged aching follows days or weeks after the onset of temperature-provoked pain. The constant ache may progress over a period of hours or days to an excruciating, intolerable, throbbing pain. Endodontic surgery or extraction may be required for pain relief. Extension of pulpal infection from the root into the periapical area can cause a *periapical abscess* visible on a dental x-ray as a radiolucent zone. Dull aching pain or minimal discomfort may be present. Gingival tenderness may be detected over a root of the affected tooth. *Pericoronitis* is due to trauma and infection of gingival tissue overlying a partially

erupted posterior molar. There is pain and tenderness behind the last fully erupted molar; trismus may be present, limiting the examination. *Endodontic surgery* may be followed by 1 to 2 days of excruciating dental pain that resolves spontaneously. *Tooth extraction* can be followed by severe pain if the clot is lost from the socket, leaving a dry socket. A dental restoration leaving a *"high bite"* can cause pulpitis-like sensitivity of the restored tooth or its opposite contact. This can be resolved by reducing the "high bite." *Vigorous brushing* of the teeth can cause a painful gingival erosion. *Acute necrotizing ulcerative gingivitis (ANUG)* causes interdental edema, hyperemia, and erosion, with local pain and bleeding. Fever and other systemic symptoms may be present. Ulcers and exudative lesions may occur in the tonsillar areas and posterior pharynx, and a painful cervical lymphadenitis may be present.

Aching pain in the upper jaw can be associated with *acute maxillary sinusitis*. Purulent nasal and postnasal discharge, cheek pain and tenderness, sore throat, and sometimes fever may be associated. Jaw and/or neck and/or arm and chest pain may be due to an *acute myocardial infarction*. *Ernest syndrome* causes jaw, posterior tooth, eye, and ear pain; it also causes limitation of jaw opening and protrusion. Local tenderness of the stylomandibular ligament is present. Lidocaine injection of this site transiently relieves all symptoms. *Trigeminal neuralgia* causes jabs of lancinating jaw and tooth pain that occur singly or as repetitive jabs. One or more oral or facial trigger points, which provoke an attack when stimulated, are present. *Sphenopalatine ganglion neuralgia* causes nasal, orbital, maxillary, and upper-jaw dental pain; ipsilateral nasal stuffiness; rhinorrhea; and lacrimation. Symptoms are relieved temporarily by cocainization of the sphenopalatine ganglion.

Primary herpes simplex infection causes gingival redness, edema, and painful ulceration. Erythema and ulceration may also occur on the labial, buccal, and lingual mucosas. Fever, chills, malaise, and headache are associated. The diagnosis depends on the clinical findings and cultures of lesion exudate. A specific direct fluorescent antibody (DFA) stain is available for H. simplex virus and can be used to stain lesion scrapings. *Stevens-Johnson syndrome* may cause fever, chills, malaise, and a generalized maculopapular eruption with target and herpes iris lesions. Oral bullae may form, rupture, and result in painful mucosal erosions. Labial mucosal and vermilion border erosions and ulcers appear and become covered with hemorrhagic crusts. *Toxic epidermal necrolysis* causes fever and diffuse skin erythema. Large flaccid bullae form on erythematous cutaneous areas and rupture, leaving painful erosions. A similar process occurs on the oral mucosa, causing pain and tenderness. Conjunctival and genital inflammation may also be present. Sensitivity to drugs is the usual cause. *Trauma* or *thermal or chemical burns* can cause painful oral ulcerations with regular or irregular, narrow, erythematous margins and surface exudate. *Herpes zoster* causes unilateral jaw and mouth pain and an eruption of small, grouped vesicles and ulcers on the ipsilateral half of the lower or upper jaw and mouth. Culture will grow varicella-zoster virus. A DFA stain for varicella-zoster virus is available. *Epstein-Barr virus* may cause oral ulcers and a gingivostomatitis. *Coxsackievirus group A* can cause painful oral and pharyngeal vesicles and small ulcers, as well as tender finger and toe vesicles and papules *(hand-foot-and-mouth disease)*. *Herpangina* causes similar faucial pillar and palatal vesicles and small, painful ulcers; it rarely affects the tongue, gingivae, or buccal mucosa. *Gonococcal infection* of the mouth and throat is usually asymptomatic, but gingivitis, stomatitis, and/or ulcerations may occur. An initial episode of *aphthous ulceration* presents with one to five ovoid to round gray-white ulcerations measuring 0.2 to 0.8 cm across. These have a regular, narrow, erythematous margin, and appear on the tongue, gingivae, and labial or buccal mucosas. There is no local adenopathy, fever, or systemic symptoms. Oral chancres and eroded secondary lesions (e.g., mucous patches) caused by *syphilis* may be pain-

ful. The diagnosis depends on a history of sexual exposure, the clinical characteristics of the oral lesions, a direct immunofluorescent antibody stain for *Treponema pallidum* in lesion exudate, and reagin and specific treponemal antibody tests.

Stomatitis presents with edema, erythema, and tenderness of the oral mucosa, and burning discomfort. *Contact stomatitis* may be localized or diffuse. A local reaction may be due to a sensitizing metal in a crown. Diffuse contact stomatitis may be caused by dentifrices, mouth washes, materials used in dentistry, chewing gum, lozenges, cough drops, candy, or food. A local or diffuse *irritant stomatitis* may be caused by irritants used in dentistry, or by therapeutic agents, such as pancreatic extract, gentian violet, and potassium chloride.

Allergic stomatitis follows oral or parenteral administration of an antibiotic, hypnotic-sedative, local anesthetic, analgesic, antimalarial, or other drug. The reaction consists of diffuse oral redness, edema, and burning discomfort. Some drugs cause a painful erosive *lichen planus*; others cause a *pemphigus-like oral reaction* (e.g., penicillamine and captopril), or a *lupus-like ulcerative stomatitis* (e.g., hydralazine, procainamide). *Cytotoxic drugs* cause burning oral pain (i.e., mucositis), thinning of the mucosa, redness, and superficial painful erosions. *Bone marrow depression* can cause acute leukopenia. This abnormality may result in deeper, painful oropharyngeal ulcers, high fever, and sepsis. *Acute myelogenous leukemia* may cause oral pain; this pain may be related to massive *infiltration and swelling of the gingiva*; oral *candidiasis*; *pulpitis*; oral *ecthyma gangrenosum* due to *Pseudomonas* sepsis; *ANUG*; *herpes simplex* or *varicella-zoster infection*; or erosive mucositis due to *cytotoxic drug therapy*. Persons with *AIDS* have oral burning pain caused by *candidiasis*, or painful *ulcers* caused by *herpes simplex virus*, *cytomegalovirus*, *varicella-zoster virus*, or *ANUG*. Ulcer biopsy and culture are required to rule out herpes simplex virus or cytomegalovirus infection. Aphthae that are biopsy-culture–negative may respond dramatically to oral prednisone. *Necrotizing stomatitis* begins as ANUG, and then spreads to the palate and other parts of the oral mucosa. Rapidly progressive *periodontal disease* may occur in AIDS, with gingival swelling, pain, tenderness, and bleeding. Oral *Kaposi's sarcoma* and *lymphoma* are usually painless unless they invade neural tissue or ulcerate. *Diabetes mellitus* may cause xerostomia, periodontal disease, and/or oral candidiasis. Glossodynia occurs in diabetics. *Uremia* may cause an erosive stomatitis.

Acute lingual pain may be caused by an infectious glossitis caused by *Neisseria gonorrhoeae*, *Chlamydia trachomatis*, or *Trichomonas vaginalis*. These infections are acquired during oral-genital sexual activity. *Staphylococcal and gram-negative infections* may cause ulceration and glossitis in immunosuppressed patients. *Pseudomonas* infection may cause ecthyma gangrenosum of the tongue. *ANUG* causes a painful, friable, erosive gingivitis and glossal ulceration. *Stevens-Johnson syndrome* and *toxic epidermal necrolysis* cause large tongue bullae that rupture, leaving painful erosions. Skin rashes are associated with both disorders.

Herpes simplex virus, cytomegalovirus, and *Coxsackievirus*

TABLE OF DISEASE INCIDENCE

INCIDENCE PER 100,000 (APPROXIMATE)

Common (>100)	Uncommon (>5–100)	Rare (>0–5)
MOUTH PAIN		
Acute pulpitis or abscess	Pericoronitis	Mimics of dental disease:
Periapical abscess	Dry socket after tooth extraction	Acute myocardial infarction
Postendodontic surgery pain	Acute necrotizing ulcerative gingivitis (ANUG)	Ernest syndrome
"High bite" restoration	Mimics of dental pain:	Pemphigus-like oral drug reaction
Toothbrush-related gingival erosion and	Trigeminal neuralgia	Lupus erythematosus–like oral drug reaction
tooth injury	Sphenopalatine ganglion neuralgia	Acute leukemia and oral lesions:
Acute maxillary sinusitis	Stevens-Johnson syndrome	Gingivitis
Primary herpetic gingivostomatitis	Toxic epidermal necrolysis	Candidiasis
Traumatic ulcers	Herpes zoster ulcers	Dental disease (pulpitis)
Burn ulcers	Epstein-Barr virus ulcers	Ecthyma gangrenosum
Aphthous stomatitis	Hand-foot-and-mouth disease	ANUG and periodontal disease
Oral drug reactions:	Herpangina	Herpes simplex virus
Allergic stomatitis (drug-related)	Gonococcal stomatitis	Varicella-zoster virus
Cytotoxic oral drug reaction	Syphilis (primary and secondary)	Idiopathic ulceronecrotic lesions
AIDS and oral lesions:	Contact stomatitis	
Candidiasis	Irritant stomatitis	
Herpes simplex	Lichenoid oral drug reaction	
Periodontal disease and ANUG	AIDS and oral lesions:	
Hairy leukoplakia	Cytomegalovirus	
Diabetic oral lesions	Idiopathic prednisone-responsive aphthae	
	Herpes zoster	
	Acute necrotizing stomatitis	
	Kaposi's sarcoma	
	Lymphoma	
	Uremic oral lesions	
TONGUE PAIN (GLOSSITIS, GLOSSODYNIA, ULCERS)		
Candidiasis	Staphylococcal glossitis	Gonococcal glossitis and ulceration
ANUG	Pseudomonas (ecthyma gangrenosum)	*Trichomonas* glossitis
Herpes simplex virus glossitis and	Gram-negative bacterial glossitis	Tularemia
ulceration	Stevens-Johnson syndrome	
Tongue bites and burns	Toxic epidermal necrolysis	
Aphthous ulcers	*Chlamydia trachomatis* glossitis	
	Cytomegalovirus ulceration	
	Syphilis (primary and secondary)	
	Contact allergy	
	Allergic glossitis	
	Ulcers from Coxsackievirus or enterovirus	
LIP PAIN (CHEILITIS AND ANGULAR CHEILITIS)		
Isotretinoin therapy	Allergic cheilitis	
Actinic cheilitis	Factitious cheilitis	
Herpes simplex virus	Stevens-Johnson syndrome	
Impetigo	Toxic epidermal necrolysis	
Angular cheilitis due to *Candida* species		
or *Staphylococcus aureus*		
Chapping from cold/wind exposure		

can cause lingual ulcerations and pain. Specific diagnosis depends on lesion biopsy and culture. *AIDS* patients may develop prednisone-responsive, nonspecific, aphthous ulcers on the tongue and oral mucosa. *Syphilis* may cause a painful lingual chancre or mucous patches. *Allergic glossitis* can be caused by a contact allergen, or by an ingested or injected allergen. *Tularemia*, occurring after eating infected rabbit meat or crushing ticks with the fingers, may cause oral mucosal and lingual ulcerations and enlarged cervical nodes. A painful *cheilitis* involving the vermilion border can be caused by *sun exposure, isotretinoin therapy, contact allergy, herpes simplex virus, impetigo, self-injury,* the *Stevens-Johnson syndrome, toxic epidermal necrolysis,* or *chapping* from cold and wind. *Angular cheilitis* (perlèche) may be caused by *candidal or staphylococcal infection. B vitamin and iron deficiencies* may also be associated with this mildly painful disorder.

☐ DESCRIPTION OF LISTED DISEASES

Mouth Pain

1. DENTAL PAIN

A. Acute Pulpitis or Pulpal Abscess   Tooth or jaw pain begins abruptly on ingestion of a cold liquid or food. Pain may be localized to the affected tooth, but more commonly the region of the jaw containing the diseased tooth becomes severely painful. Pain may be referred to the cheek, eye, and ipsilateral ear. Symptoms cease within minutes of withdrawal of the cold stimulus. Recurrent attacks occur when the patient "forgets" and ingests a cold drink or food. Soon, hot stimuli have a similar effect. Localization to a specific tooth may be difficult, since bite and percussion pain are often absent. Within a few days or weeks, attacks of sustained jaw aching occur spontaneously. The pain becomes increasingly severe and prolonged, and bite and percussion sensitivity of the involved tooth may occur. Lying down may intensify the pain and result in wider pain referral. Constant aching may progress to an excruciating throbbing pain that radiates to the upper face and frontotemporal region. Clinical examination can demonstrate the responsible carious tooth or cracked restoration. Tests of electrical, thermal, or mechanical sensitivity will usually locate the diseased tooth. Dental radiographs may be of value in evaluating the extent of the caries and in evaluating the periapical region for development of an abscess. Pulpitis usually follows extension of dental caries or a dental fracture; contiguous spread from an adjacent periodontal or periapical pocket of pus; or hematogenous seeding of a mechanically irritated pulp. Pain relief requires endodontic surgery or tooth extraction. Analgesics and antibiotics are required to control pain and infection.

B. Periapical Abscess and Dental Ulcer   Failure to treat a pulpitis may lead to necrosis of the pulp and to partial or complete relief of dental pain. Spread of infection from the root to the surrounding soft tissues leads to pain and swelling of the adjacent gum and oral mucosa and the affected region of the face. Spread into the cheek causes tenderness and marked swelling; involvement of the maxillary sinus results in an acute sinusitis; and spread into the sublingual space causes swelling, pain and tenderness of the floor of the mouth, and elevation of the tongue.

A periapical abscess may spontaneously drain through a fistula into the oral cavity below the gingival margin or, less commonly, as a cutaneous fistula over the mandible, cheek, or perinasal area. Dental radiographs will reveal periapical rarefaction. A contrast study of the fistulous tract may help confirm an odontogenic process. Fistulous tracts tend to close after extraction of the involved tooth.

Up to 50 percent of patients with a cutaneous fistula from a periapical abscess have no history of toothache. Spontaneous drainage of the abscess on the buccal or lingual side causes a painful and/or tender dental ulcer that drains pus. Root canal surgery or extraction of the involved tooth leads to resolution of the ulcer.

C. Pericoronitis   There is pain and tenderness of the gum overlying a partially erupted wisdom tooth. The pericoronal tissue becomes swollen, red, and tender, and exudate can be expressed from beneath the infected flap of tissue. The masticator space may become inflamed, leading to trismus. Painful, tender ipsilateral lymphadenopathy may develop, and the breath may be fetid. Debridement and irrigation may bring relief. If cellulitis is present with spread to one or more deep fascial spaces then incision and drainage of accumulated pus, and tooth extraction, may be required. The cause is mechanical trapping of food particles and microorganisms beneath the gum flaps of a partially erupted tooth. This is exacerbated by the tissue trauma of chewing. Pericoronitis over an impacted molar requires extraction.

D. Acute Complications of Dental Therapy

1. Post-Endodontic Surgery Pain   Severe aching pain, with wide referral to the mandible and upper face, may follow an endodontic procedure. Such pain usually lasts 24 to 48 h, and is partially relieved by oral analgesics.

2. Dry Socket   Severe continuous pain begins 2 to 3 days after a dental extraction. The pain may exceed the pain that led to tooth extraction. Dry socket occurs when the clot at the extraction site becomes infected and falls out of the socket, leaving it "dry" and empty. Treatment includes irrigation and placement of a mixture of zinc oxide and eugenol in the socket.

3. "High Bite" Pain after Dental Restoration   A "high bite" after a dental restoration may cause thermal and bite sensitivity and pain, simulating the symptoms of pulpitis. Correction of the high bite results in symptom resolution in 1 to 3 days.

4. Toothbrush-Related Gingival Erosion and Tooth Injury   Vigorous tooth brushing may abrade the gingiva, cementum, and enamel, exposing sensitive dentin. Cold-induced pain occurs. Examination may show gum recession and wedgelike cuts into the tooth at the gum margin. Gentle brushing with a toothpaste containing an anesthetic is helpful in relieving this complaint.

E. Acute Necrotizing Ulcerative Gingivitis   Patients develop painful and tender gums. The gums show swelling and hyperemia in the interdental areas, and erosions and ulcerations occur at these sites. The gum margins are red, painful, and tender, and bleed easily. The breath is fetid. Sore throat and odynophagia are caused by pharyngeal and tonsillar ulceration and exudative inflammation. Fever, chills, malaise, weakness, and inability to eat may occur, and painful bilateral cervical adenitis may develop in severe cases. Ultrasonic debridement of necrotic gum tissue and administration of the antianaerobic drug metronidazole leads to resolution.

2. MIMICS OF DENTAL DISEASE

A. Acute Maxillary Sinusitis Aching cheek pain and purulent nasal and postnasal discharge may occur. The nasal discharge may be blood-streaked, and the ipsilateral nasal cavity partially or completely obstructed. There may be malar tenderness and a low-grade fever. The upper teeth on the affected side may ache continuously until antibiotic therapy leads to resolution of the sinusitis.

B. Acute Myocardial Infarction Patients with acute myocardial infarction may rarely present with left- or right-sided jaw and dental pain. Associated substernal, left precordial, arm, or neck pain may also occur. Sweating, weakness, pallor, nausea, and vomiting suggest a more serious disorder than toothache. Physical examination may reveal tachycardia, premature ventricular contractions, a gallop rhythm, and/or distant heart sounds. The ECG and/or cardiac isozyme measurements will establish the diagnosis.

C. Ernest Syndrome Stylomandibular ligament injury causes jaw and posterior tooth sensitivity and pain. There is limitation of jaw opening and protrusion. Palpation of the mandibular insertion of the ligament provokes jaw pain and posterior tooth sensitivity; sometimes it provokes ear, eye, or throat discomfort. Injection of lidocaine and methylprednisolone into the tender area relieves facial and dental pain.

D. Trigeminal Neuralgia Trigeminal neuralgia can cause lower or upper jaw pain of a lancinating nature. The pain may radiate to the upper face or ear. Jabs of pain last only seconds to 1 min, and may occur singly or in repetitive attacks separated by seconds or minutes. A trigger point may be present in the cheek, upper lip, or mouth. Stimulation of this point provokes a typical stabbing pain; injection of an anesthetic into the trigger point prevents triggered pain. Many patients have one or more teeth extracted on account of a mistaken belief that the pain is of dental origin.

E. Sphenopalatine Ganglion Neuralgia (Sluder's Lower-Half Headache) Unilateral pain occurs in the orbit, lateral nasal cavity, frontoparietal area, cheek, and upper teeth. It is dull and aching, and may be associated with ipsilateral nasal stuffiness, lacrimation, and a transient Horner's syndrome. Pain may last for hours or days, and can be relieved for a brief period by cocainization of the ipsilateral sphenopalatine ganglion in the nasal cavity.

3. ACUTE (PRIMARY) HERPETIC GINGIVOSTOMATITIS

This disorder usually occurs in young children, but may occur in young adults. Prodromal symptoms of fever, chills, headache, malaise, and irritability occur. Gingival and oral pain occurs in association with the appearance of small gingival and oral musocal pustules and serosanguineous vesicles. These soon rupture, forming painful ulcerations 1 to 3 mm in size. The gums are usually swollen and red. Scattered single and larger confluent gray-white ulcers are present on the gingiva, and bleed easily. Painful bilateral submandibular and cervical lymphadenitis occurs. The gums and mouth are tender, and the breath foul. Spontaneous healing may take 2 to 3 weeks. The diagnosis is usually based on the clinical findings. Ulcer scrapings or biopsies may show epithelial cell swelling; ballooning degeneration; intranuclear inclusions; and multinucleated giant cells. Herpes simplex virus (HSV) types 1 or 2 can be cultured from the ulcers or detected by direct immunofluorescent staining of scrapings from an ulcer. There may be a history of exposure to a friend or relative with a recent herpes infection, or, in the case of HSV type 2 infection, recent participation in oral-genital sexual activity. Acyclovir therapy may be beneficial in severe cases.

4. STEVENS-JOHNSON SYNDROME

This disorder may present a prodrome of fever, chills, malaise, chest pain, sore throat, cough, myalgias, arthralgias, vomiting, and diarrhea. Severe oral pain may be the only manifestation of disease (25 percent of cases). Bullous lesions form on the buccal mucosa, the palate, and the vermilion border of the lips. Rupture of bullae results in the formation of painful oral mucosal erosions covered with a gray-white exudate. Hemorrhagic crusts coat lesions on the labial mucosa and vermilion border. The lips may be edematous, and a purulent conjunctivitis may occur. Keratitis, corneal ulcers, anterior uveitis, or panophthalmitis may develop in severe cases.

The oral and nasal mucosal disease may be painful enough to interfere with speech, eating, and breathing. In most cases an extensive maculopapular rash develops on the extensor surfaces, with a tendency of lesions to group around the large joints of the lower extremity. Target, polycyclic, and arcuate lesions; urticarial plaques that persist, unlike typical transient "hives"; vesicles; and bullae are the major types of skin lesions that occur in this disorder. Herpes iris lesions develop on plaques. A central bulla forms, and is ringed by small vesicles (i.e., herpes iris lesion of Bateman).

The Stevens-Johnson syndrome has been linked to infection with *Mycoplasma pneumoniae*, herpes simplex virus, histoplasmosis, adenovirus, Epstein-Barr virus, and Coxsackievirus B5. Sulfonamides and other drugs have also been associated.

Pathologic findings include a lymphohistocytic dermal vasculitis, papillary edema of the dermis, epidermal spongiosis, intraepidermal cellular necrosis, and subepidermal bullae.

5. TOXIC EPIDERMAL NECROLYSIS (TEN)

A morbilliform rash appears on the face, trunk, and extremities, and the lesions become confluent, forming large patches of erythema. Flaccid bullae form on the erythematous patches and rapidly rupture, leaving large areas of painful partial-thickness loss. The Nikolsky sign is positive in "red" areas. Mucosal involvement in the mouth and conjunctivae, genitals, and anal area may be severe. Oral bullae rupture, leaving large areas of eroded mucosa. Fever, malaise, and leukocytosis occur. The skin appears "scalded." Pathologic findings include basal cell layer vacuolization, single cell necrosis, and subepidermal bulla formation. In staphylococcal TEN, the clearage plane for bulla formation is in the granular layer of the epidermis. The endothelial cells in the dermis show edema, but there is no perivascular inflammatory infiltrate. The relationship to erythema multiforme is controversial; some authors consider TEN a variant or a similar disorder. Commonly associated conditions include drug hypersensitivity (sulfonamides, allopurinol, and phenytoin); viral infections, lymphomas and leukemias; bacteremia, and staphylococcal infection; and immunizations to tetanus, measles, and mumps. Careful attention to fluid balance, local skin care, and prompt treatment of local and generalized infection is required for recovery.

6. ACUTE ORAL ULCERS

A. Trauma   Traumatic ulcerations are usually small (i.e., less than 1 cm in greatest diameter), shallow, and tender. They are covered with a yellow-white exudate and have an irregular or regular, narrow, erythematous border. They may have a linear or oval shape. Pain is mild but may be intensified during eating or talking. The buccal mucosa may be injured by an accidental bite or a tooth left jagged by caries or trauma. Bite injuries may also cause lingual ulceration, while vigorous use of a toothbrush may result in a gingival ulcer. Dental surgery, if it involves poorly controlled hand or rotary instruments, extended impression trays with rough edges, sharp provisional crowns, or suction-related trauma, may cause oral

ulceration. Cotton roll injuries are caused by the oral surgeon's late removal of dry, adherent cotton, producing mucosal desquamation. Alveolar ridge ulcers may result from wearing a poorly fitting complete or partial denture.

B. Burns   Chemical burns can result from prolonged aspirin contact with the mucosa during self-treatment of a toothache. Other proprietary drugs held in the mouth may cause a similar injury. Chemicals used in dentistry, such as phenol and silver nitrate, may cause burns. ''Pizza palate'' is a painful, circular lesion caused by adherence of hot pizza to the roof of the mouth.

C. Viral Infections

1. Varicella-Zoster Virus   Burning or aching unilateral pain occurs in the mouth and lower jaw (e.g., mandibular division), or in the palate, upper jaw, and midface (e.g., maxillary division), for 1 to 3 days prior to the onset of oral and facial vesicular lesions. The oral mucosa is red and swollen on one side, and contains grouped ulcers and vesicles. Some become confluent and form larger ulcers on the inner lip or palate. Lesions do not cross the midline. Some red-based vesicles and ulcers may appear on the skin of the lower or midface. The unilateral dermatomal distribution of intraoral and cutaneous lesions and the associated burning pain are diagnostic. A direct fluorescent antibody stain specific for varicella-zoster virus is available for staining lesion scrapings.

2. Epstein-Barr Virus   An acute febrile gingivostomatitis occurs, with gingival edema, erythema, and ulceration. Common accompanying findings are posterior cervical lymphadenopathy; an exudative pharyngotonsillitis; splenomegaly; and an absolute lymphocytosis, with more than 10 percent atypical lymphocytes and a positive heterophil test. Painful oral ulceration at other sites may occur.

3. Hand-Foot-and-Mouth Disease   Coxsackievirus A16 causes fever, faucial and oral vesicles, and small oral ulcers and bullae. Tender papules and clear vesicles occur on an erythematous base on the fingers, palms, and toes, and on the lateral area and soles of the feet. Similar illnesses occur in children and some adults infected with Coxsackieviruses A5, A10, B2, and B5, and enterovirus 71.

4. Herpangina   Fever and sore throat are the usual complaints. Three or more (possibly as many as 15) painful, red-rimmed, 2- to 4-mm vesicles and ulcers are scattered across the faucial pillars, soft palate, tonsils, and posterior pharyngeal wall, and, sometimes, the buccal mucosa. There are usually no gingival lesions. Group A Coxsackievirus strains are causative.

D. Gonococcal Stomatitis   Gonococcal stomatitis may present with a swollen, erythematous oral mucosa and multiple superficial painful musocal ulcerations. Ulcers as large as 2 to 3 cm may be present on the tongue, buccal mucosas, gingiva, and floor of the mouth. Medium rhomboid glossitis (i.e., glossal central papillary atrophy) has been associated with oropharyngeal gonorrhea. A diffuse gingivitis may also occur. The diagnosis can be confirmed by tongue or throat culture for *Neisseria gonorrhoeae*. There is a history of oral-genital contact. Many cases of oropharyngeal gonorrhea are asymptomatic and are detected only by screening cultures taken after genital infection, or because of exposure to a proven case.

E. Aphthous Ulcers The initial episode may occur with one or as many as five small, shallow, white-based, regular-bordered circular ulcers with a narrow erythematous margin. These painful and tender lesions may be located on the labial and buccal mucosa or their vestibular reflections, as well as on the tongue, palate, or pharynx. There is mild pain that is intensified by movement of the tongue and buccal mucosa during eating and talking. The lesions are focally tender, and there is no fever or painful lymphadenopathy. Small lesions heal spontaneously within 14 days.

F. Syphilis

1. Primary Syphilis Oral chancres most frequently occur on the lip, palate, or tongue. Chancres have narrow, raised borders that are copper-colored. The base of the chancre is reddish-brown. While genital chancres are usually painless, oral chancres are not. Exudate from the lesion can be stained directly with an immunofluorescent antibody for Treponema pallidum. Darkfield examination may be falsely positive on oral lesions. The VDRL test is positive in 60 to 70 percent of cases, and the FTA-ABS test in close to 100 percent of cases. Lesions vanish with penicillin therapy.

2. Secondary Syphilis ''Snail track'' linear ulcerations and grayish mucous patches occur on the lips, tonsils, and palate. Mucous patches may become secondarily infected and painful. Most secondary lesions are asymptomatic. A generalized macular, maculopapular, or papular squamous rash usually accompanies the oral lesions. Fever, malaise, chills, arthralgias, and myalgias also occur. Direct immunofluorescent staining of exudate from a mucous patch will reveal *Treponema pallidum* in large numbers, and the VDRL and FTA-ABS tests are confirmatory (96 to 100 percent sensitive). Oral and cutaneous lesions respond rapidly to penicillin therapy.

7. STOMATITIS

A. Contact Stomatitis Diffuse or local burning oral pain, redness, edema, and tenderness occur. Severe reactions may result in mucosal erosions or ulcerations. Lo-

cal reactions may occur on the buccal and lingual mucosa or gingiva, adjacent to a fixed source of allergen (e.g., a crown containing a sensitizing metal). Labial involvement may result from the holding of nickel-containing needles, pins, bobby pins, or metal lipstick holders in the mouth. Diffuse stomatitis may result from the use of dentifrices and mouthwashes containing sensitizing agents (e.g., cinnamic aldehyde—a flavoring agent used in toothpastes). The diagnosis of contact allergy can be made by the response to removal of the sensitizing material (which usually brings rapid remission of symptoms) and by the use of patch tests. These tests may be falsely positive (i.e., elimination of the material testing positive does not relieve symptoms). The oral sensitizing agents responsible may be present in dentifrices, mouthwashes, denture powders, denture adhesives, and cosmetics.

Materials used in dentistry, such as resins, metal alloys, mercury, antiseptics, topical anesthetics, and antibiotics, are also possible sensitizing agents. Lozenges and troches may cause a generalized contact stomatitis due to contained dyes, antibiotics, coloring and flavoring agents, antiseptics, or anesthetics. Cigarette paper, cigarette holders, and pipe stems may also cause contact reactions. Candy, chewing gum, cough drops, and breath-sweetening lozenges may cause burning mouth discomfort, redness, and swelling due to flavoring agents (oil of cinnamon, oil of anise, mint). Foods such as strawberries, chicken, tomatoes, and eggs have also been associated with oral reactions; in women, these reactions may be more severe during menstrual periods.

Ulcerative reactions to contact allergens are uncommon. Aphthous-like ulcers may occur, and may become chronic if the cause is not identified and eliminated. The substances causing ulcerative reactions are among those listed above as responsible for contact stomatitis.

B. Irritant Stomatitis Failure to dilute mouthwashes properly may cause mouth discomfort, redness, and swelling due to the presence of astringents and antiseptics such as sodium perborate, hydrogen peroxide, borax, menthol, phenol, thymol, methyl salicylate, alcohol, acids and alkalis, creosol, and boric acid. Irritants used during dental procedures, such as phenol, silver nitrate, creosol, and parachlorophenol may cause a local or diffuse stomatitis. Other drugs capable of causing stomatitis and ulceration include pancreatic extracts, potassium chloride, and gentian violet.

C. Oral Drug Reactions (Stomatitis Medicamentosa)

1. Allergic Stomatitis Oral, parenteral, or aerosol administration of a drug may cause tingling and burning in the mouth and generalized erythema and edema of the mucosa. Vesicles may form and evolve into erosions or deeper ulcerations. Urticaria or a generalized macular skin rash may be associated. Common causes of generalized allergic stomatitis include antibiotics (sulfonamides, penicillin, tetracycline); anesthetics (procaine, cocaine, tetracaine, lidocaine); hypnotics, sedatives, and similar compounds (barbiturates, phenytoin, chlorpromazine); analgesics and antipyretics (aspirin); antimalarials (quinine, quinidine, quinacrine); and miscellaneous drugs (thiouracil, gold, arsenic, phenolphthalein). In cases with erosive lesions, secondary infection with oral bacteria or *Candida* species may increase the severity of the stomatitis. The offending drug should be discontinued and symptomatic mouth care provided.

2. Lichenoid Drug Reactions   A lichen planus–like inflammatory change may occur on the buccal mucosa after drug administration. Lacy white or reticular buccal mucosal striae form, and may evolve into painful, erosive mucosal lesions. Commonly used drugs associated with lichenoid drug reactions include chloroquine, furosemide, gold, methyldopa, phenothiazines, propranolol, quinidine, lithium, spironolactone, tetracycline, thiazides, and chlorpropamide. Biopsy of a plaque will confirm the diagnosis. It reveals hyperkeratosis above a thickened malpighian layer, and a bandlike infiltrate of lymphocytes at the dermoepidermal boundary. Liquefaction degeneration of basement membrane cells, Civatte bodies, and sawtooth rete pegs occur. Immunofluorescence reveals fibrinogen deposition in the basement membrane zone. Cessation of the responsible drug leads to healing in a short period.

3. Pemphigus-Like Drug Reactions   Large oral bullae form and collapse, leaving extensive painful oral ulcerations. Penicillamine and captopril have been associated with this type of reaction, that is indistinguishable from idiopathic pemphigus vulgaris.

4. Lupus Erythematosus–Like Drug Reactions   Stomatitis occurs, with erythema, mucosal edema, and painful ulceration of the mucosa. Skin rash, fever, adenopathy, pleuritis, pericarditis, arthritis, and/or arthralgias may occur in association with the stomatitis. Drugs commonly associated with this type of oral reaction include hydralazine, procainamide, isoniazid, phenytoin, gold, methyldopa, primidone, and trimethadione.

5. Cytotoxic Drug Reactions from Chemotherapy for Neoplastic Disease   Anti-tumor drugs may impair tumor cell and mucosal cell DNA synthesis and replication (cycle-dependent drugs); or may block intracellular metabolism, leading to cell death (cycle-independent drugs). Effects on the bone marrow and oral mucosa may lead to pancytopenia and intraoral ulceration, infection, and bleeding. The effects of chemotherapy on the mouth include the following:

A. MUCOSITIS   Between 4 and 10 days after a course of therapy the patient may develop a burning discomfort in the mouth, with diffuse mucosal erythema and shininess. Painful ulcers and erosions develop on the labial and lingual mucosas. The latter may lose its papillae and become diffusely tender and painful. The ulcers become covered with a whitish-yellow pseudomembrane, or they form hemorrhagic crusts. The pain may be severe enough to prevent eating and drinking. The severity of the intraoral reaction usually depends on the agent, the dosage, and the frequency of administration. Idiosyncratic reactions to low doses may occur in a small percentage of cases. Chemotherapeutic drugs commonly associated with mucositis include bleomycin, cytarabine, dactinomycin, daunorubicin, doxorubicin, 5-fluorouracil, methotrexate, and combinations of these drugs and others. Less commonly, mucositis may occur with the use of acridinyl anisidide (AMSA), cyclophosphamide, mithramycin, mitomycin, nitrosourea, procarbazine, and vincristine. Fluid replacement and the use of topical anesthetics (e.g., viscous lidocaine, dyclonine), or parenteral analgesics and "swish and swallow" antimicrobials, lead to resolution of this severe form of stomatitis within 1 to 2 weeks.

B. MUCOSITIS AND AGRANULOCYTOSIS   Chemotherapeutic agents' effects on the bone marrow reduce circulating polymorphonuclear leukocyte and platelet levels. This may allow oral and pharyngeal ulceration to occur secondarily to loss of host defenses. Gram-negative bacterial and candidal infections of mucosal ulcers and erosions may occur, resulting in more extensive ulceration and pain, as well as fever and chills due to bacteremia and/or fungemia. Parenteral antibiotic, and sometimes antifungal, therapy is necessary to permit survival until mucosal and bone marrow cells recover.

8. SYSTEMIC DISEASE AND ORAL LESIONS

A. Leukemia   Oral lesions occur primarily in acute myelogenous, acute myelomonoblastic, and promyelocytic leukemia.

1. Leukemic Gingivitis   There is marked enlargement of the gingiva due to leukemic infiltration. The gingiva becomes protuberant and mounts up around the teeth, sometimes nearly obscuring them. Leukemia cutis may be associated with gingival lesions. Pressure sensations, pain, tenderness, and bleeding may occur along the gingival margin. Chemotherapy leads to regression of the gingivitis. Local chronic dental disease, in the form of plaque, calculus, and periodontal disease, may require therapy after regression of the leukemic process.

2. Oral Candidiasis Oral candidiasis can occur before or after chemotherapy, and after prolonged use of corticosteroids and antibiotics. White, soft exudates (pseudomembranous candidiasis) may cover large areas of the tongue and buccal mucosa and fauces. Removal of this exudate leaves a red, and sometimes bleeding, surface. Burning oral discomfort that is made worse by eating may be associated with these mucosal lesions. Most pseudomembranous lesions are painless and are discovered by examination of the oral and pharyngeal mucosas. Hyperplastic candidiasis may occur with firmly adherent plaques that require biopsy for diagnosis. Pseudomembranous candidiasis responds to topical or parenteral antifungal therapy.

3. Dental Disease Gum pain and tenderness from a periodontal abscess; posterior dental pain from pericoronitis, intensified by chewing; and toothache from pulpitis and periapical disease may occur in leukemic patients.

4. Pseudomonas-Related Ecthyma Gangrenosum This disorder may occur on the mucocutaneous border of the lip or on the palate. These lesions contain a central black area of gangrene, surrounded by a red inflammatory halo. They may be painful and/or tender. In some cases *Pseudomonas* species can be cultured from the lesion.

5. Ulceronecrotic Lesions of Unknown Etiology These are painful, ulcerative, mucosal lesions, usually covered with a grayish-white pseudomembrane. They may progress to produce large destructive ulcers despite use of local and systemic antibiotics. Their etiology is unknown.

6. Acute Necrotizing Ulcerative Gingivitis (ANUG) This condition is frequently superimposed on leukemic gingivitis, but may occur in patients without leukemic gingival infiltration.

7. Herpes Simplex Virus Infection The primary form of this disorder is described above. Patients with primary herpes simplex virus infection and leukemia may develop a severe systemic illness with viremia, high fever, oral lesions, and prostration. Parenteral acyclovir therapy is required.

8. Varicella-Zoster Virus Herpes zoster of the mouth is usually unilateral and localized. It is described above.

9. Cytotoxic Drug Reactions These reactions are described above.

B. Acquired Immunodeficiency Syndrome (AIDS) Oral pain is associated with fungal, viral, and bacterial infections; neoplasms; and ulcerative lesions of unknown etiology.

1. Candidiasis Pseudomembranous candidiasis occurs as white, milk curd–like lesions on the tongue, floor of the mouth, palate, faucial pillars, and buccal mucosa. Gentle swabbing removes the soft white exudate, exposing an erythematous, and sometimes bleeding, underlying mucosa. These lesions may be painless, or may cause a mild burning discomfort on swallowing or after ingestion of acidic or spicy liquids and food. A KOH preparation of the exudate will reveal pseudohyphae and hyphae and can be confirmed by a periodic acid-Schiff stained smear. Cotton swabs of oral lesions can be cultured semiquantitatively (i.e., colony counts) on Sabouraud dextrose agar for 48 h. Positive cultures have been defined as more than 10 colonies and more than 50, variously, by different investigators. Hyperplastic lesions are less frequent; they are white oral plaques that do not wipe off. Biopsy is required for diagnosis.

Acute atrophic candidiasis causes oral mucosal and lingual erythema, and depapillation of irregular areas on the dorsum of the tongue. This lesion may represent a pseudomembranous plaque that has shed its surface exudate, or a distinct lesion. Smears, biopsies, and cultures reveal *Candida* organisms. This acute atrophic/erythematous lesion is the most consistently painful form of candidiasis. Angular cheilitis due to candida also causes pain and soreness at the corners of the mouth. The diagnosis of painful oral candidiasis is also supported by the disappearance of pain, tenderness, and visible lesions after topical, oral, or parenteral antifungal therapy. The reported prevalence of oral candidiasis in AIDS varies from 62 to 88 percent. Hyperplastic candidiasis is uncommon (2 percent of cases), while the pseudomembranous form occurs in 88 percent of cases.

2. Ulcerative Lesions Ulcerative lesions are usually painful, and require careful clinical evaluation, biopsy, and culture to establish a specific diagnosis and therapeutic plan.

A. herpes simplex virus (hsv) (labial and intraoral) This infection may cause recurrent herpes labialis, limited to the vermilion area of the lip, or painful persistent intraoral vesicles and ulcers. Localization is on the tongue, gingiva, floor of the mouth, palate, and labial mucosa. Slitlike lesions may appear on the tongue. The diagnosis can be established by a viral culture, or a Giemsa- or direct fluorescent antibody–stained smear of material taken from the ulcer. Characteristic giant cells and intranuclear inclusions are found in only 50 percent of ulcer scrapings. Response to oral or intravenous acyclovir can be dramatic, and will support the diagnosis. In some cases, biopsy and culture of the obtained material may be required for diagnosis.

B. CYTOMEGALOVIRUS (CMV) This agent produces painful punched-out ulcers with soft margins and minimal surrounding edema. Single or multiple lesions may occur, and any area of the mouth may be affected. Biopsies studied by light microscopy show ulceration and granulation tissue, containing "owl's eye" cells caused by viral intranuclear inclusions. Saliva and urine cultures may grow CMV. There is a therapeutic response to intravenous ganciclovir, but recurrence may occur. CMV is an uncommon cause of intraoral ulceration. Such lesions are often associated with disseminated CMV infection involving the esophagus, liver, and/or gastrointestinal tract.

C. IDIOPATHIC PREDNISONE–RESPONSIVE ORAL APHTHAE These lesions cause severe pain. Cervical odynophagia may be caused by associated hypopharyngeal aphthous ulcers. Biopsies and cultures are required to exclude specific pathogens. There is a dramatic response of pain, and rapid healing, after prednisone administration.

D. HERPES ZOSTER Herpes zoster may cause unilateral aching and/or burning oral, jaw, cheek, and dental pain, associated with oral vesicles and ulcers, and similar lesions on the skin of the ipsilateral lower face. Lesion cultures grow the varicella-zoster virus. There may be a response to acyclovir therapy.

E. PERIODONTAL DISEASE Rapidly progressive periodontal disease, with gingivitis or acute necrotizing ulcerative gingivitis, occurs in AIDS. This causes gingival pain, tenderness, and bleeding. There may be a loss of interdental papillae, and rapid horizontal bone loss, so that the teeth become loose and require extraction. The pain is more severe than that seen in non-HIV-associated periodontitis.

F. NECROTIZING STOMATITIS This disorder has been reported to complicate AIDS-associated periodontitis. In one case report, acute necrotizing ulcerative gingivitis (ANUG) spread from the gingival region to cause a painful necrotic ulceration of the hard palate contiguous with the involved gingiva. The underlying bone was involved and became necrotic. The teeth adjacent to the palatal ulcer became loose and sensitive. Fever to 104°F, malaise, painful and tender submandibular adenopathy, and fetor oris were other associated symptoms. Progression to cancrum oris (noma) was prevented by administration of metronidazole and surgical debridement. ANUG occurs in 9.4 percent of homosexually active men, relative to an incidence of 0.02 to 0.08 percent in the general population.

3. Neoplastic Disorders

A. KAPOSI'S SARCOMA Intraoral Kaposi's sarcoma occurs as red, blue, purple, or, less commonly, mucosal-colored flat or nodular surface lesions. These are initially painless, but they may become painful as they grow larger and invade oral nerves, or ulcerate. The diagnosis requires biopsy. Painful, tender gingival lesions may mimic periodontal disease. Lesions may occur at any intraoral site, but are most common on the palate, gingiva, and buccal mucosa. Radiation, chemotherapy, and immunotherapy have had limited effectiveness in controlling intraoral disease.

B. LYMPHOMA Lymphoma causes a firm, painless intraoral mass. Pain may occur with ulceration of an advanced lesion.

4. Hairy Leukoplakia These hairy-appearing white lesions are probably caused by Epstein-Barr virus infection, and are pathognomonic for HIV infection with immunosuppression. They are painless and are sometimes mistaken for oral candidiasis.

C. Diabetes Mellitus Oral pain is sometimes associated with xerostomia, periodontal disease, and/or oral candidiasis. Xerostomia may result in mucositis and oral ulceration. Glossodynia has also been reported to occur with increased frequency in diabetics.

D. Uremia may be associated with a diffuse stomatitis and painful oral erosions.

Tongue Pain

9. GLOSSITIS AND/OR GLOSSODYNIA

Acute glossitis causes irregular erythematous areas on the tongue, with depapillation. Burning lingual pain, intensified by contact with the teeth, or by acidic or spicy food and drink, occurs. The causes of acute glossitis and glossodynia include:

A. Candidiasis The acute atrophic (i.e., erythematous) variety causes red, irregular, depapillated lingual areas and burning pain. Pseudomembranous candidiasis is associated. The diagnosis can be made from periodic acid-Schiff stained lesion smears, and from quantitative cultures. The lesions resolve with topical or oral antifungal therapy. Antibiotic-induced glossitis can be due to allergy, as well as to candidal superinfection. Acute lingual candidiasis occurs frequently in AIDS, in patients on prolonged antibiotic and corticosteroid therapy, and in poorly controlled diabetics.

B. Gonococcal Glossitis and Ulceration This disorder may affect the mouth, tongue, and pharynx, and can be diagnosed by culture. Yellow-white patches or a gray pseudomembrane may be present in involved areas.

Sloughing of the membrane reveals a bleeding granular surface. Oral-genital sexual activity is the usual cause.

C. *Trichomonas vaginalis* Glossitis This disorder has caused pain, swelling, and redness of the tongue. Microscopic examination of a saline wet mount of surface scrapings from the tongue will establish the diagnosis. Oral-genital activity (cunnilingus) is the usual cause.

D. Staphylococcal Glossitis and Ulceration Lingual erythema and ulceration with exudate occurs. These ulcers have irregular margins and measure 0.5 to 1 cm in diameter. *Staphylococcus aureus* ulcers may be brown, and *Staphylococcus epidermidis* ulcers white. This disorder occurs in immunosuppressed and debilitated patients.

E. *Pseudomonas* Infection *Pseudomonas* infection causes black, irregular lingual lesions with surrounding erythema (i.e., ecthyma gangrenosum). These lingual infarcts are hematogenous in origin. They are tender and may be painful. They occur in leukopenic patients; *Pseudomonas* species may be grown from the lesion, even though blood cultures are negative.

F. Gram-Negative Bacterial Ulceration Gram-negative bacteria may cause secondary infection of mucosal ulcers or erosions. They produce whitish-yellow, moist, glistening, elevated lesions that cover the superficial ulcerations. These infections usually occur in immunosuppressed patients.

G. Stevens-Johnson Syndrome This syndrome causes a maculopapular skin rash and oral, conjunctival, and genital mucosal lesions (Stevens-Johnson syndrome). Glossitis with erosion and ulceration may occur. Hemorrhagic ulcerations occur at the vermilion border of the lips. This disorder is described above.

H. Acute Necrotizing Ulcerative Gingivitis This disorder may involve the tongue, causing painful ulcerations covered by a yellow-gray pseudomembrane. It also causes interdental papillary necrosis, ulceration, and bleeding. There is a good response to metronidazole therapy.

I. *Chlamydia trachomatis* This infection is associated with oral genital sexual activity. Vesicles or small bullae occur on the tongue, rupture, and produce painful gray-white ulcerations. Culture for *Chlamydia* is necessary to establish the diagnosis.

J. Tularemia Painful gray-white oral ulcerations may occur in association with painful, tender cervical adenopathy and fever. Smaller secondary lingual ulcers also may be present. The diagnosis can be made by blood culture or by demonstrating a rise in tularemia agglutinins. There is often a history of ingesting wild rabbit, or of crushing ticks with the fingers.

K. Herpes Simplex Virus Infection This infection, as a primary disorder or as a recurrent intraoral process in AIDS patients, may cause painful lingual ulcers. Confirmation of the diagnosis requires a direct fluorescent antibody stain of lesion scrapings or a viral culture.

L. Cytomegalovirus Infection This infection may also cause painful punched-out lingual ulcers. Confirmation of the diagnosis requires viral culture and/or biopsy showing "owl's eye" cells. A direct fluorescent antibody stain of lesion scrapings may also confirm the diagnosis.

M. Syphilis

1. Primary Syphilis A lingual chancre may be painless, or may occur as a painful secondarily infected ulceration, with a firm base, raised edges, and a necrotic center covered with a gray-white exudate.

2. Secondary Syphilis Mucous patches may become secondarily infected, causing lingual pain and tenderness. Both primary and secondary lesions can be diagnosed by direct immunofluorescent staining of lesion exudate, and serologically by reagin tests and specific treponemal tests. There is a rapid response to penicillin therapy.

N. Tongue Bites and Burns Tongue bites and burns from hot liquids or solid foods (e.g., pizza) may cause pain and tenderness.

O. Contact Allergy Contact allergy may cause both stomatitis and tongue pain and tenderness. This disorder is discussed above.

P. Toxic Epidermal Necrolysis This disorder causes fever, generalized skin erythema, and extensive formation of bullae. Intraoral blisters rupture, leaving superficial gray-white lingual ulcers that are painful enough to interfere with eating.

Q. Aphthous Ulcerations These lesions occur as 0.2- to 0.5 cm yellow white ulcers with a narrow red margin. They appear on the lateral border and on the underside of the tongue, and disappear spontaneously within 2 weeks. Larger, more persistent ulcers occur in AIDS and resolve with prednisone therapy.

R. Allergic Glossitis A painful, irregular red area with depapillation may occur secondarily to parenteral administration of a drug or contrast agent. Without further exposure to the allergen, symptoms resolve within 1 week.

S. Coxsackievirus or Enterovirus Infection An acute painful glossitis may occur with redness, areas of depapillation, and small ulcers. Lingual burning, intensified by tongue contact with teeth and by acid or spicy foods and liquids, occurs. Coxsackieviruses can also cause vesicular lesions on the fingers, toes, and feet (hand-foot-and-mouth disease). Cases occur in the summer and fall.

Lip Pain

10. ACUTE CHEILITIS

A. Actinic Cheilitis   Prolonged exposure to sunlight may cause edema and redness of the lower lip. Vesicles may form and rupture, leaving painful ulcers and fissures. Residual dryness and scaliness of the lip may remain as the acute inflammatory reaction resolves. Removal from sun exposure leads to rapid resolution of this disorder.

B. Isotretinoin (Accutane) Therapy   This drug reduces sebum production and increases insensible water loss from the skin, resulting in xerosis. Cheilitis occurs within a few days of initiation of therapy in a majority of recipients of this drug.

C. Allergic Cheilitis   Contact allergy to lipstick, a dentifrice, or a food may cause burning pain, pruritus, redness, and vesiculation of the lips. Involvement of adjacent skin may occur. Patch testing will confirm the diagnosis. Avoidance of the causative material leads to resolution of all symptoms and signs.

D. Herpes Simplex Virus   This virus may cause vesiculation, redness, and ulceration of the lips, with burning pain and local tenderness. Lesions crust and gradually heal within 1 to 2 weeks.

E. Impetigo   Impetigo causes erythematous, tender, mildly painful crusted lesions on the skin of the face near the lips and nares. There is a prompt response to antibiotic ointment.

F. Factitious Cheilitis   Some persons frequently lick their lips or bite them, leading to small traumatic erosions and fissures. These may be mildly painful.

G. Stevens-Johnson Syndrome   This syndrome may cause lip ulcerations and erosions that become covered with hemorrhagic crusts. A maculopapular skin rash occurs with round, ovoid, target, and herpes iris–type lesions. These are usually localized over lower extremity joints and the trunk. Similar lip lesions may occur with toxic epidermal necrolysis.

H. Angular Cheilitis (Perlèche)   Pain, redness, fissuring, and tenderness occur at the angle of the mouth on one or both sides. Local infection with *Staphylococcus aureus* or a *Candida* species is the usual cause. There is a good initial response to topical antifungal or antistaphylococcal therapy, but recurrence is frequent. B vitamin and iron deficiencies are also associated with perlèche.

I. Chapping from Exposure to Cold and/or Wind   Exposure to cold and/or wind may cause drying and chapping of the lips, with painful fissuring. Secondary infection may cause pain and edema. Treatment of infection and the use of a lip balm with paraffin and petrolatum will lead to symptom resolution and prevent recurrence.

MOUTH PAIN REFERENCES

Aphthous Ulcers

Eisenbud L, Horowitz I, Kay B: Recurrent aphthous stomatitis of the Behçet's type: Successful treatment with thalidomide. *Oral Surg Oral Med Oral Pathol* 64:289–292, 1987.

Hammond WP IV, Price TH, Souza LM, et al: Treatment of cyclic neutropenia with granulocyte colony-stimulating factor. *N Engl J Med* 320:1306–1311, 1989.

Hutton KP, Rogers RS III: Recurrent aphthous stomatitis. *Dermatol Clin* 5(4):761–768, 1987.

Malik GH, Sirwal IA, Pandit KA: Behçet's syndrome associated with minimal change glomerulonephritis and renal vein thrombosis. *Nephron* 52:87–89, 1989.

Marshall GS, Edwards KM, Butler J, et al: Syndrome of periodic fever, pharyngitis, and aphthous stomatitis. *J Pediatr* 110:43–46, 1987.

Murphy GM, Griffiths WAD: Aphthous ulcers responding to etretinate: A case report. *Clin Exp Dermatol* 14:330–331, 1989.

Rogers RS III, Hutton KP: Screening for haematinic deficiencies in patients with recurrent aphthous stomatitis. *Aust J Dermatol* 27:98–103, 1986.

Bullous Lesions

Baird BJ, DeVillez RL: Widespread bullous fixed drug eruption mimicking toxic epidermal necrolysis. *Int J Dermatol* 27(3):170–174, 1988.

Bean SF: Diagnosis and management of chronic oral mucosal bullous diseases. *Dermatol Clin* 5(4):751–760, 1987.

Brown P, Taylor B: Herpes simplex infection associated with pemphigus vulgaris: Case report and literature review. *J Am Acad Dermatol* 21:1126–1128, 1989.

David M, Weissman-Katzenelson V, Ben-Chetrit A, et al: The usefulness of immunofluorescent tests in pemphigus patients in clinical remission. *Br J Dermatol* 120:391–395, 1989.

Delattre J-Y, Safai B, Posner JB: Erythema multiforme and Stevens-Johnson syndrome in patients receiving cranial irradiation and phenytoin. *Neurology* 38:194–198, 1988.

Dolan PA, Flowers FP, Araujo OE, et al: Toxic epidermal necrolysis. *J Emerg Med* 7:65–69, 1989.

Eveson JW: Superficial mucoceles: Pitfall in clinical and microscopic diagnosis. *Oral Surg Oral Med Oral Pathol* 66:318–322, 1988.

Fine J-D, Appell ML, Green LK, et al: Pemphigus vulgaris: Combined treatment with intravenous corticosteroid pulse therapy, plasmapheresis, and azathioprine. *Arch Dermatol* 124:236–239, 1988.

Halebian PH, Shires GT: Burn unit treatment of acute severe exfoliating disorders. *Ann Rev Med* 40:137–147, 1989.

Hanson RD, Olsen KD, Rogers RS III: Upper aerodigestive tract manifestations of cicatricial pemphigoid. *Ann Otol Rhinol Laryngol* 97:493–499, 1988.

Hopkins R, Walker DM: Oral blood blisters: Angina bullosa haemorrhagica. *Br J Oral Maxillofac Surg* 23:9–16, 1985.

Kelly SE, Wojnarowska F: The use of clinically split tissue in the detection of circulating anti-basement membrane zone antibodies in bullous pemphigoid and cicatricial pemphigoid. *Br J Dermatol* 118:31–40, 1988.

Lin AYF, Baker BA: Verapamil-associated Stevens-Johnson syndrome. *DICP, Ann Pharmacother* 23:987–988, 1989.

Manton SL, Scully C: Mucous membrane pemphigoid: An elusive diagnosis? *Oral Surg Oral Med Oral Pathol* 66:37–40, 1988.

Patterson R, Dykewicz MS, Gonzalzles A, et al: Erythema multiforme and Stevens-Johnson syndrome: Descriptive and therapeutic controversy. *Chest* 98:331–336, 1990.

Ponte CD, Arbogast JG, Dattola RK: A suspected case of trimethoprim/sulfonamide-induced localized exfoliation. *DICP, Ann Pharmacother* 24:140–142, 1990.

Rasmussen JE: Causes, diagnosis, and management of toxic epidermal necrolysis. *Comp Ther* 16(3):3–6, 1990.

Rasmussen JE: Update on the Stevens-Johnson syndrome. *Cleve Clin J Med* 55(5):412–414, 1988.

Raviglione MC, Dinan WA, Pablos-Mendez A, et al: Fatal toxic epidermal necrolysis during prophylaxis with pyrimethamine and sulfadoxine in a human immunodeficiency virus-infected person. *Arch Intern Med* 148:2683–2685, 1988.

Stanley JR: Pemphigus: Skin failure mediated by autoantibodies. *JAMA* 264(13):1714–1717, 1990.

Stitt VJ Jr: Stevens-Johnson syndrome: A review of the literature. *J Natl Med Assoc* 80(1):104, 106–108, 1988.

Venning VA, Frith PA, Bron AJ, et al: Mucosal involvement in bullous and cicatricial pemphigoid: A clinical and immunopathological study. *Br J Dermatol* 118:7–15, 1988.

Ward DJ, Krzeminska EC, Tanner NSB: Treatment of toxic epidermal necrolysis and a review of six cases. *Burns* 16(2):97–104, 1990.

Williams DM: Vesiculo bullous mucocutaneous disease: Benign mucous membrane and bullous pemphigoid. *J Oral Pathol Med* 19:16–23, 1990.

Wilson EE, Malinak LR: Vulvovaginal sequelae of Stevens-Johnson syndrome and their management. *Obstet Gynecol* 71:478–480, 1988.

Wright JM: Oral manifestations of drug reactions. *Dent Clin North Am* 28(3):529–543, 1984.

Zegarelli DJ, Sabbagh E: Relative incidence of intraoral pemphigus vulgaris, mucous membrane pemphigoid and lichen planus. *Ann Dent* 42(1):5–7, 1989.

Burning Mouth Syndrome

Grushka M: Clinical features of burning mouth syndrome. *Oral Surg Oral Med Oral Pathol* 63:30–36, 1987.

Grushka M, Sessle BJ, Howley TP: Psychophysical assessment of tactile, pain and thermal sensory functions in burning mouth syndrome. *Pain* 28:169–184, 1987.

Grushka M, Sessle BJ, Miller R: Pain and personality profiles in burning mouth syndrome. *Pain* 28:155–167, 1987.

van der Ploeg HM, van der Wal N, Eijkman MAJ, et al: Psychological aspects of patients with burning mouth syndrome. *Oral Surg Oral Med Oral Pathol* 63:664–668, 1987.

Candidiasis—Oral

Budtz-Jörgensen E: Etiology, pathogenesis, therapy, and prophylaxis of oral yeast infections. *Acta Odontol Scand* 48:61–69, 1990.

Holmstrup P, Axéll T: Classification and clinical manifestations of oral yeast infections. *Acta Odontol Scand* 48:57–59, 1990.

Carcinoma—Lip

Banerjee TK, Gottschalk PG: Unusual manifestations of multiple cranial nerve palsies and manidibular metastasis in a patient with squamous cell carcinoma of the lip. *Cancer* 53:346–348, 1984.

Brufau C, Canteras M, Armijo M: Our experience in the surgical treatment of cancer and precancerous lesions of the lower lip. *J Dermatol Surg Oncol* 11:908–912, 1985.

Douglass CW, Gammon MD: Reassessing the epidemiology of lip cancer. *Oral Surg* 57:631–642, 1984.

Fitzpatrick PJ: Cancer of the lip. *J Otolaryngol* 31(1):32–36, 1984.

Lundeen RC, Langlais RP, Terezhalmy GT: Sunscreen protection for lip mucosa: A review and update. *J Am Dent Assoc* 111:617–621, 1985.

Mohs FE, Snow SN: Microscopically controlled surgical treatment for squamous cell carcinoma of the lower lip. *Surg Gynecol Obstet* 160:37–42, 1985.

Sebben JE: Wedge resection of the lip: Minimizing problems. *J Dermatol Surg Oncol* 11:60–64, 1985.

Carcinoma—Oral

Berktold RE: Carcinoma of the oral cavity: Selective management according to site and stage. *Otolaryngol Clin North Am* 18(3):445–450, 1985.

Duncavage JA, Ossoff RH: Use of the CO_2 laser for malignant disease of the oral cavity. *Lasers Surg Med* 6:442–444, 1986.

Epstein JB: Oral and maxillofacial cancer pain. *Spec Care Dentist* 6(5):223–227, 1986.

Holmstrup P, Pindborg JJ: Oral mucosal lesions in smokeless tabacco users. *CA* 38(4):230–235, 1988.

Mashberg A, Merletti F, Boffetta P, et al: Appearance, site of occurrence, and physical and clinical characteristics of oral carcinoma in Torino, Italy. *Cancer* 63:2522–2527, 1989.

Mashberg A, Samit AM: Early detection, diagnosis, and management of oral and oropharyngeal cancer. *CA* 39(2):67–88, 1989.

Dental Pain

Bell WE: Pains of dental origin, in *Orofacial Pains: Classification, Diagnosis, Management*, 4th ed. Chicago, Year Book Medical, 1989, pp 210–238.

Bell WE: Pains of muscle origin, in *Orofacial Pains: Classification, Diagnosis, Management*, 4th ed. Chicago, Year Book Medical, 1989, pp 239–284.

Bhaskar SN, Rappaport HM: Dental vitality tests and pulp status. *J Am Dent Assoc* 86:409–411, 1973.

Cameron CE: The cracked tooth syndrome: Additional findings. *J Am Dent Assoc* 93:971–975, 1976.

Clem WH: Posttreatment of endodontic pain. *J Am Dent Assoc* 81(5):1166–1170, 1970.

Evans FO, Sydnor JB, Moore WEC, et al: Sinusitis of the maxillary antrum. *N Engl J Med* 293:735–739, 1975.

Farber PA, Miller AS: Gingivostomatitis, in Schlossberg D (ed): *Infections of the Head and Neck*. New York, Springer-Verlag, 1987 pp 105–120.

Glick DH: Locating referred pulpal pains. *Oral Surg Oral Med Oral Pathol* 15(5):613–623, 1962.

Goldman HM, Ruben MP: Desquamative gingivitis and its response to topical triamcinolone therapy. *Oral Surg Oral Med Oral Pathol* 21(5):579–593, 1966.

Heir GM: Facial pain of dental origin: A review for physicians. *Headache* 27:540–547, 1987.

Held JL, Yunakov MJ, Barber RJ, et al: Cutaneous sinus of dental origin: A diagnosis requiring clinical and radiologic correlation. *Cutis* 43(1):22–24, 1989.

Klineberg I: Occlusion as the cause of undiagnosed pain. *Int Dent J* 38:19–27, 1988.

Kreisberg MK: Atypical odontalgia: Differential diagnosis and treatment. *J Am Dent Assoc* 104:852–854, 1982.

Kureishi A, Chow AW: The tender tooth: Dentoalveolar, pericoronal, and periodontal infections. *Infect Dis Clin North Am* 2(1):163–182, 1988.

Luebke RG, Glick DH, Ingle JI: Indications and contraindications for endodontic surgery. *Oral Surg Oral Med Oral Pathol* 18(1):97–113, 1964.

Marbach JJ, Hulbrock J, Hohn C, et al: Incidence of phantom tooth pain: An atypical facial neuralgia. *Oral Surg* 53(2):190–193, 1982.

Mitchell DF, Tarplee RE: Painful pulpitis: A clinical and microscopic study. *Oral Surg Oral Med Oral Pathol* 13(11):1360–1370, 1960.

Oral surgery-oral pathology conference no. 17, Walter Reed Army Medical Center: Periapical lesions: Types, incidence, and clinical features. Conducted by SN Bhaskar. *Oral Surg Oral Med Oral Pathol* 21(5):657–671, 1966.

Sessle BJ: The neurobiology of facial and dental pain: Present knowledge, future directions. *J Dent Res* 66(5):962–981, 1987.

Summers GW: The diagnosis and management of dental infections. *Otolaryngol Clin North Am* 9(3):717–728, 1976.

Suzuki JB: Diagnosis and classification of the periodontal diseases. *Dent Clin North Am* 32(2):195–216, 1988.

Walsh W: Facial pain: Is it toothache? *Aust Fam Physician* 17(4):235–238, 1988.

Glossodynia/Glossitis

Bánóczy J, Szabó L, Csiba A: Migratory glossitis: A clinical-histologic review of seventy cases. *Oral Surg* 39(1):113–121, 1975.

Bengtsson L, Ransjö U: Acute atrophic glossitis after open-heart surgery. *Scand J Thorac Cardiovasc Surg* 22:143–144, 1988.

Bloom SR, Polak JM: Glucagonoma syndrome. *Am J Med* 82(suppl 5B):25–36, 1987.

Bredenkamp JK, Castro DJ, Mickel RA: Importance of iron repletion in the management of Plummer-Vinson syndrome. *Ann Otol Rhinol Laryngol* 99:51–54, 1990.

Carethers M: Diagnosing vitamin B_{12} deficiency: A common geriatric disorder. *Geriatrics* 43:89–112, 1988.

Challacombe SJ: Haematological abnormalities in oral lichen planus, candidiasis, leukoplakia and non-specific stomatitis. *Int J Oral Maxillofac Surg* 15:72–80, 1986.

Cohen MD, Ginsburg WW, Allen GL: Facial swelling and giant cell arteritis. *J Rheumatol* 9:325–327, 1982.

Dreizen S: Systemic significance of glossitis: Decoding the tongue's medical messages. *Postgrad Med* 75(4):207–215, 1984.

Fujita J, Seino Y, Ishida H, et al: A functional study of a case of glucagonoma exhibiting typical glucagonoma syndrome. *Cancer* 57:860–865, 1986.

Gallagher FJ, Baxter DL, Denobile J, et al: Glossodynia, iron deficiency anemia, and gastrointestinal malignancy. *Oral Surg Oral Med Oral Pathol* 65:130–133, 1988.

Gallagher FJ, Weaver T, Naylor GD: Oral lesions as a cause of glossodynia. *Ear Nose Throat J* 68:740–748, 1989.

Glass BJ: Drug-induced xerostomia as a cause of glossodynia. *Ear Nose Throat J* 68:778–781, 1989.

Goodkin DA: Radiographic contrast medium-induced glossitis. *Arch Intern Med* 145:171–172, 1985.

Goren MB, Goren SB: Diagnostic tests in patients with symptoms of keratoconjunctivitis sicca. *Am J Ophthalmol* 106:570–574, 1988.

Hatch CL: Glossodynia as an oral manifestation of diabetes mellitus. *Ear Nose Throat J* 68:782–785, 1989.

Huber MA, Hall EH: Glossodynia in patients with nutritional deficiencies. *Ear Nose Throat J* 68:771–775, 1989.

Kahn D: Hypertrophic glossitis in secondary syphilis (letter to editor). *Arch Dermatol* 16:1103–1104, 1980.

Kessinger A, Lemon HM, Foley JF: The glucagonoma syndrome and its management. *J Surg Oncol* 9:419–424, 1977.

Myers A, Naylor GD: Glossodynia as an oral manifestation of sex hormone alterations. *Ear Nose Throat J* 68:786–790, 1989.

Naylor GD, Marino GG, Shumway RC: Glossodynia and radiation therapy and chemotherapy. *Ear Nose Throat J* 68:751–757, 1989.

Powell FC: Glossodynia and other disorders of the tongue. *Dermatol Clin* 5(4):687–693, 1987.

Rhodus NL: Xerostomia and glossodynia in patients with autoimmune disorders. *Ear Nose Throat J* 68:791–794, 1989.

Schmitt RJ, Sheridan PJ, Rogers RS III: Pernicious anemia with associated glossodynia. *J Am Dent Assoc* 117:838–840, 1988.

Sullivan PD: The diagnosis and treatment of psychogenic glossodynia. *Ear Nose Throat J* 68:795–798, 1989.

van der Wal N, van der Kwast WAM, van der Waal I: Median rhomboid glossitis: A follow-up study of 16 patients. *J Oral Med* 41(2):117–120, 1986.

Wysocki GP, Daley TD: Benign migratory glossitis in patients with juvenile diabetes. *Oral Surg Oral Med Oral Pathol* 63:68–70, 1987.

Intraoral Pain

Cooper BC: Intraoral pain, in Cooper BC, Lucente FE (eds): *Management of Facial, Head and Neck Pain*. Philadelphia, Saunders, 1989, pp 115–130.

Lingual Seizures

Neufeld MY, Blumen SC, Nisipeanu P, et al: Lingual seizures. *Epilepsia* 29(1):30–33, 1988.

Lip Pain—Cheilitis

Coenen C, Börsch G, Müller K-M, et al: Oral inflammatory changes as an initial manifestation of Crohn's disease antedating abdominal diagnosis: Report of a case. *Dis Colon Rectum* 31(7):548–552, 1988.

Connelly TJ, Kauh YC, Luscombe HA, et al: Leukemic macrocheilitis associated with hairy-cell leukemia and the Melkersson-Rosenthal syndrome. *J Am Acad Dermatol* 14:353–358, 1986.

Coulson IH, Marsden RA: Lupus erythematosus cheilitis. *Clin Exp Dermatol* 11:309–311, 1986.

Frankel DH, Mostofi RS, Lorincz AL: Oral Crohn's disease: Report of two cases in brothers with metallic dysgeusia and a review of the literature. *J Am Acad Dermatol* 12:260–268, 1985.

Friedman SJ, Connolly SM: Clarinettist's cheilitis. *Cutis* 38(3):183–184, 1986.

Hayakawa R, Matsunaga K, Suzuki M, et al: Lipstick dermatitis due to C_{18} aliphatic compounds. *Contact Dermatitis* 16:215–219, 1987.

Ho AD, Martin H, Knauf W, et al: Combination of low-dose cytarabine and 13-cis retinoic acid in the treatment of myelodysplastic syndromes. *Leuk Res* 11(11):1041–1044, 1987.

Lamey P-J, Lewis MAO: Oral medicine in practice: Angular cheilitis. *Br Dent J* 167:15–18, 1989.

MacPhail LA, Greenspan D, Schiødt M, et al: Acyclovir-resistant, foscarnet-sensitive oral herpes simplex type 2 lesion in a patient with AIDS. *Oral Surg Oral Med Oral Pathol* 67:427–432, 1989.

Maibach HI: Cheilitis: Occult allergy to cinnamic aldehyde. *Contact Dermatitis* 15(2):106–107, 1986.

Öhman S-C, Dahlén G, Moller DG, et al: Angular cheilitis: A clinical and microbial study. *J Oral Pathol* 15:213–217, 1986.

Öhman S-C, Jontell M: Treatment of angular cheilitis: The significance of microbial analysis, antimicrobial treatment, and interfering factors. *Acta Odontol Scand* 46:267–272, 1988.

Öhman S-C, Jontell M, Dahlén G: Recurrence of angular cheilitis. *Scand J Dent Res* 96:360–365, 1988.

Picascia DD, Robinson JK: Actinic cheilitis: A review of the etiology, differential diagnosis, and treatment. *J Am Acad Dermatol* 17:255–264, 1987.

Rademaker M, Kirby JD, White IR: Contact cheilitis to shellac, Lanpol 5 and colophony. *Contact Dermatitis* 15(5):307–308, 1986.

Reade PC, Sim R: Exfoliative cheilitis: A factitious disorder? *Int J Oral Maxillofac Surg* 15:313–317, 1986.

Shaikh AB, Arendorf TM, Darling MR, et al: Granulomatous cheilitis: A review and report of a case. *Oral Surg Oral Med Oral Pathol* 67:527–530, 1989.

Shalita AR: Mucocutaneous and systemic toxicity of retinoids: Monitoring and management. *Dermatologica* 175(suppl 1):151–157, 1987.

Shehade SA, Foulds IS: Granulomatous cheilitis and a positive Kveim Test. *Br J Dermatol* 115:619–622, 1986.

Tatnall FM, Dodd HJ, Sarkany I: Crohn's disease with metastatic cutaneous involvement and granulomatous cheilitis. *J R Soc Med* 80(1):49–50, 1987.

Whitaker DC: Microscopically proven cure of actinic cheilitis by CO_2 laser. *Lasers Surg Med* 7:520–523, 1987.

Winchester L, Scully C, Prime SS, et al: Cheilitis glandularis: A case affecting the upper lip. *Oral Surg Oral Med Oral Pathol* 62:654–656, 1986.

Young TB, Rimm EB, D'Alessio DJ: Cross-sectional study of recurrent herpes labialis: Prevalence and risk factors. *Am J Epidemiol* 127(3):612–625, 1988.

Neck-Tongue Syndrome

Bogduk N: An anatomical basis for the neck-tongue syndrome. *J Neurol Neurosurg Psychiatry* 44:202–208, 1981.

Elisevich K, Stratford J, Bray G, et al: Neck tongue syndrome: Operative management. *J Neurol Neurosurg Psychiatry* 47:407–409, 1984.

Fortin CJ, Biller J: Neck tongue syndrome. *Headache* 25:255–258, 1985.

Webb J, March L, Tyndall A: The neck-tongue syndrome: Occurrence with cervical arthritis as well as normals. *J Rheumatol* 11(4):530–533, 1984.

Necrotizing Sialometaplasia

Gahhos F, Enriquez RE, Bahn SL, et al: Necrotizing sialometaplasia: Report of five cases. *Plast Reconstr Surg* 71(5):650–657, 1983.

Odontogenic Infections

Chow AW: Odontogenic infections, in Schlossberg D (ed): *Infections of the Head and Neck*. New York, Springer-Verlag, 1987, pp 148–160.

Oral Cavity—Diseases

Shemen LJ: Benign diseases of the oral cavity, in Lee KJ (ed): *Textbook of Otolaryngology and Head and Neck Surgery*. New York, Elsevier, 1989, pp 366–375.

Shemen LJ: Malignant diseases of the oral cavity and salivary glands, in Lee KJ (ed): *Textbook of Otolaryngology and Head and Neck Surgery*, New York, Elsevier, 1989, pp 384–406.

Oral Lesions—AIDS

Barone R, Ficarra G, Gaglioti D, et al: Prevalence of oral lesions among HIV-infected intravenous drug abusers and other risk groups. *Oral Surg Oral Med Oral Pathol* 69:169–173, 1990.

Bolski E, Hunt RJ: The prevalence of AIDS-associated oral lesions in a cohort of patients with hemophilia. *Oral Surg Oral Med Oral Pathol* 65:406–410, 1988.

Greenspan D, Greenspan JS: The oral clinical features of HIV infection. *Gastroenterol Clin North Am* 17(3):535–543, 1988.

Langford A, Kunze R, Timm H, et al: Cytomegalovirus associated oral ulcerations in HIV-infected patients. *J Oral Pathol Med* 19:71–76, 1990.

Phelan JA, Saltzman BR, Friedland GH, et al: Oral findings in patients with immunodeficiency syndrome. *Oral Surg Oral Med Oral Pathol* 64:50–56, 1987.

Rosenstein DI, Eigner TL, Levin MP, et al: Rapidly progressive periodontal disease associated with HIV infection: Report of case. *J Am Dent Assoc* 118:313–314, 1989.

Schiødt M, Bakilana PB, Hiza JFR, et al: Oral candidiasis and hairy leukoplakia correlate with HIV infection in Tanzania. *Oral Surg Oral Med Oral Pathol* 69:591–596, 1990.

Schweitzer VG, Visscher D: Photodynamic therapy for treatment of AIDS-related oral Kaposi's sarcoma. *Otolaryngol Head Neck Surg* 102:639–649, 1990.

Sciubba J, Brandsma J, Schwartz M, et al: Hairy leukoplakia: An AIDS-associated opportunistic infection. *Oral Surg Oral Med Oral Pathol* 67:404–410, 1989.

Williams CA, Winkler JR, Grassi M, et al: HIV-associated periodontitis complicated by necrotizing stomatitis. *Oral Surg Oral Med Oral Pathol* 69:351–355, 1990.

Oral Pain—Review Articles

Archard HO: Stomatologic disorders of an internal and integumental nature, in Fitzpatrick TB, Eisen AZ, Wolff K, et al (eds): *Dermatology in General Medicine,* 2d ed. New York, McGraw-Hill, 1979, pp 834–907.

Oral Ulcerations

Borroni G, Pericoli R, Gabba P, et al: Eosinophilic ulcers of the tongue. *J Cutan Pathol* 11:322–325, 1984.

Chavalittamrong B, Ratanarapee S, Clovutivat V: Tuberculous ulcers of nose and tongue in children. *J Med Assoc Thailand* 67(4):249–252, 1984.

Rangedara DC, Lewis RR, Cawson RA, et al: An unusual case of chronic tongue ulceration. *J Trop Med Hyg* 88:223–226, 1985.

Woods MA, Mohammad AR, Turner JE, et al: Oral ulcerations. *Quintessence Int* 21:141–151, 1990.

Oropharyngeal, Laryngeal, and Neck Pain

Pincus RL: Oropharyngeal, laryngeal, and neck pain, in Cooper BC, Lucente FE (eds): *Management of Facial, Head and Neck Pain.* Philadelphia, Saunders, 1989, pp 131–152.

Stomatitis—Allergic

Bickley HC: A concept of allergy with reference to oral disease. *J Periodontol* 41(6):302–312, 1970.

Fisher AA: Contact stomatitis. *Dermatol Clin* 5(4):709–717, 1987.

Hogan DJ, Burgess WR, Epstein JD, et al: Lichenoid stomatitis associated with lithium carbonate. *J Am Acad Dermatol* 13:243–246, 1985.

Mountcastle EA, James WD, Rodman OG, et al: Allergic contact stomatitis to a dental impression material (letter to editor). *J Am Acad Dermatol* 15(5):1055–1056, 1986.

Perry HO: Idiopathic gingivostomatitis. *Dermatol Clin* 5(4):719–722, 1987.

Shepard FE, Grant GC, Moon PC, et al: Allergic contact stomatitis from a gold alloy-fixed partial denture. *J Am Dent Assoc* 106:198–199, 1983.

Silverman S, Lozada F: An epilogue to plasma-cell gingivostomatitis (allergic gingivostomatitis). *Oral Surg* 43(2):211–217, 1977.

White JW Jr, Olsen KD, Banks PM: Plasma cell orificial mucositis. *Arch Dermatol* 122:1321–1324, 1986.

Stomatitis—Cytotoxic

Bronner AK, Hood AF: Cutaneous complications of chemotherapeutic agents. *J Am Acad Dermatol* 9(5):645–663, 1983.

Epstein JB: The painful mouth: Mucositis, gingivitis, and stomatitis. *Infect Dis Clin North Am* 2(1):183–202, 1988.

Hood AF: Cutaneous side effects of cancer chemotherapy. *Med Clin North Am* 70(1):187–209, 1986.

Puavilai S, Timpatanapong P: Prospective study of cutaneous drug reactions. *J Med Assoc Thailand* 72(3):167–171, 1989.

Stomatitis—Denture

Arendorf TM, Walker DM: Denture stomatitis: A review. *J Oral Rehabil* 14:217–227, 1987.

Martin MV, Farrelly PJ, Hardy P: An investigation of the efficacy of nystatin for the treatment of chronic atrophic candidosis (denture sore mouth). *Br Dent J* 160:201–204, 1986.

Reeve CM, Van Roekel NB: Denture sore mouth. *Dermatol Clin* 5(4):681–686, 1987.

van Joost T, van Ulsen J, van Loon LAJ: Contact allergy to denture materials in the burning mouth syndrome. *Contact Dermatitis* 18:97–99, 1988.

Stomatitis—Gonorrheal

Escobar V, Farman AG, Arm RN: Oral gonococcal infection. *Int J Oral Surg* 13:549–554, 1984.

Stomatitis—Leukemia

Segelman AE, Doku HC: Treatment of the oral complications of leukemia. *J Oral Surg* 35:469–477, 1977.

Wahlin YB, Holm A-K: Changes in the oral microflora in patients with acute leukemia and related disorders during the period of induction therapy. *Oral Surg Oral Med Oral Pathol* 65:411–417, 1988.

Tongue—Neoplastic Lesions

Bruneton JN, Roux P, Caramella E, et al: Tongue and tonsil cancer: Staging with US. *Radiology* 158:743–746, 1986.

Callery CD, Spiro RH, Strong EW: Changing trends in the management of squamous carcinoma of the tongue. *Am J Surg* 148:449–454, 1984.

Kessler DJ, Mickel RA, Calcaterra TC: Malignant salivary gland tumors of the base of the tongue. *Arch Otolaryngol* 111:664–666, 1985.

Pickell G: Chronic glossopharyngeal neuralgic pain associated with mucoepidermoid carcinoma. *Can Med Assoc J* 133:579–580, 1985.

Shack RB: Carcinoma of the tongue and tonsil (oropharynx). *Surg Clin North Am* 66(1):83–96, 1986.

Shapiro SD, Abramovitch K, Van Dis ML, et al: Neurofibromatosis: Oral and radiographic manifestations. *Oral Surg* 58:493–498, 1984.

Spiro RH: Squamous cancer of the tongue. *CA* 35(4):252–256, 1986.

Westcott WG, Correll RW: Multiple recurrences of a lesion at the base of the tongue. *J Am Dent Assoc* 108:231–232, 1984.

8

Acute Throat Pain

☐ DIAGNOSTIC LIST

1. Exudative pharyngotonsillitis
   A. Group A streptococcal infection
      1. Without rash
      2. With rash (scarlet fever)
   B. Mimics of exudative group A streptococcal pharyngotonsillitis
      1. Group G streptococcal infection
      2. Group C streptococcal infection
      3. Epstein-Barr virus infection (infectious mononucleosis)
      4. *Corynebacterium hemolyticum* infection
      5. *Corynebacterium diphtheriae* infection
      6. Acute necrotizing ulcerative gingivitis (ANUG)
      7. Adenovirus infection
      8. Herpes simplex virus infection (primary)—
      9. Complicated pharyngotonsillitis— peritonsillar cellulitis and abscess, and postanginal sepsis (Lemierre's disease)
      10. Coxsackie A infection (herpangina)
      11. Exudative

pharyngotonsillitis without demonstrable etiology
      12. Exudative pharyngotonsillitis in viral, mycoplasmal, and chlamydial infections
   C. Rare and potentially lethal causes of exudative pharyngotonsillitis
      1. *Neisseria meningitidis* infection
      2. *Yersinia enterocolitica* infection
      3. *Franciscella tularensis* infection (oropharyngeal tularemia)
      4. *Yersinia pestis* infection
      5. *Bacillus anthracis* infection (oropharyngeal anthrax)
      6. Viral hemorrhagic fever (Lassa fever)
2. Nonexudative pharyngotonsillitis
   A. Viral, bacterial, and chlamydial species
      1. Rhinovirus and coronavirus infections
      2. Acute bacterial sinusitis
      3. Influenza and parainfluenza virus
      4. Unknown agents
      5. Chlamydial infection— *Chlamydia* strain TWAR; *Chlamydia psittaci*

6. Nonexudative
   pharyngotonsillitis caused
   by the etiologic agents of
   exudative
   pharyngotonsillitis
B. Sexually transmitted
   pharyngotonsillitis
   1. Oropharyngeal gonorrhea
   2. Secondary syphilis
   3. Primary HIV infection
   4. *Chlamydia trachomatis*
3. Impaired host defenses and sore
   throat
   A. Agranulocytosis
   B. AIDS and oropharyngeal
      ulceration
   C. *Candida* epiglottitis in acute
      myelogenous leukemia
4. Sore throat and airway obstruction

A. Acute epiglottitis
B. Lingual tonsillar infection
   1. Lingual tonsillitis
   2. Lingual tonsillar abscess
C. Ludwig's angina due to
   Hemophilus influenzae cellulitis
D. Retropharyngeal abscess
E. Acute calcific retropharyngeal
   tendinitis
F. Coagulopathy-related upper
   airway hematoma
   1. Warfarin therapy
   2. Hemophilia
5. Thyroiditis
   A. Suppurative
   B. Subacute granulomatous
6. Spontaneous pneumomediastinum
7. Laryngotracheal trauma

☐ SUMMARY

Acute sore throat may be caused by an exudative or nonexudative pharyngotonsillitis. The bacterial and viral agents that are known to cause an exudative process may also cause only erythema and edema of the tonsils and pharynx. Some viral, mycoplasmal, and chlamydial agents cause only nonexudative pharyngotonsillitis.

Group A streptococci may cause *exudative pharyngotonsillitis* and tender anterior superior cervical adenopathy, palatal petechiae, polymorphonuclear leukocytosis, a positive streptococcal screening test (65–96-percent sensitive), and a positive group A streptococcal culture (76–90-percent sensitive). *Group C and group G streptococcal infections* are indistinguishable by examination from group A infections, but the screening tests are negative, and cultures and serologic grouping establish the diagnosis. Group C or G may cause foodborne epidemics and sporadic cases of pharyngotonsillitis. *Epstein-Barr virus* causes sore throat and exudative pharyngotonsillitis. Minimally tender posterior cervical adenopathy and splenomegaly occur. The total leukocyte count may be normal or elevated, and there is a relative lymphocytosis ($\geq$50 percent) and more than 10 percent atypical lymphocytes. The monospot test and heterophile agglutinins are positive in 90 percent of cases within the first 2 weeks. Heterophile-negative cases can be confirmed by measuring Epstein-Barr virus IgM anti-VCA and IgG anti-VCA and early viral antigen antibody levels.

Corynebacterium hemolyticum may mimic streptococcal exudative pharyngotonsillitis as well as scarlet fever, since the majority of patients with this disorder have a scarlatiniform rash. *C. hemolyticum* hemolysis is more readily demonstrated on 5 percent human blood agar plates. Gram's stains of throat

swabs and hemolytic colonies reveal gram-positive bacilli. *Corynebacterium diphtheriae* causes an exudative tonsillitis that progresses rapidly to form a membrane over one or both tonsils. A membrane may also form on the posterior pharyngeal wall and in the nasopharynx and/or larynx. The membrane is dirty white and may have areas of green and/or black discoloration. Extensive cervical lymphadenopathy may occur, creating a "bull neck" appearance. Involvement of the larynx may cause hoarseness or muffled speech, dyspnea, and stridor. Gram's and methylene blue stains of the exudate demonstrate gram-positive bacilli with metachromatic staining. Culture of a fragment of membrane on Loeffler's or tellurite selective media will grow *C. diphtheriae*. Positive species identification using fluorescent antibody staining may be possible on smears made from 4-h cultures. *Acute necrotizing ulcerative gingivitis* (ANUG) causes swelling, redness, and ulceration of interdental papillae, gum soreness and bleeding, and a sore throat with tonsillar exudate and ulceration.

Adenovirus can cause an exudative pharyngotonsillitis, conjunctivitis, cervical adenitis, and gastrointestinal complaints (abdominal pain, nausea, vomiting, and diarrhea). Types 3 and 7a have been associated with swimming pool– or pond water–related epidemics.

Herpes simplex virus causes oral vesicles and ulcerations; tender, friable, gums; and an exudative pharyngotonsillitis. A *peritonsillar cellulitis or abscess* starts as a mild sore throat that soon begins to improve. After 3 or 4 days, the throat pain suddenly becomes more intense, and severe odynophagia develops and leads to drooling of saliva. The voice becomes muffled ("hot potato" voice), and trismus may occur. The tonsil bulges anteriorly and toward the midline. The uvula may be draped over the swollen tonsil or soft palate. A severe tonsillitis or tonsillar abscess may cause *septic thrombophle-*

bitis of a tonsillar vein. This may spread into the internal jugular vein (Lemierre's disease). Septic emboli to the lung arise from this site and produce nodular cavitating pulmonary lesions. The thrombophlebitis may cause a painful, tender mass in the anterior neck above the medial border of the sternocleidomastoid muscle. Fever, chills, sweats, and prostration are severe. The causative organism is *Fusobacterium necrophorum*. Antibiotics effective against anaerobic bacteria lead to resolution. *Coxsackie A virus* causes a low-grade fever and throat pain associated with 2- to 3-mm red-rimmed ulcerations of the soft palate and tonsillar pillars. Up to 25 percent of patients with tonsillar exudate have *negative viral, bacterial, mycoplasmal, and chlamydial cultures and serologic studies*. Exudative pharyngotonsillitis has been reported to occur in patients from whom *viruses, mycoplasma, and TWAR agents* have been isolated. It is not clear whether these isolates were the cause or only associated with another infection by an unidentified agent.

Neisseria meningitidis may cause meningitis without a clinically apparent pharyngitis or nasopharyngitis. In some cases, an exudative pharyngotonsillitis may be present. A lethal course may follow exudative pharyngotonsillitis secondary to infection with *Yersinia enterocolitica*. Patients who fail to respond to penicillin or who have abdominal pain or diarrhea should be cultured for this organism. *Oropharyngeal tularemia* causes exudative disease that fails to respond to penicillin. Pneumonia may follow. An association with rabbits or ticks is present. The diagnosis can be confirmed by culture or by an agglutination test.

Yersinia pestis may cause an exudative tonsillitis and/or a peritonsillar abscess. A history of crushing fleas by chewing on them is present in patients with this rare manifestation of plague. *Bacillus anthracis* infection causes edema, erythema, and ulceration of one tonsil and ipsilateral cervical adenopathy. A smear from the tonsillar ulcer reveals gram-positive bacilli. An immunofluorescent antibody stain or a culture will confirm the diagnosis. This disease arises from eating infected lamb or beef. *Viral hemorrhagic fevers* occur in Africa, Asia, and South America, but could be imported into the United States. Lassa fever virus causes an exudative tonsillitis that is associated with fever, chills, prostration, generalized cutaneous edema, an erythematous macular rash, and signs of mucous membrane and cutaneous bleeding.

Nonexudative pharyngotonsillitis may cause sore throat and odynophagia with associated redness and edema of the tonsils, soft palate, and posterior pharynx. Causes include cold and influenza *viruses, chlamydia, and unknown agents*. An *acute bacterial sinusitis* with a postnasal purulent discharge may cause throat pain with diffuse redness and edema of the pharynx. Fever, cheek and forehead pain and tenderness, and a purulent or bloody mucoid nasal discharge are associated symptoms and signs. *Chlamydia psittaci* and *Chlamydia strain TWAR* can cause a nonexudative pharyngitis, followed within 3 to 6 days by pneumonia. The diagnosis can be confirmed by serologic studies or culture. Both agents respond to doxycycline therapy.

Sore throat may be associated with *oral-genital activity*. Females and male homosexuals are at highest risk. *Chlamydia trachomatis* and *Neiserria gonorrhoeae* can cause a nonexudative pharyngotonsillitis. Small vesicles on the mucosa and erythema are associated with *N. gonorrhoeae* infection.

Syphilitic pharyngitis is a rare manifestation of secondary syphilis. Snail track ulcers and ulcerated mucous patches and erythema occur on the palate and tonsillar areas and cause throat pain. The RPR and VDRL tests are positive. Symptoms respond rapidly to penicillin therapy.

Primary HIV infection begins suddenly with fever, myalgias, and generalized aching. A nonexudative pharyngotonsillitis with mild to severe throat pain occurs. A hard palate enanthem and oral, palatal, or tonsillar aphthous-like ulcerations occur in up to 30 percent of cases. The tonsils and axillary and/or cervical lymph nodes enlarge toward the end of the first week. A maculopapular rash may occur during the first 7 days. Leukopenia and thrombocytopenia are frequent early findings.

Neurologic disease such as aseptic meningitis, encephalopathy, myelopathy, facial paralysis, and peripheral neuropathy occur in only a small percentage of cases. HIV antigen can be detected, or HIV can be cultured from the blood. Conversion to seropositivity, as evidenced by the appearance of IgM-anti-HIV, occurs during the first 3 months after onset in 98 to 100 percent of cases.

Agranulocytosis may be associated with gingival necrosis and bleeding and palatal ulcerations covered with yellow pseudomembranes. One or more oropharyngeal or hypopharyngeal ulcerations with a white shaggy base may be present. The absolute polymorphonuclear leukocyte count is usually less than 750 cells/mm^3.

AIDS may be associated with hypopharyngeal and/or oropharyngeal ulceration. The causes include herpes simplex virus, cytomegalovirus, *Candida* species, cryptosporidia, and steroid-responsive idiopathic aphthous ulcers. Determination of the cause of ulcerations in this setting may require the use of biopsy and culture as well as therapeutic trials of acyclovir for herpex simplex virus, fluconazole for *Candida,* and steroids for nonspecific aphthous ulceration.

Candida infection causes edema and redness of the epiglottis. The enlarged epiglottis becomes visible as a "thumb sign" on a lateral soft tissue radiograph of the neck. There is a response to intravenous amphotericin or oral fluconazole.

Acute bacterial epiglottitis causes hoarseness, a muffled voice, and severe throat pain that is out of proportion to the minimal erythema seen in the oropharynx and tonsillar area. Odynophagia and dysphagia may be associated with symptoms and signs of airway obstruction (e.g., dyspnea, stridor, cyanosis) as the epiglottitis becomes more severe. Epiglottic edema and redness can be visualized by indirect or direct laryngoscopy, and enlargement by a lateral radiograph of the neck. Diagnosis of a specific bacterial agent requires culture of the blood or pus draining from an epiglottic abscess. There is a good response to intravenous antibiotics.

Lingual tonsillitis may cause a severe sore throat and odynophagia, and tongue tenderness with a normal oropharyngeal examination. Lingual tonsillar enlargement, hyperemia, and exudate may be visualized with a laryngeal mirror or fiberoptic laryngoscope. A *lingual tonsillar abscess* may prevent tongue protrusion. Since the abscess can cause airway obstruction, with dyspnea and stridor, it requires immediate surgical drainage.

Ludwig's angina may begin as a sore throat with severe odynophagia. A diffuse cellulitis of the anterior neck, with brawny edema and an overlying purple, red, or red-blue skin rash, occurs. The floor of the mouth is indurated and the tongue elevated and edematous. It protrudes between the incisors and cannot be extended voluntarily or used to modulate speech. Saliva drools from the open mouth. Etiologic agents of non-odontogenic Ludwig's angina include *Hemophilus influenzae* and *Streptococcus pyogenes*. Culture of the blood or tissue fluid from the anterior neck will identify the causative agent. There is a therapeutic response to parenteral antibiotics. A *retropharyngeal abscess* causes sore throat, odynophagia, fever, and a mass in the posterior pharynx. Posterior neck pain, tenderness, and paravertebral muscle spasm are often present, and the posterior pain can be intensified by swallowing. A lateral neck radiograph confirms prevertebral soft tissue swelling. Drainage of retropharyngeal pus relieves obstructive symptoms, and culture provides an etiologic diagnosis. *Retro-calcific tendinitis* may cause fever, sore throat, posterior neck pain, odynophagia, leukocytosis, mimicking a retropharyngeal abscess. Throat examination does not reveal a mass, and a lateral neck radiograph shows retropharyngeal soft tissue swelling and an amorphous calcification opposite the body of C2. *Hemophilia* and *anticoagulant therapy* can cause throat pain and airway obstruction secondary to a sublingual and hypopharyngeal hematoma. Lateral neck radiographs or physical examination will demonstrate the hematoma.

Suppurative thyroiditis causes a high fever; chills; sweats; and a tender, firm unilateral thyroid mass. Within 1 to 2 weeks, the mass may become fluctuant. Skin erythema and pustulation may occur over the tender thyroid region, and pus may drain spontaneously through the skin. Drainage of the abscess and antibiotic therapy lead to resolution. *Subacute granulomatous thyroiditis* can cause unilateral or bilateral throat and neck pain, made worse by swallowing. Transient hyperthyroidism may occur in up to 50 percent of cases. The radioactive iodine uptake is low, and the serum T_4 and T_3 are high or normal. A needle biopsy of the thyroid will demonstrate giant cells and granulomatous tissue. Symptoms respond to corticosteroids. *Spontaneous pneumomediastinum* may cause acute sore throat, dysphagia, and anterior neck and pleuritic central or precordial chest pain. The chest pain becomes worse with lying flat, inspiration, or coughing. Subcutaneous emphysema and Hamman's sign may be present. A chest radiograph demonstrates mediastinal air. *Laryngotracheal trauma* may cause pain and tenderness over the larynx and trachea, sore throat, a hoarse or muffled voice, or aphonia. Cartilaginous crepitus may be present over the thyroid and cricoid cartilages. Subcutaneous emphysema and/or a hematoma may occur in the anterior neck. Flexible fiberoptic laryngoscopy may reveal submucosal he-

matomas and cartilage fractures, and can help in assessment of airway patency. A CT scan of the neck can define cartilage fractures and airway distortion. Airway control is essential in patients with this type of injury. Some patients can be intubated, while more severe injuries require tracheostomy.

☐ DESCRIPTION OF LISTED DISEASES

1. EXUDATIVE PHARYNGOTONSILLITIS

A. Group A Streptococcal Infection

1. Without Rash There is an abrupt onset with chills, fever to 101°F or higher, malaise, myalgias, headache, and nausea. Constant throat pain or pain only on swallowing may be present. Tenderness at the angle of the jaw may be noted. The pharynx, tonsils, or tonsillar remnants are usually hyperemic and swollen, and irregular patches of gray-white exudate may stud their surface. Petechiae may be seen on the soft palate and pharyngeal wall. Confluent exudate on the tonsils and pharynx may mimic a diphtheritic membrane, but this is uncommon. Lymph nodes at the angle of the mandible and in the submandibular region are often enlarged and/or tender. Milder forms of infection may occur without fever, without exudate (50 percent of cases), and even without throat pain. A viral cold may be mimicked, with nasal stuffiness and rhinorrhea associated with tender anterior cervical nodes. Leukocytosis ($>$12,000 cells/mm^3) with a shift to the left is commonly present. Throat cultures are usually positive, with a sensitivity of 80 to 95 percent if the culture is done by a clinical laboratory with good quality control. A single initial swab culture has a sensitivity of 90 percent (10 percent false-negative rate) when compared to use of two swabs at a single sampling, and only 76 percent if three swabs taken on three consecutive days are used as a ''gold standard.'' Cultures taken prior to tonsillectomy, compared to culture of the homogenized tonsillar tissue, have a sensitivity of 82 percent. Single cultures taken from patients with streptococcal scarlet fever are positive in only 75 percent of cases. Asymptomatic adults have a streptococcal colonization rate of only 0.84 to 1.22 percent, giving a specificity of the throat culture of 99 percent for this age group. School-age children have higher colonization rates (15 percent in winter months), giving cultures in this age group a lower specificity.

Clinical judgment identifies only 55 to 75 percent of patients with positive cultures and predicts streptococcal disease in 23 to 27 percent of the patients who have negative cultures, resulting in unnecessary treatment of this group.

TABLE OF DISEASE INCIDENCE

INCIDENCE PER 100,000 (APPROXIMATE)

Common (>100)
Group A streptococcal infection
Scarlet fever
Epstein-Barr virus
Herpes simplex virus
Exudative pharyngotonsillitis without
demonstrable etiology
Exudative pharyngotonsillitis due to viral,
mycoplasmal, or chlamydial infections
Nonexudative pharyngotonsillitis caused by
rhinoviruses and coronaviruses, acute
bacterial sinusitis, influenza and
parainfluenza viruses, unknown agents,
chlamydial strain TWAR and agents
causing exudative pharyngotonsillitis
AIDS and oropharyngeal ulceration
Subacute granulomatous thyroiditis

Uncommon (>5–100)
Group G streptococcal infection
Group C streptococcal infection
C. hemolyticum
Acute necrotizing ulcerative gingivitis
Adenovirus infection
Peritonsillar cellulitis or abscess
Coxsackie A infection (herpangina)
Gonorrhea (oropharyngeal)
Primary HIV infection
C. trachomatis infection
Acute epiglottitis
Lingual tonsillitis
Spontaneous pneumomediastinum
Laryngotracheal trauma

Rare (>0–5)
C. diphtheriae
Postanginal sepsis (Lemierre's disease)
Exudative pharyngotonsillitis caused by
*N. meningitidis, Y. enterolitica, F. tularensis, Y.
pestis, B. anthracis,* and viral hemorrhagic fever
(Lassa fever)
Nonexudative pharyngotonsillitis due to *C. psittaci*
Secondary syphilis
Agranulocytosis
Candida epiglottitis
Lingual tonsillar abscess
Ludwig's angina due to *H. influenzae*
Retropharyngeal abscess
Acute calcific retropharyngeal tendinitis
Coagulopathy and upper airway hematoma
Suppurative thyroiditis

Rapid antigen tests use antibodies for detection of group A carbohydrate antigen taken directly from a throat swab. Latex agglutination, enzyme immunoassay, and antibody-coated liposome indicator systems have been used in clinical trials and may provide results in 5 to 15 min. The reported sensitivities and specificities of these commercially available tests have varied with the number of organisms found in semiquantitative cultures and the investigative group doing the test. The Directigen 1-2-3 group A streptococcus test was positive in 26 percent of patients with 10 or fewer colonies of group A streptococci on culture and in 77 percent of those with more than 100 colonies. The latex agglutination Directogen test has reported sensitivities of 61 to 95 percent and specificities of 82 to 99 percent. The liposome-based Directogen test has a sensitivity of 65 percent and a specificity of 84 percent. Similar variable sensitivities and specificities have been noted for other antigen detection kits (e.g., Culturette 10-min group A streptococcus identification kit, sensitivity 62–95 percent and specificity 92–100 percent). To use a rapid test without sacrificing clinical accuracy, it is necessary to follow a negative rapid test with a culture, ensuring against a false-negative result. Unnecessary treatment can be reduced by selecting a highly specific rapid test and/or culturing rapid test-positive cases that do not appear to have streptococcal disease. Treatment with oral penicillin or intramuscular penicillin will decrease morbidity by 1 or 2 days if treatment is begun within 36 h of onset. Treatment is also directed at the prevention of acute rheumatic fever and its most serious sequela, class IV rheumatic valvular disease, requiring valve replacement. The risk of this is lower today than 40 years ago. Attack rates of rheumatic fever for an untreated streptococcal sore throat are 1 in 4000 to 1 in 40,000 cases. Only 2 percent of patients

with acute rheumatic fever will develop severe valvular disease, making the risk of failing to treat a streptococcal sore throat today much less than it was in the past.

2. With Rash (Scarlet Fever) Patients with streptococcal pharyngotonsillitis may develop a diffuse pink-to-red rash over the upper body that soon spreads to involve the neck and extremities. The rash is slightly elevated in some areas due to sweat gland occlusion and has a texture similar to that of sandpaper. The skin folds in the antecubital fossae, neck, groin, and popliteal areas are darker red (Pastia's lines), and there is a circumoral pallor.

The tongue may be covered with a whitish coat, with prominent red papillae ("white strawberry tongue"). After 4 to 5 days, the tongue becomes beefy red ("red strawberry" or "raspberry tongue").

After 7 days, the rash clears, and the skin may desquamate. Eosinophilia may occur during the first week.

B. Mimics of Exudative Group A Streptococcal Pharyngotonsillitis

1. Group G Streptococcal Infection Sore throat and dysphagia occurred in 100 percent of cases, tender swollen cervical nodes in 60 percent, pharyngotonsillar exudate in 46 percent, and fever in 81 percent of patients reported in a food-borne epidemic of streptococcal group G disease. Such epidemics have an abrupt onset and termination. Egg salad and hard-boiled eggs have been the usual source. Egg salad has been shown to be a good medium for growth of streptococci. The clinical illness is indistinguishable from that produced by group A streptococci. Culture on sheep blood agar, followed by serologic typing, will identify group G streptococci. Bacitracin testing of beta-hemolytic colonies misidentifies 11 percent of group G streptococci as group A. Group

G streptococcal disease is responsive to penicillin. Non-epidemic cases may also occur. The reported incidence in one survey of acute pharyngitis that included testing for *Chlamydia, Mycoplasma,* viruses, and bacteria in adults with pharyngitis was 4.6 percent.

2. Group C Streptococcal Infection   Epidemic and sporadic cases occur and mimic group A streptococcal pharyngotonsillitis. Food-borne disease has followed ingestion of contaminated milk, egg salad, and chicken salad, and recurrent group C pharyngotonsillitis has been associated with exposure to a possibly infected pet cat. Treatment of two recurrent cases required tonsillectomy. Elevation of liver enzymes and acute right upper abdominal pain have been associated with this organism. In the survey described above, nonepidemic group C infection occurred in 12 percent of adults with pharyngitis.

3. Epstein-Barr Virus   This virus causes an infectious mononucleosis syndrome. This disorder may begin abruptly or gradually, with malaise, chills, sweats, febrile episodes, anorexia, and loss of the desire to smoke. Frontal and retro-orbital headache, generalized myalgias, and abdominal fullness are other complaints. A severe sore throat and fever are the most prevalent symptoms. The throat pain may be severe enough on swallowing to prevent eating. The tonsils are enlarged and hyperemic, and gray-white patches of exudate are splattered over their surface and portions of the pharyngeal wall. There may be palatal petechiae in 25 to 60 percent of cases. The findings of the oropharyngeal examination are indistinguishable from those for acute streptococcal disease. Clinical differences between these disorders include the absence of tender anterior superior cervical nodes and the presence of prominent, minimally tender posterior cervical nodes (93–100 percent) and splenomegaly (52 percent) in Epstein-Barr virus infection. Rapid streptococcal antigen tests and throat cultures reveal group A streptococci in no more than 5 to 7 percent of cases. Hematologic examination reveals a relative and absolute lymphocytosis in 70 percent of cases at the onset of the illness, and the percentage with this finding increases during the first 2 weeks. More than 50 percent of the total white cells are mononuclear, and more than 10 percent of these are atypical lymphocytes. Heterophile antibodies to horse red blood cells are demonstrable by the monospot test in 90 percent of cases. The heterophile sheep cell agglutination titer is 40 or more after absorption of the patient's serum with guinea pig kidney. The heterophile antibodies produced in normal serum (Forssman antibody) or in serum sickness are removed by guinea pig kidney absorption. Serum alanine aminotransferase (ALT or SGPT) and/or lactic dehydrogenase activities are elevated in 90 percent of cases and the alkaline phosphatase in 60 percent. Enzyme elevations remain less than 10 times normal and are usually only 2 to 3 times the normal level. While bilirubin values exceed the normal range in 45 percent, clinical jaundice occurs in only 5 percent of patients. Cryoglobulins can be demonstrated in 90 to 95 percent, but titers are low. Heterophile-negative cases can be tested for specific Epstein-Barr virus antibodies. Several patterns of IgM anti-viral capsid antigen response may be observed in acute Epstein-Barr virus infection. Some patients have an initial low titer that rises from day 0 to day 14, while other initial titers do not change, and some fall. The reason for this heterogeneous response to Epstein-Barr virus infection is unknown. Administration of ampicillin will cause the eruption of a diffuse, pruritic, maculopapular rash in 90 to 100 percent of cases. Rash occurs in only 5 percent of patients not given ampicillin. If the rash is scarlatiniform, the clinical findings mimic streptococcal scarlet fever.

The fever and pharyngotonsillitis do not respond to penicillin and other antibiotics.

4. Corynebacterium hemolyticum Infection   Patients may have a sore throat, fever (40 percent), a scarlatiniform rash (67 percent), and cough (37 percent). Pharyngeal erythema occurs in all cases, and a patchy white exudate in up to 70 percent. Confluent pharyngeal exudates occur in 7 percent of cases and may mimic diphtheria. Lymphadenopathy occurs as bilateral tender anterior cervical and submandibular nodes (48 percent). Leukocyte counts have ranged from 7100 to 17,400 cells/mm^3, and monospot tests have been negative. A Gram's stain of pharyngeal exudate is considered consistent with *C. hemolyticum* infection if it demonstrates numerous gram-positive pleomorphic bacilli associated with polymorphonuclear leukocytes. Consistent smears were found in 68 percent of culture-positive patients tested in one reported series. Culture on 5 percent human blood agar plates is required, since hemolysis shows up poorly on sheep blood agar. This disorder occurs primarily in adolescents and young adults. The role of this organism in the causation of exudative pharyngotonsillitis has been questioned because smears and cultures have not been done in suitable control groups and cultures for viruses, *Mycoplasma* species and *Chlamydia* species have not been performed on the same patients cultured for *C. hemolyticum* and beta-hemolytic streptococci. Penicillin and erythromycin have both been effective in infections caused by this organism.

5. Corynebacterium diphtheriae Infection   There is an abrupt onset of fever, sore throat (71 percent), and malaise. A patchy, easily removable exudate can be observed during the first day on one or both tonsils. Within hours, it may be replaced by an adherent, greenish gray thick membrane. The membrane may extend to the palate, pharynx, and larynx, producing cough, hoarseness, and sometimes dyspnea and stridor. Extensive lymphadenopathy may occur in the submental and cervical region, creating a wide "bull neck" appearance. An odor described as that of a "wet mouse" has been noted in association with this disease.

Clinical clues to the diagnosis include a dirty white membrane on the tonsils and pharynx with areas of green and black discoloration, a "bull neck," cough, hoarseness and stridor, palatal weakness, and a nasal membrane with a serosanguineous discharge from one or both nares. Gram's stain of pharyngeal exudate may show polymorphonuclear leukocytes associated with gram-positive rod-shaped bacteria, and a methylene blue stain may demonstrate rod-shaped bacteria with metachromatic granules. A piece of membrane or a submembrane exudate should be cultured on Loeffler's medium and/or tellurite selective medium. Confirmation of the diagnosis may sometimes be made rapidly using immunofluorescent antibody staining of smears of 4-h cultures, but final identification, using colonial and microscopic morphology and fermentation reactions, may take 24 h or longer.

Therapy with diphtheria antitoxin and erythromycin should be initiated with the suspicion of pharyngotonsillar diphtheria and should not be delayed until laboratory confirmation is received. Epstein-Barr virus, streptococcal disease, acute necrotizing ulcerative gingivitis (ANUG), *C. hemolyticum,* and *Corynebacterium ulcerans* can produce membranous exudates. Cases caused by *C. hemolyticum* may so closely mimic diphtheria that administration of antitoxin is necessary. The membrane of Epstein-Barr virus remains adherent, stays white, and does not produce tonsillar bleeding when it is removed. There is a peripheral lymphocytosis, atypical lymphocytes, and a positive monospot test. A rapid antigen test will detect streptococcal infection, but coinfection with group A streptococci may occur in 20 to 30 percent of cases of diphtheria. In some cases, group A streptococcal and *C. diphtheria* infections are clinically indistinguishable, and treatment for both may be required before the results of the diphtheria cultures are available. ANUG causes gingival ulcerations and bleeding, as well as tonsillar ulcers, exudate, and membranes, and can be differentiated by the clinical findings described below.

6. Acute Necrotizing Ulcerative Gingivitis (ANUG)

Mild-to-severe throat pain may occur. Odynophagia may be severe, limiting ingestion of food and fluids. The tonsils may be streaked with a shaggy, gray-white exudate, and pharyngeal ulceration may be present. Rarely, membranous tonsillitis, mimicking diphtheria, occurs. The interdental papillae are swollen and hyperemic. Some of them are denuded, forming craterlike ulcers that bleed spontaneously (67 percent) or after tooth brushing (37 percent). The gums may ache, and the interdental papillae are tender. The ulcerations are covered by a loosely attached gray pseudomembrane. The breath has a fetid odor (97 percent). Fever may be present in up to 39 percent of cases but is an inconstant finding. Tender cervical lymphadenopathy occurs in 61 percent of cases. Interproximal necrosis and ulceration, local pain, and

bleeding are present in 100 percent of cases and are the major criteria for the clinical diagnosis of ANUG. Risk factors for development of this disease include fatigue, stress, physical debilitation, smoking, poor oral hygiene, trauma, and possibly AIDS. The etiologic agents of this disorder are still unknown. Candidate organisms have included *Treponema* and *Selenomonas* species, *Bacteroides intermedius,* and *Fusobacterium* species. There is usually a good therapeutic response to the antianaerobic drug metronidazole, providing evidence that one or more of the responsible organisms are anaerobes. Debridement of interdental ulcerations using a curette or ultrasound also speeds recovery.

7. Adenovirus Infection (Pharyngoconjunctival Fever)

There is an acute onset of low-grade fever, myalgias, malaise, chills, and headache. A severe sore throat with tonsillar exudate occurs and may mimic streptococcal disease. Conjunctivitis involving one or both eyes occurs in 33 to 51 percent of cases and is a useful differential finding. Cervical adenitis may be present. In one swimming pool-associated epidemic, abdominal pain (64 percent), nausea or vomiting (54 percent), diarrhea (49 percent), and cough (43 percent) were also prominent complaints. There are usually no sequelae, and spontaneous recovery occurs within 5 days. Types 3 and 7a have been associated with swimming pool- or pond water-related outbreaks.

8. Herpes Simplex Virus Infection (Primary)

Acute herpetic pharyngotonsillitis is more common in children under age 5 but may occur in adults. There may be a severe sore throat and odynophagia associated with an exudative tonsillitis that is difficult to distinguish from streptococcal infection. The presence of vesicles and ulcerations on the tongue, palate, floor of the mouth, and buccal and labial mucosa; and tender, friable gums suggest the diagnosis of herpetic infection. Fever, toxicity, and a fetid odor of the breath are common findings. Tender anterior cervical adenopathy may be present. Oropharyngeal culture will grow herpes simplex virus.

Primary herpes simplex type 2 genital infection causes severe genital pain, multiple grouped genital vesicles and ulcers, dysuria, and sometimes urinary retention. An associated exudative pharyngotonsillitis may be present.

Herpes simplex virus infection can be separated from ANUG by the lack of interdental ulceration and the presence of grouped oral ulcers, but some cases may require herpes simplex virus culture for differentiation. Treatment with acyclovir may be of benefit in primary herpes simplex virus infection.

9. Complicated Pharyngotonsillitis

Peritonsillar cellulitis and abscess follow a sore throat and fever that are present for several days. The illness seems to be improving when suddenly the throat pain becomes very severe. Rather than swallow, the patient may sit with his or her mouth open and drool saliva. The voice may be muffled and has been characterized as a "hot potato" voice. One or both tonsils may be involved. The tonsil is enlarged and displaced anteriorly, downward, and medially. The swollen and red uvula may be draped over the bulging tonsil or against the edematous soft palate. There may be a grayish white exudate studding the tonsillar surface. Extension of the infection into the lateral pharyngeal space may cause pain, swelling, and tenderness below the angle of the mandible and inability to open the jaw more than 10 to 15 mm (i.e., trismus).

Differentiation of peritonsillar cellulitis from abscess in children has not been possible on the basis of presenting symptoms and signs. Both may cause a pharyngotonsillar bulge, trismus, a "hot potato" voice, drooling, throat pain, dysphagia, fever, and an elevated leukocyte count. Twenty-three to 49 percent of patients may have only cellulitis and do not require surgery. In patients without airway obstruction, administration of intravenous antibiotics (clindamycin or a second-generation cephalosporin) for 24 to 48 h may differentiate the two processes. Patients with cellulitis or a small abscess show improvement in one or more symptoms over the first 2 days, while those with pus requiring drainage remain unchanged or become worse. This disorder may be precipitated by group A streptococcal infection, but the abscess usually contains anaerobic bacteria.

Peritonsillar abscesses may be treated by needle aspiration, open surgical drainage, or tonsillectomy and intravenous antibiotics.

Postanginal sepsis (Lemierre's disease) is a disorder of young adults and adolescents that begins with a sore throat and fever. Pharyngotonsillar exudate may be present. Within 3 to 5 days, fever, chills, and prostration become worse, and pain and tenderness may appear anterior to the border of a sternocleidomastoid muscle. A palpable tender mass may be present in the same area (36 percent) and represents a septic thrombophlebitis of the internal jugular vein. This mass arises from involvement of a tonsillar vein. Tonsillitis or, less commonly, a peritonsillar abscess (10 percent) is the initiating disorder. Septic embolization to the lung causes dyspnea (45 percent), cough, hemoptysis, and pleuritic pain (27 percent). Chest radiographs show bilateral nodular infiltrates with cavitation (90–100 percent) and effusions. Septic arthritis, splenic abscess, and osteomyelitis may also occur in a minority of cases. The jugular vein thrombophlebitis can be confirmed by an ultrasound study of the neck. Blood cultures grow *Fusobacterium necrophorum* and, less commonly, additional bacteria (peptostreptococcus and group C streptococcus). Clindamycin or cefoxitin and metronidazole therapy will lead to recovery after prolonged therapy (6 weeks).

10. Coxsackie A Infection (Herpangina)   Throat pain, with or without fever, occurs. Examination reveals 2 to 10 bilateral, small (2–3 mm), scattered, red-rimmed vesicles and ulcers on the surface of the soft palate and anterior tonsillar pillars. There is no pharyngotonsillar exudate. Some patients may have abdominal pain, tenderness, and anorexia. Cases tend to cluster in the summer and fall. No therapy is required, and the clinical appearance is diagnostic.

11. Exudative Pharyngotonsillitis without Demonstrable Etiology   In one study of pharyngitis that included cultural and serologic tests for bacteria, *Mycoplasma pneumoniae, Chlamydia,* and viruses, 25 percent of patients with pharyngotonsillar exudates had no demonstrable etiology.

12. Exudative Pharyngotonsillitis in Viral, Mycoplasmal, and Chlamydial Infections   In the above-mentioned study, exudative pharyngotonsillitis occurred in association with viral (e.g., respiratory syncytial virus, influenza A and B viruses, adenovirus, herpes simplex virus, Epstein-Barr virus, rhinovirus, parainfluenza A and B viruses, and coxsackie B4 virus), mycoplasmal, and TWAR agent infections. One-sixth to one-third of patients with these nonbacterial infections had exudative disease associated with causative agents other than those viruses commonly associated with exudative pharyngotonsillitis (i.e., herpes simplex virus, Epstein-Barr virus, and adenovirus).

It is not known whether these nonbacterial agents were causative or whether an associated unknown agent not detected was responsible.

C. Rare and Potentially Lethal Causes of Exudative Pharyngotonsillitis

1. Neisseria meningitidis *Pharyngotonsillitis*   An exudative pharyngotonsillitis similar to that caused by streptococcal disease may occasionally be seen in patients with meningococcal meningitis. In most cases, the pharynx is red without exudate or normal in appearance.

2. Yersinia enterocolitica *Pharyngotonsillitis*   This organism may cause an exudative pharyngotonsillitis, cervical lymphadenopathy, high fever and toxicity, and marked leukocytosis. Most adult patients have no abdominal pain or diarrhea, but an enterocolitis may occur. There is no response to penicillin or erythromycin. The absence of a therapeutic response, the presence of severe toxicity, and/or the deaths of one or more family members from a similar pharyngeal illness should raise the possibility of *Yersinia* infection. *Y. enterocolitica* grows as nonhemolytic colonies on blood agar and also on selective media (e.g., MacConkey's) used for stool pathogen isolation. For some strains, cold enrichment techniques or simultaneous incubation at room temperature may be required for *Yersinia* growth.

Aminoglycosides, trimethoprim-sulfamethoxazole, and/or third-generation cephalosporins are effective against this organism.

3. Franciscella tularensis *Infection (Oropharyngeal Tularemia)* This disease causes a severe sore throat, odynophagia, high fever, and a septic course. Exudative pharyngotonsillitis, peritonsillar abscess or tonsillar enlargement, and necrosis may occur. Cultures are negative for group A streptococci, and there is no response to penicillin therapy. Fever persists for 1 or more weeks, and marked enlargement of cervical and sometimes mediastinal nodes may occur. Pneumonia and pleural effusion may follow. A history of ingestion of wild rabbit or contact with ticks (e.g., crushing them with the fingers) may be obtained. The diagnosis can be confirmed by culture on cysteine-enriched media or by the agglutination test (i.e., >1/80 on a single titer or a fourfold rise in titer over time).

Streptomycin is the treatment of choice, but tetracycline is also effective.

4. Yersinia pestis *Infection* Exudative pharyngotonsillitis or a peritonsillar abscess may rarely occur and is secondary to crushing infected fleas between the teeth. Cervical adenopathy, fever, and toxicity accompany throat pain and dysphagia. Up to 10 percent of healthy contacts of plague patients may have pharyngeal colonization with *Y. pestis* without adverse effect. Such asymptomatic carriage may occur in a plague-endemic area or during a plague outbreak. *Y. pestis* grows on ordinary media and can be identified by immunofluorescent staining. Streptomycin and tetracycline in combination constitute an effective therapeutic regimen.

5. Bacillus anthracis *Infection (Oropharyngeal Anthrax)* A series of six cases with a 50 percent mortality was reported from Turkey. Severe sore throat, fever, lethargy, and toxemia occurred. One tonsil or the base of the tongue was edematous, hyperemic, and ulcerated. The lesion was usually covered by a gray or white pseudomembrane. Ipsilateral marked cervical adenopathy was present. Severe respiratory distress, cyanosis, hemorrhagic pneumonia, and extreme prostration occurred in the three fatal cases. Penicillin therapy was effective in the others. Ingestion of infected lamb or beef was the usual cause of this disorder. Gram-positive rods can be demonstrated on lesion smears, and rapid identification by a direct immunofluorescent antibody stain is possible. Culture on blood agar will grow *B. anthracis*.

6. Viral Hemorrhagic Fever (Africa) Lassa fever may present with fever, myalgias, malaise, and a severe sore throat with dysphagia. Exudative pharyngotonsillitis may be present. Chest and abdominal pain, diarrhea, and generalized puffiness of the skin of the face and limbs may occur. A macular rash may appear during the first week of illness. Hemorrhagic symptoms occur after 4 to 5 days and include hemorrhagic conjunctivitis, gingival bleeding, hematemesis, melena, epistaxis, hematuria, petechiae, and ecchymoses of the skin. The diagnosis can be confirmed by viral isolation from the blood or by sero-logic means. Ribavirin therapy is effective. Imported cases of this disorder may appear in the United States masquerading as influenza, malaria, or some nonspecific fever.

2. NONEXUDATIVE PHARYNGOTONSILLITIS

A. Viral, Bacterial, and Chlamydial Species

1. Rhinovirus or Coronavirus Infections Such infections may cause a scratchy or painful throat that is made more severe by sneezing or swallowing. Rhinorrhea, nasal stuffiness, myalgias, malaise, anorexia, and fatigue are other common complaints. Fever does not occur unless a complicating sinusitis or otitis media develop.

2. Acute Bacterial Sinusitis This disorder may follow an acute viral "cold." Pain, tenderness, and sometimes swelling may occur over one or both cheeks or the medial area of the forehead. Lateral nasal and orbital pain may also occur. Purulent drainage occurs from the nose or is delivered by hawking up material from the posterior pharynx. The discharge may be yellow-white or green and may be blood-streaked. Initially, some patients have a mucoid bloody discharge. Throat pain and dryness, worse on arising and relieved by drinking cold fluids, and a more persistent pharyngeal odynophagia may occur. The throat may be diffusely red and swollen, and strands of yellow mucopus may drape the posterior pharynx, but there is no tonsillar or pharyngeal exudate. Cough and hoarseness are common associated symptoms. Fever and chills occur in less than 50 percent of adult cases. Nasal endoscopy will reveal purulent secretion near the major sinus ostia and a hyperemic edematous mucosa. Maxillary and frontal sinus tenderness may be present. Plain sinus radiographs or a CT scan of the sinuses may detect mucosal thickening, sinus opacities, and air fluid levels. There is a prompt response to oral broad-spectrum beta-lactamase-resistant antibiotics such as cefaclor or cefuroxime.

3. Influenza or Parainfluenza Virus Patients may have high fever, weakness, malaise, myalgias, headache, and a mild scratchy or slightly sore throat with minimal erythema and no exudate. Coryza, a dry nonproductive cough, and abdominal symptoms may occur. The diagnosis is most likely during epidemic periods, but sporadic cases may occur throughout the year.

4. Unknown Agents The cause of a nonexudative pharyngitis may remain unidentified in up to 64 percent of cases, even though cultures and serologic tests for viruses, bacteria, *Chlamydia*, species, and *Mycoplasma* species are performed.

5. Chlamydial Infection *Chlamydia* strain TWAR causes acute respiratory illness in adolescents and young adults, but any adult age group can be affected. Initial symptoms include fever (56 percent), chills (39 percent), pleuritic chest pain (33 percent), headache (22 percent), and cough (61 percent). Productive cough may occur in up to 44 percent.

Sore throat and difficulty swallowing occur in 20 percent, and the pharynx and tonsils are erythematous but free of exudate. Basilar rales occur in 61 percent and rhonchi in 28 percent. Leukocytosis is present in 61 percent. Radiographs show mid- or lower lung infiltrates in most cases, and these are patchy or segmental. A throat swab smear can be stained directly for the TWAR organism using a fluorescein conjugated monoclonal antibody. A *Chlamydia* group complement fixation test and a microimmunofluorescence test for TWAR have been used for diagnostic and epidemiologic studies. The organism can be cultured in HeLa 229 cell cultures or chicken egg yolk sacs. A history of nonexudative pharyngitis followed by cough and evidence of pneumonia are suggestive of TWAR infection. Erythromycin or tetracycline may be effective against this agent. Human-to-human transmission is suspected.

In a large reported series of *C. psittaci* cases, there was an abrupt onset of fever (100 percent), rigors (61 percent), sweats (89 percent), severe headache (87 percent), myalgias (75 percent), nausea (49 percent), vomiting (38 percent), and abdominal pain (10 percent). Respiratory complaints were cough (78 percent), sputum (20 percent), hemoptysis (8 percent), dyspnea (24 percent), chest pain (17 percent), and sore throat (17 percent).

Physical signs included an erythematous pharynx (15 percent), meningismus (9 percent), altered consciousness (12 percent), and chest abnormalities such as rales (73 percent) and signs of consolidation (25 percent). Hepatomegaly and splenomegaly were present in 8 to 10 percent of cases. Chest radiographs revealed pulmonary infiltrates in 78 percent. In patients with normal chest radiographs, positive physical signs in the chest were present in 62 percent. A history of bird exposure was usually present (84 percent). The diagnosis may be confirmed by a complement fixation test. Oral doxycycline is usually administered on the basis of clinical findings and a history of bird exposure. Fever and other symptoms improve within 24 to 48 h of the start of therapy.

6. *Nonexudative Pharyngotonsillitis Caused by the Etiologic Agents of Exudative Pharyngotonsillitis* Organisms capable of causing exudative disease may sometimes cause only a mild sore throat accompanied by diffuse or patchy pharyngotonsillar erythema. Since the clinical findings are nonspecific, agent identification requires culture and serologic study, which are seldom done in patients with nonexudative disease.

B. Sexually Transmitted Pharyngotonsillitis

1. *Oropharyngeal Gonorrhea* Women and men practicing fellatio are at increased risk. Cunnilingus can lead

to pharyngeal disease or colonization, but the frequency is lower. Up to 20 percent of homosexual men and 10 percent of heterosexual women with gonorrhea at another site may have pharyngeal colonization. Most culture-positive patients are asymptomatic. Symptomatic patients may have a severe-to-mild sore throat. Severe cases have diffuse oropharyngeal erythema, mucosal edema, and small mucosal vesicles. Mild cases have patchy erythema and pinpoint-sized vesicles. Exudative tonsillitis may occur, but it is uncommon. Pharyngeal culture on chocolate agar or modified Thayer-Martin medium will isolate the organism.

2. *Secondary Syphilis* This disorder may cause a mild-to-severe sore throat with pharyngotonsillar erythema. Mucous patches may be present in the mouth and tonsillar regions and may ulcerate, causing local throat pain. ''Snail track'' ulcers, covered with mucosa, may involve the palate and fauces. Condyloma lata may involve the perineum, vaginal, and other intertriginous regions. A generalized macular, papular, maculopapular, or papulosquamous rash that involves the palms and soles may occur. There may be a low-grade fever, malaise, headache, and sometimes meningismus. The VDRL and RPR tests are positive, and the symptoms and signs rapidly resolve on penicillin therapy.

3. *Primary HIV Infection* There is an abrupt onset of fever and muscle pain in the back and/or extremities or generalized aching. A mild-to-severe sore throat occurs, and the palate and pharynx are diffusely erythematous. An enanthem on the hard palate consisting of 0.5-cm red circular patches may occur. Oral, palatal, and tonsillar aphthous-like ulcerations have been observed in up to 30 percent of cases. Tonsillar enlargement appears toward the end of the first week, but there is no exudate.

Cervical and axillary adenopathy are observed on days 5 to 7 after onset (85–95 percent), but splenomegaly occurs in only 10 percent. A maculopapular skin rash occurs in up to 75 percent of cases during the first week of illness. The rash is present on the upper trunk and neck (75 percent) and also affects the face and arms (60 percent) or the lower trunk, thighs, and forehead (15 percent). Severe odynophagia, due to esophagitis or an esophageal ulcer, may occur. Laboratory abnormalities during the first 2 weeks include leukopenia, thrombocytopenia, and abnormal liver function tests. The relative proportion of blood lymphocytes increases during the third week. Atypical lymphocytes, exceeding more than 10 percent of the circulating cells, occur in only 15 percent of cases.

HIV antigen can be detected in all patients during the first three weeks, and IgM anti-HIV antibody appears in 95 to 100 percent of cases within 3 months. Cultures of the blood will grow HIV during the first 2 weeks. Neurologic disease may occur in a small percentage of patients during the third or fourth weeks of the acute illness, taking the form of aseptic meningitis, facial paralysis on one or both sides, myelopathy, spinal myoclonus, ataxic neuropathy, sensory and motor disorders of the limbs, and/or neuralgic pain. Encephalopathy, characterized by mood and personality changes, lethargy, cognitive deficits, seizures, confusion, and coma, may begin at the onset of the primary illness. Primary HIV infection should be considered in patients who are bisexual or homosexual, intravenous drug abusers, hemophiliacs, or sexual partners of members of these risk groups who develop fever and sore throat followed by generalized lymphadenopathy (i.e., a mononucleosis-like illness).

4. **Chlamydia trachomatis** Pharyngeal and tonsillar chlamydial infection was suggested by serologic studies done in patients with throat pain. Cultures taken from tonsillar crypts led to the isolation of this organism in 26 percent of patients complaining of sore throat in a Tokyo clinic. Exudative tonsillitis did not occur. There was a history of oral-genital activity in 61 percent of patients with positive cultures. Positive cultures were associated with the presence of antibody to *C. trachomatis* in 58 percent.

3. IMPAIRED HOST DEFENSES AND SORE THROAT

A. Agranulocytosis Sore throat, odynophagia, fever, and chills are common presenting symptoms. Painful and bleeding gums may occur. Examination may reveal tonsillar swelling and exudate. There may be gingival necrosis and multiple palatal ulcerations covered with a yellow-white pseudomembrane. The oral mucosa may appear erythematous and shiny, and the breath may be fetid. One or more posterior pharyngeal ulcerations, with a white shaggy base, may be present. Neutropenia may be caused by leukemia, idiopathic aplastic anemia, or cytotoxic drugs used in the therapy of malignancy. Other drugs that may be associated with a severe depression of polymorphonuclear leukocyte concentrations are methimazole, propylthiouracil, sulfonamides (i.e., sulfasalazine), phenothiazines, phenytoin, pyrimethamine, chloramphenicol, primidone, aminopyrine, penicillin, and cephalosporins. The total leukocyte count and the absolute neutrophil count are markedly reduced. Antibiotic therapy and cessation of drug therapy will result in survival in 95 percent of cases of drug-induced neutropenia. Antileukemic therapy may induce a remission, a rise in the neutrophil count, and resolution of oral and throat symptoms.

B. AIDS and Oropharyngeal Ulceration Large, painful aphthous ulcers have been observed in the mouth, hypopharynx, and/or esophagus of patients with AIDS. These lesions caused sore throat and severe odynophagia. Hypopharyngeal and oropharyngeal ulceration may be related to infection with herpes simplex virus, cytomegalovirus, *Can-*

dida species, or cryptosporidia, or may be idiopathic. In a series of AIDS patients with severe sore throat and biopsy/culture-negative aphthous ulcerations in the hypopharynx and esophagus, there was a dramatic response to prednisone therapy.

C. Candida Epiglottitis This disorder was reported as a cause of sore throat, otalgia, and dysphagia in a patient with acute myelogenous leukemia. Indirect laryngeal examination revealed an erythematous and swollen epiglottis that was also visible on a lateral soft tissue radiograph of the neck (''thumb sign''). Intravenous amphotericin led to rapid cure.

4. SORE THROAT AND AIRWAY OBSTRUCTION

A. Acute Epiglottitis A severe sore throat (94–100 percent), a rapid onset of dysphagia (100 percent), and fever (74 percent) constitute a common presentation. Pharyngitis may be present in 38 to 53 percent, but the severity of the throat pain exceeds the pharyngeal findings and should direct attention to the supraglottic region. Other findings implicating this region include hoarseness (22 percent), a muffled voice (47 percent), and severe odynophagia. Dyspnea, stridor, aphonia, and cyanosis are late symptoms associated with respiratory obstruction. Indirect laryngoscopy will reveal a red edematous epiglottis and aryepiglottic folds. A soft tissue lateral radiograph of the neck will demonstrate epiglottic edema (''thumb sign'') in 95 percent. Edema of the aryepiglottic folds and arytenoid cartilages (5 percent), as well as the epiglottis, may be seen. An abscess of the epiglottis may form and make its presence known by failure of the epiglottic swelling to recede or by spontaneous release of pus into the pharynx. Swab cultures of the throat and epiglottis are often negative, and the etiologic diagnosis may hinge on a positive blood or abscess culture. In many cases, the pathogen is not identified. In adults, *H. influenzae type b*, *H parainfluenzae*, *Streptococcus pneumoniae*, *S. pyogenes,* and *Staphylococcus aureus* have been isolated from blood cultures. *S. aureus* has been recovered from an epiglottic abscess. Rare abscess isolates include *Klebsiella pneumoniae, Pasteurella multocida*, and *Candida albicans*. High fever and toxicity in association with epiglottitis suggest bacteremia. Airway control with an endotracheal tube or tracheostomy, and administration of intravenous antibiotics will usually result in recovery.

B. Lingual Tonsillar Infection

1. Lingual Tonsillitis Throat pain occurs with or without fever. Odynophagia may be present. The patient may sometimes note a swelling on the back of the tongue. Otalgia may occur. Pharyngeal erythema may be present, and mirror examination may reveal a 2- to 4-cm mass studded with exudate in the region of the lingual tonsil. There is usually a prompt response to antibiotic therapy.

2. Lingual Tonsillar Abscess Progression of infection may lead to abscess formation on the posterior tongue and floor of the mouth. Symptoms include severe throat pain, tongue pain on movement, hoarseness, and difficulty in protruding the tongue. Lingual tonsillar enlargement may lead to upper airway obstruction with dyspnea and stridor. The airway should be secured, the abscess drained, and antibiotics administered.

C. Ludwig's Angina Due to *Hemophilus influenzae* Cellulitis Sore throat, odynophagia, fever, chills, and malaise are the initial complaints. The submental region and the anterior neck become edematous, and the skin assumes a diffuse purple, red, or red-blue hue. The edema has a woody consistency. The floor of the mouth is swollen and indurated, and the tongue elevated. It protrudes between the incisor teeth and cannot be extended further or used to modulate speech. Words become unintelligible, and drooling occurs because of difficulty swallowing. Dyspnea and sometimes stridor and/or noisy breathing occur if the edematous pharyngeal tissues and secretions obstruct the airway. The total leukocyte count may be elevated or decreased, but there is usually a "shift to the left" irrespective of the total count. *H. influenzae* can be grown from the tissue fluids of the neck, obtained by aspiration or surgical incision, the blood, and the throat. The initiating illness may be an acute pharyngotonsillitis or epiglottitis. The airway must be controlled by intubation and intravenous antibiotics administered. An unusual case of Ludwig's angina secondary to group A streptococcal pharyngitis has also been reported. Ludwig's angina usually arises from a dental source, and in such cases sore throat occurs in only 10 percent.

D. Retropharyngeal Abscess Sore throat, dysphagia, fever, chills, sweats, noisy breathing, dyspnea, and stiff neck are common initial complaints. Examination of the throat reveals a unilateral or midline retropharyngeal mass. Widening of the retropharyngeal space can be confirmed with a true lateral radiograph of the neck. Some patients may present with posterior neck and shoulder pain, aggravated by swallowing. Fever may be low-grade or absent. Adults may develop an acute retropharyngeal abscess secondary to endoscopy, repeated suctioning, insertion of a nasogastric tube, a pharyngeal foreign body, endotracheal intubation, trauma, or osteomyelitis of the upper cervical spine. Spread from a lateral pharyngeal space infection may also occur. The latter group of patients may present initially with trismus, fever, swelling and tenderness at the angle of the jaw, and medial bulging of the lateral pharyngeal wall. Transoral or anterior cervical drainage of the abscess and intravenous antibiotic therapy will lead to resolution.

E. Acute Calcific Retropharyngeal Tendinitis This disorder may mimic a retropharyngeal abscess. There is an abrupt onset of pain and stiffness of the posterior neck, sore throat intensified by swallowing, and low-grade fever. Movements of the neck are restricted, and posterior neck tenderness and muscle spasm occur. Pain on swallowing may be referred to the posterior neck. A posterior pharyngeal mass is usually not present on inspection of the throat. A lateral neck radiograph reveals soft tissue swelling in the posterior pharynx down to the C5 level. Amorphous soft tissue calcification is present inferior to C1 and anterior to the body of C2. Leukocytosis and an elevated sedimentation rate may occur. This disorder is caused by a calcific tendinitis of the longus colli muscle at its attachment to the atlas. Indomethacin relieves symptoms within 48 h. Spontaneous resolution occurs without therapy in 2 to 3 weeks. The soft tissue calcification may resorb spontaneously over a period of 1 to 2 months, or it may remain.

F. Coagulopathy-Related Upper Airway Hematoma

1. Warfarin Therapy An acute onset of sore throat, dysphagia, stridor, and dyspnea in a patient on anticoagulant therapy may be caused by a sublingual and/or pharyngeal wall hematoma. Submucosal hemorrhage can be visualized by direct inspection and/or flexible fiberoptic laryngoscopy. Elevation of the tongue and difficulty swallowing lead to drooling. A firm mass may be palpable in the submental region, and ecchymoses may be present on the skin of the neck. Evidence of bleeding at other sites prior to onset may be present (e.g., melena, hematuria, and gingival bleeding). The prothrombin time is usually markedly prolonged (31 s and 86 s in two reported cases). Airway control and correction of the coagulopathy will lead to recovery.

2. Hemophilia Sore throat, dysphagia, dysphonia, dyspnea, and stridor may result from retropharyngeal space bleeding. A lateral neck film will confirm widening of the retropharyngeal soft tissues by a hematoma. Airway control and correction of the coagulopathy are required.

5. THYROIDITIS

A. Suppurative Suppurative thyroiditis begins with fever (92 percent), persistent anterior neck pain (100 percent), and a tender firm mass in the region of one or both thyroid lobes. Pain on swallowing occurs in 91 percent. Redness (80 percent) and sometimes pustule formation occur on the overlying skin. Throat pain occurs in 70 percent. The firm mass may become fluctuant in 1 to 3 weeks. A thyroid scan shows decreased uptake over the affected lobe(s) of the thyroid. Incision and drainage or needle aspiration reveals pus. Common isolates include *S. aureus, S. pyogenes,* and *S. pneumoniae.* There is a good response to drainage and antibiotic therapy.

B. Subacute Granulomatous Fever, chills, sore throat, and anterior neck pain with radiation to one or both ears occur. Pain in the throat and neck may be intensified by swallowing. The pharynx and tonsillar regions appear normal. The thyroid is slightly to moderately enlarged, firm, and tender. Malaise, fatigue, and myalgias in association with fever may mimic a viral pharyngitis. The paratracheal localization of pain and tenderness differentiates thyroiditis from an upper respiratory illness. Symptoms and signs of mild hyperthyroidism may be present during the first month of illness. These include nervousness, tremulousness, palpitations, and heat intolerance. The sedimentation rate is elevated (50–100 mm/h), and radioactive iodine uptake is markedly reduced due to follicular cell damage and suppression of TSH by released thyroid hormone. The initial hyperthyroid phase (e.g., T_4 and T_3 levels are elevated in 50 percent) may be followed by a euthyroid phase and in 25 percent, by a hypothyroid phase. Fine-needle aspiration biopsy reveals granulomatous tissue with giant cells. Symptoms respond dramatically to oral prednisone or salicylates. This disorder may follow an acute infection caused by coxsackie-, mumps, adeno-, measles, influenza, or Epstein-Barr viruses. In most patients, the provoking agent cannot be identified.

6. SPONTANEOUS PNEUMOMEDIASTINUM

This disorder may begin abruptly with sore throat and dysphagia severe enough to limit food intake. Fever does not occur. Anterior neck pain and/or substernal or precordial chest pain may be associated. The chest pain is sharp and sticking, and intensified by inspiration, coughing, swallowing, or lying flat. Dyspnea may be associated. The chest pain may radiate to the back or neck. Signs include subcutaneous emphysema, decreased cardiac dullness, mediastinal crepitation with cardiac contraction (Hamman's sign), and evidence of mediastinal air on a chest radiograph.

Reported causes of pneumomediastinum include bronchial asthma, diabetic hyperpnea, labor, respiratory tract infections, severe cough, emesis, pulmonary function testing, smoking marijuana and ''crack'' cocaine, heroin injection, and inhalation of nitrous oxide. Gas-forming infection in the mediastinum and esophageal and/or bronchial rupture or perforation are other causes. Disruption of the esophagus or bronchus should be excluded, since delay in treatment may lead to mediastinitis.

7. LARYNGOTRACHEAL TRAUMA

Blunt trauma may cause anterior neck pain and tenderness, intensified by neck movement and swallowing. Hoarseness, a muffled voice, or aphonia may be present. Odynophagia may result from movement of fractured laryngeal cartilages during swallowing. Hemoptysis may result from mucosal disruption. Airway obstruction can cause dyspnea; stridor; and, when very severe, cyanosis.

Neck swelling, tenderness, subcutaneous crepitus, voice changes, and loss of the cartilage landmarks (e.g., thyroid and cricoid cartilages) are frequent signs. A cross-table lateral radiograph can evaluate the cervical spine and detect radiographic signs suggestive of laryngeal fracture, including narrowing of the laryngeal air shadow, prevertebral soft tissue widening, emphysema in the soft tissues of the neck, and hyoid bone fracture. Endoscopy and/or a CT scan of the neck will identify laryngeal fractures and submucosal hematomas. Careful monitoring and control of the airway are required. Surgical repair may be necessary.

Causes of blunt laryngotracheal trauma include motor vehicle accidents with impact of the anterior neck against the steering wheel or dashboard, strangulation, fist or baseball impact, and ''clothesline injuries'' suffered by snowmobilers or bikers. Penetrating trauma includes knife, bullet, and fragment wounds.

THROAT PAIN REFERENCES

Agranulocytosis
Derry CL, Schwinghammer TL: Agranulocytosis associated with sulfasalazine. *Drug Intell Clin Pharm* 22:139–142, 1988.
Hou G-L, Tsai C-C: Oral manifestations of agranulocytosis associated with methimazole therapy. *J Periodontol* 59(4):244–248, 1988.

Chronic Fatigue Syndrome
Buchwald D, Goldenberg DL, Sullivan JL, et al: The ''chronic, active Epstein-Barr virus infection'' syndrome and primary fibromyalgia. *Arthritis Rheum* 30(10):1132–1136, 1987.
Buchwald D, Sullivan JL, Komaroff AL: Frequency of ''chronic active Epstein-Barr virus infection'' in a general medical practice. *JAMA* 257:2303–2307, 1987.

Cheney PR, Dorman SE, Bell DS: Interleukin-2 and the chronic fatigue syndrome (letter to editor). *Ann Intern Med* 110(4)321, 1989.
Holmes GP, Kaplan JE, Gantz NM, et al: Chronic fatigue syndrome: A working case definition. *Ann Intern Med* 108:387–389, 1988.
Holmes GP, Kaplan JE, Stewart JA, et al: A cluster of patients with a chronic mononucleosis-like syndrome. *JAMA* 257:2297–2302, 1987.
Komaroff AL: The chronic fatigue syndrome (letter to editor). *Ann Intern Med* 110(5):407, 1989.
Manu P, Lane TJ, Matthews DA: The frequency of chronic fatigue syndrome in patients with symptoms of persistent fatigue. *Ann Intern Med* 109:554–556, 1988.

Epiglottitis

Cole S, Zawin M, Lundberg B, et al: *Candida* epiglottitis in an adult with acute nonlymphocytic leukemia. *Am J Med* 82:662–664, 1987.

Guss DA, Jackson JE: Recurring epiglottitis in an adult. *Ann Emerg Med* 16:441–444, 1987.

Hanna GS: Acute supraglottic laryngitis in adults. *J Laryngol Otol* 100:971–975, 1986.

Muszynski MJ, Marks MI: Epiglottitis, croup, and laryngitis, in Schlossberg D (ed): *Infections of the Head and Neck*. New York, Springer-Verlag, 1987, pp 133–147.

Shih L, Hawkins DB, Stanley RB Jr: Acute epiglottitis in adults: A review of 48 cases. *Ann Otol Rhinol Laryngol* 97(5 part 1):527–529, 1988.

Singer JI, McCabe JB: Epiglottitis at the extremes of age. *Am J Emerg Med* 6:228–231, 1988.

Stanley RE, Liang TS: Acute epiglottitis in adults: The Singapore experience. *J Laryngol Otol* 102:1017–1021, 1988.

Tveteras K, Kristensen S: Acute epiglottitis in adults: Bacteriology and therapeutic principles. *Clin Otolaryngol* 12:337–343, 1987.

Peritonsillar Abscess

Brodsky, L, Sobie SR, Korwin D, et al: A clinical prospective study of peritonsillar abscess in children. *Laryngoscope* 98(7):780–783, 1988.

Pharyngitis—Adenovirus

Turner M, Istre GR, Beauchamp H, et al: Community outbreak of adenovirus type 7a infections associated with a swimming pool. *South Med J* 80(6):712–715, 1987.

Pharyngitis—Acute Necrotizing Ulcerative Gingivitis

Falkler WA Jr, Martin SA, Vincent JW, et al: A clinical, demographic and microbiologic study of ANUG patients in an urban dental school. *J Clin Periodontol* 14:307–314, 1987.

Johnson BD, Engel D: Acute necrotizing ulcerative gingivitis: A review of diagnosis, etiology and treatment. *J Periodontol* 57(3):141–150, 1986.

Melnick SL, Alvarez JO, Navia JM, et al: A case-control study of plasma ascorbate and acute necrotizing ulcerative gingivitis. *J Dent Res* 67(5):855–860, 1988.

Pharyngitis—*Chlamydia*

Grayston JT, Diwan VK, Cooney M, et al. Community- and hospital-acquired pneumonia associated with *Chlamydia* TWAR infection demonstrated serologically. *Arch Intern Med* 149:169–173, 1989.

Grayston JT, Kuo C-C, Wang S-P, et al: A new *Chlamydia psittaci* strain, TWAR, isolated in acute respiratory tract infections. *N Engl J Med* 315:161–168, 1986.

Kleemola M, Saikku P, Visakorpi R, et al: Epidemics of pneumonia caused by TWAR, a new *Chlamydia* organism, in military trainees in Finland. *J Infect Dis* 157(2):230–236, 1988.

Marrie TJ, Grayston JT, Wang S-P, et al: Pneumonia associated with the TWAR strain of *Chlamydia. Ann Intern Med* 106:507–511, 1987.

Ogawa H, Yamazaki Y, Hashiguchi K: Chlamydia trachomatis: A currently recognized pathogen of tonsillitis. *Acta Otolaryngol Suppl (Stockh)* 454:197–201, 1988.

Yung AP, Grayson ML: Psittacosis: A review of 135 cases. *Med J Aust* 148:228–233, 1988.

Pharyngitis—*Corynebacterium*

Green SL, LaPeter KS: Pseudodiphtheritic membranous pharyngitis caused by *Corynebacterium hemolyticum. JAMA* 245(22):2330–2331, 1981.

Greenman JL: *Corynebacterium hemolyticum* and pharyngitis (letter to editor). *Ann Intern Med* 106(4):633, 1987.

MacGregor RR: *Corynebacterium diphtheriae,* in Mandell GL, Douglas RG Jr, Bennett JE (eds): *Principles and Practice of Infectious Diseases,* 3d ed. New York, Churchill Livingstone, 1990, pp 1574–1581.

Miller RA, Brancato F, Holmes KK: *Corynebacterium hemolyticum*

as a cause of pharyngitis and scarlatiniform rash in young adults. *Ann Intern Med* 105:867–872, 1986.

Robinson BE, Murray DL: *Corynebacterium hemolyticum* and pharyngitis. *Ann Intern Med* 106(5):778–779, 1987.

Pharyngitis—EB Virus

Marklund G, Ernberg I, Lundberg C, et al: Differences in EBV-specific antibody patterns at onset of infectious mononucleosis. *Scand J Infect Dis* 18:25–32, 1986.

Marklund G, Lundberg C, Nord CE, et al: Evidence of tinidazole interference in the oropharyngeal inflammatory process during infectious mononucleosis. *Scand J Infect Dis* 18:503–510, 1986.

Sayre MR, Jehle D: Elevated *Toxoplasma* IgG antibody in patients tested for infectious mononucleosis in urban emergency department. *Ann Emerg Med* 18:383–386, 1989.

Pharyngitis—Gonococcal

Fiumara NJ: Pharyngeal infection with *Neisseria gonorrhoeae. Sex Transm Dis* 6(4):264–266, 1979.

Kraus SJ: Incidence and therapy of gonococcal pharyngitis. *Sex Transm Dis* 6(2):143–147, 1979.

Pharyngitis—HIV (Acute)

Denning DW: The neurological features of acute HIV infection. *Biomed Pharmacother* 42:11–14, 1988.

Denning DW, Anderson J, Rudge P, et al: Acute myelopathy associated with primary infection with human immunodeficiency virus. *Br Med J [Clin Res]* 294(6565):143–144, 1987.

Gaines H, von Sydow M, Pehrson PO, et al: Clinical picture of primary HIV infection presenting as a glandular-fever-like illness. *Br Med J [Clin Res]* 297 (6660):1363–1368, 1988.

Rustin MHA, Ridley CM, Smith MD, et al: The acute exanthem associated with seroconversion to human T-cell lymphotropic virus III in a homosexual man. *J Infect* 12:161–163, 1986.

Tindall B, Barker S, Donovan B, et al: Characterization of the acute clinical illness associated with human immunodeficiency virus infection. *Arch Intern Med* 148:945–949, 1988.

Valle S-L: Febrile pharyngitis as the primary sign of HIV infection in a cluster of cases linked by sexual contact. *Scand J Infect Dis* 19:13–17, 1987.

Pharyngitis—Rare Causes

Bassiouny A, El-Refai A, Nabi EAA, et al: *Candida* infection in the tongue and pharynx. *J Laryngol Otol* 98:609–611, 1984.

Doğanay M, Almac A, Hanağasi R: Primary throat anthrax: A report of six cases. *Scand J Infect Dis* 18:415–419, 1986.

Everett ED, Templer JW: Oropharyngeal tularemia. *Arch Otolaryngol* 106:237–238, 1980.

Morgan MC, Rice LI: Recurrent group C streptococcal tonsillopharyngitis in an adolescent. *J Adolesc Health Care* 10:421–422, 1989.

Rose FB, Camp CJ, Antes EJ: Family outbreak of fatal *Yersinia enterocolitica. Am J Med* 82:636–637, 1987.

Sureau PH: Firsthand clinical observations of hemorrhagic manifestations in Ebola hemorrhagic fever in Zaire. *Rev Infect Dis* 11(suppl 4):S790–S793, 1989.

Tacket CO, Davis BR, Carter GP, et al: *Yersinia enterocolitica* pharyngitis. *Ann Intern Med* 99:40–42, 1983.

Pharyngitis—Review Articles

Centor RM: Strategies for treating sore throat in adults. *J Fam Pract* 25(4):335–336, 1987.

Centor RM, Meier FA, Dalton HP: Throat cultures and rapid tests for diagnosis of group A streptococcal pharyngitis. *Ann Intern Med* 105:892–899, 1986.

Glezen WP, Clyde WA Jr, Senior RJ, et al: Group A streptococci, mycoplasmas, and viruses associated with acute pharyngitis. *JAMA* 202(6):119–124, 1967.

Gwaltney JM Jr: Acute laryngitis, in Mandell GL, Douglas RG Jr, Bennett JE (eds): *Principles and Practice of Infectious Diseases,* 3d ed. New York, Churchill Livingstone, 1990, p 499.

Gwaltney JM Jr: Pharyngitis, in Mandell GL, Douglas RG Jr, Bennett

JE (eds): *Principles and Practice of Infectious Diseases,* 3d ed. New York, Churchill Livingstone, 1990, pp 493–498.

Huovinen P, Lahtonen R, Ziegler T, et al: Pharyngitis in adults: The presence and coexistence of viruses and bacterial organisms. *Ann Intern Med* 110:612–616, 1989.

McMillan JA, Sandstrom C, Weiner LB, et al: Viral and bacterial organisms associated with acute pharyngitis in a school-aged population. *J Pediatr* 109:747–752, 1986.

Murtagh J, Newton-John H: The sore throat. *Aust Fam Physician* 15(12):1604–1605, 1986.

Ogino S, Notake N, Harada T, et al: Long-term observation of postoperative course of habitual tonsillitis. *Acta Otolaryngol Suppl (Stockh)* 454:299–304, 1988.

Talukder MAS: Prevalence of pathogenic bacteria in patients with sore throat. *Trop Geogr Med* 38:55–57, 1986.

Telian SA: Sore throat and antibiotics. *Otolaryngol Clin North Am* 19(1):103–109, 1986.

Todd JK: The sore throat: Pharyngitis and epiglottitis. *Infect Dis Clin North Am* 2(1):149–162, 1988.

Yoshida A, Okamoto K: Indication of tonsillectomy for recurrent tonsillitis. *Acta Otolaryngol Suppl (Stockh)* 454:305–312, 1988.

Pharyngitis—Streptococcal

Bismo AL: Streptococcal pharyngitis, in Mandell GL, Douglas RG Jr, Bennett JE (eds): *Principles and Practice of Infectious Diseases,* 3d ed. New York, Churchill Livingstone, 1990, pp 1521–1525.

Breese BB, Disney FA: The accuracy of diagnosis of beta streptococcal infections on clinical grounds. *J Pediatr* 44:670–673, 1954.

Caraco J, Arnon R, Raz I: Atrioventricular block complicating acute streptococcal tonsillitis. *Br Heart J* 59:389–390, 1988.

Cebul RD, Poses RM: The comparative cost-effectiveness of statistical decision rules and experienced physicians in pharyngitis management. *JAMA* 256:3353–3357, 1986.

Centor RM, Dalton HP, Campbell MS, et al: Rapid diagnosis of streptococcal pharyngitis in adult emergency room patients. *J Gen Intern Med* 1:248–251, 1986.

Clancy CM, Centor RM, Campbell MS, et al: Rational decision making based on history: Adult sore throats. *J Gen Intern Med* 3:213–217, 1988.

Crawford G, Brancato F, Holmes KK: Streptococcal pharyngitis: Diagnosed by Gram stain. *Ann Intern Med* 90(3):293–297, 1979.

Dans PE: The management of sore throat: Adjusting to success. *JAMA* 256(24):3392–3393, 1986.

DeNeef P: Selective testing for streptococcal pharyngitis in adults. *J Fam Pract* 25(4):347–353, 1987.

DuBois D, Ray VG, Nelson B, et al: Rapid diagnosis of group A strep pharyngitis in the emergency department. *Ann Emerg Med* 15:157–159, 1986.

Evans AS, Dick EC: Acute pharyngitis and tonsillitis in University of Wisconsin students. *JAMA* 190(8):699–708, 1964.

Fischer PM: Rapid testing for streptococcal pharyngitis. *Prim Care* 13(4):657–665, 1986.

Hedges JR, Lowe RA: Sore throat: To culture or not to culture. *Ann Emerg Med* 15:312–316, 1986.

Herz MJ: Antibiotics and the adult sore throat: An unnecessary ceremony. *Fam Pract* 5(3):196–199, 1988.

Hoffman S: Incidence and management of sore throat in general practice. *Scand J Prim Health Care* 4:143–150, 1986.

Huck W, Reed BD, French T, et al: Comparison of the Directigen 1-2-3 group A strep test with culture for detection of group A beta-hemolytic streptococci. *J Clin Microbiol* 27(8):1715–1718, 1989.

Hutten-Czapski P: Management of streptococcal pharyngitis: The conundrum of acute rheumatic fever. *Fam Pract* 5(3):200–208, 1988.

Lichter H, Ente G, Penzer P, et al: Rapid symptomatic relief of streptococcal pharyngitis in children. *Clin Ther* 8(6):658–666, 1986.

Pichichero ME, Disney FA, Talpey WB, et al: Adverse and beneficial effects of immediate treatment of group A beta-hemolytic streptococcal pharyngitis with penicillin. *Pediatr Infect Dis J* 6:635–643, 1987.

Pitts J, Vincent SH: Diagnostic labels, treatment and outcome in acute sore throat. *Practitioner* 232:343–346, 1988.

Walsh BT, Bookhcim WW, Johnson RC, et al: Recognition of streptococcal pharyngitis in adults. *Arch Intern Med* 135:1493–1497, 1975.

Pharyngitis—Streptococcal Group G

Cohen D, Ferne M, Rouach T, et al: Food-borne outbreak of group G streptococcal sore throat in an Israeli military base. *Epidemiol Infect* 99:249–255, 1987.

Pharyngotonsillitis

Brook I: Pharyngotonsillitis, in Schlossberg D (ed): *Infections of the Head and Neck.* New York, Springer-Verlag, 1987, pp 121–132.

Postanginal Sepsis—Lemierre's Disease

Moreno S, Altozano JG, Pinilla B, et al: Lemierre's disease: Postanginal bacteremia and pulmonary involvement caused by *Fusobacterium necrophorum. Rev Infect Dis* 11(2):319–324, 1989.

Sinnott JT IV, Weedon C, Schwartz M, et al: Postanginal sepsis: A pain in the neck. *Postgrad Med* 86(2):77–78, 81–82, 1989.

Sore Throat—Noninfectious

Benanti JC, Gramling P, Bulat PI, et al: Retropharyngeal calcific tendinitis: Report of five cases and review of the literature. *J Emerg Med* 4:15–24, 1986.

Bicknell JM, Kirsch WM, Seigel R, et al: Atlanto-axial dislocation in acute rheumatic fever: Case report. *J Neurosurg* 66:286–289, 1987.

Bouvet J-P, le Parc J-M, Michalski, B, et al: Acute neck pain due to calcifications surrounding the odontoid process: The crowned dens syndrome. *Arthritis Rheum* 28(12):1417–1420, 1985.

Bray G, Nugent D: Hemorrhage involving the upper airway in hemophilia. *Clin Pediatr* 25(9):436–439, 1986.

Cohen AF, Warman SP: Upper airway obstruction secondary to warfarin-induced sublingual hematoma. *Arch Otolaryngol Head Neck Surg* 115:718–720, 1989.

Pearlman NW, Stiegmann GV, Teter A: Primary upper aerodigestive tract manifestations of gastroesophageal reflux. *Am J Gastroenterol* 83(1):22–25, 1988.

Sarkozi J, Fam AG: Acute calcific retropharyngeal tendinitis: An unusual cause of neck pain. *Arthritis Rheum* 27(6):708–710, 1984.

Tonsillitis—Lingual

Puar RK, Puar HS: Lingual tonsillitis. *South Med J* 79(9):1126–1128, 1986.

PART THREE
Acute Neck Pain

Acute Anterior Neck Pain

☐ DIAGNOSTIC LIST

1. Thyroid gland
   A. Acute suppurative thyroiditis and/or abscess
   B. Subacute thyroiditis (de Quervain's thyroiditis)
   C. Hashimoto's thyroiditis
   D. Riedel's struma
   E. Hemorrhage into a thyroid nodule
   F. Thyroid malignancy
      1. Lymphoma
      2. Anaplastic carcinoma
   G. Secondary amyloidosis with a subacute thyroiditis-like syndrome (STLS)
2. Parathyroid gland—hemorrhage into an adenoma
3. Cervical lymphadenitis
4. Anterior triangle abscess
   A. Infection of a congenital cyst
   B. Infection unrelated to preexisting cysts
5. Carotodynia
   A. Migraine
   B. Eagle's syndrome (stylohyoid syndrome)

C. Hyoid bone syndrome
D. Myofascial pain disorder involving the digastric and stylohyoid muscles (pseudo-sternocleidomastoid pain)
E. Dental abscess
F. Posttraumatic dysautonomic cephalgia
6. Internal carotid artery dissection
7. Ludwig's angina
8. Trauma
   A. Blunt laryngotracheal trauma
   B. Anterior whiplash injury
9. Esophagus
   A. Pharyngoesophageal diverticulum and diverticulitis
   B. Carcinoma of the esophagus
10. Referred pain
    A. Cardiac and aortic
       1. Myocardial infarction or coronary insufficiency
       2. Acute pericarditis
       3. Dissecting aneurysm of the thoracic aorta
    B. Spontaneous pneumomediastinum

☐ SUMMARY

Suppurative thyroiditis causes aching or throbbing anterior neck pain and asymmetric firm or fluctuant tender thyroid enlargement, with overlying skin erythema, tenderness, and skin pustules. Fever, leukocytosis, and a low radioactive iodine uptake are associated findings. A CT scan can visualize a thyroid abscess. Transient mild hyperthyroidism may occasionally (2.5 percent of cases) be associated because of hormone release from disrupted follicles, but euthyroid serum levels are the rule.

Subacute thyroiditis (*de Quervain's thyroiditis*) causes unilateral or bilateral paratracheal pain, swelling, and tenderness. Pain may radiate cephalad to one or both ears. Sweating, nervousness, and palpitations (i.e., symptoms of hyperthyroidism) occur in approximately 50 percent of cases, and hyperthyroid serum hormone levels are present in 60 percent. Fever, leukocytosis, and an elevated sedimentation rate may occur. The radioactive iodine uptake is markedly depressed in most cases. Sonographic or CT scans show no evidence of a thyroid abscess. Thyroid fluctuance and skin erythema do not occur in subacute thyroiditis. The diagnosis can be confirmed by a needle biopsy. Prednisone dramatically suppresses pain, tenderness, and thyroid enlargement.

Some cases of *Hashimoto's thyroiditis* may cause a bilateral painful, tender thyroid swelling, but the vast majority of cases are not associated with pain. High titers of antithyroid antibodies are usually present (i.e., antimicrosomal and antithyroglobulin), and hyperthyroidism is uncommon. Salicylate and thyroxin administration control symptoms and may decrease the size of the goiter. Prednisone has not been effective.

Riedel's struma causes a woody, hard thyroid enlargement. A small number of patients have pain or pressure symptoms. Riedel's struma is very rare. Unilateral pain and tenderness may be secondary to *hemorrhage into a thyroid nodule*. Ultrasound and radioactive iodine scans can determine whether the nodule is cystic or solid, and functional or cold. Needle aspiration can be used to confirm hemorrhage and diagnose malignancy.

Rapidly growing *malignancies of the thyroid,* such as *lymphomas* or *anaplastic carcinomas,* may cause massive nodular enlargement of the thyroid, with associated anterior neck pain and tenderness. Biopsy will establish the diagnosis. *Secondary amyloidosis* of the thyroid may mimic subacute thyroiditis, with neck pain, swelling, and tenderness. It can be differentiated from subacute thyroiditis by recurrence of pain and tenderness at the same site in the gland; the presence of associated renal, bowel, and cardiac disease; and biopsy evidence of amyloid in the thyroid and at other sites (i.e., kidney, bowel wall, and skin).

Rarely, *hemorrhage in a parathyroid adenoma* may cause unilateral neck pain, swelling, and tenderness and abnormal serum calcium levels.

Cervical lymphadenitis causes pain and enlarged, tender lymph nodes. The primary site of infection may be the mouth, pharynx, tonsils, teeth, or skin of the face or head. There is a good response to antibiotic therapy. An *abscess in the anterior triangle* of the neck forms a unilateral firm or fluctuant tender mass, which may cause anterior neck pain. Such abscesses may form *in a preexisting congenital cyst* or arise *from suppurating lymph nodes, adjacent structures, or deep fascial space infections*. Lateral-space infections may cause trismus and dysphagia. A CT scan or MRI demonstrate the presence and extent of neck abscesses.

Carotodynia (a painful, tender carotid artery) can be a result of *migraine,* an *elongated styloid process,* an *elongated greater horn of the hyoid,* a *digastric-stylohyoid muscle myofascial syndrome,* a *dental abscess,* or an *internal carotid artery dissection. Dysautonomic cephalgia* follows anterior neck trauma. Neck pain, tenderness, and a unilateral headache are associated with ipsilateral facial sweating and pupillary dilatation, and can be prevented by the use of propranolol.

Internal carotid artery dissection causes anterior neck pain (19 percent of cases); a frontal, temporal, or orbital headache; and, sometimes, face pain. Oculosympathetic paralysis may accompany the neck and head pain. Ptosis, miosis, and visual blurring without loss of facial sweating (partial Horner's syndrome) occurs. Within minutes to hours of the onset of pain, up to 67 percent of patients may experience transient (40 percent) or sustained (42 percent) focal neurologic deficits (e.g., hemiparesis, hemihypesthesia, aphasia, and monocular visual loss). Recovery of function, arterial luminal patency, and flow occurs in up to 85 percent of cases treated with anticoagulants, antiplatelet drugs, and/or surgical therapy, or with only supportive care.

Ludwig's angina begins with dental-related mouth pain and progresses to cause upper anterior neck pain and woody swelling. The floor of the mouth and the tongue become swollen and indurated, and the tongue protrudes from the mouth. The patient drools saliva, and speech is impaired, as are swallowing and breathing. Fever, chills, and a toxic appearance are associated findings. A CT scan will localize purulent collections in the submandibular and sublingual spaces. Trismus may occur, secondary to spread of infection into a lateral pharyngeal space. There is complete resolution with antibiotic therapy, surgical drainage of purulent collections, and airway maintenance by intubation or tracheostomy.

Blunt laryngotracheal trauma may cause anterior neck pain, voice changes, dysphagia, hemoptysis, dyspnea, and stridor. Neck swelling, tenderness, skin and cartilaginous crepitus, loss of structural landmarks, and a hoarse or mumbling voice are signs associated with fracture of the thyroid cartilage.

The diagnosis of laryngeal fracture, with submucosal edema and hematoma obstructing the glottis or subglottis, can be made by a CT scan or by direct laryngoscopy. A *whiplash-type injury* can cause both posterior and anterior neck muscle pain and tenderness. The strap muscle pain can be intensified by extension of the neck.

An *esophageal diverticulum* may present with dysphagia, a reducible neck mass, gurgling neck sounds on swallowing, regurgitation of food, and coughing. Diverticulitis or leakage from the diverticulum can cause severe neck pain and tender-

TABLE OF DISEASE INCIDENCE

INCIDENCE PER 100,000 (APPROXIMATE)

Common (>100)	Uncommon (>5–100)	Rare (>0–5)
Cervical lymphadenitis	Subacute thyroiditis	Suppurative thyroiditis and abscess
Anterior whiplash injury	Hemorrhage into a thyroid nodule	Painful Hashimoto's thyroiditis
Myocardial infarction and/or coronary insufficiency	Carotodynia due to migraine	Riedel's struma
	Acute pericarditis	Lymphoma of the thyroid
		Anaplastic carcinoma of the thyroid
		Secondary amyloidosis with STLS
		Hemorrhage into a parathyroid adenoma
		Anterior triangle abscess due to preexisting cysts, infected lymph nodes, or deep-space infection
		Carotodynia due to Eagle's syndrome, hyoid bone syndrome, or dental disease
		Carotodynia due to a myofascial disorder or dysautonomic cephalgia
		Internal carotid artery dissection
		Blunt laryngotracheal trauma
		Ludwig's angina
		Esophageal diverticulum with perforation
		Esophageal carcinoma with perforation
		Dissecting aneurysm of the thoracic aorta
		Spontaneous pneumomediastinum

ness, intensified by swallowing and neck movements. Similarly, an *esophageal carcinoma* may perforate, initiating a deep neck space infection.

Myocardial infarction or coronary insufficiency may cause anterior chest, arm, and anterior neck pain. Thrombolytic agents or direct angioplasty may relieve the pain. An electrocardiogram will reveal evidence of infarction or ischemia, and the presence of the former can be confirmed by serum isozyme levels (i.e., LDH_1 and CPK-MB).

Pericarditis causes neck pain or neck and chest pain, made worse by inspiration or lying down and alleviated by sitting up or standing. The pain is sharp and stabbing, and associated with a pericardial rub and/or ST elevation in all leads except AVR and V_1. Characteristic T-wave flattening or inversion follows the return of the ST segment to the baseline during the first week of illness.

Dissecting aneurysm of the thoracic aorta causes tearing or ripping sequential anterior chest, neck, interscapular, and abdominal pain. The discomfort may be so severe that patients writhe in pain. Physical examination may reveal one or more absent extremity pulses, an aortic diastolic murmur, and gallop sounds. The mediastinum is widened on a plain chest radiograph, and the diagnosis can be confirmed by a CT scan with contrast or an aortogram.

Spontaneous pneumomediastinum causes the abrupt onset of anterior neck and throat pain, dysphagia, and/or anterior chest pain. Subcutaneous crepitus occurs in the neck and upper chest. A mediastinal crunch sound (Hamman's sign) may be heard with each heartbeat. The diagnosis can be confirmed by demonstration of mediastinal air on a plain chest radiograph. Some cases have been associated with "crack" cocaine smoking.

☐ DESCRIPTION OF LISTED DISEASES

1. THYROID GLAND

A. Acute Suppurative Thyroiditis and/or Abscess
Anterior neck pain (100 percent of cases), thyroid swelling (100 percent), tenderness (94 percent), fever (92 percent), and dysphagia (91 percent) are the major presenting complaints of a bacterial infection of the thyroid gland. Initially, the thyroid enlargement may be firm, but fluctuance, skin erythema, and/or skin pustules develop within 1 to 3 weeks. Leukocytosis (57 percent), an elevated sedimentation rate (100 percent), and a low radioactive iodine uptake (92 percent) are common associated findings. Transient hyperthyroidism or hypothyroidism may occur in 2.5 percent of cases. The abscess may be visualized by an ultrasound, a CT, or an [111]indium leukocyte scan, and confirmed by needle aspiration of infected purulent material. This disorder responds to intravenous antibiotics but may require surgical incision and drainage. The gland may be asymmetrically involved. In patients with a fistulous connection between a pyriform sinus and the thyroid, the involvement is almost always left-sided. Cases of suppurative thyroiditis have arisen from hematogenous (e.g., urinary tract) or lymphatic spread, from direct penetrating wounds, or from an infected thyroglossal duct cyst. The commonest infecting organisms are gram-positive cocci (*Staphylococcus aureus, Streptococcus pyogenes, Staphylococcus epidermidis,* or *Streptococcus pneumoniae*), but *Escherichia coli*

and other gram-negative bacteria and anaerobes may also be isolated. Cases involving the left lobe in young children or adolescents are frequently caused by a pyriform sinus thyroid fistulous tract (demonstrable by a barium swallow). Such infections tend to be polymicrobial and recurrent, and require total excision of the tract to prevent recurrence. Fever, skin erythema, leukocytosis, and fluctuance of a thyroid swelling favor a diagnosis of suppurative thyroiditis.

B. Subacute Thyroiditis (de Quervain's Thyroiditis)
Aching paratracheal neck pain that radiates cephalad toward one or both ears is associated with slight to moderate thyroid enlargement and tenderness. The thyroid swelling may sometimes be asymmetrical. There may be a sensation of a sore throat, with pain on swallowing. Severe cases have been associated with fever, chills, and marked thyroid swelling and tenderness, mimicking suppurative disease, but such presentations are uncommon.

Many cases begin with a prodromal influenza-like illness, with headache, myalgias, malaise, anorexia, nausea, and weight loss. During the first month after onset, transient hyperthyroidism may occur, secondary to follicle disruption by the inflammatory process and the release of thyroid hormone into the circulation. Palpitations, weight loss, nervousness, and sweating are associated with an elevated T_4 level and a high T_4/T_3 ratio. Radioactive iodine uptake is suppressed, in contrast to the high uptake seen in Graves' disease. An elevated leukocyte count and sedimentation rate are common. Gallium scans show increased thyroid uptake, secondary to the inflammatory process. Ultrasound studies show a homogeneous low echogenic pattern and no evidence of an abscess.

Fine-needle aspiration biopsy will show histocytes and distinctive foreign-body giant cells. Low titers of antithyroglobulin and antimicrosomal antibodies are present transiently.

This disorder may be self-limited and subside within 6 to 8 weeks, but recurrent attacks may occur for months in some patients. Viral agents such as Coxsackie virus, mumps, measles, influenza, adenovirus, and Epstein-Barr virus have been associated with this disorder, but no definite etiology has been established. Symptoms such as malaise, fever, and neck pain and swelling may be controlled or dramatically improved by salicylates or prednisone. Women in the 40- to 60-year age group are most commonly affected, and up to 71 percent of cases occur in the summer or autumn.

C. Hashimoto's Thyroiditis This disorder is usually painless, and the associated enlargement of the thyroid is nontender. A series of eight unusual patients who presented with anterior neck pain; a diffuse, tender goiter (seven cases); and pain, tenderness, and enlargement limited to one lobe (one case) has been reported. These patients had a normal sedimentation rate, a normal ^{131}I up-

take, and very high titers of antithyroid antibodies. Thyroid biopsies revealed diffuse lymphocytic infiltration, germinal centers, fibrosis, Hürthle cell change of follicular epithelial cells, follicle destruction, and an absence of granulomas and giant cells. Administration of thyroid hormone resulted in a decrease in goiter size and relief of pain in some, but not all, cases. Prednisone tended to be ineffective, while high doses of salicylates provided symptomatic relief. Patients with this disorder are at risk for developing permanent hypothyroidism.

High titers of antithyroid antibodies are an essential part of the diagnosis of Hashimoto's thyroiditis. Antibody to thyroglobulin occurs in 55 percent of cases, antimicrosomal antibody in 90 percent, and thyrotropin receptor antibody (TRAb) in 10 to 30 percent or 40 to 50 percent, depending on the assay method utilized. Aspiration biopsy is helpful in situations where the onset is acute, with a tender, swollen thyroid, and differentiation from subacute thyroiditis is required. A case of Graves' disease and Hashimoto's thyroiditis has been reported that presented with neck pain and tenderness and an elevated radioactive iodine uptake.

D. Riedel's Struma Rarely, this disorder may present acutely with anterior neck pain or pressure and symptoms of tracheal compression. It may be diffuse or unilateral. Fibrotic involvement of the recurrent laryngeal nerve may lead to hoarseness. The thyroid is usually stone hard and diffusely enlarged. Hypothyroidism frequently occurs, and radioactive iodine uptake is decreased. Antithyroid antibodies occur in only low titer and are often absent. This disorder is very rare and can be mimicked by a diffusely infiltrating carcinoma.

E. Hemorrhage into a Thyroid Nodule Acute unilateral neck pain and swelling can occur because of bleeding into a thyroid cyst, adenoma, or carcinoma. An ultrasound study can differentiate a cyst from a solid mass. An ^{131}I scan can determine whether it is functional or cold. Fine-needle aspiration is helpful in differentiating adenoma from carcinoma and in confirming the presence of hemorrhage into a cyst or tumor.

F. Thyroid Malignancy Follicular and papillary carcinomas of the thyroid are usually painless and nontender.

1. Lymphoma This rapidly growing tumor is more likely to arise in a gland involved with Hashimoto's thyroiditis. It is associated with diffuse anterior neck swelling, pain, and tenderness. It usually occurs in adults over age 50, but patients in their twenties and thirties have been reported. The diagnosis can be confirmed by needle biopsy.

2. Anaplastic Carcinoma This thyroid malignancy may form a painful, tender paratracheal neck mass. Necrosis and hemorrhage or rapid growth may cause pain and tenderness, and the diagnosis can be confirmed by needle biopsy. Metastatic carcinoma to the thyroid can also cause a painful, tender nodule, and perforation of an esophageal carcinoma has resulted in acute suppurative thyroiditis.

G. Secondary Amyloidosis with a Subacute Thyroiditis-Like Syndrome (STLS) Secondary amyloidosis has been associated with fever, anterior neck pain, tenderness, swelling of the thyroid (an elastic, firm, diffuse, tender goiter), and a low radioactive iodine uptake. This disorder may be associated with renal failure and the nephrotic syndrome. Biopsy evidence of thyroiditis is absent, and the thyroid is infiltrated with amyloid. The thyroid-related pain and tenderness are not related to an inflammatory infiltration of the gland.

2. PARATHYROID GLAND—HEMORRHAGE INTO AN ADENOMA

Spontaneous hemorrhage into a parathyroid adenoma presents with unilateral anterior neck pain, diffuse neck swelling, and tenderness. Compression symptoms related to the trachea can cause progressive dyspnea, hoarseness (recurrent laryngeal nerve compression), dysphagia, and neck vein distension. Skin ecchymoses in the anterior neck and upper chest may occur. Hypercalcemia or hypocalcemia may follow such an event. Ultrasound studies cannot differentiate hemorrhage into a thyroid cyst from bleeding into a parathyroid adenoma. Bleeding into thyroid cysts tends to remain confined to the capsule, does not cause skin ecchymoses, and does not affect the serum calcium level. A CT or MRI study of the neck will demonstrate the hematoma and any mediastinal extension. Surgery is required for compression symptoms and to control hyperparathyroidism.

3. CERVICAL LYMPHADENITIS

Unilateral or bilateral enlargement and tenderness of anterior cervical lymph nodes may be associated with aching anterior neck pain along the medial border of the sternocleidomastoid muscle from its midportion to the angle of the jaw. Fever, sore throat, and painful swallowing are associated symptoms when the cause is a pharyngitis and/or tonsillitis. Dental disease, an oral ulcer, or a skin infection of the face or scalp may also be a primary site of infection. The nodes vary in size from 1 to 6 cm and rarely may become fluctuant and discharge spontaneously through the skin. The usual isolates in throat infections include *Staphylococcus aureus* and *Streptococcus pyogenes*. Dental infections are commonly polymicrobial and are associated with anaerobic organisms, gram-negative bacteria, and streptococci. Skin infections with *S. aureus*

or *S. pyogenes* may cause cutaneous abscesses or impetiginous lesions. Painful, enlarged, tender nodes usually resolve on antibiotic therapy. Rare but important causes of painful lymphadenopathy in the neck include tularemia, bubonic plague, actinomycosis, herpes simplex, tuberculosis, and toxoplasmosis. The nodes associated with Epstein-Barr virus, human immunodeficiency virus (HIV), cytomegalovirus (CMV), and cat-scratch disease infections are usually not painful and are seldom tender.

4. ANTERIOR TRIANGLE ABSCESS

A. Abscesses Associated with Congenital Cysts Branchial cleft cyst abscesses cause pain and tender swelling anterior and medial to the anterior border of the sternocleidomastoid. These abscesses can be visualized by a CT scan or MRI, drained, and excised under cover of parenteral antibiotics. Similarly, a cervical bronchogenic cyst can become infected, producing an anterior triangle neck abscess.

Infection has also been associated with thyroglossal duct cysts, dermoids, and laryngoceles. Midline abscesses may arise from these congenital lesions. Such abscesses are painful, tender, fluctuant, and often associated with skin erythema. Thyroglossal duct cysts retain an attachment to the tongue and move upward in the neck when the tongue is protruded. Dermoids, thyroglossal duct cysts, bronchogenic cysts, and laryngoceles may occur as asymptomatic midline neck masses when not infected.

B. Abscesses Unrelated to Preexisting Cysts Abscesses may form in the anterior triangle secondary to bacterial lymphadenitis. A painful, tender mass, sometimes associated with erythema and tenderness of the overlying skin, appears medial to the anterior border of a sternocleidomastoid muscle. The abscess arises from suppuration of one or more nodes. The nodal infection may be secondary to oral, tonsillar, pharyngeal, dental, or facial skin infection. Infection of a deep neck space may also arise from suppuration in the parotid gland, mastoid process, teeth, tonsils, or an adjacent deep fascial space. The pain produced by the abscess may be mild to moderate in severity, deep and aching, and occasionally throbbing. Fever, chills, trismus, dysphagia, malaise, and weight loss may be associated. The mass may initially be firm and indurated, but over a period of days it usually becomes fluctuant. A CT scan with contrast injection or MRI will demonstrate overlying skin edema and will delineate the extent of an abscess in the lateral pharyngeal, pretracheal, submandicular, or other deep space. Fever, toxicity, pain, and swelling respond to open or catheter drainage and antibiotic therapy.

Methylphenidate (Ritalin) abuse has been associated with deep neck abscesses resulting from the use of the internal jugular vein for injection of nonsterile methylphenidate prepared from tablets. *Eikenella corrodens* and streptococci have frequently been isolated from such abscesses.

5. CAROTODYNIA (PAIN AND TENDERNESS IN THE VICINITY OF THE CAROTID SHEATH)

A. Migraine   Pain in the anterior neck medial to the sternocleidomastoid and associated with tenderness of the common and internal carotid artery has been considered to be a manifestation of migraine. Neck, face, and head pain may occur in association with nausea, vomiting, visual symptoms, and facial paresthesias. There may be a response to drugs effective in the management of migraine, such as propranolol or calcium channel blockers.

B. Eagle's Syndrome (Stylohyoid Syndrome)   Cases follow tonsillectomy, causing fibrosis in the vicinity of an elongated styloid process. Pain occurs in the upper neck near the angle(s) of the jaw. It may also involve the side of the face, ears, throat, sternocleidomastoid, and temporal region. Pain intensification may follow swallowing or talking.

Another presentation of this disorder is related to styloid impingement on the carotid vessels, resulting in anteromedial neck pain and tenderness, increased by turning the head. The diagnosis is confirmed clinically by transpharyngeal examination of the tonsillar fossa. This will provoke characteristic pain when the bony styloid process is palpated through the lateral pharyngeal wall. Surgical shortening or removal of the abnormally long or misdirected styloid relieves the pain and dysphagia.

C. Hyoid Bone Syndrome   Pain occurs over one or both carotid areas in the upper anterior neck. It is referred to the ipsilateral ear; sternocleidomastoid, temporal, or supraclavicular areas; and throat. It may be a dull ache or sharp and stabbing. The pain is provoked by swallowing or bending the head toward the painful side. The latter positional change may be accompanied by lightheadedness. Palpation of the hyoid bone and rocking it from side to side lead to reproduction of the patient's neck pain or produce a foreign-body sensation in the neck. A local injection of lidocaine at the tip of the greater horn of the hyoid relieves all symptoms. Eighty percent of patients with this disorder respond within 1 week to a nonsteroidal anti-inflammatory drug (sulindac). Those failing medical therapy may be relieved by excision of the greater horn of the hyoid.

D. Myofascial (Pseudo-sternocleidomastoid) Pain Involving the Digastric (Posterior Belly) and Stylohyoid Muscles   Pain radiates to the upper sternocleidomastoid, the anterior neck below the chin, and the occipital area on palpation of trigger points in the posterior belly

of the digastric or in the adjacent stylohyoid muscle. Pain related to digastric muscle trigger points is unmasked by anesthetic injection of sternocleiodomastoid trigger points. Digastric trigger points may be activated by bruxism, mouth-breathing, or retrusion of the mandible. An elongated styloid syndrome, as described above, may also activate digastric trigger points. Vapocoolant spray and stretch or trigger point injections of the digastric/stylohyoid muscles provide pain relief. This myofascial syndrome involves the same group of structures that have been associated with the stylohyoid and hyoid bone syndromes.

E. Dental Disease   A single case report of acute carotodynia related to a first molar dental abscess has been reported. Pain began abruptly deep beneath the clavicular insertion of the sternocleidomastoid muscle and radiated up the neck to the angle of the jaw. The initial excruciating pain lasted only minutes and was replaced by a dull ache. Tearing, lancinating, severe paroxysms of pain continued at irregular intervals. There was carotid tenderness above the anterior margin of the sternocleidomastoid. Following spontaneous rupture of the dental abscess, the pain immediately resolved. This disorder may also be mistaken for carotid artery dissection.

F. Posttraumatic Dysautonomic Cephalgia   Injury to the anterior neck may result in unilateral or bilateral aching neck pain and associated tenderness over the carotid sheath. After several weeks, attacks of severe unilateral headache occur in association with facial hyperhidrosis and mydriasis on the painful side. The pain lasts 8 to 16 h and spontaneously resolves. Following the headache, mild ptosis and miosis affect the eye on the painful side. Several such attacks may occur each month, and these can be prevented by administration of propranolol.

6. INTERNAL CAROTID ARTERY DISSECTION

Unilateral anterior neck pain and headache begin abruptly. The headache may be retro-orbital, orbital, frontal, temporal, or in the area of the ear and mastoid process. It is frequently dull, aching, and steady, but it may be throbbing. The neck pain (which occurs in up to 19 percent of cases) is localized to the upper anterior neck and may involve the mastoid region, angle of jaw, and sternocleidomastoid muscle. The face pain involves the cheek and eye. Ipsilateral ptosis, miosis, and visual blurring indicate the presence of interruption of the oculosympathetic pathway (Horner's syndrome). The Horner's syndrome is usually partial, with sparing of the external carotid sympathetic plexus vasomotor and sudomotor nerve fiber innervation of the face.

Focal neurologic abnormalities of a persistent (42 percent of cases) or transient (46 percent) nature or both (12 percent) may follow the onset of neck, face, and head pain within minutes or hours in up to 67 percent of cases. These abnormalities include contralateral hemiparesis or hemiplegia, and/or partial or complete hemisensory loss, aphasia, amaurosis fugax, ipsilateral blindness, and abducens paralysis with diplopia. Photophobia and scintillations may also occur. Subjective and/or objective bruits may accompany the other symptoms and signs. Bilateral neck pain and headache may be due to dissection of both carotids. Risk factors for dissection include hypertension (47 percent of cases), smoking (47 percent), and arterial fibromuscular dysplasia (14 percent). Other associations include Marfan's syndrome, syphilis, and cystic medial necrosis.

Rare manifestations of carotid dissection include dysgeusia, syncope, tinnitus, facial dysesthesia, scalp tenderness, and a Collet-Sicard syndrome. This syndrome causes dysfunction of nerve XII (deviation of the tongue to one side and atrophy), nerves IX and X (dysphagia and development of a dysphonic voice), and nerve XI (weakness of head rotation and sternocleidomastoid atrophy). Carotid angiography in patients with dissection of the internal carotid reveals stenosis (70 percent of cases), abrupt luminal reconstitution (48 percent), aneurysms (37 percent), intimal flaps (35 percent), complete occlusion (17 percent), and distal branch occlusion by emboli (11 percent). This disorder has been treated with anticoagulants, aspirin, extracranial-intracranial bypass, and nonspecific supportive care. Eighty-five percent of patients recover completely, and luminal narrowings usually regress, restoring a normal-sized lumen. Neck tenderness may occur along the carotid sheath, but the presence of neurologic deficits excludes other causes of carotodynia.

7. LUDWIG'S ANGINA (SUBMANDIBULAR SPACE INFECTION)

Pain occurs in the mouth, secondary to dental disease, and in the submandibular region and anterior upper neck, due to spreading deep-space infection. Infection may invade from the roots of molars 2 or 3 of the lower jaw. These teeth have roots that extend below the level of the mylohyoid muscle into the submandibular space. Since the lingual plate of the mandible is thin in this region, infection of these roots can seed the submandibular space. Dental abscess, caries, and postextraction infection account for 70 to 85 percent of cases. Ulcers or lacerations of the floor of the mouth, jagged mandibular fractures or tumors, carcinoma of the tongue, sialadenitis, lymphadenitis, peritonsillar abscess, a foreign body, or hypodermic injection into the submandibular space may also initiate this disorder.

There is a rapidly developing massive swelling of the floor of the mouth, tongue, submandibular region, and upper neck. The tongue is elevated and pushed backward.

The mouth is forced open, the tongue protrudes, and saliva drools from the mouth. Breathing becomes difficult, and speech (a muffled ''hot potato'' voice is common) and swallowing are impaired. The neck swelling is brawny and associated with skin erythema. During the first 48 h, the consistency of the tender neck edema is woody, and there is no pitting or fluctuance. Toxicity, with fever, chills, and malaise, may be severe. The presence of trismus indicates invasion of the lateral pharyngeal space, and involvement of the lateral pterygoid and masseter muscles. The floor of the mouth is usually tender, red, elevated, and indurated. The common causative organisms include *Streptococcus viridans* and other streptococci, staphylococci, oral anaerobic bacteria, and some gram-negative aerobic bacteria (e.g., *Pseudomonas aeruginosa, Haemophilus influenzae,* and *E. coli*). Polymicrobial infection is common (50 percent of cases). Death may follow from airway obstruction, aspiration, or hematogenous pneumonia. Spread of infection to the lateral pharyngeal or retropharyngeal space may occur, with complications related to structures within these spaces (e.g., septic jugular phlebitis, carotid artery erosion, and mediastinitis).

The airway must be secured by endotracheal intubation or tracheotomy. Parenteral antibiotics and surgical drainage, if required, will usually lead to resolution of this life-threatening infection. High-dose intravenous penicillin (12–20 mU/day) may be used as initial therapy, and metronidazole may be added in severe cases. Clindamycin or chloramphenicol may also be effective.

Surgical incision and drainage are used when the disease is progressing despite antibiotic therapy or when fluctuance or crepitus is noted (2 percent of cases). Despite the absence of physical findings (fluctuance), purulent collections are present in 44 to 76 percent of cases. Ultrasound or CT scans can identify these collections, allowing for carefully planned drainage. Mortality is less than 4 percent with optimum management, and the survivors usually recover completely.

8. TRAUMA

A. Blunt Laryngotracheal Trauma   Injuries to the larynx and trachea may occur in a head-on collision in which the head is thrown forward and strikes the windshield, producing neck hyperextension, and exposing the airway to compression against the dashboard or steering wheel. Other causes include a direct blow with a fist or other object, attempted strangulation, and clothesline injuries suffered by snowmobilers or trail bikers.

Anterior neck pain, a voice change (hoarseness or aphonia), dysphagia and/or odynophagia, and hemoptysis are common symptoms of laryngeal injury. Airway obstruction produced by a displaced laryngeal fracture, edema, or hematoma can produce stridor and dyspnea.

Neck swelling, subcutaneous crepitus due to air, cartilaginous crepitus due to fracture, a mumbling or hoarse voice, and loss of structural landmarks (flattening of the neck, loss of the thyroid cartilage contour, or asymmetry of that cartilage) are common signs of laryngotracheal injury.

Associated injuries of the cervical spine, face, head, and esophagus may be present, and these structures require evaluation. A lateral neck film for soft tissue details may demonstrate subcutaneous emphysema, laryngeal hematomas, and supraglottic or subglottic attenuation of the laryngeal air column. A chest film may show mediastinal emphysema in the presence of a laryngeal fracture. A CT scan of the larynx will demonstrate a cartilaginous fracture and submucosal bleeding. Direct laryngoscopy may also be used to confirm such injuries. The airway should be secured by tracheostomy, and the fracture repaired surgically with or without the use of a stent. Esophageal perforation detectable by an esophogram using a water-soluble contrast solution or by endoscopy requires repair or drainage before diffuse neck infection develops.

B. Anterior Whiplash Injury   Rear-end and front-to-side collisions may cause a whiplash injury in the occupants of the struck vehicle.

Posterior neck pain and tenderness as well as anterior strap muscle pain and tenderness, increased by neck extension, may occur. These muscle injuries of the anterior neck usually resolve spontaneously within 10 to 14 days. Posterior neck symptoms may persist for a longer period.

9. ESOPHAGUS

A. Pharyngoesophageal Diverticulum   There is a sensation of a lump or foreign body high in the throat on swallowing. A mass that the patient can empty with hand pressure may appear in the anterolateral neck. Ingestion of liquids may be associated with noisy gurgling sounds in the neck. Regurgitation of swallowed, partially digested food causes throat discomfort and disgust due to the malodorous nature of the material. Coughing can be provoked, and aspiration can lead to bronchitis and pneumonia. Stagnant food and local infection may cause an esophageal diverticulitis and/or esophagitis, resulting in neck pain and odynophagia. The diagnosis of an esophageal diverticulum can be confirmed by a barium swallow or endoscopy. Leakage of the diverticulum into the tissues of the neck may lead to a thyroid or other deep neck abscess. Surgical removal of a symptomatic diverticulum is necessary.

B. Carcinoma of the Esophagus   A cervical esophageal cancer may present with upper neck discomfort, weight loss, and dysphagia initially for solids and then

for all foods. Advanced tumors may perforate, producing fever; a painful, tender, fluctuant neck mass; and, in some cases, a draining fistula.

10. REFERRED PAIN

A. Cardiac and Aortic

1. Myocardial Infarction or Coronary Insufficiency   Substernal and/or left precordial pain of a pressure-like or constricting nature occurs. It may radiate to one or both arms and the anterior neck, where it may be felt as a tightness, an ache, or a choking sensation. Associated symptoms may include diaphoresis, weakness, light-headedness, dyspnea, nausea, vomiting, and anxiety. There is no effect from sublingual nitroglycerin, and this failure to respond usually precipitates an emergency room visit. The cardiac size may be normal or enlarged. Frequent premature contractions, a rapid regular or irregular rhythm, bradycardia, or a normal regular rhythm may be present. Auscultation may reveal normal heart sounds or a decreased first heart sound at the apex and/or an S_4 or S_3 in the mitral area. The electrocardiogram will reveal new Q waves, ST elevation, and T-wave inversion in patients with transmural infarction, and ST elevation or depression and T-wave inversion in those with coronary insufficiency or a non-Q-wave infarction. The presence of infarction can be confirmed by measuring serum isozyme levels. Reduction or resolution of pain and limitation of the extent of infarction may follow thrombolytic therapy and/or angioplasty.

2. Acute Pericarditis   Sharp, stabbing anterior chest pain, intensified by lying on the left side or supine or by a deep breath, occurs. This pain may radiate to the neck or may begin in the left anterolateral neck and spread to the chest. Sitting up or standing alleviates the chest and neck pain. Fever, diaphoresis, malaise, and a history of recent respiratory illness may be present. Examination may reveal a pericardial friction rub, and the electrocardiogram will show ST elevation of a concave upward configuration in all leads except AVR and V_1. Within 3 to 5 days, the ST segments may become isoelectric, and the T waves may or may not flatten or invert. Cardiomegaly may occur during the second week because of an associated myocarditis or pericardial effusion.

3. Dissecting Aneurysm of the Thoracic Aorta   Tearing or ripping anterior chest, neck, interscapular, and abdominal pain may occur sequentially over a period of minutes. In some cases, the pain is a severe ache or crushing discomfort and does not have a tearing quality. Acute myocardial infarction may occur by retrograde dissection to the aortic valve. Patients with this disorder may writhe in pain or lie still. Diaphoresis, faintness, nausea, and vomiting may occur. Physical examination may reveal a regular tachycardia, an S_3 gallop, and one or more absent peripheral pulses.

A new aortic diastolic murmur may appear in up to 50 percent of patients. The electrocardiogram may show a sinus tachycardia and an acute inferior wall infarction in up to 16 percent of cases. A chest film usually reveals a widened mediastinum. A CT scan with contrast, an ultrafast cine CT scan, or an aortogram will reveal evidence of dissection of the thoracic aorta.

B. Spontaneous Pneumomediastinum There is an abrupt onset of moderately severe anterior neck pain, sore throat, dyspnea, dysphagia, and/or anterior chest pain. Subcutaneous crepitus may appear in the neck, supraclavicular fossa, and anterior chest. Fever and leukocytosis may occur. Chest examination may reveal a crunching sound synchronous with each cardiac contraction (Hamman's sign). Other physical findings include loss of cardiac dullness and decreased breath sounds over one hemithorax due to an associated pneumothorax. Pneumomediastinum has been associated with asthma, marijuana or "crack" cocaine smoking, mountain climbing, diabetic hyperpnea, labor, respiratory infections, severe cough, vomiting, pulmonary function testing, and anorexia nervosa.

The substernal or precordial pain is sharp or stabbing and radiates to the back or neck. It is intensified by a deep respiration, a cough, swallowing, or lying flat or on the left side. It may be improved by sitting up or leaning forward. Radiologic evidence of pneumomediastinum includes lucencies due to tissue air along the left heart border and retrosternally. Therapy includes bed rest and analgesics. Spontaneous resolution occurs within 3 to 5 days.

Rare causes of pneumomediastinum include esophageal or tracheal perforation, peptic ulcer perforation with air in the retroperitoneal space, and neck surgery or trauma during which air enters the fascial planes in the neck.

10 Acute Lateral Neck Pain

☐ DIAGNOSTIC LIST

1. Parotid disorders
   A. Viral parotitis
   B. Sialodochitis
   C. Salivary duct stone
   D. Suppurative parotitis
   E. Iodine mumps
2. Cervical lymphadenitis
3. Lateral pharyngeal space infections
   A. Anterior compartment infections
   B. Posterior compartment infections
      1. Septic thrombophlebitis of the internal jugular vein
      2. Carotid arteritis; aneurysm formation and rupture
4. Infected cysts
   A. Cystic hygroma
   B. Branchial cleft cyst
5. Sternocleidomastoid disorders
   A. Trauma
   B. Pseudotumor
6. Myofascial syndromes of the trapezius muscle(s)
7. Referred pain
   A. Cardiac disease
      1. Acute myocardial infarction
      2. Acute coronary insufficiency
      3. Acute pericarditis
   B. Pleuritis involving the diaphragm
   C. Dissecting aneurysm of the aorta

☐ SUMMARY

Painful *parotid swelling* on one or both sides, with fever, occurring in children and young adults is usually due to *mumps virus;* but other viral agents may occasionally cause a similar disorder. *Sialodochitis* occurs in elderly, dehydrated, and debilitated patients. Parotid enlargement occurs on one side and is resolved by gland massage. It is due to temporary ductal obstruction. A *stone in the duct* may also cause intermittent painful parotid swelling on one side, provoked by eating. A stone may be palpable in the duct or visualized by x-ray. Removal of the stone leads to immediate resolution of the pain and swelling. *Suppurative parotitis* causes unilateral or bilateral parotid enlargement, pain, and tenderness. This disorder may be associated with high fever, chills, and toxicity. There

is a therapeutic response to intravenous antibiotic therapy and surgical drainage. *Ingestion of seafood or iodine-containing medications* may cause acute bilateral painful parotid swelling.

Cervical lymphadenitis secondary to a throat, dental, or skin infection causes pain, tenderness, and lymph node enlargement below the angle of the jaw on one or both sides. In some cases only node enlargement and tenderness occur. There is a prompt response to antibiotic therapy.

Lateral pharyngeal space infections, when the *anterior compartment* is infected, cause parotid area swelling, pain, and tenderness; dysphagia; trismus; fever and chills; and medial bulging of the ipsilateral tonsil. *Posterior compartment suppuration* may cause a *septic thrombophlebitis of the internal jugular vein,* with infected pulmonary emboli, local parotid space and neck tenderness, and lateral and/or cavernous sinus thrombosis. *Carotid infection* in the posterior compartment can lead to *aneurysm formation. Rupture* may occur, with severe hemorrhage from the mouth and nose.

Infected cystic hygromas or *branchial cleft cysts* cause lateral neck pain, with fluctuant swelling, skin redness, warmth, and tenderness in the lateral neck.

Local injury to the sternocleidomastoid, with torn muscle fibers and/or hematoma formation, causes local lateral neck pain and tenderness, and sometimes torticollis. Rarely, a *pseudotumor of the sternocleidomastoid* can cause localized neck pain and a tender mass in, or adjacent to, the body of that muscle. *Myofascial syndromes arising in the trapezius muscle* cause lateral neck pain and trigger point tenderness.

Referred pain from a *myocardial infarction* or an episode of *coronary insufficiency* may be felt in the left lateral neck, the shoulder, and one or both arms. The diagnosis can be confirmed by electrocardiography, by serum isozyme assays, and by coronary angiography. There may be a response of the pain to thrombolytic agents. *Acute pericarditis* causes chest and/or left lateral neck and shoulder pain that is relieved by sitting up and exacerbated by lying down and by deep inspiration. *Pleuritic neck and shoulder pain* produced by diaphragmatic inflammation is intensified by inspiration or by upper trunk and neck movements. Pleuritic-type pain of the lateral neck and shoulder may also be caused by subdiaphragmatic inflammation secondary to gallbladder disease; splenic inflammation; or a perirenal or subphrenic abscess. A *dissecting aortic aneurysm* causes stabbing or tearing sequential pain in the anterior chest, neck, interscapular area, and abdomen. The diagnosis can be confirmed by an ultrafast CT study, an aortogram, or a thoracic CT scan using contrast medium.

☐ DESCRIPTION OF LISTED DISEASES

1. PAROTID DISORDERS

A. Viral Parotitis Mumps virus causes illness in children and young adults. Infection begins with fever, chills, sore throat, and malaise; these symptoms are followed by pain and tenderness in the preauricular area, the angle of the jaw, and the upper anterolateral neck. Unilateral swelling and pain may occur initially, but within 1 to 2 days bilateral involvement is present in up to 75 percent of cases. The pain is continuous, severe, deep, and aching; it may be intensified by chewing, swallowing, and the ingestion of citrus juices or fruits. There is diffuse tender swelling in the preauricular area, upper neck, and submandibular region; the margins of the gland cannot be clearly defined by palpation, because of the edema. There is no specific therapy. The pain and tenderness subside spontaneously over a period of 5 to 7 days.

TABLE OF DISEASE INCIDENCE

INCIDENCE PER 100,000 (APPROXIMATE)

Common (>100)	Uncommon (>5–100)	Rare (>0–5)
Viral parotitis	Sialodochitis	Posterior compartment infections:
Salivary duct stone	Suppurative parotitis	Septic thrombophlebitis of the jugular vein
Cervical lymphadenitis	Iodine mumps	Carotid arteritis; aneurysm formation and rupture
Myofascial syndromes of the trapezius muscle(s)	Lateral pharyngeal space infections: Anterior compartment infections	Infected hygroma
Pleuritis involving the diaphragm	Sternocleidomastoid trauma	Infected branchial cleft cyst
	Referred cardiac pain	Pseudotumor of the sternocleidomastoid muscle
		Dissecting aortic aneurysm

The orifice of Stensen's duct may be reddened, but the saliva draining from it is clear and not purulent. Presternal edema may occur because of lymphatic obstruction. Up to 30 percent of adult males may develop unilateral or bilateral orchitis and epididymitis. Testicular involvement usually occurs 1 to 2 weeks after the onset of parotitis, but occasionally may precede it. Women may experience lower abdominal pain from oophoritis (5 percent of cases) or breast pain from mastitis. An aseptic meningitis syndrome may occur in up to 10 percent of cases, and pancreatitis in 5 percent. The serum amylase level is elevated in 90 percent of patients with mumps parotitis. The diagnosis is usually made clinically; serologic confirmation by neutralizing antibody, complement fixation, enzyme-lined immunosorbent assay (ELISA), or hemagglutination inhibition tests is seldom required. Viral parotitis has been reported secondary to infection with Coxsackie A, Epstein-Barr, influenza A, lymphocytic choriomeningitis, and parainfluenza viruses.

B. Sialodochitis This is a disorder of dehydrated and/or chronically ill elderly patients. Obstruction of Stensen's duct by a plug of mucus or fibrin leads to painful enlargement of a parotid gland. Massage of the gland or duct results in restoration of duct patency, return of the gland to normal size, and relief of pain.

C. Salivary Duct Stone A salivary duct stone may cause a similar obstruction and painful swelling, which is increased or provoked by attempts to eat. Duct massage, or incision with stone extraction, is required to return the distended parotid to a normal size and relieve the associated pain and tenderness.

D. Suppurative Parotitis   Acute suppurative parotitis occurs in elderly, dehydrated, and, often, debilitated patients, who have a low flow rate of salivary secretion—because of poor fluid intake, diuretic therapy, or secretion-inhibiting drug therapy for associated disorders (e.g., anticholinergic or antihistaminic drugs). In addition, these patients often have a focus of intraoral infection that provides a reservoir of bacteria to infect the salivary ducts. Chronic tonsillitis, dental sepsis, oropharyngeal malignancies, tracheostomy, and use of immunosuppressive drugs are some of the associated disorders. Up to one-third of cases occur in the postoperative period after major surgery.

A painful tender swelling of one (85 percent of cases) or both (15 percent) parotid glands develops. The overlying skin may become warm, red, and tender. High fever, rigors or chills, sweats, and prostration follow. There is leukocytosis with a shift to the left, and a rise in the serum amylase level. Pressure over the swollen gland will express pus from the parotid duct. Culture and Gram stain of expressed pus usually reveals infection with *Staphylococcus aureus,* but *S. pyogenes* and alpha hemolytic streptococci may also be causative. Needle aspiration of the gland and anaerobic cultures have documented less frequent infections with species of *Bacteroides, Peptostreptococcus,* and *Actinomyces.* Rarely, *Mycobacterium tuberculosis,* or fungi such as *Candida albicans,* may be isolated. Improvement follows administration of intravenous fluids and antibiotics, and relief of any ductal obstruction. Some cases progress to abscess formation; these require incision and drainage.

E. Iodine Mumps   Acute painful enlargement of both parotid glands may follow ingestion of iodine-containing seafood or expectorants. Avoidance of iodine leads to spontaneous resolution.

2. CERVICAL LYMPHADENITIS

Acute pharyngitis and/or tonsillitis may cause throat pain intensified by swallowing. Aching pain may also occur at one or both jaw angles and in the upper neck, along the upper anterior border of the sternocleidomastoid. Palpation reveals enlargement of one or more superior cervical nodes (i.e., to more than 1.5 cm in size) and nodal tenderness. Fever, chills, myalgias, coryza, and malaise may accompany the local neck pain. Small numbers of cases of cervical lymphadenitis are secondary to a root infection of a tooth, or to infection of the skin of the face and/or scalp.

Staphylococcus aureus and *S. pyogenes* are the microorganisms most commonly associated with pharyngeal and tonsillar infections. A dental source of the lymphadenitis suggests infection with anaerobes, such as *Bacteroides* and *Peptostreptococcus* species. *S. aureus* and *S. pyogenes* account for most of the cases secondary to impetigo and other skin infections.

Bilateral cervical lymphadenitis usually follows viral infections or streptococcal pharyngitis and tonsillitis. The involved nodes are located at the anterolateral aspect of the neck, between the angle of the jaw and the upper anterior border of the sternocleidomastoid muscle. Bacterial lymphadenitis resolves promptly after initiation of antimicrobial therapy.

Mildly painful and tender posterior cervical nodal enlargement may occur in Epstein-Barr virus and rubella infections. The pain produced is a constant dull ache. In many patients involved nodes are enlarged, but not painful or tender. Nontender posterior cervical and axillary adenopathy occurs frequently in patients with HIV infection.

3. LATERAL PHARYNGEAL SPACE INFECTIONS

The medial wall of the lateral pharyngeal space consists of the superior constrictor of the pharynx and its fascia. The peritonsillar space is adjacent to this medial wall. The lateral wall consists of the mandible, the internal pterygoid muscles, and the parotid gland. The styloid process of the temporal bone extends into the lateral pharyngeal space and divides it into an anterior and a posterior compartment.

A. Anterior Compartment Infections   This compartment normally contains fat, lymph nodes, muscle, and areolar tissue. Infection of this space may be secondary to a deep lymphadenitis, or to a tonsillar, dental, pharyngeal, or parotid infection. Anterior compartment infection causes pain of an aching or throbbing quality in the posterior jaw, lateral neck, and ear, as well as dysphagia and trismus. Turning the neck and head away from the painful side may cause an intensification of pain secondary to contraction of the ipsilateral sternocleidomastoid (which acts to rotate the head) against the lateral pharyngeal space. Shaking chills, fever, and dyspnea are common associated complaints. Physical examination may reveal trismus due to inflammation of the internal pterygoid muscle; induration; tenderness and swelling at the angle of the jaw, and over the parotid gland; systemic toxicity; and medial bulging of the lateral pharyngeal wall. Suppuration in the lateral pharyngeal space usually leads to abscess formation.

B. Posterior Compartment Infections   Fever and toxicity are the major findings. Swelling of the parotid space may occur, with marked local tenderness; but often no localizing symptoms occur. There may be a medial bulge of the posterolateral pharyngeal wall behind the palatopharyngeal arch. Since the posterior compartment contains cranial nerves IX to XII, the carotid sheath, and the cervical sympathetic trunk, injury to these structures occurs with posterior compartment abscesses. Complications of posterior compartment infections include:

1. Internal Jugular Vein Thrombophlebitis   Pain and tenderness at the angle of the jaw and along the upper border of the sternal head of the sternocleidomastoid are associated with rigors, high fever, and toxicity. Septic pulmonary emboli may occur, with pleuritic pain and hemoptysis. Lateral sinus thrombosis may occur, with severe headache, vomiting, and increased intracranial pressure. Cavernous sinus thrombosis, brain suppuration, and abscesses at remote sites may follow. The diagnosis of jugular venous thrombosis can be confirmed by retrograde venography or by MRI. Intravenous antibiotic therapy, and in some cases excision of the infected vein, are required.

2. Carotid Arteritis; Aneurysm Formation and Rupture Involvement of the carotid sheath and the carotid artery, secondary to a purulent arteritis, may result in aneurysm formation in the common, internal, or external carotid artery. Warning signs of an exsanguinating rupture of a carotid aneurysm related to a space infection include recurrent bleeding from the nose, mouth, or ear (''herald bleeds''); a prolonged clinical course; a neck hematoma; and falling blood pressure. Other signs of carotid sheath infection include ipsilateral peritonsillar swelling, Horner's syndrome, and dysfunction of cranial nerves IX to XII (i.e., jugular foramen syndrome). Surgical drainage of the pharyngeal space abscess and ligation of the leaking carotid vessel are required. Airway obstruction due to laryngeal swelling may also follow lateral space infections. Posterior extension can produce a retropharyngeal abscess.

Lateral space infections resulting from a dental source may be caused by penicillin-resistant *Bacteroides* species, so addition of clindamycin or metronidazole to a standard high-dose penicillin regimen is recommended.

4. INFECTED CYSTS

A. Cystic Hygroma   These cystic lesions occur in the posterior triangle of the neck and are usually asymptomatic, unless they become infected. Pain, tenderness, redness, and local warmth develop in the vicinity of the hygroma. Antibiotic therapy and excision lead to resolution of pain and tenderness.

B. Branchial Cleft Cyst   A branchial cleft fistula arising in the first branchial cleft remnant (i.e., a skin opening between the external auditory canal and the submandibular area) or in the second branchial cleft remnant (i.e., a skin opening along the anterior border of the sternocleidomastoid muscle) may become infected and cystic, causing aching lateral neck pain, swelling, tenderness, skin redness, and warmth. Cyst excision, under cover of antibiotic therapy, will lead to full resolution of symptoms.

5. STERNOCLEIDOMASTOID DISORDERS

Disorders of the sternocleidomastoid, such as torn muscle fibers, an intramuscular hematoma, or formation of an inflammatory pseudotumor, may cause muscle pain, spasm, and tenderness, as well as torticollis to the contralateral side. These disorders will usually resolve spontaneously—with the exception of a pseudotumor, which usually requires excision.

6. MYOFASCIAL SYNDROMES OF THE TRAPEZIUS MUSCLE(S)

Myofascial disorders of the trapezius muscle(s) occur with well-defined anterior and anteromedial trigger points. Pressure over one or several of these trigger points leads to reproduction of the patient's neck, ear, and shoulder pain. Trigger point injection with lidocaine, followed by muscle stretching exercises, usually results in complete or partial relief of pain and tenderness.

7. REFERRED NECK AND SHOULDER PAIN FROM VISCERAL DISORDERS

A. Cardiac Disease

1. Acute Myocardial Infarction   Pain occurs substernally, and/or in the left precordium, and/or in one or both arms, and sometimes in the anterior and/or left lateral neck. The quality of the pain is described as pressurelike, constricting, crushing, or burning. The neck pain has been variously described as ''a tightness,'' as ''suffocating,'' and as an ''ache.'' Diaphoresis, nausea, vomiting, dizziness, weakness, and dyspnea may accompany discomfort in the chest, neck, and arm. Rest, nitroglycerin, and simple analgesics fail to relieve the pain. Coronary angiography will show a complete or partial coronary artery occlusion. Intracoronary infusion or intravenous administration of a thrombolytic agent, or direct coronary angioplasty, will usually relieve pain within 1 to 2 h and preserve myocardium. Serial electrocardiograms and measurement of serum isozyme levels will establish a diagnosis of myocardial infarction. The chest and neck pains of myocardial ischemia are not affected by respiration, upper trunk movements, or jarring. Failure of thrombolytic therapy results in a more extensive myocardial infarction, with pain lasting 8 to 24 h.

2. Acute Coronary Insufficiency   Patients with this disorder are clinically similar to those with myocardial infarction. They have severe coronary spasm and/or a clot that is partly obstructing a coronary artery. The use of thrombolytic agents and/or direct angioplasty can restore coronary patency, relieve pain, and prevent myocardial infarction.

3. Acute Pericarditis   Acute pericarditis may cause substernal pain, left precordial pain, and/or left lateral neck and shoulder pain. It is usually sharp and stabbing, and intensified by the supine position, deep inspiration, coughing, swallowing, and changes in upper body position. The pain is less intense in a sitting or standing position. Fever, tachycardia, and leukocytosis may occur, but vomiting and profuse diaphoresis are uncommon. A three-component pericardial friction rub is usually audible at the onset of the pain. In patients with myocardial infarction, a pericardial friction rub is not heard until the second or third day after onset. The electrocardiogram shows ST-segment elevation in all leads except V_1 and aV_R with T-wave inversion following within 4 to 7 days in most, but not all, cases. Cardiac isozyme levels may rise, secondary to an associated myocarditis.

Viral, idiopathic, uremic, lupus-related, postmyocardial infarction, and postcardiotomy pericarditis respond dramatically to prednisone or nonsteroidal anti-inflammatory drugs; neoplastic, tuberculous, and purulent pericarditis do not. These latter disorders require pericardiocentesis and/or pericardial biopsy for diagnosis.

B. Pleuritis Involving the Diaphragm   Inflammation of the diaphragm may be secondary to bacterial pneumonia, pulmonary infarction, primary pleuritis, or a subdiaphragmatic process. Shoulder and lateral neck pain, and/or anterolateral chest pain intensified or provoked by deep inspiration occur. Within hours the neck and chest pains become constant; they may be intensified by changes of upper body position or by neck movement.

Bacterial pneumonia is suggested by a productive cough with rusty or purulent sputum; dyspnea; rigors; high fever; and a toxic appearance. Examination may reveal dullness, bronchial breath sounds, rales, and/or a pleural friction rub. A person with pulmonary infarction may present with dyspnea, cough, hemoptysis, and, sometimes, leg pain and swelling. Associated findings may include malignancy, heart failure, prolonged immobilization, recent pregnancy or surgery, leg trauma, use of oral contraceptives, or a family history of thromboembolic disease. Pleuritis occurring in patients with a facial rash, arthritis, and renal and neurologic disease suggests systemic lupus erythematosus. An elevated antinuclear antibody titer in serum and pleural fluid (i.e., >1:80) supports a diagnosis of lupus pleuritis. Fever, pleuritis, and pleural effusion in a young adult may be secondary to tuberculosis.

A severe episode of cholecystitis may cause diaphragmatic inflammation and right shoulder and neck pain. An ultrasound study of the gallbladder, and/or a DISIDA scan, will help establish a diagnosis of biliary tract disease.

Splenic inflammation secondary to trauma, infection, infarction, abscess formation, or subcapsular bleeding may cause left shoulder and neck pain that is intensified by inspiration, coughing, and bodily movement. Similarly, a perinephric abscess or a subdiaphragmatic abscess may cause diaphragmatic inflammation, pleural effusion, and shoulder and lateral neck pain with pleuritic qualities. A CT scan or MRI of the lower chest and upper abdomen will identify disorders of the spleen and the subdiaphragmatic region.

C. Dissecting Aneurysm of the Thoracic Aorta   Substernal discomfort develops abruptly and then spreads sequentially, as a sharp, tearing pain, to the lateral and posterior neck, interscapular region, low back, and abdomen. The pain is usually constant, deep, and severe-to-excruciating, causing patients to writhe in bed seeking relief. There is often a history of hypertension or Marfan's syndrome. Physical examination may demonstrate a new aortic insufficiency murmur and diminution or loss of one or more peripheral pulses. An S_3 gallop and arrhythmias may be present, because of an acute myocardial infarction resulting from retrograde dissection of the aortic arch. A plain chest radiograph will demonstrate mediastinal widening; the diagnosis of dissection can be confirmed by an ultrafast CT study with contrast medium, or by an arch aortogram.

11

Acute Posterior Neck Pain

☐ **DIAGNOSTIC LIST**

1. Acute meningitis
   A. Bacterial (cocci and bacilli)
   B. Spirochetal
      1. Lyme disease
      2. Neurosyphilis
      3. Leptospirosis
   C. Viral
   D. Drug-associated
   E. Amebic
2. Subarachnoid hemorrhage
   A. Aneurysmal leakage or rupture
      1. Sentinel bleed
      2. Major subarachnoid hemorrhage due to aneurysmal rupture
   B. Spinal subarachnoid hemorrhage and other causes
3. Meningismus
   A. With normal cerebrospinal fluid (CSF)
   B. With aseptic meningitis
4. Cervical disc degeneration
5. Cervical disc herniation and radiculopathy
6. Disorders mimicking cervical disc herniation
   A. Epidural abscess
   B. Cervical osteomyelitis with pathologic fracture
   C. Epidural hematoma
   D. Transverse myelitis
   E. Pachymeningitis cervicalis hypertrophica
   F. Lyme disease and radiculitis
   G. Myofascial syndrome and referred arm pain

H. Osteoarthritis of the spine with foraminal narrowing
7. Acute neck or chest wall infection and referred posterior cervical pain
   A. Retropharyngeal abscess
   B. Upper anterior chest wall abscess
   C. Cervical osteomyelitis
8. Calcium deposition
   A. Retropharyngeal calcific tendinitis of the longus colli muscle
   B. Crystal-induced neck pain (crowned dens syndrome)
9. Arthritis-related cervical subluxation—Atlantoaxial subluxation
   A. Rheumatoid arthritis
   B. Ankylosing spondylitis
   C. Juvenile rheumatoid arthritis
10. Neck trauma
   A. Whiplash injury
   B. Fractures
11. Acute myositis of the posterior neck muscles
12. Acute osteoarthritis of zygapophyseal joints and disc degeneration
13. Acute torticollis
14. Occipital migraine
15. Occipital neuralgia
16. Coital neck and head pain
17. Vertebral artery disorders
   A. Vertebral artery dissection
   B. Vertebral artery pseudoaneurysm

☐ SUMMARY

Acute meningitis due to *bacterial infection* causes high fever, chills, rigors, headache, nausea, vomiting, prostration, and a painful stiff neck. The patient appears severely ill and toxic and may be disoriented, stuporous, or comatose. The spinal fluid reveals a neutrophilic predominance, low sugar, and elevated protein. Cerebrospinal fluid Gram's stain, culture, and in some cases counterimmunoelectrophoresis reveal the responsible bacterial species. There is a dramatic response to intravenous antibiotic therapy. Aseptic meningitis is classically caused by *viral agents* and sometimes by *drugs.* The patient complains of a moderately severe headache, posterior neck pain, and stiffness. Fever seldom exceeds 102°F, and rigors do not occur. Most patients are mentally clear unless they have an associated encephalitis. The spinal fluid shows a pleocytosis, an elevated protein level, and usually a normal sugar level. Drug-associated meningitis may present a similar picture and resolves on discontinuing the offending drug. *Amebic meningoencephalitis* causes a clinical picture similar to that produced by bacterial pathogens but is usually unresponsive to therapy. Amebas may be detected as motile trophozoites in the cell-counting chamber.

Lyme disease and *other spirochetal disorders* may cause a mild meningitis with minimal neck pain and stiffness. *Borrelia burgdorferi* may cause meningitis, meningoencephalitis, myeloradiculitis, plexitis, or mononeuritis. Associated findings include erythema chronicum migrans, arthritis of the knees or ankles, and a myocarditis. The diagnosis can be confirmed by a serum immunofluorescent antibody (IFA) or ELISA test for *Borellia burgdorferi.* Meningovascular syphilis can be diagnosed by serologic studies. The diagnosis of leptospirosis depends on a history of exposure to infected animal urine and abnormalities of renal and hepatic function. Confirmation by serologic methods may require 2 or more weeks and will not allow early initiation of effective antibiotic therapy.

Leakage of an intracranial aneurysm may cause an abrupt onset of severe head and posterior neck pain, only occasionally associated with neck stiffness, mental confusion, weakness, photophobia, nausea, vomiting, and transient syncope. The course may mimic a severe episode of migraine.

If a CT scan and lumbar puncture are not done, such a *sentinel bleed* may go undetected. It may soon be followed by a second, more severe attack that may lead to profound neurologic damage and possibly death.

Spinal subarachnoid hemorrhage may cause posterior neck and head pain, nuchal rigidity, and fever. Radicular pain may occur at the site of the bleeding spinal lesion (e.g., tumor, arteriovenous malformation, or vasculitic lesion), giving rise to chest pain (thoracic region), sciatic pain (lumbar region), or rectal pain (sacral region).

Meningismus is a mimic of meningitis and occurs in patients with infectious diseases such as pyelonephritis, gastroenteritis, pneumonitis, and pleuritis. The *cerebrospinal fluid (CSF) is normal,* although the patients have enough neck and head pain and nuchal stiffness to warrant a lumbar puncture. The current literature also includes some noninfectious disorders as causes of meningismus, but these diseases usually cause an *aseptic inflammatory meningeal reaction,* as reflected in elevated CSF cell counts and protein concentrations (e.g., aseptic meningitis syndrome).

Cervical disc degeneration without herniation has been shown by provocative and analgesic discography to cause posterior neck and shoulder pain. *Disc herniation* may cause neck, shoulder, scapula, chest, and/or arm pain, associated with one or more specific cervical root syndromes. Symptoms and signs of *cervical radiculopathy* include weakness of specific muscles, loss of a specific reflex, and paresthesias and hypoesthesia of one or two adjacent fingers that are innervated by the involved root. The diagnosis can be confirmed by a metrizamide CT scan or MRI.

A *cervical epidural abscess* causes severe neck pain and tenderness associated with fever, chills, and toxicity. Multiple cervical roots are involved, resulting in extensive unilateral or bilateral arm pain and paresthesias, weakness of one or more extremities, lower-extremity numbness and paresthesias, and sphincter disturbances. MRI will reveal the abscess and its cephalocaudal extent. Symptom resolution follows intravenous antibiotic therapy and surgical drainage. *Cervical osteomyelitis* may cause fever and aching posterior neck pain. If a pathologic fracture occurs because of vertebral destruction, mechanical compression of the cervical cord and roots can mimic the findings of an acute epidural abscess. The diagnosis can be confirmed by a CT scan or MRI. An *epidural hematoma* may cause a rapidly progressive myelopathy and radiculopathy. There is a history of liver disease, coagulopathy, or minor neck trauma. The diagnosis can be confirmed by a metrizamide CT scan or MRI.

Cervical *transverse myelitis* causes tetraparesis and a sensory level associated with low-grade fever, spinal ache, and tenderness in the posterior neck region. The metrizamide CT scan or MRI shows no evidence of an epidural mass. The cord may appear normal or slightly enlarged, secondary to inflammatory edema.

Pachymeningitis hypertrophica of the cervical region causes neck pain, a bilateral polyradiculopathy, and sometimes a myelopathy. It may mimic a subacute epidural abscess. Root sleeve obliteration may be detected by a plain or CT-augmented myelogram. Diagnosis depends on exploration and biopsy. Resection of the thickened dura leads to symptom resolution. *Lyme disease meningitis* and *radiculitis* may cause neck and arm pain. The CSF contains an increased number of lymphocytes, and the serum IFA and ELISA antibody tests are positive. *Myofascial pain* related to a trapezius trigger point may cause unilateral posterior neck, interscapular, and arm pain. Arm pain and paresthesias may be provoked by neck rotation to the painful side or by finger pressure over the trigger point. Lidocaine injection of the trigger point temporarily relieves all complaints. Radiculopathy of a specific cervical root may be caused by foraminal narrowing due to *bony osteophytes* or *subluxation* of a facet joint.

A *retropharyngeal abscess* causes posterior neck pain and

TABLE OF DISEASE INCIDENCE

INCIDENCE PER 100,000 (APPROXIMATE)

Common (>100)	Uncommon (>5–100)	Rare (>0–5)
Bacterial meningitis	Lyme disease meningitis and radiculitis	Syphilitic meningitis
Viral meningitis	Sentinel bleed	Drug-associated meningitis
Cervical disc degeneration	Major subarachnoid hemorrhage	Amebic meningitis
Cervical disc herniation	Meningismus	Leptospiral meningitis
Osteoarthritis with foraminal narrowing	Myofascial syndrome and referred arm pain	Spinal subarachnoid hemorrhage
Rheumatoid arthritis and atlantoaxial subluxation	Cervical osteomyelitis	Epidural abscess
Whiplash injury	Ankylosing spondylitis and atlantoaxial subluxation	Cervical osteomyelitis and pathologic fracture
Cervical spine fracture or subluxation	Juvenile rheumatoid arthritis and atlantoaxial subluxation	Epidural hematoma
Myositis of the posterior neck muscles	Acute torticollis	Transverse myelitis
Osteoarthritis; Zygapophyseal joints/ disc degeneration		Pachymeningitis hypertrophica
Occipital migraine		Retropharyngeal abscess
Coital neck and head pain		Anterior chest wall abscess
		Retropharyngeal calcific tendinitis
		Crystal-induced neck pain
		Vertebral artery dissection
		Vertebral artery pseudoaneurysm
		Referred pain from an anterior chest abscess
		Occipital neuralgia

stiffness, associated with fever, sore throat, noisy respirations, dyspnea, regurgitation, and a toxic clinical appearance. Swallowing increases throat and posterior neck pain. A lateral neck film will outline the retropharyngeal abscess, which requires antibiotic therapy and drainage. *Calcific tendinitis* of the longus colli muscle may also cause sore throat and posterior neck pain and stiffness, intensified by neck movements or swallowing. Lateral neck films show calcium deposits anterior to C1 and C2, and a soft tissue swelling. This disorder responds to intravenous corticosteroids or oral nonsteroidal anti-inflammatory drugs, and drainage is not required. A similar syndrome is caused by *calcium deposition* around the odontoid, and this responds to nonsteroidal anti-inflammatory drugs. The diagnosis can be confirmed by a CT study of the cervical spine. Referred pain from an anterior upper *chest wall abscess* may irritate an intercostal nerve and produce severe posterior neck pain, tenderness, and stiffness, which resolve after treatment of the primary lesion. *Cervical osteomyelitis* causes neck pain and tenderness associated with an elevated sedimentation rate, and can be confirmed by a radionuclide scan and/or MRI of the spine.

Rheumatoid arthritis may cause *atlantoaxial subluxation* leading to a high cervical radiculopathy and a myelopathy, which may progress to tetraparesis. Many cases of rheumatoid subluxation are asymptomatic or associated with less severe neurological symptoms. Mild degrees of subluxation, with less severe neurological signs, are associated with *ankylosing spondylitis*.

A *whiplash injury* causes neck muscle pain, tenderness, and stiffness that may involve the anterior and posterior neck. The pain is intensified by cervical motion and may be felt in the shoulder, scapula, and upper arm. Persistent pain may be due to a *zygapophyseal joint fracture*, a missed *C1 fracture, C2 root injury, cervical disc degeneration,* or *other missed ligamentous tears or fractures.* Computerized tomography is not 100 percent sensitive for cervical fractures, while a single cross-table lateral radiograph of the cervical spine has a 26-percent false-negative rate. Most whiplash injuries are probably due to muscle trauma and improve within 2 months, but up to 30 percent of patients may still be symptomatic after 2 years.

Acute myositis of the posterior neck muscles may cause neck ache and brief, recurrent paroxysms of excruciating pain. These attacks gradually resolve on conservative therapy. *Acute torticollis* may accompany severe neck pain. Causes include exposure to drafts, viral agents, minor trauma, sleeping in a cramped position, excessive unaccustomed exercise involving the neck muscles, and excessive posterior rotation of the neck.

Acute osteoarthritis of an apophyseal joint or a *degenerated disc space* may cause posterior neck pain and stiffness, intensified by movement. Proof of the diagnosis may require joint or disc space injections with bupivacaine.

Acute posterior neck pain and torticollis may be caused by a large number of disorders, including a retropharyngeal abscess, cervical adenitis, atlantoaxial rotatory fixation, osteomyelitis of the upper cervical spine, accessory nerve neuritis, cerebellar herniation, hyperthyroidism, neck fractures, and subluxations.

Occipital migraine causes unilateral throbbing posterior neck and occipital pain that may be associated with visual phenomena, facial paresthesias, and limb heaviness and clumsiness. Nausea and vomiting may also occur. *Occipital neuralgia* causes aching constant posterior neck pain and occipital scalp pain, associated with paresthesias and hypoesthesia of the scalp. *Coital neck and head pain* begin during sexual intercourse and may mimic the explosive pain of a ruptured aneurysm. Most cases of this syndrome are benign and not associated with intracranial bleeding or an intracranial mass lesion.

Vertebral artery dissection causes severe posterolateral neck and/or occipital head pain. This may be associated with a lateral medullary syndrome and other acute neurologic findings. An angiogram will demonstrate the dissection. *Pseudoaneurysm* of the vertebral artery may also cause brain stem signs and an ipsilateral painful posterolateral neck mass. A CT scan and an angiogram will confirm the diagnosis. Some cases of dissection or aneurysm follow trauma, including chiropractic manipulation.

☐ DESCRIPTION OF LISTED DISEASES

1. ACUTE MENINGITIS

A. Bacterial (Cocci and Bacilli)   Acute bacterial meningitis may follow a very rapid course, progressive to coma within 24 h, or a more gradual onset over a period of several days. Rapidly progressive bacterial meningitis causes fever, severe headache, neck stiffness and pain, and diffuse myalgias that are worsened by movement. Nausea, vomiting, lethargy, and prostration often occur. Early central nervous system involvement may be signaled by seizures, mental confusion, combativeness, photophobia, dysesthesias, gait disturbances, and pareses. Neck discomfort is intensified by attempted flexion and/or rotation of the neck and lessened by restriction of movement.

A more gradual onset is characterized by fever, myalgias, and a mild headache, associated with stiffness and pain associated with neck flexion and/or rotation.

Selection of patients for lumbar puncture from the large number with acute fever, headache, and myalgias is usually dependent on the presence of meningeal findings, such as nuchal rigidity, Kernig's and Brudzinski's signs, photophobia, and eyeball tenderness, or symptoms or signs of central nervous system dysfunction. Up to .75 percent of patients over age 2 years may have meningitis without meningeal signs, and up to 50 percent of these patients may be completely alert and cooperative when first seen. The mildness of their presentation does not preclude a fulminant fatal course. These cases may not be detected until further progression directs attention to the central nervous system.

Suspected acute bacterial meningitis is a major indication for lumbar puncture. If a focal lesion, such as a brain abscess or necrotic tumor, is suspected, a pretap CT scan or MRI should be done to screen for abnormalities that would place the patient at risk for uncal or cerebellar herniation. These abnormalities include lateral shift of midline structures or symmetrically elevated supratento-

rial pressure, causing obliteration of suprasellar and circummesencephalic cisterns. These CT findings place the patient at risk for uncal herniation after lumbar puncture. The presence of a cerebellar tumor or other posterior fossa lesions may be difficult to exclude by a CT scan. Such lesions may be more easily visualized by MRI. Posterior fossa masses, shifts of midline structures, or obliteration of the fourth ventricle are pretap risk factors for cerebellar tonsillar herniation about the brain stem. It is claimed, but with little supporting data, that the CT or MRI findings described above are contraindications to lumbar puncture.

In the absence of papilledema and/or the CT or MRI findings described above, lumbar puncture should be performed in suspected cases of acute bacterial meningitis. The cell count may range from 0 to over 10,000/mm^3 (normal up to 5 mononuclear cells), with 90 to 95 percent of the cells neutrophils. Unfortunately, up to 32 percent of patients with CSF total cell counts of 1000/mm^3 or less may have spinal fluid differential cell counts, demonstrating a lymphocytosis of 58 to 90 percent. Conversely, some early cases of viral and tuberculous meningitis may demonstrate a preponderance of neutrophils instead of lymphocytes. The atypical findings in a viral meningitis may be clarified by a repeat tap after 12 h that demonstrates a definite lymphocytic predominance. Low glucose values (normal = ≥40 mg/dL or ≥50 percent of the blood sugar); protein elevations greater than 200 mg/dl (normal = 15–45 mg/dl); elevated CSF lactate levels (normal = ≤35mg/dl); and positive Gram's stains or agglutination, ELISA, or counterimmunoelectrophoresis (CIE) tests or cultures help differentiate CSF lymphocytosis associated with bacterial meningitis from that occurring with viral meningitis.

Neisseria meningitidis, Streptococcus pneumoniae, and gram-negative bacteria are the commonest bacterial causes of meningitis in adults. The sensitivity of the Gram's stain is 80 percent. Since *Hemophilus influenzae* and *N. meningitidis* may not survive preculture storage in the refrigerator, the CSF should be cultured as soon as possible. Up to 20 percent of cases of bacterial meningitis may be culture-negative because of a low concentration of organisms, prior antibiotic therapy, or a delay in culturing after the tap. Dead organisms (e.g., due to prior antibiotic therapy) can be detected by procedures dependent on the presence of antigen, such as agglutination (sensitivity, 70–90 percent), counterimmunoelectrophoresis (CIE) (sensitivity, 50–90 percent), and ELISA tests (sensitivity, 80–95 percent). Antibiotic therapy usually results in resolution of fever, neck pain and stiffness, and other symptoms within 72 h.

B. Spirochetal Meningitis

1. Borrelia burgdorferi (Lyme Disease)   Following the bite of an ixodid tick in summer or fall, an annular, slightly elevated, erythematous skin lesion develops at the bite site within 2 to 3 weeks. This lesion may expand, and secondary, smaller satellite ring lesions may occur. Four weeks (range, 0–10 weeks) after the onset of the rash, severe-to-mild headache, nausea, vomiting, and photophobia occur. Neck pain and stiffness are mild and are intensified by flexion and other movements. Kernig's and Brudzinski's signs are usually negative. CSF counts of 15 to 700 cells/mm^3 occur with 40 to 100 percent lymphocytosis. Glucose values are usually normal but may be depressed (range, 33–61 mg/dl), and protein values are normal or high (range, 8–400 md/dl). Meningitis may be accompanied by mild encephalitic symptoms such as somnolence, insomnia, irritability, disorders of memory and concentration, and emotional lability. Facial palsy on one or both sides may occur in up to 50 percent of cases, and peripheral sensory or motor radiculopathy in up to 32 percent. The diagnosis can be supported by an elevated titer detected on an ELISA or an indirect immunofluorescence antibody assay for *B. burgdorferi*. Meningitis may occur in patients without a history of a rash and in patients treated for Lyme disease with oral antibiotics weeks or months before.

2. Treponema Pallidum Syphilitic meningitis may present with headache, nausea, vomiting, neck pain and stiffness, and fever. Visual blurring and sensorineural hearing loss may be present. The neck is painful and stiff on flexion. The CSF demonstrates a lymphocytic pleocytosis, a low or normal glucose level, oligoclonal bands, an elevated protein level, positive CSF Venereal Disease Research Laboratory (VDRL) and fluorescent treponomal antibody absorption (FTA-ABS) tests, and negative cultures. Meningovascular syphilis may also occur in association with meningitis, leading to focal signs such as hemiparesis. Focal neurologic dysfunction is often reversible with high-dose intravenous penicillin therapy. An increased frequency and severity of neurosyphilis occur in AIDS.

3. Leptospirosis Patients may have a lymphocytic meningitis in association with fever, jaundice, bilirubinuria, proteinuria, cylindruria, and a rising creatinine level. These findings are rapidly reversible with intravenous penicillin. The diagnosis can be confirmed serologically and is based on clinical symptoms, signs, and a history of exposure to animal-urine-contaminated water.

C. Acute Viral Meningitis This illness begins over a period of several hours with a progressively severe headache, fever to 102°F, generalized myalgias, photophobia, pain on eye movement, and posterior aching neck pain and stiffness that is intensified by neck flexion. Occurrence in the summer or early fall is suggestive of an enteroviral infection. Frequent throat, stool, of CSF isolates include echoviruses 9, 4, 6, 11, 18, and 33 and Coxsackieviruses A9 and B4. Childhood diseases such as mumps,

measles, and varicella may rarely cause a similar aseptic meningitis syndrome. Herpes simplex types 1 and 2, adenoviruses, herpes zoster, hepatitis viruses, Epstein-Barr virus, and some arboviruses also cause a small number of cases. Lymphocytic choriomeningitis virus infection is associated with contact with mice and hamsters and should be suspected in cases occurring during the winter. The CSF in viral meningitis usually shows a pleocytosis with total counts less than 1000 cells/mm^3. During the first 12 h after onset, the differential count may reveal a predominance of neutrophils. This changes rapidly, and a repeat tap 12 h later will demonstrate over 55 percent of the cells to be lymphocytes. In doubtful cases, use of this repeat tap strategy will aid in establishing the diagnosis. The CSF glucose level may be depressed in fewer than 5 percent of cases of viral meningitis (mumps, herpes simplex, herpes zoster, lymphocytic choriomeningitis, and echoviruses are agents associated with low CSF glucose values). All bacterial cultures are negative. The association of pleocytosis (lymphocytic predominance) and a low CSF sugar (≤40 mg/dL or 50 percent of the blood sugar obtained simultaneously) may be caused by a partially treated bacterial infection and by tuberculous, fungal, spirochetal, drug-induced, lupus-associated, or neoplastic meningitis. The diagnosis of a specific viral infectious agent is dependent on viral isolation from throat washings, urine, stool, or CSF. In some cases, serologic diagnosis using acute and convalescent sera establishes the etiologic agent, but long after the patient has recovered. The exact cause of up to 70 percent of cases of aseptic meningitis remains unknown after diagnostic workup. Most patients recover completely within 2 weeks without sequelae or recurrent attacks. No specific therapy for viral meningitis is effective, except in the case of herpes viral infections, where acyclovir may be of benefit.

D. Drug-Related Meningitis There is an acute onset of allergic symptoms, such as pruritus, conjunctival injection, facial swelling, fever, chills, and myalgias. Headache, neck pain and stiffness, nausea, vomiting, and photophobia accompany the allergic manifestations. These signs and symptoms usually develop within hours of drug ingestion. The CSF cell count may range from 10 to 700 cells/mm^3, and the differential may reveal a preponderance of lymphocytes or neutrophils. CSF protein elevation may occur, but the glucose level usually remains normal. This disorder occurs in a very small percentage of patients taking the offending drug. It tends to occur in women with autoimmune or collagen vascular disorders, but it may develop in patients without a predisposing disorder. Drugs capable of causing drug-related meningitis include trimethoprim, ibuprofen, tolmetin, sulindac, azathioprine, penicillin, isoniazid, paraaminosalicylic acid, sulfonamides, and phenazopyridine.

E. Amebic Meningoencephalitis There is a rapid onset of fever, headache, myalgias, and posterior neck pain and stiffness. Infection follows 5 to 7 days after swimming in a freshwater lake, pond, or swimming pool. Some patients have aberrations of smell and taste due to invasion of the olfactory nerves by the causative organism, *Naegleria fowleri*. Myocarditis is a common associated finding. The CSF shows an increased number of polymorphonuclear leukocytes and a low sugar level. *Naegleria* organisms may be identified as highly motile trophozoites in the counting chamber. Amphotericin B is the most useful drug for this disease, but even with optimum therapy, the mortality is high.

2. SUBARACHNOID HEMORRHAGE

A. Aneurysmal Leakage or Rupture

1. Sentinel Headache   There is a sudden onset of a very severe unilateral (33 percent of cases) or focal (73 percent) headache, or facial or orbital pain. The pain is usually disabling and unlike anything the patient has ever experienced. In one series, it was occipital in 31 percent of cases, frontal in 26 percent, and retro-orbital in 14 percent. The pain may persist for only several hours or up to 14 days. Associated symptoms include nausea and vomiting (19 percent), meningismus and posterior neck pain (35 percent), syncope or brief coma (26 percent), photophobia and/or visual blurring (17 percent), and motor or sensory symptoms (20 percent). Since sentinel bleeds are usually minor, and CT scans are falsely negative in up to 55 percent of cases, a CT study cannot exclude a sentinel bleed. Lumbar puncture will usually reveal evidence of xanthochromia and red blood cells within hours of onset, and the former may persist for 30 days. The sensitivity of lumbar puncture is nearly 100 percent. Other findings include an elevated CSF protein level and a normal or low glucose level. Cerebral angiography will usually demonstrate an aneurysm or an arteriovenous malformation.

Surgical clipping of the aneurysm and administration of nimodipine prevents further bleeding and spasm-induced cerebral infarction, respectively. A sentinel bleed may occur in 30 to 60 percent of cases of aneurysm prior to major rupture.

2. Major Subarachnoid Hemorrhage due to Aneurysmal Rupture   Pain in one region or over the entire head begins abruptly. One patient experienced it while swinging a golf club, another while squatting to feed his dog. It has been described as being ''like a hammer blow to the head,'' ''tremendous,'' ''awful,'' ''bursting,'' ''crushing,'' and ''unbearable.'' In 30 percent of cases, the headache may be lateralized (frontal or frontoparietal) and associated with ipsilateral rupture of carotid-posterior communicating or middle cerebral aneurysms. Bilateral headache may be associated with rupture of anterior communicating aneurysms. Pain may begin in the occipital region or upper posterior neck and radiate frontally. Meningismus, with neck stiffness and pain on movement, occurs in most cases and is associated with nausea, vomiting, photophobia, visual blurring, and sometimes diplopia. Syncope at the onset may occur in 20 percent of cases, and grand mal seizures in a similar percentage. After an initial period of clarity, somnolence and lethargy occur, and progression to stupor or coma may occur during the first 48 h. More alert patients may be disoriented and demonstrate memory and judgment abnormalities. Pain in the low back and in a sciatic distribution in one or both legs occurs in a small percentage of cases.

Physical examination may reveal an alert, confused, or semistuporous patient who lies still with his or her eyelids closed. The neck is stiff and painful to passive or voluntary flexion. Dysphasia may occur, and fundoscopic examination may reveal subhyaloid hemorrhages fanning outward from the optic nerve. Such hemorrhages occur with rupture of carotid or anterior communicating artery aneurysms. Papilledema may occur in up to 10 percent of cases, as may bitemporal or homonymous field defects. Focal neurologic abnormalities such as hemiparesis, aphasia, bilateral blindness, or painful ophthalmoplegia may occur, depending on the location of the aneurysm. An increased incidence of ruptured intracranial aneurysm occurs in patients with coarctation of the aorta, polycystic renal disease, fibromuscular dysplasia, Marfan's syndrome, Ehlers-Danlos syndrome, and pseudoxanthoma elasticum. Increasing age, female sex, and hypertension are major risk factors for aneurysmal rupture. The diagnosis of intracranial subarachnoid hemorrhage after aneurysmal rupture may be confirmed by a CT scan or MRI. The distribution of blood within intracranial cisterns may localize the site of the aneurysm. Blood in the cistern of the lamina terminalis and the anterior interhemispheric fissure or a septum pellucidum hematoma are frequently indicative of an anterior communicating aneurysm. Angiography will reveal the aneurysm and spasm of vessels distal or adjacent to it. Localization of blood in the cisterns and fissures and the angiographic distribution of spasm have been used to localize and explore small aneurysms not visible by angiography. Administration of nimodipine to prevent spasm-related ischemic infarction and early surgical clipping of the aneurysm to prevent further bleeding constitute an approach likely to produce optimum mortality and morbidity statistics.

B. Spinal Subarachnoid Hemorrhage and Other Causes
Spinal subarachnoid hemorrhage may cause 1 percent of cases of spontaneous subarachnoid bleeding. Blood introduced at any site in the subarachnoid space may give rise to headache, stiffness, and posterior neck pain that is intensified by forward flexion.

Spinal subarachnoid bleeding may present with severe posterior neck, back, chest, or rectal pain of abrupt onset. The pain may radiate to the legs, arms, or loins and abdomen, depending on the site of the bleeding lesion. These cases may present a confusing initial picture, and the diagnosis may be missed until enough blood migrates cephalad to produce headache, meningismus, irritability, stupor, and diplopia (related to abducens parcsis). With lesions located in the lumbar area, sciatic pain, weakness, paresthesias and patchy sensory losses in the legs, and urinary retention may occur. A spinal arteriovenous malformation; spinal artery aneurysm; spinal tumor (ependymoma); vasculitis or coagulopathy; and, rarely, a vertebral artcry dissection may cause spinal subarachnoid bleeding. Specific lesions can be detected by MRI of the spinal canal.

Other relatively frequent causes of intracranial subarachnoid hemorrhage include arteriovenous malformations and anticoagulant drugs. While many episodes of bleeding resulting from these causes tend to be milder than those accompanying aneurysmal rupture, severe hemorrhage may occur, leading to death or permanent impairment. The less common causes of spontaneous subarachnoid hemorrhage include

1. Spinal subarachnoid hemorrhage
2. Leakage from an arteriovenous malformation
3. Infection-related
   A. Mycotic aneurysm (endocarditis)
   B. Brain abscess
   C. Meningitis (tuberculous, anthrax, syphilitic, or herpes simplex virus)
4. Primary or secondary intracranial tumors
5. Thrombocytopenia or other coagulopathy
6. Intracranial venous occlusion
7. Vasculitis
8. Severe hypertension
9. Rupture of an atherosclerotic vessel

3. MENINGISMUS (MENINGISM)

This disorder mimics infectious meningitis. Fever is associated with headache and aching posterior neck pain and stiffness. Kernig's and/or Brudzinski's signs may or may not be present. Symptoms and signs are so similar to those of meningitis that lumbar puncture is performed. By a strict definition of meningismus, the CSF should be normal. Current literature has also used the term to include cases of aseptic noninfectious meningitis (e.g., paramen-ingeal reactions and meningeal inflammation, secondary to the release of tumor or cyst material into the CSF, or immunological disorders).

Infectious diseases associated with meningismus include acute pyelonephritis, pneumonia, and gastrointes-tinal infections (e.g., typhoid fever). Pyelonephritis may cause fever; headache; and lumbar, interscapular, and neck pain and tenderness. Urinalysis reveals proteinuria and pyuria, and the CSF is normal. Similar neck pain, tenderness, and stiffness may occur with an acute pneumonitis and acute pulmonary histoplasmosis (10–15 percent of cases). Other disorders in which meningism with normal spinal fluid may occur include acute toxoplasmosis, brain abscess, leptospirosis, delirium tremens, and the toxic shock syndrome. Conversely, meningismus with normal cerebrospinal fluid has been reported in up to 3 percent of pediatric patients who were subsequently proven to have bacterial meningitis by culture of their CSF. Meningismus with normal spinal fluid has also occurred in adults with meningococcal meningitis, proven by CSF cultures.

Other disorders may cause meningismus in association with an increased CSF cell count and protein. These disorders include central nervous system tumors (e.g., craniopharyngioma), epidermoid cysts, Sjögren's syndrome, brain abscess with sterile CSF, and secondary syphilis.

4. CERVICAL DISC DEGENERATION

Aching unilateral or bilateral posterior neck pain with shoulder, upper arm, scapular, and/or pectoral radiation may be due to disc degeneration without herniation. Metrizamide myelography and CT scanning, and surface-coil MRI studies are usually normal. Anatomic studies have documented sinuvertebral nerve innervation of cervical discs. Provocative (injection of contrast) discography and analgesic (injection of bupivacaine or lidocaine) discography and anterior spinal fusion surgery for discogenic pain relief have incriminated the abnormal cervical disc as a source of neck pain. Controversy currently surrounds this concept, and many centers do not use discography. Pain relief after discectomy and fusion supports the concept of discogenic neck and shoulder pain.

5. CERVICAL DISC HERNIATION AND RADICULOPATHY

Thcrc may be an abrupt onset of severe posterior neck, shoulder, scapula, and arm pain following neck trauma or without a provoking event. The neck, shoulder, and scapula pain is severe, aching, and associated with diffuse or focal tenderness of neck and shoulder girdle muscles. Neck rotation to the painful side, coughing, sneezing, straining, or jarring may provoke lancinating electric-like pain that radiates down the arm into the hand. Background aching arm discomfort may become continuous. Spurling's maneuver (compression of the top of the head with the neck hyperextended and rotated to the pain-free side) elicits lancinating shoulder and arm pain. Abduction of the affected arm by placing the forearm on the top of the head often relieves the pain.

Pain radiation into the forearm and hand has poor localizing value for identifying the involved root, but paresthesias and hypoesthesia are reliable for this purpose. Ninety percent of cervical radiculopathies involve C7 (70 percent) and C6 (20 percent), and the remainder C5 and C8 (10 percent). The location of finger paresthesias and hypoesthesia, motor weakness, and reflex losses helps identify the involved level. A C7 lesion causes neck, shoulder, posterolateral arm, and hand pain. Paresthesias and hypoesthesias involve the index and middle fingers, and weakness of forearm (triceps) and wrist (extensor carpi ulnaris and radialis) extension occurs. The triceps jerk is depressed or absent. A C6 root lesion may cause posterior, lateral, medial, or anterior arm pain and paresthesias and hypoesthesia of the thumb and index finger. There is weakness of the biceps and brachialis muscles, and the biceps jerk may be impaired. The brachioradialis reflex may be absent or show inversion (the elbow fails to flex, but the fingers do).

C8 lesions cause radiating pain down the medial side of the arm and forearm into the ring and little fingers. These fingers have paresthesias and hypoesthesia, and there is weakness of the intrinsic muscles of the hands. All reflexes are normal. A C5 root lesion causes shoulder and proximal arm pain, with weakness of arm abduction (deltoid) and depression or loss of the biceps jerk. Hand pain and sensory abnormalities do not occur.

Imaging studies must be correlated with clinical symptoms and signs in order to determine whether the abnormalities detected by these sensitive techniques are responsible for the clinical findings. A rapid evolution in magnetic resonance imaging (MRI) is leading to the use of this modality instead of invasive techniques, such as myelography or CT-augmented myelography, for the initial evaluation of patients with neck pain and radiculopathy. Surface-coil MRI has replaced whole-body-coil MRI for cervical spine studies. Recent advances include limited flip-angle-gradient echo imaging and three-dimensional gradient-recalled MRI. The latter allows for acquisition of thin-section images without prolonged acquisition times. At centers where advanced MRI technology is not available, CT-augmented metrizamide myelography will visualize herniated soft discs, hard discs, and regions of foraminal stenosis, as well as MRI. Relief of pain and neurologic abnormalities may follow conservative therapy with rest, use of a collar and traction, epidural steroid injections, and administration of muscle relaxants and analgesics. Persistent disabling pain or progressive neurologic dysfunction requires root decompression by anterior discectomy and/or foraminotomy. Patients with an acute onset usually have single root involvement, but in more persistent or recurrent cases, the incidence of multiple root compression may vary from 9 to 37 percent.

6. DISORDERS MIMICKING CERVICAL DISC HERNIATION WITH RADICULOPATHY

A. Epidural Abscess There is an abrupt onset of aching posterior neck pain and stiffness, exacerbated by neck flexion or rotation. Diffuse aching pain and/or paresthesias and numbness may occur in one or both arms and hands. Fever, chills, and diaphoresis occur in 70 percent of cases. Since an underlying osteomyelitis is the cause in most cases (rare cases occur by direct metastatic spread from a skin infection or other site), a history of intermittent or constant posterior neck ache may be present.

Electric-like pains may radiate into one or both arms. Finger and forearm hypoesthesia and paresthesias indicate multiple root involvement. Paresthesias may occur in both legs and feet, and severe weakness of the legs may prevent walking. Arm paresis and sphincter disturbances may soon follow. Systemic toxicity may be marked or minimal.

Neck stiffness, pain on movement, and localized cervical spine tenderness may be present. Quadriparesis occurs as the abscess increases in size. Sensory losses in the arms may be patchy, but a definite sensory level may develop at the upper chest level or below. The reflexes may be hyperactive, and Babinski's signs may occur bilaterally. Leukocytosis and an elevated sedimentation rate are frequent findings. The spinal fluid contains an elevated protein level (120–1000 mg/dl), and up to 200 white blood cells/mm^3 (50–60 percent neutrophils). The glucose level is usually normal, but it may be low. The diagnosis may be confirmed by a myelogram, a CT-augmented myelogram, or MRI. T2-weighted images show the abscess clearly as a high-intensity collection posterior to the cord. Plain CT scans without subarachnoid contrast are too insensitive for reliable exclusion of this diagnosis. Therapy with intravenous antibiotics is required, as is surgical decompression of the spinal cord, if progressive neurologic symptoms and signs are present. Most cases are caused by *Staphylococcus aureus*, but *Pseudomonas* species (e.g., in drug addicts) and infections produced by gram-negative rods (e.g., arising in urinary tract infections) and streptococcal species also occur. Plain radiographs, as well as MRI, may demonstrate an associated osteomyelitis in the vertebral bodies adjacent to the abscess.

B. Cervical Osteomyelitis with Pathologic Fracture Midline posterior cervical ache and fever may be present intermittently or constantly for weeks or months. There may be a sudden increase in the intensity of the posterior neck pain, followed by the development of paresthesias and weakness of the arms and legs and a partial or complete sensory level. Inability to urinate or defecate, or complete incontinence, may follow. Plain radiographs will demonstrate destruction of one or more cervical vertebral bodies and discs. A resultant kyphosis and spinal instability causes cord compression, which can be relieved by prompt surgical decompression with bone grafting to prevent subsequent subluxation. Cases of cervical osteomyelitis have followed penetrating trauma and esophageal perforation, dental extraction, pharyngeal resection, and lodging of foreign bodies in the hypopharynx. Metastatic spread from distant skin, urinary tract, or pulmonary sites to the spine also occurs.

C. Epidural Hematoma There is a sudden onset of posterior neck pain and sometimes torticollis, tenderness, and stiffness. Electric-like pains, aching, and paresthesias may occur in one or both arms. The paresthesias are often diffuse, indicating involvement of more than a single root. Tetraparesis and a partial or complete sensory level may develop rapidly. Myelography reveals a cervical extradural mass and a partial block. A single case of epidural hematoma studied by MRI has been reported. The hematoma was easily demonstrated. The signal characteristics fit those of other types of hematomas. Patients with an epidural hematoma are usually afebrile and nontoxic. There is no evidence of vertebral osteomyelitis, and there are no consistent changes in the neutrophil count or sedimentation rate. This disorder occurs in patients on anticoagulants and with bleeding disorders (e.g., liver disease). It also occurs with ankylosing spondylitis, hypertension, and atherosclerosis; and after trauma. Prompt decompression of the spinal cord is necessary to preserve neurologic function.

D. Cervical Transverse Myelitis Posterior neck pain and tenderness occur, and fever may be present (50 percent of cases). Radicular pain and paresthesias may occur in the arms and hands; and paresthesias, sensory loss, and weakness of the legs soon follow. Flaccid weakness of the arms and hands develops, as do sphincter disturbances. In severe cases, a sensory level may be detected in the upper chest or at a lower level. The paresis is at first flaccid, but it then becomes spastic. The clinical picture of transverse myelitis may be confused with disc herniation, epidural abscess, or hematoma. CT or MRI will exclude an epidural mass and may detect cord enlargement due to the myelitis. This disorder is usually idiopathic but may be associated with bacterial and viral infections, multiple sclerosis, lymphomas, syphilis, Lyme disease, and postimmunization reactions involving the nervous system. The development of bilateral visual loss with central scotoma may accompany the myelitis and represent an idiopathic syndrome or a manifestation of multiple sclerosis. Spontaneous improvement may occur in up to 50 percent of cases of transverse myelitis, but there is no effective therapy.

E. Pachymeningitis Cervicalis Hypertrophica Aching pain occurs in the posterior neck and arm, associated with numbness and weakness of the affected arm and shoulder. Arm and hand paresthesias and hypoesthesia involving three or more cervical roots are usually present, and bilateral symptoms and signs eventually develop. Plain cervical radiographs may be normal, but a myelogram may demonstrate lack of filling of the dural sleeves about several cervical roots. Progression to spinal cord compression, with paresthesias and weakness in all extremities, may occur in advanced cases. CT-augmented myelography may reveal a thickened dura and a dorsal filling defect in the spinal canal. The CSF shows an elevated protein level but a normal sugar concentration and cell count. Surgical exploration reveals thickening of the spinal cord dura and nerve root sheaths. Resection of fibrous tissue and/or thickened dura provides prolonged remission of symptoms and improvement of neurologic abnormalities. This disorder may be caused by *Treponema pallidum, M. tuberculosis, Petriellidium boydii* (a fungus), *N. meningitidis* or *S. aureus* infections, trauma, injection of intrathecal steroids, myelography, spinal anesthesia, rheumatoid arthritis, and granulomatous sinusitis or mastoiditis. Involvement of three or more roots in association with a myelopathy suggests this disorder.

F. Lyme Disease Low-grade recurrent meningitis with headache and mild neck pain may occur. Associated arm pain; paresthesias; and focal weakness involving two or more cervical, and sometimes lumbar, roots, may develop. Cranial radiculopathy may cause unilateral or bilateral facial paralysis. Some, but not all, cases begin with the characteristic skin rash, erythema chronicum migrans. After several months, joint pain and swelling may accompany the neurological manifestations. Antibody levels to *B. burgdorferi* in serum can be detected by an IFA or ELISA method. The meningoencephalitis and radiculitis respond to high-dose intravenous penicillin therapy (20 million U/day for 10 days).

G. Myofascial Syndrome and Referred Arm Pain Aching pain occurs in the posterior neck and shoulder on one side and radiates down the ipsilateral arm. Persistent paresthesias may be felt in the lower arm and hand. Rotation of the head to the painful side or direct pressure over a posterior neck or shoulder trigger point precipitates arm pain and paresthesias. The production of arm symptoms on neck rotation mimics disc herniation. Plain radiographs and MRI or metrizamide CT scans are negative. Lidocaine injection of the trigger point eliminates the neck pain and allows neck rotation without producing arm symptoms.

H. Osteoarthritis of the Spine with Foraminal Narrowing Deep, aching posterior neck pain, increased by neck rotation, occurs. Pain and paresthesias may radiate down the arm in a specific dermatomal distribution. Diffuse or focal trigger-point tenderness may be present in the posterior neck on the affected side. Arm weakness and paresthesias and hypoesthesia of specific fingers and reflex loss may occur. Foraminal narrowing may be caused by osteophytes and/or subluxation of vertebral zygapophyseal joints. The diagnosis can be confirmed by an MRI or a CT study of the spine. Failure to respond to conservative therapy requires surgical decompression of the affected nerve root foramen.

7. ACUTE NECK OR CHEST WALL INFECTIONS AND REFERRED POSTERIOR NECK PAIN

A. Retropharyngeal Abscess Posterior neck pain and stiffness are associated with fever, sore throat, hoarseness, dysphagia, stridor, dyspnea, and regurgitation after eating or drinking. The neck pain may be intensified by swallowing. Some patients present initially with only posterior shoulder and neck pain exacerbated by swallowing, low-grade fever, and leukocytosis. A midline or asymmetrical pharyngeal mass may be visible and/or palpable. As the disorder progresses, breathing becomes noisy and more difficult because of progressing upper airway obstruction. A lateral neck x-ray reveals a soft tissue prevertebral space greater than 7 mm due to the abscess. Abscess drainage and intravenous administration of antibiotics relieve all symptoms. A retropharyngeal abscess may be caused by iatrogenic trauma (e.g., endoscopy, suctioning, nasogastric tube, or endotracheal intubation); an impaled pharyngeal foreign body (e.g., fish or chicken bone); esophageal rupture; penetrating neck trauma; infected retropharyngeal nodes draining a septic focus in the nasopharynx, sinuses, or ears; or spread from a contiguous lateral pharyngeal or prevertebral space infection (secondary to vertebral osteomyelitis).

B. Anterior Upper Chest Wall Abscess with Referred Neck Pain Posterior neck pain and stiffness, intensified by neck movement and fever, may accompany or precede the appearance of an anterior upper chest wall abscess. Within 2 to 3 days of onset of neck pain, the abscess appears as a red, tender, fluctuant mass over the region of the first or second rib anteriorly. Local drainage and intravenous antibiotics lead to rapid resolution of neck symptoms.

C. Cervical Osteomyelitis Aching, dull neck pain, intensified by movement and associated with low-grade fever and chilliness, may be due to cervical osteomyelitis. Spine stiffness and midline tenderness are usually present. An elevated temperature and leukocytosis are present in only 40 to 60 percent of cases. The sedimentation rate is elevated in up to 90 percent and is a useful screening test. Plain radiographs and CT scans of the neck may be normal for several weeks, but a radionuclide scan or MRI can demonstrate abnormalities within 7 to 10 days. There is an excellent response of neck pain and tenderness to a 4- to 6-week course of intravenous antibiotics. This diag-

nosis is frequently missed because of confusion with cervical osteoarthritis or a myofascial syndrome. Neck pain, associated with spine tenderness, fever, chilliness, torticollis, leukocytosis, and/or an elevated sedimentation rate, requires exclusion of osteomyelitis before treatment with anti-inflammatory drugs or corticosteroids is begun.

8. CALCIUM DEPOSITION

A. Calcific Tendinitis of the Longus Colli Muscle There is an abrupt onset of severe posterior neck pain and stiffness. Sore throat; low-grade fever; and, rarely, dyspnea may occur. Neck movement in any direction, jarring, or swallowing intensifies the posterior neck pain. Odynophagia may become so severe that swallowing becomes impossible. Leukocytosis and an elevated sedimentation rate may occur. Symptoms may begin after activities such as gymnastics or moving furniture, after a whiplash injury, or spontaneously. A lateral cervical spine radiograph will demonstrate soft tissue retropharyngeal swelling and amorphous deposits of calcium in the longus colli tendon inferior to the arch of C1 and anterior to the body of C2. These changes can also be visualized by a CT scan or MRI. Rapid relief can be obtained by the use of intravenous dexamethasone. Nonsteroidal anti-inflammatory drugs also provide effective therapy. This disorder may mimic the findings of a retropharyngeal abscess and has been confused with the latter and treated with antibiotics.

B. Crystal-Induced Neck Pain (Crowned Dens Syndrome) Acute severe posterior upper neck pain and stiffness occur and may be associated with knee and low back pain. Plain cervical radiographs of such patients may show calcium deposition about the odontoid. CT scans of the cervical spine show deposits of hydroxyapatite or calcium pyrophosphate dihydrate (CPPD) about the posterior and lateral aspects of the dens, forming a halo or crown-like configuration. CPPD crystals may be detected on analysis of synovial fluid obtained from a painful knee, and typical radiographic calcifications (chondrocalcinosis) of knee, shoulder, wrist, pubis, and other joints are often present. The neck pain resolves after treatment with nonsteroidal anti-inflammatory drugs (e.g., diclofenac). This syndrome presents a clinical picture similar to calcification of the tendon of the longus colli muscle, but the radiographic pattern of calcification is different in each disorder. Such deposits around the odontoid may persist or resorb spontaneously.

9. ATLANTOAXIAL SUBLUXATION

A. Rheumatoid Arthritis Subluxation of C1 on C2 occurs in up to 25 percent of patients with rheumatoid arthritis. Cervical involvement in this disease causes generalized aching posterior neck, shoulder, and occipital pain. Neck flexion, which increases the amount of subluxation, may intensify neck and shoulder pain. Localized spine tenderness and gibbus formation over C2 occur with neck flexion. Radicular pain and paresthesias may be present in one or both upper extremities, and these complaints may be exacerbated by neck flexion or hyperextension. Patients may complain that their head feels too heavy to hold up. Rapid progression to tetraparesis with a sensory level may occur after minor trauma or spontaneously. Spastic weakness, hyperreflexia, Babinski's signs, and incontinence may occur due to spinal cord compression. Vertebrobasilar insufficiency may also follow, with dizziness, drop attacks, dysarthria, dysphagia, ataxia, diplopia, and transient loss of vision.

The diagnosis can be confirmed by lateral cervical spine films taken with the neck in flexion and extension. Anterior or posterior subluxation may occur. Subluxation may be diagnosed if the distance between the anterior arch of the atlas and the odontoid exceeds 3 mm. MRI of the high cervical region will provide a clear demonstration of subluxation and will image soft tissue masses (pannus) adjacent to the odontoid and spinal cord. MRI appears to be superior to CT myelography for the evaluation of neck pain in patients with rheumatoid arthritis. Some patients with rheumatoid disease have neck pain secondary to zygapophyseal joint arthritis, and they may demonstrate subluxations at C2–C3 and/or C3–C4, or below. Cases with evidence of myelopathy or basilar artery compression require surgical fixation of C1 on C2 to prevent cord or brain stem injury.

B. Ankylosing Spondylitis Erosion of the odontoid or transverse ligament destruction may occur, allowing C1 subluxation on C2. Neck, occipital, and shoulder pain occur. Plain radiographs or MRI will demonstrate atlantoaxial subluxation. It is usually mild in this disorder.

C. Juvenile Rheumatoid Arthritis Bony fusion of the zygapophyseal joints and atlantoaxial subluxation may occur in association with neck pain, stiffness, and high cervical tenderness.

Patients with adult rheumatoid arthritis and neck pain may develop tetraplegia and respiratory insufficiency and die suddenly, due to brain stem compression by severe atlantoaxial subluxation.

10. NECK TRAUMA

A. Whiplash Injury Pain occurs in the posterior and sometimes the anterior neck after a motor vehicle accident. The pain may begin immediately or within 1 h (37 percent of cases), in 24 h (50 percent), or after 24 h (13 percent). Rear-end collisions (84 percent of cases) are more effective in producing this type of injury than are front or side impacts (56 percent). Front-seat (67 percent) are more likely than rear-seat passengers (48 percent) to

suffer neck pain, and use of a seat belt increases the frequency of cervical injury. Neck pain, stiffness, and tenderness are the major findings. Headaches, visual blurring, diplopia, inability to focus, tinnitus, and shoulder and interscapular pain also occur. Most cases are due to injury of the anterior or posterior neck muscles. More persistent cases may be due to cervical disc disruption, demonstrated by provocative and analgesic discography, zygapophyseal joint fractures imaged only by a CT scan, or disruption of posterior ligaments and traumatic zygapophyseal arthritis. The latter may be demonstrated by use of bupivacaine blocks of suspected zygapophyseal joints or medial branch blocks (the cervical spinal root branches innervating these joints). Rare cases of upper posterior neck and occipital pain and tenderness are due to traumatic compression of the C2 nerve root and ganglion between the laminae of the atlas and axis. Loss of skin sensation to pain and touch is present in the painful occipital area, and direct digital pressure over the C2 root increases the pain. Laminectomy and division of the C2 nerve root may be required for pain relief.

B. Fractures of the Cervical Spine Such fractures may be missed at a significant rate (26 percent false negatives) when the only cervical spine radiograph taken is a cross-table lateral. This view misses 73 percent of C7–T1 fractures. A five-view cervical spine series or a CT scan increases the sensitivity of detection of cervical spine fractures. A swimmer's view is useful for detecting C7–T1 fractures (87 percent sensitive), as is the CT scan (almost 100 percent sensitive). C1 fractures may also be easily missed on the cross-table lateral but are easily detected by a CT scan. Patients with persistent neck and head pain and tenderness after severe trauma should not be "cleared" of a cervical spine fracture until a full cervical spine series and/or a CT scan has been completed. Some patients without neck pain or tenderness may have significant cervical spine fractures and/or subluxations. In one series, 20 percent of patients with cervical spine fractures at C7–T1 had no neck pain or tenderness, casting doubt on the usefulness of neck pain and/or tenderness in an alert patient as a screening test for significant cervical spine injury.

Up to one-third of patients with nonfracture/subluxation-associated whiplash injuries may have persistent neck pain, tenderness, and stiffness 2 years after their accident. These patients may have cervical disc injuries and/or zygapophyseal joint arthritis or subluxation or ruptured posterior ligaments.

11. ACUTE MYOSITIS OF THE POSTERIOR NECK MUSCLES

Severe aching unilateral or bilateral posterior neck pain occurs on arising or gradually develops during the day. Attacks of sharp, excruciating neck and shoulder pain due to muscle spasm are superimposed on a background ache. These may be precipitated by a sudden neck movement, sneezing, or coughing. This paroxysm freezes the patient in one position until it abates spontaneously in 1 to 3 min. Torticollis may develop on the painful side with the neck hyperextended, rotated to the opposite side, and slightly flexed. This disorder may continue to disable the patient for 2 to 3 days, after which the aching pain and paroxysmal attacks spontaneously abate. Patients are fearful of examination and may have diffuse or focal areas of neck tenderness. Neck muscles show evidence of increased tension, which can most easily be palpated in the sternocleidomastoid and trapezius muscles. Heat, use of a soft cervical collar, muscle relaxants, and analgesics provide symptomatic relief. Cervical spine radiographs may show loss of the normal cervical lordosis but are otherwise negative. The leukocyte count and sedimentation rate are normal. Possible causes include minor neck trauma, an acute rotational strain, a cold draft, a viral infection, sleeping with the neck positioned in a peculiar position, or excessive use of neck or shoulder muscles in a job or athletic activity 1 to 2 days before onset. Some cases of this syndrome in older patients may be due to acute arthritis of one or more zygapophyseal joints or to degenerative changes in an intervertebral disc.

12. ACUTE OSTEOARTHRITIS

Pain in the posterior neck associated with vertebral or paraspinal tenderness and limitation of neck motion may be secondary to acute arthritis of one or more zygapophyseal joints. This can be confirmed by palpation of zygapophyseal joint tenderness and by relief after local joint injection with bupivacaine and methylprednisolone. Provocative and analgesic discography can be used to establish a diagnosis of acute posterior neck pain secondary to disc degeneration. In both these disorders, a CT scan or MRI may show minimal or no specific abnormalities of the involved structures.

13. ACUTE TORTICOLLIS

This disorder causes the head to be held rotated or flexed (antecollis) or hyperextended (retrocollis). The ipsilateral sternocleidomastoid may be in spasm. There is posterior neck pain, and the neck resists motion into a neutral position. Causes include the following:

1. Lateral pharyngeal and/or retropharyngeal space infections. Fever, posterior neck pain, torticollis, sore throat, stridor, dyspnea, and odynophagia occur. The neck pain may be intensified by swallowing or movement. A lateral space abscess can be palpated in the neck below the parotid gland, and a retro-

pharyngeal space infection can be visualized directly in the throat and palpated. A lateral neck x-ray will demonstrate a retropharyngeal mass. Both types of abscess can be imaged by a CT scan. Surgical drainage and intravenous antibiotics provide relief.

2. Cervical lymphadenitis in the anterior triangle of the neck may cause neck pain, fever, chills, and torticollis, relieved by antibiotic therapy.

3. Atlantoaxial rotatory fixation. This disorder may be caused by a blow to the neck or excessive voluntary neck rotation. The head is held in a "cock robin" position, with lateral neck flexion, rotation to the opposite side, and slight neck flexion, like a robin listening for a worm. Onset after neck rotation may begin abruptly with cervical pain, an audible click, and pain and paresthesias over the ipsilateral posterior scalp. Open-mouth odontoid views show asymmetrical atlantodental intervals. The rotatory fixation can be confirmed by a CT scan, and can be corrected if treated promptly with cervical traction.

4. Acute myositis. Excessive use, viral illness, exposure to a draft, or sleeping with the neck in cramped posture may precipitate this disorder.

5. Accessory nerve neuritis. The nerve is tender and inflamed, and it causes unilateral spasm of the sternocleidomastoid muscle. The torticollis is relieved by an anesthetic injection of the nerve.

6. Neurologic disorders such as a herniated cervical disc or syringomyelia, or a dystonic reaction after ingestion of a phenothiazine may cause torticollis.

7. Acute torticollis with neck pain may follow cerebellar tonsillar herniation about the brain stem in a patient with a cerebellar hemisphere mass (tumor or cyst). This may occur spontaneously or follow lumbar puncture. Failure to recognize this event can lead to rapid destructive compression of vital medullary structures.

8. Rare cases have been associated with zygapophyseal joint arthritis and with hyperthyroidism.

9. Severe torticollis, neck pain, and fever may result from a pyogenic or tuberculous osteomyelitis of the cervical spine. The diagnosis can be confirmed by plain cervical radiographs, a CT scan, or MRI with test sensitivity depending on the duration of symptoms. There is a good response to antimicrobial therapy.

10. Acute trauma causing vertebral fractures/subluxations or ligamentous disruption can cause posterior neck pain and torticollis.

14. OCCIPITAL MIGRAINE

Pain of a throbbing nature occurs in the occiput and posterior neck on one side. There may be mild localized tenderness of the scalp. Compression of the occipital artery may transiently relieve the pain. Anterior radiation of the pain to the temporal area or the nose and retro-orbital region may occur. Nausea and vomiting may be associated. Daily attacks can continue for days or weeks and then cease. Some patients have associated complaints such as visual scotoma and fortification spectra, shimmering, and scintillating scotomata; facial pains and paresthesias; and a clumsiness or heaviness of one leg and arm. Visual symptoms resolve within a half-hour, while the other complaints may last for hours and vary from day to day. Prophylactic therapy with beta receptor blockers or a calcium channel blocking drug may be effective.

15. OCCIPITAL NEURALGIA (SYNDROME OF THE GREATER OCCIPITAL NERVE)

Patients may experience unilateral constant posterior neck and occipital pain associated with scalp paresthesias and hypoesthesia. Pain may radiate anteriorly to the face and retro-orbital region. There may be severe tenderness over the occipital nerve when it is compressed against the skull posteriorly. Pain may be provoked by rotating the occiput toward the painful side or by hyperextending the neck. A subset of patients may have nasal stuffiness and lacrimation on the painful side during attacks of severe pain.

Occipital neuralgia may result from a whiplash injury to the ganglion and root of C2 or following a compressing blow over the occipital nerve. Degenerative arthritis of the atlantoaxial lateral joint may cause unilateral occipital neuralgia. Entrapment of the greater occipital nerve by lymphadenopathy or a vascular anomaly has also been associated with this disorder. Occupations involving neck hyperextension and rotation may cause damage to the C2 root by compressing it repeatedly between the laminae of the axis and atlas. Cases of recurrent occipital and neck pain following motor vehicle accidents or other trauma may sometimes be caused by posttraumatic migraine.

16. COITAL NECK AND HEAD PAIN

Severe neck and posterior head pain on one or both sides may begin explosively during sexual orgasm or in a preorgasmic period of sexual intercourse. The pain may cause transient nausea, vomiting, and anxiety; and it often makes continuation of the sexual act undesirable. The pain may persist for 24 h or longer, but mild cases resolve within minutes or hours. Attempts to have intercourse on subsequent days may cause recurrent pain or may be symptom-free. Alcohol, high altitude, and an unfamiliar partner increase the risk for coital neck and head pain. This disorder may mimic a sentinel subarachnoid hemorrhage, although neck stiffness, photophobia, and obtundation do not occur. Since a CT study is not sensitive enough to detect minor degrees of intracranial hemor-

rhage, a lumbar puncture may be required in cases with severe or prolonged symptoms, to exclude subarachnoid bleeding.

17. VERTEBRAL ARTERY DISORDERS

A. Vertebral Artery Dissection   There is an acute onset of severe unilateral posterior neck pain and/or occipital headache. Neck pain and stiffness may occur without headache. Other initial symptoms include vertigo and oscillopsia (20 percent of cases), and focal neurologic complaints (20 percent). Ischemic symptoms in a vertebrobasilar distribution occur in 76 percent of cases within 5 h to 14 days. Complete stroke is more common, but transient ischemic attacks also occur in up to 25 percent of patients. The most common neurologic presentation is that of a lateral medullary syndrome. This consists of the following: (1) pain, numbness, and hypoesthesia of the ipsilateral face (nerve V); (2) ataxia of limbs and gait (cerebellum and connections); (3) vertigo, nausea, and vomiting (vestibular nuclei and connections); (4) nystagmus, diplopia, and oscillopsia (vestibular nuclei and connections); (5) Horner's syndrome (descending sympathetic tract); (6) dysphagia, hoarseness, and vocal cord paralysis (nerves IX and X); (7) numbness of the ipsilateral arm, trunk, or leg (cuneate and gracile nuclei); and (8) hiccups. The lateral medullary syndrome may occur in isolation or in association with other neurologic findings such as hemiparesis, diplopia, syncope, ipsilateral facial paresis, and tinnitus (an add-on syndrome). Unusual cases may present with subarachnoid hemorrhage with head and neck pain, stiffness, and photophobia.

Severe cases may present with bilateral brain stem signs (basilar artery syndrome). These patients have quadriplegia, quadriparesis and often dysarthria, dysphagia, diplopia, visual loss, bilateral ataxia, and preserved sensation. Coma may develop initially or later in patients with a basilar artery occlusion. Rare cases presenting with a "locked-in" syndrome have been reported after neck manipulation. Vertebral artery dissection is demonstrable by angiography. Such studies may show an elongated, tapered, and/or irregular luminal stenosis; an aneurysm; an intimal flap; or an occlusion. The CT scan is often normal but may show evidence of cerebellar or occipital lobe infarction. Bilateral vertebral artery dissection and associated carotid dissection may occur. Hypertension, fibromuscular dysplasia, trauma, cystic medial necrosis, and chiropractic manipulation have been associated. Conservative therapy with heparin and warfarin leads to complete or good recovery in 85 percent of cases. The vessel may appear completely normal on repeat arteriography 4 to 6 months later.

B. Vertebral Artery Pseudoaneurysm   A painful unilateral posterolateral neck mass appears spontaneously or after blunt or penetrating trauma. Cases have been associated with chiropractic neck manipulation. The mass may be pulsatile, and a bruit and/or thrill may be detected by the patient and/or the physician. Headache in the ipsilateral occiput with anterior radiation may accompany the neck pain. Neurologic symptoms occur secondary to a mass effect or vascular insufficiency.

Patients may complain of dysphagia, arm and shoulder pain, and gait disturbances. A full-blown lateral or medial medullary syndrome may occur because of thrombosis or embolization of the vertebral or posterior inferior cerebellar arteries. CT or MRI will confirm the diagnosis. Angiography is required to identify the neck of the pseudoaneurysm and define the involvement of the vertebral and basilar arteries. Such cases have been successfully treated by occlusion of the aneurysmal neck by using detachable intravascular balloons.

NECK PAIN REFERENCES

Arthritis/Osteoarthritis—Zygapophyseal Joints

Alarcon GS, Reveille JD: Gouty arthritis of the axial skeleton including the sacroiliac joints. *Arch Intern Med* 147:2018–2019, 1987.

Bogduk N: Neck pain: An update. *Aust Fam Phys* 17(2):75–80, 1988.

Bogduk N, Marsland A: The cervical zygapophyseal joints as a source of neck pain. *Spine* 13(6):610–617, 1988.

Dvorak, J, Froehlich D, Penning L, et al: Functional radiographic diagnosis of the cervical spine: Flexion/extension. *Spine* 13(7):748–755, 1988.

Gore DR, Sepic SB, Gardner GM, et al: Neck pain: A long-term follow-up of 205 patients. *Spine* 12(1):1–5, 1987.

Hanly JG, Russell ML, Gladman DF: Psoriatic spondyloarthropathy: A long term prospective study. *Ann Rheum Dis* 47:386–393, 1988.

Moncur C, Williams HJ: Cervical spine management in patients with rheumatoid arthritis. *Phys Ther* 68(4):509–515, 1988.

Nose T, Egashira T, Enomoto T, et al: Ossification of the posterior longitudinal ligament: A clinico-radiological study of 74 cases. *J Neurol Neurosurg Psychiatry* 50:321–326, 1987.

Pettersson H, Larsson EM, Holtas S, et al: MR imaging of the cervical spine in rheumatoid arthritis. *AJNR* 9:573–577, 1988.

Semble EL, Elster AD, Loeser RF, et al: Magnetic resonance imaging of the craniovertebral junction in rheumatoid arthritis. *J Rheumatol* 15:1367–1375, 1988.

Zlatkin MB, Lander PH, Hadjipavlou AG, et al: Paget disease of the spine: CT with clinical correlation. *Radiology* 160:155–159, 1986.

Atlantoaxillary Rotatory Fixation

Fidler MW, de Lange J: Atlanto axial rotatory fixation: A cause of torticollis. *Clin Neurol Neurosurg* 81(2):114–118, 1979.

McClelland SJ, James RL, Jarenwattananon A, et al: Traumatic spondylolisthesis of the axis in a patient presenting with torticollis: A case report. *Clin Orthop* 218:195–200, 1987.

Van Holsbeeck EMA, Mackay NNS: Diagnosis of acute atlanto-axial rotatory fixation. *J Bone Joint Surg (Br)* 71B:90–91, 1989.

Carotid Dissection

Francis KR, Williams DP, Troost BT: Facial numbness and dysesthesia: New features of carotid artery dissection. *Arch Neurol* 44:345–346, 1987.

Kline LB, Vitek JJ, Raymon BC: Painful Horner's syndrome due to spontaneous carotid artery dissection. *Ophthalmology* 94:226–230, 1987.

Lepojarvi M, Tarkka M, Leinonen A, et al: Spontaneous dissection of the internal carotid artery. *Acta Chir Scand* 154:559–566, 1988.

Mokri B, Sundt TM Jr, Houser OW, et al: Spontaneous dissection of the cervical internal carotid artery. *Ann Neurol* 19:126–138, 1986.

Waespe W, Niesper J, Imhof H-G, et al: Lower cranial nerve palsies due to internal carotid dissection. *Stroke* 19:1561–1564, 1988.

Carotodynia

Blatchford SJ, Coulthard SW: Eagle's syndrome: An atypical cause of dysphonia. *Ear Nose Throat J* 68:48–51, 1989.

Lim RY: Carotodynia exposed: Hyoid bone syndrome. *South Med J* 80(4):444–446, 1987.

Wheeler DC, Calvey HD, Wicks ACB: A difficult pain in the neck. *Br Med J* 291:804–805, 1985.

Cervical and Thoracic Disc Disease—Surgical

Alberico AM, Sahni KS, Hall JA Jr, et al: High thoracic disc herniation. *Neurosurgery* 19(3):449–451, 1986.

Bernardo KL, Grubb RL, Coxe WS, et al: Anterior cervical disc herniation: Case report. *J Neurosurg* 69:134–136, 1988.

Bertalanffy H, Eggert H-R: Complications of anterior cervical discectomy without fusion in 450 consecutive patients. *Acta Neurochir (Wien)* 99:41–50, 1989.

Lesoin F, Biondi A, Jomin M: Foraminal cervical herniated disc treated by anterior discoforaminotomy. *Neurosurgery* 21(3):334–338, 1987.

Richaud J, Lazorthes Y, Verdie JC, et al: Chemonucleolysis for herniated cervical disc. *Acta Neurochir (Wien)* 91:116–119, 1988.

Smith DE, Godersky JC: Thoracic spondylosis: An unusual cause of myelopathy. *Neurosurgery* 20(4):589–593, 1987.

Cervical Disc Disease—Radiculopathy and Myelopathy

Bertalanffy H, Eggert H-R: Clinical long-term results of anterior discectomy without fusion for treatment of cervical radiculopathy and myelopathy: A follow-up of 164 cases. *Acta Neurochir (Wien)* 90:127–135, 1988.

Bogduk N, Windsor M, Inglis A: The innervation of the cervical intervertebral discs. *Spine* 13(1):2–8, 1988.

Herkowitz HN: The surgical management of cervical spondylotic radiculopathy and myelopathy. *Clin Orthop* 239:94–108, 1989.

Kiwerski J: Treatment of cervical canal stenosis by decompression and anterior fusion. *Arch Orthop Trauma Surg* 107:354–356, 1988.

Lestini WF, Wiesel SW: The pathogenesis of cervical spondylosis. *Clin Orthop* 239:69–93, 1989.

Manabe S. Tateishi A, Ohno T: Anterolateral uncoforaminotomy for cervical spondylotic myeloradiculopathy. *Acta Orthop Scand* 59(6):669–674, 1988.

Masaryk TJ, Modic MT, Geisinger MA, et al: Cervical myelopathy: A comparison of magnetic resonance and myelography. *J Comput Assist Tomogr* 10(2):184–194, 1986.

Schmidek HH: Cervical spondylosis. *Am Fam Physician* 33(5):89–99, 1986.

Uttley D, Monro P: Neurosurgery for cervical spondylosis. *Br J Hosp Med* 42(1):62–70, 1989.

Vassilouthis J, Kalovithouris A, Papandreou A, et al: The symptomatic incompetent cervical intervertebral disc. *Neurosurgery* 25(2):232–239, 1989.

Yu YL, Du Boulay GH, Stevens JM, et al: Computer-assisted myelography in cervical spondylotic myelopathy and radiculopathy: Clinical correlations and pathogenetic mechanisms. *Brain* 109:259–278, 1986.

Yu YL, Woo E, Huang CY: Cervical spondylotic myelopathy and radiculopathy. *Acta Neurol Scand* 75:367–373, 1987.

Cervical Epidural Abscess

Baker AS, Ojemann RG, Swartz MN, et al: Spinal epidural abscess. *N Engl J Med* 293(10):463–468, 1975.

Bouchez B, Arnott G, Delfosse JM: Acute spinal epidural abscess. *J Neurol* 231:343–344, 1985.

Buruma OJS, Craane H, Kunst MW: Vertebral osteomyelitis and epidural abscess due to mucormycosis. *Clin Neurol Neurosurg* 81(1):39–44, 1979.

Erntell M, Holtas S, Norlin K, et al: Magnetic resonance imaging in the diagnosis of spinal epidural abscess. *Scand J Infect Dis* 20:323–327, 1988.

Feldenzer JA, Waters DC, Knake JE, et al: Anterior cervical epidural abscess: The use of intraoperative spinal sonography. *Surg Neurol* 25:105–108, 1986.

Lasker BR, Harter DH: Cervical epidural abscess. *Neurology* 37:1747–1753, 1987.

Lownie SP, Ferguson GG: Spinal subdural empyema complicating cervical discography. *Spine* 14(12):1415–1417, 1989.

McGrath H Jr, McCormick C, Carey ME: Pyogenic cervical osteomyelitis presenting as a massive prevertebral abscess in a patient with rheumatoid arthritis. *Am J Med* 84:363–365, 1988.

Nagel MA, Taff IP, Cantos EL, et al: Spontaneous spinal epidural hematoma in a 7-year-old girl: Diagnostic value of magnetic resonance imaging. *Clin Neurol Neurosurg* 91(2):157–160, 1989.

Peterson JA, Paris P, Williams AC: Acute epidural abscess. *Am J Emerg Med* 5:287–290, 1987.

Cervical Osteomyelitis—Pyogenic

Bartal AD, Schiffer J, Heilbronn YD, et al: Anterior interbody fusion for cervical osteomyelitis: Reversal of quadriplegia after evacuation of epidural spinal abscess. *J Neurol Neurosurg Psychiatry* 35:133–136, 1972.

Craig JB: Cervical spine osteomyelitis with delayed onset tetraparesis after penetrating wounds of the neck: A report of 2 cases. *S Afr Med J* 69:197–199, 1986.

Guyer RD, Collier R, Stith WJ, et al: Discitis after discography. *Spine* 13(12):1352–1354, 1988.

Schwartz JG, Tio FO: Nocardial osteomyelitis: A case report and review of the literature. *Diagn Microbiol Infect Dis* 8:37–46, 1987.

Sinnott JT IV, Multhopp H, Leo J, et al: *Yersinia enterocolitica* causing spinal osteomyelitis and empyema in a nonimmunocompromised host. *South Med J* 82(3):399–400, 1989.

Stone JL, Cybulski GR, Rodriguez J, et al: Anterior cervical debridement and strut-grafting for osteomyelitis of the cervical spine. *J Neurosurg* 70:879–883, 1989.

Yang EC, Neuwirth MG: *Pseudomonas aeruginosa* as a causative agent of cervical osteomyelitis: Case report and review of the literature. *Clin Orthop* 231:229–233, 1988.

Cervical Pain—Review Articles

Gilbert R, Warfield CA: Evaluating and treating the patient with neck pain. *Hosp Pract* 22(8):223–232, 1987.

Goodman BW Jr: Neck pain. *Prim Care* 15(4):689–708, 1988.

MacRae DL: Head and neck pain in the elderly. *J Otolaryngol* 15(4):224–227, 1986.

Moskovich R: Neck pain in the elderly: Common causes and management. *Geriatrics* 43:65–92, 1988.

Payne R: Neck pain in the elderly: A management review: 1. *Geriatrics* 42:59–65, 1987; 2. *Geriatrics* 42:71–73, 1987.

Cervical Radiculopathy

Dillin W, Booth R, Cuckler J, et al: Cervical radiculopathy: A review. *Spine* 11(10):988–991, 1986.

Fast A, Parikh S, Marin EL: The shoulder abduction relief sign in cervical radiculopathy. *Arch Phys Med Rehabil* 70:402–403, 1989.

Grisoli F, Graziani N, Fabrizi AP, et al: Anterior discectomy without fusion for treatment of cervical lateral soft disc extrusion: A follow-up of 120 cases. *Neurosurgery* 24(6):853–859, 1989.

Herkowitz HN: A comparison of anterior cervical fusion, cervical laminectomy, and cervical laminoplasty for the surgical management of multiple level spondylotic radiculopathy. *Spine* 13(7):774–780, 1988.

Hunt WE, Miller CA: Management of cervical radiculopathy. *Clin Neurosurg* 33:485–502, 1986.

Katirji MB, Agrawal R, Kantra TA: The human cervical myotomes: An anatomical correlation between electromyography and CT/myelography. *Muscle Nerve* 11:1070–1073, 1988.

Makin GJV, Brown WF, Ebers GC: C7 radiculopathy: Importance of scapular winging in clinical diagnosis. *J Neurol Neurosurg Psychiatry* 49:640–644, 1986.

Massey EW: Hand weakness in elderly patients. *Postgrad Med* 85(4):59–60, 63–65, 70, 1989.

Quinn SF, Murtagh FR, Chatfield R, et al: CT-guided nerve root block and ablation. *AJR* 151:1213–1216, 1988.

Snyder GM, Bernhardt M: Anterior cervical fractional interspace decompression for treatment of cervical radiculopathy: A review of the first 66 cases. *Clin Orthop* 246:92–99, 1989.

Cervical Spinal Cord Tumors

Bradley WG Jr, Waluch V, Yadley RA, et al: Comparison of CT and MR in 400 patients with suspected disease of the brain and cervical spinal cord. *Radiology* 152:695–702, 1984.

Breuer AC, Kneisley LW, Fischer EG: Treatable extramedullary cord compression: Meningioma as a cause of Brown-Sequard syndrome. *Spine* 5(1):19–22, 1980.

Cooper PR, Epstein F: Radical resection of intramedullary spinal cord tumors in adults: Recent experience in 29 patients. *J Neurosurg* 63:492–499, 1985.

Copeman MC: Presenting symptoms of neoplastic spinal cord compression. *J Surg Oncol* 37:24–25, 1988.

Epstein JA, Marc JA, Hyman RA, et al: Total myelography in the evaluation of lumbar discs: With the presentation of three cases of thoracic neoplasms simulating nerve root lesions. *Spine* 4(2):121–128, 1979.

Garrido E, Stein BM: Microsurgical removal of intramedullary spinal cord tumors. *Surg Neurol* 7:215–219, 1977.

Grem JL, Burgess J, Trump DL: Clinical features and natural history of intramedullary spinal cord metastasis. *Cancer* 56:2305–2314, 1985.

Grob D, Loehr J: Osteoblastoma of the cervical spine: Case report. *Arch Orthop Trauma Surg* 108:179–181, 1989.

Hahn YS, McLone DG: Pain in children with spinal cord tumors. *Child's Brain* 11:36–46, 1984.

Heppner F, Ascher PW, Holzer P, et al: CO_2 laser surgery of intramedullary spinal cord tumors. *Lasers Surg Med* 7:180–183, 1987.

Levy WJ Jr, Bay J, Dohn D: Spinal cord meningioma. *J Neurosurg* 57:804–812, 1982.

Nicholas JJ, Christy WC: Spinal pain made worse by recumbency: A clue to spinal cord tumors. *Arch Phys Med Rehabil* 67:598–600, 1986.

Post MJD, Quencer RM, Green BA, et al: Intramedullary spinal cord metastases mainly of nonneurogenic origin. *AJR* 148:1015–1022, 1987.

Rawlings CE III, Giangaspero F, Burger PC, et al: Ependymomas: A clinico-pathologic study. *Surg Neurol* 29:271–281, 1988.

Sherk HH, Nolan JP Jr, Mooar PA: Treatment of tumors of the cervical spine. *Clin Orthop* 233:163–167, 1988.

Stein BM: Intramedullary spinal cord tumors. *Clin Neurosurg* 30:717–741, 1983.

Stern WE: Localization and diagnosis of spinal cord tumors. *Clin Neurosurg* 25:480–494, 1978.

Cervical Spine—Imaging Methods

Balériaux D, Deroover N, Hermanus N, et al: MRI of the spine. *Diagn Imag Clin Med* 55:66–71, 1986.

Chadduck WM, Flanigan S: Intraoperative ultrasound for spinal lesions. *Neurosurgery* 16(4):477–483, 1985.

Di Chiro G, Doppman JL, Dwyer AJ, et al: Tumors and arteriovenous malformations of the spinal cord: Assessment using MR. *Radiology* 156:689–697, 1985.

Kent DL, Larson EB: Magnetic resonance imaging of the brain and spine. *Ann Intern Med* 108:402–424, 1988.

Sherman JL, Barkovich AJ, Citrin CM: The MR appearance of syringomyelia: New observations. *AJR* 148:381–391, 1987.

Sze G, Krol G, Zimmerman RD, et al: Malignant extradural spinal tumors: MR imaging with Gd-DTPA. *Radiology* 167:217–223, 1988.

Cervical Spine Malformations

Eisenstat DDR, Bernstein M, Fleming JFR, et al: Chiari malformation in adults: A review of 40 cases. *Can J Neurol Sci* 13:221–228, 1986.

Herring JA: Klippel-Feil syndrome with neck pain. *J Pediatr Orthop* 9:343–346, 1989.

Cervical Osteomyelitis/Tuberculosis

Corea JR, Tamimi TM: Tuberculosis of the arch of the atlas. *Spine* 12(6):608–611, 1987.

Neal SL, Kearns MJ, Seelig JM, et al: Manifestations of Pott's disease in the head and neck. *Laryngoscope* 96:494–497, 1986.

Cervical Spine—Trauma

Bachulis BL, Long WB, Hynes GD, et al: Clinical indications for cervical spine radiographs in the traumatized patient. *Am J Surg* 153(5):473–478, 1987.

Balmaseda MT, Wunder JA, Gordon C, et al: Posttraumatic syringomyelia associated with heavy weightlifting exercises: Case report. *Arch Phys Med Rehabil* 69:970–972, 1988.

Barron MM: Cervical spine injury masquerading as a medical emergency. *Am J Emerg Med* 7:54–56, 1989.

Deans GT: Incidence and duration of neck pain among patients injured in car accidents. *Br Med J* 292:94–95, 1986.

Deans GT, Magalliard JN, Kerr M, et al: Neck sprain: A major cause of disability following car accidents. *Injury* 18:10–12, 1987.

Eckhardt WF, Doyle M, Woodward A, et al: Cervical spine fracture following a motor vehicle accident. *J Emerg Med* 6:179–183, 1988.

Gisbert VL, Hollerman JJ, Ney AL, et al: Incidence and diagnosis of C7–T1 fractures and subluxations in multiple-trauma patients: Evaluation of the advanced trauma life support guidelines. *Surgery* 106:702–709, 1989.

Kim KS, Rogers LF, Regenbogen V: Pitfalls in plain film diagnosis of cervical spine injuries: false positive interpretation. *Surg Neurol* 25:381–392, 1986.

Landells CD, Van Peteghem PK: Fractures of the atlas: Classification, treatment and morbidity. *Spine* 13:(5):450–452, 1988.

Maimaris C, Barnes MR, Allen MJ: ''Whiplash injuries'' of the neck: A retrospective study. *Injury* 19:393–396, 1988.

McNamara RM, O'Brien MC, Davidheiser S: Post-traumatic neck pain: A prospective and follow-up study. *Ann Emerg Med* 17:906–911, 1988.

Neifeld GL, Keene JG, Hevesy G, et al: Cervical injury in head trauma. *J Emerg Med* 6:203–207, 1988.

Pavlov H, Torg JS: Roentgen examination of cervical spine injuries in the athlete. *Clin Sports Med* 6(4):751–766, 1987.

Povlsen UJ, Kjaer L, Arlien-Søborg P: Locked-in syndrome following cervical manipulation. *Acta Neurol Scand* 76:486–488, 1987.

Ringenberg BJ, Fisher AK, Urdaneta LF, et al: Rational ordering of cervical spine radiographs following trauma. *Ann Emerg Med* 17:792–796, 1988.

Salomone JA III, Steele MT: An unusual presentation of bilateral facet dislocation of the cervical spine. *Ann Emerg Med* 16:1390–1393, 1987.

Swischuk LE: Neck pain after trauma. *Pediatr Emerg Care* 4(3):219–221, 1988.

Wertheim SB, Bohlman HH: Occipitocervical fusion. Indications, technique, and long-term results in thirteen patients. *J Bone Joint Surg* 69A(6):833–836, 1987.

Cervical Spondylosis and Radiculopathy—Imaging

Brown BM, Schwartz RH, Frank E, et al: Preoperative evaluation of cervical radiculopathy and myelopathy by surface-coil MR imaging. *AJR* 151:1205–1212, 1988.

Gammal TE, Mark EK, Brooks BS: MR imaging of Chiari II malformation. *AJR* 150:163–170, 1988.

Hedberg MC, Drayer BP, Flom RA, et al: Gradient echo (GRASS) MR imaging in cervical radiculopathy. *AJR* 150:683–689, 1988.

Hong C-Z, Lee S, Lum P: Cervical radiculopathy: Clinical, radiographic and EMG findings. *Orthop Rev* 15(7):433–439, 1986.

Larsson E-M, Holtas S, Cronqvist S, et al: Comparison of myelography, CT myelography and magnetic resonance imaging in cervical spondylosis and disk herniation. *Acta Radiol* 30(3):233–239, 1989.

Modic MT, Masaryk TJ, Mulopulos GP, et al: Cervical radiculopathy: Prospective evaluation with surface coil MR imaging, CT with metrizamide, and metrizamide myelography. *Radiology* 161:753–759, 1986.

Modic MT, Masaryk TJ, Ross JS, et al: Cervical radiculopathy: Value of oblique MR imaging. *Radiology* 163:227–231, 1987.

Modic MT, Ross JS, Masaryk TJ: Imaging of degenerative disease of the cervical spine. *Clin Orthop* 239:109–120, 1989.

Tsuruda JS, Norman D, Dillon W, et al: Three-dimensional gradient-recalled MR imaging as a screening tool for the diagnosis of cervical radiculopathy. *AJNR* 10:1263–1271, 1989.

———: Three-dimensional gradient-recalled MR imaging as a screening tool for the diagnosis of cervical radiculopathy. *AJR* 154:375–383, 1990.

Viikari-Juntura E, Raininko R, Videman T, et al: Evaluation of cervical disc degeneration with ultralow field MRI and discography. An experimental study on cadavers. *Spine* 14(6):616–619, 1989.

Yu YL, du Boulay GH, Stevens JM, et al: Computed tomography in cervical spondylotic myelopathy and radiculopathy: Visualisation of structures, myelographic comparison, cord measurements and clinical utility. *Neuroradiology* 28:221–236, 1986.

Epidural Spinal Cord Tumor—Metastatic

Bates DW, Reuler JB: Back pain and epidural spinal cord compression. *J Gen Intern Med* 3(2):191–197, 1988.

Ch'ien LT, Kalwinsky DK, Peterson G, et al: Metastatic epidural tumors in children. *Med Pediatr Oncol* 10:455–462, 1982.

Giannotta SL, Kindt GW: Metastatic spinal cord tumors. *Clin Neurosurg* 25:495–503, 1978.

Gilbert MR, Grossman SA: Incidence and nature of neurologic problems in patients with solid tumors. *Am J Med* 81(6):951–954, 1986.

Gilbert RW, Kim J-H, Posner JB: Epidural spinal cord compression from metastatic tumor: Diagnosis and treatment. *Ann Neurol* 3:40–51, 1978.

Kleinman WB, Kiernan HA, Michelsen WJ: Metastatic cancer of the spinal column. *Clin Orthop* 136:166–172, 1978.

Kostuik JP: Anterior spinal cord decompression for lesions of the thoracic and lumbar spine, techniques, new methods of internal fixation results. *Spine* 8(5):512–531, 1983.

Kuban DA, El-Mahdi AM, Sigfred SV, et al: Characteristics of spinal cord compression in adenocarcinoma of prostate. *Urology* 28(5):364–369, 1986.

Kuhlman JE, Fishman EK, Leichner PK. et al: Skeletal metastases from hepatoma: Frequency, distribution and radiographic features. *Radiology* 160:175–178, 1986.

Myles ST, MacRae ME: Benign osteoblastoma of the spine in childhood. *J Neurosurg* 68:884–888, 1988.

Nather A, Bose K: The results of decompression of cord or cauda equina compression from metastatic extradural tumors. *Clin Orthop* 169:103–108, 1982.

O'Neil J, Gardner V, Armstrong G: Treatment of tumors of the thoracic and lumbar spinal column. *Clin Orthop* 227:103–112, 1988.

Overby MC, Rothman AS: Anterolateral decompression for metastatic epidural spinal cord tumors. *J Neurosurg* 62:344–348, 1985.

Posner JB: Back pain and epidural spinal cord compression. *Med Clin North Am* 71(2):185–205, 1987.

Posner JB, Howieson J, Cvitkovic E: "Disappearing" spinal cord compression: Oncolytic effect of glucocorticoids (and other chemotherapeutic agents) on epidural metastases. *Ann Neurol* 2:409–413, 1977.

Rodriguez M, Dinapoli RP: Spinal cord compression with special reference to metastatic epidural tumors. *Mayo Clin Proc* 55:442–448, 1980.

Schaberg J, Gainor BJ: A profile of metastatic carcinoma of the spine. *Spine* 10(1):19–20, 1985.

Schulz U, Bamberg M: Relationship between curative radiation therapy of paravertebral tumors and the incidence of radiation myelitis. *Tumori* 64:305–312, 1978.

Scully RE (ed): Case 52-1985, Case records of the Massachusetts General Hospital. *N Engl J Med* 313(26):1646–56, 1985.

Sherman RMP, Waddell JP: Laminectomy for metastatic epidural spinal cord tumors: Posterior stabilization, radiotherapy, and preoperative assessment. *Clin Orthop* 207:55–63, 1988.

Siegal T, Siegal T: Surgical decompression of anterior and posterior malignant epidural tumors compressing the spinal cord: A prospective study. *Neurosurgery* 17(3):424–432, 1985.

Sundaresan N, Scher H, DiGiacinto GV, et al: Surgical treatment of spinal cord compression in kidney cancer. *J Clin Oncol* 4:1851–1856, 1986.

Vasilakis D, Papaconstantinou C, Aletras H: Dumb-bell intrathoracic and intraspinal neurofibroma: Report of a case. *Scand J Thorac Cardiovasc Surg* 20:171–173, 1986.

Infection—Deep Fascial Spaces of the Neck

Bello EF, Pien FD: Salmonella dublin neck abscess. *Arch Otolaryngol* 111:476–477, 1985.

Blomquist IK, Bayer AS: Life-threatening deep fascial space infections of the head and neck. *Infect Dis Clin North Am* 2(1):237–264, 1988.

Hall MB, Arteaga DM, Mancuso A: Use of computerized tomography in the localization of head-and-neck-space infections. *J Oral Maxillofac Surg* 43:978–980, 1985.

Herzon FS: Management of nonperitonsillar abscesses of the head and neck with needle aspiration. *Laryngoscope* 95:780–781, 1985.

Lerner PI. The lumpy jaw: Cervicofacial actinomycosis. *Infect Dis Clin North Am* 2(1):203–220, 1988.

McManus K, Holt R, Aufdemorte TM, et al: Bronchogenic cyst presenting as deep neck abscess. *Otolaryngol Head Neck Surg* 92(1):109–114, 1984.

Nyberg DA, Jeffrey RB, Brant-Zawadzki M, et al: Computed tomography of cervical infections. *J Comput Assist Tomogr* 9(2):288–296, 1985.

Rosenberg RA, Liu PG, Myssiorek DJ: Cervical abscess caused by *Salmonella* infection. *Am J Otolaryngol* 6:42–45, 1985.

Sacks JC, Wilmore WC: Closed percutaneous catheter drainage of a cervical abscess. *J Oral Maxillofac Surg* 43:971–973, 1985.

Silverman PM, Farmer JC, Korobkin M, et al: CT diagnosis of actinomycosis of the neck. *J Comput Assist Tomogr* 8(4):793–794, 1984.

Sinnott JT IV, Wheedon C, Schwartz M, et al: Postanginal sepsis: A pain in the neck. *Postgrad Med* 86(2):77–82, 1989.

Zemplenyi J, Colman MF: Deep neck abscesses secondary to methylphenidate (Ritalin) abuse. *Head Neck Surg* 6:858–860, 1984.

Lymphadenitis—Cervical

Barton LL: Childhood cervical adenitis. *Am Fam Physician* 29(4):163–166, 1984.

Brook I: The swollen neck: Cervical lymphadenitis, parotitis, thyroiditis, and infected cysts. *Infect Dis Clin North Am* 2(1):221–236, 1988.

Castro DJ, Hoover L, Castro DJ, et al: Cervical mycobacterial lymphadenitis: Medical vs surgical management. *Arch Otolaryngol* 111:816–819, 1985.

Deitel M, Saldanha CF, Borowy ZJ, et al: Treatment of tuberculous masses in the neck. *Can J Surg* 27(1):90–93, 1984.

Siar CH, Foo GC: Cervical toxoplasma lymphadenitis: Report of a case. *Med J Malaysia* 39(4):306–310, 1984.

Ludwig's Angina

Dolan S, Mayer K: Group A streptococcal pharyngitis and bacteremia associated with a Ludwig's angina-like syndrome. *Diagn Microbiol Infect Dis* 5:323–326, 1986.

Fridrich KL, Taylor RW, Olson RAJ: Dermatomyositis presenting with Ludwig's angina. *Oral Surg Oral Med Oral Pathol* 63:21–24, 1987.

Gridley J, Franaszek J: Ludwig's angina and pneumococcal sepsis. *J Emerg Med* 4:201–204, 1986.

Juang Y-C, Cheng D-L, Wang L-S, et al: Ludwig's angina: An analysis of 14 cases. *Scand J Infect Dis* 21:121–125, 1989.

Moreland LW, Corey J, McKenzie R: Ludwig's angina: Report of a case and review of the literature. *Arch Intern Med* 148:461–466, 1988.

Schliamser SE, Berggren DV-A, Kercoff Y: Ludwig's angina and associated systemic complications. *Scand J Infect Dis* 18:477–481, 1986.

Shaw KN, Marshall GS, Tom LWC, et al: Ludwig's angina caused by *Haemophilus influenzae* type b. *Pediatr Infect Dis J* 7(3):203–205, 1988.

Whitley BD: Ludwig's angina: A rare case of dental origin. *NZ Dent J* 82:48–50, 1986.

Lumbar Puncture—Herniation

Challa VR, Crone KR, Ferree CR, et al: Chronic vermal herniation in a case of osteosarcoma of the occipital bone. *Neurosurgery* 18(2):180–185, 1986.

Gower DJ, Baker AL, Bell WO, et al: Contraindications to lumbar puncture as defined by computed cranial tomography. *J Neurol Neurosurg Psychiatry* 50:1071–1074, 1987.

Sharp CG, Steinhart CM: Lumbar puncture in the presence of increased intracranial pressure: The real danger. *Pediatr Emerg Care* 3(1):39–43, 1987.

Sternbach G: Lumbar puncture. *J Emerg Med* 2:199–203, 1985.

Meningitis—Chronic

Rosenfeld JV, Kaye AH, Davis S, et al: Pachymeningitis cervicalis hypertrophica: Case report. *J Neurosurg* 66:137–139, 1987.

Meningitis—Recurrent: Anatomic Defects and Review Articles

Bridger MWM, Phelps PD: Recurrent meningitis due to congenital malformation of the inner ear. *Br Med J (Clin Res)* 286(6365):626–627, 1983.

Herther C, Schindler RA: Mondini's dysplasia with recurrent meningitis. *Laryngoscope* 95(6):655–658, 1985.

Hirakawa K, Kurokawa M, Yajin K, et al: Recurrent meningitis due to a congenital fistula in the stapedial footplate. *Arch Otolaryngol Head Neck Surg* 109:697–700, 1983.

Hirschel BJ, Auckenthaler R, Barenkamp SJ, et al: Recurrent meningitis in an adult due to nontypable *Haemophilus influenzae*. *J Infect Dis* 149(4):656, 1984.

Izquierdo JM, Gil-Carcedo LM: Recurrent meningitis and transethmoidal intranasal meningoencephalocele. *Dev Med Child Neurol* 30(2):248–251, 1988.

Kline MW: Review of recurrent bacterial meningitis. *Pediatr Infect Dis J* 8:630–634, 1989.

Komune S, Enatsu K, Morimitsu T: Recurrent meningitis due to spontaneous cerebrospinal fluid otorrhea. A case report. *Int J Pediatr Otorhinolaryngol* 11:257–264, 1986.

Kossak B, Kornberg AE: Spontaneous atraumatic CSF otorrhea. *Pediatr Emerg Care* 5(3):166–168, 1989.

Manning KP, Gudrun R: Recurrent meningitis secondary to concealed cerebrospinal fluid otorrhoea. *Arch Dis Child* 58(2):153–155, 1983.

Nagahiro S, Matsukado Y, Miura M, et al: Cervical dermal sinus associated with meningitis and motor paralysis. *Brain Dev* 7:504–507, 1985.

Neely JG, Kuhn JR: Diagnosis and treatment of iatrogenic cerebrospinal fluid leak and brain herniation during or following mastoidectomy. *Laryngoscope* 95(11):1299–1300, 1985.

O'Brien MD, Reade PC: The management of dural tear resulting from mid-facial fracture. *Head Neck Surg* 6:810–818, 1984.

Phillipps JJ: Bilateral oval window fistulae with recurrent meningitis. *J Laryngol Otol* 100:329–331, 1986.

Quiney RE, Mitchell DB, Djazeri B, et al: Recurrent meningitis in children due to inner ear abnormalities. *J Laryngol Otol* 103:473–480, 1989.

Rosen PR, Chaudhuri TK: Radioisotope myelography in the detection of pleural-dural communication as a source of recurrent meningitis. *Clin Nucl Med* 8(1):28–30, 1983.

Shelanski S, Zweiman B: Recurrent meningitis. *Ann Allergy* 60(4):306–7, 343–345, 1988.

Steele RW, McConnell JR, Jacobs RF, et al: Recurrent bacterial meningitis: Coronal thin-section cranial computed tomography to delineate anatomic defects. *Pediatrics* 76(6):950–953, 1985.

Meningitis—Recurrent: Immunologic Deficiencies

Castagliuolo PP, Nisini R, Quinti I, et al: Immunoglobulin deficiencies and meningococcal disease. *Ann Allergy* 57(1):68–70, 1986.

Cooke RPD, Zafar M, Haeney MR: Recurrent meningococcal meningitis associated with deficiencies of C8 and anti-meningococcal antibody. *J Clin Lab Immunol* 23:53–56, 1987.

Eby WM, Irby WR, Irby JH, et al: Recurrent meningitis with familial C8 deficiency: Case report. *Va Med* 114(2):91–94, 1987.

Hardcastle SW: Recurrent meningococcal meningitis. *S Afr Med J* 66(9):345–346, 1984.

Herva E, Leinonen M, Kayhty K, et al: Recurrent meningococcal meningitis due to partial complement defects and poor anti-meningococcal antibody response. *J Infect* 6:55–60, 1983.

Nurnberger W, Pietsch H, Seger R, et al: Familial deficiency of the seventh component of complement associated with recurrent meningococcal infections. *Eur J Pediatr* 148:758–760, 1989.

Onwubalili JK: Sickle cell disease and infection: Special review. *J Infect* 7:2–20, 1983.

Orren A, Potter PC, Cooper RC, et al: Deficiency of the sixth component of complement and susceptibility to Neisseria meningitidis infections: Studies in 10 families and five isolated cases. *Immunology* 62:249–253, 1987.

Shackelford PG, Polmar SH, Mayus JL, et al: Spectrum of IgG2 subclass deficiency in children with recurrent infections: Prospective study. *J Pediatr* 108(1):647–653, 1986.

Zimran A, Rudensky B, Kramer MR, et al: Hereditary complement deficiency in survivors of meningococcal disease: High prevalence of C7/C8 deficiency in sephardic (Moroccan) Jews. *Q J Med* 63(240)349–358, 1987.

Myofascial Pain

Bengtsson A, Bengtsson M: Regional sympathetic blockade in primary fibromyalgia. *Pain* 33:161–167, 1988.

Cooper BC, Alleva M, Cooper DL, et al: Myofascial pain dysfunction: Analysis of 476 patients. *Laryngoscope* 96:1099–1106, 1986.

Graff-Radford SB, Reeves JL, Jaeger B: Management of chronic head and neck pain: Effectiveness of altering factors perpetuating myofascial pain. *Headache* 27:186–190, 1987.

Rosomoff HL, Fishbain DA, Goldberg M, et al: Physical findings in patients with chronic intractable benign pain of the neck and/or back. *Pain* 37:279–287, 1989.

Travell JG, Simons DG: *Myofascial Pain and Dysfunction*. Baltimore, Williams & Wilkins, 1983, pp 103–164; pp 183–218; pp 305–328.

Neck Pain—Reviews and Monographs

Adams RD, Victor M: *Principles of Neurology,* 4th ed. New York, McGraw-Hill, 1989.

Cailliet R: *Neck and Arm Pain*. 2d ed. Philadelphia, F.A. Davis, 1981.

Lucente FE, Cooper DL: Perspectives in head and neck pain, in Cooper BC, Lucente FE (eds): *Management of Facial, Head and Neck Pain.* Philadelphia, Saunders, 1989, chap 1, pp 1–22.

Pincus RL: Oropharyngeal, Laryngeal and neck pain, in Cooper BC, Lucente FE (eds): *Management of Facial, Head and Neck Pain.* Philadelphia, Saunders, 1989, chap 7, pp 131–152.

Pneumomediastinum and Neck Pain

Brody SL, Anderson GV Jr, Gutman JBL: Pneumomediastinum as a complication of "crack" smoking. *Am J Emerg Med* 6:241–243, 1988.

Rose WD, Veach JS, Tehranzdeh J: Spontaneous pneumomediastinum as a cause of neck pain, dysphagia, and chest pain. *Arch Intern Med* 144:392–393, 1984.

Shahar J, Angelillo VA: Catamenial pneumomediastinum. *Chest* 90(5):776–777, 1986.

Sparacino ML, Mackay PE: Subcutaneous emphysema and pneumomediastinum complicating labor in a twin pregnancy. *J Am Osteopath Assoc* 89(2):185–187, 1989.

Repetition/Strain Disorders

Andersen HT: Neck injury sustained during exposure to high-G forces in the F16B. *Aviat Space Environ Med* 59:356–358, 1988.

Dartigues JF, Henry P, Puymirat E, et al: Prevalence and risk factors of recurrent cervical pain syndrome in a working population. *Neuroepidemiology* 7:99–105, 1988.

Hagberg M, Wegman DH: Prevalence rates and odds ratios of shoulder-neck diseases in different occupational groups. *Br J Ind Med* 44:602–610, 1987.

Knudson R, McMillan D, Doucette D, et al.: A comparative study of G-induced neck injury in pilots of the F/A-18, A-7, and A-4. *Aviat Space Environ Med* 59:758–760, 1988.

LaBan MM, Meerschaert JR: Computer-generated headache: Braciocephalgia at first byte. *Am J Phys Med Rehabil* 68(4):183–185, 1989.

Linton SJ, Kamwendo K: Risk factors in the psychosocial work environment for neck and shoulder pain in secretaries. *J Occup Med* 31(7):609–613, 1989.

Miller MH, Topliss DJ: The "repetitive strain injury syndrome" is referred pain from the neck (letter to editor). *J Rheumatol* 16(7):1007, 1989.

Sikorski JM, Molan RR, Askin GN: Orthopaedic basis for occupationally related arm and neck pain. *Aust NZ J Surg* 59:471–478, 1989.

Smythe H: The "repetitive strain injury syndrome" is referred pain from the neck (editorial.) *J Rheumatol* 15(11):1604–1608, 1988.

Tola S, Riihimaki H, Videman T, et al: Neck and shoulder symptoms among men in machine operating, dynamic physical work and sedentary work. *Scand J Work Environ Health* 14:299–305, 1988.

Tendonitis—Retropharyngeal and Crowned Dens Syndrome

Artenian DJ, Lipman JK, Scidmore GK, et al: Acute neck pain due to tendonitis of the longus colli: CT and MRI findings. *Neuroradiology* 31:166–169, 1989.

Benanti JC, Gramling P, Bulat PI, et al: Retropharyngeal calcific tendinitis: Report of five cases and review of the literature. *J Emerg Med* 4:15–24, 1986.

Bouvet J-P, Le Parc J-M, Michalski B, et al: Acute neck pain due to calcifications surrounding the odontoid process: The crowned dens syndrome. *Arthritis Rheum* 28(12):1417–1420, 1985.

Bywaters EGL, Hamilton EBD, Williams R: The spine in idiopathic haemochromatosis. *Ann Rheum Dis* 30:453–465, 1971.

Sarkozi J, Fam AG: Acute calcific retropharyngeal tendinitis: An unusual cause of neck pain. *Arthritis Rheum* 27(6):708–710, 1984.

Weinberger A, Myers AR: Intervertebral disc calcification in adults: A review. *Semin Arthritis Rheum* 8(1):69–75, 1978.

Thoracic Outlet Syndrome

Baumgartner F, Nelson RJ, Robertson JM: The rudimentary first rib: A cause of thoracic outlet syndrome with arterial compromise. *Arch Surg* 124:1090–1092, 1989.

Bilbey JH, Muller NL, Connell DG, et al: Thoracic outlet syndrome: Evaluation with CT. *Radiology* 171:381–384, 1989.

Blair SJ: Avoiding complications of surgery for nerve compression syndromes. *Orthop Clin North Am* 19(1):125–130, 1988.

Brown SCW, Charlesworth D: Results of excision of a cervical rib in patients with the thoracic outlet syndrome. *Br J Surg* 75:431–433, 1988.

Capistrant TD: Thoracic outlet syndrome in cervical strain injury. *Minn Med* 69(1):13–17, 1986.

Cherington M, Happer I, Machanic B, et al: Surgery for thoracic outlet syndrome may be hazardous to your health. *Muscle Nerve* 9:632–634, 1986.

Connolly JF, Dehne R: Nonunion of the clavicle and thoracic outlet syndrome. *J Trauma* 29(8):1127–1133, 1989.

Cuetter AC, Bartoszek DM: The thoracic outlet syndrome: Controversies, overdiagnosis, overtreatment, and recommendations for management. *Muscle Nerve* 12:410–419, 1989.

De Silva M: The costoclavicular syndrome: A ''new cause.'' *Ann Rheum Dis* 45:916–920, 1986.

Hawkes CD: Neurosurgical considerations in thoracic outlet syndrome. *Clin Orthop* 207:24–28, 1986.

Kritzer RO, Rose JE: Diffuse idiopathic skeletal hyperostosis presenting with thoracic outlet syndrome and dysphagia. *Neurosurgery* 22(6):1071–1074, 1988.

Lecour H, Miranda M, Magro C, et al: Human leptospirosis: A review of 50 cases. *Infection* 17(1):8–12, 1989.

Leffert RD, Gumley G: The relationship between dead arm syndrome and thoracic outlet syndrome. *Clin Orthop* 223:20–31, 1987.

Moore M Jr: Thoracic outlet syndrome experience in a metropolitan hospital. *Clin Orthop* 207:29–30, 1986.

Pang D, Wessel HB: Thoracic outlet syndrome. *Neurosurgery* 22(1):105–121, 1988.

Perler BA, Mitchell SE: Percutaneous transluminal angioplasty and transaxillary first rib resection: A multidisciplinary approach to the thoracic outlet syndrome. *Am Surg* 52(9):485–488, 1986.

Priest JD: The shoulder of the tennis player. *Clin Sports Med* 7(2):387–402, 1988.

Rayan GM: Lower trunk brachial plexus compression neuropathy due to cervical rib in young athletes. *Am J Sports Med* 16(1):77–79, 1988.

Selke FW, Kelly TR: Thoracic outlet syndrome. *Am J Surg* 156(1):54–57, 1988.

Sessions RT: Reoperation for thoracic outlet syndrome. *J Cardiovasc Surg* 30:434–444, 1989.

Stanton PE, Vo NM, Haley T, et al: Thoracic outlet syndrome: A comprehensive evaluation. *Am Surg* 54(3):129–133, 1988.

Takagi K, Yamaga M, Morisawa K, et al: Management of thoracic outlet syndrome. *Arch Orthop Trauma Surg* 106:78–81, 1987.

Urschel HC, Razzuk MA: The failed operation for thoracic outlet syndrome: The difficulty of diagnosis and management. *Ann Thorac Surg* 42(5):523–528, 1986.

Warrens AN, Heaton JM: Thoracic outlet compression syndrome: The lack of reliability of its clinical assessment. *Ann R Coll Surg Engl* 69(5):203–204, 1987.

Wood VE, Twito R, Verska J: Thoracic outlet syndrome: The results of first rib resection in 100 patients. *Orthop Clin North Am* 19(1):131–146, 1988.

Thoracic Outlet Syndrome—Vascular Aspects

Al-Hassan HK, Sattar MA, Eklof B: Embolic brain infarction: A rare complication of thoracic outlet syndrome. *J Cardiovasc Surg* 29(3):322–325, 1988.

Cormier JM, Amrane M, Ward A, et al: Arterial complications of the thoracic outlet syndrome: Fifty-five operative cases. *J Vasc Surg* 9:778–787, 1989.

Goadsby PJ: A subclavian bruit in the thoracic outlet syndrome (letter to editor) *Ann Intern Med* 110(4):323, 1989.

Grant DS, Shaw PJ, Adiseshia M: Vascular compression in thoracic outlet syndrome: A potentially missed diagnosis. *J R Soc Med* 81(8):476–478, 1988.

Kunkel JM, Machleder HI: Treatment of Paget-Schroetter syndrome: A staged, multidisciplinary approach. *Arch Surg* 124:1153–1158, 1989.

O'Leary MR, Smith MS, Druy EM, et al: Diagnostic and therapeutic approach to axillary-subclavian vein thrombosis. *Ann Emerg Med* 16(8):889–893, 1987.

Riddell DH, Smith BM: Thoracic and vascular aspects of thoracic outlet syndrome: 1986 update. *Clin Orthop* 207:31–36, 1986.

Scher LA, Veith FJ, Samson RH, et al: Vascular complications of thoracic outlet syndrome. *J Vasc Surg* 3(3):565–568, 1986.

Strange-Vognsen HH, Hauch O, Anderson J, et al: Resection of the first rib, following deep arm vein thrombolysis in patients with thoracic outlet syndrome. *J Cardiovasc Surg* 30(3):430–433, 1989.

Swenson WM, Rennich D, Capp KA, et al: Axillary vein thrombosis due to thoracic outlet syndrome: Correction via the supraclavicular approach. *AORN J* 46(5):878–881, 884–886, 1987.

Thyroid Neoplasms

Aozasa K, Inoue A, Yoshimura H, et al: Plasmacytoma of the thyroid gland. *Cancer* 58:105–110, 1986.

Block MA: Diagnosis and management of carcinoma of the thyroid. *Compr Ther* 13(6):48–56, 1987.

Butler JS, Brady LW, Amendola BE: Lymphoma of the thyroid: Report of five cases and review. *Am J Clin Oncol* 13(1):64–69, 1990.

Damion J, Hybels RL: The neck mass: 2. Inflammatory and neoplastic causes. *Postgrad Med* 81(6):97–103, 106–107, 1987.

Donnell CA, Pollock WJ, Sybers WA: Thyroid carcinosarcoma. *Arch Pathol Lab Med* 111:1169–1172, 1987.

Eisenberg BL, Hensley SD: Thyroid cancer with coexistent Hashimoto's thyroiditis: Clinical assessment and management. *Arch Surg* 124:1045–1047, 1989.

Higashi T, Ito K, Nishikawa Y, et al: Gallium-67 imaging in the evaluation of thyroid malignancy. *Clin Nucl Med* 13:792–799, 1988.

Hotes LS, Barzilay J, Cloud LP, et al: Case report: Spontaneous hematoma of a parathyroid adenoma. *Am J Med Sci* 297(5):331–333, 1989.

Joensuu H, Klemi PJ, Paul R, et al: Survival and prognostic factors in thyroid carcinoma. *Acta Radiol Oncol* 25:243–248, 1986.

Kawahara E, Nakanishi I, Terahata S, et al: Leiomyosarcoma of the thyroid gland: A case report with a comparative study of five cases of anaplastic carcinoma. *Cancer* 62:2558–2563, 1988.

Lee J-K, Tai F-T, Lin H-D, et al: Treatment of recurrent thyroid cysts by injection of tetracycline or minocycline. *Arch Intern Med* 149:599–601, 1989.

Makepeace AR, Fermont DC, Bennett MH: Non-Hodgkin's lymphoma of the thyroid. *Clin Radiol* 38:227–281, 1987.

Oertel JE, Heffess CS: Lymphoma of the thyroid and related disorders. *Semin Oncol* 14(3):333–342, 1987.

Shvero J, Gal R, Avidor I, et al: Anaplastic thyroid carcinoma: A clinical, histologic, and immunohistochemical study. *Cancer* 62:319–325, 1988.

Stoffer SS, Loomus M: The painful thyroid: A three-step diagnostic approach. *Postgrad Med* 81(1):161–164, 1987.

Takashima S, Ikezoe J, Morimoto S, et al: Primary thyroid lymphoma: Evaluation with CT. *Radiology* 168:765–768, 1988.

Takashima S, Morimoto S, Ikezoe J, et al: CT evaluation of anaplastic thyroid carcinoma. *AJNR* 11:361–367, 1990.

Tupchong L, Phil D, Hughes F, et al: Primary lymphoma of the thyroid: Clinical features, prognostic factors, and results of treatment. *Int J Radiat Oncol Biol Phys* 12:1813–1821, 1986.

VanRuiswyk J, Cunningham C, Cerletty J: Obstructive manifestations of thyroid lymphoma. *Arch Intern Med* 149:1575–1577, 1989.

Thyroiditis and Mimics

Alves C, Eidson MS, Zakarija M, et al: Graves disease presenting as painful thyroiditis. *Eur J Pediatr* 148:603–604, 1989.

Farrell A, McKenna J: Thyrotoxicosis, subacute thyroiditis and thyroid pain in Ireland. *Irish Med J* 80(2):55–57, 1987.

Hamburger JI: The various presentations of thyroiditis: Diagnostic considerations. *Ann Intern Med* 104:219–224, 1986.

Hay ID: Thyroiditis: A clinical update. *Mayo Clin Proc* 60:836–843, 1985.

Ikenoue H, Okamura K, Kuroda T, et al: Thyroid amyloidosis with recurrent subacute thyroiditis-like syndrome. *J Clin Endocrinol Metab* 67:41–45, 1988.

Ishihara T, Mori T, Waseda N, et al: Pathological characteristics of acute exacerbation of Hashimoto's thyroiditis: Serial changes in a patient with repeated episodes. *Endocrinol Jpn* 33(5):701–712, 1986.

Kitchener MI, Chapmann IM: Subacute thyroiditis: A review of 105 cases. *Clin Nucl Med* 14:439–442, 1989.

Strakosch CR: Thyroiditis. *Aust NZ J Med* 16:91–100, 1986.

Zimmerman RS, Brennan MD, McConahey WM, et al: Hashimoto's thyroiditis. *Ann Intern Med* 104:355–357, 1986.

Thyroiditis—Suppurative

Baker SR, van Merwyk AJ, Singh A: Abscess of the thyroid gland presenting as a pulsatile mass. *Med J Aust* 143:253–254, 1985.

Barton GM, Shoup WB, Bennett WG, et al: Case report: Combined *Escherichia coli* and *Staphylococcus aureus* thyroid abscess in an asymptomatic man. *Am J Med Sci* 295(2):133–136, 1988.

Hirata A, Saito S, Tsuchida Y, et al: Surgical management of piriform sinus fistula. *Am Surg* 50(8):454–457, 1984.

Schloss MD, Taibah K, Nogrady MB: Third branchial cleft sinus: Route of infection in deep neck abscesses. *J Otolaryngol* 15(1):56–58, 1986.

Szabo S, Allen DB: Thyroiditis: Differentiation of acute suppurative and subacute: Case report and review of the literature. *Clin Pediatr* 28(4):171–174, 1989.

Torticollis

Boisen E: Torticollis caused by an infratentorial tumour: Three cases. *Br J Psychiatry* 134:306–307, 1979.

Bolivar R, Kohl S, Pickering LK: Vertebral osteomyelitis in children: Report of four cases. *Pediatrics* 62(4):549–553, 1978.

Bolton PS: Torticollis: A review of etiology, pathology, diagnosis and treatment. *J Manipulative Physiol Ther* 8(1):29–32, 1985.

Harenko A: Retrocollis as an irreversible late complication of neuroleptic medication. *Acta Neurol Scand* 43(suppl 31):145–146, 1967.

Ho K-L, Konno ET, Chason JL: Focal myositis of the neck. *Hum Pathol* 10:353–356, 1979.

Kiwak KJ: Establishing an etiology for torticollis. *Postgrad Med* 75(7):126–134, 1984.

Mathern GW, Batzdorf U: Grisel's syndrome: Cervical spine clinical, pathologic, and neurologic manifestations. *Clin Orthop* 244:131–146, 1989.

Richardson FL: A report of 16 tumors of the spinal cord in children: The importance of spinal rigidity as an early sign of disease. *J Pediatr* 57:42–54, 1960.

Sarnat HB, Morrissy RT: Idiopathic torticollis: Sternocleidomastoid myopathy and accessory neuropathy. *Muscle Nerve* 4:374–380, 1981.

Swett C Jr: Drug-induced dystonia. *Am J Psychiatry* 132(5):532–534, 1975.

Visudhiphan P, Chiemchanya S, Somburanasin R, et al: Torticollis as the presenting sign in cervical spine infection and tumor. *Clin Pediatr* 21(2):71–76, 1982.

Webb M: Acute torticollis: Identifying and treating the underlying cause. *Postgrad Med* 82(3):121–126, 128, 1987.

Torticollis—Spasmodic

Avman N, Arasil E: Spasmodic torticollis due to colloid cyst of the third ventricle. *Acta Neurochir* 21:265–268, 1969.

Bianchine JR, Bianchine JW: Treatment of spasmodic torticollis with diazepam. *South Med J* 64(7):893–894, 1971.

Bigwood GF: Treatment of spasmodic torticollis. *N Engl J Med* 286:1161, 1972.

Cockburn JJ: Spasmodic torticollis: A psychogenic condition? *J Psychosom Res* 15:471–477, 1971.

Cooper IS, Upton ARM, Amin I: Reversibility of chronic neurologic deficits: Some effects of electrical stimulation of the thalamus and internal capsule in man. *Appl Neurophysiol* 43:244–258, 1980.

Dooley DM, Nisonson I: Treatment of patients with degenerative diseases of the central nervous system by electrical stimulation of the spinal cord. *Appl Neurophysiol* 44:71–76, 1981.

Fitz Simmons HJ: Congenital torticollis: Review of the pathological aspects. *N Engl J Med* 209(2):66–71, 1933.

Gilbert GJ: Familial spasmodic torticollis. *Neurology* 27:11–13, 1977.

Gilbert GJ: Spasmodic torticollis treated effectively by medical means. *N Engl J Med* 284(16):896–898, 1971.

Herz E, Glaser GH: Spasmodic torticollis: 2. Clinical evaluation. *Arch Neurol Psychiatry* 61(3):227–239, 1949.

Jannetta PJ: Spasmodic torticollis. *J Neurosurg* 65:725–726, 1986.

Lal S: Pathophysiology and pharmacotherapy of spasmodic torticollis: A review. *Can J Neurol Sci* 6(4):427–435, 1979.

Meares R: Natural history of spasmodic torticollis, and effect of surgery. *Lancet* 2:149–151, 1971.

Shaw KM, Hunter KR, Stern GM: Medical treatment of spasmodic torticollis. *Lancet* 1:1399, 1972.

Simpson BA: Spasmodic torticollis relieved by removal of a cervical foreign body (letter to editor). *J Neurol Neurosurg Psychiatry* 49:1208–1209, 1986.

Transverse Myelopathy

Heilbronn YD, Tovi F, Hirsch M, et al: Transverse cervical myelopathy: An unusual complication of retropharyngeal abscess. *Head Neck Surg* 6:1051–1053, 1984.

Trauma—Anterior Neck

Mace SE: Blunt laryngotracheal trauma. *Ann Emerg Med* 15(7):836–842, 1986.

Vertebral Artery Dissection

Adams RD, Victor M: Cerebrovascular Diseases, in *Principles of Neurology,* 4th ed. New York, McGraw-Hill, 1989, chap. 34, pp 617–692.

Detwiler K, Godersky JC, Gentry L: Pseudoaneurysm of the extracranial vertebral artery: Case report. *J Neurosurg* 67:935–939, 1987.

Mas J-L, Bousser M-G, Hasboun D, et al: Extracranial vertebral artery dissections: A review of 13 cases. *Stroke* 18:1037–1047, 1987.

Mas JL, Henin D, Bousser MG, et al: Dissecting aneurysm of the vertebral artery and cervical manipulation: A case report with autopsy. *Neurology* 39:512–515, 1989.

Mokri B, Houser OW, Sandok BA, et al: Spontaneous dissections of the vertebral arteries. *Neurology* 38:880–885, 1988.

PART FOUR

Acute Chest and Breast Pain

CHAPTER

12

Acute Central Chest Pain

☐ DIAGNOSTIC LIST

1. Acute myocardial infarction
2. Acute coronary insufficiency
3. Variant angina (Prinzmetal's angina)
4. A. Esophageal pain (motor disorders and gastroesophageal reflux)
   B. Infectious esophagitis
      1. *Candida* species
      2. Herpes simplex virus
      3. Cytomegalovirus
5. Chest wall musculoskeletal pain
   A. Costochondritis
   B. Pectoral myositis or trigger point
   C. Precordial catch syndrome
6. A. Anxiety-related chest pain
   B. Panic attacks
7. Hyperventilation
8. Acute pericarditis
   A. Viral and idiopathic
   B. Bacterial (pyogenic)
   C. Tuberculous
9. Acute massive pulmonary embolism
10. Acute aortic dissection (dissecting aneurysm)
11. Mediastinitis
12. Pneumomediastinum
13. Pneumothorax
    A. Simple type
    B. Tension type
14. Tracheobronchitis
15. Herpes zoster
16. Esophageal rupture—Boerhaave's syndrome and other causes

☐ SUMMARY

Acute myocardial infarction usually begins with the gradual buildup, over a 5- to 15-min period, of mild-to-severe substernal pain that may radiate to one or both breasts, the shoulders, the jaw, the neck, and one or both arms. The pain is described as a heaviness, a weight, a constriction, a viselike pain, a burning, or a peculiar feeling in the midchest. Sweating, nausea, vomiting, weakness, and faintness are common associated symptoms. Very severely ill patients, or those who have had the infarction 3 to 4 days before, may complain of shortness of breath that is due to left-sided heart failure.

Physical examination may reveal pallor, a rapid and sometimes irregular pulse, an S_3 gallop, a mitral systolic murmur, and loss of intensity of the first heart sound near the mitral area. Electrocardiograms confirm the diagnosis in only 60 to 80 percent of cases; an elevation of serum isozymes, such as lactic dehydrogenase 1 and creatine phosphokinase–MB, will establish the diagnosis in most other patients, within 14 to 24 h.

Acute coronary insufficiency causes a picture similar to that of infarction, but the pain resolves in a shorter time and there is no evidence of infarction by electrocardiogram or by enzyme assay.

Variant angina causes substernal crushing or constricting pain that occurs at rest, frequently in the early morning hours. Electrocardiograms taken during an attack show ST-segment elevation that is reversible and ventricular arrhythmias, such as ventricular tachycardia or multifocal premature ventricular contractions. Coronary angiograms reveal occluded or narrowed coronary vessels, and may demonstrate spontaneous or provoked coronary artery spasm.

Esophageal pain may mimic the pain of angina. *Motor disorders* cause spasm, which can be recorded with a balloon placed in the esophageal lumen. Esophageal spasm is not always associated with the severe anterior crushing or constricting pain described by these patients.

These patients usually have normal coronary angiograms or thallium stress tests. Rarely, the act of swallowing or the drinking of cold liquids precipitates a similar attack of crushing chest pain. Only a minority of patients with unexplained central chest pain and normal coronary arteries can be shown to have an esophageal motor disorder by manometric studies.

Gastroesophageal reflux causes a burning midline chest pain sometimes associated with regurgitation of bitter-tasting acid material into the throat and mouth. This discomfort is usually relieved promptly by antacids and H_2-blocking agents. Reflux may also cause constricting coronary-like central chest pain, which may respond to intensive antacid treatment or H_2 blockers.

Infectious esophagitis can cause aching, burning, or pressurelike lower substernal and parasternal chest pain, associated with odynophagia. A double-contrast barium study may make the diagnosis in a severe case, but is less sensitive than endoscopy. Brushing and biopsies will establish a diagnosis of either a fungal or viral etiology. This disorder occurs predominantly in patients with acquired immunodeficiency syndrome (AIDS).

Chest wall pain is often associated with local tenderness of the second to fourth left or right costal cartilages or the pectoralis muscles. Aching pain may continue for hours or days and mimic myocardial infarction. Deep inspiration—or arm and shoulder movement, in a minority of patients—reproduces the pain. In most cases only local tenderness is present, but the spontaneous pain, as usually experienced, can seldom be reproduced by provocation. Similar pain, in quality and location, can be transiently produced by direct pressure over the tender chest wall area, but this subsides as pressure is relieved. Precordial pain localized to the cardiac apex area that begins abruptly and does not radiate has been called *precordial catch*. The attacks are infrequent and can be terminated by a deep inspiration, or by straightening up, within 1 to 3 min of onset.

Panic attacks, with inner trembling, palpitations, sweating, tremulousness, fear of death, tenseness, inability to rest, and shortness of breath, may be associated with pressurelike pain beneath the sternum or at the region of the left nipple.

Hyperventilation is associated with very rapid breathing or excessively deep sighing respirations. Such breathing causes light-headedness, tingling, and paresthesias of the hands, arms, and face, and may cause substernal or parasternal pain. In some of these cases (e.g., 39 to 42 percent) the discomfort can be reproduced by asking the patient to breath rapidly and deeply for 1 to 2 min.

Acute pericarditis may mimic a myocardial infarction by causing constricting, pressurelike chest pain. More frequently, there is a different type of chest pain that involves the left anterior and central chest, the neck, and the left shoulder ridge. Right chest and shoulder pain may also occur. Deep inspiration or coughing intensifies this type of pericardial pain, while sitting up eases it. Lying supine or on the left side worsens it. The electrocardiographic pattern demonstrates the findings of acute pericarditis (i.e., ST-segment elevation in most leads except aVR, and, after 3 to 7 days, T-wave inversion).

Acute massive pulmonary embolism may cause central crushing chest pain that mimics infarction of the heart. There is severe dyspnea and a falling blood pressure. A lung scan will show a large perfusion defect affecting the circulation to more than 50 percent of the lung. This can be confirmed by a pulmonary angiogram that demonstrates major pulmonary arterial branches occluded by clot (i.e., abrupt vessel cutoffs or filling defects).

Dissection of the aorta causes severe central chest pain that begins suddenly and is described as a very severe tearing or ripping pain. It may rapidly radiate sequentially through to the upper and lower back and the midabdomen. Dyspnea, sweating, and fainting may accompany the pain. Acute aortic insufficiency occurs in 50 percent of cases, and myocardial infarction in 16 percent. A chest radiograph usually shows a widened superior mediastinum. An aortogram will confirm the diagnosis by visualizing the narrowed aortic lumen, intimal flap, and double channel in the affected aortic segment. Similarly, a contrast-enhanced CT scan can also establish the diagnosis.

Mediastinitis follows the spread of infection from the teeth, pharynx, neck, esophagus, subdiaphragmatic space (abscess), lung, pleura, or pericardium. There is severe central and left chest pain, dyspnea, fever, and chills. Swallowing, breathing, and coughing may intensify the pain. CT scans are very helpful in localizing and identifying mediastinal infections. *Pneumomediastinum* results from rupture of pulmonary alveoli into the perivascular connective tissue. Air dissects through the mediastinum, causing substernal pain that is made worse by deep inspiration and swallowing and eased by sitting up and leaning forward. A chest radiograph will confirm the diagnosis of mediastinal air. About 50 percent of patients have skin crepitus due to air in the subcutaneous tissue of the chest and neck. Hamman's sign, a crunching noise synchronous with the heart sounds, may also be present.

Pneumothorax usually results from rupture of a subpleural bleb or cyst. Chest pain begins abruptly in the anterior or lateral chest and may be intensified by deep inspiration or by movement. The affected side is hyperresonant and breath sounds are decreased. An expiratory chest radiograph will confirm the diagnosis. Tension pneumothorax causes almost total lung collapse and shift of the heart and trachea to the opposite side.

Marked tachycardia, falling blood pressure, and severe chest pain and dyspnea may occur. These abnormalities are markedly improved by needle thoracentesis or by insertion of a chest tube. Simple pneumothorax is associated with milder chest pain and shortness of breath.

Tracheobronchitis causes mild midsubsternal pain that becomes very severe and sharp during coughing. Fever and sputum production may occur in some cases.

Herpes zoster causes a burning pain in a unilateral dermatomal band over one side of the chest, associated with a pustular or vesicular rash that erupts in the painful zone.

Boerhaave's syndrome begins with substernal, left precordial aching or pleuritic pain that follows an episode of forceful vomiting. Dyspnea, mild hematemesis, dysphagia, fever, and cold-water polydipsia may be associated complaints. Subcutaneous emphysema, pneumothorax, pleural effusion, and mediastinal emphysema may be detected on physical examination and/or by a plain chest radiograph. Hamman's sign occurs in 20 percent of cases. Subcutaneous and mediastinal emphysema separate this disorder from the major thoracic catastrophes (e.g., myocardial infarction, dissecting aneurysm, pulmonary embolism) and abdominal catastrophes (e.g., perforated ulcer, acute pancreatitis, mesenteric thrombosis) that it may mimic. The diagnosis can be confirmed by a contrast esophagogram. Other causes of esophageal rupture include endoscopy, instrumentation, foreign bodies, and underlying esophageal disease.

☐ DESCRIPTION OF LISTED DISEASES

1. ACUTE MYOCARDIAL INFARCTION

This disorder begins with retrosternal chest discomfort of mild-to-moderate intensity that builds, over a period of 5 to 15 min, to a severe, and sometimes excruciating, level.

TABLE OF DISEASE INCIDENCE

INCIDENCE PER 100,000 (APPROXIMATE)

Common (>100)	Uncommon (>5–100)	Rare (>0–5)
Acute myocardial infarction	Hyperventilation	Acute bacterial or tuberculous pericarditis
Coronary insufficiency	Acute viral pericarditis	Mediastinitis
Variant angina	Acute pulmonary embolism	Pneumomediastinum
Costochondritis	Aortic dissection	Tension pneumothorax
Pectoral myositis	Simple pneumothorax	Esophageal rupture: Boerhaave's syndrome and other causes
Precordial catch syndrome	Infectious esophagitis	
Anxiety-related pain	Herpes zoster	
Panic attacks		
Tracheobronchitis		
Esophageal pain due to reflux or motility disorder		

This may or may not radiate to more distant areas, such as the right or left anterior chest; the neck, shoulders, upper and lower jaws, and teeth; and one or both arms. In some cases pain may be felt only in the central chest or in the back, between the scapulas. Inferior wall infarction may cause lower sternal or upper midabdominal pain. The pain may be mild enough to allow such activities as driving a car, climbing stairs, or taking out cans of garbage. In fact, we have seen several patients who performed such actions, in attempts to reassure themselves they were *not* having a heart attack, before reporting their chest pain.

The pain may be so intense that some patients are afraid to move for fear that they will make it worse. They sit very still, covered with cold sweat, and are afraid even to talk. On occasion we have seen patients writhing in pain and unable to find comfort in any position. Narcotic injections may fail to alleviate the discomfort; as much as 45 mg of morphine may be ineffective. The pain of infarction has been described as like a heavy weight; as viselike; as a pressure; as constricting; as expanding; as dull and boring; as a tightening, and, sometimes, as a burning pain. In milder attacks it may be described as "a funny feeling," or "something not right" beneath the central chest, and the words *pain* and *discomfort* may not be mentioned.

The chest discomfort of an infarction may pass in as short a time as 15 min, but this is unusual. In most cases the pain lasts at least 1 h, and often it lasts as long as 12 to 24 h. Residual mild discomfort may continue for 2 to 3 days.

The pain is steady and unrelenting, and is not usually relieved by antacids, change of position, lying down, rest, or nitroglycerin. Thombolysis with streptokinase (SK) or recombinant tissue plasminogen activator (rt-PA) may rapidly, and sometimes instantaneously, relieve the pain as the coronary artery–obstructing clot lyses. In most cases myocardial infarction begins at rest; but it may occur during effort, or during a heated argument or some other emotionally charged activity. Very often it occurs in the early hours of the morning, awakening the patient and preventing him or her from returning to sleep. In some cases the infarction occurs during, or shortly after, intense exercise.

The neck discomfort is frequently described as a choking or smothering sensation. Pain is more frequent in the left arm than in the right, but pain may radiate from the chest and shoulders to both arms and hands at once. Left arm pain may be localized to an elbow, forearm, or wrist. Tingling and numbness may affect the forearm and hand, and the arm may feel heavy and weak.

The presence of lower chest pressure, nausea, and vomiting persuades many wishful patients that they are suffering from "indigestion." If the attack was preceded by a large meal, such a patient is even more convinced. But vomiting and antacids fail to relieve the unrelenting pressure. Frequently, sweating and profound weakness supervene, prompting such patients to seek emergency care—sometimes hours later. Prolonged "indigestion" in a middle-aged or elderly patient should be considered to be a possible heart attack until serial electrocardiograms and serum cardiac isozyme assays rule out the possibility. Some patients believe they have the flu, because of the sweating and nausea.

Drenching cold sweats often occur in several waves. Nausea and vomiting are common. If severe cardiac damage has occurred, there may be profound weakness, prostration, and dizziness associated with a rapid, thready pulse and hypotension. Palpitations may be symptomatic of cardiac arrhythmias. Fainting may occur from severe hypotension, from heart block, or from a cardiac tachyarrhythmia (e.g., ventricular tachycardia or fibrillation).

By contrast, the general appearance of other patients with myocardial infarctions may be perfectly normal. We have seen patients with pain mild enough to allow them to come into the office and wait to be seen. These patients usually have no associated symptoms (such as sweating, weakness, and nausea or vomiting).

Sometimes, mild pain relief occurs when the patient extends his or her arms upward above the shoulders. The patient may be found lying in bed with the arms extended above, and the hands clutching the headboard. One patient was found hanging by his arms from the top of a door.

When severe myocardial damage and shock are present, the patient looks pale and is very weak, unable to sit or stand without severe dizziness or fainting. The hands, feet, and central face are cold and moist. Vocal responses are usually a little above a whisper, and are brief. In most cases, despite a barely obtainable blood pressure, thinking is clear and rational; but as time goes by, mental confusion and even uncooperative or psychotic behavior may ensue.

In patients with extensive left ventricular damage the chest pain may be accompanied by severe dyspnea and orthopnea. Both pain and a sense of suffocation may be present. Respirations are often noisy and loud. Expirations are prolonged, and coughing and wheezing occur. The material coughed up may be white, or else blood-tinged, pink, and frothy, reflecting heart failure and pulmonary edema.

The pulse is usually accelerated (in the range of 100 to 120 beats per minute). Frequent irregularities, due to premature ventricular contractions, may be present. Rates of more than 140 to 150 beats per minute suggest a paroxysmal tachycardia and require an electrocardiogram for accurate diagnosis. In inferior wall infarction the pulse rate may be slow (in the range of 45 to 60 beats per minute), and transient heart block may occur because of excessive vagal activity.

The blood pressure may be high, normal, or low. A fall in blood pressure may be due to severe loss of left ventricular muscle mass from infarction; to tachyarrhythmia; to severe acute mitral insufficiency; to an acquired intraventricular septal defect; to a vagal reflex with bradycardia and hypotension; to hypovolemia from overzealous diuretic treatment; or to infarction of the right ventricle and atrium, with release of atrial natiuretic hormone resulting in volume loss.

The respiratory rate may be elevated because of fever, pulmonary congestion and edema due to left ventricular damage, or pulmonary embolism.

Fever may occur; it represents myocardial injury and cellular death. Temperatures usually range from 100 to 102°F. The fever may last up to 7 days, but usually lasts only 2 to 3 days. Some patients never develop fever. The presence of fever and sweats also suggests to some patients that they are suffering from the flu.

The heart size is usually normal. The first heart sound may be muffled and indistinct, producing a "tic-tac" rhythm. Twenty-five to 50 percent of patients have a gallop rhythm of either the S_3 or the S_4 type. There may be very frequent ectopic beats, causing severe irregularity of the cardiac rhythm. A pericardial friction rub may appear within 2 to 3 days after the initial onset of pain (10–25 percent of cases). Fine rales are often present over the posterior bases of the lungs.

The absence of any or all of the physical signs described does not preclude the presence of an acute myocardial infarction. The white blood cell count may be elevated into the range of 10,000 to 20,000 cells per mm³. The rise may occur within hours of the onset of pain and be present for several days. The blood sedimentation rate becomes elevated after 2 to 3 days, and remains elevated for several weeks. The electrocardiogram usually is abnormal within minutes (or less) of the onset of pain, but changes may not be apparent for 24 to 48 h.

In 60 to 80 percent of cases the electrocardiogram is abnormal when the patient is first seen. Ischemia is the initial finding, with tall, peaked T waves evolving into T-wave inversions. Injury to the myocardial muscle membrane is indicated by ST-segment elevation, and infarction of the muscle wall of the heart by the development of Q waves and/or loss of more than 30 percent of R-wave amplitude. Myocardial infarction is usually due to a thrombus acutely occluding a stenotic segment of a coronary artery. If the right coronary artery is occluded, Q waves and ST-T changes occur in leads II, III, and aVF. If the main left or anterior descending coronary artery is involved, changes occur in leads V_1 to V_5. Circumflex artery closure may cause lateral wall infarction (V_5–V_6) or infarction of the inferior wall in the minority of patients whose blood supply to the inferior surface of the heart is from the circumflex artery.

A normal electrocardiogram during the attack does not rule out infarction. In some patients with lateral wall infarction, changes may be delayed for 2 days or more. Serum enzyme levels for creatine kinase-MB (CPK–MB) and serum aspartate aminotransferase (AST) are elevated within hours and stay elevated for 2 to 4 days.

In small infarctions, baseline levels of CPK may rise threefold without exceeding the normal upper limit of enzyme concentration. The problem with using total serum enzyme levels to diagnose or confirm infarction in a patient with chest pain is nonspecificity: total CPK may rise because of injections, exercise, trauma to skeletal muscle, muscle diseases, cardioversion, seizures, stroke, or surgery. Currently, serum isozymes of LDH (lactic dehydrogenase) and CPK are used as confirmatory tests, or to detect evidence of infarction when electrocardiographic abnormalities are absent or nondiagnostic. CPK-MB and LDH_1 are released into the plasma within hours of ischemic infarction of cardiac muscle. A radioimmunoassay technique for detection of CPK–MB provides greater specificity than the gel electrophoresis method. LDH_1, the cardiac isozyme, may become elevated above the level of LDH_2 ("LDH flip") even when the total serum LDH activity is not increased. In most cases the total serum LDH is elevated.

Non-Q-wave infarctions are associated with ST-segment elevations and T-wave inversions, which revert to normal after days or weeks. This form of infarction is believed to involve less muscle mass than the transmural infarction described above. Despite this, the long-term outlook for patients with non-Q-wave infarction is no better than for patients with Q-wave infarction.

Other techniques used in a minority of patients to document the presence of myocardial infarction include:

1. The use of ^{99m}Tc stannous pyrophosphate to label an infarcted area. This "hot spot" imaging gives an estimate of infarct size and localizes the infarct. Such scans become positive sometime from day 2 to day 5. Pyrophosphate scans are less sensitive for the diagnosis of infarction than a CPK–MB determination.
2. Thallium 201 imaging outlines the infarct area as a "cold spot." It is very sensitive but is not specific, and does not allow differentiation of old scars from acute infarctions. This test, like ^{99m}Tc stannous pyrophosphate imaging, can be used to diagnose a recent infarction, or to rule it out if the patient is not seen until 7 to 14 days after the onset of chest pain.
3. Cine CT also may be used to confirm a recent or healed myocardial infarction.

Myocardial infarction may be managed by one of the following strategies:

1. Supportive care: Patients may be admitted to a monitored unit and given intravenous lidocaine (to prevent lethal arrhythmias), narcotics, analgesics, and warfarin. Complications, such as arrhythmias, shock, heart failure, and embolism, are treated as they arise.
2. Intravenous thrombolysis: If a diagnosis of acute early (i.e., less than 4 h old) infarction is made, the patient is given intravenous streptokinase (SK) or recombinant tissue plasminogen activator (rt-PA). Such therapy results in dramatic pain relief as the responsible clot completely or partially lyses. It is effective in 70 to 80 percent of cases. Revascularization by percutaneous transluminal coronary angioplasty (PTCA) may be done during the next 3 days to more permanently open and dilate the affected vessel. After angioplasty, 80 percent of vessels open, and after a second procedure, a total of 95 percent of the treated arteries are patent. Surgical intervention may be required to bypass vessels that cannot be opened by angioplasty.
3. Intracoronary thrombolysis: In some centers the clot is first localized by angiography, then lysed by direct intracoronary infusion of SK or rt-PA. PTCA or a surgical bypass procedure is used to revascularize the myocardium in the bed of the narrowed and thrombosed artery.

Some cardiologists avoid the use of thrombolytic agents, in order to prevent delay and avoid bleeding. They proceed directly to angioplasty and open the thrombosed vessel mechanically. Oral aspirin helps prevent reocclusion after PTCA, and is currently being used for this purpose.

Restoration of flow by thrombolysis or angioplasty may provide rapid and dramatic relief of pain, and thus confirm the diagnosis in a highly specific manner.

2. ACUTE CORONARY INSUFFICIENCY ("INTERMEDIATE CORONARY SYNDROME"; UNSTABLE ANGINA)

Patients with this disorder develop substernal and anterior chest pain lasting 20 to 30 min or longer. These attacks occur at rest, without prior exertion or emotional aggravation. The symptoms are compatible with a diagnosis of myocardial infarction. These patients should be admitted to a coronary care unit and the diagnosis of infarction excluded as described above.

The cause of the spontaneous prolonged chest pain may be a progressively enlarging atherosclerotic plaque, further narrowing a coronary vessel; a clot superimposed on an obstructing plaque, causing more sudden narrowing of a vessel; or spasm of the arterial wall at the site of a plaque.

All studies show no evidence of infarction. Prevention of recurrent pain requires an understanding of the mechanism of the pain. If exercise tolerance is preserved and pain attacks cluster in the morning hours, coronary spasm is likely. Such patients may benefit from the use of calcium channel–blocking drugs and nitrates. The stenotic site at which increases of arterial tone cause complete obstruction can be dilated with a balloon catheter. Patients with a sudden marked decrease of exercise tolerance and frequent episodes of rest pain may have partial obstruction of a coronary vessel caused by a plaque and a super-imposed new clot. The clot and segment of narrowing can be detected by coronary angiography or angioscopy (more sensitive for clots). Clots can be lysed with intracoronary infusion of SK or rt-PA and the stenotic vessel can be dilated by PTCA. Such therapy leads to pain relief and prevents recurrence.

Attacks of chest pain, which may even go on to infarction, may occur in young adults sniffing or smoking cocaine. These patients experience chest pain, palpitations, and fainting from severe coronary spasm and, in some cases, coronary thrombosis. Such patients may develop myocardial infarction or die of fatal arrhythmias without infarction. They may respond to intracoronary infusion of nitroglycerin for intense spasm and/or SK and balloon dilatation for clots.

3. VARIANT ANGINA (PRINZMETAL'S ANGINA)

These patients usually have a normal exercise tolerance with minimal, if any, exertional pain. However, as many as 30 percent may have effort-related pain as well. Attacks of spontaneous pain occur at any time, but frequently in the early hours of the morning. Such attacks may occur in a cluster during one part of a day, and then not recur until the next day. Pain may last 10 to 20 min, clear spontaneously, and recur in 5 to 10 min. Some attacks of pain may last 1 to 2 h. The pain is severe and is located substernally; it may radiate to the anterior chest, neck, head, and arms. It is not readily relieved by nitroglycerin, but it may be after several tablets are dissolved beneath the tongue.

Palpitations, sweating, light-headedness, and nausea are frequent accompanying symptoms. Electrocardiograms taken during an attack usually show ST-segment elevation, and sometimes ST-segment depression. Extrasystoles and attacks of ventricular tachycardia during the painful period may also occur. Ambulatory electrocardiographic monitoring of coronary disease patients has demonstrated that as many as 70 percent of attacks of ischemia, as indicated by ST-segment shifts, are painless.

The cause of such spontaneous pain, with little or no effect on exercise ability, is spasm of a major coronary artery, usually at a site of arterial narrowing caused by an atherosclerotic plaque. Such lesions are usually situated proximally, in a major coronary vessel. Some patients with this disorder have only single-vessel disease, while others have disease in all three vessels. As many as 10 percent of patients with spasm-induced chest pain may have totally normal coronary vessels.

Spontaneous spasm has been documented during angiography in such cases; it can be relieved in the catheterization laboratory by the use of an intracoronary infusion of nitroglycerin. With dilation of the spastic segment, chest pain is usually relieved. Ergonovine has been given

to suspect patients during catheterization, to provoke coronary artery spasm that reproduces the patient's pain and confirms the diagnosis. This disorder yields to therapy with oral calcium channel blockers or nitrates (90 percent response rate). A stenotic site where spasm occurs may be dilated with a balloon catheter or bypassed with a surgically implanted internal mammary artery graft.

Patients with variant angina due to spasm may be made worse by the use of beta blockers (propranolol, nadolol, metoprolol), since coronary spasm is probably alpha receptor–mediated and beta blockade leaves the latter sympathetic fibers unopposed.

4. A. ESOPHAGEAL PAIN (MOTOR DISORDERS AND GASTROESOPHAGEAL REFLUX) It is estimated that 5 to 10 percent of patients admitted to coronary care units with pain compatible with a diagnosis of myocardial infarction are suffering from a motor disorder of the esophagus, or from esophageal reflux. These patients usually show no evidence of infarction by serial electrocardiograms and enzyme studies. Coronary angiograms, performed after an acute infarction has been ruled out, are usually normal.

The pain described by such patients is usually substernal or located in the left anterior chest, or over the entire chest. It is described as a heavy pressure, as a tightness, or as gripping or viselike. The pain may radiate to one or both arms, the epigastrium, the neck, the jaw, and the back. Such pain may be precipitated by exertion or emotional events, or may start spontaneously without obvious cause. In rare cases it begins during swallowing. It may be relieved by nitroglycerin, as is coronary disease-related angina. It is difficult to distinguish angina due to coronary disease from similar pain produced by esophageal motor disorders on the basis of history and physical findings.

The usual initial strategy is to refer patients with possible cardiac pain for an extensive evaluation, including treadmill electrocardiographic and thallium stress tests, echocardiography, and, in doubtful cases, coronary angiography. In addition, ambulatory electrocardiographic monitoring has been done in an attempt to record ischemic changes occurring with or without attacks of spontaneous pain. In patients with negative cardiac studies who are having frequent distressing chest pains, an esophageal cause for the pain should be sought. The tests used for this purpose have not all been carefully standardized in a large number of control patients with and without chest pain, so the diagnostic criteria proposed have not been rigorously validated.

Esophageal pressure at different levels in the esophagus can be measured for up to 24 h, by a manometric system passed down the esophagus. A pH electrode situated 5 cm above the lower esophageal sphincter can monitor a fall in pH into the acidic range, documenting reflux. A positive test using the most rigorous criteria requires that the onset and persistence of the patient's pain be related to recorded motility disorders, such as diffuse esophageal spasm, a nutcracker esophagus, lower esophageal sphincter hypertension, classic achalasia, or vigorous achalasia. Pain may also begin in association with pH-documented reflux. Since the yield of short-term manometric and pH monitoring in catching an attack of typical pain has been low, 24-h monitoring has been used to increase the likelihood of such an event.

In addition, a provocative test for reflux—such as an esophageal infusion of dilute hydrochloric acid (the Bernstein test)—has been used to provoke an attack of typical pain. Edrophonium has been used to induce an attack of angina-like pain and a recordable esophageal motility disturbance. With the use of prolonged monitoring and provocative tests, about 50 percent of symptomatic chest pain patients with normal coronary arteries by angiography may be positively diagnosed as having chest pain of esophageal origin. The presence of esophagitis on endoscopy correlates highly with the presence of reflux-induced pain or a motility disorder.

Esophagitis may be treated with antacids or H_2 blockers, or both. Lower esophageal sphincter pressure may be increased by the use of metoclopramide. Esophageal motility disorders have been treated, to good effect, with nifedipine and nitrates in patients with lower esophageal sphincter hypertension. Surgical treatment of esophageal motility disorders is still in an early phase and has not been rigorously evaluated.

Patients with short-duration angina-like pain and normal coronary arteriograms constitute a heterogeneous group. Some patients have esophageal causes of pain; others have ischemia by stress tests and ambulatory monitoring, while another group has functional, possibly psychogenic, chest pain.

Patients with gastroesophageal reflux may have no angina-like chest pain. They may complain only of a burning substernal discomfort relieved by antacids and precipitated, or made worse, by caffeinated soda, coffee, citrus juices, tomato juice, and spicy foods. There may be reflux of bitter-tasting, throat-burning fluid into the mouth and throat. Lying flat in bed after a large meal may provoke heartburn-like pain in the midchest. Nocturnal reflux and aspiration may cause coughing and wheezing that wakes the patient. Recurrent aspiration may lead to chronic bronchitis and recurrent attacks of pneumonia. Antireflux surgery may be required for patients with pulmonary complications or intractable chest pain.

Since esophageal disorders and coronary artery disease are common after age 40, it is possible that some patients have angina-like pain induced by both coronary heart disease and esophageal motor or reflux disorders.

B. Infectious Esophagitis There is intermittent or constant lower substernal and parasternal burning or aching pain intensified by each swallow. Hematemesis, melena,

and sometimes fever may be associated symptoms. The pain may begin abruptly and may recur at variable periods (i.e., weeks or months) after it has responded to therapy. Once present, the chest pain lasts for days or weeks until it is treated. The severity varies from a mild, tolerable discomfort to a severe pain requiring hospital management. This disorder commonly occurs in patients with AIDS and in other immune-suppressed patients (e.g., diabetics, malnourished elderly patients, prednisone-antibiotic-treated patients, and bone marrow transplant patients).

1. **Candida** *Species* Candidal esophagitis is associated with oral thrush in AIDS patients (90–100 percent) and others. A double-contrast esophagogram will show vertically aligned small plaques, pseudomembranes, and decreased esophageal motility. More severe cases demonstrate cobblestoning. In very advanced cases the esophageal wall has a shaggy outline related to plaques and confluent ulcers. Marked constriction of the lumen can occur in chronic candidal esophagitis, leading to severe dysphagia. Endoscopy reveals white plaques, extensive pseudomembranes, ulcers, and a bleeding, friable mucosa. Plaques and exudates can be brushed, and smears made and stained with Gram's, methenamine silver, or PAS stain. Mycelial forms and large numbers of yeast organisms (blastospores) are diagnostic. Biopsies may be taken of the mucosa and stained with methenamine silver to demonstrate mycelial forms. This disorder will respond to oral fluconazole or intravenous amphotericin.

2. **Herpes Simplex Virus (HSV)** Herpes simplex may cause an extensive esophagitis in rare normal individuals and in patients with AIDS. An esophagogram may demonstrate herpetic ulcers. Endoscopy reveals vesicles, and discrete and confluent ulcers. Herpes lesions may occur in the mouth and nose; these lesions support a herpetic etiology of the esophageal complaints. The diagnosis is made by brushing and biopsy of the ulcers, and biopsy cultures. This disorder will respond to treatment with acyclovir.

3. **Cytomegalovirus (CMV)** Cytomegalovirus esophagitis causes similar complaints. Endoscopy of a CMV esophagitis reveals serpiginous and coalescing ulcers. The diagnosis requires biopsy of the center of an ulcer and depends on immunohistology and viral cultures.

Persons with AIDS frequently develop esophagitis with associated chest pain and odynophagia. Candida, HSV, and CMV are the main etiologic agents. HSV and CMV ulcers may become secondarily infected with *Candida* species. Rarely, esophageal lymphoma may cause odynophagia and chest pain.

Central chest pain in a patient with AIDS is usually due to esophagitis. Rare cases of purulent or tuberculous pericarditis may occur in AIDS, but pericardial pain is distinctive in character and is associated with a pericardial rub and/or an effusion.

5. Chest Wall Musculoskeletal Pain

A. Costochondritis Spontaneous pain occurs in the left parasternal region over the third to fifth costal cartilages. The pain is aching, sharp, or pressurelike, and is frequently associated with localized tenderness or soreness over the affected cartilage. Rarely, the tender cartilage is actually swollen and larger than normal *(Tietze's syndrome);* usually it is only tender. Pressure from the examiner's knuckle may be required to locate the tender area, which may be confined to a site the size of a dime or a quarter. Patients may be able to precipitate the pain by walking or climbing stairs. This relationship to exertion mimics angina pectoris associated with coronary heart disease. However, exertional chest pain associated with chest wall disorders is more likely to be due to jarring; to stimulation of the tender area by arm movements during the normal arm swing of walking; to contact of the exercised heart with the inner side of the chest wall during stair climbing or to chest wall movements during the accelerated breathing associated with exertion. In other cases the pain may occur spontaneously without precipitation by exertion, lasting 4 to 5 s—or minutes, hours, or, even days. It may radiate in a narrow band to the left axilla and even down the left arm. In some patients the pain begins a few minutes after a period of exercise and lasts for hours. Many victims of this syndrome become convinced that they have severe heart disease. They may have anxiety attacks, with sweating, trembling, dizziness, and nausea, associated with episodes of severe chest pain. If hyperventilation accompanies the anxiety attacks and chest pain, the electrocardiogram may show ST- and T-wave abnormalities, thus mimicking coronary heart disease.

In some patients with chest wall pain, qualitatively similar pain can be provoked by having the patient take a deep breath, with the shoulders thrust back and the neck extended, while the examiner exerts traction on the patient's posteriorly extended arms (the "crowing rooster" maneuver).

Abduction or adduction of the left arm against resistance by the examiner may also provoke pain that is qualitatively similar to that experienced spontaneously. Crossing the arms in front of the body in a posture of extreme adduction (arms wrapped around the chest, as though hugging oneself) may also bring on the pain. The key requirement for diagnosis is that palpation of a tender area, or some movement of the chest wall or arms, brings on pain that is qualitatively similar to, and localized to the same area as, the spontaneous pain. Provoked pain does not usually persist once the stimulus is removed.

This type of pain may sometimes occur without local tenderness or the ability to precipitate it by bodily movements. In this setting it is more likely to be attributed to anxiety, hyperventilation, or some other psychogenic mechanism.

The cardiac examination is usually normal, although some patients have a midsystolic click, a systolic heart murmur, or both; these patients usually have mitral valve prolapse. There appears to be an association between mitral valve prolapse and chest wall syndromes.

In chest wall pain, the resting electrocardiogram, the electrocardiographic and thallium exercise stress tests, and the coronary arteriogram are usually normal.

Some physicians prescribe nonsteroidal anti-inflammatory drugs for this disorder, but there is no proof of their efficacy. We have witnessed a variable response to their use, with some patients improved and others made worse as they developed esophagitis or gastritis from the drug. We do not use these agents, but treat such pain with reassurance, warm moist heat, and exercise, which seems to control or eliminate the chest pain. Rarely, costochondritis with chest pain is related to more specific disorders, such as gonorrhea, rheumatoid arthritis, Reiter's syndrome, or multiple myeloma.

About 5 to 10 percent of angina patients with coronary heart disease have chest wall pain as an associated disorder. It is also common after sternal splitting surgery for coronary bypass. It is seldom seen in patients with acute myocardial infarction.

B. Pectoral Myositis This is a chest wall pain syndrome associated with marked tenderness in the body of the left pectoralis major muscle. This pain occurs spontaneously and is aching and continuous. Arm motion and deep breaths may intensify the pain. Patients with prolonged chest wall pain may be admitted to a coronary unit to rule out myocardial infarction.

C. Precordial Catch Syndrome Pain of a sharp, sticking nature begins suddenly with the patient at rest, or during mild exertion (such as while walking slowly, raking leaves, mopping a floor, bending forward to exit a car, or standing still). The pain is localized to a small area near or below the left nipple in men, or beneath the left breast in women. It does not radiate. There is a sensation described by some patients as "of something being caught" when a deep inspiration is attempted after the pain begins. Most patients "freeze in their tracks," frightened that a change of position will intensify the pain. Breathing becomes more rapid and shallow. Patients have found that forcing themselves to straighten up and throw their shoulders back may lessen the discomfort. Many find that a forced deep inspiration will terminate the pain as abruptly as it began. Attacks usually last for several minutes. They may be followed by residual aching for a variable period (usually less than a half-hour). There is usually no tenderness. Most attacks are not witnessed, and patients cannot provoke them at will. They may occur only once, but more frequently they recur at variable intervals over days or months. Most attacks have been described in patients under age 35. This disorder has occurred with equal frequency in both sexes.

One patient has described a similar pain occurring on the right side, but this is very uncommon.

Chest x-rays and electrocardiograms are usually normal. No underlying disease is associated with this syndrome. Eventually, the attacks spontaneously cease. There is no effective therapy. It is important to recognize this condition and its benign nature, so as to be able to counsel patients not to undergo exhaustive and possibly hazardous testing for heart or pulmonary disease.

In summary, the following features are associated with chest pain of musculoskeletal or chest wall origin:

1. The pain often occurs at rest and, if associated with exercise, ceases within seconds of stopping the activity.
2. There is local chest wall tenderness along the left or right side of the sternum, or at the nipple area on the left side. This is not true in patients with the precordial catch syndrome.
3. Sticking pains may occur, lasting only seconds.
4. Prolonged aching may occur, lasting for days.
5. Transient relief can be produced by heat, massage, pressure of the hand, lidocaine injection, or a change in left arm or body position (e.g., rolling over onto one side). A deep inspiration or straightening up will relieve precordial catch.
6. Pain of a qualitatively similar kind and location can be precipitated by arm or chest wall movement or pressure over a tender area.
7. The results of electrocardiographic and thallium exercise tests, chest radiographs, and coronary angiograms are usually negative.

6. A. Anxiety-Related Chest Pain Several kinds of chest pain have been associated with anxiety. Individual patients may have one or more of these types of pain:

1. Sharp or stabbing pain along the left sternal border or over the left nipple. This pain may have a rapid onset and disappearance, lasting only 2 or 3 s, and may recur several times each minute for 5 to 20 min. There may be local skin tenderness at the pain site.
2. Aching constant pain over the left breast lasting for hours or days, and unrelated to exertion.
3. Substernal constriction or pressure that mimics the complaints of patients with variant angina. These patients may complain of throat tightness and a lump

in the throat when swallowing. The discomfort may radiate to the left neck and left arm, mimicking coronary artery disease.

B. Panic Attacks Patients with panic attacks have other complaints in addition to the anxiety-related chest pains described above. These symptoms may occur in association with the chest pain, or independently. They include the following:

1. Profuse sweating. This may precede or accompany chest pain and may require the use of a towel and a change of clothes. The sweating affects the neck, axillae, chest surface, antecubital fossae, and back.
2. Palpitations—a sensation of the heart beating rapidly and forcibly against the chest wall.
3. A subjective feeling of fear and tension. There may be excessive restlessness and an inability to sleep or to remain calm. There may be a feeling of impending doom.
4. A feeling of ''inner trembling.'' The patient feels shaky, as though trembling, but the hands are not tremulous.
5. Claustrophobia—a feeling of extreme discomfort and tension from being in a closed place. Such patients wish to be sure that there is a ready way out of any room they are in.
6. Light-headedness, giddiness, or dizziness.
7. Nausea and vomiting.
8. Shortness of breath—a feeling of suffocation or a sensation of not being able to take in a deep, satisfying breath.

Any or all of these complaints may be present in individual patients or during specific attacks. Very often these patients appear anxious, and have cool, moist palms, tachycardia, premature beats, and elevated systolic pressures. The symptoms are not continuous and often occur during the night, early in the morning, or at quiet times of the day. They last from 30 to 60 min and usually have an abrupt onset.

Patients with substernal pressure or constriction may even have false-positive exercise electrocardiograms. Usually the coronary angiogram is normal.

Small numbers of patients who appear to have this disorder may have hyperthyroidism or a pheochromocytoma.

Patients addicted to diazepam (Valium) and similar drugs may have panic attack–like symptoms of a severe nature, including chest pain, nausea, and early morning sweating, if they discontinue taking the drug for 5 to 7 days. Usually they are diagnosed as having anxiety, rather than drug withdrawal, and more diazepam is administered—reestablishing the addiction.

In some instances panic attack patients have been admitted to coronary care units for observation because of crushing chest pain, but all studies have been negative. Panic attacks are more common in young adults, who have a low prevalence of heart disease.

7. HYPERVENTILATION

This is another anxiety-related symptom. These patients have attacks of rapid breathing, light-headedness, tingling, or warm sensations over the face and hands; and, sometimes, painful carpal spasms, chest pain, and abdominal pain. Other patients, who are not breathing rapidly, complain of light-headedness and episodes of chest pain. These patients do not necessarily breathe more rapidly than normal, but may take deep inspirations and long sighing expirations. We have been able to provoke left precordial and left parasternal pain in some of these patients by asking them to breathe as deeply and rapidly as they can for 1 to 2 min. Published studies report pain provocation by hyperventilation in 39 to 42 percent of such patients. Since T-wave inversion and ST-segment depression can occur with hyperventilation, some patients are diagnosed as having coronary artery disease and may be admitted to coronary care units and have coronary angiograms done on one or more occasions.

Treatment of acute hyperventilation is begun by having such a patient rebreathe his or her own CO_2-rich expired air by covering the nose and mouth with a paper bag. Reassurance and mild sedation are useful as well. Most patients with recurrent attacks do well with supportive psychotherapy and learn to control their symptoms by controlling their breathing.

This form of management is possible once the patient can consciously relate symptoms to deep or rapid breathing. This relationship is dramatically demonstrated during the 2-min hyperventilation test described above. One must be careful, however, not to dismiss symptoms hastily as due to psychogenic hyperventilation, since secondary hyperventilation can occur in patients with true organic heart disease. In a patient with known heart disease or a disease in which the heart can be affected (e.g., scleroderma or sickle cell disease), it is necessary to do a careful evaluation of any complaints of chest pain or shortness of breath. Patients with heart disease have been discharged from emergency rooms with the diagnosis of hyperventilation only to die, unattended, at home.

8. ACUTE PERICARDITIS

This disorder begins with one of two types of chest pain:

1. A central, substernal pain that is variously described as dull and pressurelike, constrictive, or squeezing, or as a tightness. Such pain mimics that of myocardial infarction.

2. A sharp, sticking pain over the left anterior and central chest, and sometimes the right anterior chest. This pain is often increased in severity and sharpness by deep inspiration, coughing, swallowing, or lying flat on the back or on the left side. It is decreased in intensity by breath-holding, by sitting and leaning forward, and by standing.

A. Viral or Idiopathic Pericarditis   One or both types of pain may be present. Fever is frequently present; it begins before, or simultaneously with, the pain. It may range from 100 to 103°F.

The pain of pericarditis may also be referred to the tip of the left shoulder, the left and/or right shoulder ridge (trapezius ridge), and the left side of the neck. In some patients the pain may be referred to the interscapular area or the epigastrum. Uncommonly, it is felt in the jaw, ear, throat, or arms.

Physical examination may reveal fever, tachycardia proportionate to the temperature rise, and a normal blood pressure. Unless there is pericardial effusion, the heart size is normal. A two- or three-component pericardial friction rub may be present at the left sternal border. It may be heard with the patient supine, or leaning forward, or on the left side. In rare cases it is heard only over the back.

The friction rub in acute viral or idiopathic pericarditis usually appears at the time of the pain, and not 2 or 3 days later as it does in patients with acute transmural myocardial infarction. Fever also begins the first day in acute pericarditis, but is usually delayed in onset for 1 to 2 days with myocardial infarction.

In unusual cases acute myocardial infarction may be painless, and the first sign of disease may be an associated pericarditis beginning on day 2 or 3 of the illness. This can clinically mimic viral pericarditis, but is usually easily differentiated by the electrocardiogram.

In most cases of acute pericarditis the electrocardiogram shows 1 to 3 mm of ST-segment elevation in leads I, II, III, aVL, aVF, and V_2 or V_3 through V_6. Depression of ST segments may occur in leads aVR and V_1, and PR-segment depression is frequently seen. T waves remain of low amplitude and may or may not invert after 5 or 6 days. In infarction, T waves invert in association with ST-segment elevation. Q waves and loss of R-wave amplitude do not occur with acute pericarditis. The T waves may never invert. In some cases with friction rubs, the electrocardiogram may remain normal. ST-segment elevations usually return to the baseline in 5 to 7 days, but T-wave inversion can persist indefinitely or revert within 2 to 4 months.

Serial serum enzyme studies may show nonspecific rises of AST and lactic dehydrogenase activity levels. Even infarction-like changes in LDH and CPK isozymes have been reported on occasion, but such cases have usually been uncommon. A recent report from Finland, however, has reported that 60 to 70 percent of soldiers with acute idiopathic pericarditis had elevated CPK–MB levels during the first 48 h of the illness. In viral or idiopathic pericarditis, the white blood cell count is usually elevated to between 12,000 and 14,000 cells per mm^3, and the sedimentation rate may be elevated. Two-dimensional (2-D) echocardiograms may show a small pericardial effusion or may be normal. An effusion can also cause globular enlargement of the heart without evidence of pulmonary congestion in the lungs. Small pleural effusions may occur in pericarditis, as may pulmonary infiltrates due to atelectasis or pneumonia.

Pericarditis may be due to a viral infection (e.g., coxsackievirus B, echovirus, influenza, Epstein-Barr), or it may be idiopathic. For the latter group, an autoimmune basis is postulated.

Infections caused by pyogenic bacteria or tuberculosis must be separated from pericarditis due to viruses or autoimmune disease.

B. Bacterial (Pyogenic) Pericarditis   Acute bacterial pericarditis is usually caused by staphylococci or enteric gram-negative rods. The pericardial space contains bacteria and purulent fluid. This disorder frequently follows chest surgery or occurs in immunosuppressed patients. Fever may precede chest pain by several days. This disease may also occur in patients with pneumonia and empyema; in patients with a history of shaking chills and fever due to bacteremia; in patients with endocarditis and myocardial abscesses; secondary to meningococcemia; and with spread from a liver abscess.

In pericarditis due to pyogenic bacteria there may be a large pericardial effusion with neck vein distension, a pericardial rub, an enlarged heart on x-ray, shortness of breath, chills, fever, hepatic enlargement, and pleural effusions. An echocardiogram confirms the presence of pericardial effusion, and a pericardiocentesis will reveal an exudative effusion with a neutrophil count exceeding 50,000 cells per mm^3. Gram stains and cultures of the fluid will reveal the causative organism.

Intravenous antibiotics and surgical drainage of the purulent pericardial fluid are required for cure. Thoracotomy and drainage of loculated pleural and pericardial pus may be necessary. Aggressive surgical and antibiotic therapy can reduce the mortality rate from 30 percent to less than 10 percent.

C. Tuberculous Pericarditis   Tuberculous pericarditis may mimic viral pericarditis, but there is often (50 percent of cases) evidence of old pulmonary or mediastinal tuberculosis. The tuberculin skin test may be falsely negative in 30 percent of cases. The diagnosis may be confirmed by culture of pericardial fluid or by biopsy of the pericardium. In some cases, antituberculous therapy is started empirically without a definitive diagnosis being made.

Other causes of acute pericarditis include malignant tumors and disseminated lupus erythematosus. Tumor may be diagnosed by cytologic study of the pericardial fluid after aspiration, or by pericardial biopsy. Lupus is associated with arthralgias, facial rash, renal disease, pleuritic pain, anemia, leukopenia and thrombocytopenia, and a positive antinuclear antibody and/or LE test.

Sensitivity to certain drugs, such as phenytoin (Dilantin), hydralazine (Apresoline), procainamide, dantrolene, methysergide and cromolyn sodium, can cause pericarditis. The therapy required is discontinuation of the offending drug.

Pericarditis may occur 1 week or more after a myocardial infarction (Dressler's syndrome), cardiac surgery, or cardiac trauma; or it may follow radiation therapy to the mediastinum.

Viral and idiopathic pericarditis, drug-related pericarditis, and post-surgery and postinfarction pericarditis all respond rapidly and dramatically to oral prednisone therapy (20–60 mg/day). Relapses and recurrences may follow reduction in dosage or discontinuation of therapy in up to one-third of patients.

Complications of pericarditis include tamponade, with signs of right-sided heart failure and falling blood pressure, and constrictive pericarditis, which may present in a similar manner. Differentiation of tamponade from constriction can be made by 2-D echocardiography. Effusion and constriction combined may cause tamponade.

Most patients with viral and idiopathic pericarditis recover without sequelae. Occasional patients develop tamponade and/or constriction; these conditions require pericardiocentesis and/or surgery. Patients with specific causes for pericarditis, such as metastatic carcinoma, mesothelioma, tuberculosis, bacterial infection, or lupus erythematosus, constitute fewer than 15 percent of all cases of acute pericarditis.

9. ACUTE MASSIVE PULMONARY EMBOLISM

Severe crushing or constricting substernal pain may accompany a massive pulmonary embolism. Such emboli arise in large thigh or pelvic veins and are big enough to occlude one or both main pulmonary arteries with clot. The volume of a thrombus extending from the calf into the thigh is approximately 100 ml. Massive embolization has been defined as a clot obstructing more than 50 percent of the pulmonary circulation. In addition to intense midsternal chest pain, such patients may develop severe dyspnea, wheezing, and a marked drop in blood pressure, which initially may return to normal, only to fall again later. In addition, neck veins may be distended and right upper abdominal pain may occur because of acute hepatic congestion. A right ventricular gallop and marked tachycardia may be present. Some patients may develop atrial tachycardia or fibrillation. An electrocardiogram may show an S_1Q_3 inverted T_3 pattern, or complete or incomplete right bundle branch block, and there may be T-wave inversion in leads V_1 to V_3. Chest radiographs may be normal or may show a unilateral hilar mass with a paucity of vascular markings on the affected side (Westermark's sign). A perfusion lung scan will show absence of perfusion to one lung and part of the other. A pulmonary angiogram may show occlusion of one main pulmonary artery or multiple lobar or segmental arteries, and partial occlusion of the circulation to the other lung. Surgical embolectomy has resulted, in the past, in a mortality rate in the range of 50 to 61 percent; it has largely been abandoned and replaced by thrombolytic therapy and administration of intravenous heparin as treatment for relatively stable patients. Embolectomy is now used only for patients with cardiac arrest or failed thrombolytic therapy. The results of such surgery have improved since the advent of extracorporeal circulation; the mortality figures reported recently are in the range of 11 to 31 percent.

Associated clinical evidence of phlebitis or lower-extremity venous thrombosis (e.g., deep leg pain and edema) occurs in only a minority of patients.

Risk factors that increase the incidence of clots in the legs or pelvis and subsequent embolization include the following:

1. Immobilization (e.g., bed rest, long auto or airplane trips, casts on legs, and paralysis of legs in stroke or spinal cord injury patients).
2. Recent surgery—30 percent of patients undergoing major abdominal surgery after age 40 develop calf vein thrombosis. One-fifth of these (6 percent overall) propagate clot to thigh veins, and 50 percent of these (3 percent overall) have pulmonary emboli. Of patients having hip surgery, 70 to 80 percent develop leg clots, as do 22 percent of patients suffering myocardial infarction.
3. Pregnancy.
4. Use of birth control pills.
5. Cancer.
6. Heart failure.
7. Massive obesity.
8. Hypercoagulable states:
   A. Antithrombin III (AT III) deficiency may account for as many as 2 percent of clinical episodes of thromboembolic disease. Estrogen-induced thromboembolism may occur because of estrogen depression of AT III production by the liver.
   B. Protein C deficiency.
   C. Protein S deficiency.

Diagnostic methods for leg thrombi and pulmonary embolization include:

1. Doppler venography and impedance plethysmography are both accurate (90–100 percent) in detecting thrombi in thigh veins. The "gold standard" test for venous thrombi in calf and thigh veins is contrast venography. Unfortunately, this test is invasive, causes pain (50 percent of cases), and may produce some leg vein thrombi in 33 percent of patients. Use of nonionic contrast media may reduce these complications. Most of these clots occur in the calf, but pulmonary emboli have occurred. The presence of thigh vein thrombi is an indication for anticoagulation, since such clots pose a high risk of embolization. Many such emboli may occur and be asymptomatic, being detectable only by lung scan. In 30 to 50 percent of patients with proven pulmonary emboli, thigh thrombi are absent; the presumption is that these have broken off and embolized entirely to the lung.

2. Lung scans. A perfusion lung scan will be normal in the absence of pulmonary emboli in patients with otherwise normal lungs, and will effectively rule out a diagnosis of embolization. In patients with other pulmonary disorders, such as asthma, emphysema, atelectasis, pneumonia, lung cancer, pulmonary vasculitis, radiation pneumonitis, or pulmonary congestion, the perfusion lung scan is frequently abnormal (falsely positive for embolization). One strategy that has been used to make lung scans more specific is to combine perfusion scans with ventilation scans using xenon 133. With pulmonary emboli, ventilation scans are usually normal when the perfusion scan is abnormal. This is called a *ventilation perfusion* or *V/Q mismatch*. Multiple segmental or lobar perfusion defects associated with a V/Q mismatch pattern are associated with angiographic evidence of pulmonary embolization in 90 percent of cases. In patients with a lung infiltrate on chest x-ray, a ^{99m}Tc perfusion defect larger than the infiltrate is associated with embolization in 89 percent of cases. Radionuclide defects smaller than the infiltrate show emboli in only 10 percent of arteriograms.

When clinical findings are considered in association with the large defects and V/Q mismatch, low-probability clinical findings drop the likelihood of finding angiographic evidence of pulmonary emboli to 54 percent.

In sick hospitalized patients, the correlation between a specific type of lung scan and evidence of pulmonary emboli by arteriography is not good.
In summary:
A. A negative perfusion scan indicates that there is no evidence of pulmonary emboli.
B. A positive perfusion lung scan with V/Q mismatch is associated with emboli in 40 to 90 percent of cases. The false-positive rate is as high as 60 percent.
C. A positive perfusion scan with V/Q match is associated with emboli in as many as 30 to 42

percent of cases. A V/Q match does not completely eliminate the possibility of embolization, so the ventilation scan has not been as useful in aiding the interpretation of abnormal perfusion scans as originally was hoped.

3. Angiography. A positive perfusion scan requires an angiogram for accurate interpretation regardless of whether there is a V/Q mismatch. In major centers, selective injections, special views, and image intensification and magnification techniques are being used to increase the sensitivity of the angiogram.

   A positive angiogram will show an abrupt vessel cutoff or a partly occluding filling defect. Rarely, it will be falsely negative in the presence of a clinically likely embolism, a positive ventilation-perfusion scan, or venous thrombosis in the leg by venography.

Massive and submassive emboli may be treated with intravenous streptokinase or urokinase. These agents will lyse emboli by producing plasmin, a fibrin-destroying enzyme. Dissolution of emboli with restoration of the pulmonary circulation occurs rapidly with these therapeutic agents. Mortality, however, remains as high as it is with heparin or warfarin therapy. Thrombolytic agents may cause bleeding (severe in 9 percent of cases), fever, and allergic reactions.

Heparin should be used intravenously. It complexes with AT III and inhibits thrombin and factor Xa to prevent fibrinogen polymerization into a thrombus. Bleeding is the major side effect, and usually occurs in patients who have abused alcohol or aspirin or who have an underlying disease such as cirrhosis or cancer. Thrombocytopenia secondary to heparin therapy may also occur and cause bleeding.

Warfarin is an oral anticoagulant that decreases the activities of thrombin factors VII, IX, and X. The recurrence rate of thromboembolism with warfarin therapy is 2 percent or less and bleeding frequency is 4 percent. It should be used after heparin therapy for long-term maintenance.

Vena cava interruption, using ligation, clipping, plication, or transvenous insertion of a filter, may be used when anticoagulation fails to prevent subsequent embolization; when bleeding occurs; when other diseases contraindicate anticoagulants; or when paradoxic embolization occurs.

Transvenous insertion of a Greenfield filter into the inferior vena cava has a lower operative mortality rate (0.6–2 percent) than open surgery, and prevents recurrent emboli and venous insufficiency.

10. ACUTE AORTIC DISSECTION

This disorder begins with the abrupt onset of severe substernal and left chest pain. The pain has been described as tearing or ripping, but this quality is often absent. The intensity of the pain reaches a maximum within seconds. It may spread rapidly to the face and jaw, the shoulders, and one or both arms, and straight through to the back. It may also radiate into the upper abdomen. The pain is usually so intense that patients are unable to lie still; they writhe and roll from side to side, seeking some position that will afford relief. In a minority of cases the pain is of moderate severity, and can be partly controlled by analgesics. It is not affected by coughing or deep breathing.

Pain in the flank suggests renal artery dissection, and pain in the epigastrum indicates involvement of the abdominal aorta. The pain pattern may change rapidly over the first 24 h.

Fainting, hemiplegia, unilateral blindness, or aphasia indicates involvement of the right innominate or left common carotid artery.

Spinal cord dysfunction secondary to dissection may develop, resulting in paralysis of one or both legs and numbness of the lower body.

Dissection of the coronary arteries may cause more intense substernal chest pain from a myocardial infarction; this will be reflected in the electrocardiogram.

Acute aortic insufficiency, from retrograde dissection of the aortic valve area, can cause dyspnea at rest and orthopnea.

Nausea, vomiting, constant severe upper abdominal pain, hematemesis, or passage of a bloody, soft, or liquid stool reflects involvement of the blood supply to the intestinal tract and ischemic infarction of the bowel. Physical signs in the abdomen may be minimal in the presence of severe ischemic pain.

Pain and progressive numbness, coldness, and pallor of a leg, with loss of pulses, may result from dissection of the length of the aorta and unilateral occlusion of a common iliac artery.

Physical examination reveals hypertension and a decrease or loss of pulses in the neck or extremities. Tachycardia is common, but fever is unusual. A shocky appearance, with pallor and cool hands and feet, may be present.

The left external jugular vein may be distended as the enlarged aorta partially obstructs venous return across the upper mediastinum. Bilateral jugular venous distension associated with a paradoxic pulse and a falling blood pressure indicates bleeding into the pericardial space and cardiac tamponade, which usually is rapidly fatal if unrelieved; it is a common cause of death with aortic dissection.

Dullness and decreased breath sounds over the left lower posterior chest indicate hemothorax resulting from leakage from the aorta.

A diastolic murmur of aortic insufficiency indicates retrograde dissection from a tear in the lining of the ascending aorta. This causes the insertions of the valve cusps into the aortic wall to become distorted and produces valvular incompetence. This is found in 50 percent of cases.

Pulsation of the sternoclavicular joint, Horner's syndrome, and a pericardial friction rub are signs uncommonly seen in aortic dissection. Abdominal tenderness and distension may occur secondary to bowel involvement. One or both lower extremities may be cold, pale, and pulseless.

Neurologic examination may reveal hemiparesis, with or without aphasia; anesthesia with a sensory level; or paraplegia.

The electrocardiogram may show evidence of left ventricular hypertrophy due to prior hypertension. In one series, 16 percent of cases showed electrocardiographic evidence of myocardial infarction. In a minority of cases, signs of pericarditis may appear in the electrocardiogram.

The chest radiograph usually shows widening of the superior mediastinum (80–90 percent of cases). A normal aorta on a chest radiograph does not completely exclude dissection. Chest radiographic findings suggestive of dissection include aortic dilatation (ascending arch or descending aorta), progressive widening of the aortic shadow on serial radiographs, a serrated margin of the aortic shadow, and detection of internal calcification more than 6 mm inside the outer aortic wall (i.e., thickened wall of the aorta).

LDH_1 and CPK–MB serum levels may be elevated when the dissection occludes a coronary artery and produces myocardial infarction.

The definitive diagnosis of dissection requires the use of catheter aortography to define the site of the intimal flap, the region of aortic narrowing, the origin and termination of the double lumen, and the presence of occlusion of aortic branches. In less severely ill patients, where the diagnosis is in doubt, a CT scan with contrast enhancement will be helpful in confirming the diagnosis. Echocardiography has a fairly high sensitivity for the diagnosis of dissection of the ascending aorta, but is not useful for more distal (type III—see below) dissections. CT scans with contrast enhancement have greater sensitivity and specificity than echocardiograms and can be done in 15 to 20 min.

Dissections of the aorta have been classified as types I, II, and III (DeBakey classification) or as types A and B (Daily et al). Type I starts in the ascending aorta and involves the entire length of the aorta; type II is limited to the ascending aorta; and type III starts just beyond the arch origin of the left subclavian artery and spares the ascending aorta and arch. In the Daily classification, type A includes all patients with involvement of the ascending aorta; type B includes all patients with dissection distal to the origin of the left subclavian artery from the arch.

Type A dissections occur in younger patients with less severe hypertension. Cases involving Marfan's syndrome and those arising in relation to aortic valvular stenosis tend to be type A dissections. Type B dissections occur in older patients with severe hypertension and generalized vascular disease.

As soon as the patient is reasonably stable, surgical treatment of type A (types I and II) dissections should be undertaken. Using newer surgical techniques, operative mortality varies from 10 to 20 percent. Recent improvements in surgical technique have also encouraged the operative treatment of type B dissections, which formerly were treated medically. Current mortality figures for surgical repair of type B dissections are 13 to 15 percent.

The major risk factors for the development of aortic dissection include hypertension (80–90 percent of cases), Marfan's syndrome (10 percent), cystic medial necrosis of the aortic wall (20 percent), bicuspid aortic valve, aortic stenosis, mitral valve prolapse, and coarctation of the aorta.

Trauma during coronary angiography, or after insertion of an aortic counterpulsation balloon to treat cardiogenic shock, has been associated with subsequent dissection. Cystic medial necrosis occurs in younger patients who have Marfan's syndrome or Ehlers-Danlos syndrome, or who are pregnant.

11. MEDIASTINITIS

These infections of the central chest begin with fever, rigors, and retrosternal pain that may be pressurelike or constricting. The pain may be intensified by coughing and deep breathing. Physical examination reveals fever, rigors, tachycardia, and rapid, shallow breathing. If the infection is secondary to chest surgery, the sternal wound may be red, tender, and fluctuant, or may be draining pus.

Mediastinal infection results from spread of infection from the head and neck, lungs, pleural or pericardial spaces, chest wall, local lymph nodes, or from perforation of the pharynx, esophagus, or trachea. Cardiac surgery is currently a frequent cause of mediastinal infection.

A chest radiograph may show a widened mediastinum with right paratracheal opacification, and air-fluid levels in mediastinal abscesses. Free air in the tissue planes of the neck and mediastinum may be visualized in some cases. In many patients, the routine posteroanterior and lateral chest radiographs are normal or show nonspecific findings. CT scans of the chest provide excellent visualization of posterior mediastinal masses (associated with rupture of the esophagus). Obliteration of mediastinal fascial planes and abscesses with air-fluid levels may be seen. An unexpected associated empyema may be detected.

Esophageal perforation may follow erosion by a tumor; it also may occur subsequent to injury to the chest or lower neck, or, rarely, during esophagoscopy. Severe vomiting and retching may result in a through-and-through tear in the esophageal wall (Boerhaave's syndrome). Other marked increases in pressure in the abdomen can cause esophageal rupture. Straining at stool or lifting a heavy weight can cause this. Air may be visualized in the mediastinum, and a left pleural effusion usually develops in association with fever and chills.

Mediastinal infections arising in the teeth often begin with dental pain or dental treatment. These infections often affect the neck, causing high fever, toxicity, neck and throat pain, and brawny edema and tenderness of the anterior neck region and upper chest. Dysphagia and odynophagia may occur, and the patient may drool. A lateral neck radiograph may show a retropharyngeal abscess. Such infections may involve the anterior, middle, or posterior mediastinum. After CT scan localization, the mediastinum can be surgically explored and drained with a large-bore soft suction catheter. Antibiotic coverage for anaerobic and aerobic bacteria is necessary.

In mediastinal infections, chest pain occurs in a setting of toxicity and fever. This condition should rarely be confused with myocardial infarction.

12. PNEUMOMEDIASTINUM

This disorder begins with substernal pain, dysphagia, sore throat, and neck pain. The chest pain is often intensified by coughing, swallowing, and deep inspiration, and by lying flat in bed; it is partly relieved by leaning forward. Dyspnea is usually mild. The chest pain, when occurring alone, may radiate to the back or neck. Physical findings include subcutaneous emphysema of the neck and chest and Hamman's sign (a precordial crunching sound), best heard along the left sternal border with the patient lying on his or her left side. Hamman's sign is synchronous with the heart sounds. It is present in 50 percent of cases.

The subcutaneous emphysema may extend to involve the face, chest, and abdominal wall. There is no fever or chills, unless esophageal leakage has occurred.

The diagnosis can be made by a plain chest radiograph, which frequently shows air surrounding the pericardium and outlines the thin dense line of the anterior mediastinal pleura. Retrosternal free air may be seen on a lateral radiograph. Air may also outline the trachea and aorta.

Pneumomediastinum may be precipitated by coughing, vomiting, or straining (e.g., lifting, straining at stool, childbirth, breath-holding, or blowing on a wind instrument). It may also follow surgery or spontaneous esophageal perforation. It may result from barotrauma related to artificial ventilation.

Patients with mediastinal air secondary to spontaneous rupture of lung alveoli do well on bed rest and O_2 therapy. No specific therapy is required. Esophageal rupture as a cause of pneumomediastinum must be ruled out, since failure to treat the esophageal lesion can result in death from infection.

With esophageal rupture, the substernal pain is very severe and there is associated fever, chills, and signs of toxicity and shock. Frequently, a chest radiograph will show a pleural effusion, mediastinal air, and pneumothorax. Endoscopy or an esophageal radiographic study with a water-soluble contrast agent is required to locate the esophageal injury.

Therapy of pneumomediastinum with 95% O_2 decreases the partial pressure of nitrogen in the blood and facilitates nitrogen reabsorption from the mediastinum. Any underlying disorder, such as atelectasis, pneumonia, asthma, or esophageal leakage, requires specific therapy. Uncomplicated cases clear in 3 to 5 days. Chest pain is usually improved in 24 h.

Tension pneumomediastinum as a result of this disorder can rarely occur; if air under high pressure dissects into the pericardial space, tamponade may occur. Tension pneumomediastinum may also impair venous return and cause a drop in systemic arterial pressure and shock. Immediate decompression is required.

13. PNEUMOTHORAX

A. Left Simple Pneumothorax Rupture of a bleb, bulla, or cyst on the pleural surface of the lung allows air to leak into the pleural space. The lung partly collapses. There is an abrupt—almost instantaneous—onset of sharp anterior and/or lateral chest pain, made worse by arm or bodily movement and/or deep inspiration. Dyspnea may also be present. The chest pain becomes constant. Examination of the chest shows decreased expansion and breath sounds over the involved side of the thorax. The percussion note is hyperresonant or tympanitic. Cardiac sounds may be distant and muffled. A chest radiograph will demonstrate air in the pleural space and atelectasis of the lung. A chest radiograph taken with the breath held at the end of expiration will aid in the demonstration of a small pneumothorax (25 percent of the hemithorax). Small pneumothoraces in otherwise healthy patients are treated with bed rest and observation. Larger pneumothoraces (i.e., 25–50 percent of the hemithorax) may be treated by removal of air through a small catheter. Very large pneumothoraces should be treated by insertion of a chest tube attached to a drainage and suction system.

Primary pneumothoraces are more common in men (male/female ratio 8 to 1), in those with a tall, thin habitus, and in smokers (92 percent of cases). In cases secondary to another disease, panacinar emphysema and interstitial lung diseases are the most common primary disorders.

Pneumothoraces secondary to trauma or other diseases (e.g., asthma, necrotizing pneumonia, tuberculosis, eosinophilic granuloma, and adult respiratory distress syndrome) require tube thoracostomy and suction drainage.

B. Tension Pneumothorax   Tension pneumothorax occurs when there is a one-way leak from the lung into the pleural space. There is intense chest pain, dyspnea, cyanosis, a weak pulse, and falling blood pressure. The trachea and apical impulse are displaced to the side opposite the pneumothorax, and there is jugular venous distension. The breath sounds are absent over the affected side of the chest, and the percussion note is hyperresonant. Blood is not delivered to the right side of the heart in amounts large enough to maintain blood pressure; hypotension develops. The blood-pressure drop occurs because the high intrathoracic pressure prevents venous inflow into the thorax, and the mediastinal shift to one side distorts the large veins entering the thorax. Coronary blood flow and oxygenation may also be affected, leading to electrocardiographic evidence of cardiac injury, with ST-segment elevations and potentially lethal arrhythmias (e.g., ventricular tachycardia). These resolve rapidly after decompression of the chest and administration of oxygen. Definitive treatment requires insertion of a chest tube and use of continuous suction to evacuate the pleural space.

14.   TRACHEOBRONCHITIS

An acute viral or bacterial infection of the trachea and larger bronchi may cause sharp substernal pain that is markedly intensified with each cough and is somewhat intensified with each inspiration. Fever and chills may be present. The cough may be nonproductive with influenza virus infection; with bacterial infections the sputum may contain mucus, bacteria, and red and white blood cells. Bacterial infection responds to antibiotics such as cefuroxime or cefaclor. The chest radiograph may be negative or may show patchy pneumonic infiltrates. Most symptoms and the substernal pain usually clear in 5 to 7 days with treatment.

15.   HERPES ZOSTER

Shingles, or herpes zoster infection, begins as a burning, aching, pruritic, or constricting discomfort in a 3- to 4-in.-wide band about one side of the chest. Within 2 to 3 days of the onset of the pain, red-based tiny vesicles and pustules appear, in groups of four or five, in the painful zone. The skin rash is confined to one side of the thorax. It may begin with grouped lesions on the back, adjacent to the spine, in the midlateral line, or on the front of the chest. The lesions soon rupture and develop a reddish-brown crust. Acyclovir, an antiviral drug, may be used to treat severe cases. Pigmentation of the skin may result after the lesions heal. In black persons depigmentation may occur.

Postherpetic neuralgic pain may persist for months after healing of the rash.

16.   ESOPHAGEAL RUPTURE—BOERHAAVE'S SYNDROME AND OTHER CAUSES

Nausea and forceful vomiting are followed within a brief period by the abrupt onset of substernal or left precordial pain (70 percent of cases). Pain may also occur in the epigastrium, left shoulder, and upper back. The substernal pain has been variously described as a tightness, a pressure, and a dull ache. The precordial and back pain may be dull and aching, or pleuritic. Associated symptoms include dyspnea (50 percent of cases) (related to pleuritis, pneumothorax, or pleural effusion), mild hematemesis (50 percent), fever (11–50 percent), odynophagia or dysphagia (<10 percent), and cold-water polydipsia (<10 percent).

Physical examination may reveal tachycardia, tachypnea, fever, and hypotension (25 percent of patients may be in a shocklike state); or all vital signs may be normal. Subcutaneous emphysema may first appear in the supraclavicular fossae in up to 33 percent of cases. It is a late sign, and develops 6 to 18 h after the onset of pain. Decreased breath sounds and/or rales may be heard over the left posterior chest because of a pneumothorax and/or pleural effusion. Hamman's sign (described as a crackling, bubbling, or crunching substernal noise, synchronous with cardiac contraction) may be heard in up to 20 percent of cases, and is related to the presence of pneumomediastinum. Rarely, a pericardial rub may be audible because of a purulent pericarditis related to mediastinal infection. Epigastric and lower chest direct tenderness, and epigastric rigidity and rebound tenderness, may occur, mimicking a perforated ulcer. To confuse the clinical picture further, up to 5 percent of patients may have free air under the diaphragm.

The plain chest radiograph may demonstrate pneumomediastinum along the left border of the heart, the aortic arch, and the descending aorta. The "V" sign of Naclerio may be present in 20 percent of cases. This is a V-shaped radiolucent shadow formed by air dissecting the fascial planes of the mediastinum and pleura. A left lower lobe infiltrate and left pleural effusion may be present, or a pneumothorax or hydropneumothorax. The presence of subcutaneous and/or mediastinal air differentiates spontaneous esophageal rupture from more common causes of anterior chest pain, such as myocardial infarction, pulmonary embolism, aortic dissection, and pericarditis. Abdominal disorders often confused with esophageal rupture include perforated ulcer, mesenteric occlusion, a ruptured subphrenic abscess, an incarcerated diaphragmatic hernia, and acute pancreatitis.

The diagnosis can be confirmed in up to 90 to 95 percent of cases by a diatrizoate meglumine (Gastrografin) swallow, which will demonstrate leakage of the contrast material into the mediastinum or left pleural cavity. Endoscopy and/or barium swallows have been used to detect rupture in suspected cases after negative Gastrografin swallows.

Pain and physical findings are usually substernal or left-sided, but right chest pain, pneumothorax, and effusion may occur in a small number of cases.

CT scanning has been used to evaluate patients too ill or uncooperative to allow contrast studies of the esophagus. The CT scan may demonstrate a mediastinal hematoma; free air and/or abscesses in the mediastinum; pleural fluid; and/or a pneumothorax. The pleural fluid is dark-brown and sometimes foul-smelling. It is an exudate with a high salivary amylase concentration (90 percent of cases) and a pH below 6 (50 percent of cases), and often contains food particles.

The classic story of postemetic chest and/or epigastric pain associated with the development of subcutaneous emphysema and/or pneumomediastinum occurs in 50 to 65 percent of cases. In other cases there may be no history of vomiting or, rarely, no pain. Some cases occur in a setting of severe asthma; childbirth; severe coughing or hiccups; weight lifting; food bingeing; during dialysis; and after a Heimlich maneuver. Some cases of esophageal rupture are related to endoscopy, esophageal instrumentation, trauma, and foreign bodies. Underlying esophageal diseases, such as stricture, carcinoma, achalasia, or a paraesophageal hernia, may lead to rupture. There is controversy as to the best therapy. Immediate surgical exploration, esophageal closure, and mediastinal lavage and drainage are advocated by some authors; others claim good results with conservative medical management using total parenteral nutrition, antibiotics, fluid replacement, and chest tube drainage.

13 Acute Right or Left Anterior or Anterolateral Chest Pain

☐ **DIAGNOSTIC LIST**

1. Pleuritic Pain
   A. Pneumonia
      1. Bacterial pneumonia (including polymicrobial aspiration pneumonia)
      2. *Mycoplasma pneumoniae* (primary atypical pneumonia)
      3. *Legionella pneumophila* (legionellosis)
      4. A. *Chlamydia psittaci* (psittacosis/ornithosis)
         B. *Chlamydia pneumoniae* (TWAR strain)
      5. Q fever
      6. Tularemia pneumonia
   B. Pulmonary embolism and infarction
   C. Tuberculosis
   D. Disorders involving the pleura and/or pericardium
      1. Systemic lupus erythematosus and drug-induced lupus
      2. Rheumatoid arthritis
      3. Postmyocardial infarction, postcardiotomy, or post-cardiac trauma syndromes
      4. Acute viral or idiopathic pericarditis
      5. Persistent pericarditis
         A. Purulent pericarditis
         B. Tuberculous pericarditis
         C. Neoplastic pericarditis
   E. Pleurodynia and other causes of "viral" pleurisy
   F. Empyema
   G. Subdiaphragmatic abscess
   H. Tumors
      1. Benign mesothelioma
      2. Malignant mesothelioma
      3. Primary or metastatic cancer involving the pleura
   I. Fitz-Hugh–Curtis syndrome
2. Pneumothorax
   A. Simple pneumothorax
   B. Tension pneumothorax
3. Chest wall pain
   A. Rib fractures (traumatic and pathologic)
   B. Costochondritis
   C. Pectoral myositis and injury (myofascial syndromes)
   D. Rib infarcts from sickle cell anemia
4. Neuritic pain
   A. Intercostal neuritis
   B. Herpes zoster
   C. Spinal disease and radiculopathy
5. Mondor's disease (thrombophlebitis of the chest wall)
6. Coronary heart disease
   A. Myocardial infarction
   B. Unstable angina
7. Rupture of the esophagus (Boerhaave's syndrome and other causes)

☐ SUMMARY

Pleuritic chest pain is a sharp or stabbing pain that is made worse by deep inspiration or by coughing, and sometimes by movement of the upper body, as in sitting up from a supine position. *Bacterial pneumonia* is associated with pleuritic pain, fever, rigors, chills, cough, and yellow-green, rust-colored, or prune-colored sputum. Streaks of blood may be mixed with purulent sputum. *Mycoplasma pneumoniae* may cause an atypical pneumonia. Only a minority of cases are associated with pleuritic pain. Intractable cough and fever are the major symptoms. *Legionella* species cause pneumonia with pleuritic pain, cough with mucoid or mucopurulent sputum, fever, and chills. Patients with this disorder often have abdominal pain, diarrhea, and mental changes; they may have renal and liver-function abnormalities. Patients with *psittacosis* seldom have pleuritic pain, but in severe cases they may. They usually have cough, fever, and headache; they may have splenomegaly and physical and radiographic evidence of pneumonia. There is a positive history of exposure to parakeets, parrots, or other birds, such as ducks or turkeys. The chest radiograph usually demonstrates pneumonic infiltrates in all of these disorders. Diagnosis depends on clinical findings and laboratory analysis of sputum or tracheal secretions and serologic studies. *Chlamydia pneumoniae* [Taiwan acute respiratory (TWAR) strain] causes an acute respiratory illness, with fever, headache, cough, and laryngitis, and x-ray evidence of subsegmental or segmental pneumonia. It is tetracycline-responsive and mimics a *Mycoplasma pneumoniae* infection. Diagnosis requires isolation of the organism or use of a specific TWAR antigen for serologic studies. Q fever and tularemia may cause penicillin-resistant pneumonias. The diagnosis is usually established by serologic studies.

Pulmonary emboli occur in persons whose legs are immobilized because of recent surgery, prolonged bed rest, casts, paraplegia, or hemiplegia. Use of contraceptive pills, a family history of phlebitis and embolism (e.g., due to antithrombin III, or to protein S or protein C deficiency), malignancy, pregnancy, and congestive heart failure also predispose patients to embolism. Pleuritic pain is usually sharp and well localized. It may be transient, vanishing within hours, or it may last for days. Fever, but not rigors, may occur. Hemoptysis of bright-red or dark blood occurs in 20 to 30 percent of cases. Purulent or rust-colored sputum is not present. Dyspnea and cough occur. The chest radiograph shows ipsilateral platelike atelectasis or a pleural-based triangular infiltrate (Hampton hump). The lung scan and pulmonary angiogram will usually confirm the diagnosis.

Tuberculosis can cause pleuritic pain, fever, and a pleural effusion discernible by physical examination and a chest radiograph. Culture of the effusion and/or pleural biopsy will confirm the diagnosis in 70 percent of cases. This disorder usually occurs in young adults. The tuberculin skin test is positive in 90 percent of patients with this disorder.

Systemic lupus erythematosus (SLE) may cause pleuritic pain, joint pain, a butterfly facial rash, renal disease, pericar-

ditis, neurologic problems (e.g., seizures and loss of memory and/or judgment), abdominal pain, alopecia, and positive antinuclear antibody (ANA) and LE cell tests. Pleuritic pain may be the sole clinical manifestation of SLE in a small percentage of cases. Five percent of patients with *rheumatoid arthritis* may have pleuritic pain associated with a generalized symmetrical arthritis, subcutaneous nodules, and a positive latex agglutination test for rheumatoid factor.

Persons with *acute pericarditis* present with chest pain made worse by lying supine or on the left side, or by deep inspiration. The pain is ameliorated by shallow breathing or by sitting up and leaning forward. A pericardial friction rub may be heard, and fever is usually present from the time of onset. The electrocardiogram shows concave-upward ST-segment elevation in all leads but aV_R and V_1. After 2 to 5 days, when the ST segment returns to the baseline, the T waves may or may not invert. This disorder is usually viral or idiopathic. An identical disorder can occur 1 to 10 weeks after a documented myocardial infarction. This syndrome, which is similar to idiopathic pericarditis, has been called *postmyocardial infarction syndrome,* or Dressler's syndrome. An identical illness may follow cardiac injury (post-cardiac trauma pericarditis) or surgery (*postcardiotomy syndrome*). *Idiopathic, viral, uremic, post–cardiac damage,* and *lupus-associated forms of pericarditis* are usually prednisone-responsive. *Purulent, tuberculous, and neoplastic pericarditis* may mimic other forms of acute pericarditis, but they are resistant to prednisone therapy.

Pleurodynia, a viral epidemic disease that occurs in the late summer and fall, causes pleuritic chest pain that sometimes occurs in paroxysms lasting 2 to 10 h. It may involve one or both sides of the chest. Abdominal pain, tenderness, and fever are common associated symptoms. The chest radiograph is normal or shows a small pleural effusion. *Empyema* follows an episode of bacterial pneumonia. Pleuritic pain, fever, and chills, associated with a pleural effusion present on a chest radiograph 1 week or more after the onset of pneumonia, suggest this diagnosis. *Subdiaphragmatic abscess* begins with abdominal surgery; after perforation of a gastric or duodenal ulcer, a gastric carcinoma, or a segment of colon involved by diverticulitis or cancer; or following blunt or penetrating trauma to the abdomen. Fever, sweats, rigors, and sometimes upper abdominal or lower chest pain and tenderness occur. A pleural friction rub and pleural fluid may be present on the affected side of the chest.

Pleural nodules or sheets of *metastatic tumor* may cause pleuritic or nonpleuritic chest pain. If a *mesothelioma* is present, a large pleural effusion may form. Thoracentesis and biopsy of the pleura will establish the diagnosis. There is often a history of asbestos exposure 20 or more years before, but this is not always obtainable. *Primary lung cancer* or *metastatic cancer from other organs* (e.g., the breast) may invade the pleura and cause pleuritic chest pain, or dull aching nonpleuritic chest pain, and an effusion. The diagnosis can be suspected from a history of a recent malignancy and can be confirmed by a chest radiograph, pleural fluid cytology, and pleural biopsy.

Lower abdominal pain due to salpingitis may be associated with right or left upper abdominal pain or diffuse upper abdominal and lower chest pain. The pain may be intensified by a deep breath or movement, and tenderness may be present over the upper abdomen and lower chest on one or both sides. Culture of the uterine cervix grows *Neisseria gonorrhoeae* or *Chlamydia trachomatis*. Laparoscopy reveals hyperemia and fibrin strands over the liver. Liver function tests may be abnormal. This gynecologic syndrome (*Fitz-Hugh–Curtis syndrome*) responds promptly to antimicrobial therapy.

Pneumothorax causes dyspnea and chest pain made worse by deep inspiration. The percussion note is hyperresonant, and breath sounds are decreased or absent. The pneumothorax can be confirmed by a chest radiograph. If *tension pneumothorax* develops, the chest pain and dyspnea become severe, the external jugular veins distend, the trachea deviates to the opposite side, and severe hypotension may follow. This diagnosis can be confirmed by inserting a needle into the chest and observing air escaping under pressure.

Chest wall pain due to *costochondritis* occurs in the area over the second, third, or fourth costal cartilages near the sternum. The pain begins spontaneously or after effort and lasts for seconds, minutes, or hours. There is localized tenderness over one or two of these cartilages. Pressure with a fingertip or knuckle causes a pain similar in quality and location to that experienced spontaneously. It is not sustained for long after pressure is removed. Some provocative arm or chest maneuvers, and walking or running, may also reproduce pain of similar quality and location. The chest radiograph and electrocardiogram are normal, as are electrocardiographic and thallium 201 stress tests. Similar pain occurs with *strains of the pectoralis major and pectoralis minor muscles* (i.e., myofascial pain) and with *myositis*. Local tenderness occurs over these muscles. *Rib fractures* cause pain worsened by movement, by deep inspiration, and by lying on the affected side. This is in contrast to patients with pleuritis, who often prefer to lie on the affected side so as to splint it. Physical examination reveals rib tenderness, skin ecchymoses, and sometimes bony crepitus at the fracture site. Special rib films or a chest radiograph will confirm the diagnosis. *Pathologic fracture of a diseased rib* will cause similar symptoms after only minor trauma or no trauma. Disorders that may cause pathologic rib fractures include metastatic carcinoma, multiple myeloma, and osteoporosis.

Sickle cell anemia can cause painful crises characterized by chest pain that is made worse by breathing and movement, as well as back, leg, and arm pains. There is a long history of episodes of a similar nature extending back to childhood.

Intercostal neuritis produces a band of lightninglike, sharp or burning pain that radiates halfway around the chest from the spine. Jarring, coughing, or sneezing may precipitate a paroxysm of pain, while respiration does not—differentiating such pain from that due to pleuritis.

Similar pain can result from a *destructive malignancy or infection of the thoracic spine*. Midline aching back pain and tenderness usually are present and precede the onset of the radiating pain. The radicular pain may have a constant aching or burning quality in association with paroxysms of lancinating pain that radiate around a hemithorax.

Herpes zoster causes unilateral burning or aching pain in a bandlike distribution around the hemithorax, followed by the eruption of clusters of tiny red-based vesicles and crusted ulcers on the skin of the painful region. Skin hyperesthesia and tenderness may be present in the area of pain.

Mondor's disease results in a painful, tender cord under reddened skin on the anterolateral chest. The cord has the diameter of a thin pencil. It is due to a clot in a superficial vein.

Coronary disease may manifest itself as a prolonged pressurelike pain in the substernal and/or anterior chest area, associated with sweating, weakness, nausea, and vomiting. Radiation of pain may occur to the neck, the jaw, and one or both arms. Tachycardia, bradycardia, or hypotension may occur. A gallop rhythm may be present. The diagnosis can be confirmed by serial electrocardiograms and by serum isozyme assays. A similar form of prolonged ischemic chest pain may occur in patients with *unstable angina;* in such cases there is no evidence of infarction, and the ischemia is reversible; it may be due to a fixed stenosis, arterial spasm, or an intraluminal clot.

Boerhaave's syndrome begins with substernal or left precordial aching or pleuritic pain that follows an episode of forceful vomiting. Dyspnea, mild hematemesis, dysphagia, fever, and cold-water polydipsia may be associated complaints. Subcutaneous emphysema, pneumothorax, pleural effusion, and mediastinal emphysema may be detected on physical examination and/or by a plain chest radiograph. Hamman's sign occurs in 20 percent of cases. Subcutaneous and mediastinal emphysema distinguish this disorder from other major intrathoracic catastrophes (e.g., myocardial infarction, dissecting aneurysm, pulmonary embolism) and abdominal catastrophes (e.g., perforated ulcer, acute pancreatitis, and mesenteric thrombosis) that it may mimic. The diagnosis can be confirmed by a contrast esophagogram. Other causes of esophageal rupture include endoscopy, instrumentation, foreign bodies, and underlying esophageal disease.

☐ DESCRIPTION OF LISTED DISEASES

1. PLEURITIS

Pleuritic pain is frequently felt over the lower anterior or anterolateral chest, and may also be felt in the shoulder. It is characteristically made sharper and more severe by a deep breath, a cough, or merely changing from a lying to a sitting position or rolling over in bed. In severe cases respirations are limited to shallow, rapid breaths, each of which may be accompanied by an audible expiratory grunt. Some patients may lie motionless with the affected side splinted

TABLE OF DISEASE INCIDENCE

INCIDENCE PER 100,000 (APPROXIMATE)

Common (>100)	Uncommon (>5–100)	Rare (>0–5)
Streptococcus pneumoniae pneumonia and pleuritis	*Staphylococcus aureus* pneumonia	Q fever pneumonia and pleuritis
Legionella pneumophila pneumonia and pleuritis	*Klebsiella pneumoniae* pneumonia and pleuritis	Tularemia pneumonia and pleuritis
Haemophilus influenzae pneumonia and pleuritis	TWAR agent pneumonia and pleuritis	Psittacosis and pleuritis
Pulmonary infarction and pleuritis	Gram-negative pneumonia and pleuritis	Subdiaphragmatic abscess
Aspiration pneumonia and pleuritis	Empyema	Benign and malignant mesothelioma
Simple pneumothorax	Lupus erythematosus pleuritis	Tension pneumothorax
Traumatic rib fracture	Drug-related lupus pleuritis	Intercostal neuritis
Costochondritis	Rheumatoid arthritis pleuritis	Spinal disease and radiculopathy
Sickle cell disease and rib infarction	Postmyocardial infarction syndrome	Mondor's disease
Coronary heart disease and myocardial infarction	Postcardiotomy syndrome	*Mycoplasma pneumoniae* pneumonia and pleuritis
Unstable angina	Post-cardiac trauma syndrome	Tuberculous pleuritis
	Viral or idiopathic pericarditis	Esophageal rupture—Boerhaave's syndrome and other causes
	Pleurodynia or viral pleurisy	Purulent pericarditis
	Pathologic rib fracture	Tuberculous pericarditis
	Herpes zoster	
	Fitz-Hugh–Curtis syndrome	
	Neoplastic pericarditis	
	Metastatic carcinoma involving the pleura	
	Pectoral myositis (myofascial syndrome)	

against the surface of the bed. Shoulder pain may progress to neck and shoulder stiffness that is made worse by movements of the neck and upper arm. Local tenderness of the chest wall, neck, or shoulder may occur and mimic musculoskeletal disease. The pain often persists between breaths as a severe aching or burning discomfort that requires analgesics. This constant pain becomes sharp and more severe at some point toward the middle or end of each inspiration.

Pleuritic pain usually begins gradually, building to peak intensity over a period of minutes to hours, but an abrupt onset is also possible. The causes of unilateral pleuritic chest pain are described below.

A. Pneumonia

1. Bacterial Pneumonia (Including Polymicrobial Aspiration Pneumonia) *Streptococcus pneumoniae* accounts for up to 75 percent of cases of community-acquired pneumonia. Risk factors for the development of pneumococcal pneumonia include age (very young or old), chronic cardiopulmonary disease, alcoholism, diabetes, hyposplenism, splenectomy, hemoglobinopathies, and immunoglobulin defects. Coryza or a flulike illness may be present for one or more days prior to onset. Classic pneumococcal pneumonia begins abruptly with a single shaking chill lasting 15 to 30 min and a rapid rise in temperature to the range of 102 to 105°F. Pleuritic pain, dyspnea, cough, and sputum production soon follow. The pain is localized to the right or left anterior and/or lateral chest, and may also be referred to the right or left shoulder. It is sharp and stabbing and is intensified by each inspiration, cough, or bodily movement. Patients may sit, or may lie with the chest splinted against the bed surface to lessen the pain; respirations are shallow and rapid. Nausea, vomiting, and upper abdominal pain may occur.

Inspiratory flaring of the alae nasi may accompany each shallow breath and be followed by an audible expiratory grunt. The sputum may have a mucopurulent, rusty, or "prune juice" appearance, and may be tenacious if there is dehydration or a high content of bacterial polysaccharide. Patients with *Klebsiella pneumoniae* infections often have purulent sputum that is blood-streaked or has a "currant jelly" or "chocolate pudding" appearance. "Apple-green" sputum has been described in some cases of *Haemophilus influenzae* pneumonia.

A single rigor at the onset of the illness is said to be characteristic of pneumococcal pneumonia, while multiple rigors suggest another etiology. Some cases of pneumococcal pneumonia occur with pleuritic pain and fever; cough and/or rigors may be absent.

On physical examination the patient may be found to be acutely ill and breathing rapidly. Tachycardia, hypotension, and central cyanosis may be present in severe cases. Herpes labialis is a common finding.

Inspection of the chest may reveal splinting, an inspiratory lag, and/or a decrease in expansion of the affected hemithorax. There may be rib and interspace tenderness in the painful area. A pleural friction rub may be palpated and heard. The ipsilateral hemidiaphragm is usually fixed and elevated; percussion dullness may be present over the anterior or posterolateral chest on the affected side. Auscultation over areas of dullness reveals decreased breath sounds and/or bronchial breathing. The latter is accompanied by confirmatory signs of consolidation, such as increased vocal fremitus, whispered voice, and egophony. Bronchial breath sounds are not specific and may occur with atelectasis and an open bronchus; with a large pleural effusion; or with a bronchopleural fistula. Cases with a poor prognosis may develop rapidly progressive consolidation of other lobes; hypotension; jaundice; and/or abdominal distension due to an ileus.

The chest radiograph reveals segmental or lobar opacities with air bronchograms in consolidated zones and/or patchy infiltrates (i.e., areas of bronchopneumonia). Pleural effusions indentifiable in the lateral decubitus position may be present in up to 50 percent of cases of pneumococcal pneumonia. Patients with pneumonia and emphysema may show areas of opacity riddled with small cystic lucencies that produce a "honeycomb" or "swiss cheese" effect. These are caused by the microcystic lung changes produced by the emphysematous process, and have been confused with necrotization. Lower-lobe spherical opacities may occur in patients with pneumococcal pneumonia; these may progress to obscure an entire lobe. Leukocytosis of up to 40,000 cells per mm^3 and a shift to the left may occur. Leukopenia is a poor prognostic sign and is associated with bacteremia.

K. pneumoniae infections occur with highest frequency in men over age 50, alcoholics, diabetics, persons with chronic cardiac or bronchopulmonary disease, and hospitalized patients. Such infections are uncommon (accounting for fewer than 1 percent of community-acquired pneumonias) and clinically may mimic pneumococcal pneumonia. The right or left upper lobe is commonly affected. A homogeneous consolidation may opacify the entire lobe and cause downward bulging of the minor fissure in the right lung. This finding, while most commonly associated with *K. pneumoniae* infection, is nonspecific; it may occur with pneumococcal and other forms of pneumonia.

Staphylococcal pneumonia usually occurs during influenza epidemics and in diabetics, immunocompromised patients, and intravenous drug abusers (hematogenous pneumonia). It accounts for 2 to 10 percent of community-acquired pneumonias. It is associated with bilaterally patchy infiltrates that progress, over 2 to 10 days, to cavitation and/or pneumatocele formation within opacified areas. Pleural effusions are common. Other organisms that may cause a necrotizing pneumonia or abscess formation include the type 3 pneumococcus, *K. pneumoniae*, anaerobes, and other gram-negative bacteria, such as *Escherichia coli* and *Enterobacter* and *Pseudomonas* species. A leukocytosis with a shift to the left is commonly present in *S. pneumoniae*, *K. pneumoniae*, *S. aureus*, and *H. influenzae* infections; leukopenia may appear as a poor prognostic sign in *K. pneumoniae* infections and in other fulminant pneumonias.

Sputum examination as a diagnostic procedure in patients with community-acquired pneumonia is not as helpful as was once believed. All Gram-stained sputum smears should be initially screened for the presence of increased numbers of squamous epithelial cells. Sputum smears in one study had a 75 percent rate of significant contamination by saliva, and such sputum was deemed unacceptable for culture. Gram stains of sputum to be used for culture should demonstrate many leukocytes, singly or in clumps and sheets, and few squamous cells. A single bacterial form, or at least a predominant organism, should be present—not diverse coccal and rod forms. Lancet-shaped gram-positive diplococci (*S. pneumoniae*); single, paired, or grapelike clusters of gram-positive cocci (*S. aureus*); short, fat, encapsulated gram-negative rods (*K. pneumoniae*); large gram-negative encapsulated rods (*E. coli*); small gram-negative coccobacilli (*H. influenzae*); or a polymicrobial spectrum of rods and cocci (aspiration pneumonia or contamination by saliva) may be present on sputum examination. Sputum Gram stain interpretation may be clouded by upper airway colonization rates of 2 to 18 percent for gram-negative bacteria and up to 50 percent for *S. pneumoniae*. In patients with proven pneumococcal pneumonia, false-negative rates of 50 percent and false-positive rates of 44 percent (i.e., implicating other microorganisms) may occur with sputum cultures. The application of immunologic techniques such as counterimmunoelectrophoresis (CIE) or coagglutination (CoA) to sputum examination can detect pneumococcal antigen in sputum (80 percent sensitivity by CIE, 94 percent by CoA). Questions about the specificity of CoA and CIE have been raised, since antigen can be detected in the sputum of patients with chronic bronchitis and no evidence of pneumonia. Immunologic testing of sputum, serum, and urine has been helpful in the early diagnosis of legionellosis.

Transtracheal aspiration provides specimens with a higher likelihood of representing the actual pulmonary pathogen in patients with community-acquired pneumonias. Sensitivity exceeds 90 percent, but false-positive results occur in up to 21 percent of patients. Interpretation is less satisfactory in patients with chronic bronchitis, who have positive cultures at an 85 percent rate in the absence of pneumonia. In one large series of patients with chronic pulmonary disease complicated by pneumonia who were subjected to this procedure, two or more organisms were isolated in the majority of cases. Common isolates in this Veterans Administration patient population consisted of *S. pneumoniae* accompanied by a gram-negative rod such as *H. influenzae*, *E. coli*, or an *Enterobacter* species. This technique is less frequently used than it used to be, because of such potentially dangerous complications as bleeding, aspiration, arrhythmias, and death. Transthoracic aspiration may provide samples of alveolar exudate with a sensitivity of 35 to 90 percent and a specificity of 88 to 100 percent. This technique requires an alert, cooperative patient, and carries with it a 20 to 30 percent risk of pneumothorax.

In up to 58 percent of cases of community-acquired pneumonia an etiologic agent may not be identified. Many cases are treated with a broad-spectrum drug, such as ceftriaxone, if the responsible organism cannot be identified by a Gram stain of sputum or a transtracheal aspirate. This drug provides coverage for *S. pneumoniae, H. influenzae, S. aureus, K. pneumoniae,* some anaerobes, and other gram-negative bacteria. Specific results on a Gram stain of a transtracheal or transthoracic aspirate, or a highly diagnostic sputum smear, allow initiation of more specific therapy (e.g., penicillin for *S. pneumoniae,* nafcillin or vancomycin for *S. aureus,* a third-generation cephalosporin for *K. pneumoniae* or *H. influenzae,* and high-dose penicillin or clindamycin for aspiration pneumonia). Pneumococcal pneumonia responds dramatically within 1 to 2 days, while the clinical response to the treatment of the other pathogens may be equivalent or delayed for 3 to 4 days.

In *aspiration pneumonia* the initial complaints may be anterior and anterolateral chest pain, and sometimes shoulder pain, of a sharp, stabbing nature; fever; and cough. In some cases cough and sputum production may be absent. Rigors do not usually occur, as they do in other bacterial pneumonias. Malaise, general weakness, and anorexia are common. The presence of pleuritic pain without cough and with minimal fever suggests the possibility of pulmonary embolism; and in many cases ventilation/perfusion (V/Q) scans are done. Aspiration pneumonia occurs 2 to 4 days after the onset of an episode of unconsciousness due to alcoholic intoxication, diabetic coma, a procedure requiring anesthesia, a seizure, a head injury, a cardiac arrest, or a drug overdose. Aspiration pneumonia may also occur in patients with achalasia, scleroderma, gastroesophageal reflux, and neurogenic dysphagia with choking and vomiting. Physical findings include fever, tachycardia, and sometimes tachypnea. Fine rales may be present posteriorly on one or both sides, sometimes in association with basilar dullness and a pleural friction rub.

The most common organisms isolated are *Fusobacterium nucleatum, Bacteroides* species, and *Peptostreptococcus* species. Chest radiographs show evidence of infiltrates in gravity-dependent segments of the lungs. Fetid sputum is helpful in confirming the diagnosis of anaerobic pneumonia, but occurs in only 5 percent of cases. Transtracheal, transthoracic, or bronchoscopic cultures are required for a specific microbiological diagnosis. There is a prompt therapeutic response to intravenous penicillin or clindamycin.

Complications include necrotizing pneumonia with cavitation and empyema; bronchogenic spread with a diffuse anaerobic pneumonia; and formation of a bronchopleural fistula with a pyopneumothorax.

2. Mycoplasma pneumoniae The major complaint of patients infected with this organism is a nagging, diffi-cult-to-control cough that troubles them day and night. Usually it is nonproductive or produces only small amounts of clear, white sputum. Occasionally pleuritic pain may occur in association with the cough. More commonly, such patients complain of a peculiar burning soreness of the anterior or anterolateral chest on one or both sides. Headache, fever, and generalized weakness and myalgias accompany the intractable cough and chest discomfort. Diarrhea and nausea may occur in this disorder and in *Legionella pneumophila* pneumonia. The physical examination reveals only fine rales, or some wheezes or rhonchi; or it is entirely normal. Patchy opacities may be present on a chest radiograph; the radiographic findings may be much more impressive than the minimal findings on physical examination. Small pleural effusions occur in 10 to 20 percent of cases. The diagnosis can be further supported by the finding of cold agglutinating antibodies in the serum and by the demonstration of a rising titer of mycoplasma-complement-fixing antibodies. A cold agglutinin titer $\geq$ 1:128 is usually caused by *M. pneumoniae* infection while lower titers are less specific. Symptoms and radiographic findings respond to therapy with erythromycin or tetracycline, but not as dramatically as they do in pneumococcal pneumonia. A response may take 4 to 7 days.

Mycoplasma infection is a frequent cause of outbreaks of epidemic pneumonia in military training camps, schools, and colleges. It is more prevalent in school age children and young adults. It spreads during bouts of coughing; entire households may become ill with "colds" and pneumonia caused by this agent. Since the incubation period is 2 to 3 weeks, household members may become sick sequentially over a period of weeks, rather than all at the same time. The complaint "My family never seems to be entirely well" may be voiced by a concerned parent. Pneumonia develops in only 3 to 10 percent of persons infected.

3. Legionella pneumophila This organism has been etiologic in as few as 1 percent (Seattle) and as many as 23 percent (Chicago) of cases of community-acquired pneumonia. There is an abrupt onset of malaise, myalgias, and severe headache. The association of cough (75–95 percent of cases), fever above 102°F (70–95 percent), chills (59–73 percent), and pleuritic pain (30–42 percent) may mimic the common bacterial pneumonias. The sputum is mucoid or mucopurulent, but is scant and may not appear until the third day of the illness. It contains neutrophils, but no predominant bacterium, on Gram stain. Clues to the diagnosis of legionellosis include the presence of risk factors, such as renal insufficiency with treatment by dialysis or transplantation; immunosuppression; chronic pulmonary disease; a history of smoking or alcoholism; diabetes; age greater than 50 years; exposure to commercial or home air conditioning, a construction or excavation site, or a resort or hotel site.

Diarrhea and/or nausea (13–54 percent of cases) and/or abdominal pain and tenderness; encephalopathy with disorientation and confusion; jaundice and/or elevated aminotransferase levels; protein, red blood cells, and casts in the urine, and/or a rising creatinine level; a relative bradycardia; and no clinical response to beta-lactam antibiotics over 48 to 72 h, and/or a response to parenteral erythromycin are clinical findings that suggest the possibility of legionellosis.

Physical examination of the chest may reveal scattered rales early in the course. After 2 to 3 days signs of consolidation, pleural effusion, and a pleural friction rub may appear on one or both sides. Prostration, toxicity, and mental confusion may be prominent findings.

Chest radiographs are nonspecific and may show patchy subsegmental infiltrates or segmental and/or lobar homogeneous opacities on one or both sides of the chest. Nodular densities are suggestive of *Legionella micdadei* infection. The radiographic picture of adult respiratory distress syndrome (ARDS) may occur in severe cases. There are no specific findings that distinguish *Legionella* pneumonia from other forms of community-acquired bacterial pneumonia. The diagnosis is primarily clinical. Rapid confirmation may be achieved, though, by noting neutrophils, but no or few bacteria, on a sputum Gram stain; and filamentous bacteria on a carbol-fuchsin, Giemsa, or Dieterle silver stain, or with a direct fluorescent antibody technique. Culture of sputum or pleural fluid on charcoal yeast extract agar (CYE) will be positive in 7 to 14 days, and indirect fluorescent antibody titers in the serum will rise, in 75 percent of cases, within 21 days. Both of these confirmatory tests require too much time to be useful for immediate diagnosis and selection of therapy. Antigen detection in sputum and urine has been used to confirm rapidly the initial clinical impression, but the sensitivity is not high enough to exclude the diagnosis. Pleuritic pain and fever usually respond to parenteral erythromycin lactobionate within 48 to 72 h. Similar sporadic illnesses caused by *L. bozemanii* and *L. micdadei* have been described in normal patients. Severe cases of *L. pneumophila* pneumonia have a tendency to relapse and may require a second course of therapy.

4. A. *CHLAMYDIA PSITTACI* *Chlamydia psittaci* infection can be responsible for an acute pneumonia capable of causing pleuritic chest pain and cough. This disorder is associated with contact with birds, such as parakeets, parrots, pigeons, ducks, or turkeys. Patients with pneumonia and histories of exposure to birds should be evaluated for psittacosis. The illness resembles legionellosis; there may be evidence of encephalopathy with delirium, renal insufficiency, and liver involvement. The cough is usually nonproductive. Chest pain due to pleuritis is uncommon but may occur, and epistaxis occurs in 25 percent of cases. Most patients have severe headache, photophobia, weakness, and a high fever. Physical findings include fever, enlargement of the liver and spleen (10–40 percent), and rales over one or more pulmonary areas. Signs of consolidation may occur. Horder's spots (similar to typhoidal rose spots) may appear, in a minority of cases, on the face or trunk. Patchy infiltrates progressive to segmental or lobar consolidation may be present on a chest radiograph. Tetracycline provides effective therapy. The diagnosis is clinical, since cultures and serologic confirmation take too long to be useful. A patient with a history of exposure to birds, clinical and radiologic evidence of pneumonia, and splenomegaly should be considered to have a high likelihood of having this disorder.

B. *CHLAMYDIA PNEUMONIAE* **(TWAR strain)** The TWAR (Taiwan acute respiratory) strain of *Chlamydia pneumoniae* causes 10 to 12 percent of community-acquired pneumonias in adolescents and young adults. It appears to be transmitted by person-to-person spread. The illness produced is clinically indistinguishable from *Mycoplasma pneumoniae* infection, and is characterized by fever, headache, nonproductive cough, laryngitis, and sometimes pharyngitis. There is nothing specific about the clinical picture or radiographic findings. The diagnosis requires cultural isolation or demonstration of a rise in antibody titer to *C. pneumoniae*. Pleuritic pain is uncommon in this disorder. The TWAR agent cannot be routinely isolated in most laboratories at present and serologic studies are available only in research laboratories. TWAR responds well to tetracycline, but erythromycin is usually ineffective.

5. *Q Fever* **(Coxiella burnetii)** Persons with this disorder present with a flulike syndrome with headache, chills, fever, diffuse myalgias, nausea, and vomiting. Cough and chest pain may occur; interstitial, patchy, and even lobar consolidation is present in up to 50 percent of patients with this disorder. The sputum is mucoid and scanty, and may be blood-tinged. Scattered rales and signs of consolidation may occur, but are uncommon. Q fever is usually seen in the western and southwestern United States, in persons exposed to livestock or to aerosols arising from livestock-raising areas. The high infectivity of this organism accounts for cases involving individuals with no direct livestock contact. There is a therapeutic response to tetracycline. Convalescence may be prolonged, with weakness and weight loss. Serologic methods are required to establish the diagnosis.

6. *Tularemia Pneumonia* This disorder may accompany ulceroglandular or oculoglandular tularemia (15 percent of cases) or typhoidal tularemia (50 percent). Dyspnea, cough, and pleuritic pain occur in association with the respective clinical signs of these forms of tularemia. Nodular densities, subsegmental or segmental homogeneous opacities, lobar pneumonia, and hilar adenopathy have been reported. The diagnosis can be made by sputum or blood culture, or by demonstration of an antibody rise. There is usually a history of contact with wild rabbits, muskrats, or opossums, or of a tick or deerfly bite. Streptomycin or doxycycline result in resolution of chest pain and fever.

Radiologic criteria cannot distinguish bacterial and nonbacterial pneumonias with a high degree of accuracy.

B. Pulmonary Embolism and Infarction   Clot embolization from a venous thrombus in a leg or pelvic vein can cause shortness of breath and sharp, stabbing chest pain associated with breathing, coughing, and/or a change of body position. Fever to 101°F may occur, but rigors do not. If cough is present, it is usually nonproductive. Hemoptysis is present in 30 percent of cases. The material produced consists of clots and liquid blood that is dark- or bright-red. There is usually no preceding upper respiratory infection. Shoulder pain and upper abdominal pain, made worse by a deep inspiration, may occur, if the surface of the lung adjacent to the diaphragm is involved. Physical examination may detect localized chest wall tenderness, a pleural friction rub, and/or a small area of dullness with rales near the painful site. With larger emboli, an entire lower lobe may show signs of consolidation. Chest radiographs may show pleural effusions and small infiltrates or zones of platelike atelectasis. Infiltrates tend to occur in the lower lobes and often are pleura-based and triangular in shape (Hampton hump). The hemidiaphragm on the affected side may be elevated and poorly mobile. Electrocardiograms should be done to rule out myocardial infarction. The transient electrocardiographic abnormalities that may occur include an $S_1Q_3T_3$ pattern, T-wave inversion in leads V_1 to V_3, right ventricular strain, right bundle branch block, and atrial arrhythmias.

Perfusion lung scans are performed by intravenous injection of technetium 99m–labeled particles. A normal perfusion scan eliminates the diagnosis of pulmonary embolism, but an abnormal perfusion scan alone neither confirms nor excludes the diagnosis.

Abnormal scans may be interpreted as being of high probability (90 percent chance of embolism), intermediate probability (30 percent chance), and low probability (10 percent chance). A high-probability scan may show a perfusion defect larger than an infiltrate visible in the same area on a chest radiograph. In addition, a high-probability scan may show absent perfusion of multiple pulmonary segments or lobes and ventilation/perfusion (V/Q) mismatch. Segmental defects with a V/Q match, or a single segmental defect with mismatch, have only a 30 percent probability of being due to pulmonary embolism. Patients with matching defects, or small subsegmental defects with mismatch, have less than a 10 percent probability of having pulmonary embolism.

The diagnosis can be ruled in or out, in cases with a high degree of uncertainty, by means of a pulmonary angiogram. This procedure will identify a subset of patients with low- or intermediate-probability scans who require anticoagulant therapy. Some physicians also do pulmonary angiograms in patients with high-probability lung scans who are not good risks for anticoagulant therapy, or who may require Greenfield filter insertion into the vena cava. Outcome studies have suggested that patients with low-probability scans do not need further study or anticoagulant therapy.

Studies of the legs for clots—using noninvasive tests such as impedance plethysmography, real-time ultrasound, Doppler techniques, and invasive tests (e.g., venograms)—if positive, will support the diagnosis in patients who do not have high-probability lung scans. Up to 30 percent of patients with abnormal perfusion scans will have one or more demonstrable femoral vein thrombi. Discovery of a femoral clot is an indication for anticoagulant therapy; in such cases pulmonary angiography is not required. Heparin is used for initial anticoagulation and is continued for 10 days at doses of 1000 to 1800 units per hour. Warfarin is started after 4 to 5 days of heparin therapy and continued for 3 to 6 months. Untreated cases have a 30 percent death rate, while diagnosed and treated cases have an 8 percent mortality. Symptoms usually clear within 2 to 3 days of starting anticoagulant therapy.

C. Tuberculosis   Pleuritic pain is associated with fever and a nonproductive cough. The chest pain may be associated with a pleural friction rub and signs of fluid. This disorder is most prevalent in persons under the age of 30. A chest radiograph may show fluid obliterating the ipsilateral costophrenic angle, and sometimes an infiltrate and/or enlarged hilar nodes on the affected side. In most cases the lung fields and hilar areas are normal. The pleural fluid usually has an elevated protein level and increased numbers of lymphocytes. The tuberculin skin test is positive in 90 percent of patients, but pleural fluid cultures are diagnostic of tuberculosis in only 20 percent. A pleural needle biopsy is positive in 50 to 60 percent of cases.

These patients usually do not have pulmonary tuberculosis, but they are at great risk of developing it within 5 years (this occurs in 65 percent of cases) unless treatment with isoniazid is initiated.

Occasionally tuberculosis will cause pleuritic pain when active pulmonary lesions are present (as in fibrocaseous and cavitary disease). The chest radiograph findings make the diagnosis straightforward and allow early initiation of antituberculous therapy.

D. Disorders Involving the Pleura and/or Pericardium

1. Systemic Lupus Erythematosus and Drug-Induced Lupus   An episode of anterior chest and/or shoulder pain that is made worse by deep inspiration and by bodily movement (i.e., pleuritis) may occur in the course of systemic (70 percent of cases) or drug-induced lupus. The pain may disappear in 1 to 2 weeks, or may require corticosteroid therapy, which rapidly and dramatically relieves the pain. Some patients with pleuritic pain develop a pleural effusion. Pericarditis also may occur in lupus; it may cause right and/or left anterior chest and shoulder pain that is made worse by deep inspiration and by lying flat. The pain is usually relieved by sitting up and leaning forward.

Clinical criteria have been developed to aid in the diagnosis of systemic lupus erythematosus. The presence of 4 or more of the 11 criteria listed below, either simultaneously or serially, strongly supports the diagnosis. The clinical findings that suggest systemic lupus are (1) malar butterfly rash; (2) discoid lupus; (3) photosensitivity; (4) oral ulcers; (5) arthritis (i.e., nonerosive arthritis involving two or more peripheral joints); (6) serositis (i.e., pleuritis or pericarditis); (7) renal disease (i.e., proteinuria or cylindruria); (8) a neurologic disorder (i.e., seizures, focal neurologic signs, delirium, or psychoses); (9) a hematologic disorder (i.e., hemolytic anemia, leukopenia, lymphopenia, or thrombocytopenia); (10) an immunologic disorder (i.e., positive LE preparation or anti-ds-DNA or anti-Sm antibodies, or a false-positive serologic test for syphilis); and (11) an abnormal serum titer of antinuclear antibody in the absence of drugs reported to cause drug-related lupus. Systemic lupus erythematosus can be treated with nonsteroidal antiinflammatory drugs or prednisone. Azathioprine and cyclophosphamide have both been used in combination with prednisone to treat severe forms of this disease.

Drugs used for the treatment of other disorders may precipitate an attack of fever, arthralgias, pleuritis, and/or pericarditis associated with a positive antinuclear antibody (ANA) test. These drugs include hydralazine, procainamide, methyldopa, isoniazid, phenytoin, chlorpromazine, and others. The disorder induced by these will usually respond to a reduction of dosage or cessation of drug use.

2. Rheumatoid Arthritis

Pleuritic pain, accompanied by the accumulation of pleural fluid, occurs in 5 percent of persons with generalized symmetric rheumatoid arthritis. Rheumatoid pleural fluid is an exudate with a low pH and a low glucose level ($\leq$15 mg/100 ml). Pleural biopsy may reveal rheumatoid nodules. While pleural effusions caused by lupus erythematosus clear rapidly, rheumatoid effusions may persist for months.

3. Postmyocardial Infarction, Postcardiotomy, or Postcardiac Trauma Syndrome

This disorder begins 1 to 16 weeks, or longer, after coronary artery occlusion and myocardial infarction, cardiac surgery, or trauma. These patients present with fever and with pleuritic and pericardial pain in the midchest and shoulders, and/or in either or both sides of the anterior chest. The anterior chest pain is intensified by breathing and by lying supine or on the left side. Tachycardia, fever, and a pleural and/or pericardial rub may be present. Radiographs of the chest usually are normal or show a transient pneumonitis, pleural fluid, and/or an enlarged heart. Pericardial fluid can accumulate, and may be hemorrhagic if anticoagulants are being used. The chest pain can be rapidly and dramatically relieved by administration of prednisone. Echocardiograms allow early detection of pericardial fluid. Rarely, the accumulation of pericardial fluid can be so rapid that cardiac tamponade and shock result.

4. Acute Viral or Idiopathic Pericarditis

This disorder begins with a sharp, stabbing chest pain that may be felt in the right or left anterior chest. The neck and/or shoulder ridges may also be painful. The pain is made worse or more intense by lying supine, lying on the left side, and respiration, and sometimes by swallowing. The pain may be eased by lying on the right side, sitting up and leaning forward, or standing. Fever and myalgias may accompany the pain. In some patients a pressurelike or constricting substernal chest pain may occur. This is similar to that occurring with a myocardial infarction, but its occurrence is uncommon. On physical examination during the first few days, there is a normal-sized heart; there may or may not be a pericardial friction rub. The electrocardiogram initially shows concave-upward ST-segment elevations in almost all leads except aV_R and V_1. T-wave inversion or flattening may occur over the next 7 days, with return of ST segments to the baseline. The serum cardiac isozyme levels and leukocyte count may be elevated. Echovirus, influenza virus, coxsackievirus, Epstein-Barr virus, and other viruses may cause this disorder, or it may be of unknown cause (idiopathic).

Patients should be kept in bed and given oral nonsteroidal anti-inflammatory drugs or prednisone. There is usually a prompt response to therapy, but relapse may occur at a variable period after the discontinuance of therapy.

5. Persistent Pericarditis

Persistent anterior chest and/or shoulder and lateral neck pain, with fever, occurring in a patient without renal failure and unresponsive to prednisone may be caused by bacterial or fungal infections, tuberculosis, or neoplasia of the pericardium.

A. PURULENT PERICARDITIS Purulent pericarditis may mimic idiopathic pericarditis. High fever, chills, rigors, generalized toxicity, and a failure to respond to prednisone make it necessary to consider bacterial or fungal infection of the pericardium. Large effusions may develop, leading to tamponade. Pericardial infection may occur by direct spread from a mediastinitis (anaerobic bacteria) or a pneumonia or an empyema (*Streptococcus pneumoniae, Haemophilus influenzae,* or *Staphylococcus aureus*); by bacteremic spread from endocarditis or some other focus of infection (e.g., *S. aureus, Neisseria meningitidis,* or *Neisseria gonorrhoeae*); after penetrating chest trauma or cardiac surgery; or, rarely, from evacuation of a hepatic, subphrenic, or perinephric abscess into the pericardium. A CT scan may sometimes be capable of differentiating a purulent from a serous effusion on the basis of fluid density. Pericardiocentesis will reveal 5000 to 90,000 neutrophils per mm^3, and positive Gram stains and/or cultures for specific bacteria or fungi. In cases caused by *S. pneumoniae*, *H. influenzae*, and *N. meningitidis* the specific agent has been rapidly identified by counterimmunoelectrophoresis. In some cases this is a difficult disorder to diagnose, since there may be no fever or chest pain to direct attention to the chest; or the underlying disorder may be so severe that attention is directed away from the pericardium. Pericardial drainage and parenteral antibiotics are required for survival. In a patient with a septic illness, purulent pericarditis may be suggested by the results of a gallium 67 or indium 111 leukocyte scan, or by echocardiographic or electrocardiographic findings.

B. TUBERCULOUS PERICARDITIS Tuberculous pericarditis may begin insidiously, with malaise, weight loss, anorexia, fever, and chilliness present for weeks before dyspnea and chest discomfort develop. Up to 10 percent of patients have an acute onset of pericardial pain and fever. Large effusions are common. Pericardial fluid culture is insensitive, while guinea pig inoculation with pericardial fluid increases the diagnostic yield. Some cases require pericardial biopsy and culture for diagnosis. The tuberculin skin test may be negative, but it is usually positive (80–90 percent of cases). A patient with persistent unexplained pericarditis, with a lymphocytic pericardial exudate, associated with a positive tuberculin test and/or evidence of granuloma on pericardial biopsy, should be given a trial of antituberculous drug therapy. Recent case reports of tuberculous pericarditis have noted its occurrence in patients with AIDS, systemic lupus erythematosus, and renal failure.

C. NEOPLASTIC PERICARDITIS This disorder may arise from a primary malignant cardiac tumor, such as a fibrosarcoma, angiosarcoma, rhabdomyosarcoma, or lymphoma. Pericardial chest pain, fever, arrhythmias, and an elevated sedimentation rate are characteristic. There is no clinical improvement of pericardial pain after initiation of prednisone therapy. The tumor can be visualized by an echocardiogram or by ultrafast CT scanning with contrast enhancement. Thoracotomy and biopsy are required to establish a specific diagnosis. Lymphomas are responsive to radiation and/or chemotherapy. Surgical removal of a cardiac sarcoma is difficult or impossible, and these tumors are not usually responsive to radiation therapy or chemotherapy.

Metastatic tumors to the heart or pericardium arise in primary lesions of the breast or lung; as distant metastases to mediastinal nodes from the bowel, kidney, or skin (melanoma); or as a primary disorder of those nodes (lymphoma). Chest pain, dyspnea, and a massive pericardial effusion may occur, causing tamponade. Retrosternal and right cardiac border dullness and a pericardial rub may be present. Imaging by echocardiography or ultrafast CT may reveal pericardial or epicardial tumor and pericardial fluid. The fluid protein and LDH levels may be very high (protein ≥ 5 g/100 ml; LDH >2500 IU/100 ml). Pericardiocentesis will reveal positive cytology for malignancy in 80 to 85 percent of cases. Pericardial biopsy may be required for cytology-negative cases. There is often a history of treatment for a carcinoma or lymphoma prior to the onset of symptoms, but pericardial disease may be the first manifestation of a previously undetected tumor.

Malignant mesothelioma may rarely begin in the pericardium. This asbestos-induced neoplasm usually starts in the pleura and may secondarily invade the pericardium. A large biopsy may be required for definitive diagnosis, since the tumor may mimic an adenocarcinoma of the lung histologically and clinically.

E. Pleurodynia and Other Causes of "Viral" Pleurisy This is a viral syndrome caused by group B coxsackievirus and some strains of echovirus. It occurs primarily in the summer and autumn. There is a sudden onset of sharp abdominal pain, often intensified by a movement or cough. The pain may begin in the lower abdomen and then move to the upper abdomen on one or both sides, simulating, in sequence, appendicitis and gallbladder disease. Pain may spread to the front or sides of one or both sides of the lower chest. This pain is made worse by coughing, moving about, and deep inspiration. The involved chest area may be tender. The pains may be continuous or may come and go in paroxysms lasting 2 to 10 h. Fever may vary from low-grade (100°F) to 103°F. The leukocyte count is usually normal or low. Virus can be cultured from the throat and stool within 7 days, and an antibody rise to a specific virus will occur within 2 weeks. The chest radiograph is negative or may show a small effusion. These findings are useful only in retrospect. The major important decision to be made in many cases is whether to explore the abdomen. Usually, despite the presence of cough and rebound tenderness, the abdomen is soft (i.e., there is minimal muscle spasm), though somewhat tender. Good surgical judgment is required to avoid unnecessary surgery. There is no specific treatment. Such patients should be kept under observation and treated with mild analgesics (acetaminophen or aspirin). Spontaneous recovery occurs in 3 to 7 days. The Fitz-Hugh–Curtis syndrome (see below) can mimic this disorder.

Patients with *viral pleurisy* have low-grade fever (or no fever), headache, malaise, and myalgias, and develop pleuritic chest pain of the anterior or lateral chest. The pain is sharp and stabbing and is made worse by deep inspiration and by movement. The chest radiograph is normal and the leukocyte count is normal or low. It is essential to differentiate these patients from those with pulmonary emboli and infarction. Viral pleurisy patients generally do not have risk factors for pulmonary embolism. In addition, they have negative perfusion lung scans. This category of diagnosis is thought by some authors to represent nonepidemic sporadic cases of pleurodynia, or subpleural bacterial bronchopneumonia in patients with chronic bronchitis or bronchiectasis. Many clinicians do not believe there is any such entity as viral pleurisy. Management is the same as for pleurodynia—rest and analgesics are the mainstays of therapy.

F. Empyema   Pleural pain, fever, chills, weight loss, cough, and night sweats occur. Purulent fluid is present in the pleural cavity, resulting from the spread of pneumonia, a lung abscess, a subdiaphragmatic abscess, or a liver abscess (bacterial or amebic) into the pleural space. Some cases follow perforation of the esophagus by trauma, a foreign body, or vomiting; others follow chest surgery.

Needle drainage of pus, cultural identification of the organism causing the infection, and antimicrobial therapy will cure many patients. Others, with thick, inspissated or walled-off loculated collections of pus, require open surgical drainage. Such purulent collections can be easily localized and identified by CT scanning of the chest.

G. Subdiaphragmatic Abscess   This disorder usually occurs in a setting of recent abdominal surgery of the gallbladder, stomach, duodenum, colon, or spleen. Bowel or gallbladder perforation can also cause this disorder. There may be spiking fevers and severe sharp chest and/or shoulder pain, made more intense by breathing, coughing, or sneezing, and/or upper abdominal pain and tenderness. A CT scan will visualize the abscess between the liver and diaphragm. A pleural effusion and basilar atelectasis may be present on the side of the subdiaphragmatic infection. Surgical drainage or percutaneous insertion of a catheter into the abscess, accompanied by antibiotic therapy, will lead to cure in most cases.

H. Nonpleuritic Pain Associated with Tumors

1. Benign Mesothelioma   This disorder follows prior exposure to asbestos. There is a latent period of 20 years or more between exposure to asbestos and the appearance of symptoms. A localized tumor appears on the pleural surface and may rarely be associated with pleuritic pain. Clubbing of the fingers, joint pain, and generalized extremity pain and swelling, with bone tenderness, may accompany this disorder (*pulmonary osteoarthropathy*). X-rays of the long bones may show periosteal elevation. This disorder can be cured by resection of the pleural lesion.

2. Malignant Mesothelioma   Malignant mesothelioma is a diffuse tumor of the pleural surfaces that results in the production of large amounts of pleural fluid. There is a history of asbestos exposure 20 or more years before. These patients may have clubbing of the fingers, joint pain and tenderness, and diffuse extremity pain and tenderness, especially over subcutaneous bony sites. Radiation and chemotherapy are relatively ineffective. Severe weakness, dyspnea, and cough are associated with a dull, aching nonpleuritic chest pain. Death occurs despite, all efforts, in 1 to 2 years.

3. Carcinoma   Carcinoma of the lung, breast, pancreas, stomach, or ovary, or lymphoma, may spread to the pleural surface and cause aching nonpleuritic or pleuritic pain and a pleural effusion. These patients usually have widespread metastatic disease. Chemotherapy may be effective in patients with small-cell carcinoma of the lung, carcinoma of the breast, and lymphoma. If fluid accumulation is a problem, then instillation of tetracycline into the pleural space will obliterate the space and prevent reaccumulation. The diagnosis of pleural metastasis can be confirmed by pleural biopsy (sensitivity = 25–40 percent of cases) and cytologic examination of the pleural fluid (sensitivity = 60 percent).

I. Fitz-Hugh–Curtis Syndrome   Fever, with lower anterior chest and upper abdominal pain and tenderness on one or both sides, may occur in female patients with perihepatitis secondary to chlamydial or gonococcal infections. Pain and tenderness in the lower abdomen is usually present, because of pelvic inflammatory disease, but may be absent. The diagnosis can be confirmed by laparoscopy and by cervical cultures. There is a prompt response to antibiotic therapy.

2. PNEUMOTHORAX

A. Simple Pneumothorax   This disorder begins abruptly with the sudden onset of sharp pain in the anterior or lateral area of one hemithorax that is made more intense by deep inspiration. The pain may localize to the axilla. There may be associated shortness of breath and rapid breathing.

Pneumothorax may begin without any precipitating event, or it may follow strenuous physical activity or a paroxysm of coughing. Penetrating or blunt trauma may also cause pneumothorax.

When the pneumothorax is spontaneous, the usual pathogenic event is the rupture of a thin-walled bleb or bulla. The physical signs include decreased expansion of the affected side of the chest, hyperresonance on percussion, and absent or markedly decreased breath sounds. Chest radiographs, with one view taken on expiration and one on inspiration, will confirm the clinical diagnosis. A 25 percent or smaller pneumothorax will usually resolve within a few days without any therapy, except rest. Larger amounts of pneumothorax require aspiration of the air from the pleural cavity, or insertion of a chest tube.

Up to 5 percent of cases of acute pneumothorax in young women may be associated with the menstrual cycle, and may be recurrent (*catamenial pneumothorax*). Hormonal suppressive therapy effectively prevents recurrence. Pneumothorax also occurs in patients with asthma, chronic obstructive lung disease, lung abscess, cystic fibrosis, eosinophilic granuloma, carcinoma, and sarcoma of the lung.

Pneumothorax in drug abusers may result from attempted subclavian injections ("pocket shots" of the supraclavicular area), and from prolonged Valsalva maneuvers performed to increase the effects of inhaled cocaine. *Pneumocystis carinii* pneumonia in AIDS patients also produces an increased incidence of pneumothorax.

Iatrogenic causes of pneumothorax include positive-pressure respiration, positive end-expiratory pressure, thoracentesis, pleural biopsy, insertion of subclavian or jugular central lines, and cardiopulmonary resuscitation.

B. Tension Pneumothorax Tension pneumothorax usually follows penetrating trauma (e.g., knife wound, gunshot, or fragment wound) or blunt trauma (e.g., falls, automobile steering wheel injuries). It may also be associated with the use of mechanical ventilators after trauma. Severe chest pain of an intense pleuritic nature, extreme shortness of breath, and central cyanosis are associated with tracheal deviation to the contralateral side, distended neck veins, tachypnea, tachycardia, and hypotension. A hyperresonant percussion note is heard on the painful side of the chest, and breath sounds are absent there. Failure to treat this major emergency, by insertion of a needle with a Heimlich valve, or a chest tube attached to an underwater seal and suction drainage system, can lead to severe circulatory compromise and death due to myocardial ischemia. Bilateral tension pneumothorax may occur in fatal cases.

3. CHEST WALL PAIN

A. Rib Fractures (Traumatic and Pathologic) Traumatic rib fractures may follow a fall, blunt trauma to the chest (as in an auto crash), or a blow to the chest. The pain is often continuous; it is made more intense by deep inspiration, by rising from a lying to a sitting position, and by coughing, and is associated with local tenderness. Lying on the affected side precipitates or intensifies the pain and may interfere with sleep. There is usually local tenderness over affected ribs; there may be skin ecchymoses and/or local bony crepitus on palpation. A secondary pneumothorax, causing more diffuse chest pain, may occur. There may be an increase of pain and tenderness after arm use, or other athletic activity, weeks after the rib has healed and the original pain has disappeared.

Pathologic rib fractures may occur spontaneously in a patient with a prior known carcinoma, an undiagnosed primary tumor with rib metastases, multiple myeloma, or severe osteoporosis. These patients develop sudden chest pain made worse by movement, breathing, coughing, and direct pressure over the involved rib. The diagnosis can be documented by rib radiographs, a radionuclide bone scan, or MRI.

B. Costochondritis Pain occurs in the parasternal region, near the junction of the costal cartilages and the sternum. It may also occur in the anterior chest, along the costal margin, and may mimic gallbladder disease on the right side, and gastric or cardiac disease on the left. Pain episodes may begin spontaneously and/or be provoked by exertion, such as walking, running, or climbing stairs or a hill. The pain may also be precipitated by turning in bed or by certain uses of the arm. Coughing, deep breaths, or sneezing may sometimes cause transient jabs of sharp pain in the same area that is affected by a dull, aching pain. In some patients sharp sticking pains or pulsating pains occur, lasting only seconds. These may recur, at intervals of minutes or hours, each day. Pain may spread from the parasternal region to the mid-anterior chest.

In patients with anterior chest pain there are often local areas of tenderness in the painful region. Pressure applied to a trigger point with a fingertip or knuckle will often give rise to pain similar in quality and location to that occurring spontaneously. Other maneuvers that may provoke the spontaneous pain include horizontal abduction or adduction of the arm against resistance, with the neck turned toward the arm being tested; traction on the patient's arms by the examiner's pulling them backward and upward, while the patient bends his or her head backward and fixes his or her eyes on the ceiling and leans forward exerting countertraction against the examiner's pull (the "crowing rooster" maneuver); the "self-hugging" maneuver, in which the patient wraps his or her arms about his or her own chest and hugs himself or herself for 30 s; a deep breath taken with the back arched backward; swinging the arms at the side for 1 to 2 min, as though actually walking; and twisting or rotation of the upper trunk backward or forward. Provocation of a pain similar to the spontaneous pain by any of these maneuvers is evidence that the cause of the pain is in the ribs, rib cartilages, small joints, ligaments, or muscles of the chest wall. The results of the chest radiograph, electrocardiogram, echocardiogram, and electrocardiographic and thallium exercise stress tests are usually within normal limits.

Uncommonly, patients have a swollen, tender, and painful costal cartilage, making easier the localization of the pain (Tietze's syndrome).

C. Pectoral Myositis (Myofascial Pain) Patients with anterior chest pain may have jobs that involve repetitive lifting, or repetitive use of the chest muscles (as in some assembly-line tasks). Prior strain of these muscles from lifting or twisting may have occurred. The pectoral muscles may be diffusely tender, or may have well-localized tender trigger points. Abduction or adduction against resistance may intensify the pain. This disorder is benign; patients should be reassured that the pain and tenderness are not due to cardiac disease, cancer, or any other serious disorder. Symptomatic treatment with oral nonsteroidal anti-inflammatory drugs and heat is usually helpful. In refractory cases, local injection of lidocaine and methylprednisolone may provide relief.

D. Sickle Cell Crisis   Patients with this disorder complain of pain on deep breathing or movement of the front or sides of the chest. Arm, leg, and/or back pain may also be present, and are intensified by movement. The chest wall may be exquisitely tender to palpation, and respirations rapid and shallow, resulting in lower-lobe atelectasis. The chest and limb pain may be accompanied by fever. In some cases the cause of the pain is not sickle cell crisis with painful rib infarctions, but rather pulmonary embolism or acute bacterial pneumonia. There is no specific therapy for a painful crisis. Bed rest, incentive spirometry, stimulation of coughing, analgesics, and intravenous fluids may prevent atelectasis and pneumonia. Episodes resolve spontaneously in 5 to 8 days, but recur at intervals of weeks or months. There is a history of limb and back pain occurring in recurrent attacks since childhood; most adult patients know that they have sickle cell anemia. Chest and abdominal pain occur less frequently than limb pain, and may not occur at all until the patient reaches adult life.

4. NEURITIC PAIN

A. Intercostal Neuritis   Pain is distributed in a band about half the chest, beginning in the midline of the back. Continuous pain of an aching or burning nature, or lightninglike jabs of sharp pain, may be caused by pressure on, or inflammation of, nerve roots in the thoracic region of the spine. These pains may be so severe that the patient remains still, afraid to move for fear that bodily movement will precipitate another sharp jab of intense pain. Jarring, coughing, or sneezing, but not inspiration, provokes the pain. Such pain can result from destructive disease of the spine (e.g., osteomyelitis or tumor), or from an osteoarthritic bony projection or a herniated disc impinging on a thoracic spinal nerve. These lesions can be detected on plain radiographs or by a CT scan or MRI. Some cases of intercostal neuritis have no apparent inflammatory or mechanical cause.

B. Herpes Zoster (Shingles)   Pain, sometimes with paresthesias, occurs in a band stretching from the back around

one side of the chest to the sternum. The pain is burning or dull and aching, and is not made more intense by breathing. It is usually followed, in 1 to 4 days, by the appearance of red-based, 2- to 3-mm vesicles that occur in several groups of 4 to 6 vesicles on the skin of the painful region. These rapidly rupture and crust. The skin of the painful zone may be hyperesthetic and tender. Herpes zoster may be treated with acyclovir, but symptom resolution is not markedly accelerated by treatment. Anterior upper abdominal and lower chest pain and associated tenderness may mimic intraabdominal disease.

C. Spine Disease Due to Tumor or Osteomyelitis Bandlike pain extending from the back around the lower chest may occur. The pain may extend anteriorly into the abdomen. It may be sharp and lancinating, occurring in paroxysms; or it may be a continuous dull ache, or a burning sensation. There is an initial history of midline back pain and tenderness preceding the chest pain. A CT scan or MRI of the spine may show lytic lesions due to tumor, pyogenic osteomyelitis, or tuberculosis. In patients without destructive changes, nerve root compression may be present from a herniated thoracic disc or an osteophyte.

Tuberculosis attacks both bony vertebrae and intervertebral discs. Because of this the spine may partly collapse, forming a tender prominence on the back (i.e., a *gibbus*). Bone biopsy and cultures are often required if the back lesion is the first apparent symptom of cancer or infection. Neoplasm may be treated by palliative local radiation therapy or resection. Pyogenic infection should be treated with antibiotics, and tuberculosis with combination chemotherapy and, sometimes, surgery.

5. MONDOR'S DISEASE

Pain, sometimes made more intense by deep inspiration, is localized to a superficial area on one side of the chest. Here, a tender cordlike structure may be felt beneath the skin. The cord has the diameter of a small pencil; the overlying skin may be tender and red. This disorder is due to thrombosis of a superficial chest wall vein. Symptoms resolve spontaneously in 1 to 4 weeks, and only rarely are serious disorders associated with this diagnosis. Forgotten trauma may be the cause.

6. CORONARY HEART DISEASE

A. Myocardial Infarction   Right or left anterior chest pain with radiation to the ipsilateral arm, neck, and jaw may be the first symptom of an acute myocardial infarction. Only a small percentage of patients have right-sided chest pain with an infarction. Most have substernal or left precordial pressurelike pain, with radiation to the neck and left arm. Sweating (52 percent of cases), weakness, pallor, nausea, and vomiting may occur. There may be a history of similar pain of milder degree and shorter duration associated with exertion, though it may have occurred in the absence of activity. Patients with acute anterior chest pain as described may have tachycardia or bradycardia, hypotension, and an accelerated respiratory rate; or the vital signs may be normal. Examination of the heart may reveal a gallop rhythm, a faint, low-pitched S_1 producing a "tic-tac" rhythm, or normal sounds—and, sometimes, frequent premature contractions or a tachyarrhythmia. The electrocardiogram confirms myocardial infarction in 80 percent of cases. Serum isoenzyme studies (LDH and CPK–MB) will raise the sensitivity of the diagnosis to over 95 percent. These enzyme levels may be elevated in myocardial infarctions that are missed by electrocardiography.

If the infarction is over 4 h old (since the onset of severe continuous pain), the patient should be admitted to a cardiac care unit and monitored. Patients whose pain has been present for less than 4 h should be given intravenous or intracoronary tissue plasminogen activator (tPA); this may be followed in hours, or during the next 3 days, by angioplasty. Thrombolysis and restoration of perfusion may be signaled by a dramatic relief or reduction in chest pain. Some cardiologists do not use thrombolytic therapy; instead, to save time, they open the occluded vessel as soon as possible by direct angioplasty. Such interventions may reduce infarct size by 25 percent, but do not usually prevent the in-progress infarction.

B. Unstable Angina   Substernal (66–72 percent of cases) pressurelike (42–50 percent) rest pain begins abruptly and may continue for 20 to 180 min. Relief may occur spontaneously, or may follow medical treatment. The pain may radiate to the jaw, neck, the left or less commonly the right precordium, and left or right arm. Reversible electrocardiographic changes may accompany the chest pain, but elevations of the serum isozymes CPK–MB and LDH-1 do not occur. These patients may have severely stenotic coronary arteries (>75 percent of cross sectional area) or partial luminal occlusion by a large intracoronary thrombus (6–37 percent). Unstable angina is associated with disruption of a coronary plaque, thrombus formation, partial clot lysis, and coronary spasm. Medical therapy is directed at disrupting the pathogenic events by decreasing platelet aggregation (aspirin) and coronary artery spasm (calcium channel–blocking drugs and nitrates). This syndrome may be treated by the use of intracoronary heparin and angioplasty to fragment, compress, and/or extrude any thrombus and dilate stenotic vessel areas. Unstable angina may mimic acute myocardial infarction clinically, but there is no electrocardiographic, enzyme, or radionuclide scan evidence of infarction.

7. ESOPHAGEAL RUPTURE (BOERHAAVE'S SYNDROME AND OTHER CAUSES)

Nausea and forceful vomiting are followed within a brief period by the abrupt onset of substernal or left precordial pain (70 percent of cases). Pain may also occur in the epigastrium, left shoulder, and upper back. The substernal pain has been variously described as a tightness, a pressure, and a dull ache. The precordial and back pain may be dull and aching, or pleuritic. Associated symptoms include dyspnea (50 percent of cases—related to pleuritis, pneumothorax, or pleural effusion), mild hematemesis (50 percent), fever (11–50 percent), odynophagia or dysphagia (<10 percent), and cold-water polydipsia (<10 percent).

Physical examination may reveal tachycardia, tachypnea, fever, and hypotension (25 percent of patients may be in a shocklike state), or all vital signs may be normal. Subcutaneous emphysema may first appear in the supraclavicular fossae in up to 33 percent of cases. It is a late sign and develops 6 to 18 h after the onset of pain. Decreased breath sounds and/or rales may be heard over the left posterior chest because of a pneumothorax and/or a pleural effusion. Hamman's sign, described as a crackling, bubbling, crunching, substernal noise that is synchronous with cardiac contraction, may be heard in up to 20 percent of cases, and is related to the presence of a pneumomediastinum. Rarely, a pericardial rub may be audible because of purulent pericarditis related to mediastinal infection. Epigastric and lower-chest direct tenderness and epigastric rigidity and rebound tenderness may occur, mimicking a perforated ulcer. To confuse the clinical picture, up to 5 percent of patients may have free air under the diaphragm.

The plain chest radiograph may demonstrate a pneumomediastinum along the left border of the heart, the aortic arch, and the descending aorta. The "V" sign of Naclerio may be present in 20 percent of cases. This is a V-shaped radiolucent shadow formed by air dissecting the fascial planes of the mediastinum and pleura. A left lower lobe infiltrate and left pleural effusion may be present or a pneumothorax or hydropneumothorax. The presence of subcutaneous and/or mediastinal air differentiates spontaneous esophageal rupture from more common causes of anterior chest pain, such as myocardial infarction, pulmonary embolism, aortic dissection, and pericarditis. Abdominal disorders often confused with esophageal rupture include perforated ulcer, mesenteric occlusion, a ruptured subphrenic abscess, an incarcerated diaphragmatic hernia, and acute pancreatitis.

The diagnosis can be confirmed in up to 90 to 95 percent of cases by a diatrizoate meglumine (Gastrografin) swallow that demonstrates leakage of the contrast material into the mediastinum or left pleural cavity. Endoscopy and/or barium swallow has been used to detect rupture in a suspected case after a negative Gastrografin swallow.

Pain and physical findings are usually substernal or left-sided, but right chest pain, pneumothorax, and effusion may occur in a small number of cases.

CT scanning has been used to evaluate patients too ill or uncooperative for a contrast study of the esophagus. The CT scan may demonstrate a mediastinal hematoma, free air and/or abscesses in the mediastinum; pleural fluid, and/or pneumothorax. The pleural fluid is dark-brown and sometimes foul-smelling. It is an exudate, and has a high salivary amylase concentration (90 percent of cases) and a pH below 6 (50 percent), and often contains food particles.

The classic story of postemetic chest and/or epigastric pain, associated with the development of subcutaneous emphysema and/or pneumomediastinum, occurs in 50 to 65 percent of cases. In other cases there may be no history of vomiting, or, rarely, no pain. Some cases occur in a setting of severe asthma, childbirth, severe coughing or hiccups, weightlifting, or food bingeing; during dialysis; or after a Heimlich maneuver. Some cases of esophageal rupture are related to endoscopy, esophageal instrumentation, trauma, and foreign bodies. Underlying esophageal diseases, such as stricture, carcinoma, achalasia, or a paraesophageal hernia, may lead to rupture. There is controversy as to the optimal therapy. Immediate surgical exploration, esophageal closure, and mediastinal lavage and drainage are advocated by some authors; others claim good results with conservative medical management, using total parenteral nutrition, antibiotics, fluid replacement, and chest tube drainage.

14 Acute Bilateral Anterior Chest Pain

☐ DIAGNOSTIC LIST

1. Acute pleuritis
   A. Bacterial pneumonia
   B. Pulmonary emboli
   C. Septic pulmonary emboli (right-sided endocarditis)
   D. Pleurodynia (devil's grippe, Bornholm disease)
2. Acute pericarditis
   A. Idiopathic and viral pericarditis
   B. Post-cardiac injury syndromes
      1. Post-myocardial infarction pericarditis
      2. Post-cardiotomy pericarditis
      3. Post-cardiac trauma pericarditis
      4. Post-cardiac radiation pericarditis
      5. Post-catheter or pacemaker-induced trauma pericarditis
      6. Post-anticoagulant–related

   intrapericardial bleeding pericarditis
   C. Collagen vascular disorders and pericarditis/pleuritis
   D. Uremic pericarditis
   E. Bacterial or fungal (purulent) pericarditis
   F. Tuberculous pericarditis
   G. Neoplastic (primary or secondary) pericarditis
   H. Intrapericardial bleeding related to a leaking aortic aneurysm
3. Acute myocardial infarction
4. Acute aortic dissection
5. Gastric distension and gastroesophageal reflux
6. Sickle cell pain crisis
7. Chest wall pain—Costochondritis and myofascial pain
8. Bilateral tension pneumothorax

☐ SUMMARY

Acute pleuritis causes sharp, stabbing pain intensified by a deep breath, cough, and change in position. It is partially relieved by analgesics, lying with the painful chest region splinted against the bed surface, and rapid shallow breathing. A persistent dull aching discomfort develops after several hours in association with severe stabbing end-inspiratory pain. *Bacte-*

rial pneumonia may present with bilateral pleuritic pain, fever, chills, cough, and purulent or rust-colored sputum. Radiographs show bilateral segmental or lobar air space filling infiltrates involving the anterior lung fields. Sputum or transtracheal aspirate smears and cultures allow selection of appropriate antibiotic therapy, which usually leads to resolution of symptoms within 1 to 4 days.

Pulmonary emboli may cause bilateral pleuritic pain, fever to 101.5°F, cough productive of scant mucoid material or blood, and moderate to severe dyspnea and cyanosis. Physical examination may reveal wheezes and rhonchi, scattered rales, and signs of small pleural effusions. The chest radiograph may show a pleural-based triangular infiltrate (Hampton hump), a large pulmonary artery with oligemic peripheral vessels (Westermark's sign), pleural effusions, and/or high fixed diaphragms. A ventilation/perfusion (V/Q) scan may show bilateral segmental or lobar defects with V/Q mismatch and/or perfusion defects larger than corresponding radiographic infiltrates. An impedence plethysmographic or Doppler ultrasound study may show thigh vein clots, and a pulmonary angiogram will show evidence of emboli. Symptoms respond to heparin-warfarin therapy.

Septic emboli occur in intravenous drug abusers with right-sided endocarditis or purulent phlebitis of an extremity vein. Such patients present acutely with high fever, chills and/or rigors, cough, severe dyspnea, and excruciating chest pain that is intensified by breathing or movement. Central cyanosis and rapid shallow breathing occur. The pulmonary examination may be negative or reveal scattered fine inspiratory rales and/or a pleural friction rub. The chest radiograph will reveal patchy, irregular subsegmental infiltrates with or without central cavitation and peripheral thin-walled ring lesions. Blood cultures are positive, and there is a prompt response of symptoms to intravenous antibiotics.

Pleurodynia causes bilateral gripping, squeezing, or stabbing lower anterior chest and upper abdominal pain, which may be intensified by breathing, coughing, laughing, and bodily movement. The pain may remain near the costal margin or it may migrate from the lower chest into the lower or upper abdomen. The chest examination is usually normal, or it may reveal a pleural friction rub and signs of a small pleural effusion. Electrocardiograms and V/Q scans are usually negative. A chest radiograph may be normal or may show unilateral or bilateral pleural effusions. This disorder is caused by a Coxsackie B or echovirus, and is most prevalent in the summer or fall months.

Acute pericarditis may cause persistent bilateral anterior chest, lateral neck, and shoulder ridge pain of an aching nature made worse by a deep breath, cough, or change in body position. Lying supine or on the left side intensifies the pain, while sitting up and leaning forward relieves it. Such patients may be encountered sitting up and leaning over the bedside table. Fever to 102°F, myalgias, arthralgias, dyspnea, and malaise may accompany the positional pain described. Physical examination reveals a pericardial friction rub and cardiomegaly in some cases. The electrocardiogram reveals concave upward ST elevation and T-wave flattening, and the echocardiogram demonstrates pericardial fluid.

Most cases have no identifiable cause *(idiopathic),* but occasionally a *viral* agent may be identified by culture of pericardial fluid, stool, or throat washings or by antibody assays. Toxoplasmosis has been associated as evidenced by changes in IgM antibody titers to that organism. Other cases have been labeled *post-cardiac injury pericarditis* because of their asso-

ciation with a previous cardiac insult. These cases include similar disorders that resemble idiopathic pericarditis and may have an associated pleuritis and pneumonitis as part of the syndrome. Post–cardiac injury syndromes include post-myocardial infarction, post-cardiac trauma, post-cardiotomy, post-catheter or -pacemaker perforation, and post-radiation, pericarditis and post–anticoagulant intrapericardial bleeding pericarditis. *Collagen vascular disorders* may present with acute pericarditis and/or pleuritis as their initial manifestation or as part of a well-developed systemic disorder involving multiple organ systems. Drug-related lupus may present as a pleuritis and/or pericarditis with or without fever. Patients with *renal failure* are subject to acute attacks of painful or asymptomatic pericarditis. The disorders described above are responsive to prednisone and nonsteroidal anti-inflammatory drugs.

Specific therapy is required for patients with *purulent, tuberculous, and neoplastic pericarditis.* Accurate diagnosis is necessary, since these forms of pericarditis do not respond to prednisone. Pericardiocentesis will provide fluid for stained smears, counterimmunoelectrophoresis, and cultures for aerobic and anaerobic bacteria, fungi and *Mycobacterium tuberculosis.* Pericardial fluid can also be submitted for cytological analysis when tumor is suspected.

Pericardial biopsies may help establish a diagnosis of fungal, tuberculous, or neoplastic pericarditis. These disorders improve completely or partially after initiation of specific therapy. A pericarditis beginning within a few days of an acute aortic dissection or in the presence of an *aortic aneurysm* suggests impending rupture and potentially fatal tamponade.

Acute myocardial infarction causes pressure-like, crushing, squeezing, or constricting anterior chest pain that may radiate to the neck, jaw, arms, or back. Dyspnea is not common unless there is pulmonary congestion secondary to myocardial damage. Breathing, changes in body position, and coughing have no effect on the pain. Associated symptoms include dizziness or faintness, paroxysms of sweating, pallor, limb coolness, nausea, and vomiting. Examination may reveal a faint or distant S_1, an S_3 or S_4 gallop and frequent premature contractions or runs of paroxysmal tachycardia, or it may be entirely normal. The electrocardiogram will show evidence of a transmural or a non–Q-wave infarction in 80 to 85 percent of cases. LDH and CPK isozyme elevations occur in the first 3 days after onset. The chest pain may be dramatically relieved by coronary thrombolysis with tissue plasminogen activator or by direct balloon angioplasty.

Aortic dissection begins abruptly with a severe tearing or ripping pain in the anterior chest that spreads within a few seconds or minutes to the mid-upper back, abdomen, and low back. Patients may writhe about in bed, in contrast to most patients with myocardial infarction, pleuritis, or pericarditis, who prefer to lie still. There may be signs of retrograde dissection of the aorta with the development of an aortic insufficiency murmur and electrocardiographic evidence of an inferior wall infarction. Hemiparesis and/or aphasia may indicate right innominate or left carotid artery involvement; loss of arm pulses, innominate or subclavian artery occlusion; and bowel

TABLE OF DISEASE INCIDENCE

INCIDENCE PER 100,000 (APPROXIMATE)

Common (>100)	Uncommon (>5–100)	Rare (>0–5)
Idiopathic pericarditis	Acute pleuritis due to pneumonia	Septic pulmonary emboli
Uremic pericarditis	Acute pleuritis due to emboli	Viral pericarditis
Neoplastic pericarditis due to metastatic tumor	Pleurodynia	Purulent pericarditis
Acute myocardial infarction	Post–cardiac injury pericarditis	Tuberculous pericarditis
Sickle cell pain crisis	Collagen vascular disorders and pericarditis/ pleuritis	Neoplastic pericarditis due to primary cardiac tumor
Chest wall pain due to costochondritis	Aortic dissection	Intrapericardial bleeding due to a leaking aneurysm
	Gastric distension	Bilateral tension pneumothorax
	Chest wall pain due to a myofascial disorder	

or spinal cord dysfunction, occlusion of branch vessels of the abdominal aorta. An aortogram or a CT scan with contrast will confirm the diagnosis.

Esophageal reflux and gastric distension may cause sticking bilateral anterior and anterolateral chest pain relieved by antacids and belching.

Sickle cell anemia may cause bilateral anterior chest pain and tenderness associated with tender, painful limbs that are made worse by active or passive movement. Some patients have only rib infarctions as a cause of their chest pain, while others develop pneumonia or a pulmonary embolus and infarction.

Costochondritis may cause bilateral parasternal chest pain and tenderness over rib cartilages 2 to 4. *Myofascial pectoral pain* is intensified by arm movements and sometimes deep breathing. There is localized pectoral muscle tenderness. Results of all laboratory studies, the chest radiograph, the resting and exercise electrocardiogram, and a thallium stress test are usually within normal limits.

Bilateral tension pneumothorax may cause severe chest pain, dyspnea, and central cyanosis with neck vein distension. Breath sounds are absent bilaterally, and the entire chest is hyperresonant. A chest radiograph or insertion of a needle with an attached Heimlich valve will confirm the diagnosis.

☐ DESCRIPTION OF LISTED DISEASES

1. ACUTE PLEURITIS

Pleuritic pain is sharp and stabbing and is felt most intensely at the end of a deep inspiration or after a cough. Changing position in bed may also worsen the discomfort during the movement. After the first hour or two, a dull aching constant pain becomes established in the affected area of the chest, often requiring narcotics for analgesia and sometimes splinting of the chest wall against the mattress or pillow. Referral to one or both shoulders and radiation to the lateral chest may occur. Pleuritic pain involving both sides of the anterior chest occurs in the following disorders.

A. Bilateral Bacterial Pneumonia Patients may present with fever; chills and/or rigors; bilateral anterior pleuritic chest pain, and cough; and rusty, prune juice, or purulent sputum, which may be streaked with blood. Examination reveals fever, tachypnea, tachycardia, and respiratory distress. Breathing may be shallow and punctuated by an audible expiratory grunt. Dullness and bronchial breath sounds may be present over the anterior and anterolateral chest bilaterally, and fine and coarse inspiratory rales may be audible over these areas and posteriorly. A pleural friction rub may be heard on one or both sides. A chest radiograph may show segmental or lobar infiltrates in the anterior and anterolateral lung fields. Sputum will reveal a neutrophilic exudate and, if free from salivary contamination (i.e., few squamous epithelial cells), may aid in identifying the etiologic agent. The presence of gram-positive lanceolate-shaped diplococci (*Streptococcus pneumoniae*); gram-negative coccobacillary organisms (*Haemophilus influenzae*); plump, encapsulated gram-negative rods (*Klebsiella pneumoniae*); or cocci in grapelike clusters (*Staphylococcus aureus*) is helpful in selection of an initial antibiotic regimen. Sputum smears are notoriously inaccurate, and in community-acquired pneumonias, use of transtracheal aspirates may provide greater sensitivity and specificity. A sputum or transtracheal aspirate smear showing neutrophils alone or associated with poorly staining filamentous gram-negative rods should suggest the possibility of *Legionella pneumophila* pneumonia. The latter disorder often begins with a prodromal illness of diarrhea and abdominal pain and/or abnormalities of renal and hepatic function, as well as an encephalopathy. A hematogenous bacterial pneumonia may present with bilateral pleuritic pain, fever, and rigors, without cough or sputum, and the chest radiograph may reveal a bilateral homogeneous ground-glass opacification of both lower anterior lung fields. In up to 58 percent of cases, despite Gram's-stained smears and cultures of sputum and/or a transtracheal aspirate, the cause of a community-acquired pneumonia remains unknown.

S. pneumoniae is the commonest cause of community-acquired bacterial pneumonia, and *L. pneumophila* is becoming more frequent and prevalent in many parts of the United States. *S. aureus* pneumonia occurs during influenza A epidemics and in diabetics, *H. influenzae* occurs in patients with chronic bronchitis and emphysema, and *K. pneumoniae* infection is most commonly associated with alcohol abuse. Aspiration pneumonia occurs in obtunded or unconscious alcoholics, drug abusers, neurologic patients, and the elderly. Bacterial pneumonia will respond within 1 to 4 days to appropriate parenteral antibiotic therapy.

B. Bilateral Pulmonary Emboli and Infarction Severe bilateral anterior pleuritic pain and chest wall tenderness may occur in association with dyspnea. Cough, fever to 101°F, and hemoptysis may also occur. A pleural friction rub, high immobile diaphragms, and scattered rales may be present on physical examination. A large infarction may result in lobar dullness, bronchial breath sounds, and signs of pleural effusion. The chest radiograph may show one or more triangular, pleural-based infarctions (Hampton hump) and pleural effusions. The major pulmonary artery on one side may be dilated, while the branching vessels to distal pulmonary segments may be oligemic or absent (Westermark's sign). These radiographic findings occur in only a small percentage of cases. Perfusion radionuclide scans will show bilateral lobar or segmental defects and mismatch with the ventilation scan. Impedence plethysmographic or Doppler ultrasound studies of the legs may show one or more thigh-level thrombi. Pulmonary angiographic studies will show bilateral intraluminal filling defects or abrupt arterial cutoffs. High-probability lung scans, showing segmental or lobar defects with mismatch or perfusion defects that are larger than radiographic opacities, are associated with a high likelihood of pulmonary embolus. The presence of risk factors and characteristic complaints in the patient being evaluated increases the likelihood that a high-probability scan represents embolism (96 percent if pretest suspicion was high). There is a current controversy about the meaning of low-probability scans, one group urging further studies, including angiographic studies, to rule out embolism (there is evidence of a 40 percent frequency of small emboli in such cases) and another taking the view that nothing further need be done to evaluate or treat a patient with such a scan. The observed benign outcome of untreated patients with low-probability scans for up to 1 year provides the major support for the latter position. Initiation of heparin-warfarin therapy usually is followed by symptom resolution.

C. Bilateral Septic Emboli and Pulmonary Infarction Severe bilateral pleuritic anterior chest pain, fever, rigors or chills, and severe dyspnea occurring in an intravenous drug abuser may be due to septic pulmonary emboli secondary to tricuspid endocarditis. The chest pain may be so severe that the patient resists movement during examination. Physical examination may reveal rapid, shallow respirations; scattered rales over both sides of the anterior chest; one or more localized pleural rubs; and, in some cases, a tricuspid systolic murmur and/or systolic pulsation of the external jugular veins and liver. Signs of intravenous drug abuse (i.e., needle tracks and thrombosed veins) are often present on the extremities. The chest radiograph may reveal multiple irregular subsegmental opacities, small infiltrates with central cavitation, and thin-walled ring lesions near the pleural surface. Blood cultures are usually positive for *S. aureus* or a *Pseudomonas* species. Intravenous antibiotic therapy leads to resolution of fever and chest pain.

D. Pleurodynia This disorder may cause gripping anterior chest pain that may be sharp and sticking. It may be intensified by inspiration, coughing, and laughing. Simultaneous lower abdominal or epigastric and hypochondriac pain may occur, and such pain may be intensified by jarring during walking or laughing. Paroxysms of pain may continue for up to 6 h or may be unremittent. A low-grade fever up to 101°F may occur. Chest examination may be normal or reveal a friction rub and/or signs of a small pleural effusion. The leukocyte count may be normal or slightly elevated. Symptoms may migrate to different abdominal or chest areas. Chest radiographs may show small bilateral effusions, or they may be normal. This disorder is caused by coxsackievirus B or an echovirus and is most common in the fall or late summer. The responsible virus can be cultured from throat washings or stool, and an antibody rise can be documented after a delay of 2 to 4 weeks. Symptoms usually abate spontaneously within 1 week. There is no specific therapy for this disorder.

2. ACUTE PERICARDITIS

Sharp, stabbing, and/or aching pain occurs on both sides of the anterior chest, in the lateral neck region, and on one or both shoulders (trapezius ridge area). The pain may be intensified by inspiration or movement of the upper body. Lying supine or on the left side also intensifies the pain, while sitting up and leaning forward or standing relieves it. Swallowing or coughing may also intensify the pain. Examination may reveal fever, tachycardia, and a three-component pericardial friction rub, heard loudest along the left sternal border. The electrocardiogram reveals elevated (1–5-mm) concave-upward ST segments in all leads except AVR and V_1. Limb-lead PR segments may be depressed. Within 3 to 7 days, the ST segments return to the baseline and the T waves remain normal, flatten, or invert. T-wave inversion may persist for weeks, months, or years. Other causes of ST elevation include acute myocardial infarction, Prinzmetal's angina, and early repolarization. In patients with ischemia, there is convex ST elevation and simultaneous T-wave inversion without a lag period after the onset of chest pain. Early repolarization in leads V_4 to V_6 is concave upward and has also been confused with acute pericarditis. The chest radiograph may be normal or show cardiomegaly resembling the configuration of a water bottle or ice bag. The echocardiogram may show evidence of a pericardial effusion. CPK-MB and LDH-1 levels may be elevated (78 percent of patients in one reported series) due to an associated myocarditis. In other series, the prevalence of isozyme elevations has been lower.

Most cases of this disorder are without any identifiable etiology *(idiopathic)*. Some patients presenting with an identical clinical picture have been shown to have a specific etiology by viral isolation from pericardial fluid, throat, or stool, and/or significant rises in serum antibody titer to a viral agent. Viral agents associated with acute pericarditis include coxsackievirus B5 and B6, influenzae A and B, echovirus 8, mumps, Epstein-Barr virus, adenovirus, hepatitis A or B, rubeola, rubella, and cytomegalovirus.

Attacks of acute pericarditis have occurred 1 to 16 weeks after an acute myocardial infarction (*post-myocardial infarction pericarditis,* or Dressler's syndrome), after cardiac surgery (*post-cardiotomy pericarditis),* after blunt or penetrating cardiac trauma (*post–cardiac trauma pericarditis),* 1 year or more after radiation therapy (*post-radiation pericarditis),* after *pacemaker or catheter perforation* of the heart, and after *anticoagulant-related pericardial bleeding.*

A similar disorder may occur as part of *multisystem disorders,* such as systemic lupus erythematosus, rheumatoid arthritis, rheumatic fever, mixed connective tissue disease, juvenile rheumatoid arthritis, and drug-related lupus. In rare cases, it may be the initial and sole presentation of a *collagen vascular disorder.* Pleuritis may occur in association with drug or systemic lupus pericarditis or it may occur without pericardial involvement. The pleuritis/pericarditis of systemic lupus erythematosis responds to prednisone and the pleuropericarditis of drug lupus resolves with discontinuance of the causative drug and prednisone therapy.

Patients presenting with *chronic renal failure* or those treated by hemo- or peritoneal *dialysis* may develop acute recurrent pericarditis. The disorders described so far in this section are usually responsive to nonsteroidal anti-inflammatory drugs or prednisone.

Steroid-resistent pericarditis may be caused by pyogenic bacteria or fungi (purulent pericarditis), tuberculosis, or primary or secondary cardiac and/or pericardial tumors.

Bacterial pericarditis usually presents with a prodrome of fever, chills, malaise, myalgias, and arthralgias. These symptoms precede more organ-specific complaints, such as pericardial chest pain and dyspnea. Physical examination may reveal a pericardial friction rub (50 percent of cases), cardiomegaly (25 percent), and signs of pleural effusion (25 percent). The chest radiograph may show cardiomegaly; pleural effusions; and, in some cases, segmental or lobar infiltrates. Patients with mediastinitis may show widening of the mediastinum. The electrocardiogram often demonstrates ST-segment elevation and T-wave flattening, but it may be normal. Echocardiographic studies reveal evidence of a pericardial effusion. Pericardiocentesis yields a purulent fluid with 5000 to 200,000 cells/mm^3 and a positive Gram's stain and/or culture. Counterimmunoelectrophoresis has been used to identify the responsible organism in cases treated with antibiotics prior to pericardiocentesis. Pericardial drainage with irrigation and intravenous administration of appropriate antibiotics is the most effective therapeutic strategy.

Bacterial pericarditis may be a primary disease caused by *Neisseria meningitidis* (15 reported cases) or *H. influ-*

enzae (8 reported cases), but primary infection is rare. Most cases of acute pericarditis arise by extension from an adjacent pneumonia or empyema *(S. pneumoniae, S. aureus,* or *H. influenzae);* a mediastinitis *(Peptococcus magnus, Eikenella corrodens);* or a subphrenic, perirenal, or liver abscess (aerobic and/or anaerobic gram-negative rods and cocci). Some cases arise in an infectious focus (i.e., osteomyelitis or skin abscess) and reach the pericardium by bacteremic spread. Cardiac surgery or penetrating trauma may also cause an acute purulent pericarditis. Bacterial pericarditis and/or a myocardial abscess may rarely complicate a myocardial infarction, usually resulting in death. It is essential to identify patients with purulent pericarditis because it is uniformly fatal without therapy. Some patients are afebrile, have no chest pain or dyspnea, and may have no symptoms related to the chest. Such patients have been discovered by detecting unexplained cardiomegaly (''water bottle'' heart) on a chest radiograph, electrocardiographic evidence of pericarditis, pericardial fluid by echocardiography, and cardiac uptake on a gallium 67 or indium 111 leukocyte scan. Pericardiocentesis performed for the relief of tamponade may yield purulent fluid and establish a diagnosis of bacterial or fungal pericarditis. *Candida tropicalis* or *Candida albicans* may cause *purulent pericarditis* in patients with a complicated course after cardiac surgery (e.g., patients requiring repeat thoracotomy for bleeding or reintubation); in patients with impaired defenses (e.g., with neutropenia, following chemotherapy for malignancy; following prolonged concurrent administration of antibiotics and corticosteroids; and in the presence of a central line); and in those with debilitating illnesses (e.g., alcoholism, renal failure, AIDS, systemic lupus erythematosus, and hematologic malignancies). The diagnosis of fungal pericarditis may be made by pericardiocentesis and culture or pericardial biopsy. Growth of the causative fungus may also be obtained from the surgical wound, blood, or pleural fluid.

Since acute pericarditis with or without tamponade may be the initial presentation of *tuberculous pericarditis* (10–44 percent of cases), this disorder must be considered in the differential diagnosis of acute disease. The tuberculin skin test may be negative in 10 to 33 percent of cases, while it may be positive (41 percent in one series) in idiopathic pericarditis. Sputum smears and cultures for tuberculosis may establish the diagnosis. Pericardiocentesis yields fluid with a low probability of demonstrating *Mycobacterium tuberculosis* on smear, while cultural evidence may sometimes be obtained after a delay of several weeks (20 percent of cases). Histopathologic examination of a diagnostic pericardial biopsy or tissue removed at pericardiectomy has a higher sensitivity than does pericardial fluid examination. In some suggestive cases with a refractory course, a trial of antituberculous therapy may be initiated if all other studies yield negative results. In one large prospective series, this strategy was not required, but it has been used in clinical practice. A response of symptoms and signs to such a trial may take 5 to 10 weeks.

Acute pericarditis and/or tamponade may be the initial presentation of a *primary cardiac tumor* (e.g., angiosarcoma or rhabdomyosarcoma) or metastatic carcinoma. Cytologic studies of pericardial fluid have a relatively high yield, while an isolated biopsy is less sensitive. Examination of a large specimen of resected pericardium will produce a high diagnostic yield in the presence of neoplastic disease. False-positive cytologic studies for neoplasia may occasionally occur in other disorders (e.g., tuberculosis). False-negative results after exmaination of pericardial fluid by culture for *M. tuberculosis* or by cytologic studies for malignancy are too common to use these tests to exclude a diagnosis of tuberculosis or tumor.

Pericardiocentesis should be performed for tamponade, suspicion of purulent or tuberculous pericarditis, or pericarditis lasting for over 1 week with evidence of pericardial effusion. Pericardial biopsy may be performed as part of a surgical drainage procedure or for patients without a diagnosis after 3 weeks. In a large prospective series from Spain, idiopathic pericarditis was present in 86 percent of cases, tuberculosis in 4 percent, neoplasia in 6 percent, purulent pericarditis in 1 percent, viral pericarditis in 1 percent, and collagen vascular disease–related pericarditis in 1 percent.

Aortic dissection commonly presents with severe tearing anterior chest pain, as described in the section on Acute Aortic Dissection, below. During the first week of this disorder, an acute pericarditis may develop, with an effusion and a pericardial friction rub due to slow *leakage of blood* into the pericardium. Acute pericarditis in a patient with aortic dissection may appear 4 to 5 days before aortic rupture into the pericardium and fatal tamponade. Typical ST-T changes of pericarditis may appear on the electrocardiogram, as may evidence of effusion by echocardiographic studies. The presence of leakage-related pericarditis is an important indication for early surgical intervention in a patient with aortic dissection to prevent rupture.

3. ACUTE MYOCARDIAL INFARCTION

Patients with this disorder may have severe central and/or bilateral anterior chest pain that may radiate to both arms, hands, neck, and jaw; or it may remain confined to the chest. The pain may be described as a dull pressure, weight, or constriction. A deep inspiration, coughing, or bodily movements have no effect on the pain. There may be some lightheadedness and shortness of breath. Sweating, nausea, vomiting, and severe weakness are associated symptoms. The cardiac examination may reveal a decrease in the intensity of the first heart sound at the apex and an S_3 gallop rhythm, or it may be entirely normal. Sustained tachycardia, ventricular premature contractions, and runs of regular or irregular tachycardia may be present. The electrocardiogram may show Q waves, ST elevation, and T-wave inversion, or only ST elevations or depressions and T-wave

inversions (non–Q-wave infarction). Serum isozymes are usually elevated. If seen within 2 to 4 h of pain onset, the patient can be treated with intravenous tissue plasminogen activator. This clot-lysing enzyme can lead to dissolution of the coronary thrombus and allow time for angioplasty or bypass to be done. In some centers, cardiologists do not use thrombolytic agents but go immediately to angioplasty. If the patient has had chest pain for over 4 to 6 h and there is electrocardiographic evidence of acute infarction, admission to a coronary care unit and supportive care are the current standards of care. Early reperfusion appears to salvage ischemic, but not yet infarcted, heart muscle, and preserves cardiac function. Such emergency therapy should be followed by an intensive medical effort to control risk factors, such as cholesterol level, hypertension, smoking, lack of exercise, obesity, and a low HDL level. Thrombolytic therapy rarely prevents myocardial infarction but does appear to decrease its size by an average of 20 to 25 percent.

4. ACUTE AORTIC DISSECTION

The pain begins abruptly and rises to a maximum intensity within seconds. It usually has a tearing or ripping quality and is felt immediately in the mid-chest with radiation to both anterior chest regions. The pain may also be felt sequentially in the interscapular area, epigastrium, and lower abdomen and back if the dissection continues into the abdominal aorta. A tearing or ripping type of pain sensation may not be experienced by some patients.

The pain associated with dissection may be so intense that patients are unable to lie still. They may writhe and roll from side to side in bed, seeking relief. The chest pain is not affected by movement, cough, or deep inspiration. Some patients with acute myocardial infarction may also writhe and turn frequently in bed.

Associated symptoms represent occlusion of the blood supply to important organs supplied by the aorta. Flank pain and hematuria may signal renal infarction. Fainting, hemiplegia, syncope, and aphasia may indicate left carotid or right innominate artery occlusion. Sudden paraplegia with a complete or partial sensory loss indicates spinal cord infarction.

Electrocardiographic evidence of an acute inferior wall infarction is most likely due to retrograde aortic dissection and coronary artery occlusion. The presence of a new aortic insufficiency murmur indicates the presence of retrograde dissection back to the aortic valve. Abdominal pain and vomiting and subsequent diarrhea, bloody stools, and distension may be caused by bowel infarction.

Leg pain and pallor, numbness, and an absent femoral pulse indicate common iliac artery occlusion, produced by the dissection. Hypertension, asymmetric loss of peripheral pulses, and cardiomegaly may be present. Cardiac tamponade, causing a paradoxic pulse, muffled heart sounds, and neck vein distension, may be present, secondary to leakage of aortic blood into the pericardium.

Dullness and decreased breath sounds at the left base provide evidence of bleeding into the left pleural space from the aorta.

The electrocardiogram may show evidence of left ventricular hypertrophy and strain and, in up to 16 percent of cases, evidence of an acute myocardial infarction. The chest radiograph shows a widened mediastinum in 80 to 90 percent of cases. Catheter aortographic studies will demonstrate the intimal flap of the aortic dissection, the region of aortic narrowing, the origin and termination of the double lumen, and the presence of branch vessel occlusions. A thoracic CT scan with contrast may also establish the diagnosis.

In patients with a proven dissection, intravenous nitroprusside or trimethaphan should be used to maintain the systolic pressure at 100 to 110 mmHg. Propranolol should be given to decrease the force of myocardial contraction. Types I and II (type A) dissection, involving the aortic arch, usually require surgery to optimize survival. Type III (type B) dissections begin distal to the left subclavian artery. These dissections may also do better with surgery than with medical management, but the use of surgery is still controversial in this group of patients.

Type I and II (type A) dissections occur in young adults with less severe hypertension. These patients may have Marfan's syndrome (10 percent of cases), cystic medial necrosis (20 percent), congenitally abnormal aortic valves, or coarctation of the aorta. Type B dissections occur in older patients with hypertension.

5. GASTRIC DISTENSION

Gastric distension associated with lower esophageal reflux may cause pyrosis and a sharp, sticking bilateral anterolateral chest pain that may be rapidly relieved by the ingestion of soluble antacids and by belching. It is probably due to gastric distension. There is no central chest pain associated with this disorder. A deep breath may make these sticking pains more intense. They are usually well-localized to one or two anterolateral interspaces.

6. SICKLE CELL ANEMIA

Patients may experience symmetric or asymmetric limb muscle and joint pains. These pains are intensified by active or passive movement of the affected limb. Small knee joint effusions may occur. Severe bilateral anterior chest pain that is intensified by breathing or by moving to turn in bed, to sit up, or to lie down may occur. The ribs, as well as the bones of the extremities, may be exquisitely tender. There is usually a history extending back to childhood of many previous attacks of similar limb, abdominal, or chest

pains. If chest pain has not been noted in previous attacks, a careful workup for pleuritis secondary to pneumonia or a pulmonary infarction should be carried out. In the absence of these disorders, the physical examination of the chest may reveal only superficial and deep tenderness and no evidence of consolidation, friction rubs, or rales. Chest radiographs may show old rib infarctions but no infiltrates or effusions. Chest pain in some patients has been so severe that atelectasis secondary to failure to expand basilar lung segments has developed. These patients may have dullness and bronchial breath sounds at one or both bases secondary to atelectasis and abnormal blood gases responsive to analgesics, incentive spirometry, and O_2 inhalation. The pulmonary findings described may mimic consolidation secondary to a pneumonia or infarction of one or both lungs. Fever may be part of a sickle cell pain crisis or may be secondary to a complication (e.g., pneumonia or pulmonary infarction).

7. BILATERAL COSTOCHONDRITIS AND MYOFASCIAL PAIN (CHEST WALL PAIN)

Pain occurs spontaneously in the parasternal regions bilaterally or in more lateral anterior chest regions. It may radiate to one or both shoulders or axillae. The pain may be described as sharp or aching, and it may persist for minutes, hours, or days. It is usually associated with localized tenderness over the second to fourth costal cartilages adjacent to both sides of the sternum or with tender trigger points in the pectoral muscles. Deep breaths, arm movements, extension of the cervical and thoracic spine, and arm abduction or adduction against resistance may intensify or precipitate pain, which is similar in quality and location to but briefer in duration than that experienced spontaneously. Use of moist heat and simple analgesics will usually relieve the symptoms of this disorder. Elimination of activities in which arm and chest muscles are used, such as on an assembly line, in lifting heaving objects, or in performing calesthenics (e.g., push-ups), may alleviate and prevent future attacks of such pain. The major confusion is with cardiac disease, but chest radiographs, electrocardiograms, and EKG and thallium stress tests are normal. Local injection of lidocaine and methylprednisolone into a tender trigger point on a costal cartilage will provide instantaneous but transient pain relief on the injected side. This procedure is not routinely recommended because the relief is usually only transient. Reassurance, use of warm, moist heat locally, and administration of nonsteroidal antiinflammatory drugs may provide symptomatic relief until spontaneous remission occurs.

8. BILATERAL TENSION PNEUMOTHORAX

This disorder may begin spontaneously or may follow severe blunt or penetrating trauma to the chest. Intense unilateral anterior chest pain and severe dyspnea occur. The blood pressure falls, the external jugular veins distend, and the trachea is shifted to the contralateral side. There are hyperresonance and absent breath sounds over the affected side. As the patient becomes more dyspneic and cyanotic and requires greater inspiratory pressure to fill the normal lung, a second pneumothorax may occur, resulting in very rapid, shallow breathing, bilateral chest pain and absent breath sounds, subcutaneous emphysema, severe cyanosis, and cardiac arrest unless the diagnosis is made and needles or chest tubes are inserted to release intrapleural air. If the diagnosis is not made promptly, the high intrathoracic pressure resulting from the pneumothorax decreases venous return and may cause shock, hypoxemia, decreased coronary perfusion, myocardial ischemia, and fatal ventricular arrhythmias.

After insertion, both chest tubes should be attached to suction to prevent reaccumulation of pleural air. A definitive prophylactic surgical procedure may be required to prevent recurrence.

CHEST PAIN REFERENCES

Angina Pectoris—Bypass Graft Surgery

Baillot RG, Loop FD, Cosgrove DM, et al: Reoperation after previous grafting with the internal mammary artery: Technique and early results. *Ann Thorac Surg* 40:271–273, 1985.

Barner HB, Standeven JW, Reese J: Twelve-year experience with internal mammary artery for coronary artery bypass. *J Thorac Cardiovasc Surg* 90:668–675, 1985.

Bashour TT, Hanna ES, Mason DT: Myocardial revascularization with internal mammary artery bypass: An emerging treatment of choice. *Am Heart J* 111:143–151, 1986.

Cote G, Myler RK, Stertzer SH, et al: Percutaneous transluminal angioplasty of stenotic coronary artery bypass grafts: 5 years' experience. *J Am Coll Cardiol* 9:8–17, 1987.

Engblom E, Arstila M, Inberg MV, et al: Early results and complications of coronary artery bypass surgery. *Scand J Thorac Cardiovasc Surg* 19:21–27, 1985.

Kamath ML, Matysik LS, Schmidt DH, et al: Sequential internal mammary artery grafts. *J Thorac Cardiovasc Surg* 89:163–169, 1985.

Kay P, Ahmad A, Floten S, et al: Emergency coronary artery bypass surgery after intracoronary thrombolysis for evolving myocardial infarction. *Br Heart J* 53:260–264, 1985.

Lolley DM, Enerson DM, Rams JJ, et al: Should coronary artery bypass be delayed following successful direct coronary artery streptokinase thrombolysis during evolving myocardial infarction? *J Vasc Surg* 3:330–337, 1986.

Loop FD, Lytle BW, Cosgrove DM, et al: Influence of the internal-mammary-artery graft on 10-year survival and other cardiac events. *N Engl J Med* 314:1–6, 1986.

Lytle BW, Loop FD, Cosgrove DM, et al: Long-term (5 to 12 years) serial studies of internal mammary artery and saphenous vein coronary bypass grafts. *J Thorac Cardiovasc Surg* 89:248–258, 1985.

Marquis J-F, Schwartz L, Brown R, et al: Percutaneous transluminal angioplasty of coronary saphenous vein bypass grafts. *Can J Surg* 28:335–337, 1985.

Orszulak TA, Schaff HV, Chesebro JH: Initial experience with sequential internal mammary artery bypass grafts to the left anterior descending and left anterior descending diagonal coronary arteries. *Mayo Clin Proc* 61:3–8, 1986.

Raess DH, Mahomed Y, Brown JW, et al: Lesser saphenous vein as an alternative conduit of choice in coronary bypass operations. *Ann Thorac Surg* 41:334–336, 1986.

Singh RN: Coronary atherosclerosis and the bypass grafts: Twenty-year follow-up of a case. *Cathet Cardiovasc Diagn* 11:505–511, 1985.

Spencer FC: The internal mammary artery: The ideal coronary bypass graft? (editorial). *N Engl J Med* 314:50–51, 1986.

Tector AJ: Internal mammary artery—Its changing role in coronary artery bypass grafting procedures (editorial). *Mayo Clin Proc* 61:72–74, 1986.

Ungerleider RM, Mills NL, Wechsler AS: Left thoracotomy for reoperative coronary artery bypass procedures. *Ann Thorac Surg* 40:11–15, 1985.

Zaidi AR, Hollman JL: Percutaneous angioplasty of internal mammary artery graft stenosis: Case report and discussion. *Cathet Cardiovasc Diagn* 11:603–608, 1985.

Angina Pectoris—Diagnosis

Brown KA, Boucher CA, Okada RD, et al: Prognostic value of exercise thallium-201 imaging in patients presenting for evaluation of chest pain. *J Am Coll Cardiol* 1:994–1001, 1983.

Chaitman BR, Brevers G, Dupras G, et al: Diagnostic impact of thallium scintigraphy and cardiac fluoroscopy when the exercise ECG is strongly positive. *Am Heart J* 108:260–265, 1984.

Currie PJ, Kelly MJ, Harper RW, et al: Incremental value of clinical assessment, supine exercise electrocardiography, and biplane exercise radionuclide ventriculography in the prediction of coronary artery disease in men with chest pain. *Am J Cardiol* 52:927–935, 1983.

DiCarlo LA Jr, Botvinick EH, Canhasi BS, et al: Value of noninvasive assessment of patients with atypical chest pain and suspected coronary spasm using ergonovine infusion and thallium-201 scintigraphy. *Am J Cardiol* 54:744–748, 1984.

Epstein SE, Quyyumi AA, Bonow RO: Myocardial ischemia: Silent or symptomatic. *N Engl J Med* 318:1038–1043, 1988.

Gibbons RJ, Lee KL, Pryor D, et al: The use of radionuclide angiography in the diagnosis of coronary artery disease: A logistic regression analysis. *Circulation* 68:740–746, 1983.

Gibbons RJ, Morris KG, Lee K, et al: Assessment of regional left ventricular function using gated radionuclide angiography. *Am J Cardiol* 54:294–300, 1984.

Goldschlager N: Use of the treadmill test in the diagnosis of coronary artery disease in patients with chest pain. *Ann Intern Med* 97:383–388, 1982.

Hickam DH, Sox HC Jr, Marton KI, et al: A study of the implicit criteria used in diagnosing chest pain. *Med Decis Making* 2:403–414, 1982.

Hickam DH, Sox HC Jr, Sox CH: Systematic bias in recording the history in patients with chest pain. *J Chron Dis* 38:91–100, 1985.

Josephson MA, Brown BG, Hecht HS, et al: Noninvasive detection and localization of coronary stenoses in patients: Comparison of resting dipyridamole and exercise thallium-201 myocardial perfusion imaging. *Am Heart J* 103:1008–1018, 1982.

Joswig BC, Glover MU, Nelson DP, et al: Analysis of historical variables, risk factors and the resting electrocardiogram as an aid in the clinical diagnosis of recurrent chest pain. *Comput Biol Med* 15:71–79, 1985.

Massie BM, Hollenberg M, Wisneski JA, et al: Scintigraphic quantification of myocardial ischemia: A new approach. *Circulation* 68:747–755, 1983.

Pryor DB, Harrell FE Jr, Lee KL, et al: Estimating the likelihood of significant coronary artery disease. *Am J Med* 75:771–780, 1983.

Salmasi AM, Nicolaides AN, Vecht RJ, et al: Electrocardiographic chest wall mapping in the diagnosis of coronary artery disease. *Br Med J* 287:9–12, 1983.

Savvides M, Froelicher V: Non-invasive non-nuclear exercise testing. *Cardiology* 71:100–117, 1984.

Selwyn AP, Ganz P. Myocardial ischemia in coronary disease (editorial). *N Engl J Med* 318:1058–1060, 1988.

Sox, HC Jr: Noninvasive testing in coronary artery disease: Selection of procedures and interpretation of results. *Postgrad Med* 74:319–336, 1983.

Sox HC Jr, Littenberg B, Garber AM: The role of exercise testing in screening for coronary artery disease. *Ann Intern Med* 110:456–469, 1989.

Willerson JT: Angina pectoris, in Wyngaarden JB, Smith LH Jr (eds): *Cecil Textbook of Medicine,* 18th ed. Philadelphia, Saunders, 1988, pp 323–329.

———: Diagnostic methods in the assessment of the patient with chest pain. *J Am Coll Cardiol* 4:1–3, 1984.

Angina Pectoris—Medical Therapy

Charap MH, Levin RI, Weinglass J: Physician choices in the treatment of angina pectoris. *Am J Med* 79:461–466, 1985.

Gottlieb SO, Weisfeldt ML, Ouyang P, et al: Effect of the addition of propranolol to therapy with nifedipine for unstable angina pectoris: A randomized, double-blind, placebo-controlled trial. *Circulation* 73:331–337, 1986.

Angina Pectoris—Unstable

de Feyter PJ, Serruys PW, van den Brand M, et al: Emergency coronary angioplasty in refractory unstable angina. *N Engl J Med* 313:342–346, 1985.

Gottlieb SO, Weisfeldt ML, Ouyang P, et al: Silent ischemia as a marker for early unfavorable outcomes in patients with unstable angina. *N Engl J Med* 314:1214–1219, 1986.

Halon DA, Merdler A, Shefer A, et al: Identifying patients at high risk for restenosis after percutaneous transluminal coronary angioplasty for unstable angina pectoris. *Am J Cardiol* 64:289–293, 1989.

Mooney MR, Mooney JF, Goldenberg IF, et al: Percutaneous transluminal coronary angioplasty in the setting of large intracoronary thrombi. *Am J Cardiol* 65:427–431, 1990.

Pathy MS: Acute central chest pain in the elderly: A review of 296 consecutive hospital admissions during 1976 with particular reference to the possible role of beta-adrenergic blocking agents in inducing substernal pain. *Am Heart J* 98:168–170, 1979.

Roberts WC: Qualitative and quantitative comparison of amounts of narrowing by atherosclerotic plaques in the major epicardial coronary arteries at necropsy in sudden coronary death, transmural acute myocardial infarction, transmural healed myocardial infarction and unstable angina pectoris. *Am J Cardiol* 64:324–328, 1989.

Sherman CT, Litvack F, Grundfest W, et al: Coronary angioscopy in patients with unstable angina pectoris. *N Engl J Med* 315:913–919, 1986.

Solomon CG, Lee TH, Cook EF, et al: Comparison of clinical presentation of acute myocardial infarction in patients older than 65 years of age to younger patients: The multicenter chest pain study experience. *Am J Cardiol* 63:772–776, 1989.

Topol EJ: Coronary angioplasty for acute myocardial infarction. *Ann Intern Med* 109:970–980, 1988.

Van der Wall EE, Kerkkamp HJJ, Lubsen J, et al: Left ventricular performance in unstable angina: Assessment with radionuclide techniques. *Intl J Cardiol* 8:287–299, 1985.

Angioplasty

Acinapura AJ, Cunningham JN, Jacobowitz IJ, et al: Efficacy of percutaneous transluminal coronary angioplasty compared with single-vessel bypass. *J Thorac Cardiovasc Surg* 89:35–41, 1985.

Detre K, Holubkov R, Kelsey S, et al: Percutaneous transluminal coronary angioplasty in 1985–1986 and 1977–1981. *N Engl J Med* 318:265–270, 1988.

Gruentzig AR, King SB III, Schlumpf M, et al: Long-term follow-up after percutaneous transluminal coronary angioplasty. *N Engl J Med* 316:1127–1132, 1987.

Kereiakes DJ, Selmon MR, McAuley BJ, et al: Angioplasty in total coronary artery occlusion: Experience in 76 consecutive patients. *J Am Coll Cardiol* 6:526–533, 1985.

McBride W, Lange RA, Hillis LD: Restenosis after successful coronary angioplasty. *N Engl J Med* 318:1734–1737, 1988.

Roberts AJ, Alexander JA, Knauf DG, et al: Clinical and angiographic experience with intraoperative transluminal balloon-catheter dilatation and coronary artery bypass graft surgery. *J Cardiovasc Surg* 26:207–211, 1985.

Ryan TJ. Angioplasty in acute myocardial infarction: Is the balloon leaking? (editorial). *N Engl J Med* 317:624–626, 1987.

Anxiety/Hyperventilation

Channer KS, Papouchado M, James MA, et al: Anxiety and depression in patients with chest pain referred for exercise testing. *Lancet,* Oct 12, 1985, pp 820–823.

Folgering H, Sistermans H: Hyperventilation and aerophagia: A negative report. *Eur J Respir Dis* 68:173–176, 1986.

Freeman LJ, Nixon PGF. Are coronary artery spasm and progressive damage to the heart associated with the hyperventilation syndrome? *Br Med J* 291:851–852, 1985.

Smith MS. Evaluation and management of psychosomatic symptoms in adolescence. *Clin Pediatr* 25:131–135, 1986.

Aortic Stenosis

Nylander E, Ekman I, Marklund T, et al: Severe aortic stenosis in elderly patients. *Br Heart J* 55:480–487, 1986.

Rackley CE, Edwards JE, Karp RB, et al: Aortic valve disease, in Hurst JW (ed): *The Heart,* 5th ed. New York, McGraw-Hill, 1982, pp 863–892.

Sherman W, Hershman R, Lazzam C, et al: Balloon valvuloplasty in adult aortic stenosis: Determinants of clinical outcome. *Ann Intern Med* 110:421–425, 1989.

Siemienczuk D, Greenberg B, Morris C, et al: Chronic aortic insufficiency: Factors associated with progression to aortic valve replacement. *Ann Intern Med* 110:587–592, 1989.

Asbestos

Faber LP. Surgical treatment of asbestos-related disease of the chest. *Surg Clin North Am* 68(3):525–543, 1988.

Boerhaave's Syndrome

Bunnell P, Richter J: Spontaneous rupture of the distal esophagus: Boerhaave's syndrome. *Tex Med* 84:34–37, 1987.

Gertler JP, Brophy C, Elefteriades J: Esophageal rupture after routine Maloney dilatation: A proposed mechanism. *J Clin Gastroenterol* 8(2):175–176, 1986.

Graeber GM, Niezgoda JA, Burton NA, et al: A comparison of patients with endoscopic esophageal perforations and patients with Boerhaave's syndrome. *Chest* 92(6):995–998, 1987.

Henderson JAM, Peloquin AJM: Boerhaave revisited: Spontaneous esophageal perforation as a diagnostic masquerader. *Am J Med* 86:559–567, 1989.

Jaworski A, Fischer R, Lippmann M. Boerhaave's syndrome: Computed tomographic findings and diagnostic considerations. *Arch Intern Med* 148:223–224, 1988.

Lucas CE, Splittgerber F, Ledgerwood AM. Conservative therapy for missed esophageal perforation after blunt trauma. *Am J Emerg Med* 4:520–522, 1986.

Pezzulli FA, Aronson D, Goldberg N. Computed tomography of mediastinal hematoma secondary to unusual esophageal laceration: A Boerhaave variant. *J Comput Assist Tomogr* 13(1):129–131, 1989.

Schwartz JA, Turnbull TL, Dymowski J, et al: Boerhaave's syndrome: An elusive diagnosis. *Am J Emerg Med* 4:532–536, 1986.

Uehara DT, Dymowski JJ, Schwartz J, et al: Chest pain, shock, and pneumomediastinum in a previously healthy 56-year-old man. *Ann Emerg Med* 16:359–364, 1987.

Ward WG: Cold water polydipsia: Unheralded marker of spontaneous esophageal rupture. *South Med J* 79(9):1161–1162, 1986.

Yellin A, Schachter P, Lieberman Y: Spontaneous transmural rupture of esophagus: Boerhaave's syndrome. *Acta Chir Scand* 155:337–340, 1989.

Bronchiectasis

Rubin EH, Rubin M: *Bronchiectasis in Thoracic Diseases: Emphasizing Cardiopulmonary Relationships.* Philadelphia, Saunders, 1962, pp 437–454.

Stockley RA: Bronchiectasis: New therapeutic approaches based on pathogenesis. *Clin Chest Med* 8(3):481–494, 1987.

Cardiac Disease—Pulmonary Complications

Remetz MS, Cleman MW, Cabin HS: Pulmonary and pleural complications of cardiac disease. *Clin Chest Med* 10(4):545–592, 1989.

Cardiomyopathy—Dilated

Stern TN: Dilated cardiomyopathy: Current concepts. *Compr Ther* 12:57–62, 1986.

Chest Pain and Chemotherapy

White DA, Schwartzberg LS, Kris MG, et al: Acute chest pain syndrome during bleomycin infusions. *Cancer* 59:1582–1585, 1987.

Chest Wall Pain

Bechgaard P: Segmental thoracic pain in patients admitted to a medical department and a coronary unit. *Acta Med Scand* 644(suppl):87–89, 1981.

Bell EJ, Irvine KG, Gardiner AJS, et al: Coxsackie B infection in a general medical unit. *Scott Med J* 28:157–159, 1983.

Caldwell DS, Kernodle GW Jr, Seigler HF: Pectoralis pyomyositis: An unusual cause of chest wall pain in a patient with diabetes mellitus and rheumatoid arthritis. *J Rheumatol* 13:434–436, 1986.

Cameron HU, Fornasier VL: Tietze's disease. *J Clin Pathol* 27:960–962, 1974.

Chicarilli ZN, Ariyan S, Stahl RS: Costochondritis: Pathogenesis, diagnosis, and management considerations. *Plast Reconstr Surg* 77:50–59, 1986.

DiTommaso S: Another look at musculoskeletal chest wall pain (letter to the editor). *Can Med Assoc J* 134:12, 1986.

Edelstein G, Levitt RG, Slaker DP, et al: Computed tomography of Tietze syndrome. *J Comput Assist Tomogr* 8:20–23, 1984.

Epstein SE, Gerber LH, Borer JS. Chest wall syndrome: A common cause of unexplained cardiac pain. *JAMA* 241:2793–2797, 1979.

Evans DW, Lum LC: Hyperventilation: An important cause of pseudo-angina. *Lancet* Jan 22, 1977, pp 155–157.

Fam AG, Smythe HA: Musculoskeletal chest wall pain. *Can Med Assoc J* 133:379–389, 1985.

Gimferrer J-M, Callejas M-A, Sanchez-Lloret J, et al: *Candida albicans* costochondritis in heroin addicts. *Ann Thorac Surg* 41:89–90, 1986.

Glazer HS, Duncan-Meyer J, Aronberg DJ, et al: Pleural and chest wall invasion in bronchogenic carcinoma: CT evaluation. *Radiology* 157:191–194, 1985.

Golding DN. What does "just muscular" chest pain signify? *Practitioner* 228:514–517, 1984.

Halle S. Tietze's syndrome: A bridge between neurocirculatory asthenia and mitral valve prolapse syndrome. *J La State Med Soc* 136:20–21, 1984.

Heinz GJ III, Zavala DC: Slipping rib syndrome: Diagnosis using the "hooking maneuver." *JAMA* 237:794–795, 1977.

Jelenko C III: Tietze's syndrome at the xiphisternal joint. *South Med J* 67:818–819, 1974.

Kantor FS, Hsiung G-D: Pleurodynia associated with ECHO virus type 8. *N Engl J Med* 266:661–663, 1962.

Kayser HL: Tietze's syndrome: A review of the literature. *Am J Med* 21:982–989, 1956.

LaBan MM, Newman JM: Occult sternal metastasis identified by laminography in patients with chest pain. *Arch Phys Med Rehabil* 65:203–204, 1984.

McCallum MID, Glynn CJ: Intercostal neuralgia following stellate ganglion block. *Anaesthesia* 41:850–852, 1986.

McElroy JB: Angina pectoris with coexisting skeletal chest pain. *Am Heart J* 66:296–300, 1963.

Miller AJ, Texidor TA: "Precordial catch": A neglected syndrome of precordial pain. *JAMA* 159:1364–1365, 1955.

Peyton FW: Unexpected frequency of idiopathic costochondral pain. *Obstet Gynecol* 62:605–608, 1973.

Raney RB Jr: Localized sarcoma of the chest wall. *Med Pediatr Oncol* 12:116–118, 1984.

Rao MV: Tietze's disease (costochondritis): Case report. *Indian J Med Sci* 27:468–470, 1973.

Sain AK: Bone scan in Tietze's syndrome. *Clin Nucl Med* 3:470–471, 1978.

Seviour PW, Dieppe PA: Sternoclavicular joint infection as a cause of chest pain. *Br Med J* 288:133–134, 1984.

Sox HC Jr, Margulies I, Sox CH: Psychologically mediated effects of diagnostic tests. *Ann Intern Med* 95:680–685, 1981.

Thompson BM, Finger W, Tonsfeldt D, et al: Rib radiographs for trauma: Useful or wasteful? *Ann Emerg Med* 15:261–265, 1986.

Wolf E, Stern S: Costosternal syndrome: Its frequency and importance in differential diagnosis of coronary heart disease. *Arch Intern Med* 136:189–191, 1976.

Wray TM, Bryant RE, Killen DA: Sternal osteomyelitis and costochondritis after median sternotomy. *J Thorac Cardiovasc Surg* 65:227–233, 1973.

Collagen Vascular Diseases

Ansari Azam, Larson PH, Bates HD: Cardiovascular manifestations of systemic lupus erythematosus: Current prospective.

Dickey BF, Myers AR: Pulmonary manifestations of collagen-vascular diseases, in Fishman AP: *Pulmonary Diseases and Disorders,* 2d ed. New York, McGraw-Hill, 1988, vol 1, pp 645–666.

Hess E: Drug-related lupus (editorial). *N Engl J Med* 318:1460–1462, 1988.

Mandel BF: Cardiovascular involvement in systemic lupus erythematosus. *Semin Arthritis Rheum* 17(2):126–141, 1987.

Coronary Heart Disease

Baim DS, Harrison DC: Nonatherosclerotic coronary heart disease (including coronary artery spasm), in Hurst JW (ed): *The Heart,* McGraw-Hill, 1982, pp 1158–1170.

Bulkley BH, Humphries JO'N: The heart and collagen vascular disease, in Hurst JW (ed): *The Heart,* 5th ed. New York, McGraw-Hill, 1982, pp 1567–1577.

Dexter L, Alpert JS, Dalen JE: Pulmonary embolism, infarction, and acute cor pulmonale, in Hurst JW (ed): *The Heart,* 5th ed. New York, McGraw-Hill, 1982, 1227–1242.

Hurst JW, King SB III, Walter PF, et al: Atherosclerotic coronary heart disease: Angina pectoris, myocardial infarction, and other manifestations of myocardial ischemia, in Hurst JW (ed): *The Heart,* 5th ed. New York, McGraw-Hill, 1982, pp 1009–1149.

Hurst JW, Morris DC, Crawley IS: The history: Symptoms due to cardiovascular disease, in: Hurst JW (ed): *The Heart,* 5th ed. New York, McGraw-Hill, 1982, pp 151–164.

Logue RB: Etiology, recognition, and management of pericardial disease, in Hurst JW (ed): *The Heart,* 5th ed. New York, McGraw-Hill, 1982, pp 1371–1393.

Ross JC: Chronic cor pulmonale, in Hurst JW (ed): *The Heart,* 5th ed. New York, McGraw-Hill, 1982, pp 1243–1249.

Coronary Heart Disease—Risk Factors

Colditz GA, Willett WC, Stampfer MJ, et al: Menopause and the risk of coronary heart disease in women. *N Engl J Med* 316:1105–1110, 1987.

Walter HJ, Hofman A, Vaughan RD, et al: Modification of risk factors for coronary heart disease: Five-year results of a school-based intervention trial. *N Engl J Med* 318:1093–1100, 1988.

Coronary Heart Disease—Thrombolytic Therapy

Ferguson DW, Dewey RC, Plante DA: Clinical pitfalls in the non-invasive thrombolytic approach to presumed acute myocardial infarction. *Can J Cardiol* 2:146–151, 1986.

Marder VJ, Sherry S: 1. Thrombolytic therapy: Current status. *N Engl J Med* 318:1512–1520, 1988: 2. Thrombolytic therapy: Current status. *N Engl J Med* 318:1585–1595, 1988.

Coronary Heart Disease—Variant Angina

Bott-Silverman C, Heupler FA Jr: Natural history of pure coronary artery spasm in patients treated medically. *J Am Coll Cardiol* 2:200–205, 1983.

Bott-Silverman C, Heupler FA Jr, Yiannikas J: Variant angina: Comparison of patients with and without fixed severe coronary artery disease. *Am J Cardiol* 54:1173–1175, 1984.

Gerry JL, Achuff SC, Becker LC, et al: Predictability of the response to the ergonovine test. *JAMA* 242:2858–2861, 1979.

Ginsburg R, Lamb IH, Bristow MR, et al: Application and safety of outpatient ergonovine testing in accurately detecting coronary spasm in patients with possible variant angina. *Am Heart J* 102:698–702, 1981.

Grollier G, Scanu P, Commeau P, et al: Role of coronary spasm in the genesis of myocardial infarction: Study of a case treated by isosorbide dinitrate *in situ* then by transluminal angioplasty. *Clin Cardiol* 8:644–648, 1985.

Isner JM, Estes NAM III, Thompson PD, et al: Acute cardiac events temporally related to cocaine abuse. *N Engl J Med* 315:1438–1443, 1986.

Madias JE: The long-term outcome of patients who suffered and survived an acute myocardial infarction in the midst of recurrent attacks of variant angina. *Clin Cardiol* 9:277–284, 1986.

Magder SA, Johnstone DE, Huckell VF, et al: Experience with ergonovine provocative testing for coronary arterial spasm. *Chest* 79:638–646, 1981.

Matsuda Y, Ozaki M, Ogawa H, et al: Coronary arteriography and left ventriculography during spontaneous and exercise-induced ST segment elevation in patients with variant angina. *Am Heart J* 106:509–515, 1983.

Mautner RK, Giles TD: Coronary artery spasm: A possible cause of graft occlusion in a patient with fixed obstructive coronary artery disease. *Arch Intern Med* 140:979–980, 1980.

Rovai D, Distante A, Moscarelli E, et al: Transient myocardial ischemia with minimal electrocardiographic changes: An echocardiographic study in patients with Prinzmetal's angina. *Am Heart J* 109:78–83, 1985.

Waters DD, Theroux P, Crittin J, et al: Previously undiagnosed variant angina as a cause of chest pain after coronary artery bypass surgery. *Circulation* 61:1159–1164, 1980.

Cystic Fibrosis

Newth CJL: Cystic fibrosis, in Wyngaarden JB, Smith LH Jr (eds): *Cecil Textbook of Medicine,* 18th ed. Philadelphia, Saunders, 1988, pp 440–442.

Deep Vein Thrombosis

Becker DM, Philbrick JT, Abbitt PL: Real-time ultrasonography for the diagnosis of lower extremity deep venous thrombosis (commentary). *Arch Intern Med* 149:1731–1734, 1989.

White RH, McGahan JP, Daschbach MM, et al: Diagnosis of deep-vein thrombosis using duplex ultrasound. *Ann Intern Med* 111:297–304, 1989.

Dissecting Aneurysm/Aorta

Clements SD Jr, Clements MH, Jones EL, et al: Abnormal aortic echocardiogram in a patient with severe retrosternal chest pain. *Arch Intern Med* 141:241–243, 1981.

Cohen LS. Diseases of the aorta, in Wyngaarden JB, Smith LH Jr (eds): *Cecil Textbook of Medicine,* 18th ed. Philadelphia, Saunders, 1988, pp 370–374.

Dalen JE: Diseases of the aorta, in Braunwald E, Isselbacher KJ, Petersdorf RG, et al (eds): *Harrison's Principles of Internal Medicine,* 11th ed. New York, McGraw-Hill, 1987, pp 1037–1040.

de Cotret PR, Sheldon H: Dilated aorta and pain in the chest in a 63-year-old man. *Can Med Assoc J* 121:1467–1473, 1979.

DeSanctis RW, Doroghazi RM, Austen WG, et al: Aortic dissection. *N Engl J Med* 317:1060–1067, 1987.

Eagle KA, Quertermous T, Kritzer GA, et al: Spectrum of conditions initially suggesting acute aortic dissection but with negative aortograms. *Am J Cardiol* 57:322–326, 1986.

Ergin MA, Galla JD, Lansman S, et al: Acute dissections of the aorta: current surgical treatment. *Surg Clin North Am* 65:721–741, 1985.

Garrett BN, Ram CVS: Acute aortic dissection. *Cardiol Clin* 2:227–238, 1984.

Greenberg DJ, Davia JE, Fenoglio J, et al: Dissecting aortic aneurysm manifesting as acute pericarditis. *Arch Intern Med* 139:108–109, 1979.

Lawson RAM, Fenn A: Dissection of an aneurysmal ascending aorta in association with coarctation of the aorta. *Thorax* 34:606–611, 1979.

Mathieu D, Larde D, Vasile N: Primary dissecting aneurysms of the coronary arteries: Case report and literature review. *Cardiovasc Intervent Radiol* 7:71–74, 1984.

Mohr R, Adar R, Rubinstein Z: Multiple aortic aneurysms in Marfan's syndrome. *J Cardiovasc Surg* 25:566–570.

Salisbury RS, Hazleman BL: Successful treatment of dissecting aortic aneurysm due to giant cell arteritis. *Ann Rheum Dis* 40:507–508, 1981.

Drug-Induced Pulmonary Disease

Fulkerson WJ Jr, Gockerman JP, Pulmonary disease induced by drugs, in Fishman AP: *Pulmonary Diseases and Disorders,* 2d ed. New York, McGraw-Hill, 1988, vol 1, pp 793–811.

Esophageal Chest Pain

Areskog M, Tibbling L: Oesophageal function and chest pain in male patients with recent acute myocardial infarction. *Acta Med Scand* 209:59–63, 1981.

Areskog M, Tibbling L, Wranne B: Non-infarction coronary care unit patients. *Acta Med Scand* 209:51–57, 1981.

Benjamin SB, Castell DO: Chest pain of esophageal origin: Where are we, and where should we go? *Arch Intern Med* 143:772–776, 1983.

Benjamin SB, Gerhardt DC, Castell DO: High amplitude, peristaltic esophageal contractions associated with chest pain and/or dysphagia. *Gastroenterology* 77:478–483, 1979.

Benjamin SB, Richter JE, Cordova CM, et al: Prospective manometric evaluation with pharmacologic provocation of patients with suspected esophageal motility dysfunction. *Gastroenterology* 84:893–901, 1983.

Brand DL, Martin D, Pope CE II. Esophageal manometrics in patients with angina-like chest pain. *Dig Dis* 22:300–304, 1977.

Castell DO: Calcium-channel blocking agents for gastrointestinal disorders. *Am J Cardiol* 55:210B–213B, 1985.

Castell DO: Esophageal chest pain (editorial). *Am J Gastroenterol* 79:969–971, 1984.

Chobanian SJ, Benjamin SB, Curtis DJ, et al: Systematic esophageal evaluation of patients with noncardiac chest pain. *Arch Intern Med* 146:1505–1508, 1986.

Chobanian SJ, Curtis DJ, Benjamin SB, et al: Radiology of the nutcracker esophagus. *J Clin Gastroenterol* 8:230–232, 1986.

Clouse RE, Eckert TC, Staiano A: Hiatus hernia and esophageal contraction abnormalities. *Am J Med* 81:447–450, 1986.

Clouse RE, Stenson WF (discussants), Avioli LV (ed): Esophageal motility disorders and chest pain. *Arch Intern Med* 145:903–906, 1985.

Cohen S: Classification of the esophageal motility disorders (editorial). *Gastroenterology* 84:1050–1051, 1983.

Cole MJ, Paterson WG, Beck IT, et al: The effect of acid and bethanechol stimulation in patients with symptomatic hypertensive peristaltic (nutcracker) esophagus: Evidence that this disorder may be a precursor of diffuse esophageal spasm. *J Clin Gastroenterol* 8:223–229, 1986.

Davies HA, Jones DB, Rhodes J: "Esophageal angina" as the cause of chest pain. *JAMA* 248:2274–2278, 1982.

DeMeester TR, O'Sullivan GC, Bermudez G, et al: Esophageal function in patients with angina-type chest pain and normal coronary angiograms. *Ann Surg* 196:488–497, 1982.

Ferguson SC, Hodges K, Hersh T, et al: Esophageal manometry in patients with chest pain and normal coronary arteriogram. *Am J Gastroenterol* 75:124–127, 1981.

Henderson RD, Marryatt GV: Transabdominal total fundoplication gastroplasty to control reflux: A preliminary report. *Can J Surg* 28:127–129, 1985.

Horton ML, Goff JS: Surgical treatment of nutcracker esophagus. *Dig Dis Sci* 31:878–883, 1986.

Janssens J, Vantrappen G, Ghillebert G: 24-hour recording of esophageal pressure and pH in patients with noncardiac chest pain. *Gastroenterology* 90:1978–1984, 1986.

Kline M, Chesne R, Sturdevant RAL, et al: Esophageal disease in patients with angina-like chest pain. *Am J Gastroenterol* 75:116–123, 1981.

Lee MG, Sullivan SN, Watson WC, et al: Chest pain: Esophageal, cardiac, or both? *Am J Gastroenterol* 80:320–324, 1985.

Little AG, Chen W-H, Ferguson MK, et al: Physiologic evaluation of esophageal function in patients with achalasia and diffuse esophageal spasm. *Ann Surg* 203:500–504, 1986.

London TL, Ouyang A, Snape WJ Jr, et al: Provocation of esophageal pain by ergonovine or edrophonium. *Gastroenterology* 81:10–14, 1981.

McCallum RW: Chest pain: When to consider esophageal spasm. *Med Times* 107:23–29, 1979.

McDonald GB: Esophageal diseases caused by infection, systemic illness, and trauma, in Sleisenger MH, Fordtran JS (eds): *Gastrointestinal Disease: Pathophysiology, Diagnoses, Management*, 4th ed. Philadelphia, Saunders, 1989, pp 640–656.

Meanock CI, Stubbs J, Thomas M: Diagnostic endoscopy in the patient with chest pain. *Eur Heart J* 2:135–137, 1981.

Mellow MH: Effect of isosorbide and hydralazine in painful primary esophageal motility disorders. *Gastroenterology* 83:364–370, 1982.

Meyer GW, Castell DO: Human esophageal response during chest pain induced by swallowing cold liquids. *JAMA* 246:2057–2059, 1981.

Mosseri M, Eliakim R, Mogle P: Perforation of the esophagus electrocardiographically mimicking myocardial infarction. *Isr J Med Sci* 22:451–454, 1986.

Narducci F, Bassotti G, Gaburri M, et al: Transition from nutcracker esophagus to diffuse esophageal spasm. *Am J Gastroenterol* 80:242–244, 1985.

Nasrallah SM, Tommaso CL, Singleton RT, et al: Primary esophageal motor disorders: Clinical response to nifedipine. *South Med J* 78:312–315, 1985.

Orlando RC, Bozymski EM: The effects of pentagastrin in achalasia and diffuse esophageal spasm. Gastroenterology 77:472–477, 1979.

Ott DJ, Richter JE, Wu WC, et al: Radiologic and manometric correlation in "nutcracker esophagus." *AJR* 147:693–695, 1986.

Rasmussen K, Ravnsbaek J, Funch-Jensen P, et al: Oesophageal spasm in patients with coronary artery spasm. *Lancet*, Jan 25, 1986, pp 174–176.

Reidel WL, Clouse RE: Variations in clinical presentation of patients with esophageal contraction abnormalities. *Dig Dis Sci* 30:1065–1071, 1985.

Richter JE, Bradley LA, Castell DO: Esophageal chest pain: Current controversies in pathogenesis, diagnosis and therapy. *Ann Intern Med* 110:66–78, 1989.

Richter JE, Castell DO: Esophageal disease as a cause of noncardiac chest pain, in Stollerman GH (ed): *Advances in Internal Medicine*, Chicago, Year Book Medical Publishers, 1988, vol 33, pp 311–335.

Richter JE, Obrecht WF, Bradley LA, et al: Psychological comparison of patients with nutcracker esophagus and irritable bowel syndrome. *Dig Dis Sci* 31:131–138, 1986.

Russell COH, Hill LD: Gastroesophageal reflux, in *Current Problems in Surgery* 20:206–275, 1983.

Spears PF, Koch KL: Esophageal disorders in patients with chest pain and mitral valve prolapse. *Am J Gastroenterol* 81:951–954, 1986.

Svensson O, Stenport G, Tibbling L, et al: Oesophageal function and coronary angiogram in patients with disabling chest pain. *Acta Med Scand* 204:173–178, 1978.

Thomas E, Witt P, Willis M, et al: Nifedipine therapy for diffuse esophageal spasm. *South Med J* 79:847–849, 1986.

Traube M, Aaronson RM, McCallum RW: Transition from peristaltic esophageal contractions to diffuse esophageal spasm. *Arch Intern Med* 146:1844–1846, 1986.

Traube M, Albibi R, McCallum RW: High-amplitude peristaltic esophageal contractions associated with chest pain. *JAMA* 250:2655–2659, 1983.

Voyles C: Esophageal angina (letter to the editor). *JAMA* 249:2640–2641, 1983.

Waterfall WE, Craven MA, Allen CJ: Gastroesophageal reflux: Clinical presentations, diagnosis and management. *Can Med Assoc J* 135:1101–1109, 1986.

Winters C, Artnak EJ, Benjamin SB, et al: Esophageal bougienage in symptomatic patients with the nutcracker esophagus: A primary esophageal motility disorder. *JAMA* 252:363–366, 1984.

Yellin A, Gapany-Gapanavicius M, Lieberman Y: Spontaneous pneumomediastinum: Is it a rare cause of chest pain? *Thorax* 38:383–385, 1983.

Hypertrophic Cardiomyopathy

Brett W, Brandt PWT, Bierre AR, et al: Progression of hypertrophic cardiomyopathy to congestive cardiomyopathy: Case report. *N Z Med J* Nov 27, 1985, pp 994–998.

Cannon RO III, Rosing DR, Maron BJ, et al: Myocardial ischemia in patients with hypertrophic cardiomyopathy: Contribution of inadequate vasodilator reserve and elevated left ventricular filling pressures. *Circulation* 71:234–243, 1985.

Johnson RA, Palacios I: Nondilated cardiomyopathies. *Adv Intern Med* 30:243–273, 1984.

Keren G, Belhassen B, Sherez J, et al: Apical hypertrophic cardiomyopathy: Evaluation by noninvasive and invasive techniques in 23 patients. *Circulation* 71:45–56, 1985.

Maron BJ, Bonow RO, Cannon RO III, et al: 1. Hypertrophic cardiomyopathy: Interrelations of clinical manifestations, pathophysiology, and therapy. *N Engl J Med* 316:780–789, 1987; 2. Hypertrophic cardiomyopathy: Interrelations of clinical manifestations, pathophysiology, and therapy. *N Engl J Med* 316:844–852, 1987.

Nicod P, Polikar R, Peterson KL: Hypertrophic cardiomyopathy and sudden death. *N Engl J Med* 318:1255–1257, 1988.

Pitcher D, Wainwright R, Maisey M, et al: Assessment of chest pain in hypertrophic cardiomyopathy using exercise thallium-201 myocardial scintigraphy. *Br Heart J* 44:650–656, 1980.

Topol EJ, Traill TA, Fortuin NJ. Hypertensive hypertrophic cardiomyopathy of the elderly. *N Engl J Med* 312:277–283, 1985.

Ischemic Heart Disease

Selwyn AP, Braunwald E: Ischemic heart disease, in Braunwald E, Isselbacher KJ, Petersdorf RG, et al (eds): *Harrison's Principles of Internal Medicine*, 11th ed. New York, McGraw-Hill, 1987, pp 975–982.

Lung Abscess

Bartlett JG: Lung abscess, in Wyngaarden JB, Smith LH Jr (eds):

Cecil Textbook of Medicine, 18th ed. Philadelphia, Saunders, 1988, pp 435–438.

Rubin EH, Rubin M: Pulmonary suppurations: Lung abscess, in *Thoracic Diseases: Emphasizing Cardiopulmonary Relationships*. Philadelphia, Saunders, 1962, pp 353–367.

Mesothelioma

Bomalaski JS, Martin GJ, Mehlman DJ: Atypical chest pain with a systolic murmur. *Arch Intern Med* 143:1583–1585, 1983.

Driscoll RJ, Mulligan WJ, Schultz D, et al: Malignant mesothelioma: A cluster in a Native American pueblo. *N Engl J Med* 318:1437–1438, 1988.

Grant DC, Seltzer SE, Antman KH, et al: Computed tomography of malignant pleural mesothelioma. *J Comput Assist Tomogr* 7:626–632, 1983.

Law MR, Gregor A, Hodson ME, et al: Malignant mesothelioma of the pleura: A study of 52 treated and 64 untreated patients. *Thorax* 39:255–259, 1984.

Metastatic Lung Disease

Filderman AE, Coppage L, Shaw C, et al: Pulmonary and pleural manifestations of extrathoracic malignancies. *Clin Chest Med* 10(4):747–807, 1989.

Miscellaneous Conditions of the Heart

Healy BP: Miscellaneous conditions of the heart: Tumor, trauma, and systemic disease, in Wyngaarden JB, Smith LH Jr (eds): *Cecil Textbook of Medicine*, 18th ed. Philadelphia, Saunders, 1988, pp 367–370.

Mitral Valve Prolapse/Disease

Devereux RB, Kramer-Fox R, Brown WT, et al: Relation between clinical features of the mitral prolapse syndrome and echocardiographically documented mitral valve prolapse. *J Am Coll Cardiol* 8:763–772, 1986.

Devereux RB, Kramer-Fox R, Kligfield P: Mitral valve prolapse: Causes, clinical manifestations, and management. *Ann Intern Med* 111:305–317, 1989.

Gottdiener JS, Borer JS, Bacharach SL, et al: Left ventricular function in mitral valve prolapse: Assessment with radionuclide cineangiography. *Am J Cardiol* 47:7–13, 1981.

Malpartida F, Arcas R, Alegria E, et al: Surgical treatment for chest pain in mitral valve prolapse. *Chest* 78:101–104, 1980.

Mautner RK, Katz GE, Iteld BJ, et al: Coronary artery spasm: A mechanism for chest pain in selected patients with the mitral valve prolapse syndrome. *Chest* 79:449–453, 1981.

Rackley CE: Valvular heart disease, in Wyngaarden JB, Smith LH Jr (eds): *Cecil Textbook of Medicine*, 18th ed. Philadelphia, Saunders, 1988, pp 340–352.

Rackley CE, Edwards JE, Karp RB, et al: Mitral valve disease, in Hurst JW (ed): *The Heart*, 5th ed. New York, McGraw-Hill, 1982, 892–927.

Reece IJ, Cooley DA, Painvin GA, et al: Surgical treatment of mitral systolic click syndrome: Results in 37 patients. *Ann Thorac Surg* 39:155–158, 1985.

Spears PF, Koch KL, Day FP. Chest pain associated with mitral valve prolapse: Evidence for esophageal origin. *Arch Intern Med* 146:796–797, 1986.

Myocardial Infarction

Cheitlin MD: Non–Q-wave infarction: Diagnosis, prognosis, and treatment, in Stollerman GH (ed): *Advances in Internal Medicine*. Chicago, Year Book Medical Publishing, 1988, vol 33, pp 267–294.

Hackett D, Davies G, Chierchia S, et al: Intermittent coronary occlusion in acute myocardial infarction: Value of combined thrombolytic and vasodilator therapy. *N Engl J Med* 317:1055–1059, 1987.

Pasternak RC, Braunwald E, Alpert JS: Acute myocardial infarction, in Braunwald E, Isselbacher KJ, Petersdorf RG, et al (eds): *Harrison's Principles of Internal Medicine*, 11th ed. New York, McGraw-Hill, 1987, pp 982–993.

Willerson JT: Acute myocardial infarction, in Wyngaarden JB, Smith LH Jr (eds): *Cecil Textbook of Medicine*, 18th ed. Philadelphia, Saunders, 1988, pp 329–337.

Wilson BC, Cohn JN: Right ventricular infarction: Clinical and pathophysiologic considerations, in Stollerman GH (ed): *Advances in Internal Medicine*, Chicago, Year Book Medical Publishing, 1988, vol. 33, pp 295–309.

Case 46-1989, Case records of the Massachusetts General Hospital. *N Engl J Med* 321(20):1391–1402, 1989.

Myocardial Infarction—Diagnosis

Fuchs R, Scheidt S: Improved criteria for admission to cardiac care units. *JAMA* 246:2037–2041, 1981.

Goldman L, Cook EF, Brand DA, et al: A computer protocol to predict myocardial infarction in emergency department patients with chest pain. *N Engl J Med* 318:797–803, 1988.

Grenadier E, Keidar S, Kahana L, et al: The roles of serum myoglobin, total CPK and CK-MB isoenzymes in the acute phase of myocardial infarction. *Am Heart J* 105:408–416, 1983.

Guerci AD, Gerstenblith G, Brinker JA, et al: A randomized trial of intravenous tissue plasminogen activator for acute myocardial infarction with subsequent randomization to elective coronary angioplasty. *N Engl J Med* 317:1613–1618, 1987.

Hackett D, Davies G, Chierchia S, et al: Intermittent coronary occlusion in acute myocardial infarction. *N Engl J Med* 317:1055–1059, 1987.

Hoffman JR, Igarashi E. Influence of electrocardiographic findings on admission decisions in patients with acute chest pain. *Am J Med* 79:699–707, 1985.

Lee TH, Cook EF, Weisberg M, et al: Acute chest pain in the emergency room: Identification and examination of low-risk patients. *Arch Intern Med* 145:65–69, 1985.

Lee TH, Rouan GW, Weisberg MC, et al: Sensitivity of routine clinical criteria for diagnosing myocardial infarction within 24 hours of hospitalization. *Ann Intern Med* 106:181–186, 1987.

Relman AS: Aspirin for the primary prevention of myocardial infarction (editorial). *N Engl J Med* 318:245–246, 1988.

Topol EJ, Burek K, O'Neill WW, et al: A randomized controlled trial of hospital discharge three days after myocardial infarction in the era of reperfusion. *N Engl J Med* 318:1083–1088, 1988.

Topol EJ, Califf RM, George BS, et al: A randomized trial of immediate versus delayed elective angioplasty after intravenous tissue plaminogen activator in acute myocardial infarction. *N Engl J Med* 317:581–588, 1987.

Tzivoni D, Chenzbraun A, Keren A, et al: Reciprocal electrocardiographic changes in acute myocardial infarction. *Am J Cardiol* 56:23–26, 1985.

White HD, Norris RM, Brown MA, et al: Effect of intravenous streptokinase on left ventricular function and early survival after acute myocardial infarction. *N Engl J Med* 317:850–855, 1987.

Zarling EJ, Sexton H, Milnor P Jr: Failure to diagnose acute myocardial infarction: The clinicopathologic experience at a large community hospital. *JAMA* 250:1177–1181, 1983.

Myocardial Infarction—Post-Myocardial Infarction Studies

Abraham RD, Freedman SB, Dunn RF, et al: Prediction of multivessel coronary artery disease and prognosis early after acute myocardial infarction by exercise electrocardiography and thallium-201 myocardial perfusion scanning. *Am J Cardiol* 58:423–427, 1986.

Castaner A, Betriu A, Roig E, et al: Clinical course and risk stratification of myocardial infarct survivors with three-vessel disease. *Am Heart J* 112:1201–1209, 1986.

DeBusk RF: Evaluation of patients after recent acute myocardial infarction. *Ann Intern Med* 110(6):485–488.

———: Specialized testing after recent acute myocardial infarction. *Ann Intern Med* 110:470–481, 1989.

Fioretti P, Sclavo M, Brower RW, et al: Prognosis of patients with different peak serum creatine kinase levels after first myocardial infarction. *Eur Heart J* 6:473–478, 1985.

Goldman L, Weinberg M, Weisberg M, et al: A computer-derived protocol to aid in the diagnosis of emergency room patients with acute chest pain. *N Engl J Med* 307:588–596, 1982.

Haines DE, Beller GA, Watson DD, et al: A prospective clinical, scintigraphic, angiographic and functional evaluation of patients after inferior myocardial infarction with and without right ventricular dysfunction. *J Am Coll Cardiol* 6:995–1003, 1985.

Hutchison SJ, McKillop JH, Hutton I: Failure of gallium-67 citrate imaging to diagnose post-myocardial infarction (Dressler's) syndrome. *Eur J Nucl Med* 13:52–53, 1987.

Jaarsma W, Visser CA, Kupper AJF, et al: Usefulness of two-dimensional exercise echocardiography shortly after myocardial infarction. *Am J Cardiol* 57:86–90, 1986.

Jerjes-Sanchez C, Ibarra-Perez A, Ramirez-Rivera A, et al: Dressler-like syndrome after pulmonary embolism and infarction. *Chest* 92:115–117, 1987.

Knight JA, Laubach CA Jr: Low-level exercise testing after myocardial infarction: A useful guide to management. *Postgrad Med* 79:123–127, 1986.

Morris KG, Palmeri ST, Califf RM, et al: Value of radionuclide angiography for predicting specific cardiac events after acute myocardial infarction. *Am J Cardiol* 55:318–324, 1985.

Murray DP, Rafiqi E, Murray RG, et al: Prognostic investigations after myocardial infarction: A comparison of radionuclide angiography and ^{201}Tl scintigraphy. *Eur J Nucl Med* 11:381–385, 1986.

Ogawa H, Hiramori K, Haze K, et al: Comparison of clinical features of non-Q wave and Q wave myocardial infarction. *Am Heart J* 111:513–518, 1986.

Powell LH, Thoresen CE: Behavioral and physiologic determinants of long-term prognosis after myocardial infarction. *J Chron Dis* 38:253–263, 1985.

Rissanen V, Ranuio J, Halinen MO, et al: Changes occurring in the post-infarction ECG in relation to age, sex, and previous myocardial infarction. *Am Heart J* 111:286–292, 1986.

Starling MR, Crawford MH, Henry RL, et al: Prognostic value of electrocardiographic exercise testing and noninvasive assessment of left ventricular ejection fraction soon after acute myocardial infarction. *Am J Cardiol* 57:532–537, 1986.

Tokuyasu Y, Endo M, Sekiguchi M, et al: Recurrent myocardial infarction showing a multiple coronary artery occlusive phenomenon in a 32-year-old male without basic coronary artery stenosis. *Heart Vessels* 1:122–123, 1985.

Myocardial Infarction—Recurrent

Ulvenstam G, Aberg A, Bergstrand R, et al: Recurrent myocardial infarction: 1. Natural history of fatal and non-fatal events. *Eur Heart J* 6:294–302, 1985.

Ulvenstam G, Aberg A, Pennert K, et al: Recurrent myocardial infarction. 2. Possibilities of prediction. *Eur Heart J* 6:303–311, 1985.

Open Heart Surgery—Infectious Complications

Miedzinski LJ, Keren G. Serious infectious complications of open-heart surgery. *Can J Surg* 30:103–107, 1987.

Osteoporosis

Riggs BL: Osteoporosis, in Wyngaarden JB, Smith LH Jr (eds): *Cecil Textbook of Medicine*, 18th ed. Philadelphia, Saunders, 1988, pp 1510–1515.

Pericardial Diseases—General

Braunwald E: Pericardial diseases, in Braunwald E, Isselbacher KJ, Petersdorf RG, et al (eds): *Harrison's Principles of Internal Medicine*, 11th ed. New York, McGraw-Hill, 1987, pp 1008–1014.

Shabetai R: Diseases of the pericardium, in Wyngaarden JB, Smith LH Jr (eds): *Cecil Textbook of Medicine*, 18th ed. Philadelphia, Saunders, 1988, pp 362–367.

Pericarditis—Collagen Vascular Disease–Associated

Alpert MA, Goldberg SH, Singsen BH, et al: Cardiovascular manifestations of mixed connective tissue disease in adults. *Circulation* 68(6):1182–1193, 1983.

Doherty NE, Siegel RJ: Cardiovascular manifestations of systemic lupus erythematosus. *Am Heart J* 110(6):1257–1265, 1985.

Solinger AM: Drug-related lupus: Clinical and etiologic considerations. *Rheum Dis Clin North Am* 14(1):187–202, 1988.

Svantesson H, Bjorkhem G, Elborgh R: Cardiac involvement in juvenile rheumatoid arthritis: A follow-up study. *Acta Paediatr Scand* 72:345–350, 1983.

Tamir R, Pick AJ, Theodor E: Constrictive pericarditis complicating dermatomyositis. *Ann Rheum Dis* 47:961–963, 1988.

Pericarditis—Constrictive

Bashi VV, John S, Ravikumar E, et al: Early and late results of pericardiectomy in 118 cases of constrictive pericarditis. *Thorax* 43:637–641, 1988.

Blake S, Bonar S, O'Neill H, et al: Aetiology of chronic constrictive pericarditis. *Br Heart J* 50:273–276, 1983.

Cameron J, Oesterle SN, Baldwin JC, et al: The etiologic spectrum of constrictive pericarditis. *Am Heart J* 113(2):354–360, 1987.

Fischbein L, Namade M, Sachs RG, et al: Chronic constrictive pericarditis associated with asbestosis. *Chest* 94:646–647, 1988.

Llewellyn MJ, Atkinson MW, Fabri B: Pericardial constriction caused by primary mesothelioma. *Br Heart J* 57:54–57, 1987.

Robertson JM, Mulder DG: Pericardiectomy: A changing scene. *Am J Surg* 148:86–92, 1984.

Shabetai R: Pathophysiology of constrictive pericarditis and cardiac tamponade, in Hurst JW (ed): *The Heart*, 5th ed. New York, McGraw-Hill, 1982, pp 1363–1371.

Pericarditis—Neoplastic

Buck M, Ingle JN, Giuliani ER, et al: Pericardial effusion in women with breast cancer. *Cancer* 60:263–269, 1987.

Dapper F, Gorlach G, Hoffmann C, et al: Primary cardiac tumors: Clinical experiences and late results in 48 patients. *Thorac Cardiovasc Surg* 36:80–85, 1988.

Davis S, Rambotti P, Grignani F: Intrapericardial tetracycline sclerosis in the treatment of malignant pericardial effusion: An analysis of thirty-three cases. *J Clin Oncol* 2(6):631–636, 1984.

Donato DM, Sevin B-U, Averette HE: Neoplastic pericarditis and gynecologic malignancies: A review of the literature. *Obstet Gynecol Surv* 41(8):473–479, 1986.

———: Ovarian adenocarcinoma complicated by malignant pericarditis. *Gynecol Oncol* 24:171–176, 1986.

Kralstein J, Frishman W: Malignant pericardial diseases: Diagnosis and treatment. *Am Heart J* 113(3):785–790, 1987.

Montalescot G, Chapelon C, Drobinski G, et al: Diagnosis of primary cardiac sarcoma: Report of 4 cases and review of the literature. *Int J Cardiol* 20:209–219, 1988.

Skhvatsabaja LV: Secondary malignant lesions of the heart and pericardium in neoplastic disease. *Oncology* 43:103–106, 1986.

Tatsuta M, Yamamura H, Yamamoto R, et al: Carcinoembryonic antigens in the pericardial fluid of patients with malignant pericarditis. *Oncology* 41:328–330, 1984.

Vesterin E, Kivinen S, Nieminen U: Cervical carcinoma complicated by malignant pericarditis. *Acta Obstet Gynecol Scand* 66:569–571, 1987.

Pericarditis—Infectious and Other Causes

Alpert MA, Goldberg SH, Singsen BH, et al: Cardiovascular manifestations of mixed connective tissue disease in adults. *Circulation* 68:1182–1193, 1983.

Arita M, Kusuyama Y, Takatsuji M, et al: Septal myocardial abscess and infectious pericarditis in a case of bacterial endocarditis. *Japanese Circ J* 49:451–455, 1985.

Bellinger RL, Vacek JL: A review of pericarditis: 1. Causes, manifestations, and diagnostic techniques. *Postgrad Med* 82:100–103, 1987; 2. Specific pericardial disorders. *Postgrad Med* 82:105–110, 1987.

Boone JL, Patrone NA, Daugherty JE: Disseminated gonococcal infection and acute pericarditis. *N C Med J* 47:466–467, 1986.

Braester A, Nusem D, Horn Y: Primary meningococcal pericarditis in a pregnant woman. *Int J Cardiol* 11:355–358, 1986.

Burma GM, Emerman CL: Pericarditis mimicking acute myocardial infarction. *Am J Emerg Med* 4:262–264, 1986.

Canas JA, Balsam D, Leggiadro RJ: Adenovirus pericarditis. *NY State J Med* 86:269–270, 1986.

Cryer PE, Kissane JM (eds): Clinicopathologic conference: Chest pain, shock, arrhythmias and death in a young woman. *Am J Med* 66:853–861, 1979.

Diamond T: The ST segment axis: A distinguishing feature between acute pericarditis and acute myocardial infarction. *Heart Lung* 14:629–631, 1985.

Farley JD, Thomson AB, Dasgupta MK: Pericarditis and ulcerative colitis. *J Clin Gastroenterol* 8:567–568, 1986.

Fowler NO, Harbin AD III: Recurrent acute pericarditis: Follow-up study of 31 patients. *J Am Coll Cardiol* 7:300–305, 1986.

Frisk G, Torfason EG, Diderholm H: Reverse radioimmunoassays of IgM and IgG antibodies to coxsackie B viruses in patients with acute myopericarditis. *J Med Virol* 14:191–200, 1984.

Gupta A, Malhotra KK, Dash SC: Late pericarditis in patients on maintenance haemodialysis. *J Assoc Physicians India* 34:857–859, 1986.

Hancock EW: Slow pulse with pleuropericarditis. *Hosp Prac* 21:63,67, 1986.

Hardy DJ, Bartholomew WR, Amsterdam D: Pathophysiology of primary meningococcal pericarditis associated with *Neisseria meningitidis* group C: A case report and review of the literature. *Diagn Microbiol Infect Dis* 4:259–265, 1096.

Houghton JL, Becherer PR: *Haemophilus influenzae* pericarditis successfully treated by catheter drainage. *South Med J* 80:766–768, 1987.

Jurik AG, Graudal H: Pericarditis in rheumatoid arthritis: A clinical and radiological study. *Rheumatol Int* 6:37–42, 1986.

Karjalainen J, Heikkil J: Acute pericarditis: Myocardial enzyme release as evidence for myocarditis. *Am Heart J* 111:546–552, 1986.

Kaufman LD, Seifert FC, Eilbott DJ, et al: *Candida* pericarditis and tamponade in a patient with systemic lupus erythematosus. *Arch Intern Med* 148:715–717, 1988.

Krainin FM, Flessas AP, Spodick DH: Infarction-associated pericarditis: Rarity of diagnostic electrocardiogram. *N Engl J Med* 311:1211–1214, 1984.

Kraus WE, Valenstein PN, Corey GR: Purulent pericarditis caused by *Candida*: Report of three cases and identification of high-risk populations as an aid to early diagnosis. *Rev Infect Dis* 10:34–41, 1988.

Kristal B, Shasha SM, Mahmoud H, et al: Management of uremic pericarditis. *Isr J Med Sci* 22:442–444, 1986.

Laaban J-P, d'Orbcastel R, Prudent J, et al: Case reports: Primary pneumococcal pericarditis complicated by acute constriction. *Intensive Care Med* 10:155–156, 1984.

Lam D, Rapaport E: Two-dimensional echocardiographic demonstration of intrapericardial fibrinous strands in rheumatoid pericarditis. *Am Heart J* 114:442–444, 1987.

Missri J, Schechter D: When pericardial effusion complicates cancer. *Hosp Pract* 15:277–281, 284–286, 1988.

Nunoda S, Mifune J, Ono S, et al: An adult case of mixed connective tissue disease associated with perimyocarditis and massive pericardial effusion. *Jpn Heart J* 27:129–135, 1986.

Patel C, Betzu R, Din I: Pericarditis and ulcerative colitis. *Am Heart J* 111:802–803, 1986.

Permanyer-Miralda G, Sagrista-Sauleda J, Soler-Soler J: Primary acute pericardial disease: A prospective series of 231 consecutive patients. *Am J Cardiol* 56:623–630, 1985.

Pohjola-Sintonen S, Totterman K-J, Salmo M, et al: Late cardiac effects of mediastinal radiotherapy in patients with Hodgkin's disease. *Cancer* 60:31–37, 1987.

Proby CM, Hackett D, Gupta S, et al: Acute myopericarditis in influenza A infection. *Q J Med* 60:887–892, 1986.

Rutsky EA, Rostand SG: Treatment of uremic pericarditis and pericardial effusion. *Am J Kidney Dis* 10:2–8, 1987.

Saner HE, Gobel FL, Nicoloff DM, et al: Aortic dissection presenting as pericarditis. *Chest* 91:71–74, 1987.

Saviolo R, Spodick DH: Electrocardiographic responses to maximal exercise during acute pericarditis and early repolarization. *Chest* 90:460–462, 1986.

Schwartz KV, Guercio CA, Katz A: *Haemophilus influenza* pericarditis. *Conn Med* 51:423–424, 1987.

Seddon DJ: Pericarditis with pericardial effusion complicating chickenpox. *Postgrad Med J* 62:1133–1134, 1986.

Shulkin BL, Wahl RL: SPECT imaging of myocarditis. *Clin Nucl Med* 12:841–842, 1987.

Skhvatsabaja LV: Secondary malignant lesions of the heart and pericardium in neoplastic disease. *Oncology* 43:103–106, 1986.

Slack JD, Pinkerton CA: The electrocardiogram often fails to identify pericarditis after percutaneous transluminal coronary angioplasty. *J Electrocardiol* 19:399–402, 1986.

Somolinos M, Violan S, Sanz R, et al: Early pericarditis after acute myocardial infarction: A clinical echocardiographic study. *Crit Care Med* 15:648–651, 1987.

Starling RC, Yu VL, Shillington D, et al: Pneumococcal pericarditis: Diagnostic usefulness of counterimmunoelectrophoresis and computed tomographic scanning. *Arch Intern Med* 146:1174–1176, 1986.

Stechel RP, Cooper DJ, Greenspan J, et al: Staphylococcal pericarditis in a homosexual patient with AIDS-related complex. *NY State J Med* 86:592–593, 1986.

Strimlan CV, Turbiner EH: Pleuropericardial effusions associated with chest and abdominal pain. *Chest* 81:493–494, 1982.

Stubbs DF: Post-acute myocardial infarction symptomatic pericarditis (PAMISP): Report on a large series and the effect of methylprednisolone therapy. *J Int Med Res* 14(suppl 1):25–29, 1986.

Suki WN: Pericarditis. *Kidney Int* (suppl 24): pp S10–S12, 1988.

Svendsen JH, Jensson V, Niebuhr U: Combined pericarditis and pneumonia caused by *Legionella* infection. *Br Heart J* 58:663–664, 1987.

Thould AK: Constrictive pericarditis in rheumatoid arthritis. *Ann Rheum Dis* 45:89–94, 1986.

Tilley WS, Harston WE: Inadvertent administration of streptokinase to patients with pericarditis. *Am J Med* 81:541–544, 1986.

Truant AL, Menge S, Milliorn K, et al: Fusobacterium nucleatum pericarditis. *J Clin Microbiol* 17:349–351, 1983.

Uhl GS, Koppes GM: Pericardial tamponade in systemic sclerosis (scleroderma). *Br Heart J* 42:345–348, 1979.

van Dorp WT, van Rees C, van der Meer JW, et al: Meningococcal pericarditis in the absence of meningitis. *Infection* 15:109–110, 1987.

Vaughan D, Warner L, Kirshenbaum JM: Myopericarditis as an initial presentation of meningococcemia: Unusual manifestation of infection with serotype WI35. *Am J Med* 82:641–644, 1987.

Wanner WR, Schaal SF, Bashore TM, et al: Repolarization variant vs. acute pericarditis. A prospective electrocardiographic and echocardiographic evaluation. *Chest* 83:180–184, 1983.

Weingarten S, Weinberg H, Fang M, et al: *Hemophilus influenzae* pericarditis in two adults. *West J Med* 145:690–694, 1986.

Weinstein L: Life-threatening complications of infective endocarditis and their management. *Arch Intern Med* 146:953–957, 1986.

White DA, Schwartzberg LS, Kris MG, et al: Acute chest pain syndrome during bleomycin infusions. *Cancer* 59:1582–1585, 1987.

Winzelberg GG, Boller M: Chest pain following aortocoronary bypass graft. *JAMA* 248:1889–1890, 1982.

Zelcer AA, LeJemtel TH, Jones J, et al: Pericardial tamponade in sarcoidosis. *Can J Cardiol* 3:12–13, 1987.

Zuckier LS, Weissmann HS, Goldman MJ, et al: Detection of postcardiotomy bacterial pericarditis with gallium-67 citrate. *Clin Nucl Med* 11:276–278, 1986.

Percarditis—Purulent

Blaser MJ, Reingold AL, Alsever RN, et al: Primary meningococcal pericarditis: A disease of adults associated with serogroup C *Neisseria meningitidis*. *Rev Infect Dis* 6(5):625–632, 1984.

Bouwels L, Jansen E, Janssen J, et al: Successful long-term catheter drainage in an immunocompromised patient with purulent pericarditis. *Am J Med* 83:581–583, 1987.

Buckingham TA, Wilner G, Sugar SJ: Hemophilus influenzae pericarditis in adults. *Arch Intern Med* 143:1809–1810, 1983.

Corachan M, Poore P, Hadley GP, et al: Purulent pericarditis in Papua, New Guinea: Report of 12 cases and review of the literature in a tropical environment. *Trans R Soc Trop Med Hyg* 77(3):341–343, 1983.

Greenberg ML, Niebulski HIJ, Uretsky BF, et al: Occult purulent pericarditis detected by indium-111 leukocyte imaging. *Chest* 85(5):701–703, 1984.

Hardy CC, Raza SN, Isalska B, et al: Atraumatic suppurative mediastinitis and purulent pericarditis due to *Eikenella corrodens*. *Thorax* 43:494–495, 1988.

Kaufman LD, Seifert FC, Eilbott DJ, et al: *Candida* pericarditis and tamponade in a patient with systemic lupus erythematosus. *Arch Intern Med* 148:715–717, 1988.

Kraus WE, Valenstein PN, Corey GR: Purulent pericarditis caused by *Candida*: Report of three cases and identification of high-risk populations as an aid to early diagnosis. *Rev Infect Dis* 10(1):34–41, 1988.

Lecomte F, Eustache M, Lemeland J-E, et al: Purulent pericarditis due to Yersinia enterocolitica. *J Infect Dis* 159(2):363, 1989.

Makó J, Jansen J, Bognár B, et al: Purulent pericarditis caused by *Staphylococcus aureus* in two patients undergoing haemodialysis. *Int Urol Nephrol* 17(1):79–83, 1985.

Morgan RJ, Stephenson LW, Woolf PK, et al: Surgical treatment of purulent pericarditis in children. *J Thorac Cardiovasc Surg* 85:527–531, 1983.

Nowicka J, Haus O, Dzik T, et al: Pericarditis in the course of acute leukemia. *Folia Haematol Leipzig* 114(2):220–233, 1987.

Olson LJ, Edwards WD, Olney BA, et al: Hemorrhagic cardiac tamponade: A clinicopathologic correlation. *Mayo Clin Proc* 59:785–790, 1984.

O'Neill D, Brebner H, Watkinson G: Purulent pericarditis following myocardial infarction. *Scott Med J* 29:191–192, 1984.

Phelps R, Jacobs RA: Purulent pericarditis and mediastinitis due to *Peptococcus magnus*. *JAMA* 254(7):947–948, 1985.

Silliman RA, Peters JD, Ginsberg MB: Infections of the heart complicating acute myocardial infarction. *South Med J* 77(7):934–936, 1984.

Sinzobahamvya N, Ikeogu MO: Purulent pericarditis. *Arch Dis Child* 62:696–699, 1987.

Starling RC, Yu VL, Shillington D, et al: Pneumococcal pericarditis: Diagnostic usefulness of counterimmunoelectrophoresis and computed tomographic scanning. *Arch Intern Med* 146:1174–1176, 1986.

Tsai J, Shands JW Jr: Staphylococcal pericarditis: An atypical presentation. *Arch Intern Med* 149:953–954, 1989.

Zuckier LS, Weissmann HS, Goldman MJ, et al: Detection of postcardiotomy bacterial pericarditis with gallium-67 citrate. *Clin Nucl Med* 11:276–278, 1986.

Pericarditis—Recurrent

Fowler NO, Harbin D III: Recurrent acute pericarditis: Follow-up study of 31 patients. *J Am Coll Cardiol* 7(2):300–305, 1986.

Ghosh SC, Larrieu AJ, Ablaza SGG, et al: Clinical experience with subxyphoid pericardial decompression. *Int Surg* 70:5–7, 1985.

Holloway JD: Post-myocardial infarction pericarditis: Chronic symptoms in a middle-aged man. *Postgrad Med* 85(3):57–60, 1989.

Laine LA, Holt KM: Recurrent pericarditis and celiac disease. *JAMA* 252(22):3168, 1984.

Palatianos GM, Thurer RJ, Kaiser GA: Comparison of effectiveness and safety of operations on the pericardium. *Chest* 88(1):30–33, 1985.

Wanner WR, Williams TE, Fulkerson PK, et al: Postoperative pericarditis following thymectomy for myasthenia gravis. *Chest* 83(4):6479, 1983.

Pericarditis—Review Articles

Permanyer-Miralda G, Sagrista-Sauleda J, Soler-Soler J: Primary acute pericardial disease: A prospective series of 231 consecutive patients. *Am J Cardiol* 56:623–630, 1985.

Sternbach GL: Pericarditis. *Ann Emerg Med* 17:214–220, 1988.

Pericarditis—Uremic or Dialysis-Associated

Kristal B, Shasha SM, Mahmoud H, et al: Management of uremic pericarditis. *Isr J Med Sci* 22:442–444, 1986.

Neff MS, Eiser AR, Slifkin RF, et al: Patients surviving 10 years of hemodialysis. *Am J Med* 74:996–1004, 1983.

Pleural Space Diseases

Brody JS: Diseases of the pleura, mediastinum, diaphragm, and chest wall, in Wyngaarden JB, Smith LH Jr (eds): *Cecil Textbook of Medicine*, 18th ed. Philadelphia, Saunders, 1988, pp 466–473.

Houston MC: Pleural fluid pH: Diagnostic, therapeutic, and prognostic value. *Am J Surg* 154:333–337, 1987.

Vukich DJ: Diseases of the pleural space. *Emerg Med Clin North Am* 7(2):309–324, 1989.

Pneumomediastinum/Mediastinal Disorders

Baur X, Hacker H, and Hauser FE: A 23-year-old female patient with precordial chest pain. *Internist* 26:357–360, 1985.

Breatnach E, Nath PH, Delany DJ: The role of computed tomography in acute and subacute mediastinitis. *Clin Radiol* 37:139–145, 1986.

Cheung EH, Craver JM, Jones EL, et al: Mediastinitis after cardiac valve operations: Impact upon survival. *J Thorac Cardiovasc Surg* 90:517–522, 1985.

Dattwyler RJ, Goldman MA, Block KJ: Pneumomediastinum as a complication of asthma in teenage and young adult patients. *J Allergy Clin Immunol* 63:412–416, 1979.

Dymowski JJ, Turnbull TL: Spontaneous pneumomediastinum (correspondence). *Ann Emerg Med* 15:761, 1986.

Halperin AK, Deichmann RE: Spontaneous pneumomediastinum: A report of 10 cases and review of the literature. *N C Med J* 46:21–23, 1985.

Hunter JG, Loy HG, Markovitz L, et al: Spontaneous pneumomediastinum following inhalation of alkaloidal cocaine and emesis: Case report and review. *Mt Sinai J Med* 53:491–493, 1986.

Khan FA, Chitkara RK: Complications of acute respiratory failure. *Postgrad Med* 79:205–214, 1986.

Krespi YP, Grossman BG, Berktold RE, et al: Mediastinitis and neck abscess following cervical spine fracture. *Am J Otolaryngol* 6:29–31, 1985.

Levine TM, Wurster CF, Krespi YP: Mediastinitis occurring as a complication of odontogenic infections. *Laryngoscope* 96:747–750, 1986.

Lewis BD, Hurt RD, Spencer Payne W, et al: Benign teratomas of the mediastinum. *J Thorac Cardiovasc Surg* 86:727–731, 1983.

Mattox KL, Allen MK: Symposium paper: Systematic approach to pneumothorax, haemothorax, pneumomediastinum and subcutaneous emphysema. *Injury* 17:309–312, 1986.

Reeder SR: Subcutaneous emphysema, pneumomediastinum, and pneumothorax in labor and delivery. *Am J Obstet Gynecol* 154:487–489, 1986.

Ribet M, Privot FR: Barotraumatic rupture of the esophagus. *J Chir* 123:164–168, 1986.

Rose WD, Veach JS, Tehranzdeh J: Spontaneous pneumomediastinum as a cause of neck pain, dysphagia, and chest pain. *Arch Intern Med* 144:392–393, 1984.

Smith PS, Roistacher K, Gordon GM, et al: Case report: Anaerobic mediastinitis complicating median sternotomy. *Am J Med Sci* 290:111–113, 1985.

Werne C, Ulreich S: An unusual presentation of spontaneous pneumomediastinum. *Ann Emerg Med* 14:1010–1013, 1985.

Pneumonias

Atmar RL, Greenberg SB: Pneumonia caused by *Mycoplasma pneumoniae* and the TWAR agent. *Semin Respir Infect* 4(1):19–31, 1989.

Carden DL, Smith JK: Pneumonias. *Emerg Med Clin North Am* 7(2):255–278, 1989.

Cotton EM, Strampfer MJ, Cunha BA: Legionella and *Mycoplasma pneumonia*: A community hospital experience with atypical pneumonias. *Clin Chest Med* 8(3):441–453, 1987.

Davis GS, Winn WC Jr: Legionnaire's disease: Respiratory infections caused by *Legionella* bacteria. *Clin Chest Med* 8(3):419–439, 1987.

Fein AM, Feinsilver SH, Niederman MS, et al: "When the pneumonia doesn't get better." *Clin Chest Med* 8(3):529–541, 1987.

Grayston JT, Diwan VK, Cooney M, et al: Community- and hospital-acquired pneumonia associated with *Chlamydia* TWAR infection demonstrated serologically. *Arch Intern Med* 149(1):169–173, 1989.

Grayston JT, Kuo CC, Wang SP, et al: A new *Chlamydia psittaci* strain, TWAR, isolated in acute respiratory tract infections. *N Engl J Med* 315(3):161–168, 1986.

Hopkins CC: Community-acquired pneumonia, in Fishman AP: *Pulmonary Diseases and Disorders*, 2d ed. New York, McGraw-Hill, 1988, vol 2, pp 1535–1542.

Huovinen P, Lahtonen R, Ziegler T, et al: Pharyngitis in adults: The presence and coexistence of viruses and bacterial organisms. *Ann Intern Med* 110(8):612–616, 1989.

Kleemola M, Saikku P, Visakorpi R, et al: Epidemics of pneumonia caused by TWAR, a new *Chlamydia* organism, in military trainees in Finland. *J Infect Dis* 157(2):230–236, 1988.

Marrie TJ, Grayston JT, Wang SP, et al: Pneumonia associated with the TWAR strain of *Chlamydia*. *Ann Intern Med* 106(4):507–511, 1987.

McKinsey DS, Bisno AL: Pneumonias caused by gram-positive bacteria, in Fishman AP: *Pulmonary Diseases and Disorders*, 2d ed. New York, McGraw-Hill, 1988, vol 2, pp 1477–1490.

Meyer RD, Edelstein PH: Legionnaire's disease, in Fishman AP: *Pulmonary Diseases and Disorders*, 2d ed. New York, McGraw-Hill, 1989, vol 2, pp 1629–1638.

Nash TW, Murray HW: The atypical pneumonias, in Fishman AP: *Pulmonary Diseases and Disorders*, 2d ed. New York, McGraw-Hill, 1988, vol 2, pp 1613–1628.

Pennza PT: Aspiration pneumonia, necrotizing pneumonia, and lung abscess. *Emerg Med Clin North Am* 7(2):279–307, 1989.

Pierce AK: Pneumonias caused by gram-negative aerobic organisms, in Fishman AP: *Pulmonary Diseases and Disorders*, 2d ed. New York, McGraw-Hill, 1988, vol 2, pp 1491–1504.

Rubin EH, Rubin M: Bacterial pneumonias, Pneumonias caused by higher bacteria, fungi and parasites and nonbacterial pneumonias: Viral, rickettsial and miscellaneous infectious diseases (concluded) in *Thoracic Diseases: Emphasizing Cardiopulmonary Relationships*. Philadelphia, Saunders, 1962, pp 277–298, 299–315, 342–352.

Tobin MJ: Diagnosis of pneumonia: Techniques and problems. *Clin Chest Med* 8(3):513–527, 1987.

Weinberg AN: Unusual bacterial pneumonias, in Fishman AP: *Pulmonary Diseases and Disorders*, 2d ed. New York, McGraw-Hill, 1988, vol 2, pp 1517–1534.

Wollschlager CM, Khan FA, Khan A: Utility of radiography and clinical features in the diagnosis of community-acquired pneumonia. *Clin Chest Med* 8(3):393–404, 1987.

Pneumothorax

Anthonisen NR, Filuk RB: Pneumothorax, in Fishman AP: *Pulmonary Diseases and Disorders*, 2d ed. New York, McGraw-Hill, 1988, vol 3, pp 2171–2182.

Case 24-1988, Case records of the Massachusetts General Hospital: Weekly clinicopathological exercises. *N Engl J Med* 318:1602–1610, 1988.

Habibzadeh MA: ECG changes associated with spontaneous left-sided pneumothorax. *Postgrad Med* 68:221–223, 1980.

Pulmonary Artery Aneurysm

Jaffin BW, Gundel WD, Capeless MA, et al: Aneurysm of the pulmonary artery as a cause of severe chest pain. *Arch Intern Med* 143:1484–1485.

Pulmonary Embolism

Alderson PO, Dzebolo NN, Biello DR, et al: Serial lung scintigraphy: Utility in diagnosis of pulmonary embolism. *Radiology* 149:797–802, 1983.

Barritt DW, Jordan SC: Clinical features of pulmonary embolism. *Lancet*, April 8, 1961, pp 729–732.

Dexter L, Alpert JS, Dalen JE: Pulmonary embolism, infarction, and acute cor pulmonale, in Hurst JW (ed): *The Heart*, 5th ed. New York, McGraw-Hill, 1982, pp 1227–1242.

Dunmire SM: Pulmonary embolism. *Emerg Med Clin North Am* 7(2):339–354, 1989.

Dunnick NR, Newman GE, Perlmutt LM, et al: Pulmonary embolism. *Curr Probl Diagn Radiol* 17:203–229, 1988.

Foley M, Maslack MM, Rothman RH, et al: Pulmonary embolism after hip or knee replacement: Postoperative changes on pulmonary scintigrams in asymptomatic patients. *Radiology* 172:481–485, 1989.

Frankel N, Coleman RE, Pryor DB, et al: Utilization of lung scans by clinicians. *J Nucl Med* 27:366–369, 1986.

Hoellerich VL, Wigton RS: Diagnosing pulmonary embolism using clinical findings. *Arch Intern Med* 146:1699–1704, 1986.

Huisman MV, Buller HR, ten Cate JW, et al: Unexpected high prevalence of silent pulmonary embolism in patients with deep venous thrombosis. *Chest* 95:498–502, 1989.

Hull RD, Hirsh J, Carter CJ, et al: Diagnostic value of ventilation-perfusion lung scanning in patients with suspected pulmonary embolism. *Chest* 88(6):819–828, 1985.

———: Pulmonary angiography, ventilation lung scanning, and venography for clinically suspected pulmonary embolism with abnormal perfusion lung scan. *Ann Intern Med* 98:981–999, 1983.

Kahn D, Bushnell DL, Dean R, et al: Clinical outcome of patients with a "low probability" of pulmonary embolism on ventilation-perfusion lung scan. *Arch Intern Med* 149:377–379, 1989.

Kelley MA, Fishman AP: Pulmonary thromboembolic disease, in Fishman AP: *Pulmonary Diseases and Disorders*, 2d ed. New York, McGraw-Hill, 1988, vol 2, pp 1059–1086.

Kipper MS, Moser KM, Kortman KE, et al: Long-term follow-up of patients with suspected pulmonary embolism and a normal lung scan. *Chest* 82(4):411–415, 1982.

Leeper KV, Popovich J, Lesser BA, et al: Treatment of massive acute pulmonary embolism: The use of low doses of intrapulmonary arterial streptokinase combined with full doses of systemic heparin. *Chest* 93(2):234–240, 1988.

Lund O, Nielsen TT, Schifter S, et al: Treatment of pulmonary embolism with full-dose heparin, streptokinase or embolectomy: Results and indications. *Thoracic Cardiovasc Surg* 34:240–246, 1986.

McCance AJ, Taylor DN: Incidence of asymptomatic pulmonary embolus following acute myocardial infarction. *Eur Heart J* 8:360–361, 1987.

Moss AA (ed): Critical review: Pulmonary angiography, ventilation lung scanning, and venography for clinically suspected pulmonary embolism with abnormal perfusion lung scan. (Hull RD, Hirsh J, Carter CJ, et al.) *Invest Radiol* 21(12):940–942, 1986.

Norris CS, Greenfield LJ, Herrmann JB: Free-floating iliofemoral thrombus. *Arch Surg* 120:806–808, 1985.

Ockelford PA, Rutland M: Evaluation of therapeutic decisions in patients with suspected pulmonary embolism and a low probability lung scan: Application of Bayes' theorem. *Aust N Z J Med* 16:216–220, 1986.

Parker JA, Markis JE, Palla A, et al: Pulmonary perfusion after rt-PA therapy for acute embolism: Early improvement assessed with segmental perfusion scanning. *Radiology* 166:441–445, 1988.

Senior RM: Pulmonary embolism, in Wyngaarden JB, Smith LH Jr (eds): *Cecil Textbook of Medicine*, 18th ed. Philadelphia, Saunders, 1988, pp 442–450.

Shaw RA, Schonfeld SA, Whitcomb ME: Pulmonary embolism presenting as coronary insufficiency. *Arch Intern Med* 141:651, 1981.

Specker BL, Saenger EL, Buncher CR, et al: Pulmonary embolism and lung scanning: Cost-effectiveness and benefit:risk. *J Nucl Med* 28:1521–1530, 1987.

Stein PD, Willis PW III, DeMets DL: History and physical examination in acute pulmonary embolism in patients without preexisting cardiac or pulmonary disease. *Am J Cardiol* 47:218–223, 1981.

Valenzuela TD: Pulmonary embolism. *Emerg Med Clin North Am* 6(2):253–266, 1988.

Vix VA: The usefulness of chest radiographs obtained after a demonstrated perfusion scan defect in the diagnosis of pulmonary emboli. *Clin Nucl Med* 8(10):497–500, 1983.

Weatherford SC, Lawrie GM. Trendelenburg pulmonary embolectomy for cardiac arrest secondary to massive pulmonary embolism. *Can J Surg* 29:383–384, 1986.

Wigton RS, Hoellerich VL, Patil KD. How physicians use clinical information in diagnosing pulmonary embolism: An application of conjoint analysis. *Med Decis Making* 6:2–11, 1986.

Woods BO'B, Beamis JF Jr, Bettencourt PE, et al: Subacute massive thromboembolic occlusion of a main pulmonary artery: Report of a case successfully treated by thrombolytic therapy and review of the literature. *Angiology* 36:58–63, 1985.

Yoo HS, Intenzo CM, Park CH. Unresolved major pulmonary embolism: Importance of follow-up lung scan in diagnosis. *Eur J Nucl Med* 12:252–253, 1986.

Pulmonary Hypertension

Fishman AP: Pulmonary hypertension, in Wyngaarden JB, Smith LH Jr (eds): *Cecil Textbook of Medicine*, 18th ed. Philadelphia, Saunders, 1988, pp 293–303.

Kuida H: Primary pulmonary hypertension, in Hurst JW (ed): *The Heart*, 5th ed. New York, McGraw-Hill, 1982, pp 1221–1227.

Pulmonary Infections

Finegold SM: Anaerobic infections of lungs and pleura, in Fishman AP: *Pulmonary Diseases and Disorders*, 2d ed. New York, McGraw-Hill, 1988, vol 2, pp 1505–1516.

Marcy TW, Reynolds HY: Pulmonary consequences of congenital and acquired primary immunodeficiency states. *Clin Chest Med* 10(4):503–519, 1989.

Rose RM, Pinkston P, O'Donnell C, et al: Viral infection of the lower respiratory tract. *Clin Chest Med* 8(3):405–418, 1987.

Shapiro MS, Dobbins JW, Matthay RA: Pulmonary manifestations of gastrointestinal disease. *Clin Chest Med* 10(4):617–643, 1989.

Skerrett SJ, Niederman MS, Fein AM: Respiratory infections and acute lung injury in systemic illness. *Clin Chest Med* 10(4):469–502, 1989.

Wiedemann HP, Matthay RA: Pulmonary manifestations of the collagen vascular diseases. *Clin Chest Med* 10(4):677–722, 1989.

Pulmonary Lesions and Tumors

Kleinerman JI: Neoplasms of the pleura, chest wall and diaphragm, in Fishman AP: *Pulmonary Diseases and Disorders*, 2d ed. New York, McGraw-Hill, 1988, vol 3, pp 2033–2044.

Ochs RH: Neoplasms of the lung other than bronchogenic carcinoma, in Fishman AP: *Pulmonary Diseases and Disorders*, 2d ed. New York, McGraw-Hill, 1988, vol 3, pp 2011–2032.

Ryan MB, McMurtrey MJ, Roth JA: Current management of chest-wall tumors. *Surg Clin North Am* 69(5):1061–1080, 1989.

Schaefer PS, Burton BS: Radiographic evaluation of chest-wall lesions. *Surg Clin North Am* 69(5):911–945, 1989.

Scoggin CH: Pulmonary neoplasms, in Wyngaarden JB, Smith LH Jr (eds): *Cecil Textbook of Medicine*, 18th ed. Philadelphia, Saunders, 1988, pp 457–466.

Pulmonary Tuberculosis

Rubin EH, Rubin M: Pulmonary tuberculosis in the adult, in *Thoracic Diseases: Emphasizing Cardiopulmonary Relationships*. Philadelphia, Saunders, 1962, pp 623–648.

Weg JG: Clinical forms of mycobacterial disease, in Fishman AP: *Pulmonary Diseases and Disorders*, 2d ed. New York, McGraw-Hill, 1988, vol 3, pp 1843–1862.

Rheumatic Fever

Barnert AL, Terry EE, Persellin RH: Acute rheumatic fever in adults. *JAMA* 232:925–928, 1975.

Sickle Cell Disease

Davies SC, Luce PJ, Win AA, et al: Acute chest syndrome in sickle-cell disease. *Lancet* Jan 7, 1984, pp 36–38.

Syndrome X

Cannon RO III, Leon MB, Watson RM, et al: Chest pain and ''normal'' coronary arteries: Role of small coronary arteries. *Am J Cardiol* 55:50B–60B, 1985.

Day LJ, Sowton E: Clinical features and follow-up of patients with angina and normal coronary arteries. *Lancet*, Aug 14, 1976, pp 334–337.

Waxler EB, Kimbiris D, Dreifus LS: The fate of women with normal coronary arteriograms and chest pain resembling angina pectoris. *Am J Cardiol* 28:25–32, 1971.

Wielgosz AT, Fletcher RH, McCants CB, et al: Unimproved chest pain in patients with minimal or no coronary disease: A behavioral phenomenon. *Am Heart J* 108:67–72, 1984.

Thrombolytic Therapy

Lee TH, Weisberg MC, Brand DA, et al: Candidates for thrombolysis among emergency room patients with acute chest pain. *Ann Intern Med* 110:957–962, 1989.

Tate DA, Dehmer GJ: New challenges for thrombolytic therapy (editorial). *Ann Intern Med* 110(12):953–955, 1989.

Tomography/MRI

Aronchick J, Epstein D, Gefter WB, et al: Evaluation of chest radiograph in the emergency department patient. *Emerg Med Clin North Am* 3:491–505, 1985.

Brown LR, Muhm JR: Computed tomography of the thorax: Current prospectives. *Chest* 83:806–813, 1983.

Brundage BH, Rich S, Spigos D: Computed tomography of the heart and great vessels: Present and future. *Ann Intern Med* 101:801–809, 1984.

Godwin JD, Korobkin M: Acute disease of the aorta: Diagnosis by computed tomography and ultrasonography. *Radiol Clin North Am* 21:551–574, 1983.

Lipton MJ, Brundage BH, Higgins CB, et al: Clinical applications of dynamic computed tomography. *Cardiovasc Dis* 28:349–366, 1986.

Margulis AR, Fisher MR: Present clinical status of magnetic resonance imaging. *Magn Reson Med* 2:309–327, 1985.

Toxoplasmosis

Leak D, Meghji M: Toxoplasmic infection in cardiac disease. *Am J Cardiol* 43:841–849, 1979.

Tuberculosis of the Pleura

Case 19-1988, Case records of the Massachusetts General Hospital: Weekly clinicopathological exercises. *N Engl J Med* 318:1257–1267, 1988.

Vasoconstriction—Cocaine Induced

Isner JM, Chokshi SK: Cocaine and vasospasm (editorial). *N Engl J Med* 321(23):1604–1606, 1989.

Lange RA, Cigarroa RG, Yancy CW Jr, et al: Cocaine-induced coronary-artery vasoconstriction. *N Engl J Med* 321(23):1557–1562, 1989.

15

Acute Breast Pain

☐ DIAGNOSTIC LIST

1. Breast abscess
   A. Peripheral abscess
   B. Subareolar abscess
   C. Puerperal mastitis
   D. Lactation-associated pain
2. Mimics of breast infection
   A. Wegener's granulomatosis
   B. Squamous carcinoma of the breast
   C. Galactocele
   D. Inflammatory carcinoma of the breast
   E. Acute fat necrosis
3. Mondor's disease
4. Infected cutaneous cyst
5. Herpes zoster
6. Costochondritis
7. Gastric distension
8. Fibrocystic disease and a rapidly enlarging cyst
9. Carcinoma of the breast
10. Early pregnancy
11. Bilateral acute breast pain

☐ SUMMARY

A *peripheral breast abscess* causes local pain, swelling, tenderness, redness, and warmth of the overlying skin. A tender, firm or fluctuant mass is palpable in the painful region. Local incision and drainage, with administration of antistaphylococcal antibiotics, usually results in resolution. Many cases occur in puerperal women who are actively breast-feeding. *Subareolar and peripheral abscesses* may occur in nonlactating, and sometimes in postmenopausal, women. There is pain, tenderness, redness, swelling, and a fluctuant mass in the subareolar area. A sinus tract from the abscess to the areola or adjacent skin may be present. Peripheral abscesses are usually caused by staphylococci or streptococci, while subareolar abscesses are usually produced by mixed infections (i.e., 3 to 5 microorganisms). These polymicrobial abscesses yield cultures containing coagulase-negative staphylococci and several anaerobes. Subareolar abscesses and mastitis are secondary to duct ectasia and epithelial metaplasia of the ducts. Duct ectasia may be stimulated by drugs or pituitary tumors that cause hyperprolactinemia. *Puerperal mastitis* may cause diffuse pain, redness, and tenderness of the entire lactating breast. This disorder may resolve with continued nursing and use of antistaphylococcal antibiotics.

Failure to nurse in the postpartum period can cause severe aching breast pain, tenderness, and swelling. This breast engorgement can be prevented by administration of bromocriptine shortly after delivery.

Mimics of a breast infection include *Wegener's granulomatosis of the breast*. A red, warm, tender, painful fluctuant mass in a localized portion of a breast can occur. Aspiration of the mass may yield sterile pus. Sinus, pulmonary, and renal involvement suggest the diagnosis, which can be confirmed by a breast, sinus mucosal, or lung lesion biopsy.

Squamous carcinoma of the breast may present as a painful, inflammatory breast mass with local tenderness, skin redness, and warmth. Needle aspiration yields inflammatory cells and sterile fluid. Biopsy establishes the diagnosis. A *galactocele* may present as a tender, painful breast mass. Mammography can confirm the diagnosis by identifying a cystic lesion with a fat/water level. Aspiration obtains milky sterile fluid.

Inflammatory carcinoma of the breast causes pain, skin warmth, edema (peau d'orange appearance), and a deep cyanotic redness and induration of the skin of the involved area. Biopsy of the skin reveals carcinoma in the dermal and subdermal lymphatics. A similar clinical presentation may be caused by *angiosarcoma of the breast* or *cystosarcoma phylloides*. *Fat necrosis* may cause local ecchymoses, swelling, pain, and a tender, hard, or firm mass. Biopsy is required to exclude abscess or carcinoma.

Mondor's disease presents with a painful, red, tender subcutaneous cordlike swelling on the anterolateral chest wall. It is due to an inflammatory phlebitis of the lateral thoracic or thoracoepigastric veins. This disorder is usually idiopathic and benign; but cases associated, variously, with carcinoma of the breast, subareolar abscess, trauma, a misdirected central venous line, filariasis, and rheumatoid arthritis have been reported. An *infected cutaneous cyst* of the breast may form a fluctuant subcutaneous abscess with overlying skin redness and warmth. *Herpes zoster* may cause unilateral burning breast pain associated with an eruption of grouped vesicles and small, red-based ulcers in the painful dermatome. *Costochondritis* causes pain and tenderness in the parasternal region and medial breast. There is usually a localized tender area over the third, fourth, or fifth costal cartilage or the adjacent chondrosternal joint on one or both sides. Pressure with a fingertip or knuckle over these tender areas may provoke pain of similar quality and location to the patient's spontaneous discomfort. *Gastric distension* may cause intermittent or constant sticking pain in one or both breasts that is relieved by belching and/or administration of antacids. Gastric disease is not usually present.

Fibrocystic disease may cause localized pain, tenderness, and a cystic mass. A dominant fluctuant mass is palpable, and the remainder of the breast may be lumpy and nodular. Mammography will reveal a smooth-bordered, round or ovoid density; ultrasonography will demonstrate the cystic nature of this lesion. Aspiration will reveal serous or, rarely, sanguineous fluid. *Cystic carcinoma* will rarely be encountered. The diagnosis of cystic carcinoma may be suspected after pneumocystography, cytologic study of the fluid, and/or recurrence or persistence of a palpable lesion after fluid aspiration. *Breast cancer* may present with localized pain and tenderness, without a palpable mass. Mammography will confirm a tumor in the painful area (2 to 10 percent of patients with persistent local breast pain and tenderness). Between 18 and 33 percent of patients with proven carcinomas may give a history, when specifically questioned, of local breast pain and tenderness preceding the appearance of a palpable mass.

TABLE OF DISEASE INCIDENCE

INCIDENCE PER 100,000 (APPROXIMATE)

Common (>100)	Uncommon (>5–100)	Rare (>0–5)
Peripheral abscess	Subareolar abscess	Wegener's granulomatosis
Puerperal mastitis	Inflammatory carcinoma of the breast	Squamous carcinoma of the breast
Lactation-associated pain	Acute fat necrosis	
Infected cutaneous cyst	Galactocele	
Costochondritis	Mondor's disease	
Fibrocystic disease and a rapidly enlarging cyst	Herpes zoster	
Carcinoma of the breast	Gastric distension	
Early pregnancy		

Early pregnancy may cause bilateral breast pain, swelling, and tenderness associated with amenorrhea, nausea, and vomiting. Some of the above-described disorders may cause acute bilateral breast pain (see Table 15-1).

☐ DESCRIPTION OF LISTED DISEASES

1. BREAST ABSCESS

Breast abscesses may be classified as subareolar (arising beneath or within 1 cm of the areola), peripheral (arising more than 1 cm from the areola), or indeterminate (arising in both areas). In one series collected over a 10-year period, 39 percent were subareolar, 46 percent peripheral, and 15 percent indeterminate.

A. Peripheral Abscess An abscess in this location is common during the puerperium, especially during lactation. Peripheral abscesses may occur in nonpregnant women as well. *Staphylococcus aureus, S. albus*, and streptococci are frequently isolated. Anaerobes occur, but are uncommon in peripheral abscesses. There is local aching and/or throbbing pain in one breast, associated with a tender, indurated or fluctuant mass, and with erythema and warmth of the overlying skin. Axillary node enlargement and tenderness may be associated. Fever, chills, myalgias, and malaise may occur in severe cases. Needle aspiration of the abscess will reveal purulent fluid. There is a good therapeutic response to incision and drainage, and to use of antistaphylococcal antibiotics. Gram stain and culture of the aspirated pus will help to guide changes in the initial antibiotic regimen. In the past, up to 3 percent of lactating women suffered from breast abscess, but that percentage has markedly decreased during the last decade.

B. Subareolar Abscess Pain, swelling, tenderness, and skin erythema are centered below the areola or adjacent to it. A tender subareolar mass, either indurated or fluctuant, is usually present, and may extend peripherally. The nipple may be inverted in up to 8 percent of cases at the time of initial presentation. This disorder is associated with duct ectasia and squamous metaplasia. Periductal inflammation may be present. These abscesses contain coagulase-negative staphylococci (60 percent) and/or anaerobes, such as *Peptostreptococcus* species (70 percent), *Propionibacterium* species (22 percent), and *Bacteroides* species (11 percent). While *Staphylococcus aureus* is usually responsible for peripheral abscesses, subareolar lesions are usually polymicrobial (83 percent); and one-third of the isolates are aerobes, and the remainder anaerobes. A mean of 3.6 species per abscess have been isolated using meticulous aerobic/anaerobic culture methods. These abscesses tend to recur with simple incision and drainage. Excision of the abscess cavity, fistulous tract(s), and diseased subareolar lactiferous duct(s) is required to prevent recurrent episodes. Subareolar abscess and duct ectasia may be associated with hyperprolactinemia. Elevated prolactin levels, secondary to subareolar inflammation, are usually transient. Persistent hyperprolactinemia is usually related to a prolactinoma of the pituitary. Nonpuerperal mastitis may be a symptom of a pituitary neoplasm.

Patients with nonpuerperal subareolar mastitis should be evaluated for hyperprolactinemia after the local breast inflammatory process has resolved. Persistence of hyperprolactinemia requires a contrast-enhanced CT scan of the brain to exclude a pituitary adenoma.

C. Puerperal Mastitis Breast infection secondary to nursing may cause pain, swelling, heat, redness, and tenderness of the affected breast. Continued nursing, or use of a breast pump, and oral antistaphylococcal antibiotics will lead to resolution of complaints, averting abscess formation and the requirement for surgical drainage.

D. Lactation-Associated Pain Lactation without nursing can cause painful swelling of both breasts, with fullness and severe tenderness. This engorgement and milk secretion can be prevented by administration of an intramuscular injection of bromocriptine mesylate (Parlodel LA) within 3 to 4 h of delivery.

2. MIMICS OF BREAST INFECTION

A. Wegener's Granulomatosis This disorder may cause a painful and tender breast mass, with warmth and erythema of the overlying skin. Aspiration will reveal sterile pus. Fever may persist despite adequate drainage of the breast lesion.

Sinusitis, with cheek and forehead pain and tenderness, cough, dyspnea, and hemoptysis, may appear and progress. Chest radiographs may demonstrate infiltrates, nodular masses, and thick-walled cavities.

Proteinuria and microhematuria may be present, and the serum creatinine concentration and sedimentation rate may be increased. Biopsy of breast and/or sinus tissue may demonstrate evidence of vasculitis and/or giant cells and a granulomatous tissue response. This disorder responds to prednisone and cyclophosphamide therapy.

B. Squamous Carcinoma of the Breast This tumor may present as a painful inflammatory breast mass with local tenderness, skin redness, and warmth. Needle aspiration may reveal only inflammatory cells; cultures are negative. Biopsy will confirm the diagnosis of carcinoma with squamous metaplasia.

C. Galactocele A galactocele may form a painful or painless, fluctuant, tender breast mass in the peripheral region of the breast. Mammography may identify a fat/water level in the breast lesion, confirming the presence of a galactocele prior to needle aspiration. Aspiration reveals milky sterile fluid. Most patients with this disorder have a history of lactation shortly before the appearance of the mass.

D. Inflammatory Carcinoma of the Breast The involved breast becomes painful, erythematous, warm, swollen, and tender. Fever may occur in up to 10 percent of cases. A peau d'orange appearance of the edematous breast skin may be present. Biopsy of the skin and subcutaneous tissue may reveal carcinoma in the dermal and subdermal lymphatics. A discrete tumor mass may not be present. Because of the diffuse redness and tenderness, this disorder has been mistaken for an infectious mastitis or a breast abscess. Angiosarcoma of the breast and some cases of cystosarcoma phylloides may present with a clinical picture similar to that of inflammatory carcinoma.

E. Acute Fat Necrosis This disorder usually follows breast trauma. The breast injury may cause skin ecchymoses, local pain, tenderness, and swelling. Skin erythema may be present. A mass may appear initially; it may remain constant or increase in size. The local pain, tenderness, and mass may mimic an abscess or carcinoma. Biopsy will establish the diagnosis of fat necrosis. Fat necrosis may also occur in patients treated for breast carcinoma with lumpectomy and radiation therapy. Fat necrosis appears between 4 and 43 months after surgical and radiation therapy, and may mimic recurrent breast cancer. Excisional biopsy is required to exclude recurrent carcinoma and confirm the diagnosis of fat necrosis. Mammography is not sufficiently sensitive or specific for this purpose.

3. MONDOR'S DISEASE

This disorder presents with unilateral anterolateral chest pain and a tender, swollen, erythematous venous cord in the subcutaneous tissue of the chest wall. The cord may have a linear or Y-shaped configuration, and may be connected to one or more small, beadlike nodules.

Trauma is believed to be the usual cause, but many cases occur in the absence of remembered injury. The underlying disorder is a phlebitis and periphlebitis of the lateral thoracic or thoracoepigastric vein. The female:male ratio is 2:1, and most cases occur in the 21- to 55-year age group. Cases of this disorder have been reported secondary to primary breast cancer and metastatic lung cancer. Palpation and/or mammography demonstrates the causative tumor, which is usually adjacent to the involved vein. Other cases have been reported 3 to 7 weeks after breast surgery [e.g., augmentation mammoplasty (5 percent), reduction mammoplasty (1.6 percent), and immediate breast reconstruction (3.4 percent)]. Mondor's disease has rarely been associated with malignancy at another site (e.g., gastric cancer), filariasis, rheumatoid arthritis, and subareolar abscess.

Mondor's disease may be mimicked by infiltrative fibromatosis, mammary arteritis, lymphangitis, fibrosarcoma, and lymphangitic carcinomatosis of the breast. Differentiation requires biopsy of the cordlike lesion. A Mondor-like disorder, with railway track–like subcutaneous cords in the axillary region, has been reported. On biopsy, these lesions showed a diffuse dermal infiltrate of lymphocytes, histiocytes, and eosinophils. No evidence of a venous thrombus or vessel involvement was present. In most cases Mondor's disease is benign and self-limited, but occasional cases may be associated with serious disease.

4. INFECTED CUTANEOUS CYST

A cutaneous sebaceous or epidermal cyst of the breast may become red, painful, and tender. The skin is fixed to the superficial fluctuant mass. Drainage of the cyst and antibiotic therapy usually lead to prompt resolution.

5. HERPES ZOSTER

Burning or aching pain and/or pruritus may affect one breast and the corresponding dermatomal region of the ipsilateral region of the back. The pain does not cross the midline. Within 3 to 4 days a rash, consisting of grouped vesicles and crusted ulcers, appears in the painful dermatomal area. The vesicles and ulcers are surrounded by erythematous, and sometimes edematous, skin.

6. COSTOCHONDRITIS

Costochondritis may cause medial breast pain that is associated with local chest wall tenderness. The tender area is usually situated over the third to fifth costal cartilages on the left or right side. Sometimes arm movements, a deep breath, or pressure from an embrace may provoke a transient episode of aching and/or sharp medial breast pain that is similar to that experienced spontaneously. The breast itself is not tender. This disorder responds to rest, local heat, and simple analgesics. In severe cases injection of lidocaine and methylprednisolone into the region of the tender costal cartilage or chondrosternal joint may relieve the pain. Exclusion of cardiac disease by use of electrocardiographic and thallium-201 imaging stress tests or coronary angiography may be required in cases simulating coronary disease.

7. GASTRIC DISTENSION

Gastric distension, with epigastric fullness and associated pyrosis, may also cause sticking, knifelike pain in one or both breasts. This may be relieved by belching or by administration of antacids. The pains are usually brief in duration and resolve when the gaseous distension, pyrosis, and epigastric distress are relieved.

8. FIBROCYSTIC DISEASE

Patients may present with lateral breast pain, tenderness, and a rapidly enlarging cyst. The diagnosis of fibrocystic disease can be established by clinical examination, mammography (80 percent sensitive), ultrasonography (80 to 90 percent sensitive), and/or breast biopsy. Acute pain results when a single cyst rapidly enlarges, causing tenderness and a palpable mass. The cystic nature of these lesions can be confirmed by ultrasonography. Aspiration of the cyst will remove the contained fluid and relieve the pain and tenderness. Cytologic analysis of the fluid should be obtained if the fluid is bloody or the patient has a high risk of developing a breast malignancy. Rarely, carcinoma may mimic a benign cystic lesion, with residual tumor in the wall of the aspirated cyst. Such a lesion may be detected by pneumocystography, cytologic analysis of aspirated fluid, or biopsy of a persistent mass at the site of the cyst.

9. CARCINOMA OF THE BREAST

A person with breast cancer may present with localized breast pain of an aching or sticking nature. The pain may be intensified by finger pressure. A palpable mass may be absent, but a tumor can be demonstrated by mammography. In one large series, 2.2 percent of patients with mastalgia and no palpable mass had mammographic evidence of carcinoma at the painful site. Fine-needle aspiration of the tender area failed to demonstrate the abnormality in 80 percent of cases.

In a large group of operable tumor patients ($N = 478$ breast cancers), localized breast pain, followed by the appearance of a palpable lump or thickening, occurred in 18 percent of cases. In a second series, 5 percent of patients had only mastalgia, while 33 percent complained of a painful lump. The mastalgia was usually localized to the site of the mammographically detected tumor. The duration of intermittent or persistent pain prior to diagnosis may exceed 4 years.

10. EARLY PREGNANCY

Bilateral breast swelling, aching outer quadrant pain and tenderness, and the appearance of prominent nipple papillae are early signs of pregnancy. Associated symptoms include amenorrhea, nausea, vomiting, hyperosmia, and light-headedness. Urine and serum pregnancy tests are positive.

11. BILATERAL ACUTE BREAST PAIN

Disorders that are likely to cause bilateral acute pain are listed in Table 15-1.

Table 15-1
CAUSES OF ACUTE BILATERAL BREAST PAIN

Puerperal mastitis
Lactation-associated pain
Costochondritis
Gastric distension
Fibrocystic disease
Early pregnancy

BREAST PAIN REFERENCES

Abscess
Rowley S, Downing R: Breast "abscess": An unusual complication of catheterisation of the subclavian vein. *Br J Radiol* 60:773–774, 1987.
Scholefield JH, Duncan JL, Rogers K: Review of a hospital experience of breast abscesses. *Br J Surg* 74:469–470, 1987.
Silverman JF, Lannin DR, Unverferth M, et al: Fine needle aspiration cytology of subareolar abscess of the breast. Spectrum of cytomorphologic findings and potential diagnostic pitfalls. *Acta Cytol* 30(4):413–419, 1986.
Walker AP, Edmiston CE Jr, Krepel CJ, et al: A prospective study of the microflora of nonpuerperal breast abscess. *Arch Surg* 123:908–911, 1988.
Watt-Boolsen S, Rasmussen NR, Bilchert-Toft M: Primary periareolar abscess in the nonlactating breast: Risk of recurrence. *Am J Surg* 153(6):571–573, 1987.
Weiss RL, Matsen JM: Group B streptococcal breast abscess. *Arch Pathol Lab Med* 111:74–75, 1987.
Yanai A, Hirabayashi S, Ueda K, et al: Treatment of recurrent subareolar abscess. *Ann Plast Surg* 18(4):314–318, 1987.

Abscess Mimics
Melamed JB, Schein M, Decker GAG: Squamous carcinoma of the breast presenting as an abscess. *S Afr Med J* 69:771–772, 1986.
Wilson ME: Wegener's granulomatosis presenting as breast abscess. *Am J Med* 83:1168, 1987.

Breast Pain—Review Articles
Rush BF Jr: Breast, in Schwartz SI, Shires GT, Spencer FC (eds): *Principles of Surgery*, 5th ed. New York, McGraw-Hill, 1989, pp 549–580.
Wilson JD: Endocrine disorders of the breast, in Braunwald E, Isselbacher KJ, Petersdorf RG, et al (eds): *Harrison's Principles of Internal Medicine*, 11th ed. New York, McGraw-Hill, 1987, pp 1837–1840.

Carcinoma—Female Breast
Benson EA: Mastalgia: Is this commonly associated with operable breast cancer? *Ann R Coll Surg Engl* 69(2):87, 1987.
Edeiken S: Mammography in the symptomatic woman. *Cancer* 63:1412–1414, 1989.
Fariselli G, Lepera P, Viganotti G, et al: Localized mastalgia as presenting symptom in breast cancer. *Eur J Surg Oncol* 14:213–215, 1988.
Harris VJ, Jackson VP: Indications for breast imaging in women under age 35 years. *Radiology* 172:445–448, 1989.
Hermansen C, Poulsen HS, Jensen J, et al: Diagnostic reliability of combined physical examination, mammography, and fine-needle puncture ("triple test") in breast tumors: A prospective study. *Cancer* 60:1866–1871, 1987.
Smallwood JA, Kye DA, Taylor I: Mastalgia: Is this commonly associated with operable breast cancer? *Ann R Coll Surg Engl* 68:262–263, 1986.

Watsky KL, Orlow SJ, Bolognia JL: Figurate and bullous eruption in association with breast carcinoma. *Arch Dermatol* 126:649–652, 1990.

Carcinoma—Male Breast

Bhagat P, Kline TS: The male breast and malignant neoplasms: Diagnosis by aspiration biopsy cytology. *Cancer* 65:2338–2341, 1990.

Davidson AT: A review of the treatment of cancer of the male breast with a case follow-up. *J Natl Med Assoc* 79(8):879–880, 1987.

Hultborn R, Friberg S, Hultborn KA: Male breast carcinoma: 1. A study of the total material reported to the Swedish Cancer Registry 1958–1967 with respect to clinical and histopathologic parameters. *Acta Oncol* 26(4):241–256, 1987.

Olsson H, Ranstam J: Head trauma and exposure to prolactin-elevating drugs as risk factors for male breast cancer. *J Natl Cancer Inst* 80:679–683, 1988.

Raviglione MC, Graham PE: Breast carcinoma in a man following local trauma. *N Y State J Med* 87(3):186–187, 1987.

Sano Y, Inoue T, Aso M, et al: Paget's disease of the male breast: Report of a case and histopathologic study. *J Dermatol* 16:237–241, 1989.

Serour F, Birkenfeld S, Amsterdam E, et al: Paget's disease of the male breast. *Cancer* 62:601–605, 1988.

Carcinoma Mimics—Female Breast

Chaudary MM, Girling A, Girling S, et al: New lumps in the breast following conservative treatment for early breast cancer. *Breast Cancer Res Treat* 11:51–58, 1988.

D'Alessandro DR, Taylor FM III: Unilateral breast enlargement due to localized fibrosis. *South Med J* 79(11):1451–1453, 1986.

Devitt JE: Benign disorders of the breast in older women. *Surg Gynecol Obstet* 162(4):340–342, 1986.

Devitt JE: False alarms of breast cancer. *Lancet* 2(8674):1257–1258, 1989.

Galea MH, Robertson JFR, Ellis IO, et al: Granulomatous lobular mastitis. *Aust N Z J Surg* 59:547–550, 1989.

Hanson PJV, Thomas JM, Collins JV: *Mycobacterium chelonei* and abscess formation in soft tissues. *Tubercle* 68:297–299, 1987.

Hines JR, Murad TM, Beal JM: Prognostic indicators in cystosarcoma phylloides, *Am J Surg* 153(3):276–280, 1987.

Kline TS: Masquerades of malignancy: A review of 4,241 aspirates from the breast. *Acta Cytol* 25(3):263–266, 1981.

Linden SS, Sickles EA: Sedimented calcium in benign breast cysts: The full spectrum of mammographic presentations. *AJR* 152:967–971, 1989.

Peterse JL, Thunnissen FBJM, van Heerde P: Fine needle aspiration cytology of radiation-induced changes in nonneoplastic breast lesions: Possible pitfalls in cytodiagnosis. *Acta Cytol* 33(2):176–180, 1989.

Pilnik S: Clinical diagnosis of benign breast diseases. *J Reprod Med* 22:277–290, 1979.

Rainwater LM, Martin JK Jr, Gaffey TA, et al: Angiosarcoma of the breast. *Arch Surg* 212:669–672, 1986.

Reddin A, McCrea ES, Keramati B: Inflammatory breast disease: Mammographic spectrum. *South Med J* 81(8):981–984, 988, 1988.

Roberts MM, Elton RA, Robinson SE, et al: Consultations for breast disease in general practice and hospital referral patterns. *Br J Surg* 74:1020–1022, 1987.

Rosen PP, Ernsberger D: Mammary fibromatosis: A benign spindle-cell tumor with significant risk for local recurrence. *Cancer* 63:1363–1369, 1989.

Fat Necrosis

Boyages J, Bilous M, Barraclough B, et al: Fat necrosis of the breast following lumpectomy and radiation therapy for early breast cancer. *Radiother Oncol* 13:69–74, 1988.

Rostom AY, El-Sayed ME: Fat necrosis of the breasts: An unusual complication of lumpectomy and radiotherapy in breast cancer. *Clin Radiol* 38:31, 1987.

Fibrocystic Disease

Deschamps M, Hislop TG, Band PR, et al: Study of benign breast disease in a population screened for breast cancer. *Cancer Detect Prev* 9:151–156, 1986.

Scott EB: Fibrocystic breast disease. *Am Fam Physician* 36(4):119–126, 1987.

Vorherr H: Fibrocystic breast disease: Pathophysiology, pathomorphology, clinical picture, and management. *Am J Obstet Gynecol* 154:161–179, 1986.

Galactocele

Gómez A, Mata JM, Donoso L, et al: Galactocele: Three distinctive radiographic appearances. *Radiology* 158:43–44, 1986.

Hall FM: Galactocele: Three distinctive radiographic appearances (letter to editor). *Radiology* 160(3):852–853, 1986.

Salvador R, Salvador M, Jiminez JA, et al: Galactocele of the breast: Radiologic and ultrasonographic findings. *Br J Radiol* 63(746):140–142, 1990.

Granular Cell Myoblastoma

Bassett LW, Cove HC: Myoblastoma of the breast. *AJR* 132:122–123, 1979.

Bonilla-Musoles F, Monmeneu S, Pardo G, et al: Granular cell myoblastoma (GCM): Contribution of three cases with genital involvement. *Eur J Gynaec Oncol* 8(2):110–114, 1987.

Gordon AB, Fisher C, Palmer B, et al: Granular cell tumour of the breast. *Eur J Surg Oncol* 11:269–273, 1985.

Löwhagen T, Rubio CA: The cytology of the granular cell myoblastoma of the breast: Report of a case. *Acta Cytol* 21(2):314–315, 1977.

McCracken M, Hamal PB, Benson EA: Granular cell myoblastoma of the breast: A report of 2 cases. *Br J Surg* 66:819–821, 1979.

Mulcare R: Granular cell myoblastoma of the breast. *Ann Surg* 168(2):262–268, 1968.

Naraynsingh V, Raju GC, Jankey N, et al: Granular cell myoblastoma of the breast. *J R Coll Surg Edinb* 30(2):91–92, 1985.

Sussman EB, Hajdu SI, Gray GF: Granular cell myoblastoma of the breast. *Am J Surg* 126(5):669–670, 1973.

Umansky C, Bullock WK: Granular cell myoblastoma of the breast. *Ann Surg* 168(5):810–817, 1968.

Vidyarthi SC: Granular cell myoblastoma of the breast. *Arch Surg* 98(5):662–667, 1969.

Gynecomastia

Bardin CW, Paulsen CA: The testes, in Williams RH (ed): *Textbook of Endocrinology*, 6th ed. Philadelphia, Saunders, 1981, pp 293–354.

Frieberg A, Hong C: Apple-coring technique for severe gynecomastia. *Can J Surg* 30(1):57–60, 1987.

Gluud C: Testosterone and alcoholic cirrhosis: Epidemiologic, pathophysiologic and therapeutic studies in men. *Dan Med Bull* 35(6):564–575, 1988.

Gooren L: Improvement of spermatogenesis after treatment with the antiestrogen tamoxifen in a man with the incomplete androgen insensitivity syndrome. *J Clin Endocrinol Metab* 68(6):1207–1210, 1989.

Grumbach MM, Conte FA: Disorders of sex differentiation, in Williams RH (ed): *Textbook of Endocrinology*, 6th ed. Philadelphia, Saunders, 1981, pp 423–514.

Kadair RG, Block MB, Katz FH, et al: "Masked" 21-hydroxylase deficiency of the adrenal presenting with gynecomastia and bilateral testicular masses. *Am J Med* 62:278–282, 1977.

Knudtzon J, Aarskog D: 45,X/46,XY mosaicism. *Eur J Pediatr* 146:266–271, 1987.

Kruss DM, Littman A: Safety of cimetidine. *Gastroenterology* 74(2):478–483, 1978.

Matsumoto AM: The testis, in Wyngaarden JB, Smith LH Jr (eds): *Cecil Textbook of Medicine*, 18th ed. Philadelphia, Saunders, 1988, pp 1410–1411.

Migeon CJ, Brown TR, Lanes R, et al: A clinical syndrome of mild androgen insensitivity. *J Clin Endocrinol Metab* 59(4):672–678, 1984.

Paulson DF, Wiebe HR, Hammond CB: Hypothalamic and pituitary function in hypogonadotropic hypogonadism. *Urology* 6(3):333–336, 1975.

Wigley KD, Thomas JL, Bernardino ME, et al: Sonography of gynecomastia. *AJR* 136:927–930, 1981.

Wurzel RS, Yamase HT, Nieh PT: Ectopic production of human chorionic gonadotropin by poorly differentiated transitional cell tumors of the urinary tract. *J Urol* 137(3):502–504, 1987.

Gynecomastia Associated with Neoplasms

Chen KTK, Spaulding RW, Flam MS, et al: Malignant interstitial cell tumor of the testis. *Cancer* 49:547–552, 1982.

Daughaday WH: The adenohypophysis, in Williams RH (ed): *Textbook of Endocrinology*, 6th ed. Philadelphia, Saunders, 1981, pp 100–114.

Davis S, DiMartino NA, Schneider G: Malignant interstitial cell carcinoma of the testis: Report of two cases with steroid synthetic profiles, response to therapy and review of the literature. *Cancer* 47:425–431, 1981.

Gabrilove JL, Nicolis GL, Mitty HA, et al: Feminizing interstitial cell tumor of the testis: Personal observations and a review of the literature. *Cancer* 35:1184–1202, 1975.

Glavind K, Søndergaard G: Leydig cell tumour: Diagnosis and treatment. *Scand J Urol Nephrol* 22:343–345, 1988.

Haas GP, Pittaluga S, Gomella L, et al: clinically occult Leydig cell tumor presenting with gynecomastia. *J Urol* 142:1325–1327, 1989.

Liddle GW: The adrenals, in Williams RH (ed): *Textbook of Endocrinology*, 6th ed. Philadelphia, Saunders, 1981, pp 285–292.

Mersey JH, Ceballos L, Levin P, et al: Estrogen-secreting adrenal tumor responsive to ACTH: Localization by adrenal venous sampling. *South Med J* 81(2):275–278, 1988.

Saadi HF, Bravo EL, Aron DC: Feminizing adrenocortical tumor: Steroid hormone response to ketoconazole. *J Clin Endocrinol Metab* 70:540–543, 1990.

Tseng A Jr, Horning SJ, Freiha FS, et al: Gynecomastia in testicular cancer patients: Prognostic and therapeutic implications. *Cancer* 56:2534–2538, 1985.

VanMeter QL, Gareis FJ, Hayes JW, et al: Galactorrhea in a 12-year-old boy with a chromophobe adenoma. *J Pediatr* 90(5):756–759, 1977.

Mammaplasty—Reduction/Augmentation

Brown FE, Sargent SK, Cohen SR, et al: Mammographic changes following reduction mammaplasty. *Plast Reconstr Surg* 80(5):691–698, 1987.

Jabaley ME, Das SK: Late breast pain following reconstruction with polyurethane-covered implants. *Plast Reconstr Surg* 78(3):390–395, 1986.

Källén R, Broomé A, Mühlow A, et al: Reduction mammaplasty: Results of preoperative mammography and patient inquiry. *Scand J Plast Reconstr Surg* 20:303–305, 1986.

Kinell I, Beausang-Linder M, Ohlsén L: The effect on the preoperative symptoms and the late results of Skoog's reduction mammaplasty: A follow-up study on 149 patients. *Scand J Plast Reconstr Hand Surg* 24:61–65, 1990.

Mastalgia—Cyclical/Noncyclical

Fentiman IS: Tamoxifen and mastalgia: An emerging indication. *Drugs* 32:477–480, 1986.

Fentiman IS, Caleffi M, Brame K, et al: Double-blind controlled trial of tamoxifen therapy for mastalgia. *Lancet* 1(8476):287–288, 1986.

Fentiman IS, Powles TJ: Tamoxifen and benign breast problems. *Lancet* 2(8567):1070–1072, 1987.

Griffith CDM, Dowle CS, Hinton CP, et al: The breast pain clinic: A rational approach to classification and treatment of breast pain. *Postgrad Med J* 63:547–549, 1987.

Hinton CP, Bishop HM, Holliday HW, et al: A double-blind controlled trial of danazol and bromocriptine in the management of severe cyclical breast pain. *Br J Clin Pract* 40(8):326–330, 1986.

Horrobin DF, Manku MS: Premenstrual syndrome and premenstrual breast pain (cyclical mastalgia): Disorders of essential fatty acid (EFA) metabolism. *Prostaglandins Leukot Essent Fatty Acids* 37:255–261, 1989.

Leinster SJ, Whitehouse GH, Walsh PV: Cyclical mastalgia: Clinical and mammographic observations in a screened population. *Br J Surg* 74:220–222, 1987.

Maddox PR, Harrison BJ, Mansel RE, et al: Non-cyclical mastalgia: An improved classification and treatment. *Br J Surg* 76:901–904, 1989.

Parlati E, Polinari U, Salvi G, et al: Bromocriptine for treatment of benign breast disease: A double-blind clinical trial versus placebo. *Acta Obstet Gynecol Scand* 66:483–488, 1987.

Parlati E, Travaglini A, Liberale I, et al: Hormonal profile in benign breast disease: Endocrine status of cyclical mastalgia patients. *J Endocrinol Invest* 11:679–683, 1988.

Sutton GLJ, O'Malley VP: Treatment of cyclical mastalgia with low dose short term danazol. *Br J Clin Pract* 40(2):68–70, 1986.

Watts JFf, Butt WR, Edwards RL: A clinical trial using danazol for the treatment of premenstrual tension. *Br J Obstet Gynaecol* 94:30–34, 1987.

Mondor's Disease

Aloi FG, Tomasini CF, Molinero A: Railway track-like dermatitis: An atypical Mondor's disease? *J Am Acad Dermatol* 20:920–923, 1989.

Bahal V, Mansel RE: Mondor's disease secondary to breast abscess in a male. *Br J Surg* 73:931, 1986.

Chiedozi LC, Aghahowa JA: Mondor's disease associated with breast cancer. *Surgery* 103(4):438–439, 1988.

Courtney SP, Polacarz S, Raftery AT: Mondor's disease associated with metastatic lung cancer in the breast. *Postgrad Med J* 65:779–780, 1988.

Green RA, Dowden RV: Mondor's disease in plastic surgery patients. *Ann Plast Surg* 20(3):231–235, 1988.

Gutman H, Kott I, Reiss R: Inflammatory carcinoma of the breast with Mondor's disease. *Practitioner* 231:1086–1088, 1987.

Hershman MJ, Archer MJ: Mondor's disease and breast cancer. *Br J Clin Pract* 41(10):979–980, 1987.

Levi I, Baum M: Mondor's disease as a presenting symptom of breast cancer. *Br J Surg* 74:700, 1987.

Nipple Discharge

Knight DC, Lowell DM, Heimann A, et al: Aspiration of the breast and nipple discharge cytology. *Surg Gynecol Obstet* 163(5):415–420, 1986.

Leis HP Jr, Greene FL, Cammarata A, et al: Nipple discharge: Surgical significance. *South Med J* 81(1):20–26, 1988.

Nipple Disease—Duct Ectasia

Browning J, Bigrigg A, Taylor I: Symptomatic and incidental mammary duct ectasia. *J R Soc Med* 79(12):715–716, 1986.

Bundred NJ, Dixon JM, Chetty U, et al: Mammillary fistula. *Br J Surg* 74:466–468, 1987.

Peters F, Schuth W. Hyperprolactinemia and nonpuerperal mastitis (duct ectasia). *JAMA* 261:1618–1620, 1989.

Raju GC, Naraynsingh V, Jankey N: Post-menopausal breast abscess. *Postgrad Med J* 62:1017–1018, 1986.

Nipple—Florid Papillomatosis

Mazzara PF, Flint A, Naylor B: Adenoma of the nipple: Cytopathologic features. *Acta Cytol* 33(2):188–190, 1989.

Piérard G: Paget's disease or erosive adenomatosis of the nipple? (letter to editor). *Dermatologica* 180(1):55, 1990.

Rosen PP, Caicco JA: Florid papillomatosis of the nipple: A study of 51 patients, including nine with mammary carcinoma. *Am J Surg Pathol* 10(2):87–101, 1986.

Nipple—Paget's Disease

Bulens P, Vanuytsel L, Rijnders A, et al: Breast conserving treatment of Paget's disease. *Radiother Oncol* 17:305–309, 1990.

Chaudary MA, Millis RR, Lane EB, et al: Paget's disease of the nipple: A ten year review including clinical, pathological, and immunohistochemical findings. *Breast Cancer Res Treat* 8:139–146, 1986.

DuToit RS, VanRensburg PSJ, Goedhals L: Paget's disease of the breast. *S Afr Med J* 73:95–97, 1988.

Fernandes FJ, Costa MM, Bernardo M: Rarities in breast pathology: Bilateral Paget's disease of the breast—a case report. *Eur J Surg Oncol* 16:172–174, 1990.

Fine RM: Paget's disease of the nipple (commentary). *Int J Dermatol* 25(5):298–299, 1986.

Fourquet A, Campana F, Vielh P, et al: Paget's disease of the nipple without detectable breast tumor: Conservative management with radiation therapy. *Int J Radiat Oncol Biol Phys* 13:1463–1465, 1987.

Menon RS, van Geel AN: Cancer of the breast with nipple involvement. *Br J Cancer* 59:81–84, 1989.

Mevorah B, Frenk E, Wietlisbach V, et al: Minor clinical features of atopic dermatitis: Evaluation of their diagnostic significance. *Dermatologica* 177:360–364, 1988.

Sanchez JA, Feller WF: Paget's disease of the breast. *Am Fam Physician* 36(2):145–147, 1987.

Pregnancy-Associated Breast Pain

Ho KY, Thorner MO: Therapeutic applications of bromocriptine in endocrine and neurological diseases. *Drugs* 36:67–82, 1988.

Matheson I, Aursnes I, Horgen M, et al: Bacteriological findings and clinical symptoms in relation to clinical outcome in puerperal mastitis. *Acta Obstet Gynecol Scand* 67:723–726, 1988.

Rolland R, Nijdam W, Weyer A, et al: Prevention of puerperal lactation with Parlodel Long-acting (Parlodel LA). *Eur J Obstet Gynecol Reprod Biol* 22:337–343, 1986.

Trauma

Dawes RFH, Smallwood JA, Taylor I: Seat belt injury to the female breast. *Br J Surg* 73:106–107, 1986.

PART FIVE

Acute Abdominal Pain

16 Acute Right Hypochondriac Pain

☐ DIAGNOSTIC LIST

1. Biliary colic
2. Acute cholecystitis
3. Acute pancreatitis
4. Acute appendicitis
5. Pain related to disorders of the liver
   A. Acute hepatitis
      1. Alcoholic hepatitis
      2. Viral hepatitis
      3. Drug-related hepatitis (toxic and idiosyncratic reactions)
         A. Acetaminophen
         B. Other drugs
      4. Toxins
         A. Mushroom poisoning
         B. Carbon tetrachloride
   B. Hepatic abscess
      1. Pyogenic abscess
      2. Amebic abscess
   C. Hepatic tumors with rapid growth, bleeding, or infarction
      1. Malignant (hepatocellular carcinoma)
      2. Benign (adenoma, focal nodular hyperplasia, hemangioma)
   D. Simple obstructive cholangitis (ascending cholangitis)
   E. Hepatic congestion
      1. Budd-Chiari syndrome
      2. Acute hepatic congestion
   F. Hepatic hemorrhage in preeclampsia
6. Gastroduodenal pain and irritable bowel
   A. Perforation of a duodenal or pyloric canal ulcer
   B. Duodenal ulcer and nonulcer dyspepsia
   C. Irritable bowel
7. Costochondritis of the lower right anterior chest and costal margin
8. Perihepatitis due to gonococcal or chlamydial infection (Fitz-Hugh-Curtis syndrome)
9. Pleuroabdominal pain due to pneumonia or pulmonary infarction
10. Disorders of the right kidney
    A. Acute pyelonephritis
    B. Acute corticomedullary abscess
    C. Cortical abscess
    D. Perinephric abscess
    E. Renal infarction
    F. Renal tumor
11. Unknown causes of acute right upper abdominal pain
12. Herpes zoster

☐ SUMMARY

Biliary colic causes constant and severe aching right hypochondriac pain that may radiate to the epigastrium and right subscapular area. The pain disappears spontaneously within 2 to 6 h or after an analgesic injection. A similar pain, lasting more than 24 h and associated with fever, tenderness, and guarding, may be due to *acute cholecystitis*. A real-time ultrasound examination will confirm the presence of gallstones, and, in the case of cholecystitis, may demonstrate a sonographic Murphy's sign, thickening of the gallbladder wall, and pericholecystic fluid. A DISIDA radionuclide scan is usually positive in cholecystitis. *Acute pancreatitis* may cause epigastric and right upper quadrant pain and tenderness, often worsened or improved by changes of body position. An elevated serum amylase level or a CT scan of the pancreas confirms the diagnosis. *Acute appendicitis* causes midepigastric pain that shifts to the right. In some cases only surgical exploration can differentiate this disorder from acute cholecystitis. In appendicitis, ultrasonography is usually negative for gallstones and may confirm the diagnosis by visualization of a diseased appendix.

Inflammation or necrosis of the liver can cause a dull and aching, or sharper, more severe, hypochondriac pain and tenderness. A history of alcohol abuse and a mild degree of aminotransferase (transaminase) elevation identifies the patient with *alcoholic hepatitis*. The enzyme levels and ratios of SGOT (AST) to SGPT (ALT) separate *viral hepatitis* from alcoholic hepatitis. Specific serologic tests can identify infection with hepatitis A or B, or delta agent. A drug history will identify causes of *toxic or idiosyncratic hepatitis;* a history of *wild mushroom ingestion* or *carbon tetrachloride exposure* will identify other causes of a painful, tender liver. Fever and hepatic pain, tenderness, and enlargement occur with *pyogenic and amebic abscesses.* These can be identified and delineated by ultrasonography or contrast-enhanced CT. Amebic abscess can be diagnosed serologically by use of an indirect hemagglutination test to *Entamoeba histolytica* in the serum (95 percent of cases) or by identifying the organism in the stool (20–30 percent). A pyogenic abscess can be aspirated and cultured. *Liver tumors* causing pain can be identified by ultrasonography, CT, or MRI; in some cases their exact nature can be determined by use of angiography (hemangioma, hepatocellular carcinoma, focal nodular hyperplasia, or adenoma) or MRI (hemangioma). Final confirmation of some lesions requires closed or open biopsy. *Ascending cholangitis* causes fever, jaundice, and constant right upper quadrant pain and tenderness in patients with common duct stones, strictures, or duct-obstructing tumors. *Acute hepatic vein occlusion* may cause a painful, tender enlargement of the liver and rapidly developing ascites. The diagnosis can be confirmed by MRI or a contrast-enhanced CT study of the liver and hepatic veins. *Acute pulmonary embolism* of massive proportions may cause dyspnea, chest pain, jugular venous distension, and sudden painful enlargement of the liver due to *acute hepatic congestion* in association with severe hypotension and cardiovascular collapse.

The sudden onset of right hypochondriac pain and tenderness in a patient with *preeclampsia* usually indicates the presence of subcapsular or parenchymal bleeding in the liver. The diagnosis can be confirmed by CT. A *perforated ulcer* may cause severe, sharp right and mid-upper abdominal pain that spreads over the entire abdomen. The physical signs include generalized direct and rebound tenderness and guarding and loss of liver percussion dullness. Free air can be detected in 70 percent of cases by a plain upright or lateral decubitus radiograph. A perforation can also be confirmed by ingestion of a water-soluble radiographic contrast dye, which can be shown to leak from the perforated ulcer. Pain due to *duodenal ulcer or nonulcer dyspepsia* may be localized to the right upper abdomen. This diagnosis can be confirmed by endoscopy or a double-contrast barium meal. *Irritable bowel* may cause aching right upper abdominal pain transiently relieved by passage of flatus or stool and sometimes associated with diarrhea and/or constipation. *Costochondritis* causes costal cartilage pain and tenderness over the right costal margin, but no other abnormalities. *Perihepatitis* (Fitz-Hugh–Curtis syndrome) causes right and mid-upper abdominal pain and tenderness that is usually, but not always, associated with lower abdominal pain, fever, and tubal inflammation on pelvic examination. *Pneumonia* and *pulmonary infarction* may cause right upper abdominal pain and tenderness, associated with abnormal physical and radiologic findings over the right lower lobe. Pleuritic pain may accompany the abdominal pain in some cases. *Renal disorders* may sometimes cause right upper abdominal pain. Such pain is usually associated with flank or lumbar pain and

TABLE OF DISEASE INCIDENCE

INCIDENCE PER 100,000 (APPROXIMATE)

Common (>100)	Uncommon (>5–100)	Rare (>0–5)
Biliary colic	Drug-related and toxic hepatitis	Hepatic abscess
Cholecystitis	Ascending cholangitis	Hepatocellular carcinoma
Acute pancreatitis	Acute pyelonephritis	Budd-Chiari syndrome
Acute appendicitis	Renal tumor	Massive pulmonary embolism with hepatic congestion
Alcoholic hepatitis	Renal infarction	
Viral hepatitis	Herpes zoster	
Hepatic hemangioma and adenoma	Active duodenal ulcer and nonulcer dyspepsia	Pleuritis from pneumonia or infarction
Focal nodular hyperplasia		Hepatic hemorrhage in preeclampsia
Irritable bowel		Perforation of a duodenal or pyloric canal ulcer
Costochondritis		Acute corticomedullary abscess
Perihepatitis (Fitz-Hugh-Curtis) syndrome		Renal cortical abscess
Unknown causes		Perinephric abscess

tenderness. In *pyelonephritis, corticomedullary abscess,* and *perinephric abscess* there is usually pyuria and bacteriuria. In *renal infarction* there is hematuria. Ultrasonography or a CT scan will detect renal and perirenal abscesses and renal cysts, and tumors. An angiogram may be required to confirm a diagnosis of renal infarction. *Renal cortical abscess* is usually associated with a normal urinary sediment and a negative urine culture.

Some patients with acute right upper quadrant pain have no identifiable cause after ultrasonography and other tests are completed. Some of these patients may have small common duct stones, strictures, sphincter of Oddi spasm, or functional disease of the bowel. *Herpes zoster* may cause a burning or aching unilateral right upper quadrant pain that persists for 2 to 3 days before the typical herpetic rash erupts on the back, lateral chest wall, and right upper abdomen. The pain usually persists for days after the rash appears, and may be accompanied by pruritus.

☐ DESCRIPTION OF LISTED DISEASES

1. BILIARY COLIC

This disorder is caused by impaction of a gallstone in the cystic duct or in the lower end of the common bile duct. The pain may begin in the mid-upper abdomen and radiate to the right hypochondrium; or it may begin in the latter area and spread to the center of the upper abdomen or to the left hypochondrium. The pain begins abruptly and rises to maximum intensity in a few seconds or minutes, and then continues for 2 to 6 h. In some cases, waves of more intense sharp pain are superimposed on the continuous pain. The pain is severe to excruciating, and may be described as sharp, aching, squeezing, or pressurelike. A few patients prefer to lie still during the attack, but most move about in bed or move from the bed to a chair, trying to become more comfortable. Sweating, weakness, light headedness, nausea, and vomiting may accompany the attack. Meperidine usually brings relief in 1 to 2 h, or the pain may stop spontaneously. During the attack the patient may be pale and clammy, and the pulse rapid. A nontender fluctuant pear-shaped mass may be palpable in the right upper abdomen. Usually, right upper abdominal tenderness and guarding are not present, but deep tenderness may be present over the gallbladder in some cases. In general the diagnosis of cholelithiasis can be confirmed by real-time ultrasonography with a sensitivity of 95 percent, but this percentage may be lower in patients with ileus or during an attack of colic, if there is only one stone and it is impacted in the neck of the gallbladder. In most cases there is more than one stone. Recurrent biliary colic is currently being treated by laparoscopic or, less commonly, by open cholecystectomy.

2. ACUTE CHOLECYSTITIS

The first episode of acute cholecystitis may begin as a typical colic, as described above. After a variable period of 2 to 6 h the pain may stop for a short time, only to begin again, in the right hypochondrium. The pain is severe and may radiate around the right lower chest to the right subscapular area, or may be referred to the right shoulder.

Fever, chills, and sweats begin within 6 to 12 h, and temperatures as high as 102°F may occur. A temperature above 102°F suggests a complication, such as perforation or gangrene of the gallbladder. Nausea, vomiting, and right upper abdominal tenderness accompany the pain. In most cases there is direct and rebound tenderness over the gallbladder region, and muscle guarding in the tender areas. Murphy's sign is positive. In 40 percent of patients the gallbladder can be palpated, or its pear-shaped profile outlined by percussion.

Jaundice, with serum bilirubin levels below 4 mg/ 100 ml, may occur in up to 20 percent of patients. If the bilirubin level is higher, a common duct obstruction should be suspected. Leukocytosis (12,000–15,000 cells per mm^3) and elevated levels of serum aminotransferases, alkaline phosphatase, and amylase may be present. Sudden cessation of pain in the right hypochondrium and the gradual spread of pain, tenderness, and distension over the entire abdomen suggest perforation of the gallbladder and spillage of bile into the peritoneal cavity. Most attacks of acute cholecystitis continue for 5 to 10 days, and then gradually resolve. Intractable cases cause persistent pain and tenderness for weeks.

The diagnosis of acute cholecystitis may be established on clinical grounds. It is supported by specific findings on ultrasonography and/or cholescintigraphy. Sonographic criteria for the diagnosis of gallbladder disease include gallstones and/or nonvisualization, wall thickening, a sonographic Murphy's sign (gallbladder tenderness when compressed with the ultrasound probe), gallbladder distension (>5 cm), round shape, and pericholecystic fluid. Wall thickening correlates best with cholecystitis. The sensitivity of ultrasonography is 90 to 98 percent, and its specificity 70 percent. Administration of a radionuclide, such as DISIDA or HIDA, and scanning of the liver, gallbladder, and common ducts can help confirm a diagnosis of acute cholecystitis. In the presence of this disorder there is nonvisualization of the gallbladder at 4 h, while the bile ducts and duodenum contain radionuclide. Cholecystectomy may be done during the first week, or it can be deferred for 6 weeks, depending on the clinical picture and initial response to conservative therapy. Laparoscopic cholecystectomy can be performed in patients with acute cholecystitis.

3. ACUTE PANCREATITIS

Epigastric and right hypochondriac pain and tenderness occur. Guarding is minimal or absent. The pain is a constant severe ache or pressurelike sensation. Lying or sitting in a flexed position may provide partial pain relief, while hyperextension of the back may intensify the pain for some patients. Meperidine or other narcotic analgesics may be required for pain relief. Light-headedness, postural dizziness, vomiting, weakness, sweating, fever, and chills may accompany the upper abdominal pain. The weakness and dizziness are secondary to fluid loss by vomiting and to third-space fluid losses in the peripancreatic tissues. Dark urine (bilirubinuria) and jaundice may occur as the swollen head of the pancreas compresses the common bile duct. The first attack of this disorder may be due to alcohol abuse, cholelithiasis, choledocholithiasis, or other obstructing lesions (strictures, choledochoceles, pancreas divisum, sphincter spasm) of the common bile or pancreatic ducts. Rare cases of pancreatitis are associated with hypercalcemia or hypertriglyceridemia. The serum amylase level is usually elevated (70–92 percent of cases), as well as the serum lipase. The amylase elevation begins within 12 h of the onset of pain and persists for 4 to 7 days. Urinary amylase excretion is also usually increased, and elevated levels may persist longer than in the serum. A CT study will show pancreatic enlargement and, if necrosis is present, poor contrast enhancement of necrotic regions of the gland. Supportive therapy, with intravenous fluids, packed red blood cells, nasogastric suction, and, when appropriate, antibiotics, will usually lead to resolution of pain and tenderness in 5 to 10 days. Careful evaluation is required to prevent recurrent disease, which may lead to a lethal outcome. Such patients require a careful search for gallstones (by means of ultrasonography or an oral cholecystogram), duct obstruction (by means of endoscopic retrograde cholangiopancreatography [ERCP]), and metabolic causes (e.g., hypercalcemia, hypertriglyceridemia, and drugs).

4. ACUTE APPENDICITIS

This common disorder usually begins with a mild aching and cramplike upper midabdominal pain. Mild anorexia, nausea, and vomiting may accompany the pain. Within 2 to 4 h the midline pain may shift into the right upper abdomen in the region below the costal margin. Local tenderness and guarding may be present in the painful area. Within hours, rebound and cough-induced localized pain develop. The leukocyte count may rise to 12,000 to 14,000 cells per mm^3, and a fever of 100 to 101°F may develop. Exploration may be done for an acute cholecystitis, only to reveal acute appendicitis.

5. PAIN RELATED TO DISORDERS OF THE LIVER

A. Acute Hepatitis

1. Alcoholic Hepatitis   There is a history of chronic alcohol abuse. Patients with this disorder may gradually develop an aching constant right upper abdominal pain, and tenderness of the liver. Epigastric pain may occur as well. Vomiting, weight loss, fever, chills, and jaundice are common associated symptoms. Tender hepatomegaly (80–98 percent of cases), jaundice (35–80 percent), fever (20–50 percent), splenomegaly (10–40 percent), and ascites (25–75 percent) may be present. The SGOT (AST) level is elevated to the range of 100 to 300 U/L. The SGOT/SGPT (AST/ALT) ratio is usually between 2:1 and 5:1 in alcoholic hepatitis, while in viral hepatitis it is close to 1. The total AST does not usually exceed 3 to 10 times normal, while in viral hepatitis total activity is much higher. The serum bilirubin level is often elevated, but seldom exceeds 5 mg/100 ml. Modest elevations of the alkaline phosphatase level (1–3 times normal) usually accompany the elevated bilirubin. Serum albumin levels may range from 1 to 4.4 g/100 ml. There may be leukocytosis or leukopenia. Anemia and thrombocytopenia are common. A liver biopsy showing hepatocellular necrosis, a neutrophil infiltrate, neutrophil rosettes, alkaline hyaline (Mallory bodies), and stellate scarring will confirm the diagnosis in a setting of alcohol abuse. Slow healing over a period of 6 weeks to 10 months follows abstinence from alcohol. During the first few weeks in the hospital, 15 to 50 percent of patients may become worse clinically and chemically despite abstinence from alcohol. Prednisone (32 mg/day for 1 month), given orally, has been shown to accelerate resolution and prevent death.

2. Viral Hepatitis   Right upper abdominal pain of a constant or aching nature may occur in up to 65 percent of icteric patients. The pain may be intensified by jarring movements, and the liver is tender. Lying prone may provoke right upper abdominal pain because of pressure against the swollen and tender liver. Anorexia, lassitude, dark urine, fever, vomiting, myalgias, and headache are common associated symptoms. Some patients lose their desire for cigarettes and develop nausea at the smell of food. Vomiting is usually mild. Arthralgias and myalgias may occur in all types of viral hepatitis. Gray or yellow stools may be seen in 20 to 40 percent of cases; such stools are uncommon in alcoholic hepatitis. True arthritis, often accompanied by skin rashes, may precede the systemic symptoms of viral hepatitis by days or weeks in a small percentage of cases. Physical examination reveals hepatic tenderness and moderate hepatic enlargement, as well as an increase in liver firmness. The spleen is palpable in 5 to 15 percent of patients, and posterior cervical nodes may be enlarged. AST and ALT levels are usually in the range of 500 to 5000 U/L. Ratios of AST to ALT are usually 1 or less. Bilirubin levels seldom exceed 10 mg/100 ml, but higher values (above 20 mg/100 ml) have been reported. Liver biopsy is usually unnecessary, and may be difficult to differentiate from some forms of drug-induced hepatitis.

Acute hepatitis A infection can be confirmed by detecting hepatitis A virus IgM antibody (anti-HAV IgM). Acute hepatitis B infection can be diagnosed by detecting anti-HB core and HBe and HB_sAg in the serum. HB_sAg may occur in the serum 1 to 10 weeks after exposure to HBV, and 2 to 8 weeks before elevated aminotransferase levels develop. Anti-HBc IgM appears early and is later replaced by anti-HBc IgG, which may persist for months or years after recovery. Anti-HBs is the last antibody to appear; it usually follows, by weeks or months, the disappearance of hepatitis B surface antigen from the serum. An ELISA test is available to test serum for hepatitis C virus (HCV) in patients with non-A, non-B hepatitis. Elevated ALT levels may precede the appearance of anti-HCV antibody by 3 to 4 weeks. The sensitivity of this test for detection of HCV infection is unknown. In one report anti-HCV antibody was detected in 56 percent of donors whose blood produced non-A, non-B hepatitis in transfusion recipients. Delta agent, an incomplete virus associated with virulent hepatitis B disease, can be detected by serologic methods.

3. Drug-Related Hepatitis

A. ACETAMINOPHEN The clinical picture may mimic a severe acute viral hepatitis in patients with an overdose, or with ingestion of moderate doses in a setting of alcohol abuse. The aspartate aminotransferase level may exceed 5000 U/L, a level seldom found in viral hepatitis. Sodium acetylcysteine, given within 10 h of ingestion, may protect the liver against lethal injury.

B. OTHER DRUGS A number of commonly used drugs can cause hepatic necrosis and right hypochondriac pain, tenderness, and sometimes liver enlargement. Fever, chills, dark urine, and jaundice, as well as leukocytosis and elevated aminotransferase and alkaline phosphatase levels, are present. These reactions may mimic viral hepatitis, cholangitis, or acute cholecystitis. Such reactions occur in fewer than 1 percent of patients taking these drugs.

Methyldopa, isoniazid, valproate sodium, phenytoin, chlorpromazine and other phenothiazines, erythromycin, and ketoconazole are the drugs that have most commonly been associated with acute hepatotoxic and idiosyncratic reactions.

4. Toxins

A. MUSHROOM POISONING (AMANITA SPECIES) After ingestion there is a latent period of 6 to 20 h, followed by the sudden onset of generalized crampy abdominal pain, diarrhea, nausea and hematemesis, and progressive cardiovascular collapse. Patients surviving for 24 to 72 h may develop right hypochondriac pain because of a tender, swollen liver. Jaundice, hypoglycemia, oliguria, and a rising creatinine level follow. The mortality rate is 50 percent during the first week.

B. CARBON TETRACHLORIDE Toxicity results from inhalation or ingestion. The immediate symptoms are light-headedness, nausea, headache, and mental confusion. During the next 24 to 48 h the liver may become painful and tender, and jaundice and other abnormalities of liver function develop. Oliguric renal failure is frequently associated with the hepatic lesion. The urine contains albumin and red cells. Death may occur from hepatic or renal injury, or from toxic effects on the heart and central nervous system.

B. Hepatic Abscess

1. Pyogenic Abscess

This disorder causes spiking fevers, shaking chills (22 percent of cases), mild right upper abdominal pain of a constant aching quality, and hepatic tenderness. The liver is enlarged in 51 percent of cases, and jaundice may occur (28 percent). Anorexia (53 percent) and weight loss (14 percent) may also be part of the clinical picture. The white blood cell count may be normal, or may be as high as 65,000 cells per mm^3. The average white blood cell counts in two series were 14,000 cells per mm^3 and 21,000 cells per mm^3. The serum albumin may be less than 3 g/100 ml, and alkaline phosphatase (74 percent of cases) and bilirubin (40 percent) levels may be elevated. Aminotransferase levels are usually normal. Single or multifocal abscesses may be detected using real-time ultrasonography. Such lesions must be differentiated from simple cysts and necrotic metastatic tumor. CT with contrast usually clearly demonstrates abscesses as small as 1 to 2 cm in diameter. The usual etiologic agents are aerobic gram-negative rods, streptococci, staphylococci, and anaerobes.

These lesions are usually secondary to an infected focus in the biliary tract, large bowel (diverticulitis, appendicitis, colitis), small bowel (Crohn's disease), or pancreas (pancreatitis, abscess), or to systemic bacteremia. Liver trauma with necrosis, tumors, or cysts may give rise to a hepatic abscess. The diagnosis of a pyogenic abscess can be confirmed by a CT-guided needle aspiration, and in some cases by catheter drainage. The latter procedure or open surgical drainage is required for cure. Parenteral antibiotics should be given prior to drainage and for 3 to 6 weeks thereafter.

2. Amebic Abscess

This form of amebic infection occurs primarily in men (male/female ratio 9 to 1) who have recently traveled to an endemic part of the world (i.e., subtropics and tropics). There is right hypochondriac pain of a constant nature, and often localized liver tenderness over the abscess. Multiple lesions may be present. The right upper abdominal pain may be dull and aching, or sharp and sticking. It may be intensified by a deep breath and may be referred to the right shoulder. Fever (50 percent of cases) and cough (50 percent), may direct attention to the base of the right lung, where diaphragmatic elevation, atelectasis, or a pleural effusion may be found in 90 percent of cases. A single abscess, or several abscesses, may be clearly demonstrated by ultrasound or CT. Abscess aspiration and drainage is not required.

The leukocyte count and serum alkaline phosphatase levels are usually elevated. Agar gel diffusion, counterelectrophoresis, or an indirect hemagglutination test for amebiasis on the patient's serum will be positive in 90 to 100 percent of cases in the presence of invasive or extra-intestinal disease. Metronidazole therapy will usually bring about clinical improvement in 2 to 3 days, and the lesions will resorb without drainage in 90 percent of cases. Only 10 to 20 percent of patients pass amaebas in their stools. In patients with very large abscesses, drainage may be required. The abscess material has an "anchovy paste" appearance and contains inflammatory cells and debris. It is difficult to demonstrate amebas in the aspirated material; the diagnosis is seldom established by this procedure.

C. Hepatic Tumors with Rapid Growth, Bleeding, or Infarction

1. Malignant Tumors (Hepatocellular Carcinoma)
This disorder may begin with the sudden or gradual onset of right upper abdominal pain of a constant nature. Movement and respiration may intensify the pain. The liver may be enlarged and tender. In other patients fever may accompany the pain, simulating an attack of acute cholecystitis. Ultrasonography of the gallbladder and liver, or a contrast-enhanced CT, will detect the tumor. The serum alkaline phosphatase and alpha-fetoprotein concentrations are usually elevated; a level of the latter above 1000 pg/ml is diagnostic. The diagnosis can also be confirmed by laparoscopic, open surgical, or CT-guided fine-needle biopsy. It is important to do other imaging studies to rule out a highly vascular benign liver lesion, such as a hemangioma, adenoma, or focal nodular hyperplasia, before a needle biopsy is attempted.

2. Benign Tumors
Adenoma and hemangioma are both highly vascular, and may sometimes cause sharp continuous right upper abdominal pain because of rapid growth or as a result of intralesional bleeding. The pain may be intensified by respiration or jarring. An MRI study will usually correctly identify a hepatic hemangioma. Such lesions do not usually enlarge when followed by ultrasound over a period of months. A cavernous hemangioma also can be identified from its highly specific pattern during dynamic contrast-enhanced computed tomography. Adenomas occur almost exclusively in young women taking contraceptive pills. They are usually 8 to 15 cm in size, and may

cause hepatic pain and tenderness because of intrahepatic or intraperitoneal bleeding (10 percent of cases). Hepatic angiography is helpful in differentiating an adenoma from focal nodular hyperplasia. Adenomas are highly vascular lesions with a peripheral blood supply and a moderate amount of capillary blush. An intralesional hematoma is a specific CT finding. These lesions are more likely to cause pain and liver tenderness than focal nodular hyperplasia (FNH), and they are usually larger in size (i.e., 8–15 cm vs. 3–7 cm). The angiogram in focal nodular hyperplasia usually shows a diffuse capillary stain with a stellate pattern. Adenomas are usually approached at open surgery, biopsied, and resected with a margin because of the small, but real, risk that these lesions are slowly growing hepatocellular carcinomas or are precursor lesions. Many adenomas decrease in size when oral contraceptives are discontinued. None of the benign tumors described are associated with elevated levels of alpha-fetoprotein. Slight elevations of serum alkaline phosphatase and aminotransferase levels may occur in patients with necrotic or hemorrhagic adenomas. Resection of focal nodular hyperplasias and most hemangiomas usually is not necessary. A choledochal cyst is a rare hepatic lesion that may require surgical exploration for identification. This lesion may be a precursor of a cholangiocarcinoma. Unfortunately, removal of the cyst may not prevent the future occurrence of this malignancy, so continued surveillance is required.

D. Simple Obstructive Cholangitis (Ascending Cholangitis)
There may be severe right hypochondriac aching pain and tenderness associated with spiking fever, chills, dark urine, and scleral and cutaneous icterus. The alkaline phosphatase and bilirubin levels are usually elevated, and marked short-lived elevations of aminotransferase levels may occur. This disorder is secondary to common duct obstruction caused by a stone, tumor, cyst, or stricture. Duct obstruction by stones is the most common cause.

The responsible lesion can usually be identified by endoscopic retrograde cholangiopancreatography (ERCP). The fever, pain, and jaundice may clear spontaneously after 2 or 3 days, or may persist for 2 weeks or more. Some cases require 1 to 2 weeks of parenteral antibiotics for resolution of symptoms. A liver biopsy usually shows many neutrophils in the portal areas. Cases may occur in the absence of the gallbladder and detectable common duct stones or other obstructing lesions.

A more severe, and often fatal, variant of this disorder is acute suppurative cholangitis. There is severe right hypochondriac pain, tenderness, fever, rigors, and progressive jaundice. Sepsis, shock, and septic coma may follow. This disorder is associated with complete bile duct obstruction. Common duct drainage by T-tube or by ERCP and parenteral antibiotic therapy will reduce the mortality rate to 35 percent.

E. Hepatic Congestion

1. Budd-Chiari Syndrome

Hepatic vein thrombosis may begin with the abrupt onset of right and mid-upper abdominal pain in association with progressive abdominal distension caused by rapidly accumulating ascites. The pain is usually mild, but it may be severe and constant. The liver is enlarged and tender, and splenomegaly and jaundice may occur in up to 30 percent of cases. Elevations of serum aminotransferase and alkaline phosphatase levels frequently occur. The hepatic pain may be ascribed to alcoholic hepatitis or cirrhosis, and the diagnosis overlooked.

Real-time ultrasonography will detect the occlusion of one or more major hepatic veins. A contrast-enhanced CT study of the liver can detect hepatic venous occlusion and may demonstrate a nonhomogeneous liver parenchyma. Recently, MRI has been reported to be a useful imaging technique for the diagnosis of venous occlusion and the identification of venous collaterals and parenchymal abnormalities. Radionuclide scans may show a "central hot spot" due to caudal lobe hypertrophy. This lobe has a separate drainage to the vena cava and may be involved if the vena cava is occluded. Acute occlusion of the hepatic veins often does not allow the development of this radionuclide sign. Selective hepatic venograms show obliteration of one or more major hepatic veins and a "spider-web-like" tangle of venous collaterals. A liver biopsy may also suggest the diagnosis (e.g., centrilobular sinusoidal congestion and extravasation of red cells into the space of Disse). This disorder occurs in patients with polycythemia vera (10 percent of cases), and in others with a subclinical form of that disorder, after sudden cessation of anticoagulants; in patients with sickle cell disease, or lupus anticoagulant; and in patients with idiopathic membranous obstruction of the inferior vena cava. Cases also occur in users of oral contraceptives; in pregnancy; in antithrombin III deficiency; and in patients with circulating antiphospholipid antibodies. Hepatic tumors, abscesses (amebic), and cysts (e.g., hydatid) may cause enough compression to occlude the hepatic veins. The inferior vena cava may be invaded and occluded by a hepatocellular or renal carcinoma. Many of these space-occupying lesions can be detected by one of the imaging techniques used to examine the hepatic venous system. The hepatic pain and tenderness is usually relieved after a side-to-side portacaval shunt or a mesocaval shunt.

2. Acute Hepatic Congestion

This rare disorder may result from an acute massive pulmonary embolus that obliterates 50 to 75 percent of the pulmonary arterial tree. Pulmonary artery pressures rise abruptly and approach 40 mmHg. This sudden rise in pulmonary artery pressure is transmitted to the right ventricle and results in acute cor pulmonale. There is dyspnea, substernal pressurelike discomfort, apprehension, and hypotension. There may be right upper abdominal pain caused by an acutely congested liver. The external jugular venous pressure is elevated and a positive hepatojugular reflux sign is present. The liver is enlarged and tender. A loud pulmonary second sound, a right ventricular gallop, or a right ventricular lift is usually present. A chest radiograph may show enlargement of the pulmonary conus; a loss of pulmonary vascular markings may be present. A ventilation/perfusion lung scan will help establish the diagnosis. Such emboli may also be easily visualized on a contrast-enhanced cine CT study or a selective pulmonary angiogram. Thrombolytic therapy may be used as the initial treatment for this life-threatening disorder. If it is unsuccessful, surgical embolectomy can be attempted, but a 25 percent mortality rate accompanies this procedure.

F. Hepatic Hemorrhage in Preeclampsia

Severe constant right upper abdominal pain and tenderness may develop days to hours before delivery, or shortly afterward. The liver may be enlarged and tender, and elevated serum levels of alkaline phosphatase and aminotransferases may be present. These patients have hypertension and edema, and may have seizures. Acute anemia and thrombocytopenia often accompany the pain. A CT study of the abdomen will demonstrate an intrahepatic subscapular hematoma or diffuse bleeding and liver necrosis. Such hemorrhages may be treated expectantly with blood and clotting factor replacement, but they should be explored if they fail to stabilize.

6. GASTROINTESTINAL PAIN AND IRRITABLE BOWEL

A. Perforation of a Duodenal or Pyloric Canal Ulcer

There is abrupt onset of excruciating sharp epigastric and right hypochondriac pain. Within minutes the pain may spread into the lower abdomen and left upper quadrant. Right shoulder pain, intensified by movement or breathing, may occur. Patients with this disorder prefer to lie quietly. Moving from the bed to a chair, or to the bathroom, intensifies the pain; a patient with this disorder will walk slowly, splinting the abdomen with the hands. Immediately after perforation, there may be nausea and clammy pallor of the skin. The respirations accelerate and the pulse becomes weak and thready. There is diffuse direct and rebound tenderness, and guarding over the entire abdomen. Free air may be detected as resonance over the normal liver dullness, or on an upright or lateral decubitus film of the abdomen (sensitivity 75 percent). After 2 h or more the initial "shocklike" state may improve, giving false reassurance that all is well. There may be a recent history of epigastric pain relieved by food or antacids, or of daily use of aspirin or a nonsteroidal anti-inflammatory drug. The perforation can also be detected using a meglumine diatrizoate (Gastrografin) swallow to visualize leakage of the contrast material through the ulcer site. Exploration should be carried out as soon as possible to maximize the opportunity for survival.

B. Duodenal Ulcer and Nonulcer Dyspepsia A duodenal ulcer causes aching, gnawing, or burning right upper abdominal pain and tenderness relieved by antacids or H_2-blocking drugs. Food may intensify or relieve symptoms. Nocturnal pain is common. The diagnosis can be confirmed by endoscopy and/or a double-contrast gastrointestinal series. Nonulcer dyspepsia may cause similar symptoms, but only a normal duodenum or duodenitis will be found at endoscopy.

C. Irritable Bowel In persons with *irritable bowel syndrome,* severe right upper abdominal pain with minimal tenderness may mimic biliary colic. This syndrome is due to spasm or distension of a segment of upper small bowel. Nausea and vomiting may accompany the pain. There is no fever; the pain may abate in several hours, or may persist for days. Lower abdominal crampy pain may occur with the right upper abdominal pain, or at other times. Passage of flatus, or belching, may temporarily relieve the pain. The stool hemoccult test, sedimentation rate, hematocrit, and leukocyte count are normal. Upper and lower tract endoscopy and contrast radiographs are within normal limits, and an abdominal ultrasound study reveals no abnormalities of the liver, gallbladder, pancreas, or retroperitoneal area.

Diarrhea or constipation, or both, may occur; stools may be ribbon-, pencil-, or pellet-shaped. Psyllium hydrophilic mucilloid (Metamucil) or dicyclomine hydrochloride (Bentyl) may provide some relief. Avoidance of milk products may relieve symptoms in some patients who have lactase deficiency. This disorder is resistant to therapy and tends to improve or worsen spontaneously.

7. COSTOCHONDRITIS OF THE LOWER RIGHT ANTERIOR CHEST AND COSTAL MARGIN

There is moderate to severe aching pain over the right lower chest and right hypochondrium. The liver and subcostal area are not tender. Pressure-induced pain is present over the cartilages of the lower right anterior chest wall. A deep breath, or arm or body movement, may intensify the pain. Hooking the fingers under the costal margin and pulling outward may reproduce or intensify the pain. Real-time ultrasonography of the gallbladder and liver and a chest radiograph are both normal. Warm, moist compresses and a brief course of a nonsteroidal anti-inflammatory drug may provide partial relief. In some cases this disorder is refractory to treatment; the pain may persist or recur over a period of months or years.

8. PERIHEPATITIS DUE TO GONOCOCCAL OR CHLAMYDIAL INFECTION

Acute upper abdominal or right hypochondriac pain may occur in women with unilateral or bilateral lower abdominal pain, and/or vaginal discharge or bleeding. The upper abdominal pain may be intensified by jarring, coughing, bodily movement, or a deep breath. There is hepatic area tenderness and guarding. An acute cholangitis may be mimicked. An oral cholecystogram may fail to visualize the gallbladder, but an ultrasound study shows a normal stone-free gallbladder. Liver function tests are normal. Pelvic examination may show a mucopurulent cervicitis and bilateral or unilateral adnexal tenderness. Fever may be related to the perihepatitis or salpingitis. In some patients the lower abdominal symptoms are minimal, but usually there is tubal tenderness on pelvic examination. Laparoscopy done during the initial days of this disorder will show redness, edema, and a fibrinous exudate over the liver surface. Most cases are associated with chlamydial salpingitis; this organism has been cultured from the surface of the liver. It is essential to consider this disorder to prevent unnecessary surgery for nonexistent gallbladder disease. It may occur in up to 5 percent of women with pelvic inflammatory disease. Rare cases have been reported in males. There is a prompt response to antibiotic therapy with ceftriaxone and doxycycline. If treatment of the right upper quadrant pain is delayed, dense ''violin-string'' adhesions form; these may give rise to a chronic recurrent form of upper abdominal pain that is precipitated by exertion.

9. PLEUROABDOMINAL PAIN DUE TO PNEUMONIA OR ACUTE PULMONARY INFARCTION

An acute pulmonary disorder may give rise to acute right upper abdominal pain, direct tenderness, and guarding, mimicking acute cholecystitis. Cough, fever, chills, and pleuritic pain may be present. The sputum may be purulent, rust-colored, or gray-white, and mucoid; or it may contain clotted blood. Tachypnea may be present, and there may be abdominal distension secondary to a paralytic ileus. Right shoulder pain, intensified by a deep breath, can be present. Physical examination may reveal only rales and rhonchi over the right lower lobe posteriorly; or there may be dullness, bronchial breath sounds, and increased transmission of the whispered voice. A chest radiograph will detect a right lower lobe segmental or lobar infiltrate. A pulmonary embolus may be associated with a wedge-shaped infiltrate with its base on the pleura. This disorder can be confirmed by a ventilation/perfusion scan or by pulmonary angiography. In some patients with pneumonia, diffuse guarding and tenderness in the entire upper abdomen may necessitate surgical exploration. In most pulmonary cases with upper abdominal pain, a lower lobe segmental or lobar consolidation is present on the chest radiograph.

Antibiotic therapy will clear abdominal complaints related to pneumonia. Heparin and warfarin will allow healing of a pulmonary infarction and will usually prevent further embolization and thrombosis.

10. DISORDERS OF THE RIGHT KIDNEY

Uncommonly, renal disease may cause right hypochondriac pain. This may occur with an acute pyelonephritis, renal abscess, or perinephric abscess. A thrombotic or embolic infarction of the kidney may also cause right upper abdominal pain. In most cases there is associated flank and right lumbar pain or, at the least, right costovertebral angle tenderness. In some cases, right flank and lumbar pain and tenderness are associated with right hypochondriac tenderness without associated pain.

A. Acute Pyelonephritis   There may be right upper abdominal pain and tenderness associated with flank pain and costovertebral angle tenderness. Fever and chills may or may not be present. Frequency, urgency, dysuria, and nocturia call attention to the urinary tract. The urine may be foul-smelling and cloudy, and microscopic pyuria, and hematuria and bacteriuria are usually present. Leukocytes in the urine occur singly, in clumps and in casts. Most cases are due to *Escherichia coli*; there is a prompt response to antibiotic therapy.

B. Acute Corticomedullary Abscess   Such lesions occur at the corticomedullary junction, secondary to renal infection, and may be single (focal) or multiple (multifocal). The clinical findings are indistinguishable from those of acute pyelonephritis. The presence of an abscess can be demonstrated by ultrasonography (i.e., a poorly marginated sonolucent mass) and by CT with contrast (i.e., a wedge-shaped hypodense lesion). These lesions generally respond to intensive parenteral antibiotic therapy. Drainage may be required if there is no clinical improvement within 5 to 7 days. The urine sediment may be normal in up to 30 percent of cases.

C. Cortical Abscess (Renal Carbuncle)   There is usually a prior history of a skin lesion (e.g., carbuncle, furuncle, paronychia, cellulitis), endocarditis, or osteomyelitis. This disorder occurs predominantly in men (male/ female ratio 3 to 1). There is an acute onset of fever, chills, and upper abdominal and flank pain. There is flank and right upper abdominal guarding and tenderness, and in some cases a flank mass may be felt. Most patients have a negative urinalysis and urine culture, since the abscess usually does not communicate with the drainage structures. Ultrasonography will demonstrate the lesion as a semisolid or liquid cortical mass. The contrast-enhanced CT scan has replaced angiography as a method for differentiating these lesions from tumors. Flank and abdominal pain usually responds promptly to antibiotic therapy. Closed or open drainage of the abscess may be required, but some cases will resolve on medical therapy alone.

D. Perinephric Abscess   These abscesses usually arise from rupture of a renal abscess into the perinephric space; by spread from an adjacent area of infection; or, rarely, by hematogenous seeding.

Flank and right upper abdominal pain and tenderness, chills, fever, dysuria, nausea, vomiting, and sometimes weight loss occur. There is flank and costovertebral angle tenderness. Abdominal tenderness occurs in up to 60 percent of cases. Pain may be referred down the leg. A mass in the flank may be present. Leukocytosis, anemia, and sometimes azotemia (25 percent of cases) may occur. Pyuria and albuminuria are commonly present. Blood cultures are positive in 40 percent of cases. The diagnosis can be confirmed with high sensitivity by the use of ultrasonography or CT. Surgical drainage under cover of parenteral antibiotics will lead to resolution.

E. Renal Infarction Due to Embolus or Thrombus
There is a sudden onset of sharp, severe, unremitting pain in the flank and right upper abdomen, associated with tenderness in those areas. Fever begins within 48 h in severe cases, and nausea and vomiting may occur. Emboli occur in a setting of cardiac disease (e.g., atrial fibrillation, mitral stenosis, atrial myxoma, infective endocarditis, or a prosthetic valve), or after aortic surgery, intraaortic catheter manipulation, or the use of an intraaortic balloon catheter. The urine may be normal or may contain increased numbers of red cells. There is no pyuria or bacteriuria. There may be a marked rise in the serum levels of LDH and AST, secondary to renal necrosis. An intravenous pyelogram shows decreased or absent renal function on the painful side, while the retrograde pyelogram reveals no obstruction or structural abnormality. Renal angiography is required to establish the diagnosis. Some lesions may be treated with thrombolytic agents; angioplasty or surgical intervention may be necessary. Without specific therapy, the pain resolves spontaneously in 3 to 4 days.

F. Renal Tumor   Large renal tumors may invade the liver, diaphragm, and retroperitoneal area, causing right hypochondriac pain as well as flank pain and tenderness. The renal mass may be as large as a football and is easily palpable. Gross or microscopic hematuria is frequently present; the diagnosis can be readily established by a fine-needle aspiration or open renal biopsy.

11. UNKNOWN CAUSES OF ACUTE RIGHT UPPER ABDOMINAL PAIN

Every series of cases of right upper quadrant pain contains a group of patients who have negative ultrasonographic and other studies. The condition of these patients mimics that of those with acute biliary colic or cholecystitis. Some cases may be caused by a passed (no longer present) gallstone; others by common duct sphincter spasm and high ductal pressures; and still others by pleurodynia or a functional bowel disturbance. Long-term follow-up may establish the correct diagnosis.

12. HERPES ZOSTER

Burning or aching unilateral pain that radiates around the upper trunk to the abdomen may be caused by herpes zoster. During the first 2 to 3 days of the illness visceral disease, such as cholecystitis, may be simulated; but the ipsilateral appearance of grouped vesicles and red-based crusted ulcers, in a band-shaped determatome at the level of the pain, establishes the diagnosis.

Acute Epigastric Pain

☐ SUMMARY

Perforation of a peptic ulcer begins with the explosive onset of severe epigastric pain, diaphoresis, pallor, and faintness. Within minutes the pain spreads over the entire abdomen; there is generalized abdominal tenderness and rigidity. Free air under the diaphragm can be detected in 60 to 85 percent of cases and is confirmatory. Leakage of swallowed diatrizoate meglumine (Gastrografin) into the peritoneal cavity will also confirm the diagnosis.

Perforation of a duodenal ulcer occurs 16 times more frequently than that of a *gastric ulcer. Stomal ulcer perforation* is rare.

Bleeding into a liver tumor (e.g., adenoma, hemangioma, carcinoma), *into the hepatic parenchyma,* and/or *into the hepatic subcapsular area in preeclampsia* causes severe constant epigastric or right upper abdominal pain and tenderness. A CT scan or MRI can help delineate the cause of hepatic hemorrhage. Confirmation may require surgical exploration or a CT-guided fine-needle biopsy of the lesion. Rupture of the hepatic capsule may unleash heavy and potentially exsanguinating hemorrhage into the free peritoneal cavity. Generalized upper abdominal tenderness may be associated with pallor and shock.

Hepatitis or *sudden vascular congestion of the liver due to acute pulmonary embolism* can cause epigastric and right hypochondriac pain and tenderness. The liver is usually firm, tender, and enlarged in hepatitis and in acute vascular congestion. When liver congestion is present, the jugular venous pressure is elevated and hepatojugular reflux can be demonstrated.

Acute pancreatitis usually occurs in patients with a history of gallstones or alcoholism. There is severe epigastric and right and/or left hypochondriac pain associated with moderate to severe tenderness, but minimal muscle guarding, in the upper abdomen. Postural dizziness and hypotension may occur. The serum and urine amylase levels are elevated, and the diagnosis can sometimes be supported by CT findings related to the pancreas.

Biliary colic causes very severe epigastric and right subcostal pain, with nausea and vomiting, that persists for up to 6 h and then spontaneously subsides. Real-time ultrasonography demonstrates *cholelithiasis.* A similar painful syndrome lasting 24 h or more and associated with fever, chills, sweats, severe right hypochondriac tenderness, and positive real-time sonographic and DISIDA studies is caused by *acute cholecystitis.*

Cholecystitis occurring in debilitated patients in an intensive care unit in the absence of gallstones (*acalculous cholecystitis*) can be detected by real-time ultrasonography or CT. *Gallbladder rupture* may occur 3 to 5 days after the onset of cholecystitis. When this complication occurs, the persistent pain of cholecystitis suddenly abates for 6 to 12 h, but the fever does not. Within 24 h, generalized abdominal pain, direct and rebound tenderness, guarding, and ileus develop because of bile—and possibly because of an infectious peritonitis. Common duct stones cause typical biliary colic, which may be associated with pruritus, jaundice, and, sometimes, chills and fever due to *ascending cholangitis.*

Acute appendicitis begins with mild aching epigastric pain, anorexia, nausea, and vomiting. The upper abdominal pain then shifts to the right lower abdomen. Well-localized tenderness is present over McBurney's point. Rebound tenderness and guarding may also occur in this area. Leukocytosis is usually, but not always, present. *Acute myocardial infarction* may cause epigastric pain and tenderness, and is associated with electrocardiographic and cardiac isozyme abnormalities.

Intestinal obstruction at the level of the proximal ileum causes true *intestinal colic* associated with vomiting, obstipa-

tion, and distension. A flat plate and upright radiograph of the abdomen will show air-fluid levels in distended loops of small bowel. There is only minimal abdominal tenderness present during bouts of colic. During each attack of pain, rushes of high-pitched bowel sounds occur; these sounds cease when the pain-free period begins. A *closed-loop obstruction* causes severe constant epigastric pain without even brief pain-free intervals. Initially, such pain is usually not associated with local tenderness or guarding. Closed-loop obstruction should be suspected when the abdominal pain is very severe relative to the physical signs. Within 8 to 24 h abdominal tenderness, a mass, and ascitic fluid may appear. *Mesenteric vascular occlusion* occurs in older patients with vascular disease or atrial fibrillation. There is a sudden onset of excruciating upper midabdominal pain and vomiting, associated with few physical findings. An aortogram and selective study of the superior mesenteric artery will reveal an occlusion due to a thrombus or an embolus, or a patent vessel (i.e., *nonocclusive ischemia*). *Mesenteric venous occlusion* causes similar symptoms, although there is an increased incidence of bloody diarrhea when the venous system is occluded. The diagnosis of mesenteric venous occlusion can be confirmed by selective arteriography. Risk factors for this disorder include use of oral contraceptives; polycythemia vera; essential thrombocytosis; abdominal sepsis; and portal hypertension.

Gastric volvulus causes extreme epigastric pain, vomiting, retching, and hematemesis. The distended stomach can be seen on a plain abdominal radiograph, straddling the diaphragm, trapped in a paraesophageal hernia.

Pyloric obstruction causes epigastric fullness, pain, and vomiting in patients with a long ulcer history. Vomiting

TABLE OF DISEASE INCIDENCE

INCIDENCE PER 100,000 (APPROXIMATE)

Common (>100)	Uncommon (>5–100)	Rare (>0–5)
Hepatitis	Perforation of a duodenal ulcer	Perforation of a gastric or stomal ulcer
Acute pancreatitis	Liver adenoma or hemangioma	Hepatic hemorrhage in preeclampsia
Biliary colic	Acalculous cholecystitis	Acute hepatic congestion
Acute cholecystitis	Rupture of the gallbladder	Acute myocardial infarction
Intestinal obstruction (open-loop)	Ascending cholangitis	Gastric volvulus
Acute indigestion	Closed-loop obstruction of small intestine	Hepatocellular carcinoma
Acute gastroenteritis	Esophageal rupture	
Drug-related gastritis	Mesenteric ischemia due to arterial occlusion	
Peptic ulcer (gastric or duodenal)	Nonocclusive mesenteric ischemia	
Nonulcer dyspepsia	Mesenteric venous occlusion	
Acute appendicitis	Pyloric obstruction	

relieves the distress. The same symptom in an older patient without a history of peptic ulcer may be caused by a gastric malignancy.

Acute indigestion causes severe epigastric pain, fullness, belching, and nausea, and is relieved by spontaneous or self-induced vomiting. *Acute gastroenteritis* is often associated with epigastric and more generalized abdominal crampy pain, fever, nausea, vomiting, and watery diarrhea. Certain drugs (e.g., nonsteroidal anti-inflammatory drugs and aspirin) cause epigastric pain that is usually made worse by eating. These drugs cause an erosive *gastritis* as well as gastric ulceration. *Ulcer and gastritis (nonulcer dyspepsia)* may cause epigastric pain relieved by food and antacids.

Boerhaave's syndrome begins with substernal or left precordial aching or pleuritic pain that follows an episode of forceful vomiting. Dyspnea, mild hematemesis, dysphagia, fever, and cold-water polydipsia may be associated complaints. Subcutaneous emphysema, pneumothorax, pleural effusion, and mediastinal emphysema may be detected on physical examination and/or by a plain chest radiograph. Hamman's sign occurs in 20 percent of cases. Subcutaneous and mediastinal emphysema separate this disorder from the major thoracic catastrophes (e.g., myocardial infarction, dissecting aneurysm, and pulmonary embolism) and abdominal catastrophes (e.g., perforated ulcer, acute pancreatitis, and mesenteric thrombosis) that it may mimic. The diagnosis can be confirmed by a contrast esophagogram. Other causes of esophageal rupture include endoscopy, instrumentation, foreign bodies, and underlying esophageal disease.

☐ DESCRIPTION OF LISTED DISEASES

1. PERFORATION OF A PEPTIC ULCER

A. Perforation of a Gastric or Duodenal Ulcer There is an abrupt onset of sharp, constant, often excruciating epigastric pain that spreads downward in a few minutes to involve the entire abdomen. Some patients may writhe in agony and cry out for relief. Faintness, pallor, weakness, sweating, and syncope may accompany the pain. Pain may be felt in one or both shoulders, and this discomfort may be intensified by a deep breath. Changing position and walking are very painful. Such patients move slowly and gingerly, splinting their abdomens with their hands. They usually prefer to lie quietly and avoid unnecessary movement. Coughing or a deep breath will usually intensify their discomfort. Up to 35 percent of patients with perforation give no history of prior epigastric pain or give only a brief history (i.e., less than 3 months) of recurrent epigastric pain that may or may not be relieved by food and antacids. A large proportion (up to 80 percent, in a series of elderly patients) have a history of ingesting nonsteroidal anti-inflammatory drugs, aspirin, or corticosteroids for the treatment of ''arthritis.''

The physical examination reveals generalized direct and rebound abdominal tenderness that is sometimes, but not always, maximal in the epigastrium. There is marked abdominal muscle spasm and rigidity, producing a ''board-like abdomen.'' Vomiting or retching is frequently present during the first hour. Rectal examination reveals generalized pelvic tenderness. The pulse and respirations are usually normal early in the course of the disorder, but in some cases they may be accelerated. During the first 12 h there is usually no fever, or only a slight one. The blood pressure may be initially normal, but with the passage of several hours it may begin to fall because of fluid losses resulting from vomiting or exudative third-space losses into the peritoneal cavity. The bowel sounds eventually become inaudible. Resonance may be detected over the region of normal liver dullness; this finding is very significant if present in the right midaxillary line, in the zone beginning at the costal margin and extending 2 to 3 in. cephalad. An upright chest or left lateral decubitus radiograph will detect ''free air'' (pneumoperitoneum) in 60 to 85 percent of cases. Some small perforations may rapidly reseal and not allow much free air to pass into the peritoneal cavity. A diatrizoate meglumine (Gastrografin) swallow will allow determination of whether the perforation is open or has already closed. In one series, 30 to 40 percent of perforations were no longer open by the time the patients were first examined.

In some cases the severe initial pain may become less intense after 1 to 2 h, and both patient and physician may be fooled into believing that all is well and that the worst has passed. The initial pallor, sweating, and skin coldness may improve. Despite these favorable changes in the skin and in the patient's overall appearance, severe generalized abdominal tenderness, muscle guarding, and an absence of bowel sounds persist as evidence of a developing peritonitis. The leukocyte count, serum amylase level, pulse, and temperature rise. Most patients reach the operating room within 12 h (mean time was 9 h in one series). Within 12 h ileus, ascites, and severe hypovolemic hypotension appear. Respirations become rapid and shallow, and the temperature rises.

Surgical risk increases with the presence of other medical conditions; preoperative shock; and delay of surgery beyond 24 h. With none of these risk factors present, the surgical mortality rate is negligible; with one risk factor present it is 10 percent; with two, it is 45 percent; and with three factors it is close to 100 percent. The mortality rate for duodenal perforation (duodenal/gastric perforation ratio, 15 to 1) is 0 to 10 percent, while the mortality rate for gastric ulcer perforation is 10 to 40 percent. Volume resuscitation to replace fluid losses and intravenous antibiotics are important supportive measures that should be initiated prior to surgery.

Duodenal ulcer perforation may be treated by closure with an omental patch and a parietal cell vagotomy to prevent ulcer recurrence. Simple closure, without a definitive anti-ulcer procedure, is frequently performed on patients with one or more risk factors, or with only brief histories of ulcer symptoms (i.e., acute ulcer).

Juxtapyloric gastric ulcers are treated by closure, truncal vagotomy, and pylorplasty, or by truncal vagotomy and resection. Ulcers at the incisura can be treated by a Billroth I gastrectomy. Prepyloric ulcers can be treated by resection and truncal vagotomy. Parietal cell vagotomy is ineffective in preventing gastric ulcer recurrence.

B. Perforation of an Anastomotic (Stomal) Ulcer
Stomal ulcers may perforate into the free peritoneal cavity. Such patients should be suspect for a gastrinoma. Simple closure should be used for high-risk, unstable patients. Others should be treated by definitive surgical procedures (i.e., vagotomy or re-vagotomy and gastric resection or re-resection) designed to prevent a future recurrence of anastomotic ulceration.

2. BENIGN AND MALIGNANT LIVER TUMORS WITH BLEEDING INTO THE TUMOR OR INTO THE FREE PERITONEAL CAVITY AND HEPATIC HEMORRHAGE DURING PREGNANCY

A. Adenoma and Other Benign Tumors   Bleeding into a hepatic tumor may be signaled by the sudden onset of moderately severe, constant aching epigastric pain. The pain may be intensified by inspiration or jarring, and there may be local epigastric tenderness. Nausea and vomiting may be associated symptoms. The pain is usually constant and may radiate to the right or left upper abdomen. Bleeding into a benign *adenoma* usually occurs in women who are taking oral contraceptives. *Focal nodular hyperplasia* and *benign hemangioma* are other benign lesions that occur predominantly in women, and may be the site of bleeding. Tumor infarction and necrosis may cause a similar pain.

B. Hepatocellular Carcinoma   Hepatocellular carcinoma is associated with the male sex (2 to 3 times more common in males than in females), a hepatitis B surface antigen carrier state (prevalence with tumors in China and Korea, 85–95 percent; in the United States, 10 percent), cirrhosis, geographic location (e.g., Asia and Africa), and age over 40. Local bleeding and/or necrosis of such tumors can also cause acute epigastric pain.

If the liver capsule ruptures, hemorrhage from a benign or malignant tumor can spill into the free peritoneal cavity, causing an exsanguinating hemoperitoneum. If this occurs, tachycardia, tachypnea, and hypotension begin abruptly in association with epigastric and generalized abdominal pain, shoulder pain, and abdominal tenderness. The abdominal examination will show rigidity and guarding, and tenderness may be present throughout the pelvis.

Rapidly bleeding tumors require immediate surgery for control. Leaking and slowly bleeding lesions can be demonstrated by ultrasonography, CT with contrast enhancement, or MRI. The latter procedure may aid in differentiating a hepatocellular carcinoma from a metastatic carcinoma or a benign hemangioma. An elevated serum alpha fetoprotein level (i.e., >20 ng/ml) provides some evidence that the bleeding lesion is a hepatocellular carcinoma. Bleeding benign lesions may require surgical resection; carcinomas may be cured if they are small or have a fibrolamellar histology.

C. Intrahepatic and Subcapsular Hemorrhage in Preeclampsia   A severe, steady right hypochondriac and/or epigastric pain may occur in women with preeclampsia, either before or shortly after delivery. The pain is associated with local guarding and tenderness, and hypertension. Shortly after the onset of pain a fall in the hematocrit and platelet count usually occurs, and liver function tests become abnormal. CT scans in such patients reveal multiple areas of intrahepatic, as well as subcapsular, hemorrhage. Such patients can be treated by careful observation and blood replacement, but surgical intervention may be required if severe bleeding continues.

3. ACUTE ENLARGEMENT OF THE LIVER DUE TO HEPATITIS OR VASCULAR CONGESTION

Pain occurs in the epigastrium and right hypochondrium. It is constant and aching and is associated with enlargement, increased firmness, and tenderness of the liver. In patients with hepatitis there is a prodromal period of several days during which fever, myalgias, anorexia, nausea, and vomiting occur. In some cases of hepatitis A, and many cases of hepatitis B, macular or urticarial rashes and joint pains precede the symptoms of liver disease by 1 to 3 weeks. Loss of appetite is often associated with a decreased desire for cigarettes and aberrations of taste and smell. Upper respiratory symptoms, such as a cough, sore throat, and coryza, may also occur. The liver ache may be intensified by jarring or coughing, but usually is not severe enough to require narcotics for analgesia. Several days after the onset of upper abdominal pain and constitutional symptoms, bilirubinuria and jaundice usually occur. The serum aminotransferase, AST (SGOT), and ALT (SGPT) levels rise initially, preceding the rise in serum bilirubin. Peak levels may range from 400 to 4000 U/L for the aminotransferases; the bilirubin level may exceed 20 mg/100 ml. Type A viral hepatitis is associated with poor hygiene, water- and food-borne epidemics, and intravenous drug abuse. Type B hepatitis is associated with blood transfusions, homosexuality, intravenous drug abuse, promiscuous heterosexual activity, and a national origin in Africa, China, Korea, or Southeast Asia. Non-A, non-B hepatitis is transmitted primarily by transfusions, but cases are associated with drug abuse, intra-family contact, occupational contact, and water-borne outbreaks in third world countries. Delta agent hepatitis has been associated with drug abuse.

Sudden acute epigastric and right hypochondriac pain, associated with liver enlargement and tenderness, severe dyspnea, neck vein distension, cyanosis, a positive hepatojugular reflux test, and sometimes a right ventricular gallop rhythm, may occur with acute pulmonary hypertension (as in acute cor pulmonale), because of massive pulmonary embolism. Recent surgery or delivery, leg immobilization, prolonged car or air travel, or a history of heart failure or malignant disease may be associated with such emboli. The diagnosis can be supported by a ventilation/perfusion scan of the lung and confirmed by a pulmonary angiogram.

4. ACUTE PANCREATITIS

Pain of a knifelike, or aching and boring, quality in the midepigastrium begins over a period of minutes and becomes constant. It may radiate to the left hypochondrium, and sometimes to the right. Referred pain may be felt in the left shoulder. Pain may also be experienced in the back, directly behind the epigastrium. Anorexia, nausea, and vomiting usually accompany the pain; there may be postural dizziness and weakness, and even transient syncope, secondary to a rapidly progressive hypovolemia. Fever may or may not be present at the onset; if not present it may soon develop. Some severely ill patients present with supine hypotension, pallor, and cyanosis, which gives them an ashen-gray appearance.

The pain may be mild, or may be so severe that an intraabdominal catastrophe is mimicked and injections of narcotics provide only partial relief. Some patients with less severe pain may note that sitting hunched forward or lying in a flexed fetal position provides partial relief, while hyperextension of the spine may intensify their discomfort. Once the pain begins, it persists for 3 to 10 days. Bouts of sharper and more severe stabbing or boring pain may be superimposed on the constant background pain. There is frequently a prior history of biliary colic, cholecystitis, asymptomatic gallstones, or alcohol abuse. A variable proportion of patients (10–30 percent) have no known risk factor for this disorder. Rare cases have been associated with hyperlipoproteinemia types I, IV, and V. Such patients develop hypertriglyceridemia prior to the attack. Such cases may be controllable by a low-fat diet and other measures. Hypertriglyceridemia may also result from pancreatitis and alcoholism; this type of secondary lipid disturbance must be differentiated from the genetic lipoprotein disorders that may precipitate acute pancreatitis.

Attacks may be precipitated by trauma; excessive ingestion of meat; gastric, biliary, or splenic surgery; and drugs, such as corticosteroids, thiazides, antimetabolites, and sulfonamides. The relationship of hyperparathyroidism to rare cases of acute pancreatitis is controversial. Some authorities consider cases with this association entirely explainable by an associated cholelithiasis or alcoholism.

The physical examination may reveal tachycardia, fever in the range of 100 to 102°F, and orthostatic or supine hypotension. There is mid- and left epigastric tenderness and, sometimes, upper umbilical area tenderness. There may be mild to moderate voluntary guarding in the tender area. The bowel sounds may be active or diminished. Moving about or changing position does not intensify the pain, as it does when a perforated ulcer is present.

The serum amylase level is usually elevated within 12 h of onset, and remains abnormal for 3 to 5 days. In some series, 8 to 32 percent of patients have had normal serum amylase levels in the presence of other evidence of pancreatitis. Amylase levels are highly variable, with one-third of the values below 200 U/L, another third between 200 and 500 U/L, and the final third with values greater than 500 U/L. Determination of the total amylase content in a 2-h urine collection is also a useful confirmatory test. The amylase/creatinine clearance ratio test, once proposed as highly specific, has been discarded because of its high false-positive rate and its lack of superiority to serum and urinary amylase determinations. Direct confirmation of pancreatic inflammation can be obtained from a CT study of the upper abdomen. However, in one study where patients were examined within 48 h of onset, only 64 percent of the CT scans provided good to excellent visualization of the pancreas. In 29 percent of these patients the pancreas appeared normal (false-negative); in 28 percent the gland alone was enlarged; and in an additional 25 percent there was pancreatic enlargement and edema of the peripancreatic fat. Eighteen percent of patients had a phlegmon (boggy, edematous, inflamed retroperitoneal connective tissue), most frequently extending into the lesser sac and left anterior pararenal space. Hemorrhagic necrotizing pancreatitis was identified by decreased pancreatic contrast enhancement during the CT scan. Other complications, such as hemorrhage, pseudocyst formation, and abscess, were also detectable by CT.

Grey Turner's sign and Cullen's sign are rare, and delayed in appearance when they do occur. Radiologic signs, such as the colon cutoff and "dilated sentinel jejunal loop," are rare. These signs are seldom of use in diagnosis, because of their low sensitivity. Hyperglycemia and glycosuria are confirmatory, but they are rarely present in the absence of an elevated amylase level.

Acute epigastric pain and hyperamylasemia may be caused by other intraabdominal disorders. An upright chest radiograph may reveal free air under the diaphragm because of ulcer perforation. An abdominal flat plate may show evidence of a closed-loop obstruction. Ultrasonography may show evidence of gallstones and enlargement of the gallbladder. Acute perforation of an ulcer, small bowel strangulation or vascular infarction, and acute cholecystitis are important mimics of pancreatitis that may be associated with hyperamylasemia.

Therapy for pancreatitis involves careful fluid, electrolyte, and colloid replacement, and administration of packed red blood cells for severe anemia. Nasogastric suction may be required for nausea, vomiting, or a developing ileus, but patients with an uncomplicated course can be treated without it. Swan-Ganz catheterization may be useful for the fluid management of patients with cardiopulmonary disorders. Hyperglycemia can be managed with regular insulin, while hypocalcemia seldom requires treatment. Early exploratory surgery may increase mortality and is now usually avoided. Fewer than 5 percent of patients with acute pancreatitis come to surgery.

5. PAIN ARISING IN THE GALLBLADDER AND BILE DUCTS

A. Acute Biliary Colic   There is a rapid increase, over a period of minutes, in the intensity of an epigastric and right subcostal aching or pressurelike pain, which soon becomes constant and severe. Superimposed jabs of sharper pain may occur at irregular intervals. The pain may radiate around the side of the lower right chest into the right subscapular area, and sometimes to the tip of the right shoulder. In up to 10 percent of cases it may radiate to the left upper abdomen. Nausea, vomiting, and diaphoresis frequently accompany the pain. Meperidine injections provide partial relief, but the pain usually subsides spontaneously in 2 to 6 h. Attacks appear to be more frequent during the night and after a large evening meal, but this is not always the case. A variable interval of weeks or months may occur between the initial attack and subsequent ones. During an attack there is epigastric tenderness and voluntary muscle guarding. These findings disappear shortly after the pain subsides.

Gallstones are present in up to 10 percent of adults. Obesity, multiple pregnancies, constitutional factors (as in Pima Indians), hemolytic anemia (i.e., pigment stones), cirrhosis, ileal resection, and ileal disease are associated with cholelithiasis. Ultrasonography will reveal evidence of cholelithiasis.

In many medical centers laparoscopic cholecystectomy has replaced open cholecystectomy for the treatment of symptomatic cholelithiasis and cholecystitis. Right upper quadrant and right shoulder pain lasting 24 to 72 h, due to retained intraperitoneal gas, occurs commonly after laparoscopic cholecystectomy. The advantages of laparoscopic cholecystectomy include low morbidity and mortality. Complications include bile duct injury, cystic duct bile leak, and abscess secondary to an intraperitoneal gallstone.

B. Acute Cholecystitis   Severe, constant, aching or pressurelike right hypochondriac and epigastric pain occurs. After 4 to 6 h this pain may abate for 2 to 3 h, only to begin again. Nausea, vomiting, chills, and fever occur, and a temperature between 100 and 102°F persists. The pain may radiate to the right subscapular and interscapular region and may be referred to the tip of the right shoulder. Dark urine (bilirubinuria) and scleral icterus may occur. There is direct and rebound tenderness and guarding in the right upper abdomen; an enlarged, tender, distended gallbladder may be palpated or percussed in 20 to 40 percent of cases. A polymorphonuclear leukocytosis, with total leukocyte counts above 12,000 cells per mm^3, is usual. Bilirubin levels are most often less than 4 mg/100 ml, and there may be a marked rise in the serum amylase level in the absence of pancreatitis (i.e., values in excess of 1000 U/L may occur).

Real-time ultrasonography is usually the initial imaging technique used to visualize the gallbladder in patients with suspected acute cholecystitis. Major criteria for an abnormal gallbladder include gallstones and nonvisualization (i.e., no fluid containing lumen and shadowing in the gallbladder fossa). Minor criteria include gallbladder wall thickening (i.e., >5 mm), tenderness of the gallbladder when compressed with the probe (sonographic Murphy's sign), gallbladder enlargement (>5 cm in any dimension), a round gallbladder shape, and evidence of fluid adjacent to the gallbladder. The use of both major and minor criteria for diagnosis increases the sensitivity of the procedure to between 90 and 98 percent. The use of only major criteria for cholecystitis increases specificity to between 94 and 98 percent. The use of both major and minor criteria decreases specificity to 70 percent.

A cholescintigram, using ^{99m}Tc disopropyl iminodiacetic acid (DISIDA), will usually fail to visualize the gallbladder in 1 to 4 h in patients with cystic duct obstruction and acute cholecystitis. This test can be used to confirm the presence of acute cholecystitis. It has a sensitivity of 95 to 97 percent and a specificity of 90 to 97 percent. False-positive results may occur in patients with prolonged fasting (e.g., patients with alcoholism or on parenteral nutrition, or those who are critically ill) and in patients with hepatitis or pancreatitis. Some authors report a high false-positive rate in patients with chronic cholecystitis.

Laparoscopic cholecystectomy can be used for the treatment of acute cholecystitis. Less than 10 percent of patients undergoing this procedure require conversion to open cholecystectomy. Criteria for preoperative endoscopic retrograde cholangiography (ERC) include a dilated common duct, jaundice, a history of cholangitis or associated acute pancreatitis, multiple small stones in the gallbladder, and an inflamed gallbladder without stones in a patient with a history of biliary colic. ERC can be used preoperatively to detect common duct stones and remove them. This procedure may also be used to remove stones detected by intraoperative cholangiography during laparoscopy.

C. Acute Acalculous Cholecystitis   This potentially lethal disorder occurs in elderly persons and in debilitated patients in intensive care units. Such patients are most commonly victims of severe trauma, extensive burns, a prolonged postoperative course after major thoracic or abdominal surgery, or a protracted medical illness (e.g., sepsis or gastrointestinal bleeding). Fever and tachycardia may be the only symptoms, or there may be epigastric and right hypochondriac pain and tenderness. It is believed that this disorder is related to an increase of bile viscosity due to stasis (e.g., from fasting), cystic duct edema and obstruction facilitated by fluid overload, a fall in oncotic pressure from hypoalbuminemia, and a decrease in gallbladder perfusion. Other cases of acalculous cholecystitis have occurred in AIDS patients and have been attributed to a combined gallbladder infection with cytomegalovirus and a cryptosporidium species. Some elderly patients may present with acute cholecystitis without stones.

Real-time ultrasonography has a sensitivity of 92 percent, and a specificity of 96 percent, for the diagnosis of this disorder. Wall thickening, pericholecystic fluid, and subserosal gallbladder edema are the major useful diagnostic findings that have been associated with positive ultrasonographic diagnoses.

In one small series, CT proved to be 100 percent sensitive and specific for the diagnosis of acalculous cholecystitis. Major criteria for the diagnosis were wall thickening beyond 4 mm; pericholecystic fluid; subserosal edema; intramural gas; and sloughed mucosa.

Aspiration of bile, and culture and a Gram-stained smear for the presence of bacteria and leukocytes, was only 33 percent sensitive in one series. Hepatobiliary scintigraphy was highly sensitive (95 percent), but had a low specificity (38 percent) because of the patients' usual state of prolonged fasting and liver dysfunction. Cholecystectomy is the treatment of choice, but many cases have required tube cholecystostomy because the former procedure would not have been tolerated. Up to 48 percent of patients may have gangrene, and 7.5 percent have perforation of the gallbladder, at the time of surgery.

D. Acute Perforation of the Gallbladder   There is an initial illness consisting of epigastric and right subcostal pain and tenderness (biliary colic and cholecystitis), fever, chills, nausea, and vomiting; this progresses over a period of 2 to 3 days. Sudden relief of the upper abdominal pain between days 3 and 6 may signal gallbladder rupture. If this has occurred, there is a continuation of fever and leukocytosis, with a gradual development over the next 12 to 24 h of generalized abdominal pain and tenderness

associated with a reflex ileus, abdominal distension, and ascites. The course of gallbladder perforation and subsequent generalized peritonitis is much slower and less dramatic than that associated with ulcer perforation. The sudden and welcome relief of the upper abdominal pain after rupture is often perceived as an improvement, until the development of generalized peritonitis becomes apparent during the subsequent 24 h.

E. Acute Choledocholithiasis, Common Duct Obstruction, and Cholangitis   Pain occurs in the epigastrium and right hypochondrium, and is often referred to the right shoulder tip and/or the right subscapular and interscapular region. This pain is similar in its severity and constancy to that produced by stone impaction in the cystic duct. Nausea and vomiting may occur; meperidine may provide temporary partial relief of the discomfort. If the common duct stone succeeds in passing through the sphincter of Oddi, the pain will dramatically vanish. If it does not, and common duct obstruction occurs, then dark amber urine, scleral icterus, and cutaneous jaundice will develop. Pruritus may be an early symptom, and the stools may take on a pale yellow-white or gray color.

The development of chills, rigors and spiking fever, generalized hepatic pain and tenderness, and more severe jaundice suggests ascending cholangitis. The diagnosis of choledocholithiasis can be suspected from the finding of a dilated common duct by ultrasonography or CT.

Endoscopic retrograde cholangiography can be used to detect common duct stones and remove them before or after laparoscopic cholecystectomy.

6. ACUTE APPENDICITIS

A diffuse epigastric or upper umbilical area ache develops. The pain is crampy or constant, and mild to moderate in intensity. Sharper, more intense pain may be superimposed for short intervals. After 3 to 4 h the midline upper abdominal pain shifts to the right lower abdomen, becomes constant, and localizes there. The upper abdominal discomfort is accompanied by loss of appetite and nausea. Vomiting may occur in some cases. Fever to 101° may begin after right lower quadrant localization has been present for several hours. The total leukocyte count is usually above 12,000 cells per mm³, but may be normal even in the presence of perforation.

Some patients do not have upper abdominal midline pain; their first symptoms are anorexia and right lower abdominal pain. In other patients the midline pain shifts to the right lumbar area (retrocecal appendicitis), hypogastrium (pelvic appendicitis), or left iliac area (long pelvic appendix).

Physical signs include direct, and sometimes rebound, tenderness at McBurney's point, with or without involuntary guarding. Coughing causes localized intensification of pain at McBurney's point, as does walking. These stimuli will also cause pain intensification at the pain sites described above for retrocecal and pelvic appendicitis. Plain radiographs may detect an appendicolith, a finding supportive of the diagnosis of appendicitis, but imaging techniques are not reliable enough for surgical decision making. The barium enema, often used to rule out appendicitis in children, may give false-negative results. A CT study may be useful to define the location and extent of a periappendiceal abscess or phlegmon. The treatment for acute appendicitis is prompt appendectomy.

7. ACUTE MYOCARDIAL INFARCTION

Steady aching discomfort begins in the upper epigastrium. Localized tenderness, without guarding, may accompany the pain. Diaphoresis, weakness, nausea, and vomiting may be present. The heart rate may be slower than 60 beats per minute; or tachycardia, frequent premature contractions, and an S_3 gallop may be present. Some patients report a history of prior episodes of substernal or epigastric pain that are precipitated by exertion or excitement and relieved, within minutes, by rest. An electrocardiogram and/or serum CPK and LDH isozyme measurements will usually confirm the diagnosis of acute myocardial infarction. If the onset of the pain was less than 4 h before arrival at the hospital, rapid pain relief may follow the use of thrombolytic therapy and/or coronary angioplasty.

8. INTESTINAL OBSTRUCTION

A. Acute Small Bowel Obstruction (Open-Loop) Obstruction of the jejunum or upper ileum can give rise to colicky epigastric pain. Initially there may be a constant epigastric discomfort, but this soon is replaced by an intermittent colic-type pain. Midepigastric pain occurs, lasting 2 to 3 min. It is associated with high-pitched, loud, metallic-sounding bowel sounds, which occur in rushes during the pain. Pain-free periods last 4 to 5 min; during this time, the bowel sounds are diminished or absent. Examination of the epigastrium during an attack of colic reveals minimal muscle guarding and tenderness. Between attacks the same area is relaxed, soft, and not tender. Vomiting begins shortly after the onset of colic and persists. Evacuation of stool and gas from the rectum may occur at first, but obstipation ensues. The vomitus in upper small bowel obstruction may contain bile, but it is

never feculent. If treatment is not initiated, the abdomen distends and a generalized constant abdominal ache replaces the attacks of intermittent colicky pain.

Strangulation and bowel perforation may occur at any time after the first 6 h. The absence of localized pain and tenderness, fever, tachycardia, and leukocytosis is no guarantee that strangulation has not occurred. On the other hand, the presence of one or more of these findings does not necessarily indicate the presence of strangulation. The accuracy of diagnosis on clinical grounds has been less than 70 percent, with many false-positive and false-negative diagnoses of bowel necrosis.

Radiologic studies are useful in establishing a diagnosis of upper small bowel obstruction. Dilated loops of small bowel, with air-fluid levels and decreased colon gas, support a diagnosis of small bowel obstruction. Differentiation of paralytic ileus from mechanical obstruction may be required in postoperative patients. Barium given by enteroclysis is very useful; it will demonstrate dilated segments and mucosal abnormalities above the point of mechanical obstruction, as well as the site of the block.

Some surgeons may treat partial or complete intestinal obstruction, when there are no clinical signs of gangrene, with a 24- to 48-h trial of tube decompression using nasogastric or long intestinal tubes. Patients less likely to progress to strangulation are those with early postoperative obstruction or obstruction that is due to adhesions or associated with Crohn's disease. Other causes of small bowel obstruction include intrinsic small bowel tumors or metastatic tumors (e.g., ovarian carcinoma) and incarcerated inguinal or femoral hernias.

B. Closed-Loop Small Bowel Obstruction with Early Strangulation Patients with this condition experience abrupt onset of severe, constant, aching epigastric or upper umbilical pain, sometimes accompanied by nausea and vomiting. The pain remains constant; there are no cycles of pain-relief-pain, as there are in patients with the usual type of open-loop intestinal obstruction. The physical examination during the first day may be unremarkable except for pallor, diaphoresis, and cool skin. The abdomen is usually nontender, and there is no voluntary or involuntary guarding. The pulse, temperature, and blood pressure are usually normal. Despite these negative findings the patient appears acutely ill, and may be writhing in pain like a victim of renal or biliary colic. During the first 12 to 24 h plain abdominal radiographs may begin to show dilated loops of small bowel, with air-fluid levels. Local tenderness in the upper abdomen, leukocytosis, and low-grade fever may develop. Ultrasonography may reveal ascitic fluid and a dilated U-shaped loop of bowel with a thickened wall. Patients with these findings should be resuscitated with fluid and electrolytes, and explored to resect the gangrenous bowel and restore the continuity of the small bowel. Bowel entrapment, in surgical adhesions, rare internal hernias, and external hernias, are the most frequent causes of closed-loop obstruction.

C. Mesenteric Vascular Occlusion

Older males (i.e., those in the 45 to 75 age range) are at highest risk for this disorder. There is often a history of coronary heart disease with angina or myocardial infarction, as well as cardiac arrhythmias (e.g., atrial fibrillation). In other cases there may be intermittent claudication, a history of abdominal angina (up to 33 percent of cases), or a prior cerebro-vascular accident or transient ischemic attack.

The onset is abrupt, with severe aching or pressurelike pain in the epigastrium or upper umbilical area. The pain may be colicky during the first hour, but then becomes very severe and constant. Vomiting occurs; diarrhea may soon follow. The stool may be grossly bloody, or may contain only occult blood. A mottled cyanosis of the limbs and abdomen may occur in some patients. During the first few hours there may be minimal abdominal tenderness or muscle guarding. Patients may writhe in pain. They have cool, clammy skin and look severely ill, yet the abdominal signs remain minimal and fail to explain the overall appearance. As gangrene progresses there appear fever, peritoneal signs, ascites, and distension due to a paralytic ileus. A tender abdominal mass may become palpable.

The leukocyte count, serum amylase level, and hematocrit may be normal or elevated. Plain abdominal radiographs may show only dilated loops of large and small bowel during the first 6 to 12 h. An aortogram and selective angiography should be done as soon as possible (i.e., within 4 to 6 h of onset) in patients with severe constant upper abdominal pain and minimal signs who are in the age- and/or disease-defined risk groups for this disorder.

Occlusion of the superior mesenteric artery by thrombus usually occurs in the proximal 3 cm of the vessel, while embolic occlusion occurs more distally. Selective study of the superior mesenteric artery may demonstrate a more distal occlusion or patent vessels (nonocclusive mesenteric ischemia). Such studies may diagnose mesenteric vein occlusions as well. Some cases of bowel infarction are due to splanchnic vasoconstriction associated with low cardiac output or hypovolemia; vasoconstricting drugs (digitalis, dopamine, diuretics, beta blockers, or vasopressin); sepsis; or recent cardiac surgery.

Thrombi and emboli require urgent surgery, bowel resection, and revascularization by embolectomy or by use of bypass procedures for proximal thrombi; these procedures should be preceded and followed by infusion of vasodilators, such as tolazoline or papaverine.

D. Nonocclusive Mesenteric Ischemia

This disorder is currently being treated by intravenous infusion of tolazoline and papavarine, with surgical exploration for patients who fail to respond clinically within 6 to 12 h.

E. Mesenteric Venous Occlusion

Venous occlusion with bowel infarction is accompanied by a severe constant epigastric midline pain like that caused by the above disorders; and by diaphoresis, weakness, vomiting, a falling blood pressure, and tachycardia. Bloody diarrhea may occur. Tenderness and distension may develop over the first 6 to 12 h. The leukocyte count and hematocrit are markedly elevated. Radiographic studies show dilated loops of small bowel with air-fluid levels and ascitic fluid. Surgical resection followed by the use of heparin is recommended. This disorder has been associated with thrombocytosis, polycythemia, the use of oral contraceptives, intraabdominal suppuration, and cirrhosis with portal hypertension.

9. ACUTE DISORDERS OF THE STOMACH

A. Volvulus

Gastric volvulus may occur as an acute disorder in persons with large paraesophageal hernias. The initial symptoms are severe epigastric pain, upper abdominal distension, retching, and sometimes hematemesis. Plain radiographs of the abdomen may show marked dilatation of the distal stomach above the diaphragm, and of the fundus below. It may be impossible to pass a nasogastric tube. If the esophagogastric area is passable, nasogastric suction or endoscopy may decompress the volvulus; but surgery is required to prevent recurrence and possible gastric strangulation and infarction. The paraesophageal hiatal hernia should be repaired to prevent life-threatening recurrence.

B. Pyloric Obstruction

This disorder produces epigastric fullness and pain after eating. Loss of appetite, nausea, and vomiting may occur; involuntary or self-induced vomiting temporarily relieves all symptoms. The patient may have a long history of duodenal ulcer disease. The onset of this symptom complex in a patient without a prior ulcer history is more ominous, and may be due to a carcinoma of the juxtapyloric region of the stomach. The cause of these obstructive symptoms can be determined by gastrointestinal contrast studies and/or endoscopy. Surgery is usually required.

C. Acute Indigestion

Severe constant epigastric distress with radiation to one or both sides of the chest, associated with nausea and frequent belching, may occur after the excessive consumption of large amounts of spicy and/or rich food, and/or alcoholic beverages. Spontaneous or self-induced vomiting usually provides nearly intantaneous relief.

D. Acute Gastroenteritis

Dull and aching, or sharp, epigastric pain, nausea, and vomiting occur. Diarrhea and crampy pains in different regions of the lower abdomen develop. Fever and chilliness, as well as headaches, myalgias, and malaise, may occur. Most of these infections are viral and occur in the summer and early fall. Symptomatic therapy is all that is required; the illness usually abates in 2 to 5 days.

E. Acute Drug-Related Gastritis Epigastric pain of a mild aching nature, sometimes intensified or precipitated by food ingestion and poorly relieved by antacids, may be caused by ingestion of an irritant drug, such as aspirin, a nonsteroidal anti-inflammatory compound, penicillin, or erythromycin. Nausea, and sometimes vomiting, may occur as an associated complaint. Withdrawal of the drug and the use of sucralfate usually relieve the symptoms.

F. Acute Ulcer Syndrome and Nonulcer Dyspepsia Epigastric pain of an aching or gnawing quality, relieved by food, milk, or antacids, may begin suddenly. Such pain usually occurs between meals and during the night, waking the patient from sleep. It may improve after several days of therapy with an H_2-blocking drug, antacids, or sucralfate.

Such pain may be caused by a duodenal ulcer, some distal gastric ulcers, and even some ulcerated carcinomas of the stomach. Many patients with this type of pain do not have an ulcer on endoscopic evaluation, but may have duodenitis or gastritis. Associated complaints can include epigastric fullness, bloating, and belching. Recent studies have related some cases of nonulcer dyspepsia to infection of the gastric mucosa with *Helicobacter pylori* (formerly *Campylobacter pylori*). In one published series, symptoms responded to a trial of bismuth and an antibiotic, both of which possessed anti–*Helicobacter pylori* activity. This organism may have a significant role in the pathogenesis of some cases of gastritis and duodenal ulcer.

10. ESOPHAGEAL RUPTURE—BOERHAAVE'S SYNDROME AND OTHER CAUSES

Nausea and forceful vomiting are followed, within a brief period, by the abrupt onset of substernal or left precordial pain (70 percent of cases). Pain may also occur in the epigastrium, left shoulder, and upper back. The substernal pain has been variously described as a tightness, a pressure, and a dull ache. The precordial and back pain may be dull and aching, or pleuritic. Associated symptoms include dyspnea (50 percent of cases—related to pleuritis, pneumothorax, or pleural effusion), mild hematemesis (50 percent), fever (11–50 percent), odynophagia or dysphagia (<10 percent), and cold-water polydipsia (<10 percent).

Physical examination may reveal tachycardia, tachypnea, fever, and hypotension (25 percent of patients may be in a shocklike state); or all vital signs may be normal. Subcutaneous emphysema may first appear in the supraclavicular fossae in up to 33 percent of cases. It is a late

sign, and develops 6 to 18 h after the onset of pain. Decreased breath sounds and/or rales may be heard over the left posterior chest because of a pneumothorax and/or a pleural effusion. Hamman's sign, described as a crackling, bubbling, or crunching substernal noise that is synchronous with cadiac contraction, may be heard in up to 20 percent of cases, and is related to the presence of a pneumomediastinum. Rarely, a pericardial rub may be audible because of a purulent pericarditis related to mediastinal infection. There may occur direct tenderness in the epigastrium and lower chest, and epigastric rigidity and rebound tenderness, mimicking a perforated ulcer. To confuse the clinical picture further, in up to 5 percent of cases there may be free air under the diaphragm.

The plain chest radiograph may demonstrate a pneumomediastinum along the left border of the heart, the aortic arch, and the descending aorta. The "V" sign of Naclerio may be present in 20 percent of cases. This is a V-shaped radiolucent shadow formed by air dissecting the fascial planes of the mediastinum and pleura. A left lower lobe infiltrate and effusion may be present, as well as a pneumothorax or hydropneumothorax. The presence of subcutaneous and/or mediastinal air differentiates spontaneous esophageal rupture from more common causes of anterior chest pain, such as myocardial infarction, pulmonary embolism, aortic dissection, and acute pericarditis. Abdominal disorders often confused with esophageal rupture include perforated ulcer, mesenteric occlusion, a ruptured subphrenic abscess, an incarcerated diaphragmatic hernia, and acute pancreatitis.

The diagnosis can be confirmed in as many as 90 to 95 percent of cases by a diatrizoate meglumine (Gastrografin) swallow, which will demonstrate leakage of the contrast material into the mediastinum or left pleural cavity. Endoscopy and/or barium swallow have been used to detect rupture in a suspected case after a negative diatrizoate meglumine swallow.

Pain and physical findings are usually substernal or left-sided, but right chest pain, pneumothorax, and effusion may occur in small numbers of cases.

CT scanning has been used to evaluate a patient too ill or uncooperative for a contrast study of the esophagus. The CT scan may demonstrate a mediastinal hematoma, air and/or abscess, pleural fluid, and a pneumothorax. The pleural fluid is dark-brown and sometimes foul-smelling. It is an exudate with a high salivary amylase concentration (90 percent of cases) and a pH below 6 (50 percent), and often contains food particles.

The classic story of postemetic chest and/or epigastric pain associated with the development of subcutaneous emphysema and/or pneumomediastinum occurs in 50 to 65 percent of cases. In other cases there may be no history of vomiting, or, rarely, no pain. Some cases of esophageal rupture occur in a setting of severe asthma, childbirth, severe coughing or hiccups, weight lifting, or food bingeing; during dialysis; or after a Heimlich maneuver. Some cases of esophageal rupture are related to endoscopy, esophageal instrumentation, trauma, and foreign bodies. Underlying esophageal diseases, such as stricture, carcinoma, achalasia, and paraesophageal hernia, may lead to rupture. Controversy exists as to the optimal therapy. Immediate surgical exploration, esophageal closure, and mediastinal lavage and drainage are advocated by some authors; others claim good results with conservative medical management, using total parenteral nutrition, antibiotics, fluid replacement, and chest tube drainage.

18 Acute Left Hypochondriac Pain

☐ DIAGNOSTIC LIST

1. Disorders of the spleen
   A. Splenic rupture
   B. Splenic infarction
   C. Splenic abscess
   D. Splenic artery aneurysm and bleeding
2. Peptic ulcer disease—gastric or duodenal ulcer, or nonulcer dyspepsia
3. Acute gastric dilatation
4. Acute gastric volvulus
5. A. Acute biliary colic
   B. Acute cholecystitis
6. Acute pancreatitis
7. Left subphrenic abscess
8. Disorders of the colon

   A. Functional disease
   B. Acute diverticulitis
   C. Carcinoma of the splenic flexure or upper descending colon
   D. Colitis
9. Disorders of the kidney
   A. Renal cortical abscess
   B. Perinephric abscess
   C. Renal infarction
10. Jejunal diverticulitis or perforation
11. Pleuritis secondary to left lower lobe pneumonia or infarction
12. Costochondritis

☐ SUMMARY

Splenic rupture causes diffuse upper abdominal pain or left hypochondriac pain and tenderness, associated with tachycardia, hypotension, and cool, pale, moist skin. Computerized tomography (CT) will confirm intraabdominal bleeding and splenic disruption. Often this is omitted, as the patient is taken directly to surgery. Sharp, sticking, left upper abdominal pain, made worse by breathing, in a patient with a myeloproliferative disorder, sickle cell disease or trait, or endocarditis, is likely to be due to *splenic infarction*. *Splenic abscess* causes left upper abdominal pain and tenderness, splenomegaly, chills, and fever. Rupture of a *splenic artery aneurysm* causes left

hypochondriac pain and tenderness, and hypovolemic shock. A CT study will visualize a splenic abscess, and may identify a splenic artery aneurysm and intraperitoneal bleeding. *Ulcer disease* and *nonulcer dyspepsia* cause left upper abdominal pain that recurs 1 or more times each day, and is relieved by food, antacids, H_2 blockers, or sucralfate. In some cases, eating intensifies or precipitates the pain. *Acute gastric dilatation* causes severe, sharp left upper abdominal pain, tenderness, tympany, and distension. A shocklike state may develop. A plain abdominal radiograph will show massive dilatation of the stomach with a gastric air-fluid level. Passage of a nasogastric tube and gastric suction reverse all symptoms and signs. *Acute gastric volvulus* causes severe left upper abdominal pain, tenderness, and distension. A water-soluble-contrast swallow shows severe distension of the stomach with both an intrathoracic and an intraabdominal portion of the organ. Symptoms and signs resolve after tube or endoscopic decompression of the obstructed stomach. *Acute biliary colic* causes constant, severe, aching left upper abdominal pain and mild tenderness. A real-time ultrasound study shows gallstones. Usually the acute pain is relieved by injectable analgesics, or resolves spontaneously within 2 to 6 h. Continuation of this pain for 1 or more days, in association with fever, chills, anorexia, and sometimes jaundice, indicates the presence of *acute cholecystitis*. Up to 10 percent of cases have left, rather than right, upper abdominal pain, with biliary colic or acute cholecystitis. *Acute pancreatitis* is usually associated with alcohol abuse or cholelithiasis. The pain is epigastric and left upper abdominal, and is associated with hypotension, nausea, and vomiting. The serum and urine amylase levels rise, and CT of the abdomen usually shows pancreatic swelling and peripancreatic edema. A *left subphrenic abscess* occurs 3 to 6 weeks after bowel or biliary surgery; splenectomy; pancreatitis; or perforation of the stomach, duodenum, or colon. There is left upper abdominal pain, tenderness, left shoulder pain, and a fixed elevated left diaphragm with atelectasis or pneumonia of the left lower lobe. Left pleuritic pain may accompany the upper abdominal pain and tenderness, and may be associated with a moderate-sized left pleural effusion.

Aching pain in the left upper abdomen, with minimal or absent tenderness, is usually due to *functional disease*. This pain may continue for many hours each day, or constantly for weeks or months. Such pain is often relieved by passage of flatus or stool. There are no associated positive findings on physical examination or on laboratory tests. *Acute diverticulitis* is very rare in the upper abdomen. It can cause pain, tenderness, and fever. The diagnosis can be confirmed by a CT scan and barium enema, done 1 week after the initiation of therapy to prevent perforation and leakage. *Carcinoma of the colon* can cause crampy upper abdominal pain due to partial obstruction, or can perforate, causing constant upper abdominal pain and tenderness and/or a tender mass. *Colitis* causes diarrhea, passage of blood or bloody mucus, and left anterolateral abdominal pain and tenderness. The various types of colitis can be differentiated by a barium enema and/or colonoscopy. A *renal cortical or perinephric abscess* may cause left upper abdominal and flank pain. The urine may or may not contain white blood cells and bacteria. A CT scan will define these lesions in the kidney or in the perinephric space. *Renal infarction* may result from emboli arising in the wall of the heart or aorta, or from an infected heart valve. There is sharp, severe left upper abdominal pain, tenderness, hematuria, and fever. An arteriogram will confirm the diagnosis, showing poor renal perfusion and an occlusion of the main renal artery or one of its branches. *Jejunal diverticuli* may become inflamed, or may perforate; they can cause constant left upper abdominal pain and tenderness. Enteroclysis will usually demonstrate the diverticulum and any perforation. Surgical exploration, resection

TABLE OF DISEASE INCIDENCE

INCIDENCE PER 100,000 (APPROXIMATE)

Common (>100)	Uncommon (>5–100)	Rare (>0–5)
Peptic ulcer and nonulcer dyspepsia	Splenic rupture	Splenic abscess
Acute biliary colic	Splenic infarction	Splenic artery aneurysm with rupture
Acute cholecystitis	Left subphrenic abscess	Acute gastric dilatation
Acute pancreatitis	Pneumonia or infarction of the left lower lobe	Acute gastric volvulus
Functional disease of the colon	Lupus pleuritis	Diverticulitis of upper descending colon
Colitis (ischemic, ulcerative *Clostridium difficile*, and granulomatous)	Pleural tuberculosis	Perinephric abscess
	Carcinoma of upper descending colon	Jejunal diverticulitis
Costochondritis (left lower chest)	Renal cortical abscess	
	Renal infarction	

of the diverticulum, and abscess drainage may be the most efficient approach to diagnosis and therapy for this disorder.

Left upper abdominal pain and tenderness, as well as guarding, may be caused by a left lower lobe *pneumonia* or *pulmonary infarction*. A careful chest examination will reveal a poorly mobile, high left diaphragm, and/or signs of consolidation at the left base. A chest radiograph will detect an infiltrate, consolidation, and/or pleural fluid in the left lower thorax. Lupus or tuberculous pleuritis may present in a similar manner. *Costochondritis* causes aching left lower anterior chest pain with no underlying pulmonary or abdominal disorder. There is marked tenderness over the affected costal cartilages; precipitation of typical pain by the hooking maneuver is highly suggestive of this disorder.

☐ DESCRIPTION OF LISTED DISEASES

1. DISORDERS OF THE SPLEEN

A. Splenic Rupture   Sharp and severe pain occurs in the upper abdomen (67 percent of cases) or in the left hypochondrium (33 percent). Usually the onset is abrupt and follows blunt or penetrating trauma. Diseased spleens may rupture spontaneously, or after trivial trauma. Left shoulder pain (Kehr's sign) may occur because of diaphragmatic irritation. Placing the patient in a Trendelenburg position may provoke left shoulder pain. Some weakness and faintness on sitting and standing, as well as pallor and sweating, accompany the pain. Moving about or coughing may intensify it. The pulse is usually rapid and thready, and the blood pressure low. Respirations may be accelerated. The skin is pale, cool, and moist. Direct and rebound tenderness, as well as guarding, is usually present in the left upper abdomen, and a vague mass may sometimes be palpable in the left subcostal region.

Splenic rupture from blunt trauma usually occurs in an automobile or motorcycle accident, or after a fall; it may occur in a sledding or bicycling mishap. A clue to splenic injury is a fracture of the lower three ribs in the left posterolateral chest. Spontaneous rupture of the spleen can occur during weeks 2 to 4 in patients with infectious mononucleosis, but this complication is very rare. The spleen may also rupture in malaria. Isolated case reports have reported spontaneous rupture in patients with large splenic abscesses, chronic leukemia, polycythemia vera, sarcoid, Gaucher's disease, and chronic hemolytic anemia. The diagnosis of rupture with intraabdominal bleeding can be confirmed by an abdominal CT study. The presence of abnormal vital signs and an acute abdomen with peritoneal signs requires surgical exploration; this is usually undertaken on clinical grounds without waiting for a CT study.

Up to 15 percent of patients with severe blunt trauma to the left upper abdomen or posterolateral chest may develop signs of rupture within 1 to 6 weeks of their injury. A CT study done after the original injury can detect a subcapsular hematoma in the spleen prior to its rupture.

B. Splenic Infarction   There is an abrupt onset of a sharp, stabbing left upper abdominal pain, sometimes with left shoulder pain, that may be intensified by breathing. The pain is mild to moderate in intensity, and is lessened by shallow breathing. Infarction occurs in patients with large spleens (e.g., patients with myeloid metaplasia or chronic myelogenous leukemia); with sickle cell disease or trait; with mural thrombi in the heart; and, in some cases, with infectious endocarditis. There may be left subcostal tenderness, with or without guarding; a tender spleen tip; and, rarely, a splenic friction rub. An infected embolus can cause fever and chills, in addition to pain. The diagnosis of infarction can be confirmed by CT or by magnetic resonance imaging (MRI).

C. Splenic Abscess   There is a gradual onset of left upper abdominal pain and tenderness, which may be intensified by deep breathing. The pain may also radiate to the left lower chest. Chills, fever, and diaphoresis occur, suggesting the presence of an infectious process. The pain may be dull and aching, but once a pleuritic component is present it becomes intense and sharp. The spleen may be palpable and tender, or there may be only vague left upper abdominal tenderness. Splenic abscess may result from generalized bacteremia, endocarditis, infected emboli, penetrating trauma, or contiguous spread from a subphrenic or perinephric abscess. Splenic abscess may be a cause of early relapse after treatment for endocarditis. The

abscess can usually be visualized on a radionuclide, ultrasound, or CT scan. Abnormal physical signs and radiographic changes may occur in the left lower chest because of diaphragmatic elevation, atelectasis, and pleural effusion. Parenteral antibiotic therapy should be initiated promptly, and should be followed by splenectomy. This disorder can be highly lethal unless it is promptly and correctly treated.

D. Splenic Artery Aneurysm and Bleeding   More than 90 percent of splenic artery aneurysms are asymptomatic and small, and are discovered only as incidental findings at autopsy. If such an aneurysm begins to bleed, there is an abrupt onset of severe, aching or sharp, left upper or generalized upper abdominal pain. Referred pain to the left shoulder may also occur. Weakness, faintness and dizziness (especially on standing), pallor, and sweating soon develop. The pain is not relieved by any specific measures, but it may be intensified by deep breathing, coughing, or movement. Bleeding from a splenic-artery aneurysm is more common in women than men, and occurs with increased frequency during pregnancy. Tachycardia, tachypnea, and orthostatic or supine hypotension rapidly develop. There is left upper abdominal tenderness and guarding, or more diffuse upper abdominal tenderness. The aneurysm may be palpable, but seldom is; splenomegaly may be present. A bruit may be audible in the left upper abdomen, but this is nonspecific and is heard most commonly because of splenic-artery tortuosity. Eggshell-thin calcification seen on a plain radiograph may outline the aneurysm in up to 15 percent of cases. A real-time ultrasound or abdominal CT scan may identify the aneurysm, or the diagnosis may go unconfirmed until laparotomy is performed. Angiography will define the aneurysm most accurately, if there is time for this study. Some aneurysms are detected during abdominal angiography performed for other reasons. Lesions of 3 cm or larger should be excised. Despite exploration, up to 75 percent of patients with ruptured aneurysms die in hemorrhagic shock. These lesions have been found in up to 10 percent of autopsies, but fewer than 10 percent of all splenic aneurysms are likely to bleed. Rupture into the free peritoneal cavity causes diffuse abdominal pain, guarding, and distension, as well as shock. Rupture into the bowel or pancreatic duct produces massive hematemesis and melena.

All hope for survival depends on prompt blood and fluid replacement, isolation and resection of the aneurysm, and/or splenectomy.

2. PEPTIC ULCER DISEASE—GASTRIC OR DUODENAL ULCER, OR NONULCER DYSPEPSIA

Pain in the left hypochondrium occurs in up to 5 percent of patients with these disorders. The pain is most often described as an aching, burning, or gnawing discomfort. Gastric ulcer and duodenal ulcer pain may be intensified within seconds after ingestion of food. Alkalis, H_2-blocking drugs, and sucralfate relieve the pain associated with these forms of peptic disease. Antacids work immediately, while improvement with the other drugs may require 2 to 3 days of therapy. Nocturnal pain occurs in one-third to one-half of all patients, and is nonspecific. Most patients find relief by ingesting milk, ice cream, or antacids, and are able to return to sleep. Pain, if relieved by food, often recurs 1 to 3 h after meals. These disorders usually occur in clusters, 1 to 3 times a year. During these periods daily pain occurs for weeks or months, or until effective therapy is begun. Anorexia, nausea, weight loss, vomiting, pyrosis, bloating, and belching occur with similar frequency in all three disorders. In some patients, epigastric and left hypochondriac pain occur together; pain radiation to the midback or left lower posterior chest may occur. The diagnosis of gastric or duodenal ulcer disease can be confirmed by a double contrast barium meal or endoscopy (sensitivities 80 to 85 percent and 95 percent, respectively). Negative studies in the presence of the above-described symptoms suggest the diagnosis of nonulcer dyspepsia.

3.   ACUTE GASTRIC DILATATION

Severe, sharp pain and distension occur in the epigastrium and left hypochondrium. The onset is sudden and may be associated with belching, nausea, and vomiting. The left upper abdomen becomes distended and tympanitic, and there is generalized upper abdominal tenderness. A succussion splash may be noted. Generalized weakness, faintness on standing, and pallor occur. Hypotension, sweating, and a fall in the serum sodium and potassium levels may develop. A plain radiograph will demonstrate massive dilatation of the stomach with an air-fluid level. If untreated, attacks of vomiting may lead to aspiration and pneumonia. This disorder follows anesthesia; surgery; trauma; the application of body casts; severe pneumonia; diabetic ketoacidosis; the use of anticholinergics; and excessive food ingestion in patients with anorexia nervosa. The marked increase in intragastric pressure results in very severe left upper abdominal pain, which, if not treated by insertion of a nasogastric tube connected to suction, can result in gangrene of the gastric wall and perforation.

4.   ACUTE GASTRIC VOLVULUS

There is severe, constant epigastric and left upper abdominal pain and distension, frequent vomiting, and retching, with delivery of saliva rather than gastric contents. It is impossible to pass a nasogastric tube past the distal esophagus. Double air-fluid levels may be seen in the left upper abdomen on a plain radiograph. A water-soluble-contrast swallow may show obstruction of the distal esophagus, or may demonstrate the volvulus, with one portion of the stomach in the chest and one in the abdomen. This condition occurs in patients with paraesophageal hernia, eventration of the left diaphragm, or left phrenic paralysis, and in patients with a high diaphragm from left pneumonectomy. Therapy requires gastric decompression, paraesophageal hernia repair, and gastropexy. Failure to diagnose and treat this disorder promptly can lead to gangrene and perforation of the stomach.

5. A. Acute Biliary Colic   Pain begins suddenly, and builds in intensity over a period of seconds or minutes. It is usually constant, but there may be superimposed jabs or surges of even more intense pain. The pain is described as aching or pressurelike. Anorexia, nausea, vomiting, and sweating accompany it. It is usually located in the epigastrium, but in 10 percent of cases the pain may occur in the left hypochondrium only, and may radiate around the side of the left lower chest to the scapular region. The pain lasts 2 to 6 h and is usually relieved by a single injection of meperidine; it may disappear spontaneously. Most patients move about, seeking relief, although a few may be found lying quietly in bed. Examination may reveal a nontender, soft right upper abdominal mass or mild epigastric or right subcostal tenderness. Real-time ultrasound will detect gallstones in up to 95 percent of patients with this disorder.

B. Acute Cholecystitis   This disorder begins as an attack of biliary colic. After 2 to 6 h the pain recedes, only to begin again 2 or more hours later. Fever, chills, sweats, vomiting, and prostration soon occur. Pain and fever may continue for 3 to 10 days. There is right and/or left upper abdominal and epigastric tenderness and guarding after the initial 10 to 12 h. A radionuclide scan with DISIDA or HIDA (^{99m}Tc-labeled N-substituted iminodiacetic acids) will show nonvisualization of the gallbladder in 95 percent of cases. A real-time ultrasound study will demonstrate a thickened gallbladder wall, gallstones, and a positive sonographic Murphy sign. The pain will be relieved by cholecystectomy.

6.   ACUTE PANCREATITIS

Mild to severe pain occurs in the epigastrium and left hypochondrium. The pain is constant and has an aching or boring quality. It may radiate directly through to the spine. It may be partly relieved by leaning forward, or by lying curled up in a fetal position. It may be intensified by lying supine or by hyperextending the back. There are frequently anorexia, nausea, vomiting, sweating, fever, and chilly sensations. Faintness, weakness, and inability to stand reflect hypovolemia. This disorder is usually caused by alcohol abuse, gallstones traversing the common duct, and obscure obstructive lesions of the lower common duct or pancreatic duct. These require endoscopic retrograde cholangiopancreatography (ERCP) for detection, and include stones, small tumors, pancreatic pseudocysts, choledochoceles, pancreas divisum, and spasm or stenosis of the pancreatic duct sphincter. Other causes include drugs, hypercalcemia, and hypertriglyceridemia. Supportive evidence for the diagnosis can be obtained by measuring the serum amylase. Elevations begin toward the end of day 1, and persist for 3 to 10 days. The sensitivity in pancreatitis is 70 to 92 percent. Lipase levels are elevated in 87 percent of cases. In the presence of normal amylase levels, a CT study may show a swollen pancreas, and peripancreatic edema, hemorrhage, and necrosis, confirming the diagnosis of acute pancreatitis.

7. LEFT SUBPHRENIC ABSCESS

Pain may be present in the left hypochondrium and may also be felt in the left shoulder. In some cases there is no pain. Fever, chills, and weight loss are usually present. Most cases follow within 3 to 6 weeks of surgery on the stomach, colon, biliary tract, or spleen. Duodenal or gastric ulcer perforation, acute pancreatitis, or acute diverticulitis may also give rise to a left subphrenic abscess. There may be tenderness and guarding in the left upper abdomen, and/or fist percussion tenderness over the lower rib interspaces. The left diaphragm may be elevated and fixed, and pleuritic pain may occur in the lower left chest and/or left shoulder, associated with a dry, nonproductive cough. Atelectasis, pneumonia, and an effusion may be present in the lower left chest. The diagnosis can be confirmed by an abdominal CT scan, and surgical drainage accomplished under cover of parenteral antibiotics.

8. DISORDERS OF THE COLON (SPLENIC FLEXURE SYNDROME)

A. Functional Disease   Aching, dull left upper abdominal pain, relieved in some cases by the passage of flatus or stool, may be due to distension or spasm of the splenic flexure of the colon (*splenic flexure syndrome*). There may be mild direct tenderness with no guarding. Food may intensify the pain, or may have no effect. Patients may have diarrhea, constipation, or both—or normal bowel frequency and form. Pellet stools, pencil stools, and ribbon stools are common, and these may alternate with stools of normal width and shape. Episodes of pain occur in clusters, continuing on a daily basis for weeks or months and then disappearing spontaneously. The pain may last for minutes or hours and then disappear,

to return again the following day. In some cases the pain persists for weeks or months without relief. Pain awakening the patient at night may occur. There is no anemia, blood in the stool, or elevation of the sedimentation rate. The use of dietary bran, Metamucil, and anticholinergics may provide symptomatic relief for a minority of patients. This condition is the most common cause of left upper abdominal pain that we see in our clinics. Balloon distension of the left colon has been shown to reproduce typical pain in these patients.

B. Acute Diverticulitis   Pain in the left hypochondrium due to this disorder is rare, since most attacks of this disease involve the sigmoid colon. There may be constant aching pain, fever, chills, alternating diarrhea and constipation, and heme-positive stools. Back pain at the same level, nausea, and vomiting may occur. There is usually left upper abdominal direct and rebound tenderness, and guarding. A leukocytosis in the range of 11,000 to 15,000 per mm^3 range may be present (36 percent of cases). CT may be used early in the course when endoscopy and barium enema are contraindicated. Localized thickening of the colon wall and increased density of the pericolic fat help establish the diagnosis. Colonoscopy is useful to exclude carcinoma, but should be done only after 1 week of therapy. A barium or water-soluble-contrast enema done during the second week may reveal diverticuli, fistulas or sinus tracts, abscesses, a pericolic mass, and leakage. Most cases can be treated by restriction of food and administration of intravenous fluids and antibiotics. Surgical intervention is reserved for patients with recurrent attacks, possible carcinoma, urinary tract symptoms, obstruction or perforation of the colon, and for patients aged under 55.

C. Carcinoma of the Splenic Flexure or Upper Descending Colon   Crampy left upper abdominal pain, associated with constipation, persistent ribbon or pencil stools, rushes of lower abdominal bowel noise, and right lower abdominal pain, may be caused by a partial obstruction due to a stenosing carcinoma, or by a stricture caused by diverticulitis or ischemic colitis. There may be lower abdominal distension. The diagnosis can be confirmed by a double contrast barium enema or colonoscopy. Acute perforation of a carcinoma in the upper left colon can cause constant, severe upper abdominal pain of a sharp or aching character; fever; chills; and signs of localized peritonitis. Free air may be seen on a plain abdominal radiograph. The barium enema may demonstrate the tumor, and colonoscopy and biopsy can be used to establish the tissue diagnosis. Resection and drainage should be performed, and a proximal colostomy with a Hartmann closure utilized. Continuity can be established at a later date.

D. Colitis   There is abrupt onset of an aching or burning pain in the left upper, and often left lower, abdomen. Diarrhea, bright red rectal bleeding or passage of bloody mucus, and abdominal tenderness may be present. Fever, chills, vomiting, and leukocytosis usually occur. Colonoscopy may reveal a diffuse, friable, bleeding mucosa with whitish-yellow exudate (ulcerative colitis), discrete ulcers with pseudomembranes (*Clostridium difficile* related colitis), polypoid and nodular blue-black lesions with ulcerations and pseudomembranes (ischemic colitis), or deep ulcers and "skip" lesions (Crohn's colitis).

A barium enema may show many nodular impressions ("thumbprinting") due to ischemic colitis; diffuse granularity and irregular serrations of the mucosa due to mucosal ulcerations (ulcerative colitis); or deep ulceration, cobblestoning of the mucosa, and "skip" areas (Crohn's disease).

9. DISORDERS OF THE KIDNEY

A. Renal Cortical Abscess   Pain in the left upper abdomen and flank may occur in some patients with this disorder. There may be left subcostal tenderness, but no guarding. Most corticomedullary abscesses are secondary to acute pyelonephritis. The urine contains white blood cells, white-cell casts, and gram-negative bacteria. If the abscess is cortical and secondary to staphylococcal bacteremia, the urine is usually normal and culture-negative. Patients with both types of abscess have fever, chills, and left upper abdominal and flank pain. If a corticomedullary abscess is present, symptoms of lower tract involvement (i.e., frequency, urgency, and dysuria) usually occur. A real-time ultrasound or CT study will identify and localize the abscess. High-dose parenteral antibiotics and percutaneous catheter drainage, or open surgical drainage, are required for cure.

B. Perinephric Abscess   Perinephric abscess usually results from rupture of a cortical abscess into the perirenal space. Left upper abdominal and flank pain, tenderness, fever, chills, and, in some cases, frequency and urgency occur. A CT scan will show a low-density perinephric mass with loss of adjacent soft tissue planes and gas-fluid interfaces. Intravenous antibiotics and open surgical drainage are usually required. The mortality rate for perirenal abscess is close to 50 percent. Kidney stones and acute pyelonephritis rarely cause left hypochondriac pain; if it does occur in these conditions, it is usually associated with left flank pain.

C. Renal Infarction   There is an abrupt onset of severe sharp pain in the left upper abdomen or left flank. Gross or microscopic hematuria, nausea, and vomiting may occur. Fever occurs on the second day, and may persist for

days. The serum LDH and AST levels may rise. Angiography is required to establish the diagnosis. Embolic occlusion of the renal artery may result from mitral stenosis with atrial fibrillation, myocardial infarction or myocarditis with mural thrombi, atheroembolism from the aorta, or endocarditis.

10. JEJUNAL DIVERTICULITIS OR PERFORATION

Jejunal diverticuli are usually asymptomatic. If inflammation or perforation occurs, there may be left upper abdominal pain and peritoneal signs. A left upper abdominal tender mass may form because of abscess formation. Enteroclysis will demonstrate the diverticulum, and may demonstrate a perforation. Surgical management, with drainage of the abscess and resection of the diverticulum, is required for cure.

11. PLEURITIS SECONDARY TO LEFT LOWER LOBE PNEUMONIA OR INFARCTION

Constant, severe, sharp or aching left upper abdominal pain develops. Left anterolateral chest and shoulder pain of a pleuritic nature may accompany the abdominal pain. Fever and cough are common associated symptoms. There may be rust-colored or purulent sputum (pneumonitis), dark-reddish hemoptysis (infarction), or mucoid sputum (*Mycoplasma* or *Legionella* species, or viral pneumonitis). The abdominal pain is not improved by any maneuver, but cough and direct palpation may intensify it. After several hours, abdominal distension due to an ileus may develop. The left upper abdomen is tender and there is muscle guarding. The left diaphragm is high; there may be bronchial breathing and dullness, as well as rales, at the left base. In some cases only rales and rhonchi are present. A chest radiograph shows evidence of consolidation of a portion of the left lower lobe, or a pleural-based triangular-shaped infiltrate. A small pleural effusion may be present. In patients with pulmonary infarction, there is a history of recent immobilization (e.g., long auto or air trip, recent surgery or parturition, casting of a leg) or of cancer or heart failure. A ventilation perfusion scan of the lungs may reveal evidence of one or more pulmonary infarcts. Antibiotic therapy will lead to resolution of the abdominal and chest pain within 48 h, if the underlying problem is bacterial pneumonia. Anticoagulant therapy will similarly benefit patients with thromboembolic disease. The major caution is not to operate on such patients on the basis of the abdominal findings, until a careful examination of the chest has been completed and the chest radiograph reviewed. Lupus pleuritis and pleural tuberculosis may present in a similar manner. In these disorders, an exudative pleural effusion usually occurs without pulmonary infiltrates.

12. COSTOCHONDRITIS

This disorder causes constant aching pain and tenderness over the costal cartilages of the left costal arch and lower parasternal region. Chest and arm movements intensify the pain. The physical examination is negative, except for local tenderness. Hooking the fingers of the left hand under the costal arch and gently pulling forward will intensify or reproduce the pain (i.e., hooking maneuver) and confirm the diagnosis. The cause of costochondritis is unknown. Some cases are repetition-strain disorders caused by excessive use of chest wall muscles in assembly-line work; other cases have no obvious origin. The remainder of the physical examination, rib and chest radiographs, and laboratory tests are all normal. This disorder may wax and wane for no apparent reason. Nonsteroidal anti-inflamatory drugs may be used as symptomatic therapy in severe cases.

Acute Unilateral Costovertebral Area and Flank Pain

☐ DIAGNOSTIC LIST

1. Pain arising in the kidney
   A. Renal colic
   B. Noncolicky renal pain
      1. Acute pyelonephritis
      2. Renal corticomedullary abscess
      3. Renal cortical abscess
      4. Perinephric abscess
      5. A. Poststreptococcal glomerulonephritis
         B. Rapidly progressive glomerulonephritis
         C. IgA nephropathy
      6. A. Acute interstitial nephritis
         B. Analgesic abuse nephropathy
         C. Loin pain hematuria syndrome
      7. Renal infarction due to emboli, renal artery dissection, or thrombi
      8. A. Polycystic kidney disease
         B. Medullary sponge kidney
      9. Renal cancer

2. Myofascial pain
3. Cough fractures
4. Pleuritis
   A. Bacterial pneumonia
   B. Pulmonary emboli
   C. Viral or bacterial pleuritis
   D. Tuberculous pleurisy
   E. Lupus pleuritis
5. Adrenal hemorrhage (i.e., apoplexy) into an adrenal tumor
6. Iliac osteomyelitis
7. Herpes zoster
8. Right-sided pain only
   A. Acute retrocecal appendicitis
   B. Pleuritic pain due to:
      1. Duodenal ulcer disease
      2. Acute cholecystitis
9. Left-sided pain only
   A. Left lumbar and iliac regions
      1. Diverticulitis
      2. Carcinoma of the colon
   B. Left lumbar and hypochondriac regions
      1. Splenic infarction
      2. Splenic abscess

☐ SUMMARY

Renal colic causes excruciating, sharp pain in the costovertebral area and flank that may radiate into the lower abdomen and beyond (i.e., into a testis, or into the perineum in women). Anorexia, nausea, and vomiting may be associated. Patients are usually in such discomfort that they writhe in bed, pace the floor, or soak in a hot bath. This is in contrast to patients with an acute inflammatory process, who prefer to lie still because of the increased discomfort associated with bodily movement. Narcotic-type analgesics are usually required for pain relief. The pain generally begins suddenly and reaches a plateau of intensity within seconds. It may increase or decrease in severity with time, but it seldom stops completely, unless the causative stone or blood clot in the ureter passes into the bladder. Such patients appear in acute distress. They usually have costovertebral-angle tenderness and lower abdominal tenderness, but no muscle guarding. Stones are frequently calcified (80–90 percent of cases) and can be seen on a plain radiograph of the abdomen. An excretory urogram will demonstrate lack of renal function on the painful side. Late dye excretion by the involved kidney (i.e., 1 to 4 h after injection) may opacify the ureter to the point of obstruction. Renal colic due to a stone or clot is associated with gross or microscopic hematuria (60 to 90 percent of cases). A sloughed renal papilla is often associated with pyuria, hematuria, and bacteriuria.

Less severe, constant, dull pain in the back, the flank, and sometimes the upper abdomen, occurs with *acute bacterial infections of the kidney*. There is local tenderness in the costovertebral angle. Fever, chills, sweats, nausea, and vomiting are common associated complaints. The urine contains white blood cells, singly or in clumps; white cell casts; and bacteria. There is usually a prompt response to intravenous antibiotics. If there is a failure of response to such therapy, then a *renal corticomedullary abscess or obstruction* should be suspected and ultrasonography or a CT scan of the kidney performed. Large abscesses may require percutaneous or open surgical drainage.

Renal cortical abscesses may arise from bloodstream dissemination of a bacterial skin or bone infection. Staphylococci lodge in the renal cortex and initiate the process. In this disorder there may be aching pain in the flank and costovertebral angle, with local muscle spasm, tenderness, chills, and high fever, and a palpable tender flank mass. The urine is usually clear (70 to 80 percent of cases) unless the abscess communicates with a calyx, spilling white cells and bacteria into the urine. Blood cultures are usually negative. The diagnosis can be confirmed by ultrasonography or a CT scan. Parenteral antibiotic therapy directed against staphylococci or other causative organisms is required, and drainage may be necessary.

A *perinephric abscess* may result from rupture of a renal abscess into the perinephric space. Flank pain, fullness, and tenderness are usually present. Chills, rigors, sweats, and fever occur. The affected side may show poor diaphragmatic excursion, dullness, and decreased breath sounds over the lower chest posteriorly. The chest radiograph may show a high diaphragm and a pleural effusion. A CT scan will show the abscess as a thick-walled mass with a fluid center adjacent to the kidney in the perinephric space. Drainage (and sometimes nephrectomy) and intravenous antibiotics are required to effectively treat this potentially lethal disorder.

Some patients present with pyelonephritis, unresponsive to therapy; with fever of unknown origin, without pain; or as very ill, with no localizing signs. In the latter situation, a gallium or indium (^{111}In) leukocyte scan will direct attention to the perinephric area.

Acute *glomerulonephritis* usually affects older children and adolescents. It begins suddenly or insidiously with brown, smoky urine, facial and hand edema, and sometimes hypertension. There may be a dull ache in one or both loins, and associated tenderness. Pain is usually mild; it does not occur in all cases. The urine commonly contains leukocytes, red cells, casts, and protein. The creatinine level rises above 2 mg/100 ml in over 50 percent of patients. Dyspnea and orthopnea may occur because of salt retention and heart failure. *Rapidly progressive glomerulonephritis* is a disorder of older adults (mean age 58 years). Aching pain in one or both sides of the back and flanks may occur, but is not uniformly present. Edema and hypertension occur infrequently. The urine is brown or smoky and contains red cell and granular casts, red cells, white cells, and protein. Oliguria may occur. A renal biopsy will show many glomeruli with crescents. *IgA nephropathy* (Berger's disease) can cause constant back and flank pain and tenderness on one or both sides. It usually begins during an upper respiratory infection or a flulike illness. Smoky urine, brown or gray, is the major symptom. Facial and hand edema and hypertension occur in fewer than 50 percent of patients. The serum creatinine level may rise above 2 mg/100ml in 25 percent of cases. The urine contains red cells and red cell casts. Renal biopsy shows deposits of IgA in the mesangial region of many glomeruli. Segments of some glomeruli, but not all, show mesengial proliferation.

Acute interstitial nephritis occurs in patients taking certain antibiotics, sulfa-containing diuretics, anticoagulants, antituberculous drugs, and other medications. Symptoms begin 3 to 35 days after the patient starts the causative drug. There may be flank and back pain and tenderness on one or both sides, and gross or microscopic hematuria. Fever, chills, a macular rash, and eosinophilia may occur. The urine contains red cells, granulocytes, and eosinophiles; urine cultures are usually negative. The serum creatinine and BUN levels may rise. Discontinuance of the causative drug leads to resolution of this disorder.

Analgesic abuse causes the insidious onset of chronic renal failure. Renal infection occurs with increased frequency in this disorder. Drug toxicity may cause sloughing of a renal papilla. Passage of tissue fragments down the ureter can cause renal colic similar to that caused by a ureteral stone. In addition, flank pain from ureteral obstruction may occur in small numbers of patients because of a transitional cell cancer of the ureter or renal pelvis. Such lesions are more common in patients with analgesic abuse.

Loin pain on one or both sides, with hematuria, sometimes occurs in young women taking *oral contraceptive drugs*. Discontinuance of this medication leads to rapid resolution of this syndrome.

Renal infarction usually begins suddenly, with sharp, severe, unremitting back and flank pain and tenderness. It may mimic ureteral colic. Microscopic hematuria occurs, but gross hematuria is rare. Serum levels of lactic dehydrogenase, alkaline phosphatase, and aspartate aminotransferase (AST) may rise to high levels, reflecting release of these enzymes by ischemic renal cells. A CT scan with dye contrast will show normal renal structures without dye excretion on the affected side. A renal arteriogram will show renal artery obstruction. Occlusion of a renal artery may be caused by emboli arising in the heart, by thrombosis, or by dissection. Patients with paroxysmal or sustained atrial fibrillation, a recent myocardial infarction, a ventricular aneurysm, endocarditis, or a cardiomyopathy are at increased risk for embolism. Sustained or transient hypertension often accompanies infarction.

Patients with *polycystic disease* present with flank pain and bilateral renal masses. There may be local tenderness. Pain caused by stones or infection is commonly present in this disorder. Gross or microscopic hematuria occurs. A renal ultrasound or CT study will confirm the clinical diagnosis, which is based on palpation of bilateral nodular masses in the upper abdomen and flanks.

Excretory urography in patients with *medullary sponge kidney* reveals small cysts in the renal medulla. These patients suffer frequently from renal colic due to stones, or flank pain and tenderness from pyelonephritis.

Carcinoma of the kidney may present with gross or microscopic hematuria (50 to 60 percent of cases), flank pain and tenderness (25 to 30 percent), or a flank mass. The diagnosis can be made by ultrasonography or contrast-enhanced CT. A small percentage of patients may also have one or more of the following: anemia or erythrocytosis, fever, pulmonary emboli, hypertension, and weight loss.

Muscular pain in the thoracolumbar area is associated with local tenderness that is diffuse or focal (i.e., related to a trigger point). Pressure over a trigger point reproduces the patient's pain. A specific movement of the back, such as flexion, extension, or upper trunk rotation, may intensify the discomfort during the motion. The urinalysis and renal radiograph studies are normal.

Cough fracture occurs from violent coughing in patients with bronchitis or pneumonia. There is local tenderness over rib 11 or 12. The pain is aching and constant, and is made worse by a deep breath or by lying on the affected side.

Pleuritis causes pain in the back of the lower chest and flank on one side; the pain is made worse by taking a deep breath and by certain body movements. A pleural friction rub may be heard over the painful area. *Pneumonia*, with cough, sputum, fever, and chills, causes some cases of pleuritis. *Pulmonary emboli and infarction* also cause pleuritis. A ventilation-perfusion lung scan and/or a pulmonary angiogram will aid in confirming the diagnosis of embolization. Pleuritis can also be caused by a *viral illness*.

In patients with a nonspecific viral cause for pleuritis, the perfusion lung scan is negative or demonstrates a low-probability pattern. *Tuberculosis* can cause fever, pleuritic pain, and an effusion in young adults. A pleural biopsy is usually necessary for the diagnosis, since tubercle bacilli are difficult to isolate from pleural fluid. Systemic lupus erythematosus may cause pleuritis with effusion. This pleural fluid may contain LE cells and/or anti-nuclear antibody in a titer greater than 1:160.

TABLE OF DISEASE INCIDENCE

INCIDENCE PER 100,000 (APPROXIMATE)

Common (>100)	Uncommon (>5–100)	Rare (>0–5)
Renal colic	Renal corticomedullary abscess	Renal cortical abscess
Acute pyelonephritis	Poststreptococcal glomerulonephritis	Perinephric abscess
Myofascial pain	IgA nephropathy	Rapidly progressive glomerulonephritis
Cough fracture	Acute interstitial nephritis	Renal infarction
Pleuritis due to pneumonia or emboli	Analgesic abuse nephropathy	Pleuritis due to tuberculosis
Pleuritis due to viral infection	Loin pain-hematuria syndrome	Adrenal tumor with hemorrhage
	Polycystic kidney disease	Iliac osteomyelitis
	Medullary sponge kidney	Retrocecal appendicitis
	Carcinoma of the kidney	Splenic infarction
	Diverticulitis	Splenic abscess
	Carcinoma of the colon with perforation	
	Herpes zoster	
	Pleuritis pain due to:	
	Duodenal ulcer	
	Acute cholecystitis	
	Pleuritis due to systemic lupus	

Right-sided pleuritic pain may occur in the right lower posterolateral chest secondary to acute peptic ulcer disease or acute cholecystitis. The chest pain responds to treatment of the ulcer with antacids and H_2 blockers, or treatment of the cholecystitis with intravenous fluids and antibiotics.

The sudden onset of severe unilateral flank and back pain and tenderness, in association with hypotension, fever, and respiratory distress from noncardiogenic pulmonary edema, may be secondary to bleeding into a pheochromocytoma (*adrenal apoplexy*). Such pain may be intensified by a deep breath or by movement, and usually requires narcotic analgesics for relief. A similar pain occurring in a male with a feminizing syndrome or Cushing's syndrome, or in a woman with virilization and Cushing's syndrome, suggests bleeding into an adrenal cortical carcinoma.

Iliac osteomyelitis causes iliac and flank pain and tenderness, high fever, chills or rigors, nausea and vomiting, and limitation of leg extension. Leg and body movements may intensify the abdominal and flank pain. Buttock and sciatic pain may also occur. Plain radiographs are often negative, but a radionuclide bone scan, a gallium scan, CT, or MRI will usually localize the inflammatory process to the ilium. Cases of subacute iliac osteomyelitis that fail to respond to intravenous antibiotics within 72 h should be biopsied to rule out Ewing's sarcoma. *Herpes zoster* causes a unilateral band of pain that involves the flank and anterior abdomen. The pain is described as aching or burning, and pruritus may be associated with it. Within 3 or 4 days of the onset of the pain, an eruption of vesicles and crusted ulcers appears in the painful area. These lesions do not extend beyond the midline.

Right-sided flank and iliac pain may be caused by *acute retrocecal appendicitis*. Midline visceral pain may not precede the right-sided pain. Tenderness may be present in the iliac area and over the flank and back above the iliac crest. Anorexia and low-grade fever occur, as well as leukocytosis.

Left-sided abdominal and flank pain associated with fever, anorexia, and vomiting may be due to *acute diverticulitis* or leakage from a perforated *carcinoma of the colon*. There may be direct tenderness over the iliac area, as well as rebound tenderness and guarding. The diagnosis can be confirmed by a CT scan or a low-pressure barium enema. Carcinoma can be detected and biopsied by colonoscopy.

Splenic infarction causes left hypochondriac and flank pain that is intensified by a deep breath or by jarring. Left shoulder pain is commonly associated. Fever, if present at all, is low-grade. This disorder most commonly occurs in patients with sickle cell disease or trait, or with *myeloproliferative* disorders, such as chronic myelogenous leukemia and myeloid metaplasia.

A *splenic abscess* can cause painful tender splenomegaly with left upper abdominal and flank pain. Fever, chills, or rigors and left upper abdominal tenderness are often present. The diagnosis can be confirmed by a gallium or CT scan or MRI.

☐ DESCRIPTION OF LISTED DISEASES

1. PAIN ARISING IN THE KIDNEY

A. Renal Colic Pain arising from a stone in the renal pelvis or ureter takes the form of *renal colic*. In contrast to the intermittent colicky pain of labor or intestinal obstruction, renal colic pain increases within seconds to high intensity (i.e., "very severe" or "excruciating") and then persists for a variable period (i.e., minutes to many hours). During that time there may be peaks of more intense pain. The pain has been described as worse than that of labor. Large doses of meperidine do not completely relieve it. The patient may writhe in bed, pace the floor, or lie in a tub of warm water with the legs extended up the wall in an attempt to find relief. This behavior is in contrast to that of the patient with an acute inflammatory process, who prefers to lie still because of the discomfort associated with bodily movement.

The pain may originate in the back and radiate anteriorly around the flank, and beyond—into the lower abdomen, testis, and penis, or into the perineum in women. Urine held up to the light in a clear glass container may be red or pink, or may be clear yellow with reddish threads floating in it. Microscopic hematuria occurs in 60 to 90 percent of patients with pain caused by a renal stone. (The absence of hematuria does not rule out this disorder.) Anorexia, nausea, and vomiting may accompany the pain. An intravenous pyelogram done while the pain is present will show no, or delayed, dye excretion into the drainage structures on the painful side (90 percent of cases). There is usually marked tenderness in the costovertebral angle. Usually this tenderness disappears within 36 h of stone passage.

Pain relief may occur spontaneously during a 1- to 3-day bout of colic. Unless the stone has passed, the pain recurs intermittently until it does pass. Most stones larger than 1 cm lodge at the uteropelvic junction and do not pass into the ureter. Smaller stones (i.e., 6 mm to 1 cm) may lodge at the point where the ureter crosses the iliac vessels, or at the ureterovesical junction. Stones that reach the bladder (i.e., those smaller than 6 mm) are generally passed to the outside, with or without mild discomfort during passage.

To confirm the diagnosis of stone-related colic, all urine should be passed through a strainer. The recovered stone proves the diagnosis; it can be analyzed by crystallography, providing information about its composition and sequence of formation.

Initial management requires narcotic administration to relieve pain until the stone is passed. Failure to pass a stone in 2 to 3 days is associated with a persistent ache, and possibly with a rise in temperature. Costovertebral angle tenderness does not subside. Impacted stones can be removed using a percutaneous nephrostomy and forceps extraction. Alternatively they can be removed by in situ shattering, by means of ultrasonic lithotripsy and ureteroscopy. With large stones (e.g., staghorn calculi), surgical removal is often necessary.

Calcium phosphate (apatite), calcium oxalate, magnesium ammonium phosphate (struvite), and cystine stones are radiopaque and are visible on a plain radiograph of the abdomen. Stones may be confused with phleboliths, calcified lymph nodes, calcified costal cartilages, gallstones, or foreign bodies.

Recurrent stone disease is most commonly due to hypercalciuria. This can be documented by a 24-h urine collection taken while the patient is on a regular diet. Urinary excretion of calcium, uric acid, phosphate, oxalate, citrate, and creatinine should be measured. If hypercalciuria is present, the patient should be placed on a low calcium (400 mg/day) and low sodium (100 mEq/day) diet for 1 week, and a second 24-h urine collection taken for measurement of calcium, phosphate, uric acid, and creatinine excretion. Serum calcium, uric acid, and creatinine levels should also be measured. Fasting and calcium-loading tests of calcium excretion should be carried out. Calcium stones occur in association with the following metabolic problems:

Absorptive hypercalciuria occurs in 60 percent of patients with calcium oxalate stones. Reduction of calcium intake to 150 mg/day, or fasting, normalizes the calcium excretion rate, but an oral calcium load increases it into the hypercalciuric range. Since the basic defect is an inherited ability of the jejunum to absorb more calcium than it should, dietary restriction of calcium, sodium, carbohydrate, and protein will reduce urinary calcium levels. In addition, ingestion of 2 to 3 liters of water per day lowers the urinary calcium concentration by dilution. Thiazide diuretics increase urinary calcium reabsorption and reduce urine calcium levels. Absorptive hypercalciuria occurs in the presence of normal serum concentrations of vitamin D.

Renal hypercalciuria occurs in 10 percent of stone-forming patients, and is due to failure of renal reabsorption of calcium. These patients maintain hypercalciuria with calcium restriction and may also show increased excretion after a calcium load. Thiazide diuretics decrease renal hypercalciuria by increasing calcium reabsorption.

Resorptive hypercalciuria is due to excessive parathormone produced by a parathyroid adenoma or carcinoma. The serum calcium level is elevated, and the phosphorous level is often depressed. Hypercalciuria responds to removal of the tumor.

Resorptive hypercalciuria may also be caused by bone invasion by tumor, hyperthyroidism, Cushing's disease, or immobilization. Sarcoid is associated with absorptive hypercalciuria, and type I renal tubular acidosis with renal hypercalciuria. Patients with the latter disorder have acidosis, an elevated alkaline phosphatase level, and decreased levels of serum potassium and bicarbonate and urinary citrate.

Some patients with hyperuricuria form calcium oxalate stones. This may be due to heterogeneous nucleation or to inhibition of stone-inhibiting urinary substances by the increased levels of urinary uric acid.

Uric acid stones are radiolucent. They may occur in patients with consistently acid urines and normal urinary uric acid concentrations. They also occur in patients with elevated urinary uric acid excretion due to primary gout, the Lesch-Nyhan syndrome, or a myeloproliferative disorder. Dehydration caused by sweating or diarrhea can produce increased urinary uric acid levels. Some patients without hyperuricemia have hyperuricuria because of excessive ingestion of purines and protein, ingestion of salicylates, or administration of thiazide diuretics. Increased fluid intake, alkalization of the urine, and purine and protein restriction constitute the initial prophylactic regimen. In difficult cases, allopurinol may be required to reduce uric acid production and excretion.

Struvite stones result from renal infection by urea-splitting organisms. The urine is alkaline. Infection stones may also be associated with any of the metabolic disorders described above. Struvite stones usually require surgical removal. Hemiacedrin irrigation of struvite stones in the renal pelvis and calices may produce stone dissolution. Concurrent antibiotic therapy is required, because stone dissolution releases pathogenic bacteria.

Elevated urinary oxalate excretion (>60 mg/day) occurs in patients with inflammatory disease of the ileum, after surgical resection of the ileum, or after an ileal bypass procedure. Intestinal calcium is bound by unabsorbed fatty acids, allowing increased oxalate reabsorption, urinary excretion, and stone formation. Administration of potassium citrate, medium-chain triglycerides, oxalate restriction, and oxalate binders (such as aluminum hydroxide, cholestyramine, and calcium) reduces urinary oxalate excretion and stone formation. Primary hyperoxaluria is a rare genetic disorder that causes increased oxalate excretion, stone formation, and renal failure in young patients.

Cystinuria is an autosomal recessive disorder (frequency 1 in 20,000) that impairs the absorption of dibasic amino acids by the kidney and bowel. It accounts for 1 to 4 percent of all stones. Homozygotes excrete 500 to 1000 mg of cystine in their urine daily; normal excretion is less than 100 mg/day. A qualitative sodium nitroprusside test performed on a 24-h urine specimen is an effective screen for this disorder. The first episode of colic usually begins during the teenage years, and multiple episodes usually follow. Other family members are commonly affected. These radiopaque stones often appear laminated when viewed radiologically. Examination of the first morning urine may demonstrate typical flat hexagonal cystine crystals. Stone analysis and the nitroprusside test will usually establish the diagnosis. Quantitative measurement of urinary amino acids should be done for confirmation. Therapy is directed at stone dissolution and prevention of recurrent stone formation. Increased fluid intake decreases urinary cystine concentration; alkalization of the urine with oral potassium citrate increases cystine solubility; and excretion may be decreased by penicillamine or alpha-mercaptopropyl glycine. In the past, a mean diagnostic delay of 6 years has been observed because of failure to investigate stone composition or do a metabolic workup.

Other causes of renal colic-like pain include:

1. Passage of clots resulting from intrarenal or pelvic bleeding from a tumor.
2. Passage of a sloughed renal papilla in a diabetic with infection, an analgesic abuser, or a sickle cell patient.
3. Passage of a sloughed portion of a carcinoma of the renal pelvis.

The incidence of renal colic caused by passage of obstructing soft tissue is low, relative to that of renal colic caused by stones.

B. Noncolicky Renal Pain Renal pain may also result from inflammation and edema of the kidney, or from vascular occlusion with ensuing ischemia and infarction. Such pain is felt as a dull ache in the back and flank. It may be transiently intensified by bending or turning, and thus may be mistaken for pain due to a local muscular problem. In some cases bodily movement may have no effect. There is usually tenderness in the flank and costovertebral angle.

Pain and muscle spasm may extend up the back to the interscapular area and neck, and may be referred to the abdomen, producing ipsilateral abdominal pain and/or tenderness.

1. Acute Pyelonephritis Infection of the bladder may precede the onset of upper urinary tract disease, or may begin with it. Irritative bladder symptoms include urinary frequency, urgency, burning discomfort during voiding, and nocturia. Suprapubic pain and tenderness may be present. Patients with renal infection may have only irritative bladder symptoms, only flank pain and fever, or both sets of complaints. Presentation of upper urinary tract disease as a case of cystitis is common in women in inner-city areas.

Fever, chills, and aching flank and costovertebral pain begin abruptly. Pain may be associated with muscle spasm and tenderness, and bending and turning often intensify it. Some patients believe they have strained a back muscle, and may seek aid from an orthopedist or chiropractor. Some patients have no fever or chills, but only back pain and pyuria. Others have fever, chills, headache, upper and lower back pain, and a stiff neck, mimicking meningitis. Flank pain has been described with lower tract infections (e.g., cystitis or urethritis); it may be due to spasm at the ureterovesical junction causing elevated ureteral back pressures. Microscopic examination of uncentrifuged urine can be performed in a hemacytometer chamber. Concentrations greater than 10 leukocytes per mm^3 are considered to be abnormal. In acute pyelonephritis, there are usually too many leukocytes to count; bacteria; red blood cells; clumps of leukocytes; and white blood cell casts. Proteinuria is scant to moderate. Bacteria can be seen as rod-shaped or coccal forms by light microscopy, and their numbers can be estimated by Gram stain. Some laboratories centrifuge 15 ml of urine and examine the sediment. More than 1 or 2 leukocytes per high-power field is considered abnormal. In community-acquired pyelonephritis, urine cultures usually grow *Escherichia coli* or another gram-negative enteric organism. In the past, *E. coli* were usually sensitive to most antibiotics; but recently 40 percent have been resistant to ampicillin. Bacterial counts in pyelonephritis usually exceed 10^5 organisms per ml, but values as low as 10^4 may be associated with renal infection.

Severely ill patients with acute pyelonephritis require hospital admission and intravenous antibiotics. Those without fever and toxicity can be treated as outpatients with oral antibiotics.

In the past, ampicillin and gentamicin were given intravenously until fever and toxicity abated. Because of *E. coli* resistance, current recommendations are to use intravenous trimethoprim-sulfamethoxazole, or a third-generation cephalosporin (e.g., ceftriaxone) or gentamicin alone. Antibiotic therapy should be continued for 2 weeks, and posttreatment cultures obtained for follow-up to detect recurrent or persistent infection. Between 96 and 100 percent of pathogens causing community-acquired pyelonephritis are sensitive to the antibiotic regimens recommended.

If fever, chills, toxicity, and back pain do not resolve in 72 h, ureteral obstruction and/or a corticomedullary renal abscess should be ruled out by ultrasonography or a CT scan.

2. Renal Corticomedullary Abscess This disorder should be considered in any patient with acute ascending pyelonephritis who fails to improve with treatment as described above. It causes severe aching thoracolumbar pain that radiates to the flank and, sometimes, into the ipsilateral upper abdomen. Fever, chills, nausea, vomiting, and irritative bladder symptoms are also often present. A tender flank mass can be felt in up to 60 percent of cases. The peripheral white blood cell count is usually elevated, but the urine may be normal in as many as 30 percent of cases because the abscess may not drain into the collecting system. When the urine is abnormal, it contains leukocytes, leukocyte clumps, red blood cells, and bacteria. *Escherichia coli, Klebsiella* species, and *Proteus mirabilis* are most frequently isolated from the urine. Blood cultures may be positive in a large percentage of cases.

Renal ultrasonography or a CT scan will clearly delineate a corticomedullary abscess. Sonography is a sensitive screening test for a focal demarcated lesion, such as an abscess. However, the sonographic appearance of an intrarenal abscess is quite variable. If there are no internal echoes in the abscess, a cyst or a caliceal diverticulum may be mimicked. Such lesions may also produce the reflective echoes of a tumor. CT is used when a sonographic study is technically inadequate because of the patient's obesity, or when the results are too ambiguous. CT is more sensitive, since it can detect abscesses smaller than 2 cm in diameter. An early abscess on CT has low attenuation and usually fails to enhance. It is sharply marginated by renal parenchymal tissue. This sharp demarcation distinguishes these lesions from the less well-defined images of a focal bacterial nephritis that has not yet gone on to liquefaction and abscess formation. The presence of gas in a focal lesion is pathognomonic for infection. A "ring sign" caused by contrast-infusion enhancement of the hyperemic capsule of the abscess is present in some cases.

Corticomedullary abscess formation occurs with ascending gram-negative infection. Patients with this complication are likely to have a history of a prior episode of pyelonephritis with scarring, renal stones, or vesicoureteral reflux. Diabetes, hyperparathyroidism, and ureteral obstruction are also predisposing conditions.

Therapy should be directed at the infection, with prolonged antibiotic treatment. Urinary tract obstruction requires decompression. If the abscess is large or has been present for a long time, or is associated with ureteral obstruction or urosepsis, then drainage may be required. This can be done percutaneously by aspiration with a needle or catheter. If obstructive uropathy is present, a nephrostomy may be required.

If percutaneous abscess drainage is not successful or feasible, then open surgical drainage should be performed. Severely damaged kidneys require removal. Ultrasonography can be used to monitor resolution. All patients should remain on antibiotic therapy for at least 2 to 3 weeks.

3. Renal Cortical Abscess (Renal Carbuncle)

This disorder begins with fever, chills, rigors, and toxicity. Pain may occur in the costovertebral area, in the flank and upper anterior abdomen, or only in the back. The pain is dull and aching, and may be intensified by bending or other movements. There may be local costovertebral-angle tenderness, with or without associated pain. Reflex muscle spasm can occur in the back, and a tender flank mass may be present. Physical examination of the ipsilateral lower posterior chest may demonstrate a high, poorly mobile diaphragm; decreased breath sounds; dullness; and rales. These findings are caused by diaphragmatic irritation secondary to the inflammatory process. Laboratory findings include leukocytosis and, in most patients, a completely negative urinalysis. In a small percentage of patients there may be proteinuria, pyuria, and hematuria. These latter patients have probably developed enough inflammation around the abscess to make the urine abnormal. Blood cultures are usually negative.

Cortical abscess results from hematogenous spread of staphylococci to the renal cortex from a focus of infection in the skin (furuncle, carbuncle, paronychia, cellulitis), in bone (osteomyelitis), or on a heart valve (endocarditis). Intravenous drug abusers, diabetics, and dialysis patients are at increased risk for this disorder.

Since the infectious agent (*Staphylococcus aureus* in 90 percent of cases) usually spreads from a remote site directly to the kidney and lodges in the outer cortex, patients with this disorder do not have frequency, urgency, or dysuria. The abscess can be identified by ultrasonography or a CT scan; the findings are similar to those for a corticomedullary abscess. Early mass lesions identified by sonography require differentiation from a renal tumor. In patients who have little toxicity and fever, renal tumor may be considered strongly enough to do a renal arteriogram.

Nafcillin or vancomycin should be administered intravenously and continued for 10 days to 2 weeks, and should be followed by antistaphylococcal oral therapy for 4 weeks. Pain resolves in 24 to 48 h, and fever resolves in 5 to 7 days. Only 3 percent of patients have abscesses simultaneously in both kidneys.

If the symptoms fail to improve within 48 h of initiating therapy, then needle or catheter drainage should be performed. If percutaneous drainage fails, open surgical drainage should be carried out.

4. Perinephric Abscess

This disorder may develop secondary to rupture of a renal abscess into the perinephric space. Smaller numbers of cases come about via hematogenous spread from a nonrenal infected site to the perinephric space. Colon lesions, adjacent infected vertebrae, an empyema, an infected gallbladder, a liver abscess, or pelvic inflammatory disease may secondarily infect the perirenal space.

This disorder most commonly develops as a complication of a renal abscess. Failure of response of a renal abscess to antibiotics and drainage should suggest the possibility of perinephric extension.

Unilateral back and flank pain occurs in 80 percent of cases, and chills and burning on urination in 40 percent. Nausea, vomiting, and weight loss occur in 25 percent of cases. Some patients have a painful, tender back and no other complaints. Flank, costovertebral-angle, or mid- or upper abdominal tenderness may occur. A flank mass is palpable in fewer than half the cases. Pain may be referred to the ipsilateral hip, thigh, and knee. Bending the back or extending the thigh on the hip during walking may intensify the back pain and associated muscle spasm, suggesting a musculoskeletal problem. Anemia (40 percent of cases) and leukocytosis occur. Pyuria and proteinuria are common; but up to 33 percent of all patients with perinephric abscesses have negative urinalyses, and 40 percent have negative urine cultures. Blood cultures may be positive in up to 40 percent of cases.

The clinical presentation described above, with fever and flank pain, is common; but some patients have only vague complaints, such as malaise, anorexia, weakness, and weight loss. The presence of a pleural effusion, or a poorly moving diaphragm and dullness at one lung base, in a patient with fever and ipsilateral flank tenderness should suggest the possibility of a perinephric lesion.

This diagnosis should also be added to the list of causes of fever of unknown origin and should be considered when there is an unexplained peritonitis, pelvic abscess, or empyema. Up to one-third of cases end in death with no diagnosis made prior to autopsy.

Ultrasonography or a CT scan will readily identify a perinephric abscess and define its extent. CT will demonstrate areas of fluid attenuation in the perirenal space surrounded by a thick-walled capsule, which usually enhances. Gas may be seen in some lesions; it confirms an abscess.

Prompt surgical drainage and broad-spectrum antibiotic therapy, using an aminoglycoside and an antistaphylococcal drug, should be initiated. The mortality rate for this disease is 20 to 50 percent; many of the deaths are due to failure to consider the diagnosis and to treat appropriately. The absence of findings on urinalysis may direct attention away from the kidney in cases of renal and perinephric abscess. In this setting, a ^{67}Ga citrate or ^{111}In leukocyte scan will detect renal and perirenal inflammation. A CT scan can be used to define the nature and anatomic location of the inflammatory process (e.g., renal and/or perinephric abscess).

5. A. POSTSTREPTOCOCCAL GLOMERULONEPHRITIS

Flank and costovertebral-angle pain of an aching nature, accompanied by tenderness, may sometimes accompany the other symptoms of this disorder. These include swelling of the hands, face, and eyelids; hypertension; and dark brown (smoky) or coffee-colored urine. Nephritic urine contains protein (.5 to >3.5 g/day), red and white cells, and red cell and granular casts. Erythrocyte casts are a frequent finding (60–85 percent of cases) and should be sought in any urine sample with a cast-preserving acid pH, using a gently centrifuged urine sediment. Poststreptococcal glomerulonephritis affects children aged from 5 to 15 years, but may also occur in adults into the sixth decade. It may follow a streptococcal sore throat within a period of 6 to 20 days, or impetigo within 14 to 21 days. Streptococcal skin infections may cause nephritic disease in as many as 25 percent of cases. Prompt penicillin therapy of a streptococcal throat or skin infection does not appear to prevent this disorder. Other findings that may be present include renal failure with a rising creatinine level (50 percent of cases) and congestive heart failure with dyspnea and orthopnea. Therapy includes salt restriction and diuretics to control edema, hypertension, and heart failure. Dialysis may be temporarily required for patients with more severe renal failure. Most patients (95 percent) heal completely and recover normal renal function.

B. RAPIDLY PROGRESSIVE GLOMERULONEPHRITIS

This disorder occurs primarily in older patients (average age 58 years). Loin and thoracolumbar pain of an aching quality may occur in some cases. Associated flank tenderness is present. Myalgia, arthralgia, and abdominal pain also occur. Some patients have hemoptysis and associated pulmonary infiltrates. The urine is brown or smoky and contains casts, red blood cells, and protein. Edema and hypertension are infrequent, but oliguria is common; it results in elevation of the serum creatinine. Renal biopsy demonstrates that more than half the glomeruli have epithelial cell crescents.

More than 75 percent of patients die, or go onto chronic maintenance dialysis, within 2 years. Prognostic indications of a poor outcome include persistent oliguria, hypertension, a creatinine level above 6 mg/dL, and a renal biopsy with more than 50 percent of the glomeruli containing crescents. Remission may occur with methylprednisolone pulse therapy or plasma exchange. The latter treatment group has also been treated with prednisone and cyclophosphamide. Fur-

ther long-term follow-up studies will be required to determine the effects of steroid pulse therapy and plasma exchange on the ultimate prognosis.

C. IgA NEPHROPATHY (BERGER'S DISEASE)

This disorder usually begins within 2 days of the onset of an upper respiratory infection (50 percent of cases), a flulike illness (15 percent), or nausea, vomiting, and diarrhea (10 percent). Gross hematuria is the predominant symptom. The urine is dark gray-brown or coffee-colored. A low-grade fever, malaise, muscle aches, and back pain and tenderness on one or both sides may occur. Dysuria may also be present. Edema of the face and hands and hypertension occur in fewer than 50 percent of cases. The creatinine level rises minimally in 25 percent of cases. Microscopic findings in the urine include red cells, red cell and granular casts, and leukocytes. Some patients have only microscopic hematuria and never have smoky-brown urine. Fifty percent of patients have recurrent attacks of gross hematuria occurring in association with acute viral infections. Microscopic hematuria may persist between attacks of gross hematuria. A renal biopsy will confirm the diagnosis. Focal glomerular lesions with mesangial proliferation and deposits of IgA are present. Only segments of individual glomeruli are involved. The disease follows an insidious course, with a poor outcome in 20 percent of cases over the first 6 months. An additional 30 percent of patients die, or go onto chronic dialysis, within 20 years of onset. There is no known therapy that can control progression.

6. A. ACUTE INTERSTITIAL NEPHRITIS

This drug-related hypersensitivity disease was originally reported in patients receiving methicillin. It has subsequently been reported with many other types of penicillin, sulfa drugs, and sulfa-containing diuretics, such as the thiazides, the cephalosporins, and rifampin.

Symptoms begin within 3 days to 5 weeks after starting the causative drug. The onset is sudden, with fever; chills; malaise; aching loin and back pain; and brown or smoky urine, or bright red, gross hematuria. Fewer than 25 percent of patients develop a generalized maculopapular rash. Microscopic hematuria and pyuria occur, but urine Gram stains and cultures are negative. A Wright-stained smear of the urine sediment may show eosinophils; such a finding strongly supports the diagnosis. Peripheral eosinophilia is present in 79 percent of cases, but may be missed if frequent blood counts are not done. Oliguria and renal insufficiency may occur. Renal salt wasting and a rise in serum potassium may occur, and a hyperchloremic acidosis may develop. In some cases, antibodies to tubule cell basement membrane are present and can be demonstrated by renal biopsy. Biopsies also show infiltration of renal interstitial tissue with lymphocytes, monocytes, and eosinophils. Treatment consists of stopping the offending drug, and a brief course of oral corticosteroids. The efficacy of steroids is uncertain, but many physicians use them. Back pain may be unilateral or bilateral, and may be mild or absent in some cases.

Rifampin is more likely to cause this disorder if it is given after a prior course of treatment or is used for intermittent therapy.

B. ANALGESIC ABUSE NEPHROPATHY Phenacetin, or acetaminophen and aspirin used in combination for pain, may produce chronic renal failure if taken in large doses over a prolonged period. A history of the use of 1 g or more of acetaminophen and aspirin per day for 3 or more years, or a total of 3 kg or more of these drugs, is required for a presumptive diagnosis of this disorder. An elevated creatinine level and hypertension (50 percent of cases) are present. Anemia is common. There is usually a history of chronic headache or back pain for which analgesics have been taken. Pyelonephritis due to infection occurs in 50 percent of cases. Analgesic abuse nephropathy is usually painless, unless a renal papilla necroses and sloughs into the urine, or infection occurs.

A sloughed renal papilla may partly or completely obstruct the ureter, giving rise to severe costovertebral angle and flank pain, which may radiate anteriorly into the lower abdomen and genitalia, mimicking renal colic produced by the passage of a stone.

Obstruction of the ureter, without colic, by such tissue can cause distension of the renal collecting system and a dull, aching discomfort in the back and loin. This may be intensified by administration of fluids if the excreted fluid further distends the renal collecting system. Localized tenderness is present with colic or with hydronephrosis. An intravenous pyelogram may demonstrate caliceal clubbing (due to obstruction), a papillary cavity, and a caliceal filling defect caused by the presence of a portion of a papilla free in a calix (ring sign).

Transitional cell cancers are more common in patients with this disorder. They can bleed or cause obstruction, with back and flank pain.

Treatment consists of stopping excessive analgesic use. Some or all of the renal failure will reverse itself. Cancer of the renal pelvis or ureter requires complete surgical resection. Renal failure requires maintenance dialysis and/or renal transplantation.

C. LOIN PAIN HEMATURIA SYNDROME This syndrome of unilateral or bilateral flank pain and tenderness, associated with gross hematuria and sometimes hypertension, has been seen in young women on contraceptive medication. While the intravenous pyelogram is usually normal, a renal arteriogram will show evidence of stenotic and spastic vessels. The pain is most likely ischemic. Cessation of contraceptive pills usually leads to resolution of the problem.

7. Acute Renal Infarction Severe, sharp, continuous pain begins suddenly in the costovertebral angle and flank on one side, and may radiate anteriorly to the upper abdomen or periumbilical region. Anorexia, nausea, and vomiting occur, but fever usually does not begin until 1 or 2 days after the onset of pain. Tenderness is present in the flank and back, as well as in the upper abdomen. Acute hypertension may develop from renal ischemia. Gross hematuria is rare, but microscopic hematuria is frequent. Proteinuria is almost universal. With necrosis of the affected kidney due to loss of its blood supply, renal enzymes are released into the blood in high concentrations. These include lactate dehydrogenase (LDH), alkaline phosphatase, and aspartate aminotransferase (AST). LDH levels may also be elevated in the urine. These enzyme elevations occur within 3 days of the onset of symptoms, but LDH levels may remain high for a longer period. An excretory urogram will show absent function on the affected side, and a retrograde pyelogram will show no evidence of structural damage of the affected kidney. A renal arteriogram will establish the diagnosis. A CT scan with contrast enhancement will demonstrate normal renal structure on the affected side with no dye excretion. The causes of acute renal infarction include the following:

Clot emboli arise from the heart in patients with atrial fibrillation. Most patients who suffer clot embolism have coronary artery disease, but some have mitral valve disease. Left ventricular clots may occur in patients with recent myocardial infarction, myocarditis, cardiomyopathy, or ventricular aneurysm. In patients with endocarditis, vegetations can obstruct the renal artery. Anticoagulants prevent clot embolism from the heart. Endocarditis requires prolonged antibiotic therapy. Thrombolytic therapy, using streptokinase intravenously, and angioplasty have not had notable success in relieving embolic renal artery occlusions.

Surgical revascularization should be avoided unless both kidneys are involved by emboli. With bilateral emboli, patients treated surgically do better than those treated with anticoagulants alone (survival 63 percent vs. 14 percent).

Arterial occlusion can also occur because of a spontaneous or trauma-related *thrombosis* or a renal artery *dissection*. A syndrome like that described above occurs. Some cases of renal artery occlusion are asymptomatic. Renal artery dissections can be differentiated from embolic occlusion by arteriography. Indications for surgical repair of a renal artery dissection include severe hypertension and deterioration of renal function. While permanent renal damage may occur abruptly, cases of complete renal arterial occlusion have been operated on, and the kidney revascularized, as long as 1 month after the occlusion, with good return of renal function. Presumably, collateral vessels have kept kidney cells viable during the delay between occlusion and definitive treatment.

8. **A. POLYCYSTIC KIDNEY DISEASE (AUTOSOMAL DOMINANT)** This disease causes flank and back pain of mild or moderate intensity. The pain is usually dull and aching. Either gross or microscopic hematuria may occur; this may be precipitated by trauma or active exercise, or may occur spontaneously. The patient may feel masses in the sides of his or her abdomen. Headache, nausea, vomiting, nocturia, and polyuria are frequent complaints. Hypertension occurs in 30 to 40 percent of patients. Renal failure occurs in 50 percent of patients who live to the age of 70.

The diagnosis can be confirmed by ultrasonography or a CT scan of the renal area. Liver cysts occur in 50 percent of cases and may enlarge the liver. These cysts have been confused with metastatic liver cancer. Cerebral aneurysms are associated with polycystic disease (10–40 percent of cases). In most centers these patients are not evaluated for aneurysms by means of radiologic studies unless they develop symptoms of headache or neurologic dysfunction.

Common problems include anemia due to chronic gross hematuria and renal failure. Pain may occur in the flank because of enlargement or rupture of cysts, or bleeding into cysts. Retroperitoneal bleeding from ruptured cysts may also occur. Polycystic kidneys often form stones, which can lead to renal colic. Cysts can also become infected and can cause flank and back pain. Trimethoprim-sulfamethoxazole has been shown to enter cyst fluid, and is effective against cyst infections.

There is no proven role for cyst puncture in preserving renal function. CT scans are used to evaluate flank pain or enlargements. Flank pain may also arise from a renal carcinoma, which occurs with increased frequency in patients with polycystic disease.

B. MEDULLARY SPONGE KIDNEY Cystic dilatation occurs in the collecting ducts of the medulla. Patients with this condition form stones and are more prone to pyelonephritis. Hematuria is common. Flank and back pain is associated with renal stones or with infection. The diagnosis can be made by an intravenous pyelogram, which shows dye-filling, 1- to 5-mm, cystlike cavities in the medulla. These have been described as forming a ''bouquet-of-flowers'' pattern in the medullary region.

Stones and calcium deposits occur in the medulla. Hyperparathyroidism is more common in this disorder, so that the serum calcium and parathyroid hormone levels should be measured to rule out a parathyroid tumor in the presence of stones or nephrocalcinosis. There may also be decreased urine concentrating ability and renal tubular acidosis.

Treatment is directed against infection and stone formation. The disorder itself is benign, and does not lead to progressive renal failure. Up to 20% of patients with renal stones may have this disorder.

9. *Renal Cancer* This disorder may cause aching back and flank pain (35–40 percent of cases), gross or microscopic hematuria (50–60 percent), and/or a mass in the side of the abdomen or flank that may be discovered by the patient (25–45 percent). Fever may be the only presenting complaint (15 percent); it may be associated with weight loss and anemia. Hypertension occurs in up to 40 percent of cases. Some patients (3–6 percent) develop a ruddy complexion and an elevated hemoglobin, presumably from bone marrow stimulation by an erythropoietin produced by the tumor. Intravenous pyelography may identify 75 percent of such cancers as mass lesions. Ultrasonography can be used to determine if the mass is solid or cystic. If it is cystic, then no further workup is done. If it is solid, a contrast-enhanced CT scan should be done. If the lesion enhances, it is likely to be a cancer, and surgery should be performed. If the solid lesion does not enhance, a renal arteriogram should be performed. If the lesion is vascularized, then surgery should be done and the kidney removed. If the lesion is avascular, a needle aspiration should be done to attempt to detect malignant cells.

The therapy of renal cancer requires careful staging by CT or MRI. If tumor extension into the renal vein is suspected, then an inferior venacavogram should be done to determine the extent of tumor growth into the inferior vena cava. Patients with stage I tumors localized to the kidney; with stage II tumors localized to the perinephric space and adrenal gland region; and with stage IIIA tumors that have extension in the renal vein or vena cava can undergo removal of the kidney, the adrenal gland, any thrombus in the vena cava, and the surrounding fat and fascia. This surgery carries with it a 50 to 70 percent likelihood of 5-year survival. However, if the nodes along the aorta or at distant sites are involved (stage IIB, IIC), then survival drops down to 15 to 35 percent at 5 years. Patients with extensive spread (stage IV) have recently responded to immunotherapy using autologous lymphocytes activated by exposure to interleukin-2 (LAK cells) in vitro. The long-term prognosis of such treated cases is unknown at present. Only 10 percent of interleukin-2–treated patients have complete remission; an additional 20 percent have partial resolution of their tumors. This therapy is still experimental, and is quite toxic.

2. MYOFASCIAL PAIN—DIFFUSE MUSCULAR PAIN AND TENDERNESS AND TRIGGER POINT TENDERNESS

Pain of a dull, aching, continuous nature occurs in the thoracolumbar area on one side. This pain may be intensified by bending, lifting, or rotating the upper body, and there is often limitation of movement. There may be a history of unaccustomed lifting, as in the case of the young mother who reaches down to lift a toddler from a crib or playpen several times a day. Examination may show generalized or focal tender spots (trigger points). Fingertip pressure over these muscle trigger points will reproduce the patient's pain, and sometimes its distant referral pattern. There may be one or more tender trigger points in a region. This syndrome may or may not respond to the use of nonsteroidal anti-inflammatory drugs. Alternatively, local injection of the trigger point with lidocaine and methylprednisolone usually provides immediate relief of the pain (because of the lidocaine), and often long-term relief as well. Trigger points in this region may arise from the multifidus, rotatores thoracis, or the longissimus thoracis muscles. Other techniques that have been reported to be effective for the treatment of trigger point myofascial pain include spraying of the skin with coolant, and stretching of the painful muscles; ischemic compression of the painful trigger point with finger pressure; and needling of the trigger point. We have found lidocaine and steroid injections to be effective, but they are seldom required, since the pain and tenderness usually respond to heat, analgesics, and exercise.

In addition to being therapeutic, the lidocaine injection is also diagnostic, since it provides immediate and rapid relief—which would not occur if the cause of the pain in this region were related to the kidney, pleural surface, or spine. The urinalysis, intravenous pyelogram, and renal ultrasonogram are usually normal.

3. COUGH FRACTURES

A respiratory illness, such as a severe bronchitis or pneumonia, may cause such violent coughing that the eleventh or twelfth rib may fracture, posteriorly in the costovertebral region, under the pull of the attached muscles. These are usually nondisplaced fractures. There is local point tenderness over the eleventh or twelfth rib. A deep breath, a cough, or lying on the painful area may intensify the pain. The use of a potent cough suppressant and an adjustable rib splint will usually provide pain relief. In some patients the pain and tenderness arise in the intercostal muscles and not in the rib, and there is local tenderness over these muscles; this pain is relieved by the same measures that are used for rib fractures.

4. PLEURITIS

Pleural pain may cause a sharp, sticking, or knifelike discomfort in the lower posterior chest. The pain is intensified at the end of an inspiration, or by coughing. Bodily movement may also aggravate it. Holding the breath and lying still with the affected side against the bed (i.e., splinting) usually brings relief, although a dull ache may persist between breaths. Many patients alter their breathing because of the pain, taking rapid, shallow breaths. The causes of pleuritis include the following.

A. Pneumonia Pneumonia due to bacterial infection is associated with pleuritic pain; cough; yellow-green, rusty, or "currant jelly" sputum; fever; chills; and, sometimes, rigors. Sputum Gram stains show many neutrophils and bacteria, and there is usually a prompt response to antibiotic therapy. The chest radiograph shows segmental or patchy opacities. *Legionella pneumophila* causes severe pneumonia, often preceded by diarrhea and abdominal pain. In addition, chemical measures of renal and hepatic function are often abnormal. This disorder usually occurs in patients with chronic pulmonary disease or immunosuppression, but may attack young adults. Therapy with erythromycin is effective.

B. Pulmonary Emboli Small pulmonary emboli may cause acute pleuritic pain. Other frequent symptoms include dyspnea, cough, hemoptysis (30 percent of cases), and syncope. On physical exam, rales and/or a pleural friction rub may be heard (28 percent), and there may be signs of pleural fluid. The lung scan will show abnormal perfusion; if this involves multiple pulmonary segments or lobes, and is associated with ventilation-perfusion (V/Q) mismatch, the diagnosis has a high probability. However, if the perfusion scan is positive with a different type of V/Q pattern (e.g., V/Q match), then a pulmonary angiogram should be done to determine the significance of the lung scan. Impedance plethysmography may establish the presence of a thigh vein thrombus in a patient with an abnormal perfusion scan, and this alone is enough to warrant the use of heparin and warfarin therapy. Chest radiographs in patients with emboli may be normal, but more often they show a pleural-based lung opacity, and, sometimes, a small pleural effusion.

Patients with emboli or a recent thigh vein thrombosis should be treated with intravenous heparin for 7 to 10 days, and then with oral warfarin therapy for 3 to 6 months.

C. Viral or Bacterial Pleuritis Viral or bacterial pleuritis related to a small subpleural bronchopneumonia may be diagnosed by a history of typical pleuritic pain, low-grade fever, and, sometimes, headache and myalgias. The chest radiograph may show a small pleural effusion, or may be entirely normal. Perfusion scans and pulmonary angiograms show no evidence of pulmonary emboli. Impedance plethysmography shows no clots in the thigh veins. This disorder can clinically mimic pulmonary infarction from emboli, requiring the use of a V/Q lung scan and/or a pulmonary angiogram to rule out pulmonary infarction. The identities of the viral agents causing this syndrome are unknown. In ambulatory patients, viral pleuritis is 3 to 4 times more common than embolic disease.

D. Tuberculous Pleurisy Patients with this disorder present with pleural pain, fever, and fluid in the chest. The tuberculin skin test is positive, or converts within weeks of the onset of this disorder. Pleural biopsies with biopsy cultures are necessary for diagnosis, since *Mycobacterium tuberculosis* is grown from pleural fluid in fewer than 20 percent of cases. Therapy is required, because a large proportion of these patients will go on to develop pulmonary tuberculosis if not treated. Therapy with isoniazid and another antituberculous drug for 1 year should be initiated once the diagnosis is confirmed.

E. Lupus Pleuritis   Systemic lupus erythematosus may present acutely with unilateral pleuritic pain in the lower posterior chest and sometimes in the ipsilateral shoulder. Fever, weakness, fatigue, and anemia may be associated. A small or moderate-sized pleural effusion may form on the painful side. The fluid is an exudate, and it may contain LE cells. The pleural fluid ANA titer is greater than 1:160 and may be equal to or greater than the serum ANA titer. There is a dramatic improvement with prednisone therapy. The ANA test in non-lupus effusions is usually negative.

5. ADRENAL TUMOR (PHEOCHROMOCYTOMA OR ADRENAL CARCINOMA) WITH ACUTE HEMORRHAGE

The sudden onset of acute flank and midback pain on one side may signal hemorrhage into an adrenal tumor. There is exacerbation of the pain by a deep breath or by movement. Narcotics are usually required for pain relief. If a pheochromocytoma is the underlying neoplasm, there may be a history of hypertension, recurrent throbbing headaches, diaphoresis, palpitations, weight loss, and chest pain. A recent myocardial infarction may have occurred. Patients with adrenal hemorrhage secondary to pheochromocytoma may present with flank pain and tenderness, tachycardia, hypovolemia-associated hypotension, and sometimes catecholamine-induced acute pulmonary edema (i.e., dyspnea, wheezing, and cough with production of pink frothy sputum). The presence of the tumor can be supported by finding elevated levels of plasma or urinary catecholamines, but the results can be normal if there has been an episode of "adrenal apoplexy." A CT scan or MRI will confirm the presence of an adrenal mass on the painful side, and may demonstrate the adrenal hemorrhage.

An adrenal scintigraphic study with [131]I- or [121]I-labeled metaiodobenzylguanidine (MIBG) is specific, but insensitive for pheochromocytoma. It is unlikely to be positive in the presence of a major adrenal hemorrhage.

Acute flank pain due to intraadrenal hemorrhage may also complicate the course of an adrenal cortical carcinoma. The sudden onset of flank discomfort in a patient with Cushing's syndrome should prompt a CT or MRI study of the adrenal region. Some adrenal carcinomas are asymptomatic until hemorrhage occurs. Other carcinomas produce a feminizing syndrome in men, or virilization and Cushing's syndrome

in women. These tumors can be detected by a CT scan or MRI.

6. ILIAC OSTEOMYELITIS

Osteomyelitis of the ilium can cause iliac pain, tenderness, and guarding, as well as groin and flank pain. The leg may be flexed and externally rotated, and abdominal and flank pain may be increased by leg movement. There may be direct abdominal and flank tenderness and guarding. High fever, chills or rigors, anorexia, vomiting, and weight loss, as well as leukocytosis may occur. Pelvic radiographs may remain normal for 2 or 3 weeks. Early diagnosis can be facilitated by a radionuclide bone scan or an MRI study of the pelvis. There is usually a response to antibiotic therapy within 48 h. Patients who have had symptoms for more than 4 weeks, have lytic lesions, and fail to respond to parenteral antibiotics within 72 h should have a bone biopsy to rule out Ewing's sarcoma. The clinical symptoms, signs, and radiologic findings of this tumor can be easily confused with subacute osteomyelitis.

7. HERPES ZOSTER

This disorder may cause a unilateral band of aching or burning pain that may precede the classic eruption by 1 to 4 days. The rash consists of clusters of small ulcers and vesicles haloed by a narrow rim of erythema. These ulcers rapidly become covered with hemorrhagic crusts. The rash may be minimal or very extensive; it is localized to the dermatomal region of pain. Acyclovir taken orally may be used in severe cases.

8. RIGHT-SIDED PAIN ONLY

A. Acute Retrocecal Appendicitis   Pain may begin in the right lower abdomen and lumbar region without any preceding midabdominal pain. There may be local right iliac and/or lumbar direct tenderness, simulating renal stone or infection. Vomiting is infrequent, and leukocytosis is usually present. Appendiceal rupture with abscess formation produces a tender right iliac mass and may cause right flank and costovertebral-area tenderness and guarding. Appendectomy should be performed prior to rupture. Antibiotic therapy and drainage are required if an abscess has already formed.

B. Pleuritic Pain Due to:

1. Duodenal Ulcer Disease   A duodenal ulcer may cause right lower posterolateral chest and flank pain. The pain may simulate pleuritic pain because of intensification by movement and respiration. The ipsilateral diaphragm may be elevated and fixed, and the breath sounds decreased. Administration of antacids and/or an H_2 blocking drug relieves the lower chest and flank pain, and leads to resolution of the abnormal pulmonary physical findings within 48 to 72 h.

2. Acute Cholecystitis Acute cholecystitis may cause fever and pleuritic pain in the right lower posterior chest and flank, and sometimes in the right shoulder, that is intensified by inspiration, coughing, and bodily movement. Administration of intravenous antibiotics or cholecystectomy relieves the pleuritic back and flank pain and leads to resolution of physical signs in the right lower chest.

9. LEFT-SIDED PAIN ONLY

A. Left Lumbar and Iliac Regions

1. Diverticulitis Diverticulitis of the descending colon may cause left lumbar and iliac pain, guarding, and tenderness. Fever, lumbar ache, nausea, vomiting, and diarrhea may also occur. Leukocytosis is common, but not always present. The diagnosis can be confirmed by a barium enema done without preparation and without a high filling pressure. A CT scan can also confirm the diagnosis. Medical therapy may lead to resolution, but some patients require exploration, abscess drainage, and resection of the diseased segment of colon.

2. Carcinoma of the Colon Perforation of a carcinoma can cause a clinical picture identical to that of diverticulitis. A prodromal history of rectal bleeding, severe constipation, and/or worsening lower abdominal pain may

be present. The diagnosis can be established by a low-pressure barium enema, colonoscopy, or laparotomy.

B. Left Lumbar and Hypochondriac Regions

1. Splenic Infarction Left hypochondriac and left flank pain may result from an acute splenic infarction. The pain is usually sharp, sticking, and intensified by respiration. Left upper abdominal and flank tenderness is frequently present. The spleen, if palpable, will also be tender. Infarction occurs in patients with large spleens secondary to chronic myelogenous leukemia and other myeloproliferative diseases. Patients with atrial fibrillation may suffer splenic infarction due to embolism. Infarction also occurs with sickle cell disease, as well as with sickle cell trait. Septic infarcts may occur secondary to endocarditis. A CT scan can confirm the diagnosis of splenic infarction.

2. Splenic Abscess Fever, chills, tender or nontender splenomegaly, and mild to severe left upper quadrant and flank pain occur. Localized left upper abdominal and flank tenderness and guarding may be present. Left shoulder pain may occur, and may be intensified by a deep breath or a cough. Rarely, a splenic friction rub may be present. The abscess may be secondary to embolization from endocarditis, or may result from salmonellosis or a streptococcal, staphylococcal, or gram-negative bacteremia. Risk factors include prior splenic infarctions, traumatic subcapsular bleeding, bacterial pneumonia and empyema, and subphrenic or other intraabdominal abscesses. The abscess can be imaged by gallium scintigraphy and/or a CT scan. Splenectomy and intravenous antibiotic therapy are essential to recovery.

Acute Umbilical Pain

☐ SUMMARY

Intestinal obstruction causes umbilical colic, with pain-free intervals of 5 to 20 min between attacks of pain. *Jejunal obstruction* causes an earlier onset of vomiting (i.e., day 1 or day 2) than *ileal obstruction*. In the latter, the vomitus may be yellow-brown or orange and may have a feculent odor. In both jejunal and ileal obstruction, distension eventually develops and the pain becomes a generalized constant ache. Plain radiographs show dilated loops of small bowel with air-fluid levels when obstruction is present. After an initial evacuation of the colon, there is no passage of stool or flatus from the rectum.

In patients with a *closed loop strangulating obstruction* there is an abrupt onset of severe, constant periumbilical or low epigastric pain, without abdominal guarding or tenderness. The patient appears ill and often writhes from side to side. Ultrasonography may demonstrate a U-shaped loop of dilated small bowel. Within 6 to 12 h, signs of localized peritonitis begin to develop, with tenderness and minimal guarding. Within 24 h a tender palpable mass may be present in the mid- or lower abdomen, and ascitic fluid may be detected.

Acute *mesenteric vascular occlusion* causes an abrupt onset of constant, severe periumbilical pain with minimal tenderness. If an *embolus* is the cause, there is usually a prior history of heart disease, arrhythmias, or endocarditis. In patients with *thrombi* there are other manifestations of generalized arteriosclerosis, and often a prior history of intestinal angina. Patients with this disorder have intense pain and appear severely ill, but usually have a soft, nontender abdomen. This clinical picture should suggest the diagnosis and lead to angiography, which can confirm the diagnosis of a superior mesenteric embolus or thrombus. In some patients with severe umbilical pain a selective arteriogram reveals no evidence of occlusion, but may show marked vasoconstriction (*nonocclusive intestinal infarction*). These patients usually have a history of heart failure, hypotension, and/or use of pressor drugs or digitalis. *Venous occlusion* causes similar symptoms, but can be detected by a

TABLE OF DISEASE INCIDENCE

INCIDENCE PER 100,000 (APPROXIMATE)

Common (>100)	Uncommon (>5–100)	Rare (>0–5)
Intestinal obstruction	Incarcerated umbilical hernia	Mesenteric vasculitis
Closed loop obstruction with gangrene	Acute mesenteric occlusion	Cecal diverticulitis
Acute appendicitis	Nonocclusive intestinal infarction	Meckel's diverticulitis
Acute gastroenteritis	Mesenteric venous thrombosis	
	Rupture of an abdominal aortic aneurysm	

CT study and by selective arteriography. *Vasculitis* can cause symptoms that mimic those of embolism or thrombosis, but patients with this cause have rheumatoid arthritis or evidence of a multisystem disease (e.g., polyarteritis nodosa).

Acute appendicitis and its mimics, *cecal diverticulitis* and *Meckel's diverticulitis,* may begin with crampy midabdominal pain that soon shifts into the right lower abdomen. A variable percentage of patients with these disorders also develop fever, nausea and vomiting, and signs of localized peritonitis in the right lower abdomen.

Acute gastroenteritis causes crampy umbilical pain with mild tenderness, nausea, vomiting, and diarrhea, and sometimes fever. *Rupture of an abdominal aortic aneurysm* may cause lower epigastric, umbilical, flank, and back pain, which may be pulsatile or constant. Often the pain is worse when the patient is supine, and is partly relieved by sitting up. A pulsatile tender abdominal mass may be felt; the diagnosis can be confirmed by CT scan or ultrasonography.

A soft but tender umbilical mass that is not reducible indicates the presence of an *incarcerated hernia*. If bowel is trapped within the sac, then colicky umbilical pain, vomiting, and distension of the abdomen may occur because of intestinal obstruction. Increasing firmness and tenderness of the mass, associated with constant severe umbilical pain, fever, toxicity, and leukocytosis suggest the diagnosis of *strangulation of the incarcerated bowel*.

☐ DESCRIPTION OF LISTED DISEASES

1. INTESTINAL OBSTRUCTION

A. Obstruction of the Proximal Small Bowel (Jejunum)

This disorder begins suddenly with constant, and then colicky, umbilical and lower epigastric pain. The initial crampy pain may persist for 15 to 30 min and abate, and then recur 4 to 5 min later. Each subsequent attack of pain lasts for 2 to 3 min and is associated with high-pitched bowel sounds during the pain. The abdomen may become tender during the painful episode. After each attack of pain subsides, there is a 4- to 5-min pain-free interval until the next attack. This pain–relief–pain cycle may continue for 12 to 24 h, and is associated with nausea and frequent vomiting. During pain-free periods the abdomen is soft and nontender. Vomiting occurs early in the course of proximal small bowel obstruction. The vomitus consists initially of watery yellow gastric juice, and somewhat later of greenish-yellow material from the upper small bowel. If the obstruction persists, the upper abdomen begins to become distended. No stool or gas is passed per rectum after one or two early evacuations. Radiographs of the abdomen show dilated loops of small bowel and air-fluid levels. Unless there is strangulation of a bowel loop, the leukocyte count, temperature, pulse rate, and abdominal examination remain within normal limits (i.e., there is no evidence of localized tenderness, guarding, or rebound). As the abdomen gradually distends, the colicky intermittent periumbilical pain ceases and is replaced by a constant generalized ache. Mechanical obstruction of the small bowel is caused by adhesions from prior surgery (74 percent of cases), incarceration in a hernia (8.1 percent), metastatic or primary cancer (8.6 percent), and Crohn's disease (5.2 percent). The nonsurgical therapy of acute intestinal obstruction is controversial. Management is governed by the inaccuracy of clinical determination of the presence of bowel strangulation.

Even if leukocytosis, localized pain, tachycardia, and fever are absent, 5 to 13 percent of patients may have strangulated bowel. In some medical centers, a trial of conservative management is attempted in selected patients. A long intestinal tube or a nasogastric tube is used to decompress the proximal bowel, and intravenous fluid and electrolytes are administered. Patients selected for a trial of nonoperative management usually have an early postoperative obstruction, obstruction secondary to adhesions, partial obstruction, or obstruction secondary to Crohn's disease. Patients in this latter group are also treated with steroids and parenteral hyperalimentation. In other medical centers, all patients with complete obstruction are treated by immediate surgical exploration, and only patients with partial obstruction are treated conservatively

B. Obstruction of the Distal Small Bowel (Ileum)

The attacks of midabdominal pain are similar to those described above, but the intervals between colics are longer (10–20 min). Vomiting may be delayed for 1 to 2 days, and it is not as frequent. The vomitus, which is initially yellow or green, soon becomes orange or brown, and has a foul, feculent odor, but does not contain feces. The abdomen remains soft and nontender between attacks of pain, but after 2 or 3 days it distends and becomes tender, and the colic is replaced by a milder, generalized, diffuse, aching pain. Plain radiographs show many dilated loops of small bowel and air-fluid levels. Surgical intervention is required to relieve symptoms and preserve life.

C. Closed Loop Obstruction and Strangulation An abrupt onset of constant, severe, aching umbilical and/or lower epigastric pain, with a soft, flat, nontender abdomen, suggests intraabdominal ischemia. Patients with this condition may writhe in pain. During the first day there is usually no fever, tachycardia, anemia, or localized tenderness or guarding. Plain abdominal radiographs may show no evidence of gas in the small bowel or of air-fluid levels. During the second 24 h, fever, leukocytosis, tachycardia, and a tender mass may appear. Repeat radiographs may show dilated loops of small bowel. Ultrasonography may demonstrate a dilated, fluid-filled, U-shaped loop of small bowel and ascites. The ascitic fluid is usually found to be foul-smelling and serosanguineous; its levels of phosphate, LDH, and amylase usually exceed serum levels. Surgical exploration is required to resect the loop of strangulated gangrenous bowel before it spills toxic, and potentially lethal, necrotic bowel contents into the peritoneal cavity. The incidence of strangulation when fibrous adhesions cause obstruction is 9 to 32 percent in various series. More than 80 percent of adhesion-related obstructions occur within 5 years of surgery; the remaining 20 percent occur between 5 and 15 years after the adhesion-producing surgery.

2. ACUTE MESENTERIC ARTERIAL OCCLUSION

A. Embolus or Thrombus There is an abrupt onset of severe, colicky umbilical or low epigastric pain. Bowel sounds are initially present, and may even be hyperactive. Over the next 4 to 5 h the pain becomes more intense and constant, and it gradually spreads over the entire abdomen. Initially the abdomen is soft and nontender, but at the end of 8 h there may be mild abdominal tenderness and leukocytosis; then bowel sounds become inactive, and early abdominal distension is evident. During the first 4 to 5 h the diagnosis of bowel ischemia should be entertained, and selective abdominal angiography performed. Prompt surgical intervention is required to remove a superior mesenteric artery embolus or thrombus and resect necrotic bowel. A second-look operation, 36 h after the first, is usually done to detect residual necrotic bowel.

Failure to intervene in the case of a patient with intense midabdominal pain with minimal physical signs, who has a history of arrhythmia, coronary or valvular heart disease, or endocarditis, will allow the development of bowel infarction and gangrene. This will develop 8 to 16 h after the onset of pain, and is signaled by abdominal distension, localized peritoneal signs, rectal bleeding or heme-positive stools, and systemic signs, such as fever, tachycardia, leukocytosis, acidosis, and ascites. The prognosis for bowel

salvage or patient survival is poor if surgery is not performed within 6 h of the onset of the pain. Angiography will localize the site of an embolus or thrombus and identify patients who have nonocclusive infarction.

B. Nonocclusive Intestinal Infarction Umbilical pain of a constant nature, indistinguishable from that seen with a superior mesenteric artery occlusion due to an embolus or thrombus, may occur in patients with cardiac output reduced by heart failure, shock, or severe hypoxemia. Confirmation of the diagnosis requires selective angiography of the superior mesenteric artery. In this syndrome, splanchnic vasoconstriction is a common angiographic finding. In addition, there is slow flow and poor filling of the intramural vessels in the bowel wall.

Nonocclusive ischemia can be associated with the administration of digitalis, catecholamines, diuretics, beta blockers, and vasopressin. Low cardiac output, hypovolemic shock, dialysis, and endotoxemia may also be associated with nonocclusive ischemia. Pharmacologic reversal of acute abdominal pain and tenderness has been demonstrated in such cases using an intraarterial bolus of tolazoline and an intravenous papaverine infusion. With pharmacologic intervention, survival has increased to 50 to 60 percent. Some surgeons recommend surgical intervention 6 to 12 h after pharmacologic therapy is initiated; others operate only if angiographic vasoconstriction persists on a follow-up angiogram, or if peritonitis begins to develop.

C. Mesenteric Venous Thrombosis This disorder begins suddenly with severe, constant midline umbilical or epigastric pain. Nausea, vomiting, and bloody or heme-positive stools and diarrhea may accompany the pain, but there are few physical findings during the first 8 h. Tenderness, guarding, and distension are minimal. Venous occlusion may occur in a setting of venous stasis (e.g., heart failure, cirrhosis with portal hypertension, or venous compression by abdominal tumor) or of abdominal inflammatory disease (peritonitis, abscess, enteritis), or in patients with a hypercoagulable state (contraceptive pill use, polycythemia, antithrombin III deficiency). Some patients have no easily discernible risk factor. Hemoconcentration and leukocytosis occur early, and a serosanguineous ascitic fluid begins to collect. Plain radiographs show small bowel distension and thickening of the bowel wall. An abdominal CT study can readily demonstrate occlusion of the superior mesenteric vein. A contrast-enhanced CT scan will reveal a high-density vein wall with a central filling defect and clearly visible collateral vessels. Plain radiographs, contrast studies, and CT may demonstrate the "rigid loop sign" and/or thrumbprinting. Selective angiography will demonstrate a thickened edematous bowel wall with a blush due to capillary opacification, stretching of small peripheral arteries due to bowel wall edema, and decreased venous return without filling of the mesenteric vein.

Venous occlusion with bowel infarction is treated by surgical resection. Anticoagulants are used postoperatively unless there is a risk in their administration (e.g., portal hypertension, tumor, severe trauma).

D. Vasculitis and Intestinal Infarction Acute arterial occlusion of large or medium-sized vessels may occur in polyarteritis nodosa or in the vasculitis associated with rheumatoid arthritis. Arteriosclerotic occlusion can be mimicked. Patients with polyarteritis may have hypertension, fever, distal gangrene, renal failure, a cerebral or myocardial infarction, mononeuritis multiplex, anemia, leukocytosis, and/or eosinophilia in addition to acute, constant abdominal distress. Patients with rheumatoid arthritis and vasculitis may have similar abdominal pain, skin nodules, extensive symmetrical arthritis, leg ulcers, and high titers of rheumatoid factor in their serum. Acute infarction of a segment of bowel requires surgical intervention and bowel resection. Initiation of therapy with cyclophosphamide and steroids may be required to prevent recurrent attacks of bowel ischemia and infarction in patients with these disorders.

3. ACUTE APPENDICITIS AND ITS MIMICS

The initial symptom is a mild, crampy or aching, low epigastric or umbilical pain, which continues, with few other symptoms, for 3 to 5 h. This pain then abates and a new, aching or burning, constant discomfort appears in the right lower abdomen. In some cases the pain shifts instead to the right lumbar region (retrocecal appendix), suprapubic area, or left lower abdomen (pelvic appendix). Nausea and vomiting soon develop; within 8 to 24 h a temperature rise, to as high as 101°F, may develop. This is usually accompanied by a leukocytosis of up to 18,000 cells per mm^3. The physical examination reveals right lower abdominal tenderness, rebound tenderness, and guarding. Coughing and bodily movements intensify the pain, which is usually well localized to a specific lower abdominal site. Surgical exploration and appendectomy will relieve all symptoms.

A. Acute Cecal Diverticulitis This disorder may mimic acute appendicitis. It usually begins as a constant mild pain in the right lower abdomen. In a minority of cases, there may be an initial brief period of periumbilical pain before pain begins on the right side. Nausea and vomiting may occur, but affect fewer than 25 percent of patients. Low-grade fever may also develop, and leukocytosis may or may not be present. This disorder behaves like a slowly progressive case of appendicitis; symptoms are often present for 3 to 30 days before medical help is sought. In up to 75 percent of cases, the patient is operated on for acute appendicitis and the true diagnosis is made at surgery. In patients with a prior appendectomy, and a palpable mass in the right-lower abdomen or heme-positive stools, a sono-

graphic or CT study may clarify the diagnosis prior to surgery and allow a course of medical management. In some cases, this disorder will resolve without need for surgery.

B. Meckel's Diverticulitis Another rare mimic of acute appendicitis is acute inflammation of Meckel's diverticulum. Such cases are usually discovered at surgery, when the appendix is found to be normal.

4. ACUTE GASTROENTERITIS

Acute gastroenteritis may cause constant or crampy periumbilical pain associated with watery diarrhea, nausea, and vomiting. The leukocyte count is usually normal or low. There may be mild umbilical tenderness or more generalized abdominal tenderness. Rebound tenderness may also occur, but involuntary guarding does not. Bowel sounds are usually hyperactive. Fever may or may not accompany the abdominal symptoms. The presence of heme-positive stools and/or fecal leukocytes suggests an infection with a *Campylobacter*, *Shigella*, or *Salmonella* species, or an initial attack of inflammatory bowel disease.

5. RUPTURE OF AN ABDOMINAL AORTIC ANEURYSM

Periumbilical throbbing or aching pain occurs, with associated flank and midback pain. The pain may be more intense when the patient is supine, and may be relieved by sitting up. Nausea and vomiting, and generalized weakness and faintness, may accompany the pain. Examination of the abdomen will reveal a midline, upper abdominal, tender pulsatile mass. A CT scan will demonstrate the aneurysm and extravasated blood in the retroperitoneum. If the aneurysm is leaking, tachycardia and hypotension will develop rapidly, and the hematocrit will fall abruptly after 2 or 3 liters of fluid resuscitation. Emergency surgery is required to prevent death.

6. INCARCERATED OR STRANGULATED UMBILICAL HERNIA

A painful mass appears at the umbilicus at the site of a known hernia. If the small bowel is incarcerated in the hernia sac, typical periumbilical colic with vomiting and retching may occur, indicating partial or complete intestinal obstruction. The mass is usually firm, tender, and not reducible, and bowel sounds may be heard within it. The skin over the hernia sac may be reddened, simulating cellulitis. If the obstructed bowel distends against a rigid hernia ring, bowel ischemia may occur, leading to gangrene. With a closed loop obstruction and gangrene, the pain becomes very severe and continuous; within 12 to 24 h, fever, leukocytosis, toxicity, and severe tenderness of the hernia mass develop. Surgical exploration is required to remove necrotic bowel, restore intestinal continuity, and repair the hernia. In some cases, especially in teenagers, only omentum is trapped in the hernia. This causes pain and tenderness, and may require surgery for relief.

Umbilical hernia incarceration and strangulation have been reported in patients with cirrhosis and ascites after rapid reduction of the amount of ascitic fluid present, whether by paracentesis, peritoneovenous shunting, or diuretic therapy. Patients undergoing continuous ambulatory peritoneal dialysis may develop umbilical, inguinal, or catheter-site hernias, which may become incarcerated or strangulated.

CHAPTER

21

Acute Right Iliac Pain

☐ DIAGNOSTIC LIST

1. Acute appendicitis
2. Nonsurgical mimics of acute appendicitis
   A. 1. Pleuritic pain
      2. Herpes zoster
   B. Mesenteric adenitis and ileitis due to *Yersinia* infection
   C. Ureteral colic
   D. Acute gastroenteritis
   E. Renal and perirenal infection
      1. Renal cortical abscess
      2. Renal corticomedullary abscess
      3. Perinephric abscess
      4. Acute pyelonephritis
   F. Crohn's disease
   G. Abdominal pain of unknown cause
   H. Amebiasis
   I. Acute osteomyelitis of the ilium
   J. Ewing's sarcoma of the right ilium
3. Surgical mimics of acute appendicitis
   A. Cecal diverticulitis
   B. Cecal carcinoma with perforation
   C. Cecal distension due to distal obstruction of the colon
   D. Meckel's diverticulitis
   E. Carcinoma of the appendix with perforation
   F. Perforation of a duodenal ulcer with leakage down the right lumbar gutter
   G. Acute cholecystitis

   H. Infarction of the greater omentum
   I. Ileocecal intussusception
   J. Psoas abscess
   K. Torsion of an intraabdominal testis and other pain of testicular origin
   L. Anisakiasis
   M. Rupture of an infrarenal aortic aneurysm
   N. Rupture or enlargement of a common iliac aneurysm
   O. Cecal volvulus
   P. Perforation of the ileum due to typhoid fever
   Q. Neutropenic enterocolitis
   R. Ileocecal tuberculosis
4. Gynecologic mimics of acute appendicitis
   A. Pelvic inflammatory disease (PID)
      1. Acute salpingitis
      2. Acute tubo-ovarian abscess (TOA)
      3. Rupture of a TOA
   B. Tubal pregnancy
   C. Mimics of tubal pregnancy, PID, and appendicitis
      1. Corpus luteum cyst with bleeding
      2. Corpus luteum cyst of pregnancy
      3. Threatened abortion
      4. Follicle cyst with intraperitoneal bleeding (mittelschmerz)
      5. Endometrioma with intraperitoneal bleeding
      6. Adnexal torsion

☐ SUMMARY

Acute appendicitis frequently begins with mild, crampy epigastric or periumbilical pain. This pain is dull and aching and is not intensified by movement or coughing. Within 4 to 5 h, this discomfort abates and a new pain begins in the right lower abdomen. At first, it is a mild, dull ache that is intensified by walking, coughing, or moving about in bed. Anorexia, nausea, and vomiting may begin. The patient can often localize the right-sided pain to an area the size of a half dollar. There may be a low-grade fever, which begins 12 to 24 h after the onset of the pain, but this seldom exceeds 101°F. Constipation and a feeling that a good bowel movement might eliminate all complaints may be experienced. Some patients develop diarrhea and are often misdiagnosed as having an enteritis. Urinary frequency and dysuria may occur because of proximity of the inflamed appendix to the bladder. There is usually direct, well-localized tenderness in or around McBurney's point (91 percent), rebound tenderness (68 percent), a leukocytosis and/or shift to the left, and a progressive course.

A number of *nonsurgical disorders* may mimic acute appendicitis because they present with right lower abdominal pain or have it as a major component of their symptom complex. *Pneumonia, pulmonary infarction,* or *pleurodynia* affecting the right lower thoracic or diaphragmatic pleura can cause right lower abdominal pain and tenderness, mimicking acute appendicitis. Review of the preoperative chest radiograph usually allows diagnosis of a pulmonary cause for the symptoms, but cases continue to occur in which a healthy appendix is removed from a patient with pneumonia because of failure to examine the chest radiograph.

Herpes zoster may cause burning or aching right posterolateral thoracolumbar pain that radiates into the right lower abdomen and a rash consisting of vesicles and crusted ulcers that appears after 2 to 3 days. The lesions are restricted to the painful area.

Mesenteric adenitis may cause a clinical picture indistinguishable from acute appendicitis with a leukocytosis and/or shift to the left and localized direct and rebound tenderness in the right lower abdomen. High-resolution compression ultrasonography studies can demonstrate the enlarged nodes and fail to demonstrate an enlarged appendix. If *ileitis* is part of the clinical picture, there may be diarrhea, and an edematous ileum may be visualized by sonography. Adenitis and ileitis are commonly caused by *Yersinia enterocolitica,* an organism that is antibiotic-sensitive in vitro. Nevertheless, the illness responds only minimally to parenteral antibiotic therapy.

Acute ureteral colic causes constant severe pain, and there is usually costovertebral-angle tenderness, as well as right lower abdominal tenderness. Gross or microscopic hematuria and demonstration of an obstructing stone in the ureter by an excretory urogram confirm the diagnosis.

Gastroenteritis causes anorexia, nausea, vomiting, fever, chills, diarrhea, and crampy or constant abdominal pain, which may localize to the right lower abdomen. This occurs commonly with *Yersinia* and *Salmonella* infections. Crampy pain may occur throughout the abdomen, and there may be localized tenderness and rebound tenderness in the right lower abdomen.

A *renal cortical abscess* causes fever, chills, and flank and abdominal pain and tenderness. Results of the urinalysis are usually negative. A *corticomedullary abscess* occurs in patients with a gram-negative urinary tract infection and partial obstruction. The diagnosis of abscess can be confirmed by sonography or a CT scan. A *perinephric abscess* usually results from rupture of a renal abscess. It may cause flank and lower abdominal pain and fever. It can be diagnosed by CT scan with contrast.

Acute pyelonephritis also may cause right lower abdominal pain with or without flank pain. There may be mild, poorly localized right lower abdominal tenderness and costovertebral-angle tenderness. The urine contains large numbers of bacteria and leukocytes and some red blood cells. There is a prompt response to parenteral antibiotic therapy.

An acute exacerbation of *Crohn's disease* may be suspected if there is a history of chronic recurrent crampy and/or constant periumbilical and right iliac pain and diarrhea.

Amebiasis causes right lower abdominal pain, fever, and diarrhea. There may be local tenderness. The diagnosis can be confirmed by microscopic stool examinations and colonoscopic biopsy of ulcers. This disorder may cause an acute abdomen that is easily confused with acute appendicitis because of its tendency to involve the cecum. The diagnosis is seldom made preoperatively.

Acute osteomyelitis of the right ilium can cause right iliac pain and tenderness. There may be a local mass and a positive radionuclide bone scan or MRI, confirming the diagnosis. Rarely, *Ewing's sarcoma* may mimic the findings of osteomyelitis.

A number of *surgical disorders* may present with similar findings in the right lower abdomen. Acute *cecal diverticulitis* may mimic appendicitis, but the pain often begins initially in the right lower abdomen without prodromal periumbilical or epigastric pain. The pain is mild, and this disorder usually progresses more gradually than appendicitis. The diagnosis is seldom made preoperatively, but it can be by use of a CT study or laparoscopy. If the diagnosis is confirmed, antibiotic therapy can resolve symptoms without need for surgery. In most cases, the diagnosis is made in the operating room. *Cecal or appendiceal carcinoma* also may provide a surprise to the operating surgeon expecting to find appendicitis. These lesions have usually perforated, forming a localized abscess. *Perforation of a duodenal ulcer* usually causes the abrupt onset of severe upper abdominal pain that may shift to the right lower abdomen. There may be epigastric as well as right lower abdominal tenderness and evidence of free air on an upright abdominal radiograph. A diatrizoate meglumine swallow can sometimes demonstrate a duodenal ulcer and leakage from the perforation if it has not already sealed.

A *distended inflamed gallbladder* may extend into the right lower abdomen, causing pain and local tenderness. The gallbladder may sometimes be detected by palpation or percussion, and can be demonstrated by sonographic studies. A history of recurrent 2- to 6-h attacks of severe epigastric pain suggests the diagnosis. A *psoas abscess* may be suspected from a history of spinal osteomyelitis, Crohn's disease, or diverticulitis. In addition, there is right lower abdominal pain and tenderness and a positive psoas sign. Most patients hold the thigh flexed on the trunk and are unable to fully extend the affected leg. The diagnosis can be confirmed by a CT study of the pelvis.

Further abdominal exploration after removal of a normal appendix may reveal *Meckel's diverticulitis,* an *omental infarction,* or an *intussusception.* Patients with the latter disorder may have hematochezia and intestinal obstruction. The diagnosis can be made by CT scan or in the operating room. *Cecal dilatation due to distal obstruction of the colon* may present with diffuse lower abdominal pain that becomes more intense in the right lower abdomen as the cecum distends. A cecum with a diameter of more than 10 cm on a plain abdominal radiograph is at risk for perforation.

Right lower abdominal pain arising in a testicle can be suspected from a history of recent vasectomy or pain and tenderness in the testicle. Torsion causes acute severe pain, swelling, and retraction of the testicle. The diagnosis can be confirmed by ultrasonography and/or a radionuclide scan. Prompt surgery to correct the torsion relieves symptoms. *Acute torsion of an intraabdominal testis* can cause severe right lower abdominal pain and peritoneal signs in association with absence of the right testis from the scrotum.

Anisakiasis of the ileocecal region may mimic acute appendicitis and is a frequent surgical finding in Japan where raw fish is frequently ingested. It is caused by a herring worm.

The sudden onset of excruciating right lower abdominal pain, with or without low back pain, in a patient over age 50 suggests the possibility of a *ruptured aortic aneurysm.* Diaphoresis, dizziness, and hypotension may result from the pain and retroperitoneal blood loss. The abdominal examination reveals a poorly defined midline pulsatile mass. The presence of an aneurysm can be confirmed by ultrasonography but this procedure is seldom necessary. Most patients are taken directly to the operating room for emergency surgery. Right lower abdominal pain associated with a psoas syndrome in the presence of a tender pulsatile lower abdominal mass may be due to an aneurysm of the right iliac artery. This diagnosis can be confirmed by a sonographic or CT study. Unless there is bleeding, emergency surgery is not required. *Cecal volvulus* may cause right lower abdominal pain and distension. Plain radiographs demonstrate cecal distension and displacement to the left. The diagnosis can be confirmed by a contrast enema or an abdominal CT scan.

Right lower abdominal pain, tenderness, and guarding occurring in the second or third week of a febrile illness typical of *typhoid* is due to ileal perforation, and immediate surgery is required to prevent spreading peritonitis.

Neutropenic enterocolitis causes generalized abdominal and right iliac pain and peritoneal signs in patients with neutrophil counts of $10^3/\text{mm}^3$ or less secondary to leukemia, aplastic anemia, cyclic neutropenia, or myelotoxic chemotherapy. The diagnosis can be confirmed by a CT scan of the abdomen. Symptoms may respond to intravenous antibiotics or surgical

resection of the right colon. A patient with *ileocecal tuberculosis* may present as having acute appendicitis after perforation of the ileocecal region.

The negative appendectomy rate for women is 35 to 45 percent, twice as high as the rate for men. Several *gynecologic disorders* are capable of mimicking acute appendicitis. The gynecologic disorders most commonly confused with acute appendicitis are acute pelvic inflammatory disease (PID), tubal pregnancy, and bleeding from a cyst. *PID* may cause right lower abdominal pain and direct and rebound tenderness. The absence of nausea and vomiting in most cases, a pain duration greater than 2 days, onset in the first week after onset of menstruation, a history of sexually transmitted diseases, cervical motion and adnexal tenderness, and abdominal tenderness outside the right lower abdomen suggest the diagnosis of PID. Sonographic studies will fail to demonstrate an enlarged, noncompressible appendix and may demonstrate dilated edematous tubes or a *tubal abscess.* Laparoscopy can confirm the diagnosis and can visualize a normal appendix. In some centers, women with a classical history of appendicitis are operated on without benefit of laparoscopy, and PID is the only operative finding.

Lower abdominal pain in a woman in the childbearing years may be due to an *ectopic pregnancy.* The pain may be colicky and mild in the early stages, but after several days or weeks it may become constant and intense. If the right tube contains the pregnancy, it may mimic acute appendicitis. There is usually a history of amenorrhea or a recent scant period. Spotting and staining may begin after one or two missed periods and persist, but simple amenorrhea may also occur.

The pregnancy can be visualized by ultrasonography as a live embryo in the tube (7–15 percent) or a noncystic mass (92 percent), and the absence of an intrauterine pregnancy can be demonstrated. The serum beta-hCG or urine ICON test is positive in 96 to 99 percent of cases. The diagnosis can be confirmed at laparoscopy or laparotomy. Cases have been treated by observation or by laparoscopic or open surgery. *Adnexal torsion* causes intermittent crampy and then constant, progressively severe, lower abdominal pain and tenderness. A tender adnexal mass may be palpable on pelvic examination. Sonographic studies show a uniformly echogenic adnexal mass. The diagnosis can be confirmed by laparoscopy or in the operating room where surgical resection of the ovary and tube or correction of the torsion may be performed.

A *corpus luteum cyst* may cause a missed or delayed period, followed by irregular bleeding and right lower abdominal pain and tenderness. Pelvic examination reveals right adnexal tenderness and, sometimes, a small mass. The pregnancy test results are negative, and laparoscopy reveals bleeding into or from a corpus luteum cyst.

A *corpus luteum cyst of pregnancy* may mimic a tubal pregnancy by causing right lower abdominal pain, tenderness, an adnexal mass, and a positive pregnancy test. Ultrasonography will confirm an intrauterine pregnancy, and laparoscopy will identify the hemorrhagic cyst and normal tubes. Similarly, laparoscopy can identify bleeding *follicle cysts* or *endome-*

triomas. *Threatened abortion* usually causes crampy, midline pain, but may cause right adnexal pain. Ultrasonography will demonstrate an intrauterine gestation. Laparoscopy can be used to demonstrate the absence of an ectopic pregnancy in the tubes or ovarian areas.

Abdominal pain of unknown cause is a "wastebasket" diagnosis. It includes patients with right lower abdominal pain and tenderness who have no abnormality detected at surgery. Some of these patients may have viral disorders such as *pleurodynia* or a very mild *salpingitis* without a grossly observable inflammation of the tube, but most cases are unexplained.

☐ DESCRIPTION OF LISTED DISEASES

1. ACUTE APPENDICITIS

Mild pain of a crampy quality begins abruptly in the epigastrium or periumbilical region. This discomfort continues for 2 to 4 h and then shifts its location to the right lower abdomen and becomes a constant ache or burning discomfort, intensified by walking, coughing, or even moving about in bed. Anorexia, nausea, and vomiting may accompany the initial pain. Patients seen within 24 h of onset frequently have well-localized tenderness over McBurney's point. Direct palpation, percussion, or cough elicit the tenderness. Between 8 and 24 h, the temperature may rise to as high as 101.5°F, but in some cases the temperature remains normal. The pulse rate usually remains in the normal range.

Guarding and rebound tenderness are late findings and may not be present during the first 18 h. Absence of these findings should not delay diagnosis and surgical intervention. Laboratory studies reveal either a moderate leukocytosis ($10–18 \times 10^3$ cells/mm^3) or a normal count with a left shift in 95 percent of cases. The urine sediment may contain white blood cells and/or red blood cells in up to 20 percent of cases. The sedimentation rate is usually normal during the first 36 h.

Alvarado has devised a ten-point scoring system that summarizes the findings described above. One point each is awarded for the presence of (1) pain shift to the right lower quadrant, (2) anorexia, (3) nausea and vomiting, (4) rebound pain, (5) fever, and (6) a shift to the left on the differential count. Two points are given for right lower quadrant tenderness and two for a leukocytosis. A score of 7 or more is associated with a correct diagnosis of appendicitis in 88 percent of cases. The presence of a tender palpable right lower quadrant mass, a temperature over 102°F, or pain for more than 30 h is suggestive of appendiceal perforation and early abscess formation.

Other symptoms may occur but are less common. Constipation and the feeling that a good bowel movement will bring relief ("gas stoppage sensation" or "downward urge") lead patients to use cathartics and enemas. Passage of stool or gas, however, does not bring relief. Diarrhea may occur if there is inflammatory irritation of the recto-

TABLE OF DISEASE INCIDENCE

INCIDENCE PER 100,000 (APPROXIMATE)

Common (>100)	Uncommon (>5–100)	Rare (>0–5)
Acute appendicitis	Meckel's diverticulitis	Pleuritis causing lower abdominal pain
Mesenteric adenitis	Acute cholecystitis	Cecal diverticulitis
Acute gastroenteritis	Adnexal or ovarian torsion	Cecal carcinoma and perforation
Abdominal pain of unknown cause	Acute pyelonephritis causing low abdominal pain	Cecal distension due to distal obstruction of the colon
Ureteral colic	Corpus luteum cyst with bleeding	Cecal volvulus
Pelvic inflammatory disease	Corpus luteum cyst of pregnancy with bleeding	Carcinoma of the appendix with perforation
Tubo-ovarian abscess (TOA)	Endometrioma with bleeding	Duodenal ulcer perforation with leakage into right lower abdomen
Ectopic pregnancy	Crohn's disease	Infarction of the greater omentum
Threatened abortion	TOA with rupture	Ileocecal intussusception
Follicle cyst with bleeding	Herpes zoster	Psoas abscess
		Testicular torsion and epididymitis
		Testicular torsion of an intraabdominal testis
		Anisakiasis of the ileocecal area
		Amebiasis
		Rupture of an infrarenal aortic aneurysm
		Rupture or enlargement of an iliac artery aneurysm
		Perforation of the ileum in typhoid fever
		Acute osteomyelitis of the ilium
		Ewing's sarcoma of the ilium
		Acute renal abscess
		Acute perinephric abscess
		Neutropenic enterocolitis (typhlitis)
		Ileocecal tuberculosis with perforation

sigmoid or ileum. Rarely, urinary frequency and dysuria result from appendiceal involvement of the right ureter, bladder, or prostate. Rare cases of obstructive appendicitis may cause severe generalized abdominal pain that mimics the colic of intestinal obstruction or the constant severe pain of mesenteric occlusion.

In some cases (e.g., retrocecal appendicitis), pain begins abruptly in the right lower abdomen, and there is no preceding midline visceral pain. In other deceptive cases, there is only right lower abdominal and/or pelvic tenderness on rectal examination, but no right-sided pain. Patients with a retrocecal or pelvic appendicitis often have poorly localized pain over the mid- or lower abdomen and may never develop localized right lower abdominal pain and tenderness. Rare presenting complaints include gross hematuria and referred testicular pain and tenderness.

Less common physical signs include right lower abdominal skin hyperesthesia associated with the area of tenderness, guarding, referred or direct rebound tenderness, rectal tenderness, and testicular tenderness or retraction. A positive psoas or obturator sign occurs in some cases.

Abdominal radiographs may demonstrate a localized ileus or a fecalith, but the accuracy of this test is too low to be of value. Barium enemas were done for diagnosis at one time because it was believed that appendiceal filling excluded the diagnosis and failure to fill supported it. However, since 10 percent of normal appendixes fail to fill and 20 percent of nongangrenous inflamed appendixes do fill, the 70 percent accuracy of the procedure is too low to be useful. In addition, the utilization of a barium enema in the setting of an acute abdomen is difficult and potentially hazardous.

Male patients with classical symptoms and signs have a negative appendectomy rate of 10 to 15 percent, while women have a rate of 30 to 45 percent. When diagnostic delay is utilized in order to improve accuracy and decrease the negative appendectomy rate, the rate of perforation tends to rise from 14 percent (accuracy, 67 percent) to 29 percent (accuracy, 89 percent). This trade-off between early operation with decreased accuracy and a lower perforation rate remains a current problem.

High-resolution ultrasonography performed with a graded compression technique has been used to detect cases of appendicitis in groups of patients with lower abdominal pain and equivocal or nonclassical clinical findings. In this group of patients, ultrasonography may detect 83 percent of patients with acute appendicitis. Diagnosis is based on sonographic visualization of an enlarged inflamed appendix with a diameter of 6 mm or more. Only a small number of normal appendixes can be visualized by ultrasound, and these have a diameter less than 6 mm. Earlier operation is a possible option for patients with dubious clinical findings but a positive sonographic study for appendicitis. A negative sonographic study does not rule out appendicitis. Ultrasonography may also be of use in confirming a diagnosis of appendiceal abscess and in identifying alternative disorders, such as salpingitis and ovarian cysts, that are responsible for the clinical symptoms and signs.

In one series, 80 percent of women with mimicking gynecologic disorders, 82 percent of patients with gastrointestinal disorders, and 33 percent of patients with urinary tract problems were detected by the use of ultrasonography. Overall, the correct alternative diagnosis to appendicitis was suggested by sonographic studies in 70 percent of those with a specific cause for their symptoms.

Laparoscopy has been utilized in female patients with an equivocal clinical picture in order to confirm a diagnosis of appendicitis without need for continued clinical observation and in order to detect and diagnose alternative causes for the clinical findings. In one study, laparoscopy did not decrease the false-negative appendectomy rate but did identify other disorders (i.e., salpingitis, ovarian cysts, and ileitis) at an earlier time.

Failure to visualize the appendix may occur in 20 percent of cases, and in this situation the decision to operate may be affected by detection of an alternative cause of symptoms. If no alternative diagnosis is discovered, surgical intervention is dependent on continued clinical appraisal. Since 25 percent of appendixes removed in women with classical symptoms and signs are normal, the use of laparoscopy in all patients with suspected appendicitis might decrease the negative appendectomy rate. A prospective study of such patients has not been done. Laparoscopy is invasive, requires anesthesia and time, and has a false-positive rate and a nonvisualization rate that may lead to surgery in women without appendicitis. A technetium 99m–albumin colloid white cell scan has been recently used to diagnose appendicitis. Use of the scan introduces a delay of 3 to 5 h in management. It has a 97 percent predictive value negative and a 93 percent predictive value positive in men. In women, the predictive value positive of only 43 percent is unreliable for diagnosing appendicitis. Too few patients have been studied to allow evaluation of this test.

Perforation remains a major problem in children under age 8 and adults above age 60, in whom rates as high as 70 percent have been reported. Delay by the patient and/or physician has been responsible for this high rate and increased morbidity and mortality in these age groups. Thus far, use of quantitative clinical scales, laboratory tests, radiologic procedures, ultrasonography or laparoscopy, or radionuclide scans for early diagnosis have not decreased the perforation rate in these patients.

The definitive treatment of acute appendicitis is amputation of the appendix and ligation of the stump without inversion. A perforated appendix with a local abscess will often resolve with intravenous antibiotic therapy. If not, abscess drainage may be required. Appendectomy after abscess drainage is usually not necessary and can be done in the 10 to 20 percent of patients who suffer recurrent symptoms.

2. NONSURGICAL MIMICS OF ACUTE APPENDICITIS

A.   *1. Pleuritic Pain*   Pneumonia or pulmonary embolism with infarction can cause right lower abdominal pain and localized tenderness that may be mistaken for acute appendicitis. Pain may also be felt in the right lower anterior chest and/or shoulder and may be intensified by a deep breath or cough. Pleuritic pain due to pneumonia may be associated with fever; chills; cough; and purulent, rusty or blood-streaked sputum. Physical examination may reveal a friction rub, dullness, bronchial breath sounds, and rales over the right lower chest. A chest radiograph will reveal a pneumonic infiltrate or consolidation on the right side. Pulmonary embolism and infarction may cause cough, dyspnea, hemoptysis, and fever. The physical examination may be negative or reveal a friction rub, signs of effusion, rales, wheezes, or rhonchi. The chest radiograph may be negative or show evidence of a pleural effusion, a pleural-based triangular opacity, a nonspecific infiltrate or consolidation, pulmonary artery enlargement, and/or loss of vascularity in portions of the right lung. A perfusion lung scan is positive, and, in patients without a ventilation scan mismatch, this finding can be supported by detecting a thigh vein thrombus by impedance plethysmography or ultrasonography. In patients with an abnormal perfusion scan and a negative impedance plethysmogram, pulmonary angiography will be required to confirm a diagnosis of pulmonary infarction. High-risk patients for embolism include those with recent trauma, surgery, pregnancy, heart failure, or malignancy; a family history of thromboembolism (i.e., families with antithrombin III, protein C, or protein S deficiencies); a previous embolism; or recent prolonged automobile or air travel and other causes of leg immobilization (e.g., paralysis, casting, severe arthritis). Antibiotic therapy for pneumonia and anticoagulant treatment for embolism usually leads to prompt resolution of symptoms. It is essential to examine the chest carefully and review a preoperative chest radiograph to rule out a pleural cause for right lower abdominal pain. Pleurodynia due to a coxsackievirus or echovirus infection may cause right lower abdominal pain and tenderness, as well as right upper abdominal pain and/or right chest pain. Cough, tenderness, and voluntary guarding may occur. This disorder clears spontaneously in 1 to 3 days.

2. Herpes Zoster   Acute appendicitis may be mimicked by herpes zoster. There is a gradual onset of aching or burning pain in the low back, right lower abdomen, and lateral abdominal wall. Within 2 to 3 days, small groups of crusted ulcers or vesicles appear in a bandlike distribution in the painful area. The skin lesions and pain are restricted to the back, side, and front of the right side of the trunk.

B.   Mesenteric Adenitis and Acute Ileitis Due to *Yersinia*

Infection   *Yersinia* species (*Y. enterocolitica* and *Y. pseudotuberculosis*) may cause an enterocolitis with abdominal pain, diarrhea, and fever. Confirmation of the diagnosis requires cultures and measurement of serum antibody levels by an ELISA method. Some patients with *Yersinia* infection develop a true appendicitis, mesenteric adenitis, and/or acute ileitis. These cases simulate the clinical picture of acute appendicitis. Nodal enlargement may suggest perforation and abscess formation.

Graded-compression ultrasonography has been successful in differentiating appendicitis from mesenteric adenitis and acute terminal ileitis. The most useful sonographic criteria for the exclusion of appendicitis have been (1) nonvisualization of an inflamed appendix, (2) mural thickening of the terminal ileum, and (3) visualization of enlarged mesenteric lymph nodes. Node enlargement occurs in up to 40 percent of patients with appendicitis, but the inflamed appendix can usually be visualized by ultrasonography. Stool cultures and serological studies have too long a turnaround time to aid in differentiating *Yersinia* infection from appendicitis. When mesenteric adenitis and ileitis are discovered at surgery, node culture or immunofluorescent antibody staining of sectioned tissue will identify *Yersinia* enterocolitica. Stool and tissue samples can be cultured on CIN (cefsulodin-irgasan-novobiocin) agar, deoxycholate-citrate agar, and cold-enrichment carried out at 22°C for 48 to 72 h. In one large sonographic study, 8 percent of 170 patients studied because of suspicion of appendicitis were found to have mesenteric adenitis, acute ileitis, and positive stool cultures. Antibiotics such as aminoglycosides, trimethoprim-sulfamethoxazole, or ceftriaxone may favorably influence the course of a severe *Yersinia*-associated sepsis, but antibiotics do not seem to reduce the moderate and limited morbidity associated with mesenteric adenitis and acute ileitis. The latter disorder does not appear to evolve into a chronic recurrent form of Crohn's disease.

C. Ureteral Colic   Pain may occur in the right lower abdomen when a renal stone, blood clot, or tissue fragment becomes lodged in the lower half of the ureter. The pain produced is severe and constant, and may radiate to the testis and penis in men and the perineum in women. Right lumbar pain may occur simultaneously or may precede the right lower quadrant pain by several hours. There is only mild poorly localized tenderness in the right lower abdomen, and this may be inconstant. Guarding is absent, but right costovertebral-angle tenderness is usually present. There may be gross hematuria (20 percent of cases) or clear yellow urine, sometimes containing fine strands of clot. Hematuria can be detected microscopically in 60 to 80 percent of cases. Ultrasonography may demonstrate the stone and a dilated proximal ureter. An emergency pyelogram may show only a nephrogram or absence of right renal function. Calyceal and ureteral filling may be delayed, but after 2 to 24 h, a dilated drainage system may be visualized up to the point of obstruction. Eighty percent of stones

6 mm or less in diameter will pass without surgical intervention, while those 8 mm or more rarely do, and intervention is required. Warm baths and the use of meperidine alleviate the severe pain until spontaneous passage occurs.

Large stones or stones that fail to pass after 72 h require urological intervention. Stones in the lower half of the ureter can usually be approached with a ureteroscope from below, and impacted stones can be fragmented and removed by ultrasound or electrohydraulic lithotripsy. Patients with ureteral stones do not usually give a history of midline visceral pain or develop fever, and the leukocyte count usually remains normal.

D. Acute Gastroenteritis There is usually generalized or localized abdominal pain associated with anorexia, nausea, vomiting, fever, and diarrhea. The pain may be intermittent or constant, and may remain localized to one area or shift in location. In some patients, the pain may localize to the right lower abdomen and mimic appendicitis. These patients may have local tenderness, voluntary guarding, and even rebound tenderness. The absence of diarrhea and the presence of leukocytosis may make the simulation of appendicitis more convincing and lead to surgery. Other patients with gastroenteritis improve under observation or develop pain at other sites in the abdomen. Failure of progression or improvement is the usual finding that leads surgeons to delay intervention or discharge the patient. The high perforation rate in patients with acute appendicitis who are discharged after an initial assessment and diagnosis of gastroenteritis or nonspecific pain is indicative of the inexactness of the clinical approach. Such cases have been the stimulus for attempts at more specific diagnosis by use of graded-compression ultrasonography and laparoscopy to increase accuracy.

Gastroenteritis, mesenteric adenitis, and abdominal pain of unknown cause are not distinguishable from appendicitis by duration of pain; the presence of appetite loss, nausea, vomiting, chills, or fever; or any other historical information. Even physical findings such as localized tenderness (91 percent in appendicitis vs. 75 percent) and rebound tenderness (68 percent in appendicitis vs. 48 percent) are too nonspecific to differentiate appendicitis from these disorders. The leukocyte count and left shift tend to be statistically greater in appendicitis than in these nonsurgical disorders, but the differences are not large enough to provide differential criteria in individual cases. In patients with well-localized right lower abdominal pain and tenderness, rebound tenderness, leukocytosis, and/or shift to the left, surgical exploration is the best course to follow. In up to 15 percent of cases with a typical history and physical findings, the appendix is normal. Failure to explore on less than complete diagnostic criteria may lead to an increased incidence of missed diagnoses and an unacceptably high rate of perforation and abscess formation.

E. Renal and Perirenal Infection Renal inflammation can present as an acute surgical abdomen. There may be an abrupt or gradual onset of right iliac or right upper abdominal pain. Right flank and posterior lumbar pain are usually present. Nausea, vomiting, fever, and chills occur in some, but not all, cases. There may be direct tenderness only in the right lower abdomen and costovertebral area. In other cases, rebound tenderness and involuntary guarding also occur in the right iliac region and sometimes higher in the abdomen. The frequency of acute anterior abdominal pain and tenderness in patients with infectious renal disorders is 15 to 60 percent. The cause is inflammatory involvement of the posterior peritoneum by the renal process.

1. Renal Cortical Abscess Fever, chills, and right lower or midabdominal and/or flank pain occur. Irritative bladder symptoms are uncommon unless the abscess erodes a calix. Urinalysis and cultures are also usually negative. Staphylococci cause 95 percent of renal cortical abscesses. Skin and sometimes staphylococcal bone infections spread to the kidney through the circulation. In a minority of cases, a tender flank mass may become palpable. An intravenous pyelogram reveals caliceal distortion from an intrarenal mass. Ultrasonography demonstrates a hypoechoic cystic mass that contains fluid. A CT scan shows a hypodense complex thick-walled cystic mass. The rim of the abscess may enhance following contrast injection. Such mass lesions can be aspirated for pus under CT guidance, confirming the diagnosis of abscess. Therapy with nafcillin or vancomycin is effective and leads to resolution within 6 days. Refractory cases may require more complete abscess drainage.

2. Renal Corticomedullary Abscess This type of abscess results from an episode of acute pyelonephritis. Irritative bladder symptoms, flank pain and tenderness, and fever may precede the formation of the abscess. A flank mass may be palpable in up to 60 percent of cases. Pain and tenderness may occur in the right lower abdomen. This disorder is more likely to occur in patients with ureteral obstruction, vesicoureteral reflux, renal stones, diabetes mellitus, and renal scarring. The urinalysis is abnormal in 70 percent, and urine cultures are positive in an equal percentage of cases. Ultrasonography in acute pyelonephritis is usually normal. An abscess is seen as a fluid-filled well-circumscribed mass in the corticomedullary region. Sonographic findings can be confirmed by CT using contrast. This procedure can detect lesions as small as 2 cm. A contrast-enhanced CT may show enhancement of the rim of the abscess and a hypodense center. Most cases resolve with intravenous antibiotics, but drainage may be required, using percutaneous CT-guided catheter placement or an open surgical approach.

3. Perinephric Abscess This lesion can result from rupture of a renal abscess into the perinephric space. Less common sources of perinephric infection include dissemination of bacteria from infected sites in the skin, hepatobiliary tree, pleura, prostate, and female pelvic organs. Spread from an area of appendicitis, diverticulitis, a perforated colon carcinoma, or an adjacent osteomyelitis may occur. Fever and right flank and low or midabdominal pain are frequent. Chills and dysuria occur in up to 40 percent of cases. Costovertebral-angle tenderness occurs in 80 to 90 percent, leukocytosis in 90 to 95 percent, and right-sided abdominal tenderness in 60 percent. Rebound tenderness and guarding may occur. A tender flank or abdominal mass may be palpable in up to 50 percent of cases. Involvement of the right pleural cavity may occur, causing pleuritic pain and/or shoulder pain. A pleural effusion, empyema, nephrobronchial fistula, or subphrenic abscess may complicate the course of this disorder. The chest radiograph is frequently abnormal, demonstrating an elevated right diaphragm, an effusion, and/or a pulmonary infiltrate. CT scan is the best imaging procedure for demonstration of a perinephric abscess. These images usually demonstrate a thick-walled mass with a liquified center in the perinephric space. Fluid may also surround the mass. Ultrasonography may show a cystic extrarenal lesion but is less specific. Perinephric abscess requires prompt drainage and broad-spectrum intravenous antibiotic therapy. In refractory cases, nephrectomy may be required.

4. Acute Pyelonephritis   In addition to a right lumbar ache and irritative bladder symptoms, acute pyelonephritis may cause mild abdominal pain and direct tenderness but is seldom associated with peritoneal signs. Cases with marked right-sided anterior abdominal tenderness may mimic acute appendicitis or cholecystitis. The urine usually contains many leukocytes, red blood cells, and bacteria.

F. Crohn's Disease   This is a chronic disorder, characterized by constant or intermittent right lower abdominal or periumbilical pain, diarrhea, weight loss, and fever. Not all symptoms are present in every case. There may be periumbilical or right lower abdominal tenderness. In some cases, a soft irregular tender mass may be palpable in the right lower abdomen. An enteroclysis or small bowel series will show inflammatory stenosis of the terminal ileum. If the onset of right lower abdominal pain and tenderness is acute, this disease may mimic appendicitis. The diagnosis is usually made at surgery. Preoperative diagnosis is very difficult. In rare cases, Crohn's disease involves the appendix and causes acute appendicitis.

G. Abdominal Pain of Unknown Cause   There are a number of patients with acute right lower abdominal pain, tenderness, and sometimes rebound tenderness and/or guarding and leukocytosis who go to surgery with a presumptive diagnosis of acute appendicitis and who, on exploration, have no observable abnormality. In some cases, viral disorders such as pleurodynia may be the cause, and

this can be confirmed by viral isolation studies and antibody assays, but in most of these cases no etiology is apparent.

H. Amebiasis   Acute amebiasis often involves the cecum and can cause right lower abdominal pain, tenderness, guarding, and diarrhea, mimicking appendicitis. The diagnosis can be made by examining passed mucus and blood for amebic trophozoites and by sigmoidoscopy. Cases taken to surgery for the erroneous diagnosis of acute appendicitis have an increased mortality.

I. Acute Osteomyelitis of the Right Ilium   This disorder may mimic acute appendicitis by causing right iliac pain and tenderness. Pain is aching and constant, and begins in the right iliac area, flank, and/or hip. It does not begin in the epigastrium or the umbilical region, as is the usual sequence in appendicitis. Pain is often present for several days before medical help is sought. High fever, rigors, anorexia, nausea, and vomiting may begin several days after the onset of pain. Local pelvic trauma and Crohn's disease are risk factors for the development of iliac osteomyelitis. Physical examination may demonstrate right iliac region tenderness and sometimes guarding, but rebound tenderness is rarely present. A tender right iliac mass may be palpable. Some patients have accompanying hip pain and a differential limitation of hip motion that superficially mimics septic arthritis of the hip. Others have buttock pain and swelling and/or sciatica. Leukocytosis and an elevated sedimentation rate are usually present. Plain radiographs are nondiagnostic during the first 2 to 3 weeks after onset, but a gallium 67-citrate and/or technetium 99m-methylene diphosphonate bone scan will show increased uptake over the right iliac area. A CT scan may show lytic changes before plain radiographs do. MRI T_1 images show bony areas of decreased or intermediate signal intensity, and T_2 images demonstrate the same areas to have an increased signal intensity. This change from a low-intensity to a high-intensity signal is characteristic of an active infectious process in bone. MRI is sensitive, and abnormalities occur long before they are apparent on plain radiographs. The signs and symptoms of acute osteomyelitis of the ilium respond to intravenous antibiotic therapy within 36 h. The change is usually dramatic and is used to support the correctness of the diagnosis. Failure of response may be due to a bone or soft tissue abscess that requires drainage or to an incorrect diagnosis (e.g., the presence of a tumor).

J. Ewing's Sarcoma of the Right Ilium   This disorder may cause bone and abdominal pain and fever, and may simulate the clinical signs and symptoms of acute osteomyelitis. If an osteomyelitis is present for 4 weeks or more, the changes in the plain radiographs may be indistinguishable from those of Ewing's sarcoma of the ilium. Failure of a prompt and dramatic response to antibiotic therapy requires multiple bone biopsies to rule out this highly malignant but treatable tumor. The presence of flank pain may simulate pyelonephritis, but the urine sediment is usually normal.

3. SURGICAL MIMICS OF ACUTE APPENDICITIS

A. Cecal Diverticulitis   The clinical picture is almost indistinguishable from acute appendicitis. Right lower quadrant pain and tenderness, low-grade fever, and leukocytosis are common to both. Nausea (27–52 percent) and vomiting (16–31 percent) are less frequent, and pain is mild and more gradual in onset in up to 41 percent of patients. A history of similar attacks, hematochezia or melena, a duration of symptoms exceeding 48 h, an initial pain onset in the right lower abdomen without prodromal midline pain, minimal toxicity, fecalith shadows on abdominal radiographs, a tender right lower abdominal mass, or a previous appendectomy are features suggestive of diverticulitis.

Barium enema is hazardous and may be nondiagnostic in 50 percent of cases. It may help confirm the diagnosis if it demonstrates a diverticulum and a normal appendix, extrinsic filling defects, absence of an intraluminal defect due to malignancy, edema or spasm, of the bowel wall, and poor distensibility and fixation of the involved portion of the cecum. Colonoscopy has been technically difficult and nondiagnostic in the small number of patients with cecal diverticulitis who have had this procedure. CT offers a noninvasive way of confirming the diagnosis, but some abnormal findings are nonspecific and require careful clinical correlation. CT may demonstrate regional thickening of the colon wall, a pericolonic soft tissue mass with or without gas, and edema of the pericolic fat. The pericolic mass is usually cephalad to the ileocecal valve but may not be. Demonstration of a cecal diverticulum is helpful but occurs infrequently. The CT findings are nonspecific, and similar findings may occur in patients with an appendiceal abscess. Too few cases have been studied by CT to evaluate the usefulness of CT in confirming the diagnosis of cecal diverticulitis and differentiating it from other disorders.

In patients identified as having cecal diverticulitis preoperatively, a course of intravenous antibiotics usually leads to resolution of symptoms and signs without surgery. Intraoperative diagnosis may be difficult in patients with a pericolic abscess. Such cases are difficult to differentiate from perforated cecal carcinomas intraoperatively. Right hemicolectomy is the recommended procedure for patients with this "hidden variant" of diverticulitis. In 65 percent of cases, the diagnosis is evident at surgery. These cases can be drained, closed, and treated with antibiotics, or a limited resection can be done, followed by antibiotic therapy. Most surgeons also do an incidental appendectomy to prevent future diagnostic confusion.

B. Cecal Carcinoma with Perforation   Cecal carcinomas are usually painless and present with iron deficiency anemia due to chronic blood loss. Such patients may complain of pallor, dyspnea, exertional chest pain, dizziness, weakness, and ease of fatigue. Stools may be normal or have a mahogany color caused by admixture with blood. An irregular, hard, nontender mass may be felt in the right lower abdomen by the patient and/or physician. If the tumor erodes through the bowel wall, it may cause right lower abdominal pain and tenderness due to the formation of a pericolic abscess. This disorder may be confused with acute appendicitis or diverticulitis with abscess formation. A barium enema or CT scan may demonstrate an intraluminal tumor mass in the cecum. Colonoscopy can confirm the diagnosis. Such lesions require right hemicolectomy and removal of the lymphatic drainage of the right colon.

C. Cecal Distension Due to Distal Obstruction of the Colon   There is usually a history of crampy lower abdominal pain, diarrhea or constipation, and the passage of blood per rectum. Stools may narrow and become pencil- or ribbon-shaped. At the onset of total obstruction of the left colon, there are attacks of lower abdominal colicky pain lasting 2 to 4 min, with pain-free intervals of 5 to 10 min. Lower abdominal distension occurs, and no stool or gas is passed per rectum. If the ileocecal valve remains competent, the cecum dilates with gas and fluid, and forms a painful, tender, tympanitic mass in the right lower abdomen. The pain is severe and constant, and may be associated with rebound tenderness. Abdominal radiographs show a cecum that is gas-filled and dilated to greater than 10 cm. Failure to operate and decompress or resect the cecum and proximal colon will lead to perforation with abscess formation and/or acute peritonitis. A contrast edema or colonoscopy will confirm the left-sided obstruction, which is usually due to carcinoma (70 percent), diverticulitis (8 percent), or volvulus (6 percent).

Subtotal colectomy, removal of the obstructing tumor and draining nodes, and immediate ileosigmoidostomy can be performed. The anastomosis uses normal ileum and collapsed distal colon. The distended cecum and the right and transverse colon are removed.

D. Meckel's Diverticulitis   Up to 2 percent of the population have a Meckel's diverticulum, which is situated within 100 cm of the ileocecal valve. Inflammation causes a syndrome indistinguishable from acute appendicitis. In some cases, the pain and tenderness are more medial in location than in appendicitis. If the appendix appears normal at operation and there is no apparent cause of the clinical picture, examination of the distal ileum may reveal Meckel's diverticulitis. The incidence of perforation and peritonitis in the presence of diverticulitis is 50 percent. Surgical resection of the diseased diverticulum is required. A perforated diverticulum may be resected and drained under antibiotic coverage.

E. Carcinoma of the Appendix with Perforation   This disorder often presents with fever, constant right lower abdominal pain, local tenderness, and/or a palpable tender mass. Perforation occurred in up to 55 percent of cases in one large series. The diagnosis is usually made at surgical exploration. In 13 percent of patients, a hard right lower quadrant or groin mass or a fistula may suggest the diagnosis of advanced malignancy. Right hemicolectomy and node resection with anastomosis of the ileum to the left transverse colon are the required procedures. Carcinoma of the appendix, although rare, is the most frequently perforating gastrointestinal malignancy.

F. Perforation of a Duodenal Ulcer with Leakage Down the Right Lumbar Gutter   There is often a history of recurrent daily bouts of gnawing or aching epigastric pain that has been relieved by food, antacids, or H_2-blocking drugs. The pain may wake the patient from sleep and return 2 to 4 h after eating relieves it. Such pain occurs on a daily basis for days or weeks and then may disappear spontaneously for months at a time. It usually responds within 1 to 7 days to an antiulcer regimen. Ulcer perforation begins suddenly, with excruciating epigastric pain and sometimes discomfort on the top of the right shoulder. Leakage of gastric content down the right lumbar gutter can cause right lower abdominal pain and tenderness. Such patients may resemble those with acute appendicitis. However, the presence of diffuse abdominal or epigastric tenderness, severe rigidity of the abdominal wall, and free intraabdominal air by physical examination and/or by abdominal radiography suggest the diagnosis. In cases where the leaking ulcer seals promptly, there may be confusion, since the pain and tenderness may be confined to the right lower abdomen. A careful history of previous abdominal complaints, a Gastrografin swallow, or upper gastrointestinal endoscopy can establish the true cause of the right lower abdominal complaints.

G. Acute Cholecystitis   This disorder can mimic acute appendicitis by producing right-sided mid- and lower abdominal pain and tenderness. There may be a history of attacks of biliary colic with 2- to 6-h periods of severe epigastric pain separated by days, weeks, or months. Similar pain with a shift to the right may occur and persist for 1 or more days. Fever, anorexia, nausea, and vomiting usually accompany the pain. On physical examination, an enlarged, tender, palpable gallbladder may be felt or percussed in the right upper abdomen. Leukocytosis and/or a shift to the left is usually present. A DISIDA scan will confirm the diagnosis, and ultrasonography can detect stones (90 percent sensitive) and reveal the presence of gallbladder wall thickening and pericholecystic fluid. Exploration for a possible appendicitis may, instead, reveal acute cholecystitis. Cholecystectomy, drainage, and intravenous antibiotic therapy usually lead to resolution of all complaints.

H. Infarction of the Greater Omentum   Pain in the epigastrium, followed by right lower quadrant pain, nausea,

and fever, occur. There may be a leukocytosis in 67 percent of patients. In some cases, there are previous prodromal attacks, and the duration of symptoms when the patient is first seen may exceed 2 days.

Localized direct and rebound tenderness mimic the findings of acute appendicitis or cholecystitis, which are the commonest preoperative diagnoses. Exploration reveals a normal appendix, cecum, small bowel and mesentery, and serosanguineous fluid. Inspection of the greater omentum reveals a wedged-shaped area of purple discoloration and induration of the right lateral dependent free edge. Resection of the infarcted omentum and incidental appendectomy lead to prompt recovery. Secondary cases of omental infarction occur in patients with severe heart failure or polycythemia vera and after portal vein occlusion.

I. Ileocecal Intussusception   Cases occurring in adults are associated with benign or malignant tumors, jejunoileal bypass, celiac disease, or Meckel's diverticulitis. The pain in the right lower abdomen may be colicky or constant and associated with vomiting and the passage of dark or bright-red stools. There are usually direct and sometimes rebound tenderness in the right lower abdomen. A mass may be palpable, and severe guarding may be present. A CT scan will confirm the diagnosis. CT can identify any mass lesions serving as a lead point and can define the level of involvement. It can also detect free air or a localized perforation, which are contraindications to the use of a barium enema.

J. Psoas Abscess   Pain occurs in the right lower abdomen. It is usually mild to moderate in intensity, and aching. It is increased by extension of the thigh on the trunk or with hyperextension of the thigh. Patients may lie in bed with the knee on the affected side flexed and the thigh externally rotated. There is tenderness in the right iliac fossa, and a mass may be palpable. Fever is common, but may be intermittent or absent in up to 75 percent of cases. Anemia and leukocytosis may occur. Weight loss is common.

Psoas abscess is caused by tuberculous or nontuberculous infections of the thoracolumbar spine or is secondary to intestinal disorders such as Crohn's disease, diverticulitis, or a perforated colon cancer. Rarely, a perinephric or pancreatic abscess invades the psoas muscle. Culture of *Staphylococcus aureus* from a psoas abscess supports the diagnosis of a primary bacteremic infection and is rare. Culture of two or more gram-negative bacteria and/or anaerobes suggests a bowel-related origin. Drainage, removal of the leaking bowel, and sustained parenteral antibiotic therapy for residual infection in the abscess cavity or in the spine are necessary for cure. An important complication of a psoas abscess is obstruction of the ureter and flank pain, and fever may occur secondary to this.

K. Torsion of an Intraabdominal Testis and Other Pain of Testicular Origin   There is an abrupt onset of severe right lower abdominal pain. It may be crampy at first, but it soon becomes constant. Nausea and vomiting occur. Right iliac tenderness, rebound tenderness, and guarding develop over a period of hours, requiring surgical exploration. The right testis is absent from the scrotum. In some cases, the inflammatory mass produced by testicular infarction may trap small bowel and cause intestinal obstruction. The involved testis may harbor a seminoma or an embryonal carcinoma, which precipitated the torsion. Surgical resection is required if infarction occurs.

A painful process in a descended testis may also cause right lower abdominal pain and tenderness. Disorders such as testicular torsion, epididymitis, and postvasectomy infarction can superficially mimic acute appendicitis. The right testis is usually exquisitely tender and may be swollen (e.g., torsion and epididymitis).

An undescended testis may also cause a mild aching right iliac fossa pain and tenderness unrelated to torsion. A clue to this diagnosis is the absence of the right testis from the scrotum.

L. Anisakiasis The herring worm may produce a granulomatous lesion in the ileocecal region and cause right lower abdominal pain and tenderness and, in some cases, a palpable tender mass, mimicking acute appendicitis. It is a common surgical mimic of appendicitis in Japan, where the ingestion of worm-bearing raw fish is highly prevalent. Peripheral eosinophilia may be present. The diagnosis is usually made at surgery.

M. Rupture of an Infrarenal Aortic Aneurysm There is an abrupt onset of very severe constant right lower abdominal pain, which may spread laterally. Associated low back pain is often present. Faintness, weakness, nausea, and sweating frequently accompany the pain. There is usually tachycardia, and hypotension may be present in up to 33 percent of cases. A pulsatile tender retroperitoneal mass (hematoma) is present (80 percent) in the midline of the abdomen above the umbilicus. Up to 80 percent of patients may be unaware of the previous presence of an aneurysm. Once the diagnosis is suspected because of the patient's age (older than 40), history, and findings, immediate laparotomy should be done and the aorta cross-clamped to prevent exsanguination and allow time for volume resuscitation and repair of the aorta. A small percentage of aneurysms are infected, and cultures of all aneurysms should be obtained in the operating room. This disorder has mimicked acute appendicitis because of right lower quadrant pain and tenderness. It has also mimicked renal colic because of pain radiation to the inguinal region, testicle, and perineum. Pain may also radiate down the leg in a sciatic distribution. Pain can be relieved by surgical repair of the aneurysm using an aortic bifurcation prosthesis.

N. Rupture or Enlargement of a Common Iliac Aneurysm Pain occurs in the right iliac fossa. There may be radiation into the anterior thigh, and the upper leg may be held flexed on the trunk and externally rotated because of psoas irritation. Extension may cause pain, and it is resisted. Aneurysmal pressure on the common iliac vein may result in thrombosis and unilateral deep leg pain, duskiness of the leg, and edema. Right flank ache may result from ureteral obstruction from the expanding aneurysm or an associated hematoma. There are right lower abdominal tenderness and guarding, and a palpable pulsatile mass may be felt in the right lower abdomen between the umbilicus and the inguinal ligament. The aneurysm can be visualized by ultrasonography or a CT study. Surgical resection and grafting will relieve pain and prevent exsanguinating rupture.

O. Cecal Volvulus The sudden onset of colicky right lower, and sometimes midabdominal, pain is followed within hours by right lower abdominal distension and tenderness. Nausea and vomiting may occur, but fever and leukocytosis are uncommon. A plain abdominal radiograph will demonstrate a dilated cecum in the mid- or left abdomen and, sometimes, a single air-fluid level in the cecum. Air-fluid levels may also be present in loops of small bowel due to complete obstruction distal to the ileocecal valve. In up to 30 percent of cases, accurate diagnosis may require a contrast enema, which will demonstrate the site of obstruction. An abdominal CT scan may also demonstrate a "whirl sign" due to twisted mucosal folds at the site of obstruction. While colonoscopy may sometimes decompress the cecum, surgical therapy is required in many cases because of inability to pass the colonoscope past the point of obstruction. In addition, cecopexy is required to prevent recurrent attacks.

P. Perforation of the Ileum Due to Typhoid Fever Typhoid fever begins with fever, headache, malaise, myalgia, lethargy, anorexia, diarrhea, or constipation. The temperature rises abruptly or in a stepwise fashion over 3 to 4 days and then ranges between 103 and 105°F. This febrile response may be sustained or intermittent. Relative bradycardia (25 percent of cases), cough (15 percent of cases), and splenomegaly occur. Rose spots occur on the trunk and are diagnostically helpful. They usually appear during the second week. The diagnosis can be made during the first week by blood culture and after that by stool or urine culture. O and H antigen titers rise after week 1 to values of 1:160 or more. In fewer than 3 percent of cases, during the third week, acute right lower quadrant pain, tenderness, and guarding occur secondary to perforation of an ileal Peyer's patch. This may be accompanied by a rise in pulse and a fall in temperature. Aggressive surgical management is recommended to prevent fatal peritonitis. This complication may occur in patients receiving antibiotic therapy.

Q. Neutropenic Enterocolitis (Typhlitis) This disorder occurs in neutropenic (white blood cell count $\leq 10^3/mm^3$) patients with acute leukemia, cyclic neutropenia, or aplastic anemia. Neutropenia may also follow a course of myelo-toxic chemotherapy. Fever, anorexia, and generalized abdominal and right lower quadrant pain occur. There may be generalized abdominal tenderness or right iliac direct and rebound tenderness and guarding, or right iliac signs may be absent in the presense of pain. Nausea, vomiting, distension, and diarrhea sometimes containing gross or occult blood may accompany the pain. The diagnosis can be confirmed by a CT scan, which shows a thick-walled edematous right colon with spiculation of pericolic fat and subcutaneous edema. All symptoms may be suppressed by steroid administration or resolve on antibiotic therapy. Recurrent or refractory attacks will cease after resection of an ulcerated or necrotic cecum (i.e., right hemicolectomy) and formation of an ileostomy.

R. Ileocecal Tuberculosis Patients may have vague right lower abdominal pain; tenderness; and a palpable, tender mass (50 percent of cases). Weight loss, fever, and malaise are commonly present. Diarrhea or constipation may occur. Some patients may present as having an acute abdomen secondary to perforation of the ileocecal region. This causes more severe right iliac pain and tenderness and peritoneal signs, and can mimic acute appendicitis. The diagnosis is usually established at surgical exploration.

4. GYNECOLOGIC MIMICS OF ACUTE APPENDICITIS

The negative appendectomy rate for women in the ovulating age group ranges between 20 and 46 percent, exceeding that for men (15 percent). The common causes of diagnostic confusion are gynecologic disorders such as acute salpingitis, ruptured ovarian cysts, and ectopic pregnancy. These may be diagnosed preoperatively on clinical, sonographic, or laparoscopic findings, but the use of these tests has thus far failed to lower the negative appendectomy rate.

A. Pelvic Inflammatory Disease (PID)

1. Acute Salpingitis This disorder is a common cause of confusion with acute appendicitis. Right lower abdominal pain and tenderness and an elevated leukocyte count may occur in both disorders. The absence of prodromal midline pain, anorexia, nausea, and vomiting; a duration of pain greater than 2 days; and onset within 7 days of the beginning of a menstrual cycle favor a diagnosis of acute salpingitis. A history of episodes of sexually transmissible disease, cervical motion and adnexal tenderness, and an area of abdominal tenderness outside the right lower abdomen also support a diagnosis of salpingitis. Upper abdominal pain may occur with salpingitis and is caused by perihepatitis (5–15 percent of cases). This pain is severe and usually pleuritic, and may also be felt in the right lower chest and/or shoulder. It may be intensified by laughing, walking, deep breathing,

and coughing. There is usually right, and sometimes left, upper abdominal tenderness. Without treatment, such pain may persist for days. The location, severity, duration, and quality of this upper abdominal pain differentiate it from the transient, crampy, midline visceral pain that occurs at the onset of acute appendicitis. High-resolution graded compression ultrasonography can make a positive imaging diagnosis of appendicitis by visualizing an appendix with a diameter of 6 mm or more. Failure to visualize the appendix by ultrasonography does not rule out appendicitis, since the sensitivity is only 75 to 89 percent. The value of ultrasonography is to allow prompt surgical intervention in cases of appendicitis with confusing or equivocal findings. When an enlarged appendix is detected by an ultrasonography, there is a high likelihood of appendicitis. This approach may also be of use in cases of possible appendicitis because ultrasonography may detect alternative causes for the symptoms. In a series of 297 patients undergoing compression sonography for possible appendicitis, such studies were able to suggest a specific alternative diagnosis in 33 percent of cases negative for appendicitis. Salpingitis and ovarian cyst rupture were the two most common gynecologic disorders, accounting for 75 percent of the ultrasonography appendicitis-negative cases due to a specific cause. Laparoscopy may also be useful in confirming appendicitis in cases that have atypical findings and in establishing a diagnosis of salpingitis, ovarian cyst rupture, or ectopic pregnancy. When the appendix cannot be visualized because of adhesions or a retrocecal location, patients must be evaluated clinically and explored if surgical indications are present. Salpingitis may respond within 2 to 4 days to antibiotics. Recently used regimens include tobramycin and clindamycin, doxycycline and metronidazole, cefoxitin and doxycycline, and aztreonam and clindamycin. Cases with severe pain and tenderness, fever, and toxicity require admission to the hospital and parenteral therapy.

2. Acute Tubo-ovarian Abscess (TOA) Pain occurs in the lower abdomen and may mimic appendicitis if it is present on the right side only. Fever is common, but 35 to 65 percent of patients may be afebrile. Nausea, vomiting, and diarrhea occur in less than 25 percent of cases. The leukocyte count is elevated in 70 percent, and the sedimentation rate in 80 percent.

Local tenderness and rebound are maximal deep in the pelvis and low in the abdomen near or below the pelvic brim. Pelvic examination reveals adnexal tenderness and a mass in less than 50 percent of cases. Ultrasonography has a high sensitivity for detection of TOA and will demonstrate a complex adnexal mass or a pure cystic lesion due to a TOA in up to 35 percent of cases of severe PID. Laparoscopy can be used for diagnostic confirmation and to lyse adhesions, drain purulent fluid, and excise necrotic lesions. Most cases will respond to intravenous antibiotic therapy within 3 to 5 days. Aztreonam and clindamycin or gentamycin and metronidazole will usually lead to resolution. Medical therapy is successful in 33 to 74 percent of cases overall.

Failure to improve on antibiotic therapy or rupture of the abscess requires immediate surgical intervention, since soiling of the peritoneum can lead to septic shock and death.

3. Rupture of a TOA   There is a 14 to 35 percent incidence of TOA in adults hospitalized with PID. It is very difficult to differentiate uncomplicated PID from a TOA without the use of ultrasonography or laparoscopy. If the abscess is on the right, it may mimic appendicitis. Rupture occurs in only a small number of cases. It may occur abruptly and explosively with the acute onset of generalized abdominal pain and peritoneal signs. A mass may be felt on pelvic examination. Fever may be low-grade or high, and severe hypotension and progression to septic shock may occur within hours. More gradual leakage results in extension of pelvic pain and tenderness into the lower, and then upper, abdomen. Rupture may occur in untreated patients or in those on intravenous antibiotics. The diagnosis of rupture can be confirmed by laparoscopy or laparotomy. Culdocentesis is useful if the results are positive, but they may be negative in the presence of abscess rupture.

Bilateral salpingo-oophorectomy and hysterectomy provide the best opportunity for cure. Surgery should be accompanied by copious saline irrigation of the abdomen and intravenous antibiotic therapy. Such abscesses contain anaerobic rods such as *Bacteroides fragilis* and *Bacteroides bivius,* gram-positive anaerobic cocci such as *Peptococcus* and *Peptostreptococcus,* and aerobes such as *Escherichia coli.* Antibiotic therapy should include tobramycin or aztreonam and an antianaerobic drug such as clindamycin or metronidazole. The mortality rate may range from 5 to 20 percent.

B. Tubal Pregnancy   More than two-thirds of patients presenting with this disorder have a history of PID, tubal ligation, tubal reconstruction, use of an IUD, or a previous ectopic pregnancy. Some patients have more than one risk factor.

Pain occurs in 98 percent of cases and may at first be intermittent and colicky and ipsilateral to the affected tube. If a hematoma forms in the wall of the tube, the pain may become a constant dull ache. Tubal rupture with bleeding is accompanied by severe, sharp, unilateral pain that spreads over the lower abdomen and then into the upper abdomen. Shoulder pain may be associated with generalized lower abdominal pain and tenderness in 10 to 15 percent of cases. One or more missed periods may occur in 50 to 60 percent of cases. The weeks following a missed period are frequently characterized by irregular spotting or staining. A scant previous menstrual period and/or contin-

ued staining or bleeding since the last period occurs in up to 43 percent of cases. Profuse vaginal bleeding with passage of clots, as occurs with an incomplete abortion, is uncommon. Amenorrhea without bleeding for 2 to 3 months may also occur in a small percentage of cases.

There may be mild or moderately severe lower abdominal tenderness on the side of the tubal pregnancy. Pelvic examination reveals pain on cervical motion and adnexal tenderness, and a tubal enlargement may be palpable (19–35 percent of cases). If significant leakage of blood has occurred, there will be tenderness and fullness in the cul-de-sac. Lower abdominal direct and rebound tenderness accompany rupture.

Endovaginal ultrasonography can rule out a tubal pregnancy by detecting an intrauterine pregnancy. This technique is more sensitive than transvesical ultrasonography for this purpose. In addition, endovaginal ultrasonography may provide positive evidence for the diagnosis of tubal pregnancy by detecting a live embryo in the adnexae (7–15 percent of cases), a noncystic adnexal mass (88–92-percent sensitive), or free fluid in the adnexal region. Older methods of urine assay for human chorionic gonadotrophin may be negative in 20 to 30 percent of cases of ectopic pregnancy, while a radioimmunoassay for serum beta-hCG is only rarely negative (99 percent sensitivity). The clinical accuracy of beta-hCG varies between 97 and 100 percent. A new enzyme-linked immunoassay urine pregnancy test (ICON) had a 96 percent sensitivity in a series of 27 cases. This test is rapid (4 min) and detects levels of 50 mIU/ml in urine. When this test is negative, the radioimmunoassay for beta-hCG can be utilized. A negative pregnancy test makes the diagnosis very unlikely. Confirmatory studies consisting of endovaginal ultrasonography and beta-hCG determination will provide a 95 to 100 percent diagnostic accuracy rate. The additional use of laparoscopy will increase this. Culdocentesis for nonclottable blood is positive in up to 90 percent of cases but is invasive, and equivalent information can be obtained from ultrasonography in the usual clinical setting. Some patients spontaneously abort down the tube and are not operated on. Nonoperative management requires hospitalization and monitoring of clinical symptoms, signs, and serum beta-hCG levels. Most patients with a mass larger than 3 cm should be treated by salpingectomy if further pregnancies are not desired. If preservation of reproductive function is desired, then tubal resection, followed by microsurgical reanastomosis of the tube at a later date, is recommended.

The diagnosis of tubal pregnancy should be suspected in any woman in the childbearing years with lower abdominal pain. The presence of abnormal menstruation and signs of peritoneal irritation (tenderness and shoulder pain) and hypovolemia (weakness, dizziness, fainting, and shock) should initiate confirmatory tests for pregnancy, adnexal mass (ultrasonography or laparoscopy), and cul-de-sac blood (ultrasonography or culdocentesis), or immediate laparotomy if the patient is unstable.

C. Mimics of Tubal Pregnancy, PID, and Appendicitis

1. Corpus Luteum Cyst with Bleeding

An ovarian cyst can cause lower abdominal pain and tenderness by rapid growth or by bleeding into the cyst or the peritoneal cavity. The pain is moderate to severe and may be associated with lower abdominal, cervical motion and adnexal tenderness, thus mimicking PID. Hemoperitoneum may be associated with low-grade fever, enhancing the simulation of infection.

Corpus luteum cysts often delay the onset of menses and cause unilateral abdominal pain and tenderness, as well as adnexal tenderness, with a palpable mass. This may simulate tubal pregnancy. The urine and serum pregnancy tests are negative, and laparoscopy can confirm the diagnosis.

2. Corpus Luteum Cyst of Pregnancy

Bleeding into a corpus luteum cyst of pregnancy may cause right lower abdominal pain and tenderness and adnexal tenderness, with a palpable mass. There is a history of amenorrhea and a positive pregnancy test, and ultrasonography usually demonstrates an intrauterine pregnancy and an adnexal mass. Laparoscopy can evaluate the tube and ovary on the affected side. Some of these cases are misdiagnosed clinically as an ectopic pregnancy and explored.

3. Threatened Abortion

A threatened abortion can cause right lower and mid lower abdominal pain and tenderness, spotting, or vaginal bleeding in a patient with one or more missed periods. The pain is often crampy and may be referred to the low back as well. The urine and serum beta-hCG tests are positive. An endovaginal sonographic study can confirm the presence of an intrauterine pregnancy, and, if fetal heart motion is detected, there is a 90 percent probability of continuation of the pregnancy. Ultrasonography may also demonstrate the absence of an adnexal mass. In difficult cases, laparoscopy may be required.

4. Follicle Cyst with Intraperitoneal Bleeding (Mittelschmerz)

Follicle cysts may cause right lower abdominal pain and tenderness. In some patients, the onset of pain is abrupt, and there may be severe disability. In other patients, the pain may be mild and easily tolerable. Examination reveals lower abdominal and pelvic tenderness on the side of the pain. Such pain usually occurs at midcycle, and previous episodes of similar discomfort on the same or the opposite side may be recalled. Culdocentesis may reveal blood, and laparoscopy will confirm the diagnosis and should be done before laparotomy.

5. Endometrioma with Intraperitoneal Bleeding

Hemorrhage into or from an endometrioma can cause similar right lower abdominal pain and tenderness. There is usually a history of secondary dysmenorrhea and dyspareunia and sometimes menstrual period-associated diarrhea, tenesmus, rectal pain, and/or bleeding; in some cases, there are irritative bladder complaints. The diagnosis of endometriosis with bleeding can be confirmed by laparoscopy.

6. Adnexal Torsion

Colicky or continuous right lower abdominal pain occurs. It becomes progressively severe and sustained. Fever is uncommon and, if present, is low-grade. Nausea, vomiting, diarrhea, constipation, and leukocytosis may occur. After 3 to 4 h, a tender adnexal mass may be detected on pelvic examination. Ultrasonography will detect an enlarged ovary, which appears as a uniformly echogenic mass that is hypoechoic to surrounding structures (ovarian torsion) or as a complex mass (associated with adnexal torsion). Laparoscopy will confirm the diagnosis and allow for early surgery. In most cases, the diagnosis is made too late to avoid surgical resection of the infarcted ovary. Such ovaries are frequently enlarged prior to the episode of torsion because of a cyst or tumor. If malignancy is present, alternative intraoperative management is required.

22

Acute Hypogastric Pain

☐ DIAGNOSTIC LIST

1. Acute prostatitis
2. Acute urinary retention
   A. Benign prostatic hypertrophy (BPH)
   B. Prostatitis
   C. Chronic prostatitis plus BPH
   D. Prostatic carcinoma
   E. Urethral stricture
   F. Retention due to neurogenic causes
3. Urinary retention in women, neurogenic and psychogenic causes
4. Acute bacterial cystitis
   A. Acute cystitis
   B. Acute cystitis with occult pyelonephritis
   C. Acute cystitis with clinical acute pyelonephritis
   D. Acute dysuria-frequency syndrome
5. Pelvic appendicitis
6. Bladder calculi
7. Disorders of the colon
   A. Obstruction
      1. Carcinoma
      2. Diverticulitis
      3. Colonic pseudo-obstruction (Ogilvie's syndrome)
      4. Fecal impaction and obstruction
      5. Sigmoid volvulus

6. Cecal volvulus
   B. Perforation of the colon
      1. Diverticulitis
      2. Carcinoma of the sigmoid colon
      3. Ischemic colitis
      4. Toxic megacolon
      5. Fecal impaction
   C. Acute infectious diarrhea
      1. *Salmonella* species
      2. *Campylobacter* species
      3. *Shigella* species
      4. Other organisms
      5. Initial attack of ulcerative colitis or Crohn's disease
8. Incarcerated or strangulated ventral or spigelian hernia
9. Gynecologic causes for hypogastric pain
   A. Endometritis
   B. Septic abortion
   C. Uterine myoma with necrosis and/or bleeding
   D. Acute spontaneous abortion
   E. Tubal pregnancy
   F. Bleeding from a follicle or a corpus luteum cyst
   G. Endometriosis and intraabdominal bleeding
   H. Intracystic hemorrhage

☐ SUMMARY

Acute prostatitis may produce suprapubic pain as well as perineal, scrotal, and low back pain. Irritative and obstructive bladder symptoms are usually present, as well as systemic symptoms such as fever, chills, and malaise. The urine contains leukocytes, red blood cells, and bacteria, and there is a good response to antibiotic therapy.

Acute urinary retention causes a dull, hypogastric ache associated with a desire to void. In men, *acute prostatitis* with fever and chills can cause this syndrome, but it is more commonly seen after years of obstructive symptoms (*benign prostatic hypertrophy,* or BPH, with or without *chronic prostatitis* or *urethral stricture*) or after months of rapidly progressive complaints (*carcinoma of the prostate*) of an obstructive nature (e.g., diminished stream, dribbling, incomplete emptying, hesitation, split stream, or need to strain). *Retention in women* is rare and usually has a *psychogenic basis,* but *carcinoma of the urethra or vagina* or *neurogenic causes* may be responsible.

Acute bacterial cystitis causes suprapubic discomfort of an aching or burning nature, which decreases after voiding. Pyuria, gross or microscopic hematuria, frequency, urgency, and dysuria are associated complaints. There are no systemic symptoms. Up to 40 percent of these patients do not have a bacterial infection on culture and appear to have the nonspecific *dysuria-frequency syndrome.* These women have negative urine Gram stains and cultures, or they may have low-grade bacterial infections with low colony counts or intermittently positive cultures. Many do not have white or red blood cells in the urine. Fewer of these women than those with positive Gram stains and cultures are sexually active, and many of them have a vaginal discharge. Some women who present with acute cystitis have an associated *occult pyelonephritis.* This is more common in patients with a history of 7 days or more of symptoms; relapse after previous short-course antibiotic therapy; or a history of pyelonephritis, diabetes, immunosuppression, pregnancy, failure of a therapeutic response within 3 days, or onset of urinary infections before age 12 or over age 65. These patients can be identified by bladder washout cultures or by detecting antibody-coated bacteria. Acute cystitis can accompany classical pyelonephritis, with flank pain and tenderness, fever, and chills. Acute cystitis can also be the first manifestation of a colovesical fistula due to Crohn's disease or diverticulitis. Pneumaturia and fecal contamination of the urine may accompany irritative bladder symptoms.

Pelvic appendicitis may begin with crampy, upper or midabdominal pain followed by a shift of pain and tenderness to the hypogastrium and pelvis. Nausea, vomiting, fever, and leukocytosis are frequent, and rectal examination reveals pelvic tenderness and may detect a pelvic mass. Peritoneal signs indicate the need for laparotomy. The diagnosis can also be aided by use of sonographic or laparoscopic studies to visualize the abnormal appendix. *Bladder calculi* cause irritative bladder symptoms, made worse by exercise and jarring. Acute shutoff of urine flow during voiding may occur, as well as terminal dysuria and hematuria. Cystoscopic studies may be required to visualize all stones, since some are radiolucent.

Colon obstruction causes hypogastric and sometimes unilateral or bilateral iliac pain; lower abdominal distension; obstipation; and, later, feculent vomiting. *Carcinoma, diverticulitis, fecal impaction,* and *stenosing lesions* due to inflammatory bowel disease or ischemic colitis can produce obstruction. *Pseudo-obstruction (Ogilvie's syndrome)* can mimic this problem and can be diagnosed by a contrast enema or colonoscopic studies that exclude mechanical obstruction of the colon. In several series, 35 to 37 percent of patients with a presumptive diagnosis of colon obstruction were not obstructed and resolved without surgery. *Sigmoid and cecal volvulus* may cause marked lower abdominal distension, obstipation, and pain that can usually be diagnosed by a plain abdominal radiograph, but confirmation of the diagnosis may require a contrast enema or a CT scan of the abdomen in up to 36 percent of cases.

Perforation of the colon may cause constant hypogastric pain and localized or more diffuse peritoneal signs. *Diverticulitis, carcinoma of the colon, ischemic colitis,* and *inflammatory bowel disease* or *impaction* can lead to perforation. With distal colon obstruction and distension of the cecum beyond a diameter of 12 cm, cecal perforation may occur.

Acute infectious colitis causes lower abdominal pain, fever, and watery or bloody diarrhea. Lower abdominal pain related to defecation, and tenesmus may occur. *Salmonella, Campylobacter,* and *Shigella* species are the common bacterial causes, and *amebic colitis* is the most important parasitic cause.

Ischemic colitis and *ulcerative colitis* can mimic acute infectious colitis. Contrast enemas in ischemic colitis show thumbprinting and ulcerations, and colonoscopic studies may demonstrate blue-black submucosal nodules. A first attack of ulcerative colitis may only be differentiated from an acute infectious diarrhea on the basis of negative microscopic examinations of stool for entamoeba histolytica and negative cultures for bacterial pathogens and progression to chronicity or a tendency to recurrence.

An *incarcerated ventral hernia* causes localized hypogastric pain and a tender mass, and may cause generalized abdominal colicky pain, nausea, and vomiting due to intestinal obstruction.

Acute hypogastric pain in women may be related to gynecologic causes. *Endometritis* may occur in a patient with an IUD, causing fever, deep dyspareunia, suprapubic pain and tenderness, and uterine enlargement and tenderness. There is a therapeutic response to IUD removal and antibiotic therapy. A similar illness can occur in a setting of early pregnancy after an attempt to induce an *abortion* by introduction of a foreign body into the uterus. Fever; chills; lower abdominal pain, and a tender, boggy uterus with a bloody vaginal discharge are part of the clinical picture. Clot and membranes may be trapped in the os.

Hypogastric crampy pain and bleeding may signal the onset

of a first-trimester abortion. Some patients complete the abortion, while others cease to have pain and bleeding. In patients who are likely to complete the abortion, the os is usually patulous, and products of conception may protrude into the vagina.

A *uterine myoma* may necrose or hemorrhage into itself, causing hypogastric pain and tenderness. Examination reveals a large myomatous uterus with a localized tender nodular area. The diagnosis can be aided by sonographic studies.

Tubal pregnancy in the proximal tube or isthmus can cause crampy or constant hypogastric pain, one or more missed periods, spotting, or vaginal bleeding. Pelvic examination may reveal a palpable tubal mass. Sonographic or laparoscopic studies and a urine or serum pregnancy test will confirm the diagnosis.

Bleeding from an ovarian cyst or a cyst arising from an implant of endometriosis can cause severe lower abdominal pain of a constant nature. Localized or diffuse lower abdominal direct and rebound tenderness may occur, as well as guarding. Pelvic tenderness may be present. A bleeding *corpus luteum cyst* may mimic a ruptured ectopic pregnancy because it can cause amenorrhea, irregular vaginal bleeding, and lower abdominal peritoneal signs. Bleeding from a follicle cyst occurs at midcycle (Mittelschmerz), and usually all symptoms resolve in 24 to 72 h. *Bleeding from an endometrioma* occurs in a setting of chronic secondary dysmenorrhea, menorrhagia, and/or infertility. Sonographic studies are helpful in detecting cysts, and laparoscopic examination will confirm intraabdominal bleeding. *Bleeding into cystic lesions* may also occur without leakage into the free peritoneal cavity. This causes a dull, constant lower abdominal pain and a tender localized adnexal mass.

☐ DESCRIPTION OF LISTED DISEASES

1. ACUTE PROSTATITIS

Dull, aching discomfort occurs in the suprapubic region and is transiently relieved by voiding. Low back and perineal aching may also occur. During and/or after urination, a sharp, burning pain may sometimes be felt in the perineum and penis. Excruciating pain due to cystourethral spasm (strangury) may occur without warning in the suprapubic region and radiate into the penis and perineum. A small amount of urine may be expressed involuntarily during such an attack. Strangury lasts only seconds or minutes, but may recur until antibiotic therapy reduces the acute inflammatory response.

Chills and/or rigors, temperature elevations to 105°F, malaise, anorexia, myalgias, and arthralgias reflect the systemic nature of this disorder. Irritative bladder symptoms such as frequent small voidings, nocturia, urgency, a sensation of incomplete emptying, and incontinence are common associated complaints. Urinary obstructive symptoms occur because of prostatic edema and urethral inflammation. These include a marked decrease in the size, force, and velocity of the stream; difficulty initiating voiding; dribbling; a split stream; and partial or complete urinary retention.

Physical findings include fever; tachycardia; and an enlarged, soft, tender prostate. The urine is usually turbid and

TABLE OF DISEASE INCIDENCE

INCIDENCE PER 100,000 (APPROXIMATE)

Common (>100)	Uncommon (>5–100)	Rare (>0–5)
Acute urinary retention in men due to BPH or BPH and prostatitis	Acute prostatitis	Acute prostatic abscess
Acute bacterial cystitis	Acute urinary retention due to: carcinoma of the prostate; acute prostatitis or prostatic abscess; urethral stricture	Acute urinary retention in women
Acute cystitis and pyelonephritis		Cecal volvulus
Dysuria-frequency syndrome	Acute prostatitis or stricture of the penile urethrae	Perforation due to toxic megacolon or fecal impaction
Colon obstruction due to carcinoma	Pelvic appendicitis	Incarcerated ventral hernia
Perforation of the colon due to diverticulitis	Bladder calculi	Septic abortion
Acute infectious diarrhea	Colon obstruction due to diverticulitis or fecal impaction	Acute urinary retention in men due to neurogenic or drug-related causes
Uterine myoma with necrosis and/or bleeding	Pseudo-obstruction of the colon	
Nonseptic abortion	Sigmoid volvulus	
Tubal pregnancy	Perforation due to carcinoma or ischemic colitis	
Hemorrhage from an ovarian cyst	Ischemic colitis	
	Initial attack of inflammatory bowel disease	
	Endometritis due to IUD	
	Intracystic hemorrhage	
	Endometrioma with intraperitoneal hemorrhage	

contains leukocytes and bacteria. A two-glass test may show more turbidity and leukocytes in the initial 10 ml of voided urine than in a midstream specimen. Prostatic massage or compression should be avoided because it can initiate bacteremia. Diagnosis of the causative organism can be achieved by culture of the urine. These patients require hospital admission, intravenous fluids, and antibiotics. Urinary retention can be relieved by catheterization or suprapubic cystotomy. If there is no response to antibiotic therapy within 48 h, the prostate should be reevaluated by rectal examination or rectal sonographic studies for a prostatic abscess that may require drainage. After recovery, a thorough urologic evaluation for obstructing urethral lesions should be done.

2. ACUTE URINARY RETENTION

There is a desire to urinate but an inability to do so. As the bladder distends with urine, a sense of lower abdominal pressure, and then discomfort, develops, associated with a desire to void. The bladder is palpable as a compressible suprapubic mass. It may distend to the level of the umbilicus. The mass and the discomfort vanish with bladder catheterization and the removal of 700 to 1500 ml of urine. There are several causes of acute urinary retention.

A. Benign Prostatic Hypertrophy (BPH)　There is a long history of nocturia and small frequent voidings with a weak and narrow stream. Initiating urination may be delayed, and there may be dribbling and stuttering urination. The patient may have to strain to keep the urinary stream flowing. The prostate is moderately firm but compressible and enlarged. If the gland is not enlarged to examination, the presence of an obstructing median bar should be suspected.

B. Prostatitis　Acute inflammation causes suprapubic, perineal, and lumbosacral back pain; fever; chills; frequent, small voidings; dysuria; a diminished stream; and, in some cases, urinary retention.

C. Chronic Prostatitis Plus Benign Prostatic Hypertrophy　Chronic prostatitis causes glandular swelling with dysuria, frequency, a diminished stream, and suprapubic aching or burning that is relieved by voiding. The presence of a moderate amount of prostatic hypertrophy and an associated prostatitis may lead to urinary retention related to a component of obstruction introduced by each of these disorders.

D. Prostatic Carcinoma　Acute retention may be caused by prostatic carcinoma. A short and rapidly progressive history of increasing frequency, nocturia, and diminished force and size of the stream is characteristic of malignancy. The development of such complaints may progress over a period of months, rather than years, as occurs with prostatic hypertrophy. Weight loss, anorexia, and lumbosacral back pain may develop. On examination, the prostate is enlarged and contains stony hard tissue in one or both lobes. Serum acid and alkaline phosphatase and prostate specific antigen (PSA) levels may be increased.

E. Urethral Stricture　Cases of urethral stricture are usually secondary to a gonococcal urethritis. There is a history of a progressive decrease in the force and size of the stream before retention occurs.

F. Retention Due to Neurogenic Causes　Bladder contractility may be impaired by spinal cord disease. Retention also occurs after trauma; surgery; anesthesia (e.g., spinal); the use of certain drugs, such as anticholinergics and meperidine.

3. URINARY RETENTION IN WOMEN

This condition may rarely be caused by *obstructive lesions* such as urethral carcinoma, stricture, or invasion by a tumor in the vagina or cervix. *Neurogenic* factors and *psychogenic* causes account for most cases of acute retention in women.

4. ACUTE BACTERIAL CYSTITIS

A. Acute Cystitis　Suprapubic aching pain accompanied by internal dysuria, frequency, urgency, and sometimes incontinence, occurs. The urine is often malodorous and cloudy because of increased numbers of neutrophils and/or bacteria. Only small amounts of urine are passed at each voiding, and there is often a sensation of incomplete bladder emptying. Gross hematuria may occur in up to 50 percent of women with this disorder. Sexual intercourse plays a role in causation in women, and use of a diaphragm increases the risk in sexually active women. The periurethral area is often colonized by the same organism that causes the cystitis. Bacterial vaginosis may be associated with urinary infection and *Escherichia coli* colonization. This condition causes a vaginal pH greater than 5; colonization of the vagina with *Gardnerella vaginalis, Mycoplasma hominus,* and anerobes including *Bacteroides, Mobiluncus,* and *Peptostreptococcus* species; and decreased numbers of lactobacilli. Chills, fever, malaise, nausea, and vomiting are not usually present unless there is an associated pyelonephritis.

Suprapubic discomfort is partially and temporarily relieved by passage of urine. There may be suprapubic tenderness. An unspun drop of urine contains more than 10 white blood cells/mm^3 when counted in a hemacytometer. This method of counting correlates better with an elevated 24-h leukocyte excretion rate than does wet-mount counting of leukocytes in a centrifuged urine specimen.

A Gram stain of unspun urine will detect one or more bacteria per oil field in 90 percent of patients with at least 10^5 colony-forming units (CFU)/ml. Up to 33 percent of women with bacterial cystitis caused by *E. coli, Proteus* species, or *Staphlococcus saprophyticus* have only 10^2 to 10^4 CFU/ml, while the others have at least 10^5 CFU/ml. An initial urine culture can be done; or therapy with amoxicillin, trimethoprim-sulfamethoxasole, or ciprofloxacin may be initiated without a culture. Sensitive organisms will disappear from the urine rapidly, and clinical and laboratory abnormalities will revert to normal in 1 to 3 days. In patients without complicating factors, single-dose or 3-day short-course therapy can be used. Seven or more days of treatment can be reserved for patients with acute cystitis and complicating factors, such as the presence of symptoms for over 7 days, pregnancy, diabetes, urinary tract abnormalities, and suspected occult upper tract infection.

B. Acute Cystitis with Occult Pyelonephritis These patients present with suprapubic pain and symptoms of inflammatory irritability of the bladder. They do not usually have fever, chills, or flank pain and tenderness. Certain risk factors, such as a relapse after treatment for cystitis, recent antibiotic use, diabetes, immunosuppression, onset of infection before age 12 or after age 65, pyelonephritis within the previous 12 months, symptoms for at least 7 days before therapy, pregnancy, and failure to respond to therapy in 3 days, make it likely that a patient with acute cystitis has occult pyelonephritis. Patients with simple cystitis associated with these risk factors have been shown to harbor upper tract bacterial infection. This has been demonstrated using techniques such as bladder washout cultures, selective ureteral catheterization cultures, or the demonstration of antibody-coated urinary bacteria. A urine culture and sensitivity should be obtained, and the patient treated for at least 14 days. Posttreatment cultures should be done to evaluate the effectiveness of therapy.

C. Acute Cystitis with Clinical Acute Pyelonephritis Symptoms of cystitis frequently precede upper tract involvement by 2 to 8 days. Evidence of upper tract disease includes chills, fever, vomiting, malaise, an ache in one or both flanks, and costovertebral-angle tenderness. Patients who develop symptoms in a setting of a recent urethral catheterization, urologic surgery, obstructive lesions, or recent hospitalization deserve readmission and parenteral antibiotic therapy with drugs such as ceftriaxone or trimethoprim-sulfamethoxazole. Short-term catheterization (<3 days) is associated with infection by *E. coli, Proteus mirabilis, Pseudomonas aeruginosa, Klebsiella pneumoniae, Staphylococcus epidermidis,* and enterococci. Long-term catheterization is associated with infection by the same organisms, as well as *Providencia stuartii* and *Morganella morganii.*

D. Acute Dysuria-Frequency Syndrome Symptoms of acute cystitis, such as frequency, urgency, and dysuria, are present, but cultures for urinary pathogens are negative. Compared to women with positive cultures, such patients are less likely to have leukocyturia (45 percent vs. 80 percent), hematuria (6 percent vs. 24 percent), and a positive Gram stain (13 percent vs. 89 percent). Women with negative cultures are also more likely to have vaginal discharge (52 percent vs. 31 percent) and a longer duration of complaint (5.6 $\pm$ 3.5 days vs. 3.7 $\pm$ 3.5 days) and are less likely to be sexually active (69 percent vs. 87 percent). Such patients without positive urine findings may sometimes have a sexually transmitted infection with *Neisseria gonorrhoeae, Chlamydia trachomatis,* or *Herpes simplex*; very low colony counts; inconstantly present positive cultures; or a disorder of unknown etiology. Many such patients receive an initial trial of antibiotics and either respond promptly (i.e., false-negative bacterial culture group) or do not respond. Positive cultures (i.e., low colony count) usually are caused by *E. coli* (55 percent); *Staphylococcus* species (10 percent); and *Klebsiella, Proteus,* and enterococcal species (29 percent).

5. PELVIC APPENDICITIS

Acute pelvic appendicitis begins with transient periumbilical crampy dull pain that vanishes after 4 to 6 h. Suprapubic pain, and sometimes pain in the right iliac fossae, then develops and persists. Walking and coughing intensify this pain. Inflammatory irritation of the bladder may cause urinary frequency, urgency, dysuria, and sterile pyuria. Rectal involvement may result in frequent bowel movements, diarrhea, or tenesmus. Urinary symptoms are less frequently seen in women. Anorexia, nausea, vomiting, low-grade fever, and leukocytosis soon develop. The abdominal examination reveals tenderness at the pelvic brim, in the mid-lower abdomen, or on the right, without guarding. An obturator sign is often present. Rectal examination reveals pelvic tenderness. A sonographic or a laparoscopic study may aid in establishing a diagnosis of appendicitis by direct imaging of the appendix.

A sudden improvement in the pain may initially suggest spontaneous resolution, but if this relief is subsequently followed by a rise in temperature and worsening pain, then appendiceal perforation is likely. Rectal or pelvic examination may reveal a tender fluctuant abscess along the right pelvic wall. Alternatively, diffuse lower abdominal direct and rebound tenderness, guarding, and distension may signal free perforation and peritonitis. The diagnosis of a pelvic abscess can be confirmed by sonographic studies or a CT scan. The abscess can be drained percutaneously or surgically under an umbrella of intravenous antibiotics. Whether appendectomy is required in addition to abscess drainage is still controversial, since the risk for recurrence without appendectomy is less than 10 to 20 percent.

6. BLADDER CALCULI

There may be dull suprapubic discomfort, with sharper pain precipitated by jarring and exercise. During voiding, the stone may obstruct the urethra abruptly, diminishing or stopping the stream. Terminal hematuria may also occur. Frequency, urgency, and internal dysuria also may accompany obstructive symptoms, such as a diminished stream and hesitation. Cystoscopic studies may be required for diagnosis, since many bladder stones (e.g., uric acid) are radiolucent. Other stones found in the bladder contain calcium oxalate or struvite. Bladder stones are usually secondary to chronic obstruction and/or residual bladder urine produced by prostatic disease, urethral stricture, or a neurogenic bladder. Foreign bodies such as long-term catheters predispose to the formation of vesical calculi. Ultrasonic or mechanical lithotripsy may be used to remove bladder stones, but surgery may be required. Treatment of infection, stasis, metabolic errors, and foreign body removal are helpful in preventing recurrent stone formation.

7. DISORDERS OF THE COLON

A. Obstruction

1. Carcinoma Luminal stenosis secondary to carcinoma accounts for 67 percent and cicatrizing occlusion due to diverticulitis for 7 percent of cases of large bowel obstruction. Colicky pain in the hypogastrium, and sometimes the iliac areas or perineum, is an early complaint. Such pain lasts for 2 to 3 min and then remits for relatively long intervals (10 to 20 min). Nausea and anorexia occur, and the lower abdomen becomes distended. If the ileocecal valve is incompetent (20 percent of patients), then upper abdominal distension and feculent vomiting may occur. Over a period of 8 to 24 h, the intermittent pain becomes constant as the abdomen distends. Initially, the rectum may empty itself of gas and feces in one or two movements, and then complete obstipation occurs. Physical examination usually demonstrates lower abdominal distension and tenderness. Muscle guarding may occur during attacks of colic. Bowel sounds become bursts or rushes of high-pitched metallic noises coincident with attacks of colic. In cases of distal obstruction, abdominal radiographs demonstrate proximal dilatation of the colon; air-fluid levels; cecal distension; and, in the 20 percent of patients with an incompetent ileocecal valve, fluid- and gas-filled loops of small bowel.

A water-soluble contrast enema should be performed before surgical intervention in patients with suspected large bowel obstruction. In two reported series, 34 and 37 percent of such cases had no obstruction and did not require surgery.

Patients with mechanical obstruction of the colon have been temporarily decompressed endoscopically by passing tubes retrograde past the obstruction or by the use of laser photocoagulation to recanalize the colon lumen.

Optimal operative treatment is controversial. Many surgeons advocate resection of an obstructing malignancy and primary anastomosis. The danger is the development of postoperative anastomotic leaks and peritonitis. Alternatively, a proximal decompressing colostomy can be done, and the distal lesion can be resected and an anastomosis completed at a second stage, utilizing the decompressed proximal bowel. Primary resection and anastomosis in patients with malignancy allows for superior 5-year survival rates (48 percent vs. 21 percent) compared to treatment by a two-stage procedure.

Other causes of large bowel obstruction include fecal impaction (5 percent), cicatrization caused by ulcerative colitis (<1 percent), intestinal pseudo-obstruction, and sigmoid volvulus (9 percent).

2. Diverticulitis With pericolonic inflammation or cicatrizing intraluminal changes, diverticulitis can cause partial or complete large bowel obstruction and produce a clinical picture indistinguishable from that resulting from an obstructing carcinoma. Bowel resection with proximal colostomy and a Hartmann closure is the safest operative procedure. Differentiation of carcinoma from diverticulitis in the obstructed segment may not be possible until the operative specimen is studied.

3. Colonic Pseudo-obstruction (Ogilvie's Syndrome) Painless lower abdominal distension develops, followed by the development of nausea and vomiting. Obstipation occurs in half the patients, while others continue to pass gas and liquid stool. As the distension increases, up to 80 percent of patients develop a lower abdominal constant dull pain. Direct and rebound tenderness may occur in the lower abdomen because of the marked distension of the cecum and colon up to the splenic flexure, where the distension usually appears to end. Bowel sounds are seldom absent, and they may be hyperactive. Fever and marked leukocytosis may occur. Colonic perforation can occur because of cecal distension. Plain abdominal radiographs demonstrate proximal colon dilatation and a possible distal obstruction. The dilated colon of pseudo-obstruction has visible septa, distinct haustral markings, and less striking gas-fluid levels. A water-soluble contrast enema will demonstrate the absence of mechanical obstruction. This can be confirmed by colonoscopic studies, and the proximal colon can be decompressed by this procedure without surgery. To maintain decompression, a long radiopaque tube can be left in place beyond the hepatic flexure as the colonoscope is withdrawn. After decompression, most patients improve, and colon function normalizes in 3 to 6 days.

In one small series of 12 cases, with an initial diagnosis of pseudo-obstruction, 2 were found to have true mechanical obstruction requiring operation. It is clear that without a contrast enema or colonoscopic studies, pseudo-obstruction and mechanical obstruction of the large bowel may be indistinguishable. Colonic pseudoobstruction may be idiopathic or related to retroperitoneal involvement of autonomic ganglia by tumor, surgery, or trauma; a retroperitoneal inflammatory process or infection; radiation therapy; drugs (e.g., narcotics, anticholinergics, and antidepressants); severe cardiac disease; neurologic disorders (e.g., Parkinson's disease, multiple sclerosis, and myotonic dystrophy); respiratory failure; diabetes; uremia; hypothyroidism; pheochromocytoma; and collagen vascular disorders (e.g., systemic sclerosis, systemic lupus erythematosus, and dermatomyositis). Treatment of these underlying disorders does not usually relieve the pseudo-obstruction without mechanical decompression.

4. Fecal Impaction and Obstruction   This multifactorial disorder has its highest prevalence in the elderly and the demented. Certain drugs contribute to the risk of developing an impaction. These include narcotics, anticholinergic tricyclic antidepressants, phenothiazines, antihypertensives, diuretics, sucralfate, iron, and antacids. Laxative abuse may damage the myenteric plexus and cause the "cathartic syndrome."

Decreased activity, dementia, dehydration, and poor dentition increase the risk. Patients with chronic renal failure, diabetes with autonomic neuropathy, and spinal cord metastases have an increased incidence of impaction. Neurologic patients with weakness and immobility (e.g., patients with stroke, multiple sclerosis, or amyotrophic lateral sclerosis) suffer from this disorder. It is also a common complication of Parkinson's disease, spinal cord injury, and tumor.

Impaction in young adults may be due to Hirschsprung's disease, Chagas' disease, the cathartic syndrome, or idiopathic megacolon.

Obstruction is signaled by a history of obstipation for 3 or more days and/or paradoxical diarrhea, lower abdominal discomfort, distension, anorexia, and nausea. Fever and tachycardia may occur. Urinary frequency, retention, and overflow incontinence may be present due to bladder compression by the distended colon. The diagnosis can be made by rectal examination or by sigmoidoscopic or colonoscopic studies in those uncommon cases in which the rectal vault is empty and there is a "high" impaction. Such cases are seen with adenocarcinomas and with pathologic conditions of the cervical and thoracic spinal cord. Manual removal and enemas usually break up the impaction and relieve the obstruction. High impactions may require sigmoidoscopically directed lavage or use of hyperosmotic water-soluble contrast media to stimulate peristalsis and lubricate the fecal mass. Surgical removal of the obstructed colon may be required if all else fails.

5. Sigmoid Volvulus   There is an abrupt onset of constant or crampy mid-lower abdominal pain, which may spread to the left iliac area. Distension of the lower abdomen develops and increases rapidly. Nausea, vomiting, and obstipation occur. The abdomen is distended, tender to palpation, and tympanitic. Plain abdominal radiographs show a greatly dilated ahaustral sigmoid loop (bent inner tube or omega loop sign). The convexity of the loop points away from the site of obstruction. The "bird's beak"–like narrowing of the distal air column identifies the obstruction. In 30 to 40 percent of cases, the plain radiograph is nondiagnostic, and a CT scan showing the "whirl sign," or contrast studies will be required to confirm the diagnosis. A Gastrografin enema may demonstrate stenosis of the upper rectum. The site of obstruction shows a bird's beak sign and corkscrew or spiral mucosal folds. If there is no fever, leukocytosis, or abdominal guarding, prompt sigmoidoscopic passage of a well-lubricated rectal tube will usually decompress the colon, with a sudden release of fluid and gas. The success rate for nonsurgical decompression is 70 to 90 percent, but since recurrence is common (30–60 percent), elective resection of the redundant colon should be done within 7 days. Careful observation of the stool for blood and of the abdomen for signs of peritonitis is required after decompression to detect early evidence of bowel necrosis. Failure of decompression by rectal tube or colonoscopic studies requires immediate surgical exploration and decompression, with resection of any gangrenous bowel. This disorder tends to occur in the elderly as well as in pregnant women. Chronic constipation and a redundant sigmoid are associated. There is an increased frequency of volvulus in patients with Chagas' disease, Parkinson's disease, spinal cord paraplegias and quadriplegias, or ischemic colitis. Sigmoid volvulus is a common cause of intestinal obstruction in pregnant women.

6. Cecal Volvulus   Mild right lower abdominal and/or hypogastric crampy pain or severe colic may occur. Lower abdominal distension develops, along with tenderness over the distended cecum. A plain radiograph will show a markedly dilated ovoid or circular gas-filled shadow in the midabdomen (cecum). A Gastrografin enema will demonstrate the site of cecal obstruction. Colonoscopic studies may successfully decompress the volvulus, but open surgery may be required to prevent cecal gangrene and/or perforation. Cecopexy or cecostomy after correction of the volvulus is necessary to prevent recurrence.

Failure to operate before the onset of gangrene increases the operative mortality rate to 55 percent because of an increased incidence of postoperative peritonitis, abscess formation, and sepsis.

B. Perforation of the Colon   This may occur as a complication of diverticulitis of the cecum or rectosigmoid; carcinoma; or ischemic colitis. Less commonly, it follows volvulus, fecal impaction, and amebic or ulcerative colitis.

When perforation occurs, peritoneal soiling may produce acute suprapubic and/or iliac pain. This pain is constant and intensified by coughing, laughing, jarring, or movement. There is usually direct and rebound tenderness, involuntary guarding, pelvic pain and tenderness, and lower abdominal distension. Low back pain, nausea, vomiting, fever, and leukocytosis may also occur. The history may provide information as to the cause of the perforation and localized or generalized peritonitis. Surgical exploration is usually required to resect perforated bowel and/or ischemic bowel and decompress the colon with a proximal colostomy. Primary anastomosis should be avoided because of peritoneal soilage, which can lead to dehiscence of the anastomosis.

The clinical findings of the disorders associated with colon perforation are discussed below.

1. Diverticulitis   Pain of a constant aching or burning nature occurs in the hypogastrium and at times in the left lower abdomen with diverticulitis of the sigmoid. Cecal diverticulitis may be associated with right lower abdominal pain and hypogastric pain. Low back pain may occur simultaneously with the abdominal pain. Fever, nausea, vomiting, diarrhea, or constipation may occur. Leukocytosis is commonly present.

Associated urinary frequency and urgency may result from inflammatory involvement of the bladder. Localized direct and rebound tenderness, as well as guarding, may be present in the hypogastrium and right or left lower abdomen. A tender left iliac or hypogastric mass may be palpable.

In many medical centers, contrast barium enemas are deferred for fear of precipitating perforation from increased colonic pressures during the procedure. In other centers, barium studies have been done without complication. In a recent comparative study, contrast enemas and CT studies were compared for usefulness in the diagnosis of acute diverticulitis. Contrast enema studies had a 77 percent sensitivity for diagnosis. CT studies demonstrated specific diagnostic findings such as a pericolonic mass or gas collection in 41 percent of cases and findings consistent with diverticulitis in another 38 percent (i.e., bowel wall thickening and mesenteric or fascial soft-tissue stranding). In many centers, CT scans are being used instead of contrast enemas to confirm acute diverticulitis. Since there is a significant false-negative rate with both procedures (10–15 percent), negative studies do not rule out the diagnosis. CT scans have the advantage of being able to detect localized abscesses in the lower abdomen and pelvis and at more remote sites, such as the liver and subdiaphragmatic space. Therapy for perforation requires administration of parenteral antibiotics (antiaerobic and antianaerobic drugs) and percutaneous catheter or open surgical drainage of localized abscesses. At surgery, proximal colostomy, resection of the diseased area, and a Hartmann closure of the distal bowel are the preferred procedures.

A colovesical fistula may occur in 2 to 4 percent of cases. It can be associated with suprapubic discomfort, frequency, urgency, dysuria, pyuria, and bacteriuria, as well as pneumaturia and fecaluria. The diagnosis can be made by a CT scan showing air in the bladder, cystoscopic studies, or a water-soluble contrast enema that opacifies the bladder immediately after administration. A fistulogram performed during cystoscopy has a high sensitivity, while a contrast enema detects only 25 percent of colovesical fistulas. Charcoal ingestion followed by examination of the urine may confirm the diagnosis, but false-positive results may occur in women because of fecal contamination of the periurethral area.

2. Carcinoma of the Sigmoid Colon   Patients can experience perforation adjacent to the tumor or a blowout perforation of the cecum. Crampy lower abdominal (suprapubic and/or iliac) pain may occur in discrete episodes and precede the perforation. Signs of localized peritonitis accompany perforation, as do fever and chills. There may be a history of constipation and/or diarrhea, hematochezia, and ribbon- or pencil-shaped stools. The diagnosis can be confirmed by colonoscopic studies, and the extent of the abscess defined by a CT scan. Proximal colostomy, diseased segment resection, and a Hartmann closure under an antibiotic umbrella constitute the preferred method of treatment.

3. Ischemic Colitis   This disorder occurs in patients over age 50 who have a significant history of cardiovascular disease (e.g., angina, myocardial infarction, stroke, or lower limb amputation for gangrene). Fulminant ischemic colitis begins with crampy, and later constant, hypogastric and left lower abdominal pain, distension, fever, nausea, vomiting, and severe constipation or diarrhea. The stools are formed or loose, and contain bright red or occult blood. Lower abdominal direct and rebound tenderness, guarding, and distension are present after 8 to 24 h. The diagnosis can be supported by colonoscopic studies that reveal an absence of lesions until the 15-cm level of the rectosigmoid (i.e., rectal sparing). Above 15 cm, ulcerations, bleeding, and blue-black submucosal nodules are frequently present. Plain radiographs show gaseous dilatation of the colon with distension stopping at the involved colon segment. Air bubbles may be detected in the infarcted bowel wall. Barium enemas are usually deferred for fear of producing a perforation. A contrast enema performed when pain, tenderness, and fever have abated may show thumb printing and saw tooth ulcerations. Angiograms usually fail to reveal arterial obstruction, are not helpful diagnostically, and are seldom used. Surgery is required for perforation and spillage of feces into the free peritoneal cavity. Most episodes of ischemia cause only lower abdominal pain, tenderness, and mild bloody diarrhea that usually clears with supportive care. The colonoscopic findings may mimic Crohn's disease or ulcerative colitis, and the clinical picture may mimic diverticulitis. An initial attack of acute ulcerative colitis in an elderly patient may actually be due to ischemic colitis.

In patients with perforation or bowel gangrene, resection of the necrotic colon, a proximal colostomy, and a Hartmann closure provide the best opportunity for survival.

This disorder occurs in arteriosclerotic individuals, with localized disease in the inferior mesenteric artery, after rupture of an aneurysm, in severe heart failure with a low output state, after aortic aneurysm surgery, and after abdominoperineal resection for rectal cancer. Rare cases occur secondary to vasculitis; amyloidosis; hypercoagulable states; colorectal cancer; and the use of ergot preparations, vasopressin, or oral contraceptives.

4. Toxic Megacolon   Ischemic, amebic, or bacterial colitis; ulcerative colitis; and Crohn's disease may cause toxic megacolon, with severe abdominal pain and distension, ending in perforation and generalized peritonitis.

5. Fecal Impaction   This disorder can cause stercoral ulcers, which can perforate, or obstructive perforation of a distended cecum.

C. Acute Infectious Colitis   Crampy abdominal pain occurs in the periumbilical and hypogastric areas. Right lower abdominal pain (i.e., pseudoappendicitis) is common with *Salmonella* and *Yersinia* infections, as well as with ileocecal amebiasis. The abdominal pain and rectal discomfort may begin or intensify with the desire to defecate and are temporarily relieved by passage of stool and gas. Tenesmus may occur. The stool may be watery green or brown, or it may be flecked with mucus and blood. In severe cases, there is gross bleeding, with the passage of clots. The clinical picture produced by one enteric pathogen may be indistinguishable from that of another without cultures or microscopic stool studies. The agents capable of producing acute infectious diarrhea are discussed below.

1. Salmonella Species   These organisms cause 2.3 percent of all severe gastroenteritis in the United States. Pain is usually present in the hypogastrium and sometimes in the periumbilical area and right lower abdomen. Diarrhea may be watery or dysenteric. Fever to 102°F occurs in up to 50 percent of cases. Abdominal tenderness may be mild, or it may simulate an acute surgical abdomen. The stool usually contains increased fecal leukocytes and occult blood. If fever persists beyond 3 to 4 days, a bacteremic or metastatic infection should be considered. *Salmonella* gastroenteritis should not be treated with antibiotics unless the patient is above age 50; has leukemia, lymphoma, underlying vascular disease, severe arthritis, a joint replacement, sickle cell disease, or AIDS; or is a transplant recipient. Such patients can be treated with amoxicillin or chloramphenicol. Resistant

strains of *S. typhi* may require treatment with quinolones or third-generation cephalosporins.

2. Campylobacter Species   Diarrhea and fever, accompanied by mid- and low abdominal pain, occur in 70 to 90 percent of cases. Systemic symptoms such as myalgias, arthralgias, chills, anorexia, and vomiting often precede the diarrhea.

The pain is crampy and usually intensifies before defecation and is relieved afterward. Stools contain increased leukocytes and gross or occult blood, and a wet stool preparation may show comma-shaped bacteria with darting motility. The diagnosis is confirmed by culture on selective media at 42°C (e.g., modified Butzler medium). *Campylobacter* account for 5 to 7 percent of cases of severe gastroenteritis in the United States. Erythromycin or ciprofloxacin are effective against *Campylobacter* infections.

3. Shigella Species   Initially, copious watery diarrhea may occur, followed by bloody dysentery. Up to 33 percent of patients have fever. Lower abdominal pain and tenesmus may accompany the diarrhea. Trimethoprim-sulfamethoxazole or ciprofloxacin are effective against shigellosis.

4. Other Organisms   *Yersinia* species, *Clostridium difficile* (after antibiotic therapy), *E. coli* (0157:H7), *Vibrio parahemolyticus* (after ingesting raw shellfish), and *Entamaeba histolytica* are also capable of producing similar attacks of fever, abdominal pain, and diarrhea. The stool may contain gross or occult blood, mucus, and increased numbers of leukocytes with each of these agents.

5. Initial Attack of Ulcerative Colitis or Crohn's Disease   An acute bacterial diarrheal illness or amebiasis may mimic an initial attack of ulcerative colitis or Crohn's disease. In patients with inflammatory bowel disease, stool cultures are negative for pathogenic bacteria and microscopy reveals no evidence of parasites (e.g., ameba).

8. INCARCERATED OR STRANGULATED VENTRAL OR SPIGELIAN HERNIA

These lower midabdominal hernias can contain loops of bowel that may become incarcerated or strangulated, giving rise to a local mass, constant aching hypogastric pain, tenderness, and induration. If incarceration or strangulation is complete, obstruction occurs. Then vomiting, generalized colic, and abdominal distension follow. Strangulation may be signaled by the development of more severe direct and rebound tenderness in the lower abdomen, fever, and leukocytosis. Surgical reduction, resection of gangrenous bowel, and repair of the hernia will relieve all symptoms.

9. GYNECOLOGIC CAUSES FOR HYPOGASTRIC PAIN

A. Endometritis   Aching constant or crampy mid-lower abdominal pain is associated with a leukocyte-containing vaginal discharge. There may be fever and chills and direct abdominal tenderness in the area of pain. The uterus is slightly enlarged, and cervical motion and palpation of the corpus elicits pain. Adnexal tenderness on one or both sides may also be present. Culture of the cervix may reveal *Neisseria gonorrhoeae*, *Chlamydia trachomatis*, gram-negative rods, or enterococci.

The presence of an IUD doubles the risk of endometritis and salpingitis.

A rare type of endometritis and tubal infection caused by *Actinomyces israeli* has been associated with the presence of an IUD. In this disorder, lower abdominal and pelvic pain and fever are associated with a tubo-ovarian abscess and sometimes with metastatic infection to other regions of the abdomen, chest, or brain. The pain and other symptoms associated with endometritis resolve with antibiotic therapy. Removal of an IUD may be necessary to control endometrial infection.

B. Septic Abortion   A severe form of acute endometritis may occur in a patient subjected to a nonsterile attempt at abortion. Chills, fever, and prostration are associated with hypogastric aching or crampy pain and tenderness. There may be lower abdominal signs of peritonitis and abdominal distension. The uterus is usually enlarged, soft, and tender. A bloody vaginal discharge is present. The cervix is open and soft. Necrotic decidua or membranes may be trapped in the os. There is often tenderness in the broad ligaments bilaterally. Leukocytosis and anemia may be present. In severe cases associated with *Clostridium perfringens* infection, jaundice, shock, and severe hemolytic anemia progress to rapid death.

Septic abortion is a life-threatening emergency requiring early evacuation of the uterus, high doses of parenteral antibiotics, and an emergency hysterectomy for patients who fail to improve promptly.

C. Uterine Myoma with Necrosis and/or Bleeding
Hemorrhage into or necrosis of a uterine myoma may cause the sudden onset of mid-lower abdominal pain and tenderness. Pelvic examination reveals an enlarged, knotty uterus with a localized tender nodule at the site of maximal pain. Sonographic studies may help confirm the diagnosis. The pain may continue as a dull, constant ache for up to a week and then abate. This disorder can be treated expectantly, and surgery is seldom required. Large myomatous uteri are uncommon before age 35.

Surgery for a myomatous uterus is usually performed because of rapid growth, massive size with pressure symptoms affecting the bladder and rectum, dragging lower abdominal discomfort, and excessive menstrual and/or intermenstrual bleeding.

D. Acute Spontaneous Abortion   Amenorrhea of 1- to 3-month's duration, followed by vaginal staining or bleeding, is suggestive of threatened abortion. In some cases the bleeding stops spontaneously, but in others it is accompanied by hypogastric and lumbosacral cramping pain and the passage of clots and products of conception.

Mid-lower abdominal pain associated with vaginal bleeding in early pregnancy is a poor prognostic sign. The pains may be laborlike or dull and persistent. If bleeding ceases without passage of a fetus or membranes, pregnancy viability can be assessed by serial hCG testing, estimation of uterine size on pelvic examination, and examination of the uterus for a viable pregnancy by ultrasonography. If the pregnancy is nonviable, it should be terminated.

E. Tubal Pregnancy   Pain of an aching or crampy quality occurs slightly to one or the other side of the midline. There may be a history of one or more missed or scant periods. Staining, spotting, or frank bleeding is commonly present after the first missed period. If a hematoma forms in the tube, the lower abdominal pain usually becomes constant.

Severe knifelike pain in the lower abdomen, followed by more generalized abdominal pain and tenderness, shoulder pain, pallor, and dizziness, is suggestive of rupture of the pregnant tube with intraabdominal bleeding. In up to 5 percent of cases, cold, pale, sweaty extremities are present, in addition to tachycardia, hypotension, and tachypnea. Such patients require immediate volume resuscitation and operation to prevent exsanguination.

Pelvic examination done before rupture may reveal adnexal tenderness close to the body of the uterus and, in some cases, a palpable mass. The urine and serum pregnancy tests are positive. Ultrasonography will reveal a complex or noncystic tubal mass and absence of an intrauterine gestation. Laparoscopy can be used to visualize the tubal pregnancy and to evaluate it. At open surgery, salpingectomy can be done, or the pregnancy can be resected and the tube repaired immediately or at a second procedure.

F. Bleeding from a Follicle or a Corpus Luteum Cyst
Bleeding from a cystic lesion can cause explosive mid-lower abdominal pain and tenderness. Follicle cysts bleed at midcycle (mittleschmerz). Corpus luteum cysts can mimic an ectopic pregnancy because they cause lower abdominal pain and can cause a delay in the onset of the next period. Spotting or staining may follow the amenorrhea. Severe intraabdominal bleeding with diffuse lower abdominal pain and tenderness may occur from a luteal cyst. There may be diffuse rebound tenderness in the lower abdomen and guarding. Sonographic or laparoscopic studies can confirm the presence of the luteal cyst, and the urine and serum hCG tests remain negative. These cysts can be

treated expectantly, unless there is severe bleeding requiring laparotomy for control.

A corpus luteum cyst of pregnancy is associated with a positive hCG test. Ultrasonography reveals an intrauterine gestation, and laparoscopy can identify the luteal cyst and normal tubes.

G. Endometriosis and Intraabdominal Bleeding Lower abdominal, midline and pelvic pain beginning several days before every period and continuing into it or throughout the cycle is characteristic of endometriosis. Deep dyspareunia, pain on defecation, diarrhea, and hematochezia, as well as frequency and dysuria, may occur due to rectal and bladder involvement. The pelvic examination may reveal tenderness and fine granular lesions or small nodules on the uterosacral ligaments, adnexal areas, and rectovaginal septum.

The sudden onset of severe lower midabdominal and sometimes iliac pain, direct and rebound tenderness, and guarding may be caused by rupture and bleeding of a cystic lesion caused by this disorder. The diagnosis can be confirmed by laparoscopy, and treatment to control bleeding and relieve pain can be initiated. Laser photocoagulation of lesions with a laparoscope can be used, but if bleeding is massive, open surgery is required for control.

H. Intracystic Hemorrhage Bleeding directly into an ovarian cyst or endometrioma without leakage into the free peritoneal cavity can cause less severe localized constant lower abdominal pain and tenderness. A tender adnexal mass may be palpable on pelvic examination. The diagnosis can be confirmed by laparoscopy.

Acute Left Iliac Pain

☐ **DIAGNOSTIC LIST**

1. Acute diverticulitis
2. Mimics of acute diverticulitis
   A. Acute appendicitis
   B. Acute perforation of a carcinoma of the left colon
   C. Acute intestinal obstruction secondary to carcinoma of the colon
   D. Ischemic colitis
   E. Acute infectious colitis
   F. Acute ulcerative colitis
   G. Small bowel ischemia and necrosis with secondary sigmoiditis
   H. Inflammation and/or compression of the sigmoid secondary to disease in other organs
   I. Ruptured aneurysm of the infrarenal aorta
   J. Psoas abscess
   K. Psoas syndrome secondary to an expanding left common iliac artery aneurysm
   L. Sigmoid volvulus
   M. Torsion of an intraabdominal testis
   N. Renal and perinephric abscess and pyelonephritis
      1. Acute renal cortical abscess
      2. Acute corticomedullary abscess

   3. Perinephric abscess
   4. Acute pyelonephritis
   O. Herpes zoster
   P. Diverticulosis with negative pathologic evidence of inflammation
   Q. Acute osteomyelitis of the left ilium
3. Ureteral colic
4. Pneumonia or a pulmonary infarction
5. Gynecologic disorders
   A. Pelvic inflammatory disease (PID)
      1. Acute salpingitis
      2. Tuboovarian abscess
      3. Tuboovarian abscess with rupture
   B. Tubal pregnancy
   C. Mimics of tubal pregnancy and PID
      1. Corpus luteum cyst with bleeding
      2. Corpus luteum cyst of pregnancy with bleeding
      3. Threatened abortion
      4. Follicle cyst with intraperitoneal bleeding (mittelschmerz)
      5. Endometrioma with intraperitoneal bleeding
      6. Adnexal torsion

☐ SUMMARY

Acute diverticulitis causes crampy or constant aching pain and tenderness in the left iliac area. Fever, chills, nausea, vomiting, and leukocytosis may also occur in some cases. A contrast enema can demonstrate diverticuli, tracking of contrast medium, an extrinsic mass, bowel stenosis, colonic fold thickening, and one or more fistulas. A CT scan may show bowel wall thickening, mesenteric stranding, and pericolic collections of fluid and/or gas. There is a good therapeutic response to antibiotic therapy. *Acute appendicitis* may rarely cause localized left iliac and hypogastric pain associated with peritoneal signs, fever, nausea, vomiting, and leukocytosis. The diagnosis can be made by laparoscopy or at surgery. *Perforation of a colon carcinoma* can mimic diverticulitis, producing a pericolic abscess, a sinus tract, and in some cases a fistula. A patient with colon carcinoma may present with a history of *obstructive symptoms,* including crampy left lower abdominal pain, pencil or ribbon stools, and episodes of lower abdominal distension and constipation. Hematochezia and/or anemia, secondary to gross or occult bleeding, may occur in some cases. A contrast enema reveals a stenotic area that can best be evaluated by colonoscopic biopsy. In up to 15 percent of cases, the presence of cancer can be verified only after colon resection. Colon cancer is the most common cause of large bowel obstruction in the United States. Complete obstruction may lead to right lower abdominal pain due to cecal distension. A contrast enema can confirm obstruction, and colonoscopy can be used to decompress the proximal colon and confirm the diagnosis by biopsy.

Ischemic colitis usually occurs in a patient over age 50 with a history of cardiovascular disease. Left lower abdominal pain and bloody diarrheal or semiformed stools are common complaints. Severe cases, with bowel infarction, may become febrile and toxic. The diagnosis can be supported by endoscopy with visualization of dusky edematous mucosa, blue-black submucosal nodules, and a bleeding, friable mucosal surface with ulcerations. Eighty-five percent of cases resolve with expectant treatment; such cases are often misdiagnosed as diverticulitis. More severely ill patients are febrile and toxic, and have peritoneal signs and abdominal distension, resulting from gangrene and perforation of the colon wall.

Infectious colitis causes aching and/or crampy left iliac, hypogastric, and often right iliac pain; fever; chills; myalgias; arthralgias; and headache. Up to 25 watery or bloody stools may be passed per day, and tenesmus may occur. Severe sharp lower abdominal pain may accompany the urge to defecate, and may be relieved by the passage of gas and stool. Leukocytes are present in the stool, usually accompanied by a positive test for blood. Epidemiologic data provide some clinical clues to the causative organism, but careful microscopic study of the stool and bacteriologic cultures are required for a specific diagnosis. An initial attack of *ulcerative colitis* may mimic infectious colitis. The radiologic and endoscopic findings in idiopathic ulcerative colitis may mimic those of infection or ischemia. The absence of amebas in the stool by microscopy, the absence of anti-ameba antibody in the serum (indirect hemagglutination test), and negative cultures for *Salmonella, Shigella, Campylobacter, Clostridia, Yersinia,* and other pathogenic species, are required before such a case can be considered to be due to idiopathic ulcerative colitis. The subsequent course of idiopathic ulcerative colitis may include an initial response to steroids or a protracted period of illness, neither of which is seen in the infectious diarrheas. *Small bowel ischemia* can cause periumbilical or generalized abdominal pain, vomiting, and distension. *Adherence of ischemic inflamed bowel to the sigmoid* can cause left iliac pain and tenderness, and mimic diverticulitis. Surgical exploration will reveal a mass of ischemic small bowel adherent to the sigmoid. Other inflammatory processes, such as a perinephric abscess or an infarcted intraabdominal testis, can cause a sigmoid serositis by direct spread. A *ruptured aortic aneurysm* may cause the abrupt onset of left lower abdominal and back pain, collapse, weakness, and sweating. A midline, pulsatile, tender, poorly defined mass may be identified in the umbilical area in over 90 percent of cases. Plain abdominal radiography is reported to be 76 to 83 percent sensitive, and ultrasonography close to 100 percent sensitive, for the diagnosis of aneurysm. Aneurysmal rupture is a clinical diagnosis and requires immediate surgery. A rare form of aneurysmal rupture, with formation of an aortoduodenal fistula, causes pain, hematemesis, and melena; in such cases the aneurysm can be detected by physical examination (25 percent) or by ultrasonography (97–100 percent).

A *psoas abscess* causes left iliac, groin, and anterior thigh pain and tenderness; fever; chills; impaired walking; and a tendency to keep the left thigh flexed and externally rotated. The diagnosis can be confirmed by CT. The abscess is usually secondary to a bowel perforation resulting from Crohn's disease, colon carcinoma, or diverticulitis. It can also occur secondary to pyogenic or tuberculous osteomyelitis of the lower thoracic or lumbar vertebrae. A similar, painful syndrome, caused by pressure necrosis of the psoas muscle, occurs with an *expanding common iliac artery aneurysm.* The aneurysm can usually be palpated or demonstrated by ultrasonography. *Sigmoid volvulus* causes severe left lower abdominal pain, marked distension, and obstipation. The diagnosis can be suspected from plain abdominal radiographs, which demonstrate the "bent inner tube" sign and the "bird's beak" sign. In up to 30 percent of cases, diagnostic confirmation requires a contrast enema or a CT scan. Rectal tube decompression of the volvulus can also confirm the diagnosis.

Torsion of a left intraabdominal testis causes left iliac pain, nausea, and vomiting, with associated left lower abdominal and rectal tenderness. The left testis is absent from the scrotum. This disorder may cause localized left lower abdominal peritoneal signs. The diagnosis is usually made at surgery. *Renal abscess* may cause flank and left lower abdominal pain and tenderness. Local peritoneal signs may be present. The diagnosis can be confirmed by ultrasonography or CT. A renal *cortical abscess* caused by staphylococci is usually associated with a normal urinalysis and a negative urine culture, while the opposite is true for a *corticomedullary abscess* caused by gram-negative bacteria. A *perinephric abscess* usually begins by extension from a renal abscess. There may be spiking fever, chills and rigors, lower abdominal pain and tenderness, a tender flank or abdominal mass, and leukocytosis. The diagnosis can be confirmed by a contrast-enhanced CT study. *Acute pyelonephritis* may cause left iliac and lumbar pain and tenderness, fever, chills, and pyuria, which respond dramatically to antibiotics. *Herpes zoster* causes a left lower abdominal burning bandlike pain and an associated herpetic rash in the painful zone. Irritable bowel may cause constantly aching or crampy pain and tenderness in the left lower abdomen in a patient with *diverticulosis,* giving rise to an erroneous diagnosis of diverticulitis—resulting in unnecessary medical or surgical therapy. *Acute osteomyelitis* of *the left ilium* can cause left iliac pain, a tender mass, and direct left lower abdominal tenderness. Fever, chills, and malaise also occur, leading to confusion with acute diverticulitis. MRI or a radionuclide bone scan will localize the process to the ilium. Cases with lytic lesions that do not improve clinically within 36 h after the initiation of antibiotic therapy should be biopsied, since *Ewing's sarcoma* may be present.

A *renal stone traversing the ureter* may give rise to a constant severe pain in the left lumbar area and left iliac area. Direct iliac area tenderness may be detected, and costovertebral angle tenderness is usually present. The urine contains red cells and small clots, and the diagnosis can be confirmed by an excretory urogram, which will demonstrate the obstructing ureteral stone on a delayed film.

Pneumonia or a pulmonary infarction may cause pain in the left chest, shoulder, and upper or lower abdomen. In addition, a *subdiaphragmatic lesion,* like a renal, pancreatic, or subphrenic abscess, can cause clinical and radiologic pulmonary findings and left lower abdominal pain.

Pelvic inflammatory disease (PID) can cause left iliac pain in various ways.

Acute salpingitis causes left lower abdominal pain and tenderness, cervical motion, and adnexal tenderness. Deep dyspareunia is commonly present. Purulent vaginal discharge may be present in 30 to 40 percent of cases, and fever and leukocytosis in 50 percent. Endocervical cultures reveal *Chlamydia trachomatis* or *Neisseria gonorrhoeae* in 50 to 75 percent of cases. There is a response to antibiotic therapy in 90 percent of cases.

Up to 40 percent of patients hospitalized with PID have a *tuboovarian abscess.* This can be diagnosed by pelvic-exam detection of a tender adnexal mass, or by ultrasonography or CT. *Rupture of a tuboovarian mass* is signaled by spreading lower abdominal pain and peritoneal signs. Surgical exploration is required for pain relief and recovery. *Tubal pregnancy* may begin with left lower abdominal pain and tenderness preceded by amenorrhea, spotting, or frank vaginal bleeding. Physical examination may reveal an adnexal mass (30–40 percent of cases). The urine or serum tests for human chorionic gonadotropin (β-hCG) are positive, and transvaginal ultrasonography may reveal an empty uterus and/or an adnexal mass. Laparoscopy can be used to confirm the diagnosis in doubtful cases. PID and tubal pregnancy can be mimicked by a *bleeding ovarian cyst.* A persistent corpus luteum cyst may cause left lower abdominal pain, tenderness, and amenorrhea, simulating a tubal pregnancy; but the pregnancy test is negative.

Hemorrhage into a corpus luteum cyst of pregnancy causes left lower abdominal pain and tenderness associated with amenorrhea and spotting, and a positive pregnancy test. Ultrasonography and/or laparoscopy will usually differentiate this disorder from a tubal pregnancy.

Bleeding from an ovarian cyst or endometrioma into the peritoneal cavity causes the sudden onset of spreading left lower abdominal pain and peritoneal signs. A *threatened abortion* may cause left hypogastric and left iliac pain and tenderness, and profuse vaginal bleeding with clots, in association with a positive pregnancy test. Ultrasonography will help in

---

TABLE OF DISEASE INCIDENCE

INCIDENCE PER 100,000 (APPROXIMATE)

Common (>100)	Uncommon (>5–100)	Rare (>0–5)
Acute diverticulitis	Carcinoma of the colon with obstruction	Acute appendicitis
Acute infectious colitis	Ischemic colitis	Carcinoma of the colon with perforation
Irritable bowel with diverticulosis and negative pathologic evidence of inflammation	Acute ulcerative colitis	Small bowel ischemia with sigmoiditis
	Ruptured aortic aneurysm	Sigmoiditis secondary to an adjacent infectious process
Ureteral colic	Psoas abscess	Psoas syndrome due to a left iliac artery aneurysm
Follicle cyst with bleeding (mittelschmerz)	Sigmoid volvulus	
Acute salpingitis	Acute pyelonephritis	Torsion of an intraabdominal testis
Acute tuboovarian abscess	Renal abscess	Perinephric abscess
Tubal pregnancy	Herpes zoster	Pneumonia or pulmonary infarction
Threatened abortion	Corpus luteum cyst with bleeding	Adnexal torsion
	Corpus luteum cyst of pregnancy with bleeding	Aortoduodenal fistula
	Endometrioma with bleeding	Subdiaphragmatic abscess
	Acute tuboovarian abscess with rupture	Acute osteomyelitis of the ilium
		Ewing's sarcoma of the ilium

the diagnosis of threatened abortion by detecting an intrauterine pregnancy and excluding tubal pregnancy by imaging of the tubes. Laparoscopy can be used directly to visualize the tubes to rule out tubal pregnancy. *Adnexal torsion* causes a rapidly progressive increase in left iliac pain and tenderness. Pelvic examination and ultrasound will demonstrate an enlarged, tender ovary. Laparoscopy may be used for diagnostic confirmation. Immediate surgery is required; many such ovaries harbor tumors that predispose them to torsion.

☐ DESCRIPTION OF LISTED DISEASES

1. ACUTE DIVERTICULITIS

Crampy, intermittent left iliac pain may be the initial symptom. More constant aching or burning left lower abdominal pain soon develops. Left lower back pain may accompany the iliac pain or may precede it by several hours. Coughing, jarring, and palpation by the physician may intensify the pain, while quiet rest in bed prevents sharp twinges of increased discomfort. Nausea and vomiting (20 percent of cases), diarrhea (53 percent), and constipation (7 percent) may accompany the pain. Fever and chills occur in 50 to 75 percent of cases, and leukocytosis in 60 to 70 percent. Physical examination reveals fever, tachycardia, left iliac direct tenderness (and sometimes rebound tenderness), and guarding. A left lower abdominal or pelvic mass may be palpable. The majority of cases will respond to home care with a liquid diet, bed rest, and a 7- to 10-day course of tetracycline therapy. Patients with signs of sepsis, gram-negative shock, peritonitis, an abdominal mass, extreme age, and comorbid conditions such as renal failure, severe diabetes, and/or immunosuppression should be admitted to the hospital and treated with parenteral antibiotics (e.g., clindamycin or metronidazole, and an aminoglycoside).

Imaging studies are useful for confirming the diagnosis of diverticulitis in those who fail to respond to medical therapy, in detecting complications, and in diagnosing other disorders that may mimic diverticulitis. Plain radiographs may detect free air, an air-fluid level in an abscess, or gas-fluid patterns of small and/or large bowel obstruction.

A contrast enema with barium may be given if administered *without* pressure or prior preparation with enemas, and *without* use of double-contrast technique. Some centers use only water-soluble contrast media for fear of spilling barium into the peritoneal cavity, but such studies are not always technically adequate.

The diagnosis of diverticulitis by contrast enema may be made by demonstration of two or more of the following: localized extravasation of contrast medium (i.e., tracking); markedly distorted colonic fold thickening; a localized mass and tethering of the mucosa. Other possible findings include diverticula, narrowing of the lumen of the colon (caused

by spasm or an intramural abscess), fixation of the affected colon segment, and a fistula to the bladder, ureter, vagina, bowel, or skin. Differentiation from carcinoma by contrast enema is unreliable; in one study, 30 to 69 percent of associated carcinomas were missed. Colonoscopy is more accurate in determining the nature of a colonic obstruction, since it allows direct visualization and biopsy. In up to 20 percent of cases, it is not technically possible to reach the lesion with the colonoscope.

The role of CT in the diagnosis and management of diverticulitis is still controversial. CT scans are considered to be diagnostic of diverticulitis if a pericolic fluid or gas collection (e.g., abscess) is found in conjunction with one or more of the following: bowel wall thickening to more than 4 mm; mesenteric soft tissue stranding; or fascial soft tissue stranding. In one series, CT was diagnostic in 47 percent of cases and consistent in 39 percent, for a combined sensitivity of 86 percent. CT was less sensitive (70 percent) in milder forms of disease. CT findings may be nonspecific, since a thickened colon wall may be caused by cancer, inflammatory bowel disease, or ischemia. However, CT has the advantage of detecting more remote collections of pus (e.g., in the subdiaphragmatic areas and pelvis), and in diagnosing other disorders that may mimic diverticulitis, such as a perinephric or psoas abscess or a ruptured aneurysm.

Pain related to diverticulitis may spread, within hours, from the left iliac area to include the right side and upper abdomen. Such pain is usually accompanied by severe direct and rebound tenderness; guarding or rigidity; and high fever and toxicity. It usually indicates perforation and spillage of feces from the colon, or pus from a pericolic abscess, into the peritoneal cavity. Free air may be present in up to 50 percent of cases. Surgical intervention is required.

Colicky pain, lower abdominal distension, and obstipation indicate either functional obstruction (spasm) or mechanical obstruction (intramural or pericolic abscess) of the colon. Carcinoma may be ruled out or diagnosed by colonoscopy; if it is diagnosed, surgical therapy will be required. A contrast enema or colonoscopy may be helpful in identifying patients without true mechanical obstruction.

2. MIMICS OF ACUTE DIVERTICULITIS

A. Acute Appendicitis Epigastric or periumbilical pain of a crampy nature begins gradually and continues for 4 to 6 h. This pain abates, and a dull ache or burning discomfort appears in the hypogastric and left iliac areas. Nausea, vomiting, and low-grade fever may occur. Left lower abdominal direct and rebound tenderness, with or without guarding, develop. Rectal tenderness may be present. Leukocytosis or a shift to the left of the differential count is present in over 80 percent of cases. The diagnosis may not be made until surgical exploration for perforation; sometimes it can be made earlier on clinical findings or by laparoscopy. Left iliac pain is a rare manifestation of acute appendicitis.

B. Acute Perforation of a Carcinoma of the Left Colon

Aching or burning left iliac pain, fever, chills, nausea, and vomiting occur. There are localized signs of peritonitis in the painful area. There may be a history of weeks or months of crampy or dull left lower abdominal pain, intermittent hematochezia, loose stools, constipation, or an alteration of stool size and shape (i.e., pencil- or ribbon-shaped stools). With perforation, a leukocytosis and/or a shift to the left of the differential count is usually present. A hypochromic anemia may be detected (27 percent of cases); if present, it is secondary to chronic blood loss from the tumor. A contrast enema with mucosal detail may detect the carcinoma, but is hazardous with a free perforation. Colonoscopy allows for direct observation and biopsy. A CT scan may be useful to determine the limits of extracolonic disease (e.g., abscesses, fistulas, sinus tracts, and metastases). Spreading peritonitis requires immediate surgical exploration.

C. Acute Intestinal Obstruction Secondary to Carcinoma of the Colon

This condition may cause crampy hypogastric and left iliac pain, lower abdominal distension, obstipation, and, sometimes, right iliac pain due to cecal distension. Feculent vomiting may occur after 24 to 48 h. Plain abdominal radiographs show cecal and proximal colon distension with a cutoff in the left colon. The cecum may be distended to more than 10 cm in diameter. In the 20 percent of patients with incompetent ileocecal valves there will be air-fluid levels in the small bowel. A contrast enema will demonstrate mechanical obstruction, and colonoscopy can visualize the obstructed area and allow for biopsy.

D. Ischemic Colitis

Eighty-five percent of cases are mild and self-limited. Involvement of the descending colon and sigmoid causes dull, constant, and/or crampy left iliac pain, with bloody diarrhea or passage of blood and clots. Nausea and low-grade fever may occur. Direct tenderness is usually mild, and peritoneal signs are frequently absent. Leukocytosis is uncommon, unless there is significant gangrene. Most cases resolve spontaneously in 1 or 2 weeks after a course of bed rest, intravenous fluids, and antibiotics. Cases with localized peritoneal signs may be misdiagnosed as diverticulitis. Ischemic colitis occurs in persons over age 50 with a history of cardiovascular disease, atherosclerosis, hypotension, arrhythmias, or prior embolization. Some cases are associated with hypercoagulable states, such as polycythemia; with use of oral contraceptives; with protein C or S deficiency, amyloidosis, or vasculitis; or with use of ergotomine or vasopressin. Ischemic colitis is a relatively common complication of ruptured aortic aneurysm and aortic replacement surgery. It may occur with advanced colon cancer.

Colonoscopy reveals cyanotic edematous mucosa, generalized mucosal bleeding and friability, large irregular ulcers, pseudomembranes, and, in some cases, blue-black submucosal nodules. Biopsy of the boundary zone between normal and ischemic colon mucosa facilitates pathologic diagnosis. The endoscopic findings may mimic idiopathic inflammatory bowel disease and/or clostridial toxic colitis. Rectal sparing occurs in 95 percent of cases, but may also occur in Crohn's disease (45 percent of cases). Contrast enema shows thumbprinting and ulcerations; the findings may mimic those of inflammatory bowel disease or pseudomembranous colitis. All cultures for stool pathogens, microscopic studies for *Entamoeba histolytica*, and tests for *Clostridium difficile* by culture and toxin assay are negative.

Up to 15 percent of cases may be severe, with acute onset and a rapidly progressive course. These cases have severe left lower abdominal pain and bloody diarrhea. Diffuse left lower abdominal direct and rebound tenderness and guarding develop, and spread over the abdomen. Fever and leukocytosis suggest bowel necrosis and leakage.

Prompt surgical intervention to resect necrotic bowel and lavage the abdomen is required.

E. Acute Infectious Colitis

Pain in the left lower abdomen may be aching, burning, or crampy. There may also be superimposed episodes of sharper, severe, hypogastric and left iliac pain, associated with an urge to defecate. This pain is completely or partly relieved by passage of stool and flatus. Tenesmus may be present. Watery diarrhea—up to 20 bowel movements per day—may continue for several days. In some cases the initial watery diarrheal stools are passed with mucus streaked with blood, or with liquid pools of blood. In severe cases, stools consisting only of dark red blood and clots are passed. Systemic symptoms, such as fever, chills, myalgias, arthralgias, headache, prostration, weakness, and light-headedness, reflect the toxic and dehydrating aspects of these illnesses. There is a wide spectrum of symptomatology: a single pathogen may cause only mild watery diarrhea in one case, bloody stools without systemic symptoms in another, and, in a third, a full-blown clinical picture like that described above.

Usually stools are positive for occult or gross blood and contain increased numbers of leukocytes when stained with methylene blue. Sigmoidoscopy reveals mucosal petechial hemorrhages, friability, and bleeding. Sloughing of the mucosa and pseudomembrane formation may be found. Fecal leukocytes may be present in patients with watery diarrhea, as well as in those with dysentery. The clinical picture and sigmoidoscopic and laboratory findings described above may be caused by *Shigella, Salmonella,* or *Campylobacter* species; enteroinvasive *Escherichia coli; Vibrio parahaemolyticus; Plesiomonas shigelloides; Entamoeba histolytica;* inflammatory bowel disease; or ischemic colitis. A specific diagnosis depends on microscopic analysis of stool (for such findings as the darting mobility of *Campylobacter* species and the trophozoites and cysts of *E. histolytica*) and stool cultures.

Certain epidemiologic clues may predict the occurrence of individual species. *Campylobacter* species are spread by ingestion of untreated surface water, unpasteurized milk, and inadequately cooked poultry; and by direct contact between humans and household pets with diarrhea, between mothers and babies, between children in day-care centers, and between male homosexuals. Infection with *Campylobacter* species often begins with a prodrome of fever, chills, headache, malaise, and myalgias lasting up to 24 h before diarrhea starts. A remittent diarrhea with a biphasic course follows.

Salmonellosis is associated with ingestion of contaminated milk products, eggs, meat, and poultry; with flooding; and with contact with turtles and birds. Contamination of food and drink by human carriers, and fomite infection in hospitals, may occur. Salmonellosis may cause an appendicitis-like syndrome, as does infection with *Yersinia enterocolitica*.

Shigellosis is spread within families and other groups by person-to-person contact (67 percent of cases); by common-source outbreaks caused by contamination of water or food; and by person-to-person transmission between homosexually active males. This agent is most common in severely ill patients with diarrhea, who require hospitalization. Flies also appear to be capable of causing spread of this infection.

Amebiasis has been associated with recent travel or residence in an endemic area; with homosexual activity between males; and, in a unique outbreak, with contaminated enema equipment used for giving "high colonics" in a chiropractic clinic. Spread within families may occur.

Enteroinvasive *E. coli* infection is associated with food or water ingestion, and may occur in epidemics. *Vibrio parahaemolyticus* causes a brief epidemic diarrheal illness in groups of people ingesting raw seafood. Crampy abdominal pain (82 percent of cases), nausea (71 percent), vomiting (52 percent), and fever (27 percent) accompany diarrheal stools that contain leukocytes and blood. *Plesiomonas shigelloides* causes a similar dysentery-like illness after ingestion of shellfish.

Clostridium difficile causes aching left lower abdominal pain, and watery stools and/or passage of blood and mucus during a course of antibiotic therapy (or within 3 weeks of completing it). Most cases of *C. difficile* infection begin after 5 to 10 days of oral or intravenous antibiotic therapy. The most commonly associated drugs are clindamycin, ampicillin, and the cephalosporins.

F. Acute Ulcerative Colitis A severe case may present initially with a brief history of diarrhea with frequent watery and/or bloody stools, aching and/or cramping left iliac and hypogastric pain, anorexia, vomiting, and fever to 105°F. Ten or more stools per day, a temperature exceeding 104°F, tachycardia, anemia, leukocytosis, nocturnal diarrhea, and tenesmus may occur in severe cases. Bloody mucus or gross

blood and clots are passed, resulting, in some cases, in the rapid development of hypovolemia and anemia. The abdomen may be diffusely tender, or there may be localized tenderness over the left lower abdomen. Proctosigmoidoscopy reveals a diffusely involved mucosa from the rectum up to the 65 cm level, and higher. Petechiae, friability, and granularity of the mucosa, and bleeding ulcerations occur, and pseudomembranes may be present. It is important to eliminate an infectious cause for this disorder, since the use of corticosteroids (e.g., as therapy for ulcerative colitis) in the presence of certain infectious organisms can lead to disseminated invasive disease and a lethal outcome. Crohn's disease usually has a chronic insidious onset and rarely presents as an acute colitis. The stool should be stained with Loeffler's methylene blue for fecal leukocytes, and a wet drop studied by phase contrast for the darting motility of *Campylobacter* species. A Gram stain of the feces should be done to detect cocci in grapelike clusters (e.g., staphylococcal enterocolitis). A fresh piece of stool can be emulsified in saline solution, and/or saline solution with iodine, to detect amebas in the form of trophozoites or cysts. If amebic trophozoites are present, then staining of a stool preparation with buffered methylene blue or trichrome stain may help in their detection. In addition, the serum indirect hemagglutination test for amebiasis may help to exclude this disorder, since the test has a high predictive value negative. Stool should be used for cultures, although rectal swabs are satisfactory for shigella isolation. Stool specimens should be plated as soon as possible or stored at 4°C. Isolation of pathogenic Enterobacteriaceae such as *Salmonella* or *Shigella* species, or enteroinvasive *E. coli* and *Yersinia entercolitica*, can be accomplished on eosin-methylene blue (EMB) agar and on MacConkey's agar. The latter medium also permits growth of *Vibrio parahaemolyticus*, *Aeromonas* species, and *Plesiomonas shigelloides*.

Salmonella-Shigella (SS) agar will grow the same pathogens as EMB. Samples possibly containing *Campylobacter jejuni* should be inoculated into a liquid medium and then onto a selective medium containing antibiotics. Incubation at 42°C in a 6% O_2, 8% CO_2 atmosphere enhances isolation of *Campylobacter jejuni*.

Alkaline or cold enrichment aids in the isolation of *Yersinia enterocolitica*. Cefsulodin-irgasan-novobiocin (CIN) agar is a useful selective medium for isolation of this organism. *Clostridium difficile* can be isolated from stool using a selective medium with an egg yolk–fructose base with added cycloserine and cefoxitin. *Clostridium difficile* toxin can be detected using a fibroblast target cell cytotoxicity assay. Isolation of the organism has a greater sensitivity than the toxin assay.

Finally, ulcerative colitis follows a chronic recurrent or persistent course over a period of years. Infection with almost all of the pathogens described is self-limited, and symptoms, signs, and endoscopic findings resolve over a period of weeks or, rarely, months. Amebiasis may take a more chronic course; since it can be exacerbated by cortico-

steroid therapy, testing serum by an indirect hemagglutination test for anti-ameba antibodies is a sensitive and useful
procedure for excluding amebic infection before initiating
such therapy.

**G. Small Bowel Ischemia and Necrosis with Secondary
Sigmoiditis**   Occlusion of the superior mesenteric artery
or its branches may cause a person to present with left iliac
pain and tenderness, associated with fever, vomiting, and
localized signs of peritonitis in the left lower abdomen.
Diarrhea and gross bleeding do not occur. Distension is
commonly present, and plain radiographs reveal evidence
of small bowel dilatation and air-fluid levels. Contrast enemas provide evidence of an extrinsic mass compressing the
sigmoid, with thumbprinting and spiculation of the sigmoid
border adjacent to the mass. A small bowel series reveals
stenotic or obstructed small bowel. At surgical exploration,
necrotic small bowel may be found adherent to an inflamed
sigmoid surface. In one series, three cases were related to
a vascular thrombus or embolus, while a fourth was caused
by small bowel strangulation in an internal hernia. Surgical
resection and anastomosis of the necrotic small bowel is
required. Most such patients are over age 50 and have a
history of atherosclerotic disease, arrhythmias, hypotension, or use of vasoconstricting drugs such as ergotamine,
vasopressin, or parenteral digitalis.

**H. Inflammation and/or Compression of the Sigmoid
Secondary to Disease in Other Organs**   Pelvic inflammatory disease may cause compression and inflammation
of the sigmoid, causing localized left lower abdominal pain
and peritoneal signs with fever. Torsion of an intraabdominal testis can cause severe left lower abdominal pain, tenderness, and an inflammatory mass that compresses the colon.
A perinephric abscess may also affect the sigmoid, causing
constant, aching, left lower abdominal pain and tenderness.

I. Ruptured Aneurysm of the Infrarenal Aorta   There
is abrupt onset of very severe left lower abdominal pain,
sometimes in association with excruciating ipsilateral lumbar or midline lumbosacral pain. Pain radiation to one or
both testes can mimic renal colic, and posterior leg radiation
can be mistaken for sciatica. Profound weakness, faintness,
collapse, and diaphoresis may accompany the pain. Other
complaints include nausea, vomiting, and anuria. Physical
examination reveals hypotension in 35 percent of cases, and
a tender, midline, ill-defined umbilical-area mass, which is
pulsatile, in 75 percent. Obesity may interfere with the
examination. Rare associated findings may include mottling
of the skin of the abdomen and legs (2 percent of cases)
and of the flank (2 percent), and perianal and scrotal ecchymosis (1 percent). Plain radiographs confirm the presence of an aneurysm in 76 to 83 percent of cases. Physical
examination detects a ruptured aneurysm with a sensitivity
of 91 to 100 percent. Diagnostic confirmation and accurate
sizing can be obtained by ultrasonography or CT, but these
procedures are seldom performed in a setting of rupture.

Such patients should be started on volume replacement and
taken immediately to the operating room before resuscitation is complete, and the aneurysm replaced with an aortoiliac bifurcation prosthesis. The remains of the aneurysm
and left colon mesentery are then sutured over the graft to
prevent bowel adherence. Some cases, with pain and aneurysmal tenderness, may be related to aneurysmal expansion,
since there is no evidence of rupture at surgery. Fever,
chills, positive blood cultures, and local pain and tenderness
suggest an aneurysmal infection, requiring antibiotic therapy and graft replacement of the infected aneurysm. Cultures of all resected aneurysms should be obtained, since a
small proportion will be infected without characteristic
symptoms.

Aortoduodenal fistula is an uncommon complication of
infrarenal aortic aneurysm. Evidence of bleeding, in the
form of hematemesis or melena, occurs in 64 percent of
cases as an initial symptom (''herald bleed''). Lower right
or left abdominal pain, and lumbar or flank pain, may occur
in 32 percent of patients, but fewer than 25 percent have a
palpable pulsatile mass. Presentation with hypovolemic
shock is uncommon (5 percent), indicating that most initial
bleeds are limited. The diagnosis of aneurysm is rarely
considered in this setting. Endoscopy is seldom useful,
since the fistula is usually between the second or third portion of the duodenum and the aorta. A plain radiograph
may demonstrate an aneurysm in 58 to 91 percent of cases.
Barium meal studies are rarely useful. Arteriography has
not been used for diagnosis. Only 28 percent of patients
with this disorder have been operated upon. The surgical
mortality rate is 36 percent. One major review recommends
screening of the aorta with ultrasonography in all patients
with upper gastrointestinal bleeding who have nondiagnostic endoscopic findings.

J. Psoas Abscess   Pain occurs in the left iliac area, and
sometimes in the left anterior thigh, groin, and hip region.
The left leg is held flexed at the hip and externally rotated;
or, in less severe cases, the patient's main difficulty is an
inability to completely extend the left thigh on the trunk
and rest the left popliteal fossa flat on the bed. The left
psoas sign is positive. Left iliac tenderness and, less commonly, an inguinal mass, may be present. Skin crepitus
may be palpable in the groin or upper leg. Spiking fevers,
chills, malaise, myalgias, difficulty in walking, and weight
loss may be present. Cases secondary to pyogenic or tuberculous osteomyelitis have upper lumbar–lower thoracic
midline back pain and tenderness.

Microbiological analysis of abscess cultures may be helpful in pointing to a bowel lesion as a cause. Isolation of
Enterobacteriacae and anaerobes suggests a diagnosis of
abscess secondary to Crohn's disease, diverticulitis, or colorectal carcinoma. Osteomyelitis, however, may also be
caused by gram-negative rods. Primary psoas abscesses are
rare, and are caused by staphylococci. Uncommon causes
of a psoas abscess include perinephric or pancreatic ab-

scesses that rupture into the psoas sheath. CT is excellent for the diagnosis and follow-up of this disorder.

Psoas abscesses, secondary to bowel disease, require drainage and resection of the involved bowel, and parenteral administration of appropriate antibiotics.

K. Psoas Syndrome Secondary to an Expanding Left Common Iliac Artery Aneurysm   Pain occurs in the left iliac area and groin, and may be felt in the anterior thigh. The left leg may be kept partly flexed at the hip, and externally rotated. It resists extension (positive psoas sign). There is direct tenderness in the left iliac area, and a pulsatile mass is usually present to the left and below the umbilicus. The left leg may be swollen secondary to iliac vein compression or occlusion, and flank pain may occur on the left side because of ureteral compression. A sonographic or CT study will identify the aneurysm and its extent. Repair of the aneurysm is required for symptomatic relief. The psoas muscle shows signs of hemorrhage and necrosis secondary to pressure from the aneurysm.

L. Sigmoid Volvulus   There is abrupt onset of left iliac and, sometimes hypogastric pain and lower abdominal distension. Nausea, vomiting, and obstipation may be associated complaints. The lower abdomen is distended, tympanitic, and tender. Distension may be localized to the left lower abdomen or may be more widespread. There is no fever or leukocytosis, unless gangrene has occurred. Plain abdominal radiographs show the colon to be markedly distended (bent inner tube or omega loop sign). The convexity of the bowel loop is opposite the site of the obstruction, and a narrow, tapered distal colon (bird's beak sign) points toward the site of obstruction. This can be better demonstrated by a contrast enema or a CT study in that minority of cases (up to 30 percent) that may have inconclusive physical and radiographic findings. Many cases can be decompressed by passage of a rectal tube or by sigmoidoscopy. Others require surgical exploration. A definitive procedure to prevent recurrence should be done within a week of decompression, because the recurrence rate may exceed 40 percent. This disorder is a common cause of large bowel obstruction in Scandinavia, in Eastern Europe, and in underdeveloped countries in Asia and Africa. In the United States it is seen primarily in the elderly, some of whom also have psychiatric disorders. It is also the most common cause of intestinal obstruction during pregnancy. Volvulus is associated with Chagas' disease, Parkinson's disease, spinal cord pathology with paralysis, and ischemic colitis, and is probably related to the increased colon redundancy found in these disorders.

M. Torsion of an Intraabdominal Testis   Pain begins abruptly in the left lower abdomen. It may be crampy or constant, and it becomes progressively severe. Nausea and vomiting occur; there is left iliac, and sometimes rectal, tenderness. Cases on the left side have mimicked acute diverticulitis. A helpful clue is the absence of the left testicle from the scrotum. In some cases, the inflammatory mass caused by the infarcted testicle may produce small bowel obstruction. In one review, 45 percent of patients presenting with torsion of an intraabdominal testis had a seminoma or an embryonal carcinoma in that testis. Resection of an infarcted intraabdominal testis is required.

N. Renal and Perinephric Abscess and Pyelonephritis   Moderate to severe left iliac pain of a constant aching or burning quality may occur alone, or in association with left flank pain. Nausea and vomiting are frequent associated symptoms. These patients also have high fevers, chills, and rigors. The abdominal pain may be intensified by jarring or coughing. Local abdominal tenderness is present in the painful area, and rebound tenderness and guarding may occur in some cases. The frequency of abdominal pain and tenderness varies between 15 and 60 percent in different series; it appears to be due to inflammatory involvement of the posterior parietal peritoneum by a renal or perinephric abscess, and is less common with uncomplicated pyelonephritis.

1. Acute Renal Cortical Abscess   These patients usually present with fever, chills, and abdominal and/or flank pain. There are usually no irritative bladder symptoms, although these may occur if the abscess erodes into a calix. Consequently, analysis of the urine sediment and cultures are usually negative. There is usually an antecedent staphylococcal skin, bone, or cardiac valve infection, or a primary bacteremia. Staphylococci are seeded to the renal cortex, producing a multiloculated abscess. A tender flank may be present, as well as abdominal signs, such as tenderness and guarding. An excretory urogram shows caliceal distortion from an intrarenal mass. Ultrasonography and CT will both display the lesion; CT allows clear-cut differentiation from a neoplasm and serves to guide needle aspiration for culture. Therapy with nafcillin or vancomycin is usually effective, and leads to resolution within 6 days. Cases failing to respond may require percutaneous or open drainage.

2. Acute Corticomedullary Abscess   This disorder is a complication of an ascending type of pyelonephritis produced by gram-negative bacteria. There is usually an associated urinary tract obstruction, urinary stones, or vesicoureteral reflux. Irritative bladder symptoms, an abnormal urinary sediment (leukocytes, erythrocytes, bacteria) and positive cultures are usually present (70 percent of cases). A flank mass is palpable in 60 percent of cases, and the liver enlarges in 30 percent. Fever, chills, and flank and abdominal pain occur.

Ultrasonography or CT with contrast enhancement will demonstrate unifocal or multifocal bacterial nephritis. Sonography shows a sonolucent mass at the corticomedullary junction. In acute focal bacterial nephritis, contrast-enhanced CT shows one or more wedge-shaped hypodense areas in the kidney. An abscess appears as a hypodense, sharply demarcated parenchymal lesion that fails to enhance with contrast. Most patients respond to parenteral antibiotics, but some require percutaneous or open drainage.

3. Perinephric Abscess   Either type of intrarenal abscess may rupture into the perinephric space to form a secondary abscess. This type of abscess can also arise by hematogenous or local spread from infection in an adjacent organ (e.g., liver, pancreas, pleura, gallbladder). There is usually an insidious onset, with fever, malaise, weight loss, anorexia, and nausea, which may not be associated with localizing symptoms and signs for 7 to 21 days. Left flank and left iliac pain and tenderness may eventually direct attention to the left renal area. A flank or abdominal mass may be felt in up to 50 percent of cases. Spiking fever, leukocytosis, and anemia reflect the infectious nature of this disorder. The urine sediment and cultures may be negative in 30 percent of cases. Ultrasonography and CT can confirm the diagnosis. A thick-walled extrarenal mass with a liquid density center may be seen on contrast-enhanced CT. Secondary tissue planes may be thickened or obliterated. Immediate surgical intervention, with drainage and sometimes nephrectomy, is required under an umbrella of intravenous antibiotics.

4. Acute Pyelonephritis   Acute pyelonephritis with flank pain and irritative bladder symptoms may cause mild abdominal pain and direct tenderness, but it seldom mimics an acute abdomen as do the disorders described above.

O. Herpes Zoster   Burning or aching pain may occur in the left lower abdomen, flank, and back. Within 1 to 4 days an eruption of grouped vesicles and small, crusted ulcers occurs in the painful abdominal, flank, and back regions. The eruption appears in a zone no more than several inches wide and does not cross the midline.

P. Diverticulosis with Negative Pathologic Evidence of Inflammation   Sigmoid resection has been advocated for initial attacks of diverticulitis in patients under age 55, if there are urinary symptoms, bowel obstruction, or perforation. Other reasons for surgery have been recurrent attacks and inability to rule out carcinoma. Prior to the mid-1970s, up to 33 percent of patients whose colons were resected for diverticulitis had only diverticulosis and no evidence of inflammation. These patients may have had severe irritable-bowel symptoms of pain and bowel disturbance. In the present era, the rate of resection of pathologically normal colons is much lower, but exact percentages are unknown. Documentation of inflammation by barium enema or CT prior to surgery should lower the percentage of uninflamed colons resected.

Q. Acute Osteomyelitis of the Left Ilium   Local pelvic trauma and Crohn's disease are risk factors for the development of iliac osteomyelitis. This disorder may mimic a paracolic abscess secondary to carcinoma or diverticulitis. There may be left lower abdominal pain and tenderness, fever, chills or rigors, nausea, and vomiting. The white blood cell count and sedimentation rate are elevated. A tender left iliac mass may be present. Many patients have hip or buttock pain. There may be pain on active and passive hip motion. In contrast to patients with septic arthritis of the hip, there is limitation of motion in only one or two directions of movement, not in all. Plain radiographs are normal or nondiagnostic until several weeks have elapsed; bone scans are sensitive, but nonspecific.

MRI usually demonstrates a low-intensity signal on T_1 images and a high-intensity signal of the corresponding area on a T_2 image—a sequence characteristic of active bone infection. Symptoms and signs respond to intravenous antibiotics within 36 h. The presence of flank pain may raise the question of pyelonephritis, but the urine sediment is usually normal.

Ewing's sarcoma of the left ilium can cause similar, but less acute, complaints, with hip and abdominal pain and fever. Plain radiographs of osteomyelitis after 4 weeks may be indistinguishable from plain radiographs of sarcoma. Failure of such a case to respond promptly to antibiotics (i.e., within 36 h) necessitates biopsy without delay, to rule out tumor.

3. URETERAL COLIC

This disorder begins with severe left-sided lumbar pain, with radiation into the left lower abdomen. The pain builds to a severe level within minutes and remains constant and very severe. Patients may writhe in pain or get up and walk about, in distinction to patients with an acutely inflamed abdomen. Some patients soak in a warm tub, trying to find relief. Gross or, more commonly, microscopic hematuria is present (90 percent of cases). There is usually left costovertebral angle tenderness and direct iliac tenderness without rebound tenderness or guarding. An intravenous pyelogram may demonstrate a dense nephrogram, followed by delayed ureteral opacification in 1 to 4 h. These late films demonstrate dilatation of the ureter and upper tract and identify the site of the obstruction in the ureter. Common sites are the ureterovesical junction, the pelvic brim, and the ureteropelvic junction. Pain continues constantly or intermittently until the stone passes. Stones smaller than 6 mm usually pass, while those larger than 8 mm usually do not. Pain relief can be obtained by administration of nonsteroidal anti-inflammatory drugs or narcotics. If the stone remains impacted, after 72 h ultrasonic ureteroscopy can be used to fragment and remove it.

4. PNEUMONIA OR A PULMONARY INFARCTION

Pneumonia or a pulmonary infarction can cause pleuritic pain, which can refer to the left lower abdomen, producing local tenderness. Pulmonary findings, such as dullness, bronchial breath sounds, rales, or a friction rub, direct attention to the chest. A chest radiograph will document the presence of pneumonia, while a ventilation-perfusion lung scan is useful for excluding pulmonary infarction. The presence of a high left hemidiaphragm, an infiltrate, or a pleural effusion on a chest radiograph may direct attention to the chest when the real problem is in the kidney, pancreas, or subphrenic region. Some of these disorders may also cause left lower abdominal pain and tenderness (e.g., perinephric abscess).

The clinical examination and the chest radiograph may provide localization of the inflammatory process to the chest or upper abdomen. In difficult cases, CT or ultrasonography may help identify a subdiaphragmatic process.

5. GYNECOLOGIC DISORDERS

A. Pelvic Inflammatory Disease (PID)

1. Acute Salpingitis   Constant, aching left iliac pain, and sometimes hypogastric pain, occurs. A left lumbosacral ache may be associated. The pain may be intensified by walking, stair climbing, jarring, or sexual intercourse. Purulent vaginal discharge may be present in up to 40 percent of patients. Fever is infrequent, with only 33 to 50 percent of cases manifesting this sign. Leukocytosis occurs in 50 percent of cases, and an elevated sedimentation rate (>15 mm/h) in 55 to 75 percent. Dependence on the presence of discharge, fever, and laboratory abnormalities can lead to missed diagnoses.

Proposed clinical criteria for the diagnosis of salpingitis require all of the following to be present: direct tenderness, with or without rebound tenderness, in the lower abdomen; cervical motion tenderness; and adnexal tenderness. In addition, one or more of the following findings are required: fever (>100.4°F); leukocytosis; leukocytosis in culdocentesis fluid; a positive Gram stain of the cervix for intracellular gram-negative cocci; or discovery of a pelvic or adnexal mass by physical examination or ultrasonography.

Ultrasonography is useful for detecting the presence of a tuboovarian abscess in the 30 to 40 percent of hospitalized patients who have this complication.

In many centers, laparoscopy has become a standard procedure for establishing the diagnosis of recurrent pelvic inflammatory disease. It has been demonstrated in several large series that only 52 to 72 percent of patients with clinical PID have this disorder. Up to 37 percent of patients may have normal tubes and ovaries when ex-

amined, and 10 to 25 percent have another disorder with clinical findings indistinguishable from PID. These include ovarian cysts, ruptured ovarian cysts, ectopic pregnancy, adnexal torsion, and pelvic bleeding from cysts.

Pelvic inflammatory disease is more likely to occur in sexually active adolescents than in older women; in those with multiple partners; in IUD users, as opposed to those using barrier methods; and in women with a prior history of sexually transmitted disease. Black race and low socioeconomic status may increase risk, but this is still controversial.

In the United States, endocervical isolation rates for *Neisseria gonorrhoeae* (39–80 percent) are higher than those for *Chlamydia trachomatis* (8–34 percent) in cases of PID. In Scandinavia, the situation is reversed; *C. trachomatis* infection is most prevalent (23–46 percent, vs. 5–28 percent for gonococci). Studies have shown higher isolation rates for *C. trachomatis* in black women and adolescents in the United States. While not absolutely specific, the onset of symptoms within 1 week of the initial day of the period favors a diagnosis of gonococcal infection. Laparoscopic cultures of purulent material from the fimbrial lumen of the tube have detected *C. trachomatis* in 12 percent of cases, but *N. gonorrhoeae* in only 1 percent. *Actinomyces israelii*, *Gardnerella vaginalis*, and *Ureaplasma urealyticum* have each been isolated with a frequency below 3 percent.

Various antibiotic drug regimens are effective in the treatment of acute salpingitis. The combination of intramuscular ceftriaxone and oral doxycycline is effective in mild cases. Severe cases respond within 3 to 4 days to parenteral drug treatment with one of the following combinations: cefoxitin plus doxycycline; clindamycin plus gentamicin; doxycycline plus metronidazole; and aztreonam plus clindamycin. The response rate usually exceeds 90 percent in acute uncomplicated cases.

2. Tuboovarian Abscess   The clinical and laboratory findings may be indistinguishable from those of uncomplicated acute salpingo-oophoritis, with the exception that a tender adnexal mass may be felt in up to 40 percent of patients. Pain occurs in 88 to 94 percent of cases, subjective fever and chills in only 35 to 50 percent, vaginal discharge in 28 percent, and abnormal uterine bleeding in 21 percent. Temperature elevation is recorded in 60 to 80 percent, and leukocytosis in 66 to 80 percent. Ultrasonography is 99 to 100 percent sensitive for the detection of an adnexal mass in a patient with a tuboovarian abscess. It will usually detect a complex mass (93 percent of cases), or a simple cystic mass (7 percent). CT and laparoscopy are 95 to 100 percent sensitive and are highly specific for the diagnosis of a tuboovarian abscess. Up to 70 percent of cases will respond to a regimen of intravenous antibiotics. These abscesses contain a mixture of aerobic gram-negative rods, such as

Escherichia coli; aerobic streptococci; and anaerobes, such as *Bacteroides fragilis*, *Bacteroides bivius*, *Peptococcus* species, and *Peptostreptococcus* species. Antianaerobic drugs, such as clindamycin or metronidazole, are required, as well as drugs effective against gram-negative aerobic bacteria, such as aminoglycosides, aztreonam, or the third-generation cephalosporins. Surgical removal of the abscessed tube and pelvic abscess drainage is required in patients who fail to respond to therapy within 3 or 4 days, or in the presence of signs of rupture.

3. Tuboovarian Abscess with Rupture   Symptoms of PID, such as localized left lower abdominal pain and tenderness, deep dyspareunia, fever and chills, vaginal discharge or bleeding, and nausea, vomiting, and diarrhea, usually precede rupture by several days. In some cases there is abrupt onset of generalized abdominal pain and peritoneal signs involving the entire abdomen; in others there is gradual spread of pain and tenderness throughout the entire abdomen over a period of hours. Culdocentesis is useful in confirming the diagnosis, as is laparoscopy. Rupture is an important indication for surgical exploration. Optimal treatment requires continuation of intravenous antibiotics and surgical removal of one or both tubes and ovaries, with or without hysterectomy. An attempt is often made, in women of reproductive age, to preserve childbearing function. Extensive intraoperative peritoneal lavage should also be done to remove pus and bacteria. Subphrenic abscess is an important complication of this disorder. A small minority of patients (5–10 percent) develop gram-negative septic shock; this group is at greatest risk. Conservative surgical management after abscess drainage and removal of the affected tube does not increase the mortality rate above the current level of 4 to 7 percent.

At exploration for spreading pain and peritoneal signs, the operating surgeon may find only salpingitis or an unruptured abscess with pelvic peritonitis. Such unnecessary explorations might be avoided by preoperative laparoscopy.

B. Tubal Pregnancy   Pain in the left lower abdomen may initially be crampy and intermittent; later it may become constant, as a hematoma develops in the wall of the tube containing the pregnancy. Fever and chills are seldom present. Amenorrhea precedes pain in 50 to 60 percent of cases, and is often followed, after a variable interval (7 days to 14 weeks), by frank vaginal bleeding or spotting. Up to 40 percent of patients do not recall a missed period; but they may give a history of spotting since their last period, or of more severe intermenstrual bleeding. The lower abdomen on the affected side may show localized or diffuse direct tenderness, and sometimes rebound tenderness. Cervical motion tenderness may occur in 50 percent

of cases, and a tender palpable adnexal mass in 25 to 35 percent.

A urine pregnancy test (ICON) is 96 to 100 percent sensitive, highly specific, and rapid (<4 min). Rare cases of tubal pregnancy, with no detectable serum β-hCG, have been reported. Transvaginal ultrasonography is more sensitive than transabdominal ultrasonography for the detection of a very early intrauterine pregnancy (100 percent vs. 20 percent). The scan may show a gestational sac, yolk sac, fetal pole, or heart motion in the uterine cavity. The presence of an intrauterine pregnancy essentially rules out a tubal pregnancy, while absence of an intrauterine pregnancy is supportive of the diagnosis of a tubal pregnancy in a patient with a positive urine pregnancy test. In patients with a serum β-hCG titer above 3600 mIU/ml, transvaginal ultrasonography should be able to identify an intrauterine pregnancy. Most patients presenting with the signs and symptoms of ectopic pregnancy have β-hCG titers below 3600 mIU/ml; in such cases, failure to detect an intrauterine pregnancy can be explained by either early gestational age or ectopic location. Transabdominal ultrasonography should be able to demonstrate an intrauterine pregnancy when the menstrual age of the fetus is 40 days or more. The β-hCG titer becomes positive at 23 days, and there is a period between 23 and 40 days when transvaginal ultrasonography has superior sensitivity for detection of an intrauterine pregnancy. The ability of ultrasonography to demonstrate an adnexal mass in such cases provides positive supportive evidence for the diagnosis of tubal pregnancy. In one report, transvaginal ultrasonography detected an adnexal mass in 91 percent of cases, while transabdominal ultrasonography was able to demonstrate a mass in only 50 percent. Laparoscopy may be used to view the affected tube directly in cases where the diagnosis is in doubt.

Rupture of an ectopic pregnancy may be signaled by spreading pelvic, abdominal, and, sometimes, shoulder pain, and diffuse lower abdominal direct and rebound tenderness. Tachycardia and hypotension reflect significant hemorrhage. Ultrasonography can confirm blood in the cul-de-sac and/or generalized hemoperitoneum. Culdocentesis will usually confirm intraabdominal bleeding (sensitivity 70–97 percent), and laparotomy may be required to prevent exsanguination.

Early diagnosis of tubal pregnancy is desirable in order to prevent extensive bleeding and to allow preservation of the affected tube and its function. Surgical management includes total salpingectomy, segmental resection of the pregnancy and reanastamosis of the tube, or incision (salpingostomy) and removal of the pregnancy. Laparoscopic surgery has also been successful.

Tubal pregnancy usually occurs in the setting of one or more established risk factors. These include prior salpingitis (found in 50 percent of cases where tubes are surgically resected), tubal ligation, tubal repair surgery, the presence of an IUD, and a prior ectopic pregnancy (10 percent risk in a subsequent pregnancy).

C. Mimics of Tubal Pregnancy and PID

1. Corpus Luteum Cyst with Bleeding An ovarian cyst can cause lower abdominal pain and tenderness by rapid growth or as a result of bleeding into the cyst or into the peritoneal cavity. The pain is moderate to severe, and may be associated with lower abdominal, cervical-motion, and adnexal tenderness, thus mimicking PID. Hemoperitoneum may be associated with low-grade fever, enhancing the simulation of infection.

Corpus luteum cysts often delay the onset of menses and cause unilateral abdominal pain and tenderness, as well as adnexal tenderness, with a palpable mass. This may simulate a tubal pregnancy. The urine and serum pregnancy tests are negative, and laparoscopy can confirm the diagnosis.

2. Corpus Luteum Cyst of Pregnancy Bleeding into a corpus luteum of pregnancy may cause unilateral lower abdominal pain and tenderness, and adnexal tenderness, with a palpable mass. There is a history of amenorrhea and a positive pregnancy test, and ultrasonography usually demonstrates an intrauterine pregnancy and an adnexal mass. Laparoscopy can be utilized to evaluate the tube and ovary on the affected side. Some of these cases are misdiagnosed as ectopic pregnancies, and are explored.

3. Threatened Abortion A threatened abortion can cause left lower and midline abdominal pain and tenderness, spotting, or vaginal bleeding in a patient with one or more missed periods. The pain is often crampy, and may be referred to the low back as well. The uterus is enlarged and may be tender. The urine and serum β-hCG titers are positive. Endovaginal ultrasonography can confirm the presence of an intrauterine pregnancy; if fetal heart motion is detected, there is a 90 percent probability of continuation of the pregnancy. Ultrasonography may also demonstrate the absence of an adnexal mass. In difficult cases, laparoscopy may be required.

4. Follicle Cysts with Intraperitoneal Bleeding (Mittelschmerz) Follicle cysts may cause unilateral lower abdominal pain and tenderness. The onset of pain is often abrupt, and there may be severe disability. In some cases, though, the pain may be mild and easily tolerable. Examination reveals lower abdominal and pelvic tenderness on the side where the pain occurs. Such pain usually occurs at midcycle; prior episodes of similar discomfort on the same or the opposite side may be recalled. Culdocentesis may reveal blood; laparoscopy will confirm the diagnosis, and should be done before laparotomy.

5. Endometrioma with Intraperitoneal Bleeding Hemorrhage into, or from, an endometrioma can cause lower abdominal pain and tenderness similar to that described above. There is usually a prior history of secondary dysmenorrhea and dyspareunia; sometimes there is a history, also, of period-associated diarrhea, tenesmus, rectal pain and/or bleeding, and, in some cases, irritative bladder complaints. The diagnosis of endometriosis with bleeding can be confirmed by laparoscopy.

6. Adnexal Torsion Colicky or continuous lower abdominal pain occurs. It becomes progressively severe and sustained. Fever is uncommon, and, if present, is low-grade. After 3 or 4 h, a tender adnexal mass may be detected on pelvic examination. Ultrasonography will detect an enlarged ovary, which appears as a uniformly echogenic mass or as a complex mass (adnexal torsion). Laparoscopy will confirm the diagnosis and allow early surgery. In most cases the diagnosis is made too late to avoid surgical resection of the infarcted ovary. Such ovaries are frequently enlarged prior to the episode of torsion, because of a cyst or tumor. If malignancy is present, alternative intraoperative management is required.

24

Acute Bilateral Upper Abdominal Pain

☐ DIAGNOSTIC LIST

1. Epidemic pleurodynia
2. Acute bilateral pleuritis
3. Bilateral costochondritis
4. Acute pancreatitis with or without associated acute cholecystitis, cholangitis, or hepatitis
   A. Acute cholecystitis and pancreatitis
   B. Ascending cholangitis and pancreatitis
   C. Alcoholic hepatitis and pancreatitis
5. Acute volvulus of the stomach

6. Perforation of a gastric or duodenal ulcer
7. Acute cholecystitis with perforation and leakage of bile
8. Acute gastric dilatation
9. Acute aerophagia
10. Acute hepatic congestion secondary to acute massive pulmonary embolism
11. Alcoholic hepatitis and acute gastritis and/or ulcer disease
12. Fitz-Hugh–Curtis syndrome (perihepatitis)

☐ SUMMARY

Epidemic pleurodynia is a febrile epidemic disease that causes episodes of upper abdominal and lower chest pain. The pain may last 2 to 10 h, remit, and then recur. There may be some upper abdominal tenderness and guarding during each painful episode, but this abates with the pain. Severe pain may lead to surgery in as many as 20 percent of cases. *Pleuritis* may cause chest pain and upper abdominal pain similar to that caused by pleurodynia. Chest radiographs may show bilateral infiltrates caused by pneumonia or pulmonary infarction. *Costochondritis* produces tender, painful lower parasternal and costal-arch cartilages. There may be upper abdominal pain, but minimal abdominal tenderness. *Acute pancreatitis* causes upper abdominal pain and tenderness, faintness, and fever. It may be associated with *acute gallbladder disease, ascending cholangitis,* or *alcoholic hepatitis.* The diagnosis is confirmed by a serum amylase and isoamylase test. Cholangitis is sug-

gested by the presence of chills, fever, and jaundice. Alcoholic hepatitis is associated with a tender, enlarged liver, elevated serum aminotransferase and gamma glutamyl transferase levels, and bilirubinuria. *Volvulus of the stomach* causes severe upper abdominal distension, pain, and retching; usually it is not possible to pass a nasogastric tube into the stomach. A barium swallow will show obstruction. Surgical exploration will reveal the problem. Often there is a history of a preexisting paraesophageal hernia. *Rupture of a peptic ulcer* causes diffuse upper abdominal pain and tenderness, and free air under the diaphragm. There is usually a prior history of daily epigastric pain that is temporarily ameliorated by food or antacids, or, in some cases, exacerbated by food. *Acute cholecystitis* causes right upper and midabdominal pain, and sometimes left upper abdominal pain. Ultrasonography may demonstrate a thickened gallbladder wall and one or more stones. A ^{99m}Tc DISIDA scan will reveal no radioactivity in the gallbladder at 1 h after isotope injection. *Perforation of the gallbladder* may be signaled by the abrupt onset of pain relief, followed within 24 h by more widespread pain, tenderness, and guarding in the upper abdomen.

Acute gastric dilatation causes upper abdominal pain, fullness, and tympany. Severe cases are cool, sweaty, and hypotensive, and are in early shock. An abdominal radiograph shows massive gastric dilatation and an air-fluid level in the stomach. Passage of a nasogastric tube relieves most complaints as the stomach is decompressed.

Similar, but less severe, complaints occur with *aerophagia;* these can be relieved with reassurance and soluble antacids—or with nasogastric intubation, if dilatation of the stomach is extreme.

Acute congestion of the liver with pain and tenderness may occur with submassive pulmonary embolism. The high pressures in the pulmonary artery produced by the clot may be transmitted back to the liver. The diagnosis of pulmonary embolism can be confirmed by a radionuclide ventilation-perfusion scan or by a pulmonary angiogram. *Alcoholic hepatitis* may cause right upper abdominal and epigastric pain and a tender liver. Patients with this condition may also have epigastric and left hypochondriac pain from gastritis or ulcer disease, and may require endoscopy if hematemesis or melena occurs. The *Fitz-Hugh–Curtis syndrome (perihepatitis)* can cause diffuse upper abdominal pain, tenderness, and fever associated with pelvic pain, adnexal tenderness, and cultural evidence of chlamydial or gonococcal infection.

☐ DESCRIPTION OF LISTED DISEASES

1. EPIDEMIC PLEURODYNIA

There is an abrupt onset of upper abdominal and lower chest pain on both sides. The pain has been described, variously, as "stabbing," "viselike," "catching," and "crushing." Rapid, shallow breathing and a feeling of shortness of breath may accompany the pain. The pain may last 2 to 10 h and then remit, only to recur in a milder form hours later. Superficial chest muscle tenderness may occur over the painful area. If guarding occurs, some patients may be explored (20 percent of patients may have a laparotomy) despite a usually normal or low white blood cell count. A deep breath or movement of the patient in bed often intensifies the pain, so the patient tends to lie still while in pain. Walking, laughing, and coughing intensify the pain for a few seconds with each step, laugh, or cough. Between bouts of pain the patient feels well. Fever, from 100.5°F to 104°F, is usually present. Chest radiographs are usually negative, but pleural effusions can occur. Electrocardiograms are usually negative. Shoulder pain is uncommon. Isolation of group B coxsackievirus or echovirus from throat washings

TABLE OF DISEASE INCIDENCE

INCIDENCE PER 100,000 (APPROXIMATE)

Common (>100)	Uncommon (>5–100)	Rare (>0–5)
Bilateral costochondritis	Epidemic pleurodynia	Acute gastric volvulus
Acute pancreatitis with alcoholic hepatitis	Bilateral pleuritis due to pneumonia or pulmonary infarction	Perforation of a duodenal or gastric ulcer
Alcoholic hepatitis and acute gastritis or ulcer disease	Acute pancreatitis with ascending cholangitis	Acute gastric dilatation
	Acute pancreatitis with acute cholecystitis	Acute hepatic congestion secondary to acute massive pulmonary embolism
	Acute cholecystitis with perforation	
	Acute aerophagia	
	Fitz-Hugh–Curtis syndrome	

or stools, or demonstration of an antibody rise, will confirm the diagnosis. Pleurodynia usually occurs in epidemics in the late summer or early fall, and tends to occur in outbreaks involving family groups or larger groups of children and adults. No specific therapy is available. This disorder clears in 1 to 6 days without specific therapy.

2. ACUTE BILATERAL PLEURITIS

Pain may occur in both sides of the upper abdomen and in the epigastrium, and may also involve the shoulder on one or both sides. Such pain is made worse by a deep breath and by bodily movement (e.g., moving from a lying to a sitting position). Fever to 104.5°F, chills, and cough, with rusty, yellow-green, or bloody sputum, may occur if the pleuritis is caused by pneumonia. Fever to 101.5°F, dyspnea, and hemoptysis occur with pulmonary embolism and infarction. Physical examination in both disorders may reveal basilar rales, friction rubs, dullness, and, sometimes, bronchial breathing bilaterally. Chest radiographs show lower lobe infiltrates with irregular margins or consolidations, and/or pleural fluid. There may be abdominal distension and absent bowel sounds due to a secondary ileus. The upper abdomen may be directly tender and there may be involuntary guarding and rebound tenderness, suggesting a surgical abdomen. Blood cultures and sputum smears and cultures, and/or transtracheal aspirate smears and cultures, are helpful in determining the cause of a bacterial pneumonia. In less cooperative patients shielded-tip bronchoscopy can be used to obtain tracheal secretions for Gram stain and culture.

A pulmonary angiogram may be necessary to confirm pulmonary emboli and infarction. Antibiotic therapy will lead to resolution of pain related to bacterial pneumonia, and anticoagulants will facilitate the resolution of pleuritic pain related to emboli. Patients with bilateral lower lobe pneumonias may have so much upper abdominal pain, tenderness, and guarding that they come to laparotomy, while pneumonic infiltrates present on a chest radiograph are ignored or are first noted postoperatively.

3. BILATERAL COSTOCHONDRITIS

There is aching pain and tenderness, localized to the lower costal cartilages on each side. The upper abdomen shows no guarding or tenderness. Pain is often increased by a deep breath or by body and arm movements. There is no shoulder pain. Physical examination reveals moderate to exquisite tenderness over the costal cartilages of the lower chest on both sides, but the pulmonary examination is normal, as is the chest radiograph. The pain and tenderness respond to moist heat and nonsteroidal anti-inflammatory drugs or aspirin.

4. ACUTE PANCREATITIS WITH OR WITHOUT ASSOCIATED ACUTE CHOLECYSTITIS, CHOLANGITIS, OR HEPATITIS

Patients with severe pancreatitis may present with diffuse, mid-upper abdominal pain that may extend into both the left and right upper abdomen. There is local direct tenderness and mild to moderate muscle guarding. Nausea, vomiting, and loss of appetite occur. There is often weakness, dizziness on standing, fever, and sweating. Hypotension and a rapid pulse accompany the fever. The white blood cell count is usually elevated, and both the total serum amylase and isoamylase values usually exceed twice normal. Treatment involves the use of nasogastric suction, intravenous fluids, and replacement of blood lost into the retroperitoneum. Meperidine injections are used for pain, and antibiotics are used for intraabdominal abscesses related to the pancreatitis. Complications include pancreatic necrosis, formation of pancreatic pseudocysts or abscesses and pulmonary atelectasis, pleural effusions, and pneumonia, usually involving the lower lobes. Surgical intervention is required only in severe cases of pancreatitis, for debridement of necrotic pancreatic tissue or to drain a pancreatic abscess. Pancreatitis is common in alcoholics and also occurs with an increased incidence if gallstones are present.

A. Acute Cholecystitis and Pancreatitis Acute cholecystitis may occur in association with pancreatitis, causing diffuse upper abdominal pain and tenderness. Stones may lodge in the common bile duct, resulting in acute pancreatitis and ascending cholangitis, with right upper abdominal pain and hepatic tenderness, jaundice, shaking

chills, and fever. Removal of common duct stones and the gallbladder in this situation has a high priority and should not be delayed. Common duct stones trapped in the sphincter of Oddi may be removed by endoscopic methods. The diagnosis of acute cholecystitis can be documented by a ^{99m}Tc DISIDA scan. A positive scan is one in which radioactivity has failed to collect in the gallbladder at 1 h.

B. Ascending Cholangitis and Pancreatitis Cholangitis is associated with right upper abdominal pain, a tender liver, high fever, shaking chills, jaundice, an elevated white blood cell count, and an elevated alkaline phosphatase level. Treatment requires biliary tract drainage and intravenous antibiotics. Epigastric and left hypochondriac pain are caused by an associated pancreatitis.

C. Alcoholic Hepatitis and Pancreatitis Alcoholics often present with right upper abdominal pain, a tender, enlarged liver and elevated aminotransferase levels from alcoholic hepatitis, and also with midabdominal and left upper abdominal pain from alcohol-induced pancreatitis. The resultant pain may extend over the entire upper abdomen. In alcoholic hepatitis the ratio of SGOT (AST) to SGPT (ALT) ranges between 2 to 1 and 5 to 1; in viral hepatitis this ratio seldom exceeds 1. The SGOT levels seldom increase to more than 10 times normal in alcohol-related hepatitis. Abstinence from alcohol, combined with nasogastric intubation and the administration of intravenous fluids, usually results in relief of pain and resolution of these disorders in 1 to 2 weeks.

5. ACUTE VOLVULUS OF THE STOMACH

There is constant, severe upper abdominal pain, retching with little vomitus, and difficulty in passing a nasogastric tube past the lower esophagus. The upper abdomen becomes greatly distended and tender, and the lower abdomen remains soft and nontender. A history of a paraesophageal hernia may be obtained. A barium swallow will demonstrate tapering of the lower esophagus. Endoscopy is not helpful in complete obstruction, since the scope will not pass. Surgical correction of the volvulus and anterior gastropexy to fix the stomach in position is the usual therapy for this disorder. A stomach that is gangrenous from strangulation of its blood supply requires resection.

6. PERFORATION OF A GASTRIC OR DUODENAL ULCER

There is usually a history of daily recurrent upper abdominal pain that is often partly relieved by food or antacids, only to recur 1 to 3 h later. In some cases the ingestion of food precipitates or worsens the pain. If such an ulcer leaks gastric contents into the peritoneal cavity, severe upper abdominal pain, tenderness, and muscle rigidity may occur. Free air may collect under the diaphragm and be visualized on a plain upright or lateral decubitus radiograph of the abdomen. A swallow of water-soluble contrast medium will provide evidence of leakage into the abdominal cavity, and may be tried if free air is not visible on plain radiographs. After fluid resuscitation, surgical exploration and closure of the leaking ulcer is required.

7. ACUTE CHOLECYSTITIS WITH PERFORATION AND LEAKAGE OF BILE

Gallbladder colic begins as epigastric pain of a severe, constant, aching quality, associated with nausea and vomiting. Occasional patients have true colic with symptom-free periods between episodes of pain lasting from 10 to 15 min. Colic pain usually lasts 1 to 5 h, and then abates spontaneously. After an episode of colic, a pain-free period of 2 to 3 h may be followed by constant right-sided upper and midabdominal pain in association with fever and abdominal tenderness. The pain may radiate to the back beneath the right scapula and be associated with right shoulder pain. A deep breath may intensify the pain. The pain may also radiate to the left. A ^{99m}Tc DISIDA scan will fail to visualize the gallbladder at 1 h. Perforation of the gallbladder, with leakage of infected bile into the upper abdomen, may provide sudden relief of continuous right upper abdominal pain, only to be followed within hours by more generalized upper abdominal pain and tenderness. This complication of acute cholecystitis usually occurs 3 to 4 days after the onset of persistent upper abdominal pain and fever. Such cases require broad coverage with intravenous antibiotics and surgical removal or drainage of the gallbladder. Patients with gallbladder perforation require copious lavage and drainage of the abdomen.

8. ACUTE GASTRIC DILATATION

Acute gastric dilatation may cause severe upper abdominal pain and distension, associated with retching. There may be sweating, hypotension, and a rapid pulse. Profound cardiovascular collapse may follow. An abdominal radiograph shows massive dilatation of the stomach and an air-fluid level. Such severe distension requires immediate insertion of a nasogastric tube. There is usually no gastric outlet obstruction. This is a common postoperative complication in abdominal surgery, and can be prevented by preoperative nasogastric intubation and suction. Acute gastric dilatation may occur in patients who have been immobilized in body casts; who have diabetic ketoaci-

dosis; or who are taking anticholinergic drugs. It may also occur with severe pneumonia, after upper abdominal trauma, or because of an embolus to the celiac artery.

9. ACUTE AEROPHAGIA

Patients who are highly tense may swallow large amounts of air and develop acute dilatation of the stomach. The pain is located in the epigastrium and is continuous; it may spread to the whole upper abdomen. Attempted belching is frequent, and relief may be obtained after a large belch, after administration of sodium bicarbonate in water, or by intubation. The upper abdomen may become visibly distended, tympanitic, and tender prior to treatment. Such habits as gum chewing and the drinking of carbonated beverages should be discontinued. Endoscopy or an upper gastrointestinal series should be done to exclude significant gastric outlet obstruction.

10. ACUTE HEPATIC CONGESTION SECONDARY TO ACUTE MASSIVE PULMONARY EMBOLISM

Severe upper abdominal pain can result from acute congestion of the liver. This may occur after a large embolus obstructs enough of the pulmonary vascular bed to produce acute pulmonary hypertension and failure of the right ventricle. The elevated pressure is transmitted to the liver from the right side of the heart. Shortness of breath and chest pain may occur with the embolism; or it may cause few, if any, pulmonary symptoms. The liver becomes enlarged and tender and the jugular venous pressure rises. A lung scan or pulmonary angiogram will confirm the diagnosis. Therapy can be initiated with an infusion of tissue-plasminogen activator (tPA) into the pulmonary artery to lyse the clot, but surgical removal may be required. Heparin therapy, to prevent recurrence or clot propagation, should be started as soon as the diagnosis is confirmed.

11. ALCOHOLIC HEPATITIS AND ACUTE GASTRITIS AND/OR ULCER DISEASE

Fever, chills, and right upper abdominal aching pain occur. The liver is enlarged, tender, and moderately firm, and ascites may be present. The serum bilirubin level and leukocyte count may be increased and the aminotransferase levels altered, as described above. Gastritis and ulcer disease may cause associated left epigastric and hypochondriac pain, nausea, vomiting, and hematemesis. Esophagogastroduodenoscopy may reveal erosive gastritis and/or one or more gastric or duodenal ulcers. The ulcer disease or gastritis responds to abstinence from alcohol and to the use of sucralfate or an H_2 blocker. Alcoholic hepatitis requires discontinuation of alcohol. In severe cases of alcoholic hepatitis survival may be enhanced by a 1-month course of prednisone therapy.

12. FITZ-HUGH–CURTIS SYNDROME (PERIHEPATITIS)

Diffuse upper abdominal pain and tenderness, with fever, may result from gonococcal or chlamydial perihepatitis. There may be upper abdominal direct and rebound tenderness and guarding, and hepatic tenderness. A friction rub may occasionally be heard over the liver. Respiration, coughing, and bodily movement can intensify the pain.

Elevation of liver enzyme levels may occur. Lower abdominal pain in one or both sides usually accompanies the upper abdominal pain, but cases have been reported without lower abdominal complaints. Pelvic examination may reveal cervical-motion and adnexal tenderness on one or both sides. *Chlamydia trachomatis* or *Neisseria gonorrhoeae* can be cultured from the cervix or urethra. Laparoscopy may reveal evidence of fibrin deposition over the liver and, after several weeks, "violin-string" adhesions. Visualization of the fallopian tubes usually reveals evidence of acute inflammation and purulent tubal discharge. There is a prompt response to specific antibiotic therapy. This disorder may rarely occur in men because of bacteremic spread of *N. gonorrhoeae*.

25 Acute Bilateral Lower Abdominal Pain

☐ DIAGNOSTIC LIST

1. Acute colitis
2. Free perforation of the colon
3. Duodenal ulcer with perforation
4. Obstruction of the colon
   A. Carcinoma of the colon or diverticulitis
   B. Sigmoid or cecal volvulus
   C. Fecal impaction
5. Toxic megacolon
   A. Inflammatory bowel disease
   B. Ischemic colitis and infectious colitis

6. Rupture of an infrarenal aortic aneurysm
7. Gynecologic disorders
   A. Pelvic inflammatory disease
   B. Intraperitoneal bleeding due to:
      1. Tubal pregnancy
      2. Corpus luteum cyst of pregnancy
      3. Corpus luteum cyst
      4. Follicle cyst
      5. Endometriosis
   C. Adnexal or ovarian torsion

☐ SUMMARY

Patients with *acute colitis* may present with constant lower abdominal aching or burning pain and/or crampy bilateral lower abdominal pain associated with food ingestion and with the urge to defecate. Frequent diarrheal stools are passed in association with bloody mucus, pools of blood, or clots. Fever, chills, arthralgias, myalgias, and headaches may accompany the abdominal complaints. Idiopathic *inflammatory bowel disease,* or a specific *colonic infection with pathogenic bacteria or Entamoeba histolytica,* may cause an identical clinical picture. Differentiation of one disorder from another depends on stool cultures, and on microscopic examination of stool and/ or samples from ulcer exudates and biopsies taken during sigmoidoscopy. *Free perforation of the colon* causes an abrupt onset of diffuse lower abdominal pain and peritoneal signs. Free air may be demonstrable on a plain abdominal radiograph. Perforation may follow the left lower abdominal pain and tenderness of diverticulitis, the right-sided pain of appendicitis or a carcinoma of the appendix, the obstructive symptoms of a distal carcinoma of the colon, the left lower quadrant pain

and bloody diarrhea of ischemic colitis, the chronic diarrhea and crampy pain of Crohn's disease, or the diffuse lower abdominal pain, distension, and systemic toxicity of toxic megacolon.

The course of a chronic *duodenal ulcer,* with epigastric gnawing or aching pain, may suddenly change with the development of acute right lower abdominal pain and tenderness, followed by more diffuse lower abdominal pain and peritoneal signs. Perforation may be demonstrated by detecting free air on a plain abdominal radiograph or by an oral diatrizoate meglumine study. *Colon obstruction* may be due to a distal stenosis caused by *carcinoma* or *divertulitis with scarring.* Crampy lower abdominal pain, distension, and obstipation occur. There may be direct and rebound tenderness in the presence of colonic dilatation. Right lower abdominal pain and tenderness reflect cecal distension due to distal colon obstruction. The diagnosis of obstruction can be confirmed by a contrast enema, and the malignant nature of the obstruction confirmed by colonoscopic biopsy. Closed loop obstruction of the colon, with diffuse lower abdominal pain, tenderness, and distension, may be caused by a *sigmoid or cecal volvulus.* The plain radiograph in sigmoid volvulus demonstrates a ''bent inner tube'' and a ''bird's beak'' narrowing of the colon gas shadow at the point of obstruction. The diagnosis may require a barium contrast enema or CT study for confirmation in up to 30 to 40 percent of cases. Cecal volvulus is likely if there is leftward displacement of a dilated, kidney-shaped cecum in a patient with lower abdominal pain, obstipation, and distension. Contrast enemas may be required for confirmation of the diagnosis. Obstruction due to *impaction of feces* can be confirmed by a rectal examination, and relieved by removal of the fecal mass.

Toxic megacolon is a potentially lethal complication of *inflammatory bowel disease,* as well as of rare cases of *infectious colitis.* Toxic symptoms include fever, chills, sweats, delirium, and weakness. There is diffuse lower abdominal pain and tenderness, and marked lower or generalized abdominal distension. A supine abdominal radiograph demonstrates dilatation of the transverse colon beyond a diameter of 6 cm. Colonoscopy reveals evidence of acute colonic inflammation, with a friable mucosa, ulcerations, and luminal mucopus and blood. The presence of pseudopolyps in the wall of the gas-distended colon favors a diagnosis of Crohn's disease of the colon or ulcerative colitis. Amebic colitis should be carefully ruled out by stool and ulcer biopsy examinations, and by a serologic test for amebiasis, before corticosteroids are used for therapy. *Ischemic colitis* with toxic megacolon is rare, but should be considered in an older patient with a history of cardiovascular disease and no prior history of colitis.

The sudden onset of lower abdominal pain (and sometimes lumbosacral pain), weakness, sweating, and faintness in the presence of a tender, pulsatile midlower abdominal mass is diagnostic of a *ruptured aortic aneurysm.*

Pelvic inflammatory disease may cause bilateral lower abdominal pain and tenderness. Some, but not all, patients also have low back pain, fever and chills, vaginal discharge, vaginal bleeding, and dysuria. Pelvic examination reveals cervical-motion and adnexal tenderness, and, in some cases, a sausage-shaped adnexal mass on one or both sides. Ultrasonography will confirm a *tuboovarian abscess,* as will laparoscopy. There is usually a prompt response to antibiotic therapy. Rupture of a tuboovarian abscess causes the sudden onset of sharp, diffuse lower abdominal pain and tenderness, with rapidly spreading peritoneal signs. The signs of peritonitis spread toward the upper abdomen. Shock may ensue, secondary to bacteremia. The diagnosis of rupture of a tuboovarian abscess can be confirmed by culdocentesis, ultrasonography, or laparoscopy.

Sudden, sharp lower abdominal pain, accompanied by tenderness and then rapidly developing peritoneal signs, may be caused by *bleeding* from a *tubal pregnancy* or an *ovarian cyst.* Culdocentesis usually reveals nonclotting blood; ultrasonography will confirm the presence of blood in the abdomen and cul-de-sac.

A tubal pregnancy usually begins with amenorrhea, followed by staining, spotting, or frank vaginal bleeding. Crampy or constant lower abdominal pain occurs on one side. Rupture or profuse bleeding is signaled by the abrupt onset of sharp, stabbing, diffuse lower abdominal pain, and direct and rebound

TABLE OF DISEASE INCIDENCE

INCIDENCE PER 100,000 (APPROXIMATE)

Common (>100)	Uncommon (>5–100)	Rare (>0–5)
Bacterial colitis	Ulcerative colitis	Duodenal ulcer with perforation
Colon obstruction due to carcinoma	Crohn's disease of the colon	Toxic megacolon due to ischemia, amebiasis, or bacillary dysentery
Pelvic inflammatory disease	Amebic colitis	
Intraperitoneal bleeding due to: corpus luteum cyst follicle cyst endometriosis	Ischemic colitis	Free perforation of the colon due to carcinoma of the appendix
	Free perforation of the colon	
	Colon obstruction due to diverticulitis	
	Colon obstruction due to volvulus or fecal impaction	
	Toxic megacolon due to inflammatory bowel disease	
	Rupture of an aortic aneurysm	
	Adnexal or ovarian torsion	
	Tubal pregnancy	
	Corpus luteum cyst of pregnancy with intraperitoneal bleeding	

tenderness. The pregnancy test is positive; ultrasonography may demonstrate absence of an intrauterine gestation and may visualize an adnexal mass. Laparoscopy can be diagnostic of tubal pregnancy or may detect a bleeding *corpus luteum cyst of pregnancy.* Similarly, other bleeding cystic ovarian lesions (*follicle cysts, endometriomas,* and *corpus luteum cysts*) can be detected by the use of the laparoscope.

Adnexal or ovarian torsion causes progressively severe unilateral lower abdominal pain that soon spreads to both sides. There is an enlarging tender adnexal mass. An sonographic study will demonstrate a uniformly echogenic adnexal mass; the diagnosis can be confirmed by laparoscopy or at exploration.

☐ DESCRIPTION OF LISTED DISEASES

1. ACUTE COLITIS

Aching lower abdominal pain and tenderness may occur in association with fever and watery or bloody diarrhea. Constant right lower abdominal pain and tenderness is associated with *Yersinia enterocolitica* and some salmonella infections. Crampy, sticking lower abdominal pain may be superimposed on a dull, constant discomfort, or may be the only type of pain present. Crampy pain may appear spontaneously, or may be associated with food intake or the desire to defecate. It is often improved transiently after passage of stool or flatus. Tenesmus and the frequent passage of small-volume stools and blood indicate the presence of an acute proctosigmoiditis. Blood-tinged mucus, gross liquid blood, or dark clots may be passed. Abdominal tenderness is usually most marked over the course of the colon, and rebound tenderness may be present. Guarding is usually voluntary. A methylene blue stain of the feces or mucus shows an increased number of stool neutrophils.

Acute inflammatory bowel disease (ulcerative colitis) and specific infectious forms of colitis produced by species of *Campylobacter, Salmonella,* and *Shigella,* and by *Clostridium difficile, Escherichia coli* O157:H7, *Vibrio parahaemolyticus,* and *Yersinia enterolitica* may cause similar clinical pictures. Sigmoidoscopy reveals mucosal friability, granularity, mucopus, ulcerations, erythema, and sometimes pseudomembranes. Rectal biopsies may show crypt abscesses, a lamina propria infiltrated with polymorphonuclear leukocytes, and, in some cases, pseudomembranes. Sigmoidoscopy in *Yersinia* infections is usually normal, since this organism localizes to the cecum and terminal ileum. *C. difficile* causes a toxic colitis, with early lesions appearing as volcanolike papules covered with pseudomembranes and separated by a normal intervening mucosa. More severe cases show diffuse friability, ulcerations, bleeding, and diffuse mucosal necrosis in some regions.

Sigmoidoscopy in patients with amebic colitis may be entirely negative if only the cecum and ascending colon are involved. When amebic proctosigmoiditis is present, small, punched-out ulcers with clear margins and slightly raised undermined edges are present, surrounded by normal mucosa. They are usually covered with a yellow-white exudate. In severe cases the rectosigmoid may show a diffusely ulcerated, friable mucosa that mimics ulcerative or bacterial colitis. Microscopic examination of ulcer exudate or an ulcer margin biopsy may identify trophozoites. Cysts and trophozoites may be detected in the stool. Serologic studies should be done to rule out amebiasis. Travel to an endemic region, or a history of homosexual activity in a male patient, makes a diagnosis of amebic colitis more likely. Detection of *Entamoeba histolytica* in male homosexuals may be misleading since many of these patients are asymptomatic carriers and amebic infection may not be the cause of their dysentery.

Recent or current antibiotic use is an indication for a stool culture for *C. difficile* and a stool toxin assay. Stool leukocytes may occur with inflammatory bowel disease, and with ischemic colitis. Stool cultures will identify specific bacterial agents. Acute ulcerative colitis may mimic amebic or bacillary dysentery, but stools are negative for *Entamoeba histolytica* and bacterial pathogens. Amebic infections respond to diiodohydroxyquin, to metronidazole, and to diloxanide furoate. *C. difficile* responds to discontinuation of antibiotic therapy and oral administration of vancomycin. Bacterial pathogens such as *Campylobacter* spe-

cies respond to erythromycin; *Shigella* species to sulfamethoxazole-trimethoprim; and both to norfloxacin. *Salmonella* colitis is usually not treated with antibiotics, but in special circumstances such therapy is indicated. Chloramphenicol and ampicillin are both effective. Nonspecific inflammatory bowel disease responds to sulfasalazine and to prednisone.

2. FREE PERFORATION OF THE COLON WITH PERITONITIS

Perforation of the colon secondary to inflammatory bowel disease, diverticulitis, appendicitis, appendiceal carcinoma, ischemic colitis, or toxic megacolon may cause bilateral lower abdominal aching pain that is intensified by jarring, walking, coughing, sneezing, and abdominal palpation. There is diffuse lower abdominal direct and rebound tenderness, along with involuntary guarding, lower abdominal distension, and a loss of bowel sounds. Diffuse pelvic tenderness is present on rectal examination. The bowel is paretic, so constipation ensues. Fever and chills accompany the abdominal findings. Radiologic evidence of free air may be present (up to 50 percent of cases of diverticulitis); this finding is an indication for surgical exploration. Leukocytosis and/or a shift to the left of the differential count is usually present.

Diverticulitis begins with left lower abdominal pain, low back pain, fever, and local tenderness. Free perforation of a diverticulum or a pericolic abscess may occur.

Acute appendicitis begins as a midline crampy pain that shifts to the right lower abdomen and is associated with direct tenderness and frequently rebound tenderness, and guarding. Fever, nausea, and vomiting may occur. Free perforation or rupture of an appendiceal abscess may also occur.

Carcinoma of the appendix is rare, but it frequently perforates and produces an abscess or diffuse peritonitis. The preoperative diagnosis is usually acute appendicitis.

Colon cancer may perforate into the free peritoneal cavity, or a small initial perforation may produce an abscess that later ruptures. This acute peritonitis may be preceded by weeks or months of increasing constipation or diarrhea, crampy lower abdominal pain, narrowing of stools to a pencil or ribbon shape, hematochezia, and anemia.

Ischemic colitis may cause left lower abdominal pain and tenderness, and bloody diarrhea, prior to perforation. A contrast enema may show thumbprinting. Sigmoidoscopy may show edematous cyanotic mucosa and blue-black submucosal nodules, and sometimes ulcerations, with or without pseudomembranes.

Crohn's disease of the colon may cause weight loss, diarrhea, crampy lower abdominal pain, and rectal bleeding. Free perforation rarely occurs.

Toxic megacolon caused by inflammatory bowel disease or by amebic, bacillary, or ischemic colitis may give rise to free perforation. Surgical exploration is required in the presence of free air or diffuse peritoneal signs.

3. DUODENAL ULCER WITH PERFORATION

Leakage of gastric juice down the right lumbar gutter, through a perforated duodenal ulcer, causes right lower quadrant pain and peritoneal signs that may spread to the pelvis and left lower abdomen. Rectal and/or pelvic tenderness is present. Physical examination reveals tachycardia, bilateral lower abdominal direct and rebound tenderness, and involuntary guarding. Liver dullness may be obscured by tympany. A plain abdominal radiograph may show free air. There is usually a long history of epigastric pain of a gnawing or aching nature that is relieved by food or antacids and recurs on a daily basis. In the absence of free air, the perforation may be documented by a diatrizoate meglumine contrast study of the duodenum.

4. OBSTRUCTION OF THE COLON

Pain of a colicky type occurs in the lower abdomen. These pains are brief in duration (i.e., 2–4 min), and are separated by pain-free periods of 10 to 20 min. High-pitched bowel sounds are associated with the discomfort. Pain may begin in the right lower abdomen and move to the left with each attack of colic. Abdominal distension and obstipation soon develop. Constant, more severe pain may occur in the right lower abdomen as the cecum distends beyond 9 to 10 cm because of distal obstruction. The cecum may perforate, causing diffuse lower abdominal pain and peritoneal signs spreading from the right lower abdomen.

A. Carcinoma of the Colon or Diverticulitis Large bowel obstruction is most frequently caused by a distal obstructing carcinoma (70 percent of cases). There may be a history of weeks or months of increasingly severe constipation, gripping lower abdominal pain, narrow pencil-shaped or ribbon stools (e.g., ribbonlike stools are usually associated with anorectal lesions or functional disorders), and rectal bleeding. Prior transient attacks of lower abdominal colicky pain and distension may have occurred. The diagnosis requires a contrast enema to confirm true obstruction, because up to 35 percent of patients with a clinical picture of colon obstruction may have unobstructed colons. Identification of the abnormal segment may be followed by colonoscopic inspection and biopsy. A clinically indistinguishable picture may be caused by diverticulitis, with pericolic or intramural abscesses, and/or fibrosis of the colon wall. Some cases of Crohn's disease may also obstruct. This is uncommon with the stenotic lesions produced by ischemic colitis, since the scarring is not usually severe.

B. Sigmoid or Cecal Volvulus Sigmoid volvulus may cause diffuse lower abdominal pain and tenderness, obstipation, and marked distension. A plain abdominal radio-graph will demonstrate a "bent inner tube" sign and "bird's beak" deformity of the colon gas column at the site of the obstruction. For up to 30 percent of patients, a barium enema (bird's beak) or CT study (spiral mucosal folds producing a "whirl sign") may be required to demonstrate the presence of a volvulus. Decompression by means of a rectal tube or colonoscope results in a rush of gas on passage of the tube through the obstructed site, confirming the diagnosis.

Cecal volvulus causes the sudden onset of mild right lower abdominal and/or hypogastric pain of a crampy or colicky nature. Lower abdominal distension, obstipation, and a constant lower abdominal ache soon follow. Right lower abdominal tenderness and tympany develop. A plain radiograph shows the markedly distended cecum as a kidney-shaped gas shadow displaced to the left in the mid- and left upper abdomen. Distended loops of small bowel are usually visible on the right, and a single air-fluid level may be visualized in the cecum. The distal colon does not usually contain gas, but it may. A contrast enema will confirm the diagnosis. Colonoscopy can be used to decompress the cecum, but most cases require surgery. Attempts to decompress a cecal volvulus may result in perforation.

C. Fecal Impaction Obstruction may also be caused by fecal impaction. This can be relieved by removal of feces manually and/or with irrigation and enemas.

5. TOXIC MEGACOLON

A. Inflammatory Bowel Disease Patients appear toxic with high fever, tachycardia, diaphoresis, rigors and chills, extreme weakness, and mental confusion. There is diffuse lower abdominal pain and distension. Diarrhea and rectal bleeding may be present, or a decrease in the number of passed stools may be noted. There is localized direct tenderness and tympany over the lower, or the entire, abdomen. Bowel sounds are usually decreased or absent. Rebound tenderness and guarding may be present in the absence or presence of free perforation. Percussion resonance or tympany over the normal liver dullness suggests free perforation. An abdominal supine radiograph shows a transverse colon distended beyond a diameter of 6 cm. Positioning the patient prone shifts the transverse colon gas to the descending colon. Leukocytosis beyond 20,000 cells per mm^3, anemia, hypoalbuminemia, and low serum sodium and potassium levels are commonly present. Perforation may occur at any time when the colon is markedly distended, leading to diffuse lower abdominal peritoneal signs and pain that spread throughout the abdomen. Detection of free air under the diaphragm may be the first sign of leakage from the colon. There is usually a prior history of crampy lower abdominal pain and bloody diarrhea in ulcerative colitis, and of right lower abdominal pain and watery diarrhea in Crohn's disease.

B. Ischemic Colitis and Infectious Colitis Rarely, toxic megacolon complicates ischemic colitis or infectious colitis caused by *Campylobacter* species, *Entamoeba histolytica*, or *Clostridium difficile*. Sigmoidoscopic findings may not distinguish severe inflammatory bowel disease from these other disorders. Detection of amebas or serologic evidence of amebiasis, or evidence of a *Campylobacter* or clostridial infection, may allow more specific therapy. There may be a good initial response to fluid and electrolyte therapy, and to administration of antibiotics and prednisolone intravenously. A therapeutic response usually occurs within 48 h. Persistence of symptoms and signs beyond this time increases the risk of free perforation, and requires subtotal colectomy or proctocolectomy and ileostomy. Delay of surgery until perforation occurs increases the mortality rate from 10 percent to 50 percent. Toxic megacolon may occur with an initial attack of inflammatory bowel disease. Up to 10 percent of patients with ulcerative colitis or Crohn's disease who require hospitalization may develop this problem. The relationship of the onset of toxic megacolon to the use of contrast enemas, anticholinergics, opiates, and steroids is controversial. Up to 80 percent of patients with toxic megacolon require surgery during their initial hospitalization.

Several other disorders may cause marked distension of the transverse and proximal left colon that may radiologically mimic toxic megacolon. These include distal colonic obstruction due to carcinoma or diverticulitis, closed loop colonic obstruction due to cecal or sigmoid volvulus, ischemia of the colon secondary to superior mesenteric artery obstruction, acute pancreatitis, and pseudoobstruction due to abnormalities of the neural innervation of the bowel wall. Pseudoobstruction may be confirmed by a contrast enema, which shows no obstruction, and/or colonoscopy, which reveals luminal patency and an absence of inflammatory mucosal change.

6. RUPTURE OF AN INFRARENAL AORTIC ANEURYSM

Aneurysmal rupture usually occurs in patients older than age 50; the majority of patients are older than 70. There is an abrupt onset of very severe lower abdominal pain, which may be unilateral or bilateral. It may spread rapidly to involve the lumbosacral area and/or the entire abdomen. Diaphoresis, profound weakness, faintness, and collapse occur in fewer than 30 percent of cases, and reflect hypovolemia secondary to retroperitoneal bleeding. Uncommon symptoms include urinary retention, leg weakness, numbness and paresthesias, vomiting, and sciatic and testicular pains. Physical examination reveals a tender, pulsatile lower midabdominal mass caused by the ruptured aneurysm with associated retroperitoneal hematoma. A diffuse mass is present on examination—rather than a clearly definable aneurysm—because of the associated retroperitoneal bleed-

ing. A pulsation is palpable in 75 percent of patients with a mass. Rare physical findings include mottling of the extremities, flank ecchymoses, and perianal and scrotal ecchymoses. The diagnosis should be made clinically, and the patient taken to the operating room for graft replacement of the aneurysmal segment. Confirmation of clinical findings can be obtained by plain abdominal radiographs (sensitivity 56–89 percent) or bedside ultrasonography. Once rupture has occurred, surgical mortality rises from 5 percent to 50 percent.

7. GYNECOLOGIC DISORDERS

A. Pelvic Inflammatory Disease Acute bilateral lower quadrant and midline pain may occur, often in association with low back pain. The pain is constant and aching, and may be intensified by walking, ascending or descending stairs, and sexual intercourse (deep dyspareunia). Vaginal discharge occurs in 30 to 40 percent of cases, and is usually purulent. Fever and chills are variable, and may be absent in up to 60 percent of cases. Other complaints include dysuria and vaginal bleeding. There is bilateral lower abdominal and adnexal tenderness, and increased pain on cervical motion. If an adnexal mass is palpable on one or both sides, a tuboovarian abscess should be suspected, and its presence confirmed by ultrasonography or laparoscopy. Salpingitis may be associated with diffuse lower abdominal rebound tenderness and guarding, and may simulate an acute abdomen. Laparoscopy can confirm the diagnosis of acute salpingitis, thus avoiding laparotomy. Rupture of a tuboovarian abscess is signaled by the onset of sharp, intense lower abdominal pain; fever; chills; and upward spread of abdominal peritoneal signs. Hypotension and septic shock may ensue. Leukocytosis, and/or a shift to the left of the differential count, and an elevated sedimentation rate occur in some, but not all, cases of pelvic inflammatory disease. Mild cases of pelvic inflammatory disease, with only lower abdominal pain and tenderness, without systemic toxicity, respond to a regimen of intramuscular ceftriaxone and oral doxycycline. Others require hospitalization and intravenous antibiotics. Failure of a tuboovarian abscess to resolve, or abscess rupture, requires surgical drainage and/or salpingectomy, or hysterectomy and bilateral salpingo-oophorectomy. The usual causes of acute salpingitis are *Neisseria gonorrhoeae* and *Chlamydia trachomatis*. Cases of salpingitis yield gram-negative aerobic bacteria, anaerobic gram-negative rods, and gram-positive cocci when tubal exudate is cultured. It is believed that the sexually transmitted organisms produce an initial mucosal insult that paves the way for superinfection of the fallopian tubes by these latter organisms.

At laparoscopy, culture of tubal pus reveals *N. gonorrhoeae* in only 1 to 3 percent of cases and *C. trachomatis* in only 10 to 12 percent.

B. Intraperitoneal Bleeding   There is usually an abrupt onset of unilateral, and then diffuse, lower abdominal pain and tenderness. Diffuse lower abdominal direct and rebound tenderness and guarding develop rapidly. Pain may also be felt in one or both shoulders. Intraabdominal bleeding in the lower abdomen may arise from a tubal pregnancy, a bleeding ovarian cyst, or a cystic lesion caused by endometriosis.

1. Tubal Pregnancy   Tubal pregnancy begins with amenorrhea (60 percent of cases), followed by vaginal staining, spotting, or frank bleeding. There is usually a history of crampy or constant unilateral lower abdominal pain, beginning several weeks after the onset of menstrual irregularities. The sudden onset of more diffuse lower abdominal pain and spreading peritoneal signs signals tubal bleeding and possible tubal rupture. The urine and serum β-hCG titers are positive, and ultrasonography or laparoscopy can detect the adnexal mass. Exploration is required for tubal pregnancy with bleeding to prevent exsanguinating hemorrhage. Severe bleeding with hypotension occurs in 5 percent of cases as an initial presentation.

2. Corpus Luteum Cyst of Pregnancy   A corpus luteum cyst of pregnancy may bleed intraperitoneally and simulate a bleeding ectopic pregnancy, since the pregnancy test is positive and diffuse lower abdominal pain and tenderness occur, accompanied by diffuse lower abdominal peritoneal signs. Ultrasonography can demonstrate an intrauterine pregnancy, as well as the corpus luteum cyst. Laparoscopy will reveal the cyst to be the source of the bleeding, and will demonstrate the absence of ectopic pregnancy. Expectant treatment without surgery is the preferred method of management of this mimic of tubal pregnancy.

3. Corpus Luteum Cyst   A corpus luteum cyst in a nonpregnant patient may rupture and bleed. Such cysts may cause a brief period of amenorrhea or a scant period, followed by spotting or staining. The pregnancy test is negative; the diagnosis can be confirmed by laparoscopy.

4. Follicle Cyst   Pain related to bleeding from a follicle cyst usually occurs at midcycle (mittelschmerz), and has a sudden onset with unilateral or diffuse lower abdominal aching and the development of unilateral or diffuse bilateral peritoneal signs. The diagnosis can be confirmed by laparoscopy.

5. Endometriosis   Bleeding from an endometrial cystic implant on the serosal surface of the pelvic organs may produce clinical findings indistinguishable from those of other bleeding lesions. There is often a prior history of severe secondary dysmenorrhea, deep dyspareunia, and infertility (up to 40 percent of cases).

C. Adnexal or Ovarian Torsion   There is gradual onset of aching unilateral lower abdominal pain that soon worsens, and that becomes progressively severe over a period of several hours. Lower abdominal and adnexal tenderness are present on the painful side. A tender mass soon becomes palpable. As the disorder progresses, the pain and tenderness may spread across the midline. Ultrasonography will detect the enlarged ovary as a uniformly echogenic mass that is hypoechoic to surrounding structures. Adnexal torsion produces a complex mass on sonography. Laparoscopy will confirm the diagnosis. Surgical intervention is required to salvage the ovary, or to remove it if it is necrotic. Such ovaries often harbor a large cyst or tumor; the presence of an ovarian malignancy requires hysterectomy and bilateral salpingo-oophorectomy.

26

Acute Bilateral Costovertebral Area and Flank Pain

☐ DIAGNOSTIC LIST

1. Pain of renal origin
   A. Acute pyelonephritis
   B. Renal cortical abscesses
   C. Acute glomerulonephritis
      1. Acute post-streptococcal glomerulonephritis (PSGN)
      2. Acute postinfectious glomerulonephritis
      3. IgA nephropathy (Berger's disease)
      4. Idiopathic nephrotic syndrome
         a. Mesangial proliferative glomerulonephritis
         b. Bilateral renal vein thrombosis
      5. Rapidly progressive glomerulonephritis (RPGN)
         a. Idiopathic RPGN
         b. Anti-glomerular basement membrane (GBM) antibody-mediated RPGN

   c. RPGN due to immune complex deposition
   d. Vasculitis-associated RPGN
   D. Acute interstitial nephritis due to drugs—hypersensitivity nephropathy
   E. Loin pain hematuria syndrome
   F. Bilateral renal infarction
      1. Embolic
      2. Thrombotic
2. Myofascial pain
3. Pleuritis
   A. Bilateral bacterial pneumonia
   B. Multiple pulmonary emboli
   C. Bilateral pleuritis due to systemic lupus erythematosus
   D. Drug-induced lupus
4. Spinal osteomyelitis with radicular involvement

☐ SUMMARY

Acute pyelonephritis may cause bilateral aching flank pain and costovertebral area tenderness. Fever, chills or rigors, vomiting, and irritative bladder symptoms frequently accompany the pain. The urine contains leukocytes, singly, in clumps, and in casts, and bacteria in large numbers. There is a prompt resolution of pain and other symptoms with intravenous antibiotic therapy. *Bilateral renal cortical abscesses* cause flank pain,

chills, fever, and leukocytosis. There is usually a history of a recent skin, bone, or heart valve infection, but there may not be. Microscopic examination and culture of the urine is usually negative, but a small percentage of cases may show abnormalities. The diagnosis can be established by a CT scan with contrast. *Acute glomerulonephritis* may present in a minority of cases with bilateral flank pain, costovertebral angle tenderness, fever, and gross or microscopic hematuria. The urine sediment is nephritic (dysmorphic red blood cells, red blood

311

cell and pigment casts, and leukocytes), and proteinuria is less than 3 g/day. This syndrome may follow *streptococcal* pharyngeal or skin infections, and the diagnosis can be established by detection of nephritogenic streptococcal strains on culture and/or an antibody response to streptococcal exoenzymes frequently associated with a low serum level of C3. An identical clinical picture can be associated with *other viral or bacterial* (endocarditis, "shunt" infections, and intraabdominal or intrathoracic sepsis) *infections. Berger's disease* may begin with loin pain and gross or microscopic hematuria. Urinalysis reveals a nephritic sediment, and IgA deposition is demonstrable in the mesangial areas on renal biopsy. Some patients with Berger's disease may develop massive proteinuria (i.e., a nephrotic syndrome) and bilateral aching dull flank pain. Patients with the *idiopathic nephrotic syndrome* may rarely present with flank pain, but proteinuria ≥ 3.5 g/1.73 M^2/day, and generalized edema are usually present. Up to 10 percent of patients with the idiopathic nephrotic syndrome have mesangial proliferative glomerulonephritis on renal biopsy. This diagnosis is suggested by a urinalysis with nephritic characteristics. The abrupt onset of marked bilateral flank pain and tenderness, fever, and hematuria in a patient with the nephrotic syndrome suggests the possibility of *bilateral renal vein thrombosis*. This can also cause an acute left varicocele, oliguria, and an abnormal venous pattern on the anterior abdominal wall (i.e., if the inferior vena cava has also occluded), as well as evidence of pulmonary embolization. The diagnosis can be confirmed by an abdominal CT scan or MRI or by selective renal venography.

Rapidly progressive glomerulonephritis (RPGN) leads to early-onset renal failure. There are many etiologies, including *idiopathic RPGN, anti-basement membrane antibody* or *immune complex* deposition, and *systemic vasculitis*. The diagnosis should be suspected in a case of acute nephritis with an elevated creatinine level and oliguria. It may be confirmed by a renal biopsy demonstrating cellular glomerular crescents in 50 percent or more of the glomeruli sampled.

Acute interstitial nephritis may be associated with bilateral flank pain and tenderness, fever, eosinophilia, a truncal upper body rash, eosinophiluria, a rising creatinine level, and a prompt response to discontinuance of the offending causative drug. Antibiotics, diuretics, allopurinol, and antihypertensives have all caused this disorder. *Loin pain and hematuria* occur in some women taking oral contraceptives, and symptoms are relieved on discontinuance of this method of birth control. *Bilateral renal infarction* may result from *emboli* or *thrombosis* of both renal arteries or the lower aorta. There is an abrupt onset of bilateral loin pain, either simultaneously or sequentially, and gross or microscopic hematuria. The diagnosis can be confirmed by a CT scan with contrast or by renal angiography. There may be a prompt response to thrombolytic therapy, or surgical intervention may be necessary to preserve renal function. *Myofascial pain* is intensified by certain bodily movements. Pain may affect both sides of the thoracolumbar area and the flanks. Results of all renal imaging studies, the chest radiograph, and urinalysis are negative. There is a response to analgesic drugs, trigger-point injection, and avoidance of muscle-straining activities. *Pleuritic reaction* at the base of both hemithoraces may cause sharp, sticking lower chest and flank discomfort intensified by breathing, movement, and coughing. Signs of consolidation, friction rubs, fever, and cough characterize patients with *bilateral bacterial pneumonia,* and there is a prompt response to intravenous antibiotics. Dyspnea, hemoptysis, and fever associated with pleural effusions and pleuritic pain may be caused by *multiple pulmonary emboli*. The diagnosis can be established by a radionuclide lung scan, color duplex flow imaging of the femoral veins, or a pulmonary angiogram. There is improvement after initiation of anticoagulant therapy. *Bilateral pleuritis associated with systemic lupus* is usually associated with other evidence of that disorder, and it is responsive to prednisone. Drugs such as hydralazine or procainamide can cause a *drug-induced lupus syndrome,* with fever, bilateral pleuritis, and sometimes pericarditis, that clears when the drug is withheld. *Spinal osteo-*

TABLE OF DISEASE INCIDENCE

INCIDENCE PER 100,000 (APPROXIMATE)

Common (>100)	**Uncommon (>5–100)**	**Rare (>0–5)**
Acute pyelonephritis	Post-streptococcal glomerulonephritis	Bilateral renal cortical abscesses
Myofascial pain	IgA nephropathy	Postinfectious glomerulonephritis
	Idiopathic nephrotic syndrome	Idiopathic nephrotic syndrome with mesangial proliferative glomerulonephritis
	Loin pain hematuria syndrome	Bilateral renal vein thrombosis
		Rapidly progressive glomerulonephritis
		Acute interstitial nephritis due to drugs
		Bilateral renal infarction
		Pleuritic pain due to:
		Bilateral bacterial pneumonia
		Pulmonary infarction
		Lupus pleuritis
		Drug-induced lupus pleuritis
		Spinal osteomyelitis with radicular flank pain

myelitis can cause a midline spinal ache and flank pain with or without fever. A spine radiograph, a radionuclide scan, or MRI may establish the diagnosis. There is a good response to parenteral antibiotic therapy within 5 to 7 days.

☐ DESCRIPTION OF LISTED DISEASES

1. PAIN OF RENAL ORIGIN

A. Acute Pyelonephritis   Pain begins in one lumbar area and spreads a short time later to the other, or begins simultaneously on both sides. The pain is dull and aching, and it may be intensified by bodily movements and jarring. Fever to 103°F or higher, chills or rigors, anorexia, nausea and vomiting, and malaise are usually present, but cases without fever or gastrointestinal symptoms occur. Irritative bladder symptoms may precede the onset of flank pain by 1 to 7 days, or may begin later. In some cases, these complaints are absent. Paraspinal muscle spasm and tenderness may be severe and may extend as far cephalad as the cervical region, causing headache, upper back and neck pain, and stiffness, mimicking the findings of bacterial meningitis. Bilateral costovertebral, and sometimes upper abdominal, tenderness are present. The urine is usually turbid and contains leukocytes singly, in clumps, and in casts, as well as red cells and bacteria. Urine cultures are positive for gram-negative bacteria [$\geq 10^5$ colony forming units (CFU)/ml] or for enterococci ($\geq 10^4$ CFU/ml). Blood cultures may be positive in up to 25 percent of cases. Most cases of acute pyelonephritis occurring in the absence of prior urinary tract instrumentation or surgery are caused by *Escherichia coli*, 30 to 40 percent of which are drug-resistant. *Klebsiella* and *Proteus* species are responsible for the majority of other initial attacks.

Infections caused by *Proteus, Klebsiella, Enterobacter, Pseudomonas, enterococci,* and *staphylococci* are more often present in patients who have had invasive urinary tract procedures.

Acute pyelonephritis responds to intravenous antibiotic therapy within 24 to 48 h. Failure of a clinical response to occur within 72 h may be related to a complication or an underlying disorder. Complications include pyonephrosis due to ureteral obstruction by a stone, a renal cortico-medullary abscess, or a perinephric abscess.

The excretory urogram is normal in 70 percent of cases of acute pyelonephritis. Delayed and decreased calyceal opacification, dilatation of the collecting system, and renal enlargement are the most common abnormalities reported in acute pyelonephritis. Fever persisting beyond 72 h in a patient treated for pyelonephritis has been associated with

excretory urographic findings of obstructive stone disease, an infected renal cyst, an abscess, or xanthogranulomatous pyelonephritis. The sonogram is usually normal in acute pyelonephritis. When the sonogram is abnormal in acute pyelonephritis, it may demonstrate renal enlargement, loss of parenchymal echoes, and corticomedullary differentiation. Ultrasonography can detect the presence of a renal or perirenal abscess. The CT scan with contrast is usually abnormal in patients with acute pyelonephritis. Nephrographic defects are usually present. Acute focal bacterial nephritis (AFBN) produces low-density striated wedge-shaped parenchymal defects extending from the cortex to the hilus. CT is more sensitive than ultrasonography for demonstrating nonabscess parenchymal infections. AFBN on CT can be mimicked by a carcinoma, a chronic inflammatory process, or a renal infarction. Delayed-contrast CT films demonstrating functioning parenchyma exclude abscess and neoplasm from the differential. An indium 111–labeled leukocyte scan can identify a renal CT mass lesion as inflammatory.

Ultrasonography may be used to follow the resolution of such an inflammatory renal mass. This practice will prevent missing the rare neoplasm that mimics AFBN. Imaging studies are also useful for detecting abnormalities that may increase susceptibility to pyelonephritis, such as a bifid collecting system, medullary sponge kidney, polycystic disease, nonobstructive stones, or ureteral stenosis. Males with a single attack of acute pyelonephritis should have a thorough urologic evaluation, including a search for chronic prostatitis. Women with uncomplicated cystitis or pyelonephritis usually respond promptly to antibiotic therapy and do not usually relapse. The absence of a therapeutic response or early relapse in a woman requires urologic evaluation.

B. Renal Cortical Abscesses   Three percent of cases involve both kidneys. Bilateral flank and back pain may begin simultaneously or sequentially. It is associated with a high fever, chills or rigors, drenching sweats, and prostration. There are bilateral costovertebral angle tenderness, and sometimes anterior upper abdominal tenderness, as well as paraspinal muscle spasm in the thoracolumbar area. A flank bulge may be noted on one or both sides. Chest examination may reveal basilar dullness due to diaphragmatic elevation or pleural fluid, with decreased breath sounds and rales present over the lower lobes posteriorly. Leukocytosis with a shift to the left of the differential count occurs in 95 percent of cases, and the urine is usually normal, but may contain leukocytes, red blood cells, and protein if the abscess has eroded into the renal medulla and/or calyces. This disorder usually arises as a result of hematogenous dissemination of staphylococci (90 percent of cases) from an infected skin site, bone, or heart valve. Trauma to the renal area, renal failure treated by hemodialysis, and diabetes mellitus are risk factors for cortical abscess. In up to one-third of cases, the prior infection is not remembered or noticed. The time interval from the initial infection to the onset of fever and flank pain may vary from a few days to several months (mean period, 7 weeks). Excretory urography may reveal bilateral intrinsic renal masses with caliceal distortion, but without renal displacement. Ultrasonography will demonstrate a thick-walled, fluid-filled parenchymal mass. An early renal carbuncle may resemble a neoplasm by ultrasonography if internal echoes are present. CT with contrast will usually define an abscess and differentiate it from a neoplasm. The presence of fever and rigors, and bilateral intrinsic masses, makes a diagnosis of neoplasm unlikely. Therapy involves administration of intravenous antibiotics. CT-guided percutaneous abscess aspiration or open drainage should be done if there is no response to antibiotic therapy within 2 to 3 days.

C. Acute Glomerulonephritis Bilateral flank pain may occur in a setting of acute nephritis. The urine may be grossly red, but it is usually smoky or gray-brown (i.e., coffee-colored). Malaise, fatigue, anorexia, nausea, and vomiting frequently accompany the urinary abnormalities. Only a minority of patients complain of flank discomfort, but bilateral costovertebral angle tenderness may be present in some patients without pain.

Microscopic examination of the urine demonstrates dysmorphic red blood cells (under phase microscopy, more than 80 percent of the red blood cells are distorted in size and shape, possibly resulting from passage through openings in the walls of damaged glomerular capillaries), red blood cell casts, pigment casts, and sometimes hyaline or granular casts. Daily proteinuria is in the .5- to 3-g range. Leukocytes and leukocyte casts reflect the level of renal inflammation.

During the first week of illness, hypertension, facial and peripheral edema, orthopnea, and dyspnea may develop. Creatinine elevation may occur with or without oliguria.

1. Acute Post-Streptococcal Glomerulonephritis (PSGN) Onset follows an episode of acute streptococcal pharyngitis within 6 to 10 days, or an episode of pyoderma within 10 to 14 days. Both types of infection are caused by nephritogenic streptococcal serotypes. A typical nephritic syndrome, as described above, may occur, or there may be few or no symptoms. The ratio of asymptomatic to symptomatic episodes is 3 to 1. Establishment of the diagnosis depends on isolation of a nephritogenic streptococcal serotype from the pharynx or a skin lesion, and/or demonstration of a significant antibody rise in one or more of the streptococcal exoenzymes [i.e., anti-streptolysin O (ASO); anti-streptokinase (ASK) anti-deoxyribonuclease B; anti-hyaluronidase (AH); or anti-nicotinyl adenine dinucleotidase (ANAdase)]. The sensitivity of testing for multiple antibodies (Streptozyme test) will exceed 90 percent if several serum samples are tested. A decline of serum C3 levels also occurs in this disorder, while C4 is

depressed minimally or not at all. Serum may test positive for cryoglobulins, immune complexes, and high-molecular-weight fibrinogen. Proteinuria is nonselective, and the urine contains high concentrations of fibrinogen degradation products and C3. Ultrasonography or a CT scan will show enlarged kidneys. Renal biopsy reveals a diffuse endocapillary proliferative glomerulonephritis, sometimes with leukocyte infiltration. Immunofluorescence studies demonstrate deposition of C3, properdin, and IgG in the glomerular capillary loops and mesangial regions. Sporadic episodes of this disorder in adults may lead to persistent renal insufficiency in up to 50 percent of cases. Flank or back pain is infrequently present in acute post-streptococcal glomerulonephritis, and when it is, it tends to resolve spontaneously within the first week of the illness.

Supportive therapy with rest, sodium restriction, loop diuretics, and antihypertensives will improve or prevent encephalopathy and pulmonary congestion. Dialysis may be required. If streptococcal infection is documented, it should be treated with penicillin or erythromycin.

2. Acute Postinfectious Glomerulonephritis Infection with viruses, other bacteria, or parasites may rarely be complicated by an acute nephritis, which is indistinguishable clinically from PSGN. The incidence of disease is low, relative to that associated with streptococcal infection. Infection with influenza virus, adenovirus, hepatitis B, Epstein-Barr virus, mumps, HIV, dengue, measles, varicella, echovirus, *Mycoplasma pneumoniae,* and coxsackievirus have been followed by acute glomerulonephritis. Infections with *Staphylococcus epidermidis* in patients with ventriculojugular or ventriculoatrial shunts, *S. aureus* or *Streptococcus viridans* in patients with endocarditis, and gram-negative intraabdominal infections have also been associated with this disorder. Case reports of occurrence after typhoid fever and secondary syphilis, and in association with sepsis have appeared. Toxoplasmosis and malaria may also give rise to glomerulonephritis. The nephritis associated with intraabdominal sepsis, endocarditis, and shunt infection will usually resolve after antibiotic therapy of the primary infection.

3. IgA Nephropathy (Berger's Disease) Bilateral dull loin pain and gross hematuria may occur. This disorder is more common in males (3 to 1) and is most frequently seen in the second and the fourth decade. The urine contains dysmorphic red blood cells, red blood cell and pigment casts, protein (up to 2 g/day), and sometimes leukocytes. Hypertension and renal insufficiency may develop in a minority of cases, but acute renal failure is uncommon. The hematuria and flank pain begin with, or follow, within 48 hours the onset of an upper respiratory illness (50 percent), influenza-like illness (15 percent), or gastroenteritis (10 percent). Patients with hypertension and nephrotic levels of protein loss are more likely to develop chronic renal failure. Renal biopsy is required for diagnosis, and it will demonstrate a focal glomerulonephritis with mesangial deposits of IgA and lesser amounts of IgG, C3, and properdin. Up to 50 percent of patients develop end-stage renal failure within 5 years of the first sign of disease. There is no effective therapy.

A similar form of nephritis occurs with Schönlein-Henoch purpura in association with a lower extremity erythematous maculopapular rash and/or palpable purpura, and, in some cases, joint pain and swelling; and abdominal pain.

4. Idiopathic Nephrotic Syndrome

There is heavy proteinuria (3.5 g/1.73 M^2/day) often, but not invariably, accompanied by hypoalbuminemia and generalized edema. Hyperlipidemia (i.e., elevated low-density lipoproteins and cholesterol) follows stimulation of liver lipoprotein synthesis by the low plasma oncotic pressure.

A. MESANGIAL PROLIFERATIVE GLOMERULONE-PHRITIS   Up to 10 percent of adults with the idiopathic nephrotic syndrome demonstrate mesangial proliferative glomerulonephritis on renal biopsy. Bilateral dull, aching flank pain, accompanied by gross hematuria, may occur. The urine may contain nephritic components (i.e., red blood cell casts, pigment casts, dysmorphic red blood cells, leukocytes, and leukocyte casts) and nephrotic elements (i.e., lipid bodies and casts, oval fat bodies, and protein). This combination has been described as "a telescoped urine" sediment. Renal biopsy demonstrates increased glomerular capillary cellularity on light microscopy. Immunofluorescent studies may identify various types of mesangial antigen deposits. Some patients have mesangial deposits of IgA, C3, and fibrin reacting antigens (i.e., Berger's disease), while others may demonstrate granular IgM deposits, C3 antigen, scattered deposits of IgG, or no demonstrable deposits. Mesangial proliferative glomerulonephritis may occur with postinfectious glomerulonephritis, hereditary nephritis, Schönlein-Henoch purpura, systemic lupus, and some forms of vasculitis. Bilateral flank pain may occur with any form of the idiopathic nephrotic syndrome, but is more common in patients with immunopathologic evidence of Berger's disease. Steroid responsiveness is associated with a benign course. Nonresponders have a greater tendency to progress to renal failure. This is more certain if there is a significant amount of focal glomerulosclerosis present on renal biopsy.

B. BILATERAL RENAL VEIN THROMBOSIS   Patients with the nephrotic syndrome may develop the sudden onset of bilateral severe aching flank pain, gross hematuria, a left-sided varicocele, and sometimes pulmonary emboli and infarction. Oliguria and progressive renal failure usually follow. There are bilateral costovertebral angle tenderness, fever, and evidence of venous collaterals on the abdomen if the vena cava

is also occluded. The diagnosis can be established by selective venography or by an abdominal CT scan or MRI. Therapy with tissue plasminogen activator, followed by the use of heparin, may relieve all complaints and restore the patency of the renal veins.

5. Rapidly Progressive Glomerulonephritis (RPGN)

A. IDIOPATHIC RPGN   This syndrome occurs in older adults (mean age, 58), with a slight male predominance. The initial prodrome resembles influenza, with arthralgias, myalgias, fever, and bilateral aching flank and abdominal pain. Sometimes hemoptysis and transient pulmonary infiltrates occur. An acute nephritic syndrome then develops, with gross or microscopic hematuria, proteinuria, and a rapid rise in creatinine. Oliguria is present in 50 percent of cases at presentation. Renal biopsy reveals that more than 50 percent of the glomeruli have prominent cellular crescents. Immunofluorescence studies reveal an absence of glomerular antibody deposits of the linear or granular type. No anti-basement membrane antibody is present in the serum, and there is no clinical or laboratory evidence of a systemic disorder. "Pulse" steroid therapy or plasma exchange may reverse deterioration of renal function in up to 75 percent of early cases, but the long-term preservation of renal function is not assured.

B. ANTI-GLOMERULAR BASEMENT MEMBRANE (GBM) ANTIBODY-MEDIATED RPGN   This disorder may begin with pulmonary symptoms such as hemoptysis and dyspnea, associated with fleeting pulmonary alveolar infiltrates (Goodpasture's syndrome) or without them. Acute nephritis soon follows the pulmonary symptoms, and may present with fever, bilateral flank pain of a dull, aching quality, and gross hematuria. The urine contains a nephritic sediment and protein. The creatinine level is elevated in 50 percent of cases when first seen. An anti-GBM antibody can be demonstrated with renal biopsy as a linear capillary immunofluorescent deposit in all glomerular capillary walls, and the presence of the anti-GBM antibody in serum can be detected by an indirect immunofluorescence test or by a radioimmunoassay. The renal lesion can be reversed by plasma exchange therapy, and the pulmonary lesion can be controlled with steroid "pulse" therapy. Some patients require dialysis and/or renal transplantation. Up to one-third of patients with anti-GBM-mediated disease do not have pulmonary symptoms, and may mimic idiopathic RPGN, but can be differentiated by renal biopsy and/or a serum anti-GBM antibody assay.

C. RPGN DUE TO IMMUNE COMPLEX DEPOSITION   This syndrome can be associated with granular IgG-C$_3$ deposits in glomeruli. It may occur in patients with postinfectious glomerulonephritis, systemic lupus erythematosus, Schönlein-Henoch purpura, and mixed cryoglobulinemia; and in the presence of an antigen derived from a carcinoma or lymphoma. Some primary renal diseases, such as idiopathic immune complex nephritis and membranoproliferative glomerulonephritis, may cause RPGN.

D. VASCULITIS-ASSOCIATED RPGN RPGN may occur in association with polyarteritis nodosa, hypersensitivity angiitis, or Wegener's granulomatosis in the absence of immune complex deposition.

D. Acute Interstitial Nephritis Due to Drugs—Hypersensitivity Nephropathy

There is an abrupt onset of fever, chills, malaise, and bilateral lumbar and costovertebral area pain and tenderness. The urine is coffee-colored or smoky, and may contain eosinophils and neutrophils, as well as red blood cells and protein. Up to 25 percent of patients have a maculopapular rash on the trunk, and peripheral eosinophilia may be present. Eosinophiluria has been associated with postinfectious glomerulonephritis and RPGN, and these disorders must be ruled out if this finding is present. Oliguria and renal failure are associated. Renal biopsy reveals increased numbers of interstitial mononuclear cells and eosinophils. This disorder begins within 3 days to 5 weeks after ingestion of a specific drug. In the past, methicillin was the most frequent offender, but many varieties of penicillin, the cephalosporins, and anti-tuberculous drugs; vancomycin, sulfonamides, and diuretics (e.g., thiazides, furosemide, chlorthalidone, and acetazolamide); allopurinol; nonsteroidal anti-inflammatory drugs; phenytoin; methyldopa; captopril; cimetidine; and others have been associated. Most cases respond clinically to discontinuance of the offending drug. With rare exceptions, laboratory evidence of renal failure is usually reversible.

E. Loin Pain Hematuria Syndrome

Bilateral dull, aching flank pain and gross hematuria, with or without associated hypertension, have been reported in young women taking oral contraceptives. The excretory urogram is usually normal, but a selective renal arteriogram may demonstrate stenosis and spasm of intrarenal vessels. Discontinuance of oral contraceptives leads to rapid resolution of symptoms.

F. Bilateral Renal Infarction

1. Embolic This disorder may follow showers of emboli arising in the heart (e.g., recent myocardial infarction, myocarditis, cardiomyopathy, atrial fibrillation, ventricular aneurysm, mitral stenosis, or bacterial endocarditis) or aorta (e.g., aneurysm or ulcerated atheroma). There is a simultaneous or sequential onset of pain in both flanks. It may be dull and aching, or severe and excruciating, as in renal colic. Pain may spread to the upper abdomen on one or both sides. Gross or, more commonly, microscopic hematuria and proteinuria are associated. Fever occurs after a 1- to 2-day latent period.

Elevation of serum LDH, AST, and alkaline phosphatase activities secondary to enzyme release from infarcted renal tissue may occur. With extensive bilateral infarction, oliguria and anuria develop, in association with a rising creatinine level. The diagnosis can be confirmed by observing failure of renal dye excretion during excretory urography or a CT scan, and preservation of normal renal structure imaged by retrograde pyelography or a CT scan. A renal arteriogram can provide specific evidence of renal artery occlusion. Use of thrombolytic therapy and anticoagulants may restore renal artery patency. In some cases, open surgery is required. Bilateral renal emboli may occur in up to 33 percent of cases.

2. Thrombotic Renal artery thrombosis rarely causes renal infarction on both sides within a brief time interval unless there is occlusion of the lower aorta. With aortic occlusion, there may be severe bilateral leg pain and weakness. The leg pain is sharp and severe, and affects the legs from the buttocks to the ankles. Lower extremity paresthesias and numbness may accompany the pain. Involvement of the kidneys is signaled by bilateral aching flank pain and tenderness, gross or microscopic hematuria, and oliguria. Absent femoral pulses provide evidence of aortic obstruction. Aortography will confirm the diagnosis and determine the extent of the process. Surgical intervention is often attempted for this disorder, and renal revascularization may restore impaired renal function partly or completely.

2. MYOFASCIAL PAIN

Bilateral flank and back pain occur, with diffuse or localized focal muscle tenderness in the affected region. In many patients, no tenderness is present. There may be precipitation of pain or pain intensification with specific flexion, extension, or rotational movements of the upper body. The pain may vary in intensity from hour to hour or over a period of days. Sneezing, coughing, or jarring can intensify the pain, but commonly have no effect. The urinalysis is normal, as are renal and spine imaging studies. Some cases are associated with an old or recent back injury, or repetitive strain of the affected back and flank muscles related to lifting or frequent bending during daily work.

Discontinuation or modification of the causative activity, use of nonsteroidal anti-inflammatory drugs, or injection of trigger points with lidocaine and methylprednisolone may bring partial or complete relief.

3. PLEURITIS

Pleuritis arising in both posterior hemithoraces may cause bilateral thoracolumbar and flank pain. At onset, sharp, sticking pain may be felt at the end of a deep inspiration or during coughing. Within 2 to 3 h, this pain appears earlier in the inspiratory phase, so that patients develop rapid, shallow breathing. The pain soon becomes a dull, constant ache that may still be intensified by a deep breath. Referral to the shoulder on one or both sides is common. Moving from a sitting to a lying position or in the reverse direction may intensify the pain. Bilateral pleuritic pain may be associated with the following.

A. Bilateral Bacterial Pneumonia Fever, chills or rigors, cough; and purulent, rusty (*Streptococcus pneumoniae*), mucoid, or currant-jelly sputum (*Klebsiella pneumoniae*) often accompany the pleuritic pain. Physical examination reveals bilateral basilar dullness, diminished bronchial breath sounds, one or more pleural friction rubs, and rales over the areas of basilar lung dullness. A chest radiograph will show bilateral lower lobe segmental or lobar consolidations and possibly a pleural effusion. A leukocytosis is usually present. Sputum Gram stains show gram-positive diplococci (*S. pneumoniae*), encapsulated gram-negative rods (*K. pneumoniae*), short pleomorphic gram-negative rods (*Haemophilus influenzae* strains), or no organisms (possibly *Legionella*). There is a prompt response of fever and pleuritic pain to appropriate parenteral antibiotic therapy.

B. Multiple Pulmonary Emboli Pleuritic pain at both lung bases posteriorly and laterally is frequently accompanied by dyspnea and sometimes by hemoptysis and fever. Physical examination may reveal tachycardia, fever, pleural friction rubs, rales, and signs of segmental or lobar consolidation and/or pleural fluid. The diagnosis may be confirmed by a ventilation-perfusion scan; color duplex flow imaging of a thigh vein thrombus; or a pulmonary angiogram. Heparin, followed by warfarin, therapy will usually lead to the resolution of symptoms and signs, and prevent recurrence. Risk factors associated with the occurrence of pulmonary emboli and infarction include immobilization; heart failure; malignancy; surgery; pregnancy; sickle cell disease; polycythemia; deficiency of anti-thrombin III, protein C, or protein S; paroxysmal nocturnal hemoglobinuria; drug abuse and tricuspid endocarditis; and the use of oral contraceptives.

C. Bilateral Pleuritis Due to Systemic Lupus Erythematosus This disorder may be associated with bilateral pleuritic thoracolumbar pain. Evidence of pleural fluid (i.e.,

dullness and decreased breath sounds) and pleuritis (i.e., pleural friction rubs) may be present on physical examination. The pleural fluid contains <3000 mononuclear cells/mm^3, decreased complement levels, and sometimes LE cells. An ANA titer $\geq$160 and a pleural fluid/serum ANA ratio >1 may occur. Criteria have been developed for the diagnosis of systemic lupus erythematosus. The presence of four or more of the following 11 criteria, either serially or simultaneously, allow the diagnosis with a high degree of probability. These include (1) malar rash; (2) discoid rash; (3) photosensitivity; (4) mouth ulcers; (5) non-erosive arthritis; (6) serositis (pleuritis or pericarditis); (7) renal disease (proteinuria, cylinduria, and/or azotemia); (8) neurologic disorder (seizures, psychoses, cognitive loss, or focal neurologic lesions); (9) hematologic disease (hemolytic anemia, leukopenia, and/or thrombocytopenia); (10) immunologic disorder [positive LE preparation (73 percent), anti-ds-DNA antibody (67 percent), or anti-Sm antibody] or a chronic biologic false-positive test for syphilis; and (11) an abnormal titer of antinuclear antibody. Using a requirement of four positive criteria, a small number of false-negative and false-positive diagnoses occur. Lupus-related pleuritic thoracolumbar pain will usually respond within 24 to 48 h to oral prednisone therapy.

D. Drug-Induced Lupus Bilateral pleuritic chest and flank pain, and sometimes pericarditis, may occur in association with fever and a positive ANA titer. Drugs commonly associated with this disorder include hydralazine, procainamide, isoniazid, chlorpromazine, methyldopa, and phenytoin. Discontinuance of the offending drug usually results in cessation of symptoms and signs within 1 to 3 weeks.

4. Spinal Osteomyelitis with Radicular Involvement

Pyogenic or tuberculous spinal osteomyelitis may cause midline thoracolumbar spinal ache, intensified by jarring or activity, and relieved by rest. Fever and malaise may accompany the pain. Radicular involvement may be signaled by unilateral and then bilateral paraspinal and flank pain of a dull or sharp quality. Leukocytosis and/or an elevated sedimentation rate are usually present. The diagnosis can be established by plain spine radiographs but confirmation may require a radionuclide scan or MRI. Relief of symptoms results from appropriate antimicrobial therapy.

CHAPTER

27

Acute Constant Generalized Abdominal Pain

☐ **DIAGNOSTIC LIST**

1. Perforation of the stomach or duodenum
2. Perforation of the gallbladder
3. Perforation of the small intestine
4. Perforation of the colon
   A. Ulcerative colitis
   B. Toxic megacolon and perforation
   C. Diverticulitis and perforation
   D. Ischemic colitis with perforation
   E. Carcinoma of the colon with perforation
   F. Appendicitis and perforation
5. Rupture of an abdominal abscess
   A. Subphrenic abscess
   B. Hepatic abscess
      1. Amebic
      2. Pyogenic
   C. Splenic abscess
   D. Perinephric abscess
   E. Tuboovarian abscess
   F. Rupture of a pericolic abscess resulting from perforation of a colonic diverticulum
6. Infarction of the small intestine
7. Obstruction of the small intestine
   A. Nonstrangulating
   B. Strangulating
8. Acute pancreatitis
9. Severe intraabdominal bleeding
   A. Ruptured ectopic pregnancy or ovarian cyst
   B. Rupture of the spleen, a splenic artery aneurysm, or the gallbladder

C. Rupture of a hepatic adenoma and anticoagulant-related bleeding
D. Abdominal apoplexy
E. Rupture of an abdominal aortic aneurysm
F. Dissecting aneurysm
10. Peritonitis in patients with ascites
    A. Spontaneous bacterial peritonitis
    B. Secondary bacterial peritonitis in cirrhotic patients with ascites
    C. Hemochromatosis
11. Peritonitis secondary to venous occlusion or arteritis
    A. Acute vascular catastrophes (venous occlusion)
    B. Arteritis involving the mesenteric vessels
       1. Polyarteritis nodosa
       2. Rheumatoid arthritis
       3. Schönlein-Henoch purpura
       4. Systemic lupus erythematosus
12. Peritonitis associated with neutropenic enterocolitis and acute leukemia (typhlitis)
13. Nonsurgical disorders causing generalized abdominal pain
    A. Acute intermittent porphyria
    B. Ketoacidosis
       1. Diabetic ketoacidosis
       2. Alcoholic ketoacidosis
    C. Black widow spider bites
    D. Lead poisoning
    E. Sickle cell pain crisis

F. Hemolytic crisis
G. Hyperparathyroid and
   hypercalcemic crisis
H. Addisonian crisis
14. Diffuse abdominal pain associated
    with specific infectious diseases

A. Tuberculosis of the ileocecal
   region and tuberculous
   peritonitis
B. Rocky Mountain spotted fever
C. Patients with AIDS and CMV
   enteritis

☐ SUMMARY

Perforation caused by peptic ulcer disease or malignancy *in the stomach* or ulcer disease *in the duodenum* releases an acidic solution of gastric enzymes into the peritoneal cavity. This material is extremely irritating to the peritoneum and causes immediate diffuse generalized abdominal pain, tenderness, rigidity of the abdominal wall muscles, faintness, and a shock-like state. Over the next 1 to 2 h, the pain lessens, and the shocklike state improves, but the abdominal tenderness and rigidity persist. Within 6 to 12 h after the onset of the initial pain, an infectious peritonitis begins, with more tenderness, pain, and abdominal distension. Many patients with duodenal ulcers have a long history of epigastric pain, partially or completely relieved by antacids and food. Some, with gastric ulcer or cancer, have a history of pain beginning soon after eating, and/or of weight loss. An upright radiograph of the abdomen or a left lateral decubitus view will show free air in 70 to 80 percent of cases.

Perforation of an infected gallbladder is preceded by right upper abdominal pain, tenderness, guarding, fever, and chills. On day 2 or 3 of the illness, there is a sudden improvement in the right-sided pain. During the next 24 h, generalized abdominal pain and tenderness, and finally peritoneal signs, develop, caused by leakage of chemically irritating and infected bile.

Crohn's disease may cause lower and midabdominal pain of a constant or intermittent nature, diarrhea, and fever. Attacks last for weeks or months, and often improve on prednisone or sulfasalazine. *Carcinoma of the small bowel* may cause anemia related to loss of blood in the stool, as well as colicky, midabdominal pain due to partial intestinal obstruction. Small bowel lymphoma may also cause bleeding and obstruction. If an area involved with Crohn's disease or a small bowel tumor perforates, intestinal content leaks into the free peritoneal cavity, producing generalized abdominal pain, fever, direct and rebound tenderness, and guarding due to peritonitis.

Perforation of the colon initially causes lower abdominal pain, tenderness, guarding, and a high fever. A painful tender lower abdominal mass may form. This almost always occurs in a colon in which there is an underlying disorder.

Ulcerative colitis causes frequent diarrheal stools, rectal bleeding, pain associated with defecation, and fever. When perforation occurs, generalized abdominal pain and tenderness develop over a 12- to 24-h period if not masked by prednisone therapy. Diffuse abdominal distension, pain, and tenderness in patients with ulcerative colitis may signal acute *dilatation of the colon* (i.e., *toxic megacolon*). Such patients are febrile and

toxic and may actually have fewer diarrheal stools than usual, or they may fail to pass stool at all. Abdominal radiographs show a markedly dilated colon. Such patients have a high risk of perforation, but the majority of episodes of colon leakage in ulcerative colitis occur in the absence of toxic megacolon. *Diverticulitis* usually causes left lower or mid-lower abdominal pain and tenderness, and fever. If a diverticulum perforates, or a *pericolic abscess* resulting from a previous perforation ruptures, generalized lower, and then upper, abdominal pain, tenderness, and guarding may occur. Abdominal pain associated with diverticulitis is often increased by defecation.

Ischemic colitis may cause lower abdominal pain, tenderness, diarrhea, bloody stools, and fever. Such patients are elderly and often have heart disease or a history of a stroke. Colonic perforation causes localized or diffuse lower abdominal pain, which spreads over the abdomen within a day. *Carcinoma of the colon* may begin with crampy, lower abdominal pain, new-onset constipation, frequent stools or diarrhea, and/or gross or chemically detectable blood in the stool. Free perforation adjacent to the carcinoma or secondary rupture of an abscess surrounding the tumor may cause a rapidly developing, generalized peritonitis. Distal obstruction may cause cecal distension, perforation, and localized right lower abdominal pain followed by generalized pain due to peritonitis.

Acute appendicitis usually begins as a midabdominal or epigastric pain, shifts to the right lower abdomen after 2–5 h, and is associated with well-localized direct and rebound tenderness. When the right, lower abdominal tenderness becomes more diffuse and/or a mass is felt, appendiceal perforation has probably already occurred. This inflammatory process may spread, to cause a generalized peritonitis.

Rupture of a formerly well-localized abscess into the free peritoneal cavity can cause rapidly spreading abdominal pain, diffuse direct and rebound tenderness, and guarding. Previous pain and tenderness in the right or left upper abdomen, spiking temperature elevations, and chills suggest a diagnosis of a subphrenic abscess. A chest radiograph may show an elevated diaphragm, a pleural effusion, and/or an air-fluid level in the abscess.

A CT scan will localize the abscess to one of four *subphrenic* spaces. A *liver abscess* may cause liver enlargement, tenderness, and fever. A CT scan will identify one or more abscesses in the liver. A *splenic abscess* causes fever, chills, left upper abdominal tenderness and pain, and splenic enlargement. A CT scan should confirm the abscess. A *perinephric abscess* causes fever, chills, flank pain, and sometimes pyuria. There is local tenderness over the affected kidney, and a chest radiograph may show a high diaphragm and/or pleural fluid on the side of the abscess. *Tuboovarian abscesses* (TOAs) cause lower abdominal pain on one or both sides, fever and chills, and pain during sexual intercourse. Tender enlargement of one or both tubes may be felt on pelvic exam. If a TOA ruptures, there is an abrupt onset of diffuse pelvic and lower abdominal pain and tenderness, and a fall in blood pressure. With massive spillage of pus, severe generalized abdominal pain and tenderness develop rapidly, accompanied by profound shock with skin pallor and coldness, tachycardia, and hypotension. The diagnosis can be confirmed by culdocentesis, laparoscopy, or laparotomy.

Infarction of the small bowel causes severe, colicky, and then constant periumbilical and epigastric pain, with only minimal tenderness and guarding during the first few hours after onset. Diarrhea develops, and the stool may contain gross or occult blood. Abdominal radiographs may be normal or may show one or more dilated loops of small bowel and air-fluid levels. Within 12 to 36 h, diffuse abdominal tenderness, guarding, and distension develop. In the elderly, this disorder may result from progressive stenosis of the superior mesenteric artery. Fifty percent of patients with occlusive disease due to thrombosis give a prior history of midabdominal pain after meals (abdominal angina) associated with weight loss and voluntary dietary restriction to small meals. The sudden onset of diffuse abdominal pain in a patient with atrial fibrillation and heart disease may be due to a mesenteric artery embolus. A number of patients with bowel infarction have no major vessel occlusions and are not candidates for arterial reconstruction. Nonocclusive infarction can be identified before exploration by an arteriogram. Infarction may be followed by transmural necrosis, perforation, leakage, and a localized or generalized peritonitis.

Obstruction (nonstrangulating) of the small intestine begins with intermittent, colicky, midabdominal pain, vomiting, and abdominal distension. If a loop of bowel is trapped by adhesions or in an internal hernia, the blood supply of the bowel can be occluded, resulting in severe, constant abdominal pain. In many cases, distension, tenderness, and guarding do not occur until after many hours, and plain abdominal radiographs may initially be negative. *Strangulation of bowel* may first cause localized tenderness without guarding. A tender mass may be felt. Perforation of the gangrenous loop leads to fever and other signs of an acute generalized peritonitis.

Acute pancreatitis begins with upper abdominal pain, tenderness, guarding, and fever. These signs may spread over the entire abdomen, resulting in generalized tenderness and distension. Elevated serum amylase and lipase levels are helpful in confirming the diagnosis.

Bleeding from intraabdominal vessels may cause the rapid onset of generalized abdominal pain and tenderness. A *tubal pregnancy* may cause lower abdominal pain on one side of the abdomen before rupture. There is often a history of a missed period and/or recent spotting. A similar history may be obtained in patients with a *corpus luteum cyst* of the ovary. Patients with a tubal pregnancy have positive pregnancy test results, while patients with a luteal cyst do not. Bleeding may

begin rapidly, causing generalized abdominal pain, tenderness, and shock.

Rupture of the spleen or a splenic artery aneurysm causes left upper abdominal pain and tenderness, shock, and sometimes left shoulder pain. *Rupture of the gallbladder,* as described above, can be associated with generalized abdominal pain and tenderness related to bleeding and bile leakage.

In some cases, the cause of the abdominal bleeding is not identified until surgery [e.g., bleeding tumor of the *liver (adenoma)* or *abdominal apoplexy* (a seemingly normal intraabdominal vessel begins to bleed)]. Patients on heparin or warfarin therapy may develop acute intraabdominal hemorrhage.

Patients with abdominal aortic *aneurysms* who bleed into the free peritoneal cavity usually die rapidly. Prior to the fatal hemorrhage, there may have been a history of lower or midabdominal, flank and/or lumbosacral pain associated with a midline abdominal pulsatile mass.

A *dissecting aneurysm* may cause "ripping" chest, upper back, and abdominal pain. A radiograph of the chest reveals a widened mediastinum, and the diagnosis can be confirmed by an aortogram or by a CT scan with contrast injection.

Spontaneous bacterial peritonitis occurs in patients with Laennec's cirrhosis with ascites. Fever, generalized abdominal pain, and tenderness are the common presenting findings. Peritoneal signs occur in less than half the cases. Paracentesis is required for diagnosis. An absolute neutrophil count exceeding 500 cells/mm^3 and pH <7.32 of the ascitic fluid are highly suggestive of the disease. Cultures are positive in 70 percent of cases and usually demonstrate a single aerobic pathogen. Identical clinical findings in a cirrhotic patient may result from bowel or gastric perforation. In these cases, the fluid leukocyte counts are very high, and polymicrobial isolates are common, but single isolates and low counts do not rule out an underlying gastrointestinal lesion. Acute abdominal pain and tenderness in a patient with *hemochromatosis* is most commonly due to spontaneous bacterial peritonitis.

Occlusion of the mesenteric and/or portal vein may cause generalized abdominal pain and tenderness, bloody diarrhea, and fever, and may result in peritonitis. The diagnosis can be confirmed by visualization of venous thrombi by a contrast CT scan or MRI. *Arterial occlusions* may result from vasculitis in multisystem disorders such as *polyarteritis nodosa, rheumatoid arthritis, Schönlein-Henoch purpura, systemic lupus erythematosus,* Behçet's syndrome, and Wegener's granulomatosis. Pain in the abdomen is caused initially by bowel ischemia and necrosis. Perforation may lead to generalized peritonitis.

Patients neutropenic from *acute leukemia,* aplastic anemia, cyclic neutropenia, or chemotherapy may develop generalized abdominal pain and right lower abdominal peritoneal signs, secondary to ulcerative mucosal disease of the cecum and ascending colon (i.e., *neutropenic enterocolitis*). This may progress to cecal gangrene, perforation, and peritonitis.

A number of nonsurgical disorders may mimic an acute surgical abdomen and lead to unnecessary laparotomy.

Acute intermittent porphyria causes generalized severe ab-

TABLE OF DISEASE INCIDENCE

INCIDENCE PER 100,000 (APPROXIMATE)

Common (>100)
Perforation of acute appendicitis
Infarction and necrosis of bowel secondary to an arterial embolus or thrombus
Rupture of tubal pregnancy or ovarian cyst with generalized intraabdominal hemorrhage
Spontaneous bacterial peritonitis associated with cirrhosis and ascites
Sickle cell crisis
Intestinal obstruction with strangulation of bowel
Intestinal obstruction without strangulation

Uncommon (>5–100)
Perforation of gastric ulcer or carcinoma
Perforation of duodenal ulcer
Perforation of gallbladder
Perforation of colon from:
    Ulcerative colitis
    Toxic megacolon secondary to ulcerative colitis
    Carcinoma of the colon
    Diverticulitis
    Ischemic colitis
Rupture of an intraabdominal abscess producing acute peritonitis:
    Tuboovarian abscess
    Pericolic or mesenteric abscess
Nonocclusive infarction of bowel
Acute pancreatitis with generalized peritonitis
Diabetic ketoacidosis
Secondary bacterial peritonitis associated with cirrhosis and ascites

Rare (>0–5)
Perforation of small bowel
Cecal rupture secondary to distal colon obstruction
Rupture of an intraabdominal abscess causing acute peritonitis:
    Hepatic abscess
    Splenic abscess
    Perinephric abscess
    Subphrenic abscess
Severe generalized intraabdominal bleeding due to:
    Rupture of spleen
    Rupture of gallbladder
    Rupture of splenic artery aneurysm
    Rupture of hepatic adenoma
    Abdominal apoplexy
    Anticoagulant therapy
    Free rupture of an abdominal aneurysm into the peritoneal cavity
    Dissecting aneurysm
Hemochromatosis and spontaneous bacterial peritonitis
Venous occlusions of mesenteric or portal veins
Bowel infarction and perforation secondary to:
    Schönlein-Henoch purpura
    Systemic lupus erythematosus
    Polyarteritis nodosa
    Rheumatoid arthritis
Hemolytic crisis
Hypercalcemic crisis
Addisonian crisis
Acute intermittent porphyria
Alcoholic ketoacidosis
Black widow spider bite
Lead colic
Ileocecal tuberculosis with perforation and acute peritonitis
Neutropenic enterocolitis
Rocky Mountain spotted fever and abdominal vasculitis
AIDS and CMV infection with bowel perforation and acute peritonitis and/or abscess formation

dominal pain with or without tenderness. Nausea, vomiting, and constipation are common accompaniments. Fever, hypertension, and tachycardia occur, and there may be evidence of a painful peripheral sensorimotor neuropathy and an encephalopathy with delirium or psychotic behavior. The diagnosis can be confirmed by detecting an elevated urinary excretion of porphobilinogen. *Diabetic ketoacidosis* may cause postural hypotension, nausea, vomiting, and generalized abdominal pain and tenderness, mimicking an acute surgical abdomen. The symptoms and signs clear within hours of initiating intravenous fluid and insulin therapy. Similar abdominal pain, tenderness,

and nausea and vomiting, may result from *alcoholic ketoacidosis,* and these complaints respond to rehydration and administration of glucose. There is usually a long history of alcohol abuse and an immediate history of heavy drinking, followed by 2 to 3 days of abstinence and starvation.

Black widow spider bites occur during the warm months of the year. The bite may sting or go unnoticed. Within an hour, there is an abrupt onset of generalized abdominal, back, and limb pains. Nausea, vomiting, muscle spasms, sweating, salivation, and tremors are commonly present. The abdominal muscles may become tender and rigid. Intravenous calcium or

10 percent methocarbamol provide symptomatic relief. *Lead poisoning* may cause crampy, generalized abdominal pain. Other findings include a wrist or foot drop, pallor, a lead line on the gingiva, and encephalopathy. Serum and urine lead levels are elevated.

Sickle cell anemia usually causes limb, back, and chest pain and tenderness, made worse by movement. Upper or diffuse abdominal pain and tenderness may occur. There is usually a long history of recurrent painful crises. *Hemolytic crises* in patients with red blood cell disorders may result in generalized abdominal pain, anemia, and high serum levels of bilirubin and LDH.

Hypercalcemia, secondary to *hyperparathyroidism,* malignancy, sarcoidosis, and other disorders may cause generalized abdominal pain and tenderness, lethargy or agitation and confusion, hypertension, constipation, nausea, and vomiting. Reduction of the serum calcium by fluid and diuretic therapy or the use of mithromycin results in symptom resolution. *Addisonian crisis* may result from idiopathic, tuberculous, or fungal disease of the adrenal gland or from withdrawal of steroid therapy. Patients have generalized constant or crampy abdominal pain, nausea and vomiting, confusion, and weakness. The serum sodium level may be normal or low, and the serum potassium level elevated or normal. The plasma cortisol level is very low. Symptoms respond to administration of corticosteroids. The diagnosis can be confirmed by measuring the plasma cortisol response to ACTH infusion.

Abdominal tuberculosis may cause ileocecal infection, resulting in acute perforation and a generalized bacterial peritonitis, or it may cause dense adhesions or scarring of the bowel lumen, leading to acute intestinal obstruction. A tender right iliac mass may be present and should raise the question of tuberculosis. *Rocky Mountain spotted fever* may present with localized or generalized signs of acute peritonitis, high fever, and headache, with or without the characteristic rash. History of a tick bite or exposure to ticks is helpful in establishing the diagnosis. Rare cases of *AIDS with CMV infection* of the bowel may result in perforation through a CMV-infected area. The resultant leakage leads to the development of an acute bacterial peritonitis and/or local abscess formation.

☐ DESCRIPTION OF LISTED DISEASES

1. PERFORATION OF THE STOMACH OR DUODENUM

Perforation of a gastric carcinoma or ulcer or a duodenal ulcer into the free peritoneal cavity causes the sudden onset of excruciating generalized abdominal pain as acidic enzyme-rich gastric juice spills into the abdominal cavity. Reflex-mediated shock occurs, with cold, clammy skin and a rapid, thready pulse. The body temperature may fall to as low as 95°F. The initial location of the pain is usually in the upper right or midabdomen. It spreads within minutes to involve the lower midabdomen and then the entire abdomen. The rapidity of spread is due to the fact that the insult is chemical and not dependent on the development of an acute inflammatory response to bacterial spillage. The latter reaction takes 6 to 24 h before it causes significant pain and tenderness. This acute period of severe pain and shock lasts for up to 2 h. Syncope may occur soon after the pain begins. When the intense pain secondary to spillage of gastric juice begins, the patient may writhe and roll from side to side, and sometimes curl up in the fetal position. Inspiring deeply and bodily movement increase the pain, so that patients breathe with rapid, shallow respirations; and as the initial severe pain subsides they lie quietly in bed without moving.

An hour or two after the onset, the pain improves. The temperature rises to normal, the pulse rate slows, and the pulse volume normalizes. The patient may say that he feels better. However, respirations remain shallow and rapid. Movements or jarring still intensify the pain, and the patient prefers to lie still in bed. During the first 2 h, the abdomen is diffusely tender, with boardlike rigidity of the abdominal muscles. These abdominal findings persist. The pelvic or rectal examination causes exacerbation of the pain in the lower abdomen. There is usually resonance due to free air that can be percussed over the liver area. If distinct resonance is found over the midaxillary line, 2 inches above the costal arch, free air is more likely to be present than if resonance is present only anteriorly. Bowel sounds are usually absent. Surgery should be performed within the first 6 h. If the diagnosis is missed and surgery delayed, the initial chemical peritonitis is soon replaced by an infectious form of this disorder. Pain and tenderness become more intense after 12 h, and vomiting, distension, and fever occur. Abdominal rigidity may decrease as distension progresses.

Free air under the diaphragm occurs in 75 to 85 percent of cases. Sixteen percent may have an elevated serum amylase level. The white blood cell count is usually elevated.

Referred pain may be felt in the right shoulder at the time of perforation and spillage when the perforation is in the duodenum or pyloric region of the stomach. Pain felt in both shoulders simultaneously usually arises from an ulcer of the anterior wall of the stomach.

Many patients presenting with the dramatic clinical findings described above will give a history of weeks or months of multiple daily episodes of gnawing or aching epigastric pain relieved by food or antacid ingestion. In others, there will be a history of food ingestion precipitating epigastric pain. Previous work-ups may have documented gastric or duodenal ulcers.

In summary, perforation, with spillage of chemically irritating and infectious material, causes severe pain almost instantaneously. If only infectious material spills, the onset of pain is more gradual before maximum intensity is reached (e.g., perforation of the colon).

Smaller leaks of gastric juice cause only local upper abdominal pain and tenderness if they are limited and walled off. It is possible to fail to appreciate the critical nature of this situation if the patient is seen during the remission period after the first 2 h. Even though the pain and pulse improve, there is still a tender, rigid abdomen, and the patient cannot move without increasing the amount of discomfort. These findings should support the decision to operate during the first 6 h.

At surgery, the abdomen should be suctioned and lavaged, and the perforated ulcer closed or resected. Patients with chronic duodenal ulcer disease may benefit from a selective vagotomy. The presence of gastric carcinoma requires more extensive surgery.

2. PERFORATION OF THE GALLBLADDER

This disorder usually begins as an attack of biliary colic with persistent mid-upper abdominal pain, nausea, and vomiting. Within 6 to 8 h, pain begins in the right upper abdomen and may radiate to the right shoulder or to the right subscapular region. Fever and shaking chills occur. There are tenderness and guarding, and sometimes an enlarged gallbladder can be felt or percussed in the right upper abdomen. In 1 to 2 percent of patients with acute inflammation of the gallbladder, perforation of the distended gallbladder, with spillage of bile and bacteria into the free peritoneal cavity, occurs on day 2 or 3 of the illness.

With perforation, there may be a dramatic decrease in right upper abdominal pain and tenderness. This relief lasts up to 1 or 2 days, but after this brief period, the previous pain is replaced by more generalized constant abdominal pain, tenderness, and distension. The temperature may rise to 103–105°F, and rigors and severe vomiting may occur. Abdominal radiographs may show dilatation of both the small and large bowel. Surgical exploration, with lavage and gallbladder drainage or removal, is required. The development of generalized abdominal pain is more gradual after leakage from the gallbladder than it is with perforation of an ulcer.

Antibiotic therapy and fluid replacement are essential in the postoperative period. Despite surgical intervention, the mortality rate is 30 percent.

3. PERFORATION OF THE SMALL INTESTINE

Crohn's disease causes abdominal pain, usually in the right lower abdomen, associated with fever and diarrhea. It is a chronic disease, and these symptoms may occur on a daily basis unless controlled by drug therapy. Sometimes drug-induced or spontaneous remission occurs. Free perforation is an uncommon event, since most perforations of the small bowel result in the formation of a fistula that joins the perforated bowel with adjacent small bowel, colon, or bladder.

With free perforation, generalized peritonitis develops over a 12- to 24-h period, with fever, generalized abdominal pain, direct and rebound tenderness, muscle guarding, distension, decreased or absent bowel sounds, nausea and vomiting, and sometimes signs of shock and dehydration. The white blood cell count is usually >20,000/mm^3. Plain abdominal radiographs show dilatation of the small and large bowel, and edema of the bowel wall. Diagnostic paracentesis may demonstrate intraperitoneal fluid containing neutrophils and bacteria. The development of a generalized peritonitis in a patient with a history of Crohn's disease indicates free perforation.

Small bowel perforation may also occur as the initial symptom in patients with *carcinoma* or *lymphoma* of the small bowel. In addition, patients with ischemia of the small bowel from embolic or thrombotic occlusion of the blood supply to the bowel wall may also perforate. Leakage of small bowel contents causes a generalized infectious peritonitis. Small bowel perforation due to disease is unusual and is more common after penetrating or blunt trauma.

4. PERFORATION OF THE COLON

The symptoms of free perforation are generalized abdominal pain and tenderness, associated with lower and midabdominal distension, vomiting, fever, and chills. These symptoms develop during a period of 6 to 24 h after the perforation and do not begin explosively, as do the pain and abdominal rigidity of a perforated ulcer.

It takes time for infectious agents to reproduce and initiate the intense inflammatory process on the peritoneal surface that causes the pain and distension. Abdominal radiographs show dilatation of the small and large intestines. The white blood cell count is usually elevated above 20,000/mm^3. Aspiration of peritoneal fluid reveals several types of bacteria and large numbers of polymorphonuclear leukocytes. Disorders associated with free perforation of the colon are discussed below.

A. Ulcerative Colitis This is a chronic diarrheal disease with a long history of lower abdominal, crampy pain associated with the desire to defecate, which is often relieved in part or totally by passage of solid or liquid stool. The stool may contain blood and mucus. Patients with severe degrees of colitis may spontaneously perforate, causing generalized infectious peritonitis. Up to 3 percent of patients with ulcerative colitis perforate in the absence of toxic megacolon. Perforation leads to the presence of free air under the diaphragm, generalized abdominal pain, distension, and direct and rebound tenderness associated with absent bowel sounds. Because of steroid therapy, direct and rebound tenderness and a rigid abdomen may not develop. Clues to perforation included a marked deterioration of the patient's general condition, an increase in the severity of abdominal pain, marked distension due to ileus and/or leakage of free air, and a decrease in bowel movement frequency. Perforation tends to occur in fulminating cases.

B. Toxic Megacolon and Perforation   This severe complication of colonic inflammation usually occurs in 1 to 2.5 percent of patients with ulcerative colitis. It can also occur in severe cases of Crohn's disease, bacterial dysentery, amebic colitis, ischemic colitis, and sometimes in typhoid fever and cholera.

These patients are very ill and toxic, with high fevers (up to 105° F), and chills. There are generalized abdominal pain; a protuberant, distended abdomen; and pain intensification with movement in bed. The pulse is rapid and of low volume, and there are profound weakness and usually some degree of mental confusion or clouding. Sweating may be profuse. The abdomen is tympanitic. Bowel sounds are absent or markedly decreased. There are usually low serum albumin and hemoglobin concentrations, and a white blood cell count >20,000 cells/mm^3.

Plain abdominal radiographs show dilatation of the entire colon or a segment, such as the transverse or ascending colon. The dilatation is >6 cm, measured in the mid-transverse or other dilated segments. Air may outline irregular ulcerations in the colon wall and may be present in the colon wall because of deep ulcerations in the mucosa. Some dilated loops of small bowel are usually present. If perforation has occurred, free air will be found beneath the diaphragm on an upright or right lateral decubitus radiograph.

The cause of this potentially lethal complication of severe colitis is unknown, but there is usually extensive necrotizing inflammation of the entire thickness of the colon wall.

Toxic megacolon secondary to severe ulcerative colitis may be treated with fluid and electrolyte replacement, transfusion, nasogastric suction, use of the prone position to decrease colon gas accumulation, withdrawal of opiates and anticholinergics, and intravenous administration of prednisolone and antibiotics (e.g., ampicillin, an aminoglycoside, and metronidazole).

Improvement results in a decrease in pain, distension, colonic dilatation, fever, and the signs of·prostration and shock. Only a minority of patients have such a therapeutic response, and most of these responders will need a colectomy within a year. Those who fail to improve in 48 to 72 h or who get worse within that time require surgery. If surgery is done before perforation, the mortality is 10 percent. If it is done after perforation, the mortality is 30 to 50 percent. A careful search for free air and worsening pain and tenderness should be conducted frequently to detect perforation as soon as it occurs, since corticosteroids (prednisolone) may mask the symptoms of this event. In many cases, a falling blood pressure, profuse sweating, and rapid pulse and respiratory rates may be the only signs of this catastrophic and highly lethal event. One-third of all deaths from ulcerative colitis result from perforation of the colon.

C. Diverticulitis and Perforation   Perforation of a colonic diverticulum may occur suddenly with minimal or no prodromal lower abdominal symptoms. There may be an abrupt onset of left lower or left upper abdominal pain. Uncommonly, the initial pain begins in the right lower or mid-lower abdomen. This pain and associated abdominal tenderness may spread over the entire abdomen during the next 12 to 24 h. Other signs, such as rebound tenderness, muscle guarding, loss of bowel sounds, and resonance over the liver, may occur. An upright radiograph of the abdomen may show free air under the diaphragm (50–60 percent). Abdominal distension develops as the peritonitis spreads. Fever, chills, vomiting, sweating, and a high leukocyte count complete the clinical picture of free perforation of a colonic diverticulum. Therapy requires the use of an aminoglycoside (for aerobic bacteria) and clindamycin or metronidazole (for anaerobic bacteria), intravenous fluids, nasogastric suction, and surgical intervention to create a colostomy and resect the perforated area of colon.

D. Ischemic Colitis with Perforation   Patients with this disorder are usually elderly. They may develop ischemia of the left colon with crampy and then steady left-sided abdominal pain, fever, and bloody diarrhea.

The use of sigmoidoscopy early in the course demonstrates ulcerations and blue-black nodules of the bowel wall. Plain radiographs show ''thumbprinting'' and mucosal ulcers. With gangrene of the bowel wall, perforation occurs and may cause generalized peritonitis and/or abdominal abscess formation.

E. Carcinoma of the Colon with Perforation   Patients with carcinoma may give a background history of recurrent lower abdominal crampy pain; rectal bleeding; narrow, pencil-sized stools; change of bowel habit, with increasing constipation or increasing stool frequency; rectal gas; or diarrhea. An iron deficiency anemia may occur secondary to right colon tumors.

If a tumor causes a perforation, it often occurs adjacent to or at the site of the carcinoma. Perforation into the free peritoneal cavity, to produce generalized abdominal pain and tenderness and fever, is uncommon. Usually, the perforation is small and leakage of colon content minimal, producing an abscess adjacent to the colon wall near the tumor. Such an abscess may increase in size and can later rupture into the free peritoneal cavity, causing generalized infection with severe pain, direct and rebound tenderness, and distension.

An obstructing carcinoma beyond the cecum may cause crampy lower abdominal pain, which may radiate across the abdomen from the right to the left side. In some patients, this pain is felt to end at about the point in the abdomen where the tumor is subsequently found to be located. Loud bowel noises may be heard by the patient in this region of the abdomen in association with brief episodes of pain. If the colon becomes completely obstructed and the ileocecal valve remains functional (80 percent of patients), the cecum may dilate as a result of tumor-related distal obstruction. If the cecum reaches a diameter of 10 cm, there is danger of cecal gangrene and perforation. This will cause the onset of acute right lower abdominal pain, free air under the diaphragm, and spreading generalized abdominal pain and tenderness due to polymicrobial peritonitis.

If complete distal colonic obstruction occurs, a dilated cecum should be decompressed. This can be done by performing a cecostomy or colostomy. The tumor and involved nodes should be resected.

F. Appendicitis and Perforation Acute appendicitis begins with epigastric or periumbilical pain, which lasts for 3 to 4 h and then ceases. Pain then appears in the right lower abdomen, associated with localized tenderness, nausea, vomiting, and fever to 100.5°F. If the appendix becomes perforated, there is often an increase of the temperature to 101 to 103°F, and the well-localized abdominal tenderness then becomes more diffuse in the right lower abdomen. If free perforation has occurred, pain and tenderness begin to spread over the left and mid-lower abdomen, and then up the left side, to involve the entire abdomen.

The pelvic or rectal examination may reveal generalized or localized pelvic tenderness, and bowel sounds are usually absent. The abdomen becomes distended and diffusely tender. The patient appears toxic and very weak. The temperature may rise to 104°F, and rigors and/or chills may occur. Sweating may be profuse. In some patients, a tender mass appears in the right lower abdomen or pelvis. Perforation is likely if symptoms have been present for more than 36 h, the temperature is over 101°F, the abdominal tenderness is no longer well-localized, and/or the white blood cell count is over 20,000/mm³.

Perforation can cause diffuse peritonitis, abscess formation, or both. Children and the elderly perforate before a diagnosis is made in the majority of cases. If surgery is performed within 12 h of onset, perforation is rare but can occur. Antibiotic therapy for appendicitis with generalized peritonitis requires the use of intravenous aminoglycosides, antianaerobic drugs (e.g., clindamycin or metronidazole) and ampicillin to eradicate enterococci, intravenous fluid infusion, nasogastric suction, abscess drainage, appendectomy, and delayed wound closure to prevent wound infection.

Patients treated medically may rquire subsequent surgery to drain the abscess in 13 to 33 percent of cases. If the abdominal mass and symptoms resolve in a few days, an elective appendectomy can be done in 5 or 6 weeks or postponed, since only 10 to 20 percent of cases of appendicitis recur if appendectomy is not performed.

The presence of chills, fever, and jaundice in a patient with appendicitis suggests that the infection has involved the portal vein. This complication requires intensive prolonged antibiotic therapy.

Peritonitis may resolve completely with antibiotic therapy, abscess drainage, and removal of the appendix. In some cases, the peritonitis clears but new abscesses form that require drainage. This is signaled by persistent spiking temperature elevations and sweats. These abscesses can be located by CT scan and may be drained percutaneously.

Rarely, a spreading peritonitis can result from rupture of a Meckel's diverticulum.

5. RUPTURE OF AN ABDOMINAL ABSCESS

A. Subphrenic Abscess An abscess beneath the diaphragm may cause right or left upper abdominal pain and/or flank pain, spiking fevers, rigors, chills, drenching sweats, and tenderness over the upper abdomen and the lower chest. Some abscesses are painless and do not cause tenderness of the chest wall. A plain abdominal radiograph may show a gas-fluid level beneath one diaphragm, and a pleural effusion may appear on the affected side. The diaphragm, on physical examination and by fluoroscopy, may be high and fixed. A CT scan will localize the abscess, allowing for surgical or catheter drainage. If a subphrenic abscess ruptures into the free peritoneal cavity, generalized pain, diffuse direct and rebound tenderness, and toxicity will occur, due to acute bacterial peritonitis.

B. Hepatic Abscess

1. Amebic Pain occurs in the right upper abdomen, and is usually constant and aching. Sometimes it may be sharp and stabbing, and made worse by a deep breath. Fever, chills, and malaise occur. Nausea and vomiting, and weight loss are often present, but jaundice is infrequent. There usually is liver enlargement and localized tenderness in the right upper abdomen or the midabdomen if the left lobe is involved. The tenderness is often well-localized. The ipsilateral hemidiaphragm is usually elevated and a hepatic friction rub may sometimes be audible. A sonographic or CT scan will demonstrate the abscess. If a right hepatic abscess ruptures into the right pleural cavity it produces a painful pleuritis. Rupture into the free peritoneal cavity causes generalized peritonitis with a 75 percent mortality rate. Amebiasis can also cause death by rupture of the colon secondary to deep ulceration or toxic megacolon. Some amebic liver abscesses resolve without drainage if metronidazole (750 mg, three times a day) is taken for 10 days.

2. Pyogenic   This type of abscess may arise in a setting of gallbladder disease, following trauma, another focus of abdominal infection (e.g., diverticulitis, appendicitis, and cancer with perforation of the colon or stomach), or disseminated bloodstream infection. The clinical picture is one of spiking fevers and chills, weakness, malaise, and weight loss. Some patients present with pleuritic chest pain, hemoptysis, and dyspnea. Right upper abdominal pain, hepatic enlargement, and tenderness also occur (50 percent), but in many cases the only symptom is a low-grade fever.

Jaundice, due to bile duct obstruction related to the abscess, may occur. The serum alkaline phosphatase level may be elevated and the albumin level decreased in up to 75 percent of cases. Bilirubin levels are elevated in 50 percent of patients, while the AST and ALT levels are usually normal. Some patients may have an abnormal chest radiograph (i.e., pleural effusion, pulmonary infiltrate, atelectasis, and/or an elevated hemidiaphragm). A pyogenic liver abscess can be visualized by ultrasonography, CT, or MRI. Treatment consists of surgical or percutaneous catheter drainage under CT guidance and antibiotic therapy.

Amebic abscess is more likely if the patient is under 50, there is a history of bloody diarrhea, ameba are found in the stool, and there is no underlying reason for a pyogenic abscess. Patients with an amebic abscess have a positive indirect hemagglutination test for amebiasis in up to 95 percent of cases.

Rupture of a pyogenic liver abscess into the free peritoneal cavity causes generalized peritonitis with diffuse abdominal pain, tenderness, guarding and toxicity.

C. Splenic Abscess   Fever and left upper abdominal pain and/or tenderness occur. The pain may also be felt in the left lower chest and is usually increased by a deep breath. Left shoulder pain from subdiaphragmatic irritation may occur. The spleen is usually enlarged and may be tender. An elevated left diaphragm and a left pleural effusion may be present on a chest radiograph. A left upper quadrant soft tissue mass, gas in the spleen, or displacement of the colon or stomach may be seen on a plain abdominal radiograph. A radionuclide, sonographic, or CT scan or MRI can confirm the diagnosis. Intravenous antibiotic therapy and splenectomy are required for cure.

Rarely, a splenic abscess may rupture into the free peritoneal cavity, causing generalized pain, tenderness and guarding, and toxicity.

D. Perinephric Abscess   Pain occurs in one flank, with local tenderness, fever, and chills. Frequent and burning urination may occur, and a tender flank mass may develop. The chest radiograph may show lower lobe infiltrates, atelectasis, a pleural effusion, and/or an elevated hemidiaphragm on the affected side. An intravenous pyelogram will show poor visualization of the kidney, distorted calyces, and displacement of the kidney anteriorly. A sonographic or CT scan will identify the abscess. Treatment requires the use of parenteral antibiotics, drainage of the abscess, and relief of urinary obstruction. Such abscesses may rarely rupture and drain into the free peritoneal cavity, causing a generalized peritonitis.

E. Tuboovarian Abscess (TOA)   This disorder may begin with fever, vaginal discharge, and lower abdominal pain on one or both sides. The pain may be intensified by walking or by sexual intercourse, so that intercourse is avoided. Tenderness occurs on movement of the cervix and palpation of the lower abdomen and the adnexae. Either one or both tubes may be enlarged to the width of a thumb or sausage. A TOA may rupture spontaneously or following sexual activity or a pelvic examination. This causes the sudden onset of lower abdominal and pelvic pain and tenderness, rigors, chills, and high fever. Such patients may become severely hypotensive, with a rapid, thready pulse, and severe prostration. Within hours, a generalized peritonitis may develop. Abdominal distension due to paralytic ileus develops, and the patient may appear near death. Temperature elevations to 107 to 108°F have been observed in some patients.

Surgical intervention for rupture should be initiated without delay, under cover of intravenous antibiotics and fluids. Hysterectomy, with removal of both tubes and ovaries, should be performed; large collections of pus removed; and the pelvis lavaged.

F. Rupture of a Pericolic Abscess Resulting from Perforation of a Colonic Diverticulum   Diverticulitis usually involves only one diverticulum. Once inflamed, this diverticulum may leak intestinal bacteria into the free peritoneal cavity or into a walled-off area adjacent to the perforation forming a pericolic abscess. Left, and rarely right, lower abdominal pain, tenderness and guarding, and fever occur, and a tender mass may be felt on abdominal or rectal examination. If a pericolic abscess ruptures into the free peritoneal cavity, generalized abdominal pain, direct and rebound tenderness, guarding, distension, and profound prostration occur over a period of several hours. Surgery to drain the abscess and resect the involved portion of the colon is necessary.

6. INFARCTION OF THE SMALL INTESTINE

Acute loss of the blood supply to part or all of the small intestine initially produces crampy midabdominal pain.

Within a period of hours, the pain becomes more severe and constant and is felt over most of the abdomen. In up to 50 percent of cases, the symptoms may be so mild that there is a delay of several days before medical care is sought. Bowel sounds may be present early in the course of this disorder, and when colicky pain is present, they may be loud and hyperactive.

Despite the presence of constant pain during the early phase of this illness, the abdominal examination may reveal only a flat abdomen with minimal or no tenderness. As the disorder progresses, the abdomen becomes more distended and tender, and the vital signs begin to reflect the severity of the illness, as fever, tachycardia, tachypnea, and hypotension occur. The leukocyte count becomes markedly elevated (to >30,000).

If bowel necrosis occurs, signs of peritonitis with direct and rebound tenderness, muscle guarding, and abdominal distension appear. Bowel sounds become muted. Plain radiographs show many dilated segments of small bowel with gas-fluid levels indicating intestinal stasis. Stool may contain gross or occult blood. The serum amylase and alkaline phosphatase levels may be elevated.

In up to 50 percent of the patients with infarction secondary to occlusion of the superior mesenteric artery, a history of intestinal angina is present. Most patients with small bowel infarction are over 60 and have a history of angina, myocardial infarction, stroke, or peripheral vascular disease.

At surgery, the bowel looks pale white from ischemia. Extensive bowel resection and arterial reconstruction are required. Since delayed infarction of the nonresected bowel may occur, many surgeons operate again at 24 h to determine if further resection is necessary. The mortality rate is very high. Elderly patients with intestinal angina should have an angiogram of their celiac and superior mesenteric arteries in the hope of finding a stenotic vessel that can be dilated or bypassed before an abdominal catastrophe occurs.

As many as 65 percent of patients with bowel infarction have intense vasoconstriction without occlusion of a major intestinal artery. In such cases, arterial bypass or angioplasty is of no help in revascularizing the bowel. The use of digitalis or diuretics may play a contributory role in precipitating this disorder. If the angiogram is negative for large vessel occlusion, vasodilator drugs may be tried to limit bowel ischemia and necrosis. Severe heart failure, shock, and hypovolemia may also cause small bowel vasoconstriction and ischemia.

In patients with a history of myocardial infarction, cardiomyopathy, valvular disease, or arrhythmias, embolic occlusion of a normal artery may occur. In such cases, early removal of the embolus and resection of the injured bowel results in a high rate of survival. Preoperative angiograms may be done to confirm the diagnosis of embolism, but they are seldom useful.

7. OBSTRUCTION OF THE SMALL INTESTINE

A. Nonstrangulating Small intestinal obstruction causes midabdominal colic, with each pain period lasting 2 to 5 min. The pain may be accompanied by loud, high-pitched bowel sounds. Each attack is separated from the next by a 5- to 10-min pain-free interval. With time, abdominal distension, hiccups, nausea, and vomiting occur. At first, the vomitus is yellow or green-tinged. After several hours, it may become orange-brown and feculent if the obstruction involves the lower small bowel. As the small intestine distends, the soft, minimally sensitive abdomen of early obstruction becomes tender, and the colicky pain becomes more generalized and constant. Fever, tachycardia, peritoneal signs, and an elevated white blood cell count suggest the possibility of strangulation. In one study, 90 percent of patients with strangulation had two or more of these findings.

Failure to pass feces and gas may be a late symptom of obstruction. During the first few hours, the colon may empty spontaneously, passing gas and feces, but after the first 6 h, no gas or feces is passed in a complete obstruction. The diagnosis of small bowel obstruction can be supported by abdominal plain radiographs that show small bowel dilatation, gas-fluid levels, and a colon with absent or few gas shadows.

B. Strangulating The onset of severe, diffuse, and constant abdominal pain, with a soft, nontender, nondistended abdomen, is suggestive of closed-loop obstruction of the small bowel or ischemic infarction. Nausea, vomiting, and distension develop over the next 6 to 18 h. A dilated small bowel with gas-fluid levels may not occur in up to 50 percent of cases of strangulated bowel, since such changes are late findings in this form of obstruction. A general haze (due to free fluid) and a coffee bean–shaped mass (due to edematous necrotic bowel) may be seen on plain abdominal radiographs in some cases.

If intestinal obstruction appears likely because of clinical findings and the abdominal radiographs are normal, there is a strong likelihood of the presence of intestinal strangulation and gangrene. It is important that the diagnosis of obstruction not be dismissed in the presence of clinical findings because of normal radiographs.

Some cases of simple obstruction seen early in their course may also have normal abdominal radiographs, since bowel distension may not have had enough time to develop.

Complete obstruction requires surgery, unless tube decompression over a 6-h period relieves it. The danger in delay is related to the presence of gangrenous bowel. Gangrene can result in perforation and generalized peritonitis. Persistent abdominal pain and tenderness after gastric or long intestinal tube decompression; and/or fever, tachycardia, and hypotension indicate a need for immediate surgery.

In nonstrangulating obstruction, the death rate is 5 to 10 percent, while in strangulating obstruction, it is 2 to 7 times higher.

8. ACUTE PANCREATITIS

This disorder occurs in patients with alcohol abuse, gallstones, or elevated serum triglyceride levels.

Pain begins in the epigastrium and left upper abdomen, and is associated with upper abdominal tenderness and, in 50 percent of cases, upper lumbar back pain. There are fluid losses from fever; sweating; vomiting; and into the retroperitoneum near the pancreas, the abdominal cavity, and the bowel lumen. The resultant hypovolemia causes faintness, weakness, and dizziness on standing.

The abdominal cavity may fill with enzyme-rich pancreatic fluid, producing a diffuse chemical peritonitis. The patient may appear pale or ashen gray and tachypneic. Vomiting and retching are frequent. Temperature ranges from 100 to 103°F. Tachypnea and hypotension may be present, as well as generalized abdominal tenderness and signs of ascites. After 3 to 5 days, green-brown discoloration of the flanks or umbilicus may occur, as intraabdominal blood seeps into the tissues of the abdominal wall.

The serum amylase is usually 2 or more times the normal level. This enzyme can increase in the serum in patients with diabetic ketoacidosis or other types of acidosis; with bowel perforation or infarction; or after a tubal pregnancy ruptures. Serum isoamylase levels are abnormal in pancreatitis and are less likely to be so in the other disorders.

An elevated serum lipase level in a clinical setting compatible with a diagnosis of pancreatitis is confirmatory of the diagnosis. Measurements of lipase levels are not sensitive enough to rely on in all cases. Plain abdominal radiographs may show some or all of the following findings in acute pancreatitis:

1. A "sentinel loop" (a gas-filled loop of small bowel near the pancreas)
2. The "colon cut-off sign" (an irritative spasm of the splenic flexure of the colon with absence of gas beyond this point in the colon)
3. Paralytic ileus
4. Diffuse haziness from pancreatic ascites
5. Gastric displacement
6. Pancreatic calcifications (due to chronic inflammation)
7. "Gas bubbles" or gas-fluid levels in pancreatic tissue related to an abscess

In 20 to 30 percent of patients, cough, shortness of breath, and pleuritic chest pain occur. Chest radiographs may demonstrate pleural effusions, elevated hemidiaphragms, atelectasis, and lower lobe infiltrates.

Therapy for acute alcoholic pancreatitis consists of restriction of oral intake, nasogastric suction, meperidine, and intravenous crystalloid-containing fluids. Antibiotics should be used if infection is likely, and blood transfused for anemia and a severe decrease in blood volume.

For patients with an irritating pancreatic ascites, peritoneal lavage may be helpful. A percutaneous catheter can be used and lavage carried out over a 3-day period. Surgery has been advocated to debride necrotic pancreatic tissue, drain abscesses or pseudocysts, relieve duodenal obstruction, or control extensive bleeding. If pancreatitis is related to gallstone impaction in the distal end of the common duct, its endoscopic removal within 24 to 36 h will facilitate recovery.

9. SEVERE INTRAABDOMINAL BLEEDING

A. Ruptured Ectopic Pregnancy or Ovarian Cyst Patients may have generalized abdominal pain and tenderness, and, in some cases, bilateral or unilateral shoulder pain. Cold clammy skin, a rapid, thready pulse, and hypotension are common associated findings.

Early manifestations of *ectopic pregnancy* include unilateral crampy lower abdominal pain; a missed period and/or spotting or staining; a positive pregnancy test; and a tender, enlarged tube. If the diagnosis is not made prior to rupture, rapid blood loss and life-threatening shock may occur.

Ovarian cysts, such as follicle or luteal cysts, can cause the sudden onset of lower abdominal pain, which can become generalized. Severe bleeding is associated with tachycardia and hypotension. In the presence of massive uncontrolled bleeding, volume replacement with crystalloid and blood, and immediate anesthesia and surgery are required.

B. Rupture of the Spleen, a Splenic Artery Aneurysm, or the Gallbladder Spontaneous *rupture of the spleen* may occur in patients with malaria, infectious mononucleosis, or myeloproliferative disorders. This may cause left upper abdominal and shoulder pain, and hypovolemic shock. Rapid surgical intervention is required. *Rupture of an aneurysm of the splenic artery* can also cause severe intraabdominal bleeding. Such patients may have a vague history of left upper abdominal pain, and a bruit may be audible in that area. Rarely, profuse bleeding may occur after *gallbladder rupture* secondary to cholecystitis. There is a history of 2 to 3 days of fever and constant right upper abdominal pain and tenderness, followed by abrupt pain relief as the gallbladder ruptures. Extensive bleeding resulting from these disorders may cause diffuse abdominal pain and direct and rebound tenderness over the entire abdomen.

C. Rupture of a Hepatic Adenoma and Anticoagulant-Related Bleeding Drugs may lead to intraabdominal bleeding. Young women using oral contraceptives may develop benign liver tumors (adenomas) that may bleed extensively into the free peritoneal cavity, producing generalized abdominal pain, accompanied by shoulder pain, generalized tenderness, and shock. Patients taking warfarin or heparin may bleed into the free peritoneal cavity with the development of generalized pain and tenderness.

D. Abdominal Apoplexy Some patients develop generalized abdominal pain, tenderness, pallor, and shock due to spontaneous intraabdominal hemorrhage. They are often hypertensive and elderly. Surgical exploration and ligation of the bleeding point is the procedure of choice. In cases where the bleeding point is elusive, the mortality rate is higher. The vessels involved are the gastric arteries or a branch of the superior mesenteric artery. No aneurysms are present, but extensive atherosclerosis usually involves the responsible vessel.

E. Rupture of an Abdominal Aortic Aneurysm Most aneurysms are asymptomatic until they begin to bleed. Mild bleeding may cause a throbbing or aching epigastric pain. Pain may also be felt in one or both flank areas, the lower quadrants, and/or the back. A pulsating, poorly defined, tender mass of diameter >4 cm is present just above the umbilicus in the midline.

Such aneurysms may rupture and bleed into the free peritoneal cavity, causing rapid exsanguination and generalized pain. The only hope for salvage is immediate surgery. The presence of an aneurysm can be confirmed by use of a sonographic or CT scan.

Aneurysms may also bleed into the retroperitoneum, causing a painful, pulsating left flank mass, or right lower abdominal pain. The pain from a leaking aneurysm may be worse when the patient lies down and improve when he sits up and leans forward (14 percent of cases), thus mimicking the pain relief seen with pancreatic disease.

The mortality of elective surgery of aneurysms is 10 percent. The expected rupture rate for 4- to 6-cm aneurysms over a 10-year period is 20 percent, while larger aneurysms have a 50 percent rupture rate.

F. Dissecting Aneurysm The attack usually begins with a tearing, sharp chest pain that radiates successively into the neck, back, and abdomen in rapid sequence. The pain is often so severe that the patient finds no relief even with narcotics. Such a patient may writhe about in bed. There is often a history of hypertension. Pulses in the limbs may be unequal. A new aortic diastolic murmur appears in 50 percent of cases due to retrograde dissection of the aortic valve, and the electrocardiogram may show

evidence of an inferior wall myocardial infarction (10 to 15 percent of cases). Involvement of the right innominate or left carotid artery can cause hemiparesis and/or aphasia. Dissection in the region of the renal arteries may cause flank pain and hematuria. A chest radiograph will show mediastinal widening. The diagnosis can be confirmed by a catheter aortogram or by a CT scan with contrast infusion.

Blood pressure should be lowered and propranolol given to reduce the force of myocardial contraction, since this may aggravate the dissection. Dissection of the ascending aorta requires surgical correction. Type 3 dissections, beginning below the left subclavian artery, cause chest and abdominal pain, and have a better outcome. Surgery should be performed if symptoms progress despite medical management. The abdominal pain may be due to bleeding into the aortic wall or to bowel ischemia and necrosis resulting from interruption of nutrient vessels by the dissection. In contrast to abdominal aortic aneurysms, rupture of a dissecting aortic aneurysm into the retroperitoneum is rare.

10. PERITONITIS IN PATIENTS WITH ASCITES

A. Spontaneous Bacterial Peritonitis This disorder occurs in patients with Laennec's cirrhosis and ascites. Fever occurs in 50 to 80 percent, diffuse abdominal pain in 27 to 72 percent, and direct or rebound tenderness in more than 50 percent of cases. Hypotension occurs in 5 to 14 percent of early, and in 70 to 100 percent of late cases. Up to 48 percent of patients with peritoneal infection may have no abdominal pain or tenderness. Patients developing this disorder usually have severe portal hypertension with ascites and hepatic dysfunction. The onset of diarrhea, a rising creatinine level, hypothermia, or worsening mental function may result from intraperitoneal infection.

Diagnostic paracentesis reveals ascitic fluid with an absolute polymorphonuclear (PMN) leukocyte count >500 mm^3 (sensitivity, 86 percent; specificity, 98 percent). Patients with a PMN count >1000 mm^3 should be treated regardless of culture results, since up to 35 percent of cases may be ascitic fluid culture negative. Patients with counts >250 and <1000 PMN cells/mm^3 should be treated with parenteral antibiotics, pending culture results and changes in clinical findings. Other tests that help support a diagnosis of infection include an ascitic fluid lactate level of >25 mg/dl (81 percent sensitive, 94 percent specific) and an arterial-ascitic fluid pH gradient >0.1. Combinations of findings such as a PMN count >500/mm^3 and/or a fluid pH <7.35 are 100 percent sensitive and 96 percent specific. A PMN count >500/mm^3 appears to be the best single predictor of bacterial infection. *Escherichia coli* (47 percent), *Klebsiella* species (11 percent), and other gram-negative enteric bacteria (11 percent) account for 69 percent of infections, and gram-positive bacteria [*Streptococcus pneumoniae* (8 percent), enterococci (5 percent), streptococci (12 percent), and staphylococci (5 percent)] cause 30 percent. Polymicrobial infection (8 percent) is uncommon, and most cases yield a single isolate. Anaerobic and microaerophilic organisms are seldom cultured (5 percent). In patients with clinical findings, an ascitic fluid PMN count $>500/mm^3$, and negative cultures (16 to 35 percent), the clinical and ascitic fluid white blood cell count responses to antibiotic therapy are helpful in management.

While spontaneous bacterial peritonitis in adults is most commonly associated with alcoholic cirrhosis and ascites, it has been reported in other types of liver disease, including postnecrotic cirrhosis, chronic active hepatitis, acute viral hepatitis, hemochromatosis, and metastatic liver disease. Rare cases have been reported in patients with cardiac ascites and in patients with systemic lupus erythematosus. The three cases associated with cardiac ascites were caused by an enterococcus (1) and *S. pneumonia* (2). The presence of ascites appears to be essential for the development of this disorder.

A Gram stain of centrifuged ascitic fluid may guide therapy. The presence of two or more types of bacteria indicates a requirement for anaerobic coverage. Intravenous use of a third-generation cephalosporin, and metronidazole or clindamycin when required, usually eradicates the infection, but mortality remains high (48 to 57 percent), and is usually due to the associated liver disease. Only 20 to 29 percent of deaths are due to peritonitis.

B. Secondary Bacterial Peritonitis in Cirrhotic Patients with Ascites The clinical picture of fever, diffuse abdominal pain and tenderness, and clinical deterioration may be identical to that produced by spontaneous bacterial peritonitis. The presence of free air on a plain abdominal radiograph suggests the diagnosis of a perforated viscus (e.g., duodenum or stomach). An ascitic white blood cell count $>10,000/mm^3$, a protein level >2.5 g/dl, an LDH level >225 IU/ml, and a glucose level <50 mg/dl are suggestive of secondary peritonitis caused by leakage of bacteria into the peritoneal cavity from a perforated viscus.

Ascitic fluid cultures usually grow multiple bacterial pathogens, including anaerobes, but in some series cultures have yielded only a single organism in the presence of gallbladder perforation or empyema, perforated gastric or duodenal ulcers, or ischemic colitis. In alcoholic patients, ulcer perforation is the most common cause of secondary peritonitis.

In one small series, ascitic fluid protein levels (4.4 ± 1.5) were greater in secondary peritonitis than in spontaneous bacterial peritonitis (SBP, 0.81 ± 0.4 g). There is considerable overlap in ascitic fluid leukocyte counts between cases of SBP and secondary peritonitis. The white blood cell count in SBP can range from 40–27,000/mm^3, with a mean of 6084/mm^3. In one series, the ascitic fluid white blood cell count was 23,756 ± 11,000 in patients with secondary peritonitis.

Cirrhotic patients without peritonitis have a mean ascitic fluid white blood cell count of 150 ± 100/mm^3, with a range of 28 to 1800/mm^3 and a mean percentage of PMNs of 43 percent. Diuretic therapy may increase the ascitic fluid white blood cell count to concentrations $>2000/mm^3$. The increase in cell count during diuresis is usually due to an increment in mononuclear cells. Because of this overlap in white blood cell concentrations between infected and uninfected fluids, Gram stains and cultures are important confirming tests when counts are in the overlap range (500–1000 PMN cells/mm^3).

Secondary peritonitis in patients without ascites is associated with polymicrobial infection and a high prevalence of anaerobes (81 percent). Polymicrobial infection may also occur in patients with ascites, but the prevalence of anaerobes may be lower because of the relatively high Po$_2$ of ascitic fluid. The presence of single aerobic isolates does not rule out a primary intraabdominal lesion requiring surgical management. In suspected cases, clinical findings and use of CT or sonographic scans, contrast bowel studies, laparoscopy, or endoscopy will usually identify the underlying disorder. Unless timely surgical intervention is undertaken, secondary peritonitis has a uniformly fatal outcome.

C. Hemochromatosis This disorder of iron metabolism causes hyperpigmentation of the skin, diabetes mellitus, and cirrhosis of the liver. The serum iron level is elevated, and the serum ferritin level markedly increased. Rarely, these patients may develop the abrupt onset of diffuse generalized abdominal pain and tenderness, shock, and a rapidly downhill clinical course. Some authorities believe that the abdominal pain and tenderness are caused by the sudden release of ferritin into the peritoneal cavity. It appears more likely that these patients develop spontaneous bacterial peritonitis that goes undetected until it is far advanced. Immediate diagnostic paracentesis and initiation of antibiotic therapy may salvage patients who develop acute peritonitis.

11. PERITONITIS SECONDARY TO VENOUS OCCLUSION OR ARTERITIS

A. Acute Vascular Catastrophes (Venous Occlusion) Occlusion of the superior mesenteric or portal vein by a clot causes diffuse abdominal pain with minimal tenderness and guarding during the first few hours after onset. Distension, watery or bloody diarrhea, and fever soon follow. The pain is severe, aching, and constant. Ascites may develop rapidly or increase in amount, and the spleen may enlarge progressively. Disorders associated with venous occlusion include polycythemia vera; essential thrombocythemia; carcinoma of the colon, stomach, or pancreas; oral contraceptive use; estrogen therapy; antithrombin III deficiency; protein C or protein S deficiency; portal hypertension secondary to cirrhosis; inflammatory bowel disease; and sickle cell anemia. The diagnosis can be confirmed by a CT scan or MRI with direct visualization of the thrombosed vein.

B. Arteritis Involving the Mesenteric Vessels

1. Polyarteritis Nodosa   There is ischemic pain in the abdomen due to vasculitic occlusion of moderate-sized intestinal blood vessels. The pain may be localized or generalized; constant; severe; and aching. Few physical findings may be present, and peritoneal signs are conspicuously absent. Within 1 or 2 days, progressive irreversible changes are signaled by the onset of fever, direct and rebound tenderness, and guarding due to perforation and leakage of bowel content into the free peritoneal cavity. Such cases require immediate surgical intervention, peritoneal lavage, intravenous antibiotics, and resection of the perforated bowel. The sequence of ischemia, bowel necrosis, perforation, and peritonitis also occurs in the other forms of vasculitis discussed below. Abdominal pain may be the initial manifestation of polyarteritis, but more commonly it occurs in a setting of other abnormalities such as hypertension, asthma, peripheral gangrene of fingers or toes, fever, renal infarction, liver function abnormalities, neurologic disorders (e.g., mononeuritis multiplex and hemiparesis), or myocardial infarction. Focal abdominal disorders such as acute cholecystitis, acute pancreatitis, and duodenal ulcer may also cause abdominal pain in patients with polyarteritis. Some attacks of abdominal pain may improve after intravenous bolus steroid therapy.

2. Rheumatoid Arthritis   Vasculitic involvement of the mesenteric arterial bed is signaled by the onset of severe diffuse abdominal pain with few signs. The abdomen may be soft and nontender. Rheumatoid arthritis has usually been present for 2 or more years prior to the onset of abdominal pain. Within 24 to 48 h, fever and peritoneal signs develop. Infarction may involve the large or small bowel or both. Bowel necrosis or open perforation occurs, resulting in acute peritonitis. The mortality is high (67 percent) and approaches 100 percent if surgical intervention is not attempted.

3. Schönlein-Henoch Purpura   Patients have purpuric maculopapular lesions on the lower extremities, arthralgias and arthritis, nephritis, and abdominal pain secondary to vasculitic ischemia and bowel wall hemorrhage. In up to 6 percent of cases, abdominal pain can be the initial symptom. Signs of peritonitis may develop in the presence of multiple hemorrhagic serosal lesions of the small and/or large bowel without necrosis or perforation of the bowel wall. In contrast to polyarteritis, perforation is rare in this disorder.

4. Systemic Lupus Erythematosus   Severe vasculitis involving the bowel is uncommon in this disorder, but bowel ischemia, infarction, and perforation may occur. In patients with perforation and spreading peritonitis, surgical exploration is required.

12. PERITONITIS ASSOCIATED WITH NEUTROPENIC ENTEROCOLITIS AND ACUTE LEUKEMIA (TYPHLITIS)

In patients with acute leukemia and severe neutropenia secondary to the disease or drug therapy, generalized abdominal pain, fever, vomiting, and diarrhea develop abruptly and persist. The liquid stools may be grossly bloody or test positive for occult blood. Within 2 or 3 days, peritoneal signs appear in the right lower abdomen. These symptoms may respond to intensive intravenous antibiotic therapy, but recurrent episodes or progression of peritonitis requires surgical removal of the right colon. The resected cecum and right colon demonstrate extensive mucosal ulceration and, in severe cases, may show bowel wall gangrene and perforation. Attacks of neutropenic enterocolitis may be recurrent and responsive to antibiotic therapy. Surgery is indicated for signs of imminent perforation, spreading peritonitis, or sepsis with vascular instability. This disorder may also occur in patients with aplastic anemia or cyclic neutropenia. The diagnosis can be supported by an abdominal CT scan.

The significant CT findings include an edematous thick-walled cecum and right colon, spiculation and inflammatory changes in the pericolic fat, and pneumatosis. Some patients with acute leukemia may develop upper abdominal pain from acute pancreatitis or from ulcerative gastroduodenal disease; and severe lower and midabdominal pain from salpingitis and endometritis, or from an antibiotic-induced pseudomembranous enterocolitis.

13. NONSURGICAL DISORDERS CAUSING GENERALIZED ABDOMINAL PAIN

A. Acute Intermittent Porphyria   This disease begins in adolescence or early adulthood. It is more common in women, and attacks may occur during menstrual periods and pregnancy and with the use of contraceptive pills.

The abdominal pain is usually crampy, but may be constant, and may be moderate to extremely severe in intensity. It may be localized or generalized. There may be some associated direct tenderness, but there is usually no muscle guarding. A plain radiograph may show a dilated stomach. The abdominal pain is usually due to autonomic neuropathy. Pain may at times radiate to the back and may be associated with fever, vomiting, constipation, and an elevated white blood cell count. The bowel may show areas of spasm or distension. These patients may have multiple surgeries because of the severity of their abdominal pains. Porphyria has been most commonly confused with intestinal obstruction or acute appendicitis.

The history or an observed attack has several other components that may aid the physician in making a diagnosis of porphyria. There may be evidence of a painful peripheral neuropathy in the form of disordered sensation involving the extremities and sometimes the face (e.g., lancinating neuritic pains, numbness and tingling, and pins-and-needles sensations) and/or weakness of the limbs in the form of foot or wrist drop, paraparesis, or quadriparesis. If the cranial nerves are involved, difficulty with speech and swallowing, diplopia, and loss of vision may occur. The blood pressure may be elevated and the heart rate rapid, due to release of catecholamines.

Mental disturbances in the form of severe anxiety, bizarre personality characteristics, restlessness, visual hallucinations, delusions, and disorientation can occur. A low serum sodium level may cause weakness and delirium, and a low serum magnesium level may cause tetany. The urine may rarely appear burgundy red on voiding, but may change color to dark red or black on standing. Elevated levels of porphobilinogen and δ-aminolevulinic acid occur during pain attacks, and the level of porphobilinogen deaminase in red blood cells or lymphocytes is decreased. The disease tends to be recurrent and can be precipitated by fasting; dehydration; alcohol; and drugs such as barbiturates, phenytoin, and contraceptive pills.

Treatment requires drug withdrawal and the use of phenothiazines, and meperidine for pain. Infusion of 20 g of glucose per hour intravenously may rapidly abort an attack. Administration of hematin every 12 h, up to 48 h, can be used if there is no response to glucose.

Prophyria should be considered in a patient with a history of recurrent episodes of abdominal pain associated with psychiatric problems, and a severe painful peripheral sensorimotor neuropathy.

B. Ketoacidosis

1. Diabetic Ketoacidosis This disorder can begin with severe nausea, vomiting, and generalized abdominal pain. The abdomen may be tender and rigid. Such patients often breathe deeply and rapidly, and, because of severe dehydration, complain of light-headedness and weakness when asked to sit or stand. If there are high blood sugar levels and ketoacidosis, the administration of insulin will rapidly lead to remission of the abdominal complaints.

If the abdominal symptoms and signs persist after insulin therapy has resolved the ketoacidosis, a surgical disorder may be present, and further evaluation is required.

2. Alcoholic Ketoacidosis A similar syndrome with nausea, vomiting, generalized abdominal pain and tenderness, and mental changes may occur in alcoholics after cessation of drinking followed by starvation for 2 or 3 days. Symptoms and signs resolve after infusion of intravenous fluids and glucose. These patients have an anion-gap acidosis caused by keto and hydroxy acids in the absence of hyperglycemia.

C. Black Widow Spider Bites Most bites occur during the warm months of the year. The initial bite may cause a stinging pain and local redness and swelling, or minimal discomfort. Within 15 to 60 min, generalized abdominal, back, and extremity pains occur in waves. These may be so severe that patients writhe and cry out. Nausea, vomiting, sweating, salivation, tremors, muscle twitching, and tingling of the hands and feet may occur. The blood pressure and temperature usually rise. The abdominal muscles become rigid, but there is usually minimal direct, and no rebound, tenderness. Pain may persist for as long as 3 days.

Intravenous calcium or 10% methocarbamol will relieve muscle spasms and pain. Antivenin can be used for young children and elderly patients, who are most at risk for a fatal outcome. This syndrome has been confused with a perforated ulcer, pancreatitis, and acute appendicitis, but the presence of generalized abdominal pain in the absence of tenderness makes a surgical diagnosis very unlikely.

D. Lead Poisoning Crampy abdominal pain occurs in association with constipation or diarrhea. There may be evidence of a motor neuropathy such as a wrist or foot drop. Pallor may occur secondary to lead-induced anemia. A blue lead line may be observed on the gingiva. Encephalopathy, with mental changes, seizures, and cerebellar ataxia or hemiplegia, usually occurs in infants and small children. The serum lead level is elevated and urine excretion high. Therapy with EDTA, D-penicillamine, or dimercaprol has been used to increase the urinary excretion of lead and relieve symptoms.

The source of lead intoxication should be identified and exposure discontinued.

E. Sickle Cell Pain Crisis Attacks of limb, back, head, chest, and sometimes abdominal pain occur on a variable schedule beginning in childhood. The abdominal pain may be intensified by movement and jarring. There may be localized or diffuse direct abdominal tenderness and voluntary guarding. Fever may also be present. Usually the abdominal pain is accompanied by painful, tender limb muscles and joints. Chest wall tenderness may also be present. Nausea and vomiting are infrequent. The presence of localized right hypochondriac pain and tenderness suggests acute cholecystitis, a common disorder in these patients. The hemogram reveals a significant anemia and a leukocytosis, which is commonly present in this disease. Conservative supportive therapy will lead to resolution of symptoms in 3 to 7 days unless acute cholecystitis is present. This disorder requires surgical intervention. In general, limb and chest pains are more common than abdominal pain in patients with a sickle cell pain crisis.

F. Hemolytic Crisis Hereditary spherocytosis and other hemolytic disorders may be associated with generalized abdominal pain without peritoneal signs during periods of hemolysis. Rising serum bilirubin, LDH, and reticulocyte counts provide evidence of the hemolytic events.

G. Hyperparathyroid and Hypercalcemic Crisis Severe hypercalcemia (14–20 mg/dl) may be associated with mental confusion, obtundation and agitation, nausea, vomiting, severe constipation, and generalized abdominal pain and tenderness. Limb pains, polyuria, and polydypsia may also occur. The serum calcium elevation may be accompanied by hypo- or hyperphosphatemia, elevated PTH levels, and a hyperchloremic acidosis. The abdominal pain may be due to peptic ulcer disease or its complications, acute pancreatitis, or passage of a ureteral stone; and/or it may be nonspecific and related to hypercalcemia. Diffuse abdominal pain and tenderness, mimicking an acute surgical abdomen, may also be caused by hypercalcemia related to sarcoidosis or malignancy. Reduction of the serum calcium level leads to remission of all symptoms. Patients with hyperparathyroidism require removal of the causative parathyroid adenoma or carcinoma.

H. Addisonian Crisis Patients develop weakness, fatigue, nausea, vomiting, and severe constant diffuse or sometimes colicky abdominal pain unaccompanied by tenderness. Apathy, confusion, and a high fever may develop. The serum sodium level is decreased (88 percent), and the potassium level is elevated (64 percent) in chronic Addison's disease; but in acute adrenal failure only 45 percent of patients have hyponatremia, and the potassium level is usually normal. Administration of saline solution and dexamethasone usually relieves the abdominal pain and other symptoms. The clinical response to dexamethasone suggests Addisonian crisis and this diagnosis can be confirmed by measuring the serum cortisol response to an ACTH infusion.

14. DIFFUSE ABDOMINAL PAIN ASSOCIATED WITH SPECIFIC INFECTIOUS DISEASES

A. Tuberculosis of the Ileocecal Region and Tuberculous Peritonitis Up to 40 percent of patients may present with an acute surgical abdomen due to perforation of the ileocecal region (i.e., bacterial peritonitis) or because of fibrous adhesions or strictures causing intestinal obstruction. Such patients may have a tender right lower abdominal mass and localized or diffuse peritoneal signs. Patients with intestinal obstruction have nausea, vomiting, obstipation, abdominal distension, and abdominal radiographs demonstrating dilated fluid-filled loops of small bowel. Such cases require definitive surgery. Culture and histopathologic examination of the resected ileocecal region or biopsies of serosal nodules usually establish the diagnosis of tuberculosis. This disorder responds to triple drug antituberculous therapy. In England, most patients are Asian or elderly. Of interest is the acute presentation of abdominal tuberculosis, since it is usually thought of as a chronic, slowly progressive disorder.

B. Rocky Mountain Spotted Fever A potentially lethal infectious disease, Rocky Mountain spotted fever begins with high fever, headache, extremity and back myalgias, and a maculopapular rash that begins on the wrists and lower legs and spreads centrally. The rash may begin 1 to 3 days after the fever, may be delayed, or may never appear. Rickettsial vasculitis may cause crampy or constant localized or generalized abdominal pain. Acute appendicitis or cholecystitis may be mimicked, or central abdominal pain and tenderness may be present because of small bowel ischemia. The abdomen may be soft and nontender, or peritoneal signs may be present locally or diffusely. A history of tick bite or exposure (e.g., camping or playing in an endemic area) or any severe febrile illness with headache in the summer or fall in an endemic area should raise the possibility of this disorder. A trial of doxycycline therapy entails minimal risk and is justified in the settings described. Unnecessary surgical intervention increases the mortality rate sevenfold.

C. Patients with AIDS and CMV Enteritis CMV infection of the small or large bowel can cause fever, abdominal pain, and diarrhea. Rarely, single or multiple perforations of the bowel wall secondary to CMV, may occur, giving rise to an acute bacterial peritonitis requiring surgical intervention.

CHAPTER

28

Acute Generalized Crampy Abdominal Pain

☐ DIAGNOSTIC LIST

1. Gastrointestinal infections
   A. Viral
   B. Bacterial
   C. Protozoal
2. Food poisoning
   A. Illness beginning after 1 to 6 h after ingestion
   B. Illness beginning between 6 to 16 h after ingestion
   C. Illness beginning after 16 h after ingestion
3. Mushroom poisoning
4. Drugs causing crampy abdominal pain
   A. Antibiotics
   B. Quinidine
   C. Propranolol
   D. Antacids
   E. Potassium chloride
   F. Narcotics
5. Constipation
6. Food allergy
   A. Eosinophilic enteritis

   B. Other forms of food allergy
7. Intestinal obstruction
8. Intestinal ischemia and infarction
9. Poisoning with heavy metals
   A. Arsenic
   B. Lead
   C. Mercury
10. Diabetic and alcoholic ketoacidosis
11. Black widow spider bite (*Latrodectus mactans*)
12. Hyperparathyroid or hypercalcemic crisis
13. Addisonian crisis
14. Acute intermittent porphyria
15. Hereditary angioedema
16. Cocaine ingestion
17. Pregnancy-associated pain
    A. False labor
    B. True labor
    C. After pains
    D. Abruptio placentae
    E. Rupture of the uterus

☐ SUMMARY

Generalized crampy abdominal pain, nausea, and diarrhea may result from infection with *rotaviruses* or *Norwalk-like agents*. Fever is low-grade, and leukocytes and blood are not present in the stool. This disorder may occur in sporadic cases but often occurs in epidemic form. *Salmonella, Shigella,* and *Campylobacter* species may cause fever, chills, crampy generalized abdominal pain, and diarrhea. Lower and midabdominal and rectal pain may precede and/or accompany each bowel movement. Such pain usually is relieved by the bowel movement. *Escherichia coli* and *Yersinia* species may cause a similar ill-

ness. *Vibrio parahemolyticus* can cause generalized abdominal pain and watery diarrhea, and such infections usually occur after ingestion of contaminated seafood. Leukocytes and blood are usually present in the stool in the majority of patients with these illnesses, except for infections with enteropathogenic *E. coli* and viral agents.

Dysentery, with crampy abdominal pain, bloody diarrhea, and tenesmus, may be caused by *Salmonella* and *Shigella* species, *Campylobacter jejuni*, invasive *E. coli* (0157:H7), *V. parahaemolyticus, Yersinia enterocolitica,* and *Entamoeba histolytica*.

These organisms can be identified by stool culture on special media, with the exception of amebic infection, which requires microscopic examination of stool. *Giardia lamblia* infection may cause crampy abdominal pain, watery diarrhea, excessive flatus, nausea, vomiting, and distension. Microscopic examination of the stool is required for identification. *Cryptosporidium* infection causes crampy abdominal pain and diarrhea. Iodine wet mounts of stool and/or acid-fast stains of stool identify this parasite. Diarrhea in AIDS patients is frequently due to this organism.

Food poisoning causes an illness that affects two or more individuals eating a common food at a family, group, or restaurant meal. Severe generalized abdominal crampy pain, diarrhea, and vomiting, beginning *1 to 6 h* after eating, is usually due to a *Staphylococcus aureus* or a *Bacillus cereus* toxin. *B. cereus* usually contaminates boiled and fried rice, meats, and vegetables. *S. aureus* may contaminate ham, canned meat, custard, cream pastries, poultry, potato salad, and mayonnaise. These organisms can be identified by study of the uneaten portion of the ingested food.

Symptoms beginning between *6 and 16 h* involve food contamination by *Clostridium perfringens* or *B. cereus. C. perfringens* usually contaminates meat and poultry that has been cooked and then allowed to cool slowly at room temperature. *B. cereus,* present in smaller amounts, may cause symptoms between 6 and 16 h by actually proliferating and producing toxin in the host's intestinal tract. These organisms can be cultured from the contaminated food.

Illness beginning after an incubation period of *16 to 72 h* may be caused by infections with toxin-producing strains of *E. coli, Vibrio cholerae,* or *V. parahaemolyticus;* or *Salmonella, Shigella,* or *Campylobacter* species. The diagnosis can be made by stool culture. *Campylobacter* and the other vibrios require the use of a selective culture media for isolation.

Nausea, vomiting, abdominal pain, and diarrhea may be the earliest symptoms of botulism. Diplopia, blurred vision, dysphagia, a painful throat, and a dry mouth occur. Progressive weakness of the arms, legs, and respiratory muscles follows. The diagnosis can be confirmed by assaying for botulinum toxin in serum, stool, and the uneaten food.

Mushroom poisoning follows ingestion of wild mushrooms and causes crampy abdominal pain and diarrhea associated with increased tearing, salivation, sweating, wheezing, cough, and blurred vision. Gastrointestinal symptoms usually precede a marked decrease in urine flow (i.e., oliguric renal failure) and hepatic failure (jaundice, liver enlargement) with some types of mushroom poisoning (*Amanita, Galerina*).

Medications, such as erythromycin, may cause abdominal pain and gas after 2 to 5 days. Other *antibiotics* given for 4 or more days may cause severe crampy abdominal pain and diarrhea. Such symptoms are often due to overgrowth in the colon of a toxin-producing anaerobic bacterium, *Clostridium difficile. C. difficile* toxin causes pain and watery diarrhea, followed by bloody diarrhea. Pseudomembranes covering small ulcers may be found in the colon on sigmoidoscopy. Other drugs that can cause crampy abdominal pain and diarrhea

include *quinidine, propranolol,* probucol, and clofibrate. *Antacids* containing magnesium may cause abdominal cramps and diarrhea in patients under treatment for ulcer disease. *Potassium* given in capsule form may cause small bowel ulceration and abdominal pain. *Codeine and other opiates* can cause severe constipation and impaction of stool in the rectum. This can cause severe constant and/or crampy abdominal pain relieved by enemas or manual removal of stool from the rectum. Intestinal obstruction, with colicky abdominal pain, vomiting, and distension, may occur with a colon packed with hard, dry feces.

Food allergy or intolerance results in generalized crampy abdominal pain when the causative food is ingested. Such symptoms are reproducible and are not relieved by antacids and antispasmodics. In some cases, other allergic symptoms accompany the abdominal pain, such as nausea, vomiting, urticaria, angioedema, wheezing, hypotension due to third-space fluid losses, and diarrhea.

Eosinophilic enteritis may cause crampy, generalized abdominal pain, nausea, and vomiting. Eosinophils are prominent in biopsies of the stomach and intestine, and an increased number of eosinophils are present in the blood. This disorder may mimic Crohn's disease. Some cases are associated with malabsorption (i.e., abdominal pain; diarrhea; and soft or loose foul-smelling, greasy stools) or with ascites. An allergic etiology is present in 20 percent of cases.

Intestinal obstruction causes colicky abdominal pain (e.g., 2–3 min of pain, 5–10 pain-free min, followed by pain, in a repeating cycle). The painful episodes are associated with audible high-pitched bowel sounds. Soon nausea, vomiting, obstipation, and distension of the abdomen occur. Plain abdominal radiographs show dilated loops of small bowel and air-fluid levels. The large bowel does not contain air.

Intestinal ischemia initially causes colicky abdominal pain and grossly bloody or watery diarrhea containing occult blood. After several hours, the pain becomes constant, and dilated small bowel and air-fluid levels become visible on abdominal radiographs. During the first few hours, the abdomen may be soft and nontender despite severe pain, but soon distension, muscle guarding, and tenderness occur. Management may require surgical exploration. Angiograms may show patency of the large vessels supplying the small and large bowel associated with small vessel vasoconstriction, ischemia, and/or infarction. In a minority of cases, the angiogram will localize the site of arterial obstruction to a major vessel.

Arsenic ingestion can cause severe crampy generalized abdominal pain, burning lips and throat, and difficulty swallowing. Vomiting and diarrhea occur, and the breath may smell of garlic. A plain abdominal radiograph may show dense white opacities due to ingested arsenic in the stomach and bowel, like residual barium from an upper gastrointestinal series. A fall in urine output may follow, and red blood cells and protein may appear in the urine. Anemia and leukopenia follow during the first few days and, later, a profound sensorimotor neuropathy may develop. The diagnosis can be confirmed by measuring blood and urine arsenic levels.

TABLE OF DISEASE INCIDENCE

INCIDENCE PER 100,000 (APPROXIMATE)

Common (>100)	**Uncommon (>5–100)**	**Rare (>0–5)**
Norwalk or rotavirus infection	*Yersinia enterocolitica* infection	*Vibrio cholerae* enteritis
Salmonella species infection	*Entamoeba histolytica* colitis	Botulism (*Clostridium botulinum*)
Shigella species infection	*Cryptosporidium* enteritis	Mushroom poisoning
Campylobacter species infection	*Vibrio parahaemolyticus* enterocolitis	Food allergy
Escherichia coli (toxigenic)	Propranolol and potassium chloride-related pain	Eosinophilic enteritis
Giardia lamblia enteritis	*Clostridium difficile* enterocolitis	Arsenic poisoning
Food poisoning due to *Staphylococcus aureus*	Intestinal ischemia and infarction	Lead poisoning
Food poisoning due to *Bacillus cereus*	Diabetic ketoacidosis	Mercury poisoning
Food poisoning due to *Clostridium perfringens*	Black widow spider bite	Alcoholic ketoacidosis
Antibiotic-induced enterocolitis	Abruptio placentae	Hyperparathyroid crisis, hypercalcemic crisis due to other disorders
Quinidine diarrhea		Addisonian crisis
Antacid-related diarrhea		Acute intermittent porphyria
Codeine-related constipation and pain		Hereditary angioedema
Constipation-related pain		Cocaine ingestion
Intestinal obstruction		Uterine rupture
Labor pains		
False labor pains		
Afterpains		

Lead colic is a true intestinal colic (e.g., there is a cycle of pain, for 2 to 5 min, and a pain-free period, of 5 to 10 min). When pain occurs, there is muscle guarding and direct tenderness, but these findings vanish or become difficult to elicit during the pain-free interval. Constipation, wrist drop, a lead line on the gums, and an anemia with basophilic stippling of the red blood cells may be present. Cylindruria, hematuria, and proteinuria are common findings. The diagnosis can be confirmed by measuring blood and urine lead levels. *Mercury poisoning* causes generalized abdominal pain and bloody diarrhea in association with acute renal failure. The diagnosis can be confirmed by measuring serum and urine mercury levels.

Diabetic ketoacidosis may cause generalized abdominal pain, tenderness and guarding, Kussmaul's respiration, dizziness, and dehydration. Elevated blood glucose and ketone levels and metabolic acidosis are present, and the pain responds promptly to several hours of insulin therapy. Alcoholic ketoacidosis can cause similar abdominal symptoms. Attacks follow 2 to 3 days after cessation of drinking.

A *black widow spider bite* may cause severe generalized abdominal pain and rigidity, but the abdomen remains nontender. Painful cramps usually occur in the extremities, chest, and back; and there may be tremors, paresthesias, and weakness of the arms and legs. There may be a history of a stinging bite on the buttocks, genitalia, or legs; and there may be local redness and swelling at the bite site. In some cases, there is no pain or local reaction in the area of the bite. This lack of reaction makes the diagnosis more difficult, since the patient may be unaware of having been bitten.

Crampy abdominal pain may occur with *hypercalcemia* (14–20 mg/dl) in association with vomiting, lethargy, or agitation. Other complaints include mental confusion, constipation, and polyuria. *Addisonian crisis* may cause aching or crampy abdominal pain, vomiting, and fever. Mental confusion and lethargy may be associated. Low levels of serum cortisol may occur but are not diagnostic. Symptoms respond promptly to dexamethasone administration. The diagnosis can be confirmed by measuring the serum cortisol response to an injection of cosyntropin (i.e., a synthetic form of ACTH).

Acute intermittent porphyria causes generalized abdominal pain with minimal or no tenderness. A painful sensorimotor neuropathy may affect the limbs. Delirium or psychotic symptoms may also accompany the abdominal complaints. Elevated urinary levels of porphobilinogen are usually present during an attack.

Hereditary angioedema may cause colicky abdominal pain, nausea, and vomiting that resolve spontaneously in 1 to 3 days. Angioedema may occur on the face, hands, and feet simultaneously with the abdominal pain or at other times. Low serum C4 and C1 esterase inhibitor levels are diagnostic. *Ingestion of cocaine* can cause severe colicky pain due to bowel ischemia and necrosis.

True and false *labor pains* occur in the third trimester and are episodic, lasting up to 90 s, with variable pain-free intervals. True labor pains affect the back and/or the abdomen and usually occur at regular intervals. False labor pains affect the lower abdomen and groin region and are seldom regular. Abruptio placentae causes severe constant generalized abdominal pain and tenderness, and vaginal bleeding. Uterine rupture usually occurs during labor, causing a sharp, tearing generalized pain during a uterine contraction. After the tear, labor ceases, and signs of hypovolemia develop.

☐ DESCRIPTION OF LISTED DISEASES

Crampy abdominal pain occurs in a local area of the abdomen in attacks that last a variable period of time, usually measured in seconds or minutes. The location of the pain may shift over a period of minutes or hours from one part of the abdomen to an adjacent or more distant area. Pains may also occur simultaneously at one or more sites. Loud bowel sounds audible to the patient may occur in association with the crampy pain.

Examination may reveal direct tenderness over the painful area and, in some patients, rebound tenderness. Muscle guarding does not usually occur, nor does distension, unless intestinal obstruction is the cause of the pain.

Pain is usually of a mild to moderate severity, but severe attacks may cause the patient to double up, grasp the abdomen with both hands, and cry out. Such pain may be relieved by passage of stool or flatus, but such relief is often only transient.

The causes of generalized crampy abdominal pain, as described above, occurring suddenly in a previously well person and then remitting over a period of hours or days, are discussed here.

1. GASTROINTESTINAL INFECTIONS

A. Viral Rotaviruses primarily cause disease in infants and small children, but they may affect adults. Norwalk-like agents affect adults. Nausea, vomiting, and diarrhea accompany crampy lower or generalized abdominal pain. Some patients also have a low-grade fever, headache, myalgias, weakness, and malaise. The illness lasts 1 to 3 days. There may be direct and even rebound abdominal tenderness, but this disappears in 2 to 3 days. Examination of the stool for leukocytes and blood is negative. Viral gastroenteritis often occurs in community-wide outbreaks. Since Norwalk epidemics are more common in the winter months, Norwalk-like agent-related disease has been called winter vomiting disease. Stool cultures for bacterial pathogens are negative, and there is no evidence of Entamoeba histolytica or *Giardia lamblia* on microscopic examination of the stool.

Since identification of Norwalk-like agents requires immune electron microscopy of a stool sample or radioimmunoassay for serum antibody, these tests are rarely done on individual patients. They may be done as part of the investigation of a large epidemic by clinical epidemiologists.

Therapy for viral gastroenteritis includes oral fluid replacement and antimotility agents such as paregoric, codeine, loperamide, or diphenoxylate with atropine. Nausea and vomiting are treated with antiemetics, such as prochlorperazine or trimethobenzamide.

B. Bacterial Infection with a *Salmonella* species causes crampy lower or generalized abdominal pain and loose, watery diarrheal stools, often associated with the passage of mucus and blood. Fever to 102°F and chills may occur. Direct and rebound abdominal tenderness may be observed without true peritonitis being present. If the colon is severely involved, the passage of grossly bloody stools is more frequent, and tenesmus occurs. Without therapy, such an illness will clear in 2 to 5 days, but cases may remain symptomatic for up to 2 weeks. Stool cultures will identify *Salmonella,* and Gram or methylene blue stains of stool or adherent mucus reveal increased numbers of leukocytes.

Very severe cases of *Salmonella* gastroenteritis may be associated with sustained fever; crampy abdominal pain and diarrhea; the appearance of a rash consisting of small pink macules on the back, chest, and abdomen (rose spots); enlargement of the spleen; and leukopenia.

Rose spots appear during the beginning of the second week of illness. Blood and stool cultures grow a *Salmonella* species. This form of illness has been called paratyphoid fever, and it is not possible to distinguish it from typhoid fever, unless cultures and antibody studies are performed.

Supportive care with oral fluid replacement is all that is required to treat uncomplicated gastroenteritis. Antibiotic therapy does not accelerate the remission of abdominal symptoms and can prolong the time it takes for the *Salmonella* carrier state to clear. Patients older than 50, with aneurysms, or known valvular, or coronary heart disease should be treated with antibiotics, as should patients with paratyphoid fever. Drugs useful for treating *Salmonella* infections include chloramphenicol, ampicillin, trimethoprim-sulfamethoxazole and ciprofloxacin.

Shigella infections cause crampy lower or generalized abdominal pain, watery and sometimes bloody diarrhea, and fever up to 105°–106°F. Other symptoms include myalgias, chills, headache, and back pain. When distal colon involvement is severe, tenesmus occurs. Stools contain leukocytes and blood. Abdominal tenderness usually occurs in painful areas. Bowel sounds are hyperactive and may be clearly audible. Sigmoidoscopy reveals erythema, edema, and superficial ulceration of the colon mucosa.

Without therapy, fever usually clears in 3 to 4 days, but diarrhea may continue for 2 weeks. Confirmation of the diagnosis depends on culturing shigella from the stool using an enteric medium [MacConkey or *Salmonella-Shigella* (SS) agar]. The stool culture is usually positive during the first week.

Fever is present in only 40 percent, and passage of blood and mucus in only 33 percent of cases. The majority of patients present with cramps and watery diarrhea.

A single stool culture may miss 33 percent of patients with *Shigella* infection. If this disorder is considered, daily cultures for 3 days should be done to increase the likelihood of a positive culture.

Mild cases are not usually treated with antibiotics. Moderate to severe cases should receive antibiotics such as trimethoprim sulfamethoxazole, amoxicillin, or ciprofloxacin.

Campylobacter infection also causes fever, chills, myalgias, watery diarrhea, and generalized abdominal crampy pain, often associated with a frequent or constant desire to defecate. In severe cases, the diarrhea becomes bloody within 1 or 2 days. Gross bright or dark red blood and clots may be passed as frequently as once every hour. Isolation of *C. jejuni* from stool requires the use of a 42°C incubator and agar containing several antibiotics. Oral administration of erythromycin may shorten the course of the illness. Severe cases with gram-negative sepsis may require parenteral antibiotic therapy.

E. coli may cause crampy abdominal pain and watery diarrhea. Strains producing enterotoxins cause inhibition of water reabsorption in the bowel, leading to diarrhea. Toxigenic *E. coli* are a common cause of traveler's diarrhea.

Strain 0157:H7 of *E. coli* can cause a disease clinically similar to the bacillary dysentery caused by *Shigella, Salmonella,* or *Campylobacter* species. The hemorrhagic colitis produced by *E. coli* 0157:H7 is not associated with fever or the presence of stool leukocytes. The absence of these findings may be helpful in distinguishing this disorder from other causes by dysentery. Cultures with typing of stool isolates are required to identify this organism. Trimethoprim-sulfamethoxazole may provide rapid relief from the diarrheal symptoms. Other bacterial agents capable of causing bloody diarrhea and fever include *Yersinia* species and *Vibrio parahaemolyticus*. Isolation of these organisms from a case of dysentery requires the use of selective media.

In patients with bacterial gastroenteritis, with stools positive for leukocytes and blood, antimotility drugs should not be used.

C. Protozoal Mild *intestinal amebiasis* causes crampy lower abdominal pain and one to four watery stools per day, associated with the passage of increased amounts of flatus. Mild abdominal tenderness may be present. The diagnosis requires microscopic examination of the stool for amebic trophozoites and cysts. Sigmoidoscopy shows numerous flask-shaped ulcers with normal intervening mucosa. The serum indirect hemagglutination test for amebiasis may be positive.

Severe attacks are characterized by fever to 104–105°F, crampy generalized abdominal pain, tenesmus, and the frequent passage of bloody stools. Abdominal tenderness, both indirect and rebound, may be marked. The liver may enlarge. Trophozoites can be detected in the passed stool. Amebiasis will respond to metronidazole and a course of iodoquinol to eradicate the intestinal phase.

One to 3 weeks after exposure to contaminated water or food, *Giardia lamblia* infection may cause crampy gen-

eralized or mid-upper abdominal pain and watery diarrhea. The stool is bulky and may not clear the toilet bowl with one flush. It may appear greasy and be foul-smelling. There may be a great deal of belching and flatus, and bowel gas may cause bloating and distension. In some patients, there is loss of appetite, nausea, vomiting, and a low-grade fever. In most cases, symptoms improve within 5 to 7 days, and complaints vanish in 1 to 4 weeks.

A small percentage of patients continue to have mushy diarrheal stools, gas, and crampy upper or generalized abdominal pain. Fever and weight loss may continue. Some patients become unable to drink milk because they develop lactase deficiency. Lactase deficiency may also produce crampy abdominal pain, diarrhea, and rectal gas after ingestion of dairy products. The diagnosis of giardiasis can be made by microscopic examination of the stool for *Giardia* trophozoites or by a formalin-ether stool concentration and examination for cysts. In cases with repeatedly negative stool examinations, a nylon string (Enterotest) can be passed into the duodenum (i.e., where *Giardia* attaches to the duodenal wall) and then drawn back for examination under the microscope. Some patients develop duodenitis and have ulcerlike pain. Duodenal aspirates taken during endoscopy for possible ulcer disease may reveal the organism. A new ELISA test detects *Giardia* antigen in stool and is probably more sensitive than microscopy. The specificity of this test has not yet been fully evaluated. Treatment with quinacrine or metronidazole is effective. *Giardia* is the most frequently identified intestinal parasite in the United States.

Giardia infection has occurred with increased incidence in male homosexuals and travelers to Aspen, Colorado, or St. Petersburg, Russia. It may contaminate municipal water systems, leading to major outbreaks of illness. The cysts resist chlorine, which is the cidal agent in municipal water supplies, and may pass defective filter systems.

The parasitic infection *cryptosporidiosis* causes watery diarrhea, crampy generalized abdominal pain, nausea, and low-grade fever. Bowel sounds are hyperactive. There may be generalized abdominal tenderness. Stools may be bulky and foul-smelling. There is little or no rectal gas. Symptoms may continue for up to 4 weeks and then disappear. This is an important infection in patients with AIDS. Diarrhea is more severe than in immune-competent patients, and it may result in fluid losses of 1 to 10 liters per day. This may lead to dehydration and weight loss, and contribute to the death of the patient. Diarrheal stools contain oocysts. Concentrated (10% formalin or 2.5% dichromate) stools should be studied if routine stool examinations are negative. Stool leukocytes and red blood cells are usually not present.

Cryptosporidial oocysts in stool do not take up iodine in a wet mount preparation of stool as do yeast organisms, and this property allows differentiation from yeast organisms, which they resemble. Acid-fast stains of stool will also identify them. These stains may be used with or without concentration techniques (sugar flotation or for-malin-diethyl-ether sedimentation). Some patients respond to treatment with spiramycin or furazolidine, but most patients fail to respond. Alpha-difluoromethylornithine (DFMO) is a new agent that has not been used enough to evaluate its efficacy.

The causes of crampy abdominal pain, diarrhea, fever, and the passage of blood and mucus include species of *Salmonella, Shigella, Campylobacter,* and *Yersinia*; and *E. coli, V. parahaemolyticus,* and *Entamoeba histolytica*. If oral antibiotics have been used during the 4 weeks prior to, or during the onset of, diarrhea, intestinal overgrowth of *Clostridium difficile*, with toxin production, becomes a likely possibility. Outside the United States, bloody diarrhea may occur as a symptom of malaria, schistosomiasis, or kala azar.

2. FOOD POISONING

Food poisoning should be considered when two or more people become ill within 72 h of ingesting a common food served at home, in a restaurant, or at a picnic or other group gathering. Illness symptoms commonly include fever, nausea, vomiting, crampy abdominal pain, diarrhea, and excessive flatus. In some cases, tingling paresthesias, dizziness, weakness, and difficulty breathing may occur.

The time from ingestion to first symptoms helps in identifying the type of food poisoning present. The symptom pattern may also be helpful in suggesting a causative microorganism or toxin. The nature of the contaminated food may also provide a clue as to the causative agent.

A. Illness Beginning 1 to 6 h after Ingestion   Illness results from ingestion of preformed *Staphylococcus aureus* enterotoxin already present in the food. Symptoms include severe vomiting and retching, intolerable nausea, crampy generalized abdominal pain, and diarrhea. Fever may occur but is uncommon. The duration of illness is usually <10 h but may be up to 2 days. Failure to refrigerate food contaminated by an infected food handler is the usual cause. Common foods causing this illness include ham, canned meats, custard, cream pastries, poultry, potato salad, mayonnaise, and egg salad.

Vomiting, nausea, crampy abdominal pain, and diarrhea occur with *Bacillus cereus* (short incubation emetic syndrome). Symptoms are produced by an enterotoxin synthesized by *B. cereus*. Common foods contaminated by *B. cereus* include fried rice, rice in Chinese restaurants, meats, and vegetables.

These organisms and preformed toxins can be isolated from samples of the contaminated food.

B. Illness Beginning 6 to 16 h after Ingestion   *Clostridium perfringens* and *B. cereus* begin to multiply in the gastrointestinal tract of the host soon after ingestion

and produce toxin. The need to first synthesize toxin accounts for the longer incubation period before illness begins, since contaminated foods contain little preformed toxin.

C. perfringens causes nausea, generalized crampy abdominal pain, and diarrhea. Vomiting and fever are uncommon. Meat and poultry products and gravy are commonly involved. If these are allowed to cool at room temperature for 12 to 24 h after removing them from the oven, spore germination and then growth of the causative bacterium up to large numbers can occur in the gradually cooled food.

B. cereus may cause generalized abdominal cramps and diarrhea. Vomiting, nausea, and mild fever may also occur. The usual food source is contaminated boiled or fried rice or vegetables.

C. Illness Beginning 16 h after Ingestion   Bacterial proliferation and toxin production in the gastrointestinal tract occur prior to the onset of symptoms. *Salmonella, Shigella,* and *Campylobacter* species and *V. parahaemolyticus* may cause generalized or localized crampy abdominal pain and watery or bloody diarrhea with or without fever and chills.

Salmonella infections are associated with contaminated dairy, meat, poultry, and egg products. Unusual outbreaks have been associated with manure-contaminated marijuana and pasteurized milk. Transmission occurs from pet turtles and other animals, as well as from person to person. Shigellosis is generally a disease of small children, and spread is by person-to-person contact. Adults typically acquire this disorder from an infected child. In developing countries, food, water, and flies may serve as vehicles of transmission. *Campylobacter jejuni* is spread by contaminated poultry, beef, eggs, water, and dairy products. *V. parahaemolyticus* contaminates shellfish, and *V. cholerae* shellfish and water. Enterotoxigenic *E. coli* infections occur in travelers to developing countries. Crampy abdominal pain is associated with watery diarrhea, and sometimes fever and a prompt response to trimethoprim-sulfamethoxasole. Infection is spread by fecally contaminated food and water. Enterohemorrhagic *E. coli* outbreaks have involved inadequately cooked hamburgers at fast-food restaurants, raw milk, and person-to-person transmission.

Salmonella and *Shigella* species grow on SS or MacConkey agar, and *V. parahaemolyticus* and *V. cholerae* on citrate-bile-salt-sucrose agar. Culture of *C. jejuni* requires an atmosphere of 5% O_2 and 5 to 10% CO_2, a temperature of 42°C, and a special culture medium containing several antibiotics. Enterotoxigenic *E. coli* produce a toxin that can be identified by stimulation of adenyl cyclase production in a cell culture or animal preparation. Enterohemorrhagic *E. coli* (0157:H7) can be identified by serotyping of stool isolates.

Yersinia enterocolitica can cause the abrupt onset of

nausea, vomiting, generalized crampy abdominal pain, watery diarrhea and sometimes bloody diarrhea, as well as fever. Constant right lower abdominal pain and tenderness may develop, simulating an acute appendicitis in adolescents and young adults. The stool frequently contains leukocytes and red blood cells. Water or food (e.g., milk products) contamination is the usual cause. Storing of stool specimens at 4 to 25°C for 2 weeks prior to culture (i.e., cold enrichment) enhances the isolation of *Y. enterocolitica.*

Botulism may begin 18–36 h or longer (up to 14 days) after ingestion of contaminated food. Nausea, vomiting, and retching affect 50 percent of patients, and abdominal pain of a generalized crampy type and diarrhea affect 25 percent. Neurologic symptoms begin soon after the abdominal complaints. Double or blurred vision, weakness of the voice, slurred speech, difficulty swallowing, sore throat, and a dry mouth occur. Progressive symmetrical weakness of the arms, legs, and respiratory muscles follow. Physical findings include ptosis; weakness or paralysis of eye muscles; and dilated, poorly reactive pupils. There may be generalized flaccid weakness involving the tongue, larynx, and extremities, but no loss of sensation. The tendon reflexes are depressed. Food, stool, and serum can be assayed for botulinum toxin using a mouse bioassay. Food should be cultured anaerobically in order to isolate the organism. Therapy includes cathartics and enemas to facilitate removal of unabsorbed toxin, administration of antitoxin, intubation and assisted ventilation, and bladder catheterization.

3. MUSHROOM POISONING

Symptoms of mushroom poisoning may begin within 2 h of ingestion. Diffuse abdominal crampy pain and diarrhea may be associated with excessive salivation, tearing, sweating, blurred vision, wheezing, and a slow pulse (e.g., muscarinic symptoms caused by *Inocybe* and *Clitocybe* species). These symptoms can be controlled with atropine.

Nausea, vomiting, crampy generalized abdominal pain, and diarrhea may also occur within 2 h of mushroom ingestion without any other symptoms.

Mushroom poisoning, with onset 6 to 24 h after ingestion, begins with nausea, vomiting, continuous diarrhea, and crampy abdominal pain and thirst, and is followed in 24 to 48 h by hepatic and renal failure. Death rates after this type of poisoning approach 30 to 50 percent. *Amanita* and *Galerina* species cause this severe form of toxicity. *A. phalloides* causes 90 percent of deaths.

Liver toxicity produces hepatic enlargement; dark, cola-colored urine; jaundice; and hypoglycemia. Oliguria and proteinuria reflect renal toxicity. Severe headache, seizures, disorientation, and coma are common neurotoxic symptoms.

There is no specific therapy for this type of severe poisoning. Early in the course, hemoperfusion may be attempted to remove lethal phallotoxins and amatoxins. Fatalities usually occur within 3 to 8 days. Liver transplantation may result in survival after *A. phalloides* poisoning.

4. DRUGS CAUSING CRAMPY ABDOMINAL PAIN

A. Antibiotics These drugs may cause nausea, vomiting, and diarrhea with or without generalized abdominal pain. Some may cause abdominal pain within 1 or 2 days and excessive rectal gas (i.e., erythromycin).

Patients on antibiotics for 4 to 10 days or patients who have discontinued a course of antibiotics as long as 4 weeks before may develop crampy and constant abdominal pain and watery or bloody diarrhea. Sigmoidoscopy demonstrates erythema, edema, friability of the colorectal mucosa, and sometimes pseudomembranes (i.e., 1–5-mm yellow-white plaques covering small mucosal ulcers). This type of diarrhea may mimic bacterial or amebic dysentery. Therapy may only require stopping the offending drug (e.g., clindamycin, cefaclor, or ampicillin) for mild cases or oral therapy with vancomycin for severe cases. Clostridial toxin is found in stool in 95 percent of those with pseudomembranous colitis; an in vitro cell culture assay may be used to detect this toxin.

For most antibiotic-related complaints, symptoms will continue until the drug is discontinued and several days of recovery time elapse.

B. Quinidine Abdominal pain is a common initial reaction to this drug, which is usually used for cardiac rhythm disturbances. Thirty-three percent of patients may be unable to tolerate quinidine because of abdominal pain and diarrhea. These symptoms may begin after only one or two doses in some patients.

C. Propranolol Patients may develop cramping abdominal pain, diarrhea or constipation, nausea, and vomiting. Drugs used to lower cholesterol, such as probucol or clofibrate, may also cause abdominal cramps and diarrhea.

D. Antacids Those containing magnesium can cause crampy abdominal pain, increased rectal gas, and diarrhea due to the laxative effect of the magnesium.

E. Potassium Chloride This drug can cause crampy or constant abdominal pain, nausea, vomiting, and diarrhea. Potassium may cause small bowel ulceration if given in capsule form.

F. Narcotics Codeine, morphine, methadone, meperidine, heroin, and other opium derivatives may cause severe constipation with accumulation of hard stool in the left colon. There may be a lower abdominal aching pain and more generalized crampy abdominal pain. Direct abdominal tenderness may occur over painful areas, but rebound tenderness does not. Coughing or jarring does not intensify the pain.

Passage of stool after enemas or laxatives usually relieves the pain and confirms the diagnosis. Other drugs that can cause severe constipation include calcium and aluminum antacids, bismuth (e.g., PeptoBismol), barium used in radiographic studies, anticholinergics (e.g., atropine and propantheline), antidepressant drugs, drugs used for Parkinson's disease [e.g., benztropine meslate (Cogentin)], and diuretics used for hypertension.

5. CONSTIPATION

Crampy generalized abdominal pain may be associated with constipation. There may be a tender, descending colon and a rectum filled with firm or hard feces.

Constipation may be associated with disorders of the endocrine system. It occurs with hypothyroidism, hyperparathyroidism with hypercalcemia, pheochromocytoma, and panhypopituitarism. Renal failure, hypokalemia, and autonomic neuropathies caused by diabetes, amyloidosis, or porphyria also cause constipation. Obstruction of the colon by tumors or inflammatory strictures and disorders such as irritable bowel, diverticulosis, and scleroderma may lead to constipation. In addition, it may occur with rectal and anal disorders such as fissures, painful hemorrhoids, and proctitis. It can be treated symptomatically with dietary changes, laxatives, or enemas. In many of these disorders, specific medical or surgical treatment is required. There is a large group of patients over age 60 with constipation of unknown cause (idiopathic constipation).

6. FOOD ALLERGY

A. Eosinophilic Enteritis This disorder may present in at least three clinical forms. With *muscle layer disease,* patients have nausea, vomiting, and crampy generalized abdominal pain that is not relieved by antacids or anticholinergic drugs. Forty percent have an allergic history. Eosinophilia is usually present. A barium study of the stomach may demonstrate narrowing of the distal third of the stomach (i.e., antrum) with decreased muscular contractility and the presence of polyps. The diagnosis can be established by gastric and small bowel biopsy. Therapy involves the use of prednisone and surgery. Elimination diets generally are ineffective, but since they may work in some patients, they should be tried. This disorder may be confused with Crohn's disease if it involves the colon

and ileum. Detection of large numbers of eosinophils in bowel biopsies and the blood confirms the diagnosis.

With *mucosal disease,* patients have nausea, back pain, generalized abdominal pain made worse by eating certain foods, weight loss, iron deficiency anemia, and hypoalbuminemia from exudation of serum proteins into the bowel.

With *subserosal disease,* patients have eosinophilic ascites in association with generalized abdominal pain and symptoms of gastric or intestinal obstruction. Combined forms of this disorder may occur with subserosal and muscle layer symptoms.

B. Other Forms of Food Allergy If a patient has reproducible symptoms after eating a specific food, food intolerance or allergy exists.

To diagnose food allergy, there should be food intolerance with the immediate onset of symptoms (in <1 h). In addition, symptoms should include crampy pain, nausea, vomiting or diarrhea, and allergic symptoms such as angioedema of the face, urticaria, asthma, wheezing, and/or rapidly developing hypotension with presyncope or syncope. These symptoms will usually recur each time the offending food is ingested.

Food allergy may be diagnosed and managed with an elimination diet. Milk, eggs, seafood, meats, seeds, chocolate, oranges, tomatoes, onions, chives, garlic, scallions, cucumbers, and other possible responsible foods are deleted from the diet for 3 weeks and then added back one by one to determine the offending food. The value of this approach depends on the ability of the elimination diet to eradicate symptoms. Food intolerance may be nonallergic, such as milk intolerance due to lack of intestinal lactase. This deficiency leads to abdominal pain, explosive diarrhea, and passage of excessive gas after milk ingestion and can be ameliorated by ingestion of lactase-containing tablets with dairy products.

7. INTESTINAL OBSTRUCTION

Pain occurs in the midabdomen but may be generalized. It is of a colicky nature (e.g., pain sustained for 2–3 min, with a pain-free interval of 5–8 min), and these cycles of pain and relief go on for up to 6 h. In high intestinal obstruction, vomiting occurs early in the course. During paroxysms of pain, the patient may draw his legs up, curl into a ball, cry out, and/or writhe in bed. Abdominal distension may soon occur. In low, small bowel obstruction, vomiting begins after pain has been present for several hours, and colic occurs less frequently (e.g., every 10–12 min). Loud bowel sounds, audible to the patient, may accompany each episode of pain. After an initial bowel movement or two, there is failure to pass stool or gas by rectum.

Vomitus is usually yellow or green in upper small intestinal obstruction. In low, small intestinal obstruction, the vomitus may become orange-brown and have a feculent or putrid odor. Physical examination may reveal distension and direct and sometimes rebound tenderness. If surgery is not performed or successful tube decompression accomplished in complete intestinal obstruction, the pain becomes constant within 6 to 12 h, and fever and an elevated white count may develop.

Plain abdominal radiographs may show gas-filled dilated loops of small bowel, with little gas in the colon unless the obstruction is in the colon. An obstructed large bowel fills with gas to the point of stenosis, and no gas is present beyond this region. Upright abdominal radiographs may show small bowel air-fluid levels and edematous thickening of the wall and mucosal folds of the small intestine in small bowel obstruction or in large bowel obstruction with an incompetent ileocecal valve. Complete intestinal obstruction requires resuscitation with intravenous crystalloid and surgical correction of the obstruction as soon as the patient is able to tolerate anesthesia.

Small bowel obstruction in adults is usually due to adhesions (71 percent) resulting from prior abdominal or pelvic surgery. Carcinoma of the small intestine may obstruct the bowel lumen (9 percent). Hernias in the inguinal or femoral region or within the abdomen account for 8 percent, and Crohn's disease accounts for 4 percent of cases. Carcinoma of the colon causes 67 percent of the cases of large bowel obstruction. Other causes include volvulus of the sigmoid colon (9 percent), strictures from diverticulitis (7 percent), and fecal impaction (5 percent).

8. INTESTINAL ISCHEMIA AND INFARCTION

Crampy generalized abdominal pain occurs with mild nausea and vomiting. Frequent bowel movements or frank, watery diarrhea and the passage of gross or occult blood may occur. Food may intensify the pain, the abdomen may become distended, and bowel sounds may become infrequent or inaudible.

Early in the course of this disorder, the bowel sounds may be easily heard and the abdomen may be soft, without muscle guarding and tenderness. Later, with the onset of distension, there may be direct and rebound tenderness. If surgery is delayed beyond a few hours, pain becomes severe and continuous. Soon distension, fever, a rising pulse rate, and a falling blood pressure occur. These patients often give a history of weeks or months of recurrent attacks of crampy midabdominal pain beginning 15 to 30 min after meals. Such discomfort may be so regular and distressing that patients avoid eating large meals and eat more frequently in order to maintain their weight (i.e., small meal syndrome). This symptom complex may precede a major attack by several months. Early association

of this history of recurrent meal-associated pain with vascular disease should lead to arteriographic study of the mesenteric and celiac vessels. Early detection of a stenotic superior mesenteric artery will provide an opportunity for a vascular surgeon to correct the obstruction and prevent future intestinal ischemia. Most patients with this disorder are elderly and may have a history of angina pectoris, claudication, myocardial infarction, or stroke.

An embolus to the superior mesenteric artery causes similar symptoms to thrombotic occlusion but tends to occur in patients with heart disease and rhythm abnormalities (e.g., atrial fibrillation). Patients with valvular heart disease or subacute bacterial endocarditis are also at increased risk. Emboli may also arise in ulcerated atherosclerotic aortic plaques.

With arterial occlusion, the small bowel becomes pale, green-white, and paralyzed. It distends with gas and fluid. These findings are evident on plain abdominal radiographs, which show small bowel distension and mucosal fold and wall thickening with air-fluid levels. Accurate diagnosis may require surgical exploration, since ischemia and infarction may occur with a normal angiogram (i.e., nonocclusive ischemia) of the major mesenteric vessels. At surgery, it may be necessary to remove a vascular obstruction and resect necrotic and/or ischemic bowel. Many surgeons reoperate within 24 h to resect any bowel that has become nonviable since the first operation.

9. POISONING WITH HEAVY METALS

A. Arsenic Ingestion of arsenic is usually accidental, suicidal, or homicidal. As_2O_3 has been a common source of poisoning. It is a tasteless, white powder.

Crampy generalized and upper abdominal pain, burning lips, throat constriction, and difficulty swallowing may begin within 1 h of ingestion or may be delayed for up to 12 h. Severe thirst, vomiting, and diarrhea may occur. A plain radiograph of the abdomen taken within a few hours of ingestion may show contrast material (i.e., arsenic) in the stomach and small bowel. It may appear as though the patient had recently swallowed barium for an upper gastrointestinal series. There may be a garlic-like odor to the breath.

Urine output decreases to <400 ml/day, and proteinuria and hematuria occur. Severe arm and leg cramps may be present.

A hemolytic anemia occurs, and leukopenia may develop within 2 to 4 days. Shortness of breath, cyanosis, and a fall in blood pressure occur in severe poisonings. Mental confusion, seizures, coma, and death may follow in 1 to 24 h. A severe sensory and motor neuropathy may develop 7 to 21 days after the onset of the initial symptoms.

Acute ingestion of arsenic requires gastric lavage or the use of syrup of ipecac to induce vomiting if the patient is alert. Dimercaprol (3–5 mg/kg) is used to bind ingested arsenic and may aid survival and prevent toxicity to the nervous system. The normal blood level for arsenic is ≤3 μg/dl and the normal urinary excretion is <100 μg/24 h.

B. Lead Abdominal symptoms are an early manifestation of lead poisoning. Lead colic causes a severe generalized colicky abdominal pain with pain-free periods. During the periods of pain, there is muscular guarding and abdominal tenderness. Loss of appetite, a metallic taste, and constipation occur. The abdominal pain is thought to be caused by intestinal spasms.

Other manifestations of lead poisoning include wrist or foot drop; encephalopathy (vertigo, ataxia, headache, restlessness, and seizures); hypochromic anemia with basophilic stippling of the red blood cells; and renal injury with proteinuria, casts, and hematuria. Renal failure and/or gout may result from lead intoxication, and both are reversible if lead can be removed by chelation therapy. A lead line (black or gray) may occur on the gum line just below the teeth. Serum lead levels exceed 40 μg/dl, free erythrocyte protoporphyrin values are increased, and urinary lead excretion exceeds 100 μg/24 h. Chelating agents such as EDTA, dimercaprol, and D-penicillamine may be used for treatment. These drugs accelerate lead removal from the body by increasing urinary excretion.

Lead poisoning may occur from retained bullets, working in a pistol range, drinking ''moonshine,'' ingestion of old house paint, artists' ingestion of paint from their brushes or hands, lead waterpipes, lead type, and burning discarded battery casings. Workers in lead smelters and storage-battery factories are also at risk. One of the most important aspects of therapy is to define the source of exposure and eliminate it.

C. Mercury Immediately after ingestion, mouth, throat, and laryngeal pain is severe. Severe generalized crampy abdominal pain and watery, bloody diarrhea follow; and tenesmus is frequently present. Nausea, vomiting, and hematemesis occur. Renal failure due to tubular necrosis may develop rapidly. Blood mercury levels are elevated, and urinary excretion exceeds 100 μg/day. Acute poisoning should be treated by inducing vomiting with syrup of ipecac or by gastric lavage. Polythiol resins may bind mercury if given before it is absorbed. Dimercaprol or acetyl DL-penicillamine should be used for chelation therapy to remove mercury from the body. Intensive fluid therapy should be initiated early to maintain a diuresis and reduce mercury levels in renal tubular fluid.

10. DIABETIC AND ALCOHOLIC KETOACIDOSIS

Severe generalized or localized crampy abdominal pain and vomiting may occur. There may be direct abdominal tenderness, orthostatic hypotension with postural dizziness, lethargy, and malaise. Excessive urination and thirst are usually present. Breathing is rapid and deep (Kussmaul's respiration). The urine contains high concentrations of glucose and ketones.

Abdominal symptoms usually lessen and then disappear after initiation of adequate insulin therapy and hydration with intravenous fluids. Failure of the pain and tenderness to disappear when ketoacidosis is controlled suggests that the pain is caused by another disorder. Surgical consultation and laboratory and radiologic investigation are then necessary, since a disorder requiring surgical intervention may be present.

Alcoholic ketoacidosis may cause abdominal symptoms similar to those associated with diabetic ketoacidosis. These patients usually develop abdominal pain 2 to 3 days after they stop drinking. A history of minimal food ingestion for 1 to 2 days prior to onset is commonly present. Symptoms resolve with infusion of fluids and glucose.

11. BLACK WIDOW SPIDER BITE (LATRODECTUS MACTANS)

Bites often occur on the genitalia, buttocks, or thighs when the victim is sitting in a privy. Other bites may occur in the vicinity of piles of rocks or lumber and commonly occur on the legs or arms. Within 15–60 min, painful cramps occur near the site of the bite and in the back, arms, and legs. Generalized crampy abdominal pain may occur, associated with a rigid but nontender abdominal wall. Chest pressure or pain may be present. The abdominal pain is often so severe that patients may writhe about in bed, roll from side to side, and cry out.

Nausea, vomiting, sweating, salivation, and systolic hypertension may develop. Low-grade fever and leukocytosis are frequent findings. Tremors and paresthesias affect the arms and legs, and muscle weakness may begin in the legs and ascend to involve the trunk and arms. Death may occur in children or the elderly. The pain may last for 12 to 24 h.

Painful cramps in the extremities and abdomen may be relieved by intravenous injection of 10% calcium gluconate or 10% methocarbamol. One vial of specific antivenin given intravenously shortens the duration of symptoms and decreases the severity of the painful limb and abdominal wall spasms. Antivenin is used primarily in young children and the elderly, who are most at risk of dying.

12. HYPERPARATHYROID AND HYPERCALCEMIC CRISIS

High levels of serum calcium (14–20 mg/dl) can cause diffuse colicky abdominal pain, vomiting, lethargy, agitation, mental confusion, hypertension, severe constipation, nocturia, polyuria, and polydypsia. Peptic ulcer disease, ureteral calculi, or pancreatitis may be responsible for some component of the abdominal pain, but a less specific variety occurs that resolves when the serum calcium returns toward normal. Hypercalcemia, whether associated with parathyroid hyperplasia or tumor, sarcoidosis, or malignancy, produces similar complaints. Up to one-third of cases of hyperparathyroid crisis have been associated with acute pancreatitis.

13. ADDISONIAN CRISIS

Patients present with vomiting, high fever, and crampy abdominal pain. Mental confusion, extreme weakness, and lethargy may be associated findings. Skin and scar pigmentation may be increased with adrenal disease secondary to tuberculosis, fungus, or idiopathic destruction of the adrenal gland. Some cases result from abrupt withdrawal of corticosteroid therapy. Postural hypotension, hypoglycemia, hyponatremia, and weight loss may be present. Patients with chronic Addison's disease often have hyperkalemia (64 percent of cases), but potassium and sodium levels may be normal in acute adrenal failure. Infusion of saline and dexamethasone will relieve gastrointestinal and other complaints within 12 to 36 h. A clinical diagnosis based on the response to dexamethasone therapy can be confirmed by measuring the serum cortisol response to an injection of cosyntropin (Cortrosyn), a synthetic form of ACTH.

14. ACUTE INTERMITTENT PORPHYRIA

Patients may experience a severe initial attack of acute generalized abdominal pain with minimal or no tenderness or guarding. Distension due to ileus, vomiting, fever, tachycardia, and leukocytosis may occur, producing a clinical picture simulating an intraabdominal vascular catastrophe. Vomiting associated with severe constipation mimics mechanical intestinal obstruction.

Isolated attacks of abdominal pain and vomiting may occur, or they may be accompanied by painful paresthesias and motor weakness in the limbs, foot or wrist drop, a flaccid paraplegia, quadriplegia, and/or respiratory muscle weakness. Signs of an acute delirium with agitation and disorientation or a depressive or delusional-hallucinatory psychosis may occur in up to 35 percent of cases. Inappropriate ADH secretion produces hyponatremia and hypomagnesemia, and can cause tetany. Fasting or alcohol or a specific drug ingestion may precipitate an attack. The Watson-Schwartz screening test will be positive for urinary porphobilinogen during an acute attack and can be confirmed by quantitative urinary delta-aminolevulinic acid and porphobilinogen measurements. Measurement of red blood cell or lymphocyte porphobi-

linogen deaminase activity may be performed in asymptomatic patients between episodes of pain and neurologic dysfunction, but the specificity of this test is not sufficient to establish a diagnosis in some cases.

Symptom response to oral or intravenous carbohydrate loading or hematin infusion may be life-saving and may provide support for the diagnosis. Attacks tend to begin near or after puberty and may occur frequently or only rarely. Variegate porphyria and hereditary coproporphyria can cause similar clinical syndromes as well as skin photosensitivity. Elevated urinary levels of porphobilinogen also occur in these disorders.

15. HEREDITARY ANGIOEDEMA

This disorder begins with central or generalized colicky abdominal pain, bloating, nausea, and vomiting. Local direct tenderness may accompany the pain, but peritoneal signs and fever are usually absent. There is usually a family history, involving one parent and/or siblings, of similar attacks of abdominal pain. Untreated, the abdominal pain and associated symptoms resolve in 1 to 3 days. Loose stools may follow relief of the pain and nausea. Nonpitting brawny angioedema of the face, hands, feet, or trunk may occur simultaneously with the abdominal pain or at other times. Severe upper respiratory obstruction due to laryngeal edema may be life-threatening. The abdominal pain is due to partial intestinal obstruction from bowel wall edema, but a minority of cases may have more persistent abdominal pain from acid hypersecretion. Abdominal radiographs may show a ''stacked coin'' or thumbprinting pattern of the small bowel. Severe intravascular fluid leakage into tissue may cause leukocytosis and increase the hematocrit to as high as 65 percent. Postural hypotension may result from third-space fluid losses. Low serum C4 and C1 esterase inhibitor activities are diagnostic and revert to normal with androgen (danocrine) therapy. Cases of angioedema are often mislabeled as irritable bowel syndrome. Gastrointestinal complaints may predate cutaneous involvement or occur as the only manifestation of this disorder. Until the diagnosis is made, these patients may undergo repeated exploratory surgery for small bowel obstruction. Attacks occur spontaneously or may be initiated by menses; oral contraceptive use; an emotional upset; or a minor trauma, such as venipuncture, squeezing pimples, puncture wounds, prolonged standing, sexual intercourse, horseback riding, or typing.

16. COCAINE INGESTION

Acute ingestion of cocaine can cause diffuse colicky and then constant abdominal pain with few physical findings except mild tenderness. This pain is due to bowel ischemia and may progress to produce severe generalized abdominal pain, nausea, vomiting, distension, and signs of acute peritonitis due to bowel necrosis and perforation. Surgical exploration and bowel resection may be required.

17. PREGNANCY-ASSOCIATED PAIN

A. False Labor The pain is brief (30–90 s) and is felt in the lower abdomen and inguinal areas. It is seldom felt in the back. Episodes occur at intervals of 15 to 30 min or longer and may continue for days. The uterine contractions associated with these false labor pains are not usually very forceful. These pains may begin in the middle of the third trimester and continue until true labor starts.

B. True Labor Pains begin in the low and midback and over the fundus of the term uterus and radiate over the whole abdomen anteriorly, following the contour of the uterus. In some patients, the pain is most severe in the back. Strong uterine contractions can be felt. The pain lasts 30–90 s and comes every 10 to 15 min when labor begins, and, as it progresses, the period between contractions shortens to as little as 1 to 2 min. "Bloody show," or drainage of amniotic fluid following rupture of the membranes, may precede or occur shortly after the onset of labor. Forceful regular contractions associated with diffuse abdominal and/or back pain are likely to represent true labor.

C. Afterpains During the first week postpartum, lower abdominal and midline pains are usually due to uterine contractions. There is an increased frequency of such pains in women who are breastfeeding.

D. Abruptio Placentae This condition may begin with profuse vaginal bleeding in the last half of pregnancy. There may be diffuse severe constant abdominal pain, increased uterine firmness and tenderness, and absent fetal heart sounds. Tachycardia and hypotension may be present. In severe cases, the generalized abdominal pain may be excruciating and the uterine tenderness marked. An extreme form of this disorder has been called uteroplacental apoplexy (Couvelaire uterus). Correction of hypovolemia is essential. If the fetus is viable, cesarean section is usually required.

E. Rupture of the Uterus During labor, there may be a sudden sharp pain that occurs during a typical labor pain. The sharp pain affects the upper and lower abdomen and may be described as tearing or ripping.

When this happens, uterine contractions cease and pain stops. Bleeding from the tear may cause diffuse abdominal and shoulder pain that may have a pleuritic component. These pains are due to the irritating effects of blood and may take several hours to develop. The fetus may be extruded from the uterus and may be palpated in an extra-uterine position. A tear in the uterine wall may be palpable on vaginal examination. Hemoperitoneum, detected by culdocentesis, will confirm the clinical diagnosis. Hypovolemia must be corrected, the fetus delivered by cesarean section, and the uterus removed or repaired. Uterine rupture may be caused by cephalopelvic disproportion, fetal malpresentation, instrumentation, oxytocin administration during labor, or obstetrical trauma due to podalic version.

UPPER ABDOMINAL PAIN REFERENCES
(Chapters 16 to 18 and Chapter 24)

Abdominal Pain—Psychogenic
Blendis LM, Hill OW, Merskey H: Abdominal pain and the emotions. *Pain* 5:179–191, 1978.
Gomez J, Dally P: Psychologically mediated abdominal pain in surgical and medical outpatient clinics. *Br Med J* 1:1451–1453, 1977.

Bezoars
Raffin SB: Bezoars, in Sleisenger MH, Fordtran JS (eds): *Gastrointestinal Disease: Pathophysiology, Diagnosis, Management,* 4th ed. Philadelphia, Saunders, 1989, pp 741–745.

Cholangitis
Chan F-L, Man S-W, Yeong LLY, et al: Evaluation of recurrent pyogenic cholangitis with CT: Analysis of 50 patients. *Radiology* 170:165–169, 1989.
Cooper JF, Brand EJ: Symptomatic sclerosing cholangitis in patients with a normal alkaline phosphatase: Two case reports and a review of the literature. *Am J Gastroenterol* 83(2):308–311, 1988.

Kaufman SL, Kadir S, Mitchell SE, et al: Left lobe of the liver: Percutaneous biliary drainage. *Radiology* 170:191–194, 1989.
Skolkin MD, Alspaugh JP, Casarella WJ, et al: Sclerosing cholangitis: Palliation with percutaneous cholangioplasty. *Radiology* 170:199–206, 1989.
Way LW, Sleisenger MH: Biliary obstruction, cholangitis, and choledocholithiasis, in Sleisenger MH, Fordtran JS (eds): *Gastrointestinal Disease: Pathophysiology, Diagnosis, Management,* 4th ed. Philadelphia, Saunders, 1989, pp 1714–1729.

Cholecystitis
Bowen JC, Brenner HI, Ferrante WA, et al: Gallstone disease: Pathophysiology, epidemiology, natural history and treatment options. *Med Clin North Am* 76: 1143–1157, 1992.
Fink-Bennett D, Freitas JE, Ripley SD, et al: The sensitivity of hepatobiliary imaging and real-time ultrasonography in the detection of acute cholecystitis. *Arch Surg* 120:904–906, 1985.

Freitas JE, Mirkes SH, Fink-Bennett DM, et al: Suspected acute cholecystitis. Comparison of hepatobiliary scintigraphy versus ultrasonography. *Clin Nucl Med* 7:364–367, 1982.

Glenn F: Acute cholecystitis. *Surg Gynecol Obstet* 143:56–60, 1976.

Glenn F: Cholecystostomy in the high risk patient with biliary tract disease. *Ann Surg* 185(2):185–191, 1977.

Hinnant K, Schwartz A, Rotterdam H, et al: Cytomegaloviral and cryptosporidial cholecystitis in two patients with AIDS. *Am J Surg Pathol* 13(1):57–60, 1989.

Holzbach RT: Pathogenesis and medical treatment of gallstones, in Sleisenger MH, Fordtran JS (eds): *Gastrointestinal Disease: Pathophysiology, Diagnosis, Management,* 4th ed. Philadelphia, Saunders, 1989, pp 1668–1691.

Jacobson MA, Cello JP, Sande MA: Cholestasis and disseminated cytomegalovirus disease in patients with the acquired immunodeficiency syndrome. *Am J Med* 84:218–224, 1988.

Jurkovich GJ, Dyess DL, Ferrara JJ: Cholecystostomy: Expected outcome in primary and secondary biliary disorders. *Am Surg* 54:40–44, 1988.

Krasna MJ, Flancbaum L, Trooskin SZ, et al: Gastrointestinal complications after cardiac surgery. *Surgery* 104:773–780, 1988.

Marton KI, Doubilet P: How to image the gallbladder in suspected cholecystitis. *Ann Intern Med* 109:722–729, 1988.

Mentzer RM Jr, Golden GT, Chandler JG, et al: A comparative appraisal of emphysematous cholecystitis. *Am J Surg* 129:10–15, 1975.

Mirvis SE, Vainright JR, Nelson AW, et al: The diagnosis of acute acalculous cholecystitis: A comparison of sonography, scintigraphy, and CT. *AJR* 147:1171–1175, 1986.

Parekh D: Acute acalculous cholecystitis. *S Afr J Surg* 26:16–19, 1988.

Ralls PW, Colletti PM, Lapin SA, et al: Real-time sonography in suspected acute cholecystitis. Prospective evaluation of primary and secondary signs. *Radiology* 155:767–771, 1985.

Schneiderman DJ: Hepatobiliary abnormalities of AIDS. *Gastroenterol Clin North Am* 17(3):615–630, 1988.

Sharp KW: Acute cholecystitis. *Surg Clin North Am* 68(2):269–279, 1988.

van der Linden W, Sunzel H: Early versus delayed operation for acute cholecystitis. A controlled clinical trial. *Am J Surg* 120:7–13, 1970.

Worthen NJ, Uszler JM, Funamura JL: Cholecystitis: Prospective evaluation of sonography and ⁹⁹ᵐTc-HIDA cholescintigraphy. *AJR* 137: 973–978, 1981.

Cholelithiasis

French EB, Robb WAT: Biliary and renal colic. *Br Med J,* July 20, 1986, pp 135–138.

Hayek T, Kleinhaus U, Hashmonai N, et al: Case report: Preoperative diagnosis of Mirizzi syndrome. *Am J Med Sci* 296(1):74–75, 1988.

Laing FC, Federle MP, Jeffrey RB, et al: Ultrasonic evaluation of patients with acute right upper quadrant pain. *Radiology* 140:449–455, 1981.

Reid MH, Phillips HE: The role of computed tomography and ultrasound imaging in biliary tract disease. *Surg Clin North Am* 61(4): 787–825, 1981.

Sackmann M, Delius M, Sauerbruch T, et al: Shock-wave lithotripsy of gallbladder stones. The first 175 patients. *N Engl J Med* 318(7): 393–397, 1988.

Wegge C, Kjaergaard J: Evaluation of symptoms and signs of gallstone disease in patients admitted with upper abdominal pain. *Scand J Gastroenterol* 20:933–936, 1985.

Way LW, Sleisenger MH: Cholelithiasis; Chronic and acute cholecystitis, in Sleisenger MH, Fordtran JS (eds): *Gastrointestinal Disease: Pathophysiology, Diagnosis, Management,* 4th ed. Philadelphia, Saunders, 1989, pp 1691–1714.

Extracorporeal shock-wave lithotripsy for gallbladder stones. *Medical Lett,* 31(785):9–10, 1989.

Diagnostic Methods—Epigastric Pain

Brown P, Salmon PR, Burwood RJ, et al: The endoscopic, radiolog-

ical, and surgical findings in chronic duodenal ulceration. *Scand J Gastroenterol* 13:557–560, 1978.

Colin-Jones DG: Endoscopy or radiology for upper gastrointestinal symptoms? *Lancet,* May 3, 1986, pp 1022–1023.

Dooley CP, Larson AW, Stace NH, et al: Double-contrast barium meal and upper gastrointestinal endoscopy. A comparative study. *Ann Intern Med* 101:538–545, 1984.

Kahn KL, Kosecoff J, Chassin MR, et al: The use and misuse of upper gastrointestinal endoscopy. *Ann Intern Med* 109:664–670, 1988.

Kahn K, Greenfield S: Endoscopy in the evaluation of dyspepsia. *Ann Intern Med* 102:266–269, 1985.

Kahn KL, Greenfield S: The efficacy of endoscopy in the evaluation of dyspepsia. A review of the literature and development of a sound strategy. *J Clin Gastroenterol* 8(3):346–358, 1986.

Kogan FJ, Sampliner RE, Feldshon SD, et al: The yield of diagnostic upper endoscopy: Results of a prospective audit. *J Clin Gastroenterol* 7(6):488–491, 1985.

Marton KI, Doubilet P: How to study the gallbladder. *Ann Intern Med* 109:752–754, 1988.

Morrissey JF: The problem of the inappropriate endoscopy (editorial). *Ann Intern Med* 109(8):605–606, 1988.

Talley NJ, McNeil D, Hayden A, et al: Prognosis of chronic unexplained dyspepsia: A prospective study of potential predictor variables in patients with endoscopically diagnosed nonulcer dyspepsia. *Gastroenterology* 92:1060–1066, 1987.

Diagnostic Methods—Right Upper Abdominal Pain

Kingham JGC, Dawson AM: Origin of chronic right upper quadrant pain. *Gut* 26:783–788, 1985.

McCarthy S, Hricak H, Cohen M, et al: Cholecystitis: Detection with MR imaging. *Radiology* 158:333–336, 1986.

Marton KI, Doubilet P: How to image the gallbladder in suspected cholecystitis. *Ann Intern Med* 109:722–729, 1988.

Shuman WP, Mack LA, Rudd TG, et al: Evaluation of acute right upper quadrant pain: Sonography and ⁹⁹ᵐTc-PIPIDA cholescintigraphy. *AJR* 139:61–64, 1982.

Valberg LS, Jabbari M, Kerr JW, et al: Biliary pain in young women in the absence of gallstones. *Gastroenterology* 60(6):1020–1026, 1971.

Duodenal Ulcer

Donahue PE, Yoshida J, Richter HM, et al: Proximal gastric vagotomy with drainage for obstructing duodenal ulcer. *Surgery* 104:757–764, 1988.

Earlam RJ: Production of epigastric pain in duodenal ulcer by lower oesophageal acid perfusion. *Br Med J* 4:714–716, 1970.

Pounder R: Silent peptic ulceration: Deadly silence or golden silence? *Gastroenterology* 96:626–631, 1989.

Soll AH: Duodenal ulcer and drug therapy, in Sleisenger MH, Fordtran JS (eds): *Gastrointestinal Disease: Pathophysiology, Diagnosis, Management,* 4th ed. Philadelphia, Saunders, 1989, pp 814–879.

Esophageal Disorders

Hogan WJ, Dodds WJ: Gastroesophageal reflux disease (reflux esophagitis), in Sleisenger MH, Fordtran JS (eds): *Gastrointestinal Disease,* 4th ed. Philadelphia, Saunders, 1989, pp 594–619.

McDonald GB: Esophageal diseases caused by infection, systemic illness, and trauma, in Sleisenger MH, Fordtran JS (eds): *Gastrointestinal Disease,* 4th ed. Philadelphia, Saunders, 1989, pp 640–656.

Pope CE II: Heartburn, dysphagia, and other esophageal symptoms, in Sleisenger MH, Fordtran JS (eds): *Gastrointestinal Disease,* 4th ed. Philadelphia, Saunders, 1989, pp 200–203.

Gallbladder—Carcinoma

Katoh T, Nakai T, Hayashi S, et al: Noninvasive carcinoma of the gallbladder arising in localized type adenomyomatosis. *Am J Gastroenterol* 83(6):670–674, 1988.

Nishino H, Satake K, Kim E-C, et al: Primary carcinoma of the gallbladder. *Am Surg* 54:487–491, 1988.

Way LW, Altman DF: Neoplasms of the gallbladder and bile ducts, in Sleisenger MH, Fordtran JS (eds): *Gastrointestinal Disease:*

Pathophysiology, Diagnosis, Management, 4th ed. Philadelphia, Saunders, 1989, pp 1734–1740.

Wilbur AC, Gyi B, Renigers SA: High-field MRI of primary gallbladder carcinoma. *Gastrointest Radiol* 13:142–144, 1988.

Gallbladder Disease

Malet PF, Soloway RD: Diseases of the gallbladder and bile ducts, in Wyngaarden JB, Smith LH Jr (eds): *Cecil Textbook of Medicine,* 18th ed. Philadelphia, Saunders, 1988, pp 859–872.

McPhee MS, Greenberger NJ: Diseases of the gallbladder and bile ducts, in Braunwald E, Isselbacher KJ, Petersdorf RG, et al (eds): *Harrison's Principles of Internal Medicine,* 11th ed. New York, McGraw-Hill, 1987, 1358–1368.

Gastric Carcinoma

Carter KJ, Schaffer HA, Ritchie WP Jr: Early gastric cancer. *Ann Surg* 199:604–609, 1986.

Chia MM, Langman JM, Hecker R, et al: Early gastric cancer: 52 cases of combined experience of two South Australian teaching hospitals. *Pathology* 20:216–226, 1988.

Davis GR: Neoplasms of the stomach, in Sleisenger MH, Fordtran JS (eds): *Gastrointestinal Disease: Pathophysiology, Diagnosis, Management,* 4th ed. Philadelphia, Saunders, 1989, pp 745–772.

Deakin M, Colin-Jones DG, Vessey MP: Routine practice in the diagnosis of adenocarcinoma of the stomach: A survey of tumours diagnosed in the Portsmouth and Oxford Health Districts 1979–1980. *Postgrad Med J* 64:33–37, 1988.

Goldin E, Zimmerman J, Okon E, et al: Should we worry about gastric cancer in duodenal ulcer patients? *J Clin Gastroenterol* 7(3):227–231, 1985.

Podolsky I, Storms PR, Richardson CT, et al: Gastric adenocarcinoma masquerading endoscopically as benign gastric ulcer. A five-year experience. *Dig Dis Sci* 33(9):1057–1063, 1988.

Sheward SE, Davis M, Amparo EG, et al: Intramural hemorrhage simulating gastric neoplasm. *Gastrointest Radiol* 13:102–104, 1988.

Vyberg M, Hougen HP, Tønnesen K: Diagnostic accuracy of endoscopic gastrobiopsy in carcinoma of the stomach. A histopathological review of 101 cases. *Acta Path Microbiol Immunol Scand* sect. A 91:483–487, 1983.

Winawer SJ: Neoplasms of the stomach, in Wyngaarden JB, Smith LH Jr (eds): *Cecil Textbook of Medicine,* 18th ed. Philadelphia, Saunders, 1988, pp 709–714.

Gastric Ulcers

Adkins RB, DeLozier JB III, Scott HW Jr, et al: The management of gastric ulcers. A current review. *Ann Surg* 201:741–751, 1986.

Graham DY: Prevention of gastroduodenal injury induced by chronic nonsteroidal antiinflammatory drug therapy. *Gastroenterol* 96:675–681, 1989.

Griffin MR, Ray WA, Schaffner W: Nonsteroidal anti-inflammatory drug use and death from peptic ulcer in elderly persons. *Ann Intern Med* 109:359–363, 1988.

Hjortrup A, Kjersgaard P, Bredesen J: Medical treatment of stomal ulcers. *Ann R Coll Surg Engl* 70:340–341, 1988.

Kang JY, Wu AYT, Sutherland IH, et al: Prevalence of peptic ulcer in patients undergoing maintenance hemodialysis. *Dig Dis Sci* 33(7):774–778, 1988.

Marks IN, Shay H: Observations on the pathogenesis of gastric ulcer. *Lancet,* May 30, 1959, pp 1107–1111.

McGuigan JE: Peptic ulcer, in Braunwald E, Isselbacher KJ, Petersdorf RG, et al (eds): *Harrison's Principles of Internal Medicine,* 11th ed. New York, McGraw-Hill, 1987, pp 1239–1253.

Richardson CT: Gastric ulcer, in Sleisenger MH, Fordtran JS (eds): *Gastrointestinal Disease: Pathophysiology, Diagnosis, Management,* 4th ed. Philadelphia, Saunders, 1989, pp 879–909.

Robert A, Kauffman GL Jr: Stress ulcers, erosions, and gastric mucosal injury, in Sleisenger MH, Fordtran JS (eds): *Gastrointestinal Disease: Pathophysiology, Diagnosis, Management,* 4th ed. Philadelphia, Saunders, 1989, pp 772–792.

Roth SH: Nonsteroidal anti-inflammatory drugs: Gastropathy, deaths,

and medical practice (editorial). *Ann Intern Med* 109(5):353–354, 1988.

Gastric Volvulus

Ahmed AF, Bediako AK, Rai D: Agenesis of the left hepatic lobe with gastric volvulus. *NY State J Med,* June 1988, pp 327–328.

Raffin SB: Diverticula, rupture, and volvulus, in Sleisenger MH, Fordtran JS (eds): *Gastrointestinal Disease: Pathophysiology, Diagnosis, Management,* 4th ed. Philadelphia, Saunders, 1989, pp 735–740.

Robbins SM, Tuten TU, Clements JL, et al: Angiographic diagnosis of gastric volvulus with report of a complication following left gastric artery embolization. *Gastrointest Radiol* 13:112–114, 1988.

Yin RL, Nowak TV: Familial occurrence of intrathoracic gastric volvulus. *Dig Dis Sci* 33(11):1483–1487, 1988.

Glomerulopathies

Glassock RJ, Brenner BM: Glomerulopathies associated with multisystem diseases, in Braunwald E, Isselbachen KJ, Petersdorf RG, et al (eds): *Harrison's Principles of Internal Medicine,* 11th ed. New York, McGraw-Hill, 1987 pp 1183–1189.

Glassock RJ, Brenner BM: The major glomerulopathies, in Braunwald E, Isselbacher KJ, Petersdorf RG, et al (eds): *Harrison's Principles of Internal Medicine,* 11th ed. New York, McGraw-Hill, 1987, pp 1173–1183.

Hepatic Disease

Ockner RK: Toxic and drug-induced liver disease, in Wyngaarden JB, Smith LH Jr (eds): *Cecil Textbook of Medicine,* 18th ed. Philadelphia, Saunders, 1988, pp 826–830.

Hepatic Lesions

Alpert E, Isselbacher KJ: Tumors of the liver, in Braunwald E, Isselbacher KJ, Petersdorf RG, et al (eds): *Harrison's Principles of Internal Medicine,* New York, McGraw-Hill, 1987, pp 1351–1353.

Scharschmidt BF: Hepatic tumors, in Wyngaarden JB, Smith LH Jr (eds): *Cecil Textbook of Medicine,* 18th ed. Philadelphia, Saunders, 1988, pp 856–859.

Shorey J: Evaluation of mass lesions in the liver, in Sleisenger MH, Fordtran JS (eds): *Gastrointestinal Disease: Pathophysiology, Diagnosis, Management,* 4th ed. Philadelphia, Saunders, 1989, pp 467–487.

Hepatic Pain

Ishak KG: Benign tumors and pseudotumors of the liver. *Appl Pathol* 6:82–104, 1988.

Manas KJ, Welsh JD, Rankin RA, et al: Hepatic hemorrhage without rupture in preeclampsia. *N Engl J Med* 312(7):424–426, 1985.

Nokes SR, Baker ME, Spritzer CE, et al: Hepatic adenoma: MR appearance mimicking focal nodular hyperplasia. *J Comput Assist Tomogr* 12(5):885–887, 1988.

Rummeny E, Weissleder R, Stark DD, et al: Primary liver tumors: Diagnosis by MR imaging. *AJR* 152:63–72, 1989.

Rustgi VK: Epidemiology of hepatocellular carcinoma, in Di Bisceglie AM (moderator): Hepatocellular carcinoma. *Ann Intern Med* 108:390–391, 1988.

Vecchio FM: Fibrolamellar carcinoma of the liver: A distinct entity within the hepatocellular tumors. A review 6. *Appl Pathol* 6:139–148, 1988.

Case 52-1988, Case records of the Massachusetts General Hospital. *N Engl J Med* 319(26):1718–1725, 1988.

Hepatitis

Dienstag JL, Wands JR, Koff RS: Acute hepatitis, in Braunwald E, Isselbacher KJ, Petersdorf RG, et al (eds): *Harrison's Principles of Internal Medicine,* 11th ed. New York, McGraw-Hill, 1987, pp 1325–1338.

Ockner RK: Acute viral hepatitis, in Wyngaarden JB, Smith LH Jr (eds): *Cecil Textbook of Medicine,* 18th ed. Philadelphia, Saunders, 1988, pp 818–826.

Nonulcer Dyspepsia—Duodenitis

Aase ST, Liavag I, Roland M: Proximal gastric vagotomy in dyspeptic patients without an ulcer. *World J Surg* 8:303–307, 1984.

Cheli R: Is duodenitis always a peptic disease? *Am J Gastroenterol* 80(6):442–444, 1985.

Christiansen J, Aagaard P, Koudahl G: Truncal vagotomy and drainage in the treatment of ulcer-like dyspepsia without ulcer. *Acta Chir Scand* 139:173–175, 1973.

Cotton PB, Price AB, Tighe JR, et al: Preliminary evaluation of "duodenitis" by endoscopy and biopsy. *Br Med J* 3:430–433, 1973.

Krag E: The pseudo-ulcer syndrome. A clinical, radiographic and statistical follow-up study of patients with ulcer symptoms but no demonstrable ulcer in the stomach or duodenum. *Dan Med Bull* 16(1):6–9, 1969.

Sircus W: Duodenitis: A clinical, endoscopic and histopathologic study. *Q J Med* 221:593–600, 1985.

Venables CW: Duodenitis. *Scand J Gastroenterol* 20(suppl 109):91–97, 1985.

Nonulcer Dyspepsia—Food Intolerance

Cohen S: Pathogenesis of coffee-induced gastrointestinal symptoms. *N Engl J Med* 303:122–124, 1980.

Friedlander PH: Food and indigestion. An investigation of possible relationships. *Br Med J,* Dec 25, 1959, pp 1454–1458.

Heyman MB: Food sensitivity and eosinophilic gastroenteropathies, in Sleisenger MH, Fordtran JS (eds): *Gastrointestinal Disease: Pathophysiology, Diagnosis, Management,* 4th ed. Philadelphia, Saunders, 1989, pp 1113–1134.

Koch JP, Donaldson RM Jr: A survey of food intolerances in hospitalized patients. *N Engl J Med* 271(13):657–660, 1964.

Taggart D, Billington BP: Fatty foods and dyspepsia. *Lancet,* August 27, 1966, pp 464–466.

Nonulcer Dyspepsia—Gastritis/*Helicobacter Pylori* (formerly *Campylobacter Pylori*)

Blaser MJ, Brown WR: Campylobacters and gastroduodenal inflammation, in Stollerman GH (ed): *Advances in Internal Medicine.* Chicago, Year Book, 1988, vol 33, pp 21–42.

Borody TJ, Carrick J, Hazell SL: Symptoms improve after the eradication of gastric *Campylobacter pyloridis* (letter to the editor). *Med J Aust* 146:450–451, 1987.

Dooley CP, Cohen H: The clinical significance of *Campylobacter pylori. Ann Intern Med* 108:70–79, 1988.

Dooley CP, Cohen H, Fitzgibbons PK, et al: Prevalence of *Helicobacter pylori* infection and histologic gastritis in asymptomatic persons. *N Engl J Med* 321(23):1562–1566, 1989.

Goodwin CS, Blincow E, Peterson G, et al: Enzyme-linked immunosorbent assay for *Campylobacter pyloridis*: Correlation with presence of *C. pyloridis* in the gastric mucosa. *J Infect Dis* 155(3):488–494, 1987.

Marshall BJ, Surveyor I: Carbon-14 urea breath test for the diagnosis of *Campylobacter pylori* associated gastritis. *J Nucl Med* 29:11–16, 1988.

Marshall BJ, Armstrong JA, Francis GJ, et al: Antibacterial action of bismuth in relation to *Campylobacter pyloridis* colonization and gastritis. *Digestion* 37(suppl 2):16–30, 1987.

Paull G, Yardley JH: Gastric and esophageal *Campylobacter pylori* in patients with Barrett's esophagus. *Gastroenterology* 95:216–218, 1988.

Perez-Perez GI, Dworkin BM, Chodos JE, et al: *Campylobacter pylori* antibodies in humans. *Ann Intern Med* 109:11–17, 1988.

Villako K, Ihamaki T, Tamm A, et al: Upper abdominal complaints and gastritis. *Ann Clin Res* 16:192–194, 1984.

Weinstein WM: Gastritis, in Sleisenger MH, Fordtran JS (eds): *Gastrointestinal Disease: Pathophysiology, Diagnosis, Management,* 4th ed. Philadelphia, Saunders, 1989, pp 792–813.

Nonulcer Dyspepsia—Irritable Bowel

Lasser RB, Bond JH, Levitt MD: The role of intestinal gas in functional abdominal pain. *N Engl J Med* 293:524–526, 1975.

Moriarty KJ, Dawson AM: Functional abdominal pain: Further evidence that whole gut is affected. *Br Med J* 284:1670–1672, 1984.

Thompson WG: Gastrointestinal symptoms in the irritable bowel compared with peptic ulcer and inflammatory bowel disease. *Gut* 25:1089–1092, 1984.

Nonulcer Dyspepsia—Motility Disorders

Clouse RE: Motor disorders, in Sleisenger MH, Fordtran JS (eds): *Gastrointestinal Disease: Pathophysiology, Diagnosis, Management,* 4th ed. Philadelphia, Saunders, 1989, pp 559–593.

Jian R, Ducrot F, Piedeloup C, et al: Measurement of gastric emptying in dyspeptic patients: Effect of a new gastrokinetic agent (cisapride). *Gut* 26:352–358, 1985.

McCallum RW: Motor function of the stomach in health and disease, in Sleisenger MH, Fordtran JS (eds): *Gastrointestinal Disease: Pathophysiology, Diagnosis, Management,* 4th ed. Philadelphia, Saunders, 1989, pp 675–713.

Nonulcer Dyspepsia/Ulcer

Crean GP, Card WI, Beattie AD, et al: Ulcer-like dyspepsia. *Scand J Gastroenterol* 9(suppl):9–14, 1982.

Earlam R, Chir M: A computerized questionnaire analysis of duodenal ulcer symptoms. *Gastroenterology* 71:314–317, 1976.

Edwards FC, Coghill NF: Clinical manifestations in patients with chronic atrophic gastritis, gastric ulcer, and duodenal ulcer. *Q J Med* 146:337–360, 1968.

Horrocks JC, De Dombal FT: Clinical presentation of patients with 'dyspepsia.' Detailed symptomatic study of 360 patients. *Gut* 19:19–26, 1978.

MacDonald WC, Rubin CE: Gastric tumors, gastritis, and other gastric diseases, in Braunwald E, Isselbacher KJ, Petersdorf RG, et al (eds): *Harrison's Principles of Internal Medicine,* 11th ed. New York, McGraw-Hill, 1987, pp 1253–1260.

Nyrén O, Adami H-O, Gustavsson S, et al: The "epigastric distress syndrome." A possible disease entity identified by history and endoscopy in patients with nonulcer dyspepsia. *J Clin Gastroenterol* 9(3):303–309, 1987.

Richardson CT: Gastritis, in Wyngaarden JB, Smith LH Jr (eds): *Cecil Textbook of Medicine,* 18th ed. Philadelphia, Saunders, 1988, pp 689–692.

Spiro HM: Moynihan's disease? The diagnosis of duodenal ulcer. *N Engl J Med* 291:567–569, 1974.

Talley NJ, Phillips SF: Non-ulcer dyspepsia: Potential causes and pathophysiology. *Ann Intern Med* 108:865–879, 1988.

Talley NJ, Piper DW: Comparison of the clinical features and illness behaviour of patients presenting with dyspepsia of unknown cause (essential dyspepsia) and organic disease. *Aust N Z J Med* 16:352–359, 1986.

Walan A, Bader J-P, Classen M, et al: Effect of omeprazole and ranitidine on ulcer healing and relapse rates in patients with benign gastric ulcer. *N Engl J Med* 320:69–75, 1989.

Pancreas—Carcinoma

Cello JP: Carcinoma of the pancreas, in Sleisenger MH, Fordtran JS (eds): *Gastrointestinal Disease: Pathophysiology, Diagnosis, Management,* 4th ed. Philadelphia, Saunders, 1989, pp 1872–1884.

Cello JP: Carcinoma of the pancreas, in Wyngaarden JB, Smith LH Jr (eds): *Cecil Textbook of Medicine,* 18th ed. Philadelphia, Saunders, 1988, pp 781–784.

Gowland M, Warwick F, Kalantzis N, et al: Relative efficiency and predictive value of ultrasonography and endoscopic retrograde pancreatography in diagnosis of pancreatic disease. *Lancet,* July 25, 1981, pp 190–193.

Mackie CR, Blackstone MO, Dhorajiwala J, et al: Value of new diagnostic aids in relation to the disease process in pancreatic cancer. *Lancet,* August 25, 1979, pp 385–388.

Manabe T, Miyashita T, Ohshio G, et al: Small carcinoma of the pancreas. Clinical and pathologic evaluation of 17 patients. *Cancer* 62:135–141, 1988.

Mitchell ML, Bittner CA, Wills JS, et al: Fine needle aspiration cytology of the pancreas. A retrospective study of 73 cases. *Acta Cytol* 32(4):447–451, 1988.

Nix CAJJ, Van Overbeeke IC, Wilson JHP, et al: ERCP diagnosis of tumors in the region of the head of the pancreas. Analysis of criteria and computer-aided diagnosis. *Dig Dis Sci* 33(5):577–586, 1988.

Pilotti S, Rilke F, Claren R, et al: Conclusive diagnosis of hepatic and pancreatic malignancies by fine needle aspiration. *Acta Cytol* 32(1): 27–38, 1988.

Pancreas—Pancreatitis

Andersen BN, Pedersen NT, Scheel J, et al: Incidence of alcoholic chronic pancreatitis in Copenhagen. *Scand J Gastroenterol* 17: 247–252, 1982.

Becker JM, Pemberton JH, DiMagno EP, et al: Prognostic factors in pancreatic abscess. *Surgery* 96(3):455–460, 1984.

Beger HG, Bittner R, Block S, et al: Bacterial contamination of pancreatic necrosis. A prospective clinical study. *Gastroenterol* 91:433–438, 1986.

Berk JE, Simon D, Fridhandler L: Inhibitor test for amylase isoenzymes. Comparison with a simplified chromatographic method. *Am J Gastroenterol* 75(2):128–131, 1981.

Crass RA, Meyer AA, Jeffrey RB, et al: Pancreatic abscess: Impact of computerized tomography on early diagnosis and surgery. *Am J Surg* 150:127–131, 1985.

Eggink WF, Schattenkerk ME, Obertop H, et al: The role of early surgery in the treatment of acute hemorrhagic necrotizing pancreatitis (AHNP). *Neth J Surg* 36(1):6–9, 1984.

Greenberger NJ, Toskes PP, Isselbacher KJ: Diseases of the pancreas, in Braunwald E, Isselbacher KJ, Petersdorf RG, et al (eds): *Harrison's Principles of Internal Medicine,* 11th ed. New York, McGraw-Hill, 1987, pp 1372–1384.

Grendell JH, Cello JP: Chronic pancreatitis, in Sleisenger MH, Fordtran JS (eds): *Gastrointestinal Disease: Pathophysiology, Diagnosis, Management,* 4th ed. Philadelphia, Saunders, 1989, pp 1842–1872.

Kivisaari L, Somer K, Standertskjold-Nordenstam C-G, et al: Early detection of acute fulminant pancreatitis by contrast-enhanced computed tomography. *Scand J Gastroenterol* 18:39–41, 1983.

Levitt MD: Pancreatitis, in Wyngaarden JB, Smith LH Jr (eds): *Cecil Textbook of Medicine,* 18th ed. Philadelphia, Saunders, 1988, pp 774–781.

Nordback IH, Auvinen OA: Long-term results after pancreas resection for acute necrotizing pancreatitis. *Br J Surg* 72:687–689, 1985.

Osborne DH, Imrie CW, Carter DC: Biliary surgery in the same admission for gallstone-associated acute pancreatitis. *Br J Surg* 68:758–761, 1981.

Pemberton JH, Becker JM, Dozois RR, et al: Controlled open lesser sac drainage for pancreatic abscess. *Ann Surg* 203:600–604, 1986.

Potts JR III: Acute pancreatitis. *Surg Clin North Am* 68(2):281–299, 1988.

Reid BG, Kune GA: Accuracy in diagnosis of acute pancreatitis. *Med J Aust* 1:583–587, 1978.

Rotman N, Bonnet F, Larde D, et al: Computerized tomography in the evaluation of the late complications of acute pancreatitis. *Am J Surg* 152:286–289, 1986.

Silverstein W, Isikoff MB, Hill MC, et al: Diagnostic imaging of acute pancreatitis: Prospective study using CT and sonography. *AJR* 137:497–502, 1981.

Soergel KH: Acute pancreatitis, in Sleisenger MH, Fordtran JS (eds): *Gastrointestinal Disease: Pathophysiology, Diagnosis, Management,* 4th ed. Philadelphia, Saunders, 1989, pp 1814–1842.

Spechler SJ, Dalton JW, Robbins AH, et al: Prevalence of normal serum amylase levels in patients with acute alcoholic pancreatitis. *Dig Dis Sci* 28(10):865–869, 1983.

Steckman ML, Dooley MC, Jaques PF, et al: Major gastrointestinal hemorrhage from peripancreatic blood vessels in pancreatitis. Treatment by embolotherapy. *Dig Dis Sci* 29(6):486–497, 1984.

Trapnell JE, Rigby CC, Talbot CH, et al: A controlled trial of Trasylol in the treatment of acute pancreatitis. *Br J Surg* 61:177–182, 1974.

Trapnell JE, Duncan EHL: Patterns of incidence in acute pancreatitis. *Br Med J* 2:179–183, 1975.

Warshaw AL: Inflammatory masses following acute pancreatitis. Phlegmon, pseudocyst, and abscess. *Surg Clin North Am* 54(3): 621–636, 1974.

Warshaw AL: The kidney and changes in amylase clearance (editorial). *Gastroenterology* 71:702–704, 1976.

Postoperative Syndromes

Way LW, Sleisenger MH: Postoperative syndromes, in Sleisenger MH, Fordtran JS (eds): *Gastrointestinal Disease: Pathophysiology, Diagnosis, Management,* 4th ed. Philadelphia, Saunders, 1989, pp 1729–1733.

Renal Vascular Injury

Brenner BM, Hostetter TH: Tubulointerstitial diseases of the kidney, in Braunwald E, Isselbacher KJ, Petersdorf RG, et al (eds): *Harrison's Principles of Internal Medicine,* 11th ed. New York, McGraw-Hill, 1987, pp 1195–1200.

Hollenberg NK: Vascular injury to the kidney, in Braunwald E, Isselbacher KJ, Petersdorf RG, et al (eds): *Harrison's Principles of Internal Medicine,* 11th ed. New York, McGraw-Hill, 1987, pp 1200–1205.

Williams RD: Tumors of the kidney, ureter, and bladder, in Wyngaarden JB, Smith LH Jr (eds): *Cecil Textbook of Medicine,* 18th ed. Philadelphia, Saunders, 1988, pp 650–655.

Sphincter of Oddi

Geenen JE, Hogan WJ, Dodds WJ, et al: The efficacy of endoscopic sphincterotomy after cholecystectomy in patients with sphincter-of-Oddi dysfunction. *N Engl J Med* 320:82–87, 1989.

Ulcer Perforation

Boey J, Lee NW, Wong J, et al: Perforations in acute duodenal ulcers. *Surg Gynecol Obstet* 155:193–196, 1982.

Boey J, Branicki FJ, Alagaratnam TT, et al: Proximal gastric vagotomy. The preferred operation for perforations in acute duodenal ulcer. *Ann Surg* 208:169–174, 1988.

Dasmahapatra KS, Suval W, Machiedo GW: Unsuspected perforation in bleeding duodenal ulcers. *Am Surg* 54:19–21, 1988.

Feliciano DV, Bitondo CG, Burch JM, et al: Emergency management of perforated peptic ulcers in the elderly patient. *Am J Surg* 148:764–767, 1984.

Graham DY: Complications of peptic ulcer disease and indications for surgery, in Sleisenger MH, Fordtran JS (eds): *Gastrointestinal Disease: Pathophysiology, Diagnosis, Management,* 4th ed. Philadelphia, Saunders, 1989, pp 925–938.

Jordan PH Jr, Morrow C: Perforated peptic ulcer. *Surg Clin North Am* 68(2):315–329, 1988.

Miller TA: Emergencies in acid-peptic ulcer. *Gastroenterol Clin North Am* 17(2):303–315, 1988.

Rees JR, Thorbjarnarson B: Perforated gastric ulcer. *Am J Surg* 126:93–97, 1973.

Rogers FA: Elevated serum amylase. A review and an analysis of findings in 1,000 cases of perforated peptic ulcer. *Ann Surg* 153:228–240, 1961.

Stringer MD, Cameron AEP: Surgeons' attitudes to the operative management of duodenal ulcer perforation and haemorrhage. *Ann R Coll Surg Engl* 70:220–223, 1988.

Urinary Tract Infection

Stamm WE, Turck M: Urinary tract infection, pyelonephritis, and related conditions, in Braunwald E, Isselbacher KJ, Petersdorf RG, et al (eds): *Harrison's Principles of Internal Medicine,* 11th ed. New York, McGraw-Hill, 1987, pp 1189–1195.

Vascular Diseases of the Bowel

Grendell JH, Ockner RK: Vascular diseases of the bowel, in Sleisenger MH, Fordtran JS (eds): *Gastrointestinal Disease: Pathophysiology, Diagnosis, Management,* 4th ed. Philadelphia, Saunders, 1989, pp 1903–1932.

Zollinger-Ellison Syndrome

McGuigan JE: The Zollinger-Ellison syndrome, in Sleisenger MH, Fordtran JS (eds): *Gastrointestinal Disease: Pathophysiology, Diagnosis, Management,* 4th ed. Philadelphia, Saunders, 1989, pp 909–925.

Richardson CT: Zollinger-Ellison syndrome, in Wyngaarden JB, Smith LH Jr (eds): *Cecil Textbook of Medicine,* 18th ed. Philadelphia, Saunders, 1988, pp 708–709.

UMBILICAL PAIN REFERENCES (Chapter 20)

Crohn's Disease

Bayerdorffer E, Hochter W, Schwarzkopf-Steinhauser G, et al: Bioptic microbiology in the differential diagnosis of enterocolitis. *Endoscopy* 18:177–181, 1986.

Greenberger N: Regional enteritis. *Ala J Med Sci* 22(1):61–67, 1985.

Itzkowitz SH: Conditions that mimic inflammatory bowel disease. *Postgrad Med* 80(6):219–231, 1986.

Lubat E, Balthazar EJ: The current role of computerized tomography in inflammatory disease of the bowel. *Am J Gastroenterol* 83(2):107–113, 1988.

Pera A, Bellando P, Caldera D, et al: Colonoscopy in inflammatory bowel disease: Diagnostic accuracy and proposal of an endoscopic score. *Gastroenterology* 92:181–185, 1987.

Perzin KH, Peterson M, Castiglione CL, et al: Intramucosal carcinoma of the small intestine arising in regional enteritis (Crohn's disease): Report of a case studied for carcinoembryonic antigen and review of the literature. *Cancer* 54:151–162, 1984.

Rickert RR: The important "imposters" in the differential diagnosis of inflammatory bowel disease. *J Clin Gastroenterol* 6:153–163, 1984.

Turse JC, Schuman BM, Tedesco FJ: Differentiating Crohn's colitis from ulcerative colitis. A rundown of likenesses and dissimilarities. *Postgrad Med* 83(4):323–330, 1988.

Hernias

Lemmer JH, Stroder WE, Eckhauser FE: Umbilical hernia incarceration: A complication of medical therapy of ascites. *Am J Gastroenterol* 78(5):295–296, 1983.

O'Connor JP, Rigby RJ, Hardie IR, et al: Abdominal hernias complicating continuous ambulatory peritoneal dialysis. *Am J Nephrol* 6:271–274, 1986.

Intestinal Angina

Beal JM, Conn J Jr (contributing eds): Intestinal angina. Chronic mesenteric ischemia. *Ill Med J,* April 1983, pp 272–277.

Jager KA, Fortner GS, Thiele BL, et al: Noninvasive diagnosis of intestinal angina. *J Clin Ultrasound* 12:588–591, 1984.

Lawson JD, Ochsner JL: Median arcuate ligament syndrome with severe two-vessel involvement. *Arch Surg* 119:226–227, 1984.

Odurny A, Sniderman KW, Colapinto RF: Intestinal angina: Percutaneous transluminal angioplasty of the celiac and superior mesenteric arteries. *Radiology* 167:59–62, 1988.

Stanton PE Jr, Hollier PA, Seidel TW, et al: Chronic intestinal ischemia: Diagnosis and therapy. *J Vasc Surg* 4:338–344, 1986.

Lymphoma

Aquilar FP, Alfonso V, Rivas S, et al: Jejunal malignant lymphoma in a patient with adult-onset hypo-gamma-globulinemia and nodular lymphoid hyperplasia of the small bowel. *Am J Gastroenterol* 82(5):472–475, 1987.

Al-Bahrani ZR, Al-Mondhiry H, Bakir F, et al: Clinical and pathologic subtypes of primary intestinal lymphoma. *Cancer* 52:1666–1672, 1983.

Al-Mondhiry H: Primary lymphomas of the small intestine: East-West contrast. *Am J Hematol* 22:89–105, 1986.

Aozasa K, Ueda T, Kurata A, et al: Prognostic value of histologic and clinical factors in 56 patients with gastrointestinal lymphomas. *Cancer* 61:309–315, 1988.

Collier PE: Small bowel lymphoma associated with AIDS. *J Surg Oncol* 32:131–133, 1986.

Megibow AJ, Balthazar EJ, Naidich DP, et al: Computed tomography of gastrointestinal lymphoma. *AJR* 141:541–547, 1983.

ReMine SG, Braasch JW: Gastric and small bowel lymphoma. *Surg Clin North Am* 66(4):713–722, 1986.

Sartoris DJ, Harell GS, Anderson MF, et al: Small-bowel lymphoma and regional enteritis: Radiographic similarities. *Radiology* 152:291–296, 1984.

Tabbane F, Mourali N, Cammoun M, et al: Results of laparotomy in immunoproliferative small intestinal disease. *Cancer* 61:1699–1706, 1988.

Theros EG: RPC of the month from the AFIP. *Radiology* 92:1363–1368, 1969.

Mimics of Crohn's Disease

Cappell MS, Mandell W, Grimes MM, et al: Gastrointestinal histoplasmosis. *Dig Dis Sci* 33(3):353–360, 1988.

Gallego MS, Pulpeiro JR, Arenas A, et al: Primary adenocarcinoma of the terminal ileum simulating Crohn's disease. *Gastrointest Radiol* 11:355–356, 1986.

Haddad FS, Ghossain A, Sawaya E, et al: Abdominal tuberculosis. *Dis Colon Rectum* 30:724–735, 1987.

Zimbalist E, Gettenberg G, Brejt H: Ileocolonic schistosomiasis presenting as lymphoma. *Am J Gastroenterol* 82(5):476–478, 1987.

Vasculitis

Baxter R, Nino-Murcia M, Bloom RJ, et al: Gastrointestinal manifestations of essential mixed cryoglobulinemia. *Gastrointest Radiol* 13:160–162, 1988.

Camilleri M, Pusey CD, Chadwick VS, et al: Gastrointestinal manifestations of systemic vasculitis. *Q J Med* 206:141–149, 1983.

Carlson HC: Perspective: The small bowel examination in the diagnosis of Crohn's disease. *AJR* 147:63–65, 1986.

Jacobsen SEH, Peterson P, Jensen P: Acute abdomen in rheumatoid arthritis due to mesenteric arteritis: A case report and review. *Dan Med Bull* 32:191–193, 1985.

Keshavarzian A, Saverymuttu SH, Chadwick VS, et al: Noninvasive investigation of the gastrointestinal tract in collagen-vascular disease. *Am J Gastroenterol* 79(11):873–877, 1984.

Miller GW Jr, Ruiz JD: Henoch-Schönlein purpura. *Am Fam Physician* 28(4):237–240, 1983.

Prouse PJ, Thompson EM, Gumpel JM: Systemic lupus erythematosus and abdominal pain. *Br J Rheumatol* 22:172–175, 1983.

Roth DA, Wilz DR, Theil GB: Schönlein-Henoch syndrome in adults. *Q J Med* 217:145–152, 1985.

Shepherd HA, Patel C, Bamforth J, et al: Upper gastrointestinal endoscopy in systemic vasculitis presenting as an acute abdomen. *Endoscopy* 15:307–311, 1983.

LUMBAR PAIN REFERENCES
(Chapters 19 and 26)

Adrenal Disorders

Libertino JA: Surgery of adrenal disorders. *Surg Clin North Am* 68(5):1027–1056, 1988.

Rao RH, Vagnucci AH, Amico JA: Bilateral massive adrenal hemorrhage: Early recognition and treatment. *Ann Intern Med* 110:227–235, 1989.

Cystic Diseases of the Kidney

Gabow PA: Cystic disease of the kidney, in Wyngaarden JB, Smith LH Jr (eds): *Cecil Textbook of Medicine,* 18th ed. Philadelphia, Saunders, 1988, vol I, pp 644–648.

Glomerulopathies

Couser WG: Glomerular disorders, in Wyngaarden JB, Smith LH Jr (eds): *Cecil Textbook of Medicine,* 18th ed. Philadelphia, Saunders, 1988, vol I, pp 582–602.

Glassock RJ, Brenner BM: The major glomerulopathies and Glomerulopathies associated with multisystem diseases, in Braunwald E, Isselbacher KJ, Petersdorf RG, et al (eds): *Harrison's Principles of Internal Medicine,* 11th ed. New York, McGraw-Hill, 1987, pp 1173–1183 and pp 1183–1189.

Whitley K, Keane WF, Vernier RL: Acute glomerulonephritis: A clinical overview. *Med Clin North Am* 68(2):259–279, 1984.

Nephropathy

McKinney TD: Tubulointerstitial diseases and toxic nephropathies, in Wyngaarden JB, Smith LH Jr (eds): *Cecil Textbook of Medicine,* 18th ed. Philadelphia, Saunders, 1988, vol I, pp 602–614.

Rector FC Jr: Obstructive nephropathy, in Wyngaarden JB, Smith LH Jr (eds): *Cecil Textbook of Medicine,* 18th ed. Philadelphia, Saunders, 1988, vol I, pp 614–617.

Pyelonephritis

Kanel KT, Kroboth FJ, Schwentker FN, et al: The intravenous pyelogram in acute pyelonephritis. *Arch Intern Med* 148:2144–2148, 1988.

Renal Calculi

Abraham PA, Smith CL: Medical evaluation and management of calcium nephrolithiasis. *Med Clin North Am* 68(2):281–299, 1984.

Brown RD, Preminger GM: Changing surgical aspects of urinary stone disease. *Surg Clin North Am* 68(5):1085–1104, 1988.

Coe FL, Favus MJ: Nephrolithiasis, in Braunwald E, Isselbacher KJ, Petersdorf RG, et al (eds): *Harrison's Principles of Internal Medicine,* 11th ed. New York, McGraw-Hill, 1987, pp 1211–1215.

Pak CYC: Renal calculi, in Wyngaarden JB, Smith LH Jr (eds): *Cecil Textbook of Medicine,* 18th ed. Philadelphia, Saunders, 1988, vol I, pp 638–644.

Spirnak JP, Resnick MI: Urinary stones. *Prim Care* 12(4):735–759, 1985.

Stewart C: Nephrolithiasis. *Emerg Med Clin North Am* 6(3):617–630, 1988.

Renal Inflammatory Disease

Piccirillo M, Rigsby C, Rosenfield AT: Contemporary imaging of renal inflammatory disease. *Infect Dis Clin North Am* 1(4):927–964, 1987.

Renal Tumors

Bosniak MA, Megibow AJ, Hulnick DH, et al: CT diagnosis of renal angiomyolipoma: The importance of detecting small amounts of fat. *AJR* 151:497–501, 1988.

Garnick MB, Brenner BM: Tumors of the urinary tract, in Braunwald E, Isselbacher KJ, Petersdorf RG, et al (eds): *Harrison's Principles*
of *Internal Medicine,* 11th ed. New York, McGraw-Hill, 1987, pp 1218–1221.

Huben RP, Mounzer AM, Murphy GP: Tumor grade and stage as prognostic variables in upper tract urothelial tumors. *Cancer* 62:2016–2020, 1988.

Kendall AR, Senay BA, Coll ME: Spontaneous subcapsular renal hematoma: Diagnosis and management. *J Urol* 139:246–250, 1988.

Medeiros LJ, Gelb AB, Weiss LM: Renal cell carcinoma. Prognostic significance of morphologic parameters in 121 cases. *Cancer* 61:1639–1651, 1988.

Nielsen K, Ostri P: Primary tumors of the renal pelvis: Evaluation of clinical and pathological features in a consecutive series of 10 years. *J Urol* 140:19–21, 1988.

Ramos IM, Taylor KJW, Kier R, et al: Tumor vascular signals in renal masses: Detection with Doppler US. *Radiology* 168:633–637, 1988.

Williams RD: Tumors of the kidney, ureter and bladder, in Wyngaarden JB, Smith LH, Jr (eds): *Cecil Textbook of Medicine,* 18th ed. Philadelphia, Saunders, 1988, vol I, pp 650–655.

Renal and Perirenal Abscesses

Patterson JE, Andriole VT: Renal and perirenal abscesses. *Infect Dis Clin North Am* 1(4):907–926, 1987.

Tubulointerstitial Diseases of the Kidney

Brenner BM, Hostetter TH: Tubulointerstitial diseases of the kidney, in Braunwald E, Isselbacher KJ, Petersdorf RG, et al (eds): *Harrison's Principles of Internal Medicine,* 11th ed. New York, McGraw-Hill, 1987, pp 1195–1200.

Urinary Tract Infections

Andriole VT: Urinary tract infections and pyelonephritis, in Wyngaarden JB, Smith LH Jr (eds): *Cecil Textbook of Medicine,* 18th ed. Philadelphia, Saunders, 1988, vol I, pp 628–632.

Johnson JR, Stamm WE: Urinary tract infections in women: Diagnosis and treatment. *Ann Intern Med* 111:906–917, 1989.

Johnson JR, Stamm WE: Diagnosis and treatment of acute urinary tract infections. *Infect Dis Clin North Am* 1(4):773–791, 1987.

Nicolle LE, Ronald AR: Recurrent urinary tract infection in adult women: Diagnosis and treatment. *Infect Dis Clin North Am* 1(4):793–806, 1987.

Shea DJ: Pyelonephritis and female urinary tract infection. *Emerg Med Clin North Am* 6(3):403–417, 1988.

Stamm WE, Turck M: Urinary tract infection, pyelonephritis, and related conditions, in Braunwald E, Isselbacher KJ, Petersdorf RG, et al (eds): *Harrison's Principles of Internal Medicine,* 11th ed. New York, McGraw-Hill, 1987, pp 1189–1195.

Warren JW: Catheter-associated urinary tract infections. *Infect Dis Clin North Am* 1(4):823–854, 1987.

Urologic Causes of the Acute Abdomen

Koch MO, McDougal WS: Urologic causes of the acute abdomen. *Surg Clin North Am* 68(2):399–413, 1988.

Vascular Disorders of the Kidney

Cohen JJ: Vascular disorders of the kidney, in Wyngaarden JB, Smith LH Jr (eds): *Cecil Textbook of Medicine,* 18th ed. Philadelphia, Saunders, 1988; vol I, pp 632–634.

Hollenberg NK: Vascular injury to the kidney, in Braunwald E, Isselbacher KJ, Petersdorf RG, et al (eds): *Harrison's Principles of Internal Medicine,* 11th ed. New York, McGraw-Hill, 1987, pp 1200–1205.

LOWER ABDOMINAL PAIN REFERENCES
(Chapters 21 to 23 and Chapter 25)

Abdominal Catastrophes

Young GP: Abdominal catastrophes. *Emerg Med Clin North Am* 7(3):699–720, 1989.

Abdominal Pain

Purcell TB: Nonsurgical and extraperitoneal causes of abdominal pain. *Emerg Med Clin North Am* 7(3):721–740, 1989.

Silen W: *Cope's Early Diagnosis of the Acute Abdomen,* 17th ed. New York: Oxford University Press, 1987, pp 66–106; pp 209–241.

Way LW: Abdominal pain, in Sleisenger MH, Fordtran JS (eds): *Gastrointestinal Disease: Pathophysiology, Diagnosis, Management,* 4th ed. Philadelphia, Saunders, 1989, pp 238–250.

Abdominal Wall

Adams JT: Abdominal wall, omentum, mesentery, and retroperitoneum, in Schwartz SI, Shires GT, Spencer FC (eds): *Principles of Surgery,* 5th ed. New York, McGraw-Hill, 1989, pp 1491–1524.

Morton JH: Abdominal wall hernias, in Schwartz SI, Shires GT, Spencer FC (eds): *Principles of Surgery,* 5th ed. New York, McGraw-Hill, 1989, pp 1525–1544.

Acute Abdomen—Gynecologic Causes

Burnett LS: Gynecologic causes of the acute abdomen. *Surg Clin North Am* 68(2):385–398, 1988.

Acute Abdomen—Toxicologic Causes

Mueller PD, Benowitz NL: Toxicologic causes of acute abdominal disorders. *Emerg Med Clin North Am* 7(3):667–682, 1989.

Adhesions—Pelvic

Fayez JA, Schneider PJ: Prevention of pelvic adhesion formation by different modalities of treatment. *Am J Obstet Gynecol* 157(5):1184–1188, 1987.

Jansen RPS: Early laparoscopy after pelvic operations to prevent adhesions: Safety and efficacy. *Fertil Steril* 49:26–31, 1988.

Aneurysms—Aortic

De Bakey ME, Crawford ES, Cooley DA, et al: Aneurysm of abdominal aorta. Analysis of results of graft replacement therapy one to eleven years after operation. *Ann Surg* 160(4):622–639, 1964.

Fielding JWL, Black J, Ashton F, et al: Diagnosis and management of 528 abdominal aortic aneurysms. *Br Med J* 283:355–359, 1981.

Jenkins AMcL, Ruckley CV, Nolan B: Ruptured abdominal aortic aneurysm. *Br J Surg* 73:395–398, 1986.

Johnson G Jr, McDevitt NB, Proctor HJ, et al: Emergent or elective operation for symptomatic abdominal aortic aneurysm. *Arch Surg* 115:51–53, 1980.

Jones CS, Reilly MK, Dalsing MC, et al: Chronic contained rupture of abdominal aortic aneurysms. *Arch Surg* 121:542–546, 1986.

Lawrie GM, Morris GC Jr, Crawford ES, et al: Improved results of operation for ruptured abdominal aortic aneurysms. *Surgery* 85(5): 483–488, 1979.

Mannick JA, Whittemore AD: Management of ruptured or symptomatic abdominal aortic aneurysms. *Surg Clin North Am* 68(2):377–384, 1988.

Ottinger LW: Ruptured arteriosclerotic aneurysms of the abdominal aorta. Reducing mortality. *JAMA* 233:147–150, 1975.

Rutherford RB, McCroskey BL: Ruptured abdominal aortic aneurysms. Special considerations. *Surg Clin North Am* 69(4):859–868, 1989.

Sweeney MS, Gadacz TR: Primary aortoduodenal fistula: Manifestation, diagnosis, and treatment. *Surgery* 96(3):492–497, 1984.

Appendicitis—Acute

Adams DH, Fine C, Brooks DC: High-resolution real-time ultrasonography. A new tool in the diagnosis of acute appendicitis. *Am J Surg* 155:93–97, 1988.

Campbell JPM, Gunn AA: Plain abdominal radiographs and acute abdominal pain. *Br J Surg* 75:554–556, 1988.

Doherty GM, Lewis FR Jr: Appendicitis: Continuing diagnostic challenge. *Emerg Med Clin North Am* 7(3):537–553, 1989.

Gaensler EHL, Jeffrey RB Jr, Laing FC, et al: Sonography in patients with suspected acute appendicitis: Value in establishing alternative diagnoses. *AJR* 152:49–51, 1989.

Henneman PL, Marcus CS, Butler JA, et al: Appendicitis: Evaluation by Tc-99m leukocyte scan. *Ann Emerg Med* 17:111–116, 1988.

Hickey MS, Kiernan GJ, Weaver KE: Evaluation of abdominal pain. *Emerg Med Clin North Am* 7(3):437–452, 1989.

Jeffrey RB Jr, Laing FC, Townsend RR: Acute appendicitis: Sonographic criteria based on 250 cases. *Radiology* 167:327–329, 1988.

Jones WG, Barie PS: Urological manifestations of acute appendicitis. *J Urol* 139:1325–1328, 1988.

Kang W-M, Lee C-H, Chou Y-H, et al: A clinical evaluation of ultrasonography in the diagnosis of acute appendicitis. *Surgery* 105:154–159, 1989.

Malt RA: The perforated appendix. *N Engl J Med* 315(24):1546–1547, 1986.

Ng PCH: Pseudo-appendicitis presenting after vasectomy. A case report. *Int Urol Nephrol* 19(2):215–216, 1987.

Schrock TR: Acute appendicitis, in Sleisenger MH, Fordtran JS (eds): *Gastrointestinal Disease: Pathophysiology, Diagnosis, Management,* 4th ed. Philadelphia, Saunders, 1989, 1382–1389.

Silen W: Acute appendicitis, in Braunwald E, Isselbacher KJ, Petersdorf RG, et al (eds): *Harrison's Principles of Internal Medicine,* 11th ed. New York, McGraw-Hill, 1987, pp 1304–1306.

Whitworth CM, Whitworth PW, Sanfillipo J, et al: Value of diagnostic laparoscopy in young women with possible appendicitis. *Surg Gynecol Obstet* 167:187–190, 1988.

Appendix—Adenocarcinoma

Cerame MA: A 25-year review of adenocarcinoma of the appendix. A frequently perforating carcinoma. *Dis Colon Rectum* 31:145–150, 1988.

Appendix—General

Altschuler E: A diagnostic sign for retrocaecal appendicitis. *Lancet* 1:891–892, 1938.

Schwartz SI: Appendix, in Schwartz SI, Shires GT, Spencer FC (eds): *Principles of Surgery,* 5th ed. New York, McGraw-Hill, 1989, 1315–1326.

Vanek VW, Spirtos G, Awad M, et al: Isolated Crohn's disease of the appendix. Two case reports and a review of the literature. *Arch Surg* 123:85–87, 1988.

Bowel Disease—General

Cheadle WG, Garr EE, Richardson JD: The importance of early diagnosis of small bowel obstruction. *Am Surg* 54:565–569, 1988.

Drossman DA: A questionnaire for functional bowel disorders. *Ann Intern Med* 111(8):627–629, 1989.

LaMont JT, Isselbacher KJ: Diseases of the small and large intestine, in Braunwald E, Isselbacher KJ, Petersdorf RG, et al (eds): *Harrison's Principles of Internal Medicine,* 11th ed. New York, McGraw-Hill, 1987, pp 1290–1302.

Talley NJ, Phillips SF, Melton LJ III, et al: A patient questionnaire to identify bowel disease. *Ann Intern Med* 111:671–674, 1989.

Colitis

Cello JP, Schneiderman DJ: Ulcerative colitis, in Sleisenger MH, Fordtran JS (eds): *Gastrointestinal Disease: Pathophysiology, Diagnosis, Management,* 4th ed. Philadelphia, Saunders, 1989, 1435–1477.

Earnest DL, Trier JS: Radiation enteritis and colitis, in Sleisenger MH, Fordtran JS (eds): *Gastrointestinal Disease: Pathophysiology, Diagnosis, Management,* 4th ed. Philadelphia, Saunders, 1989, 1369–1382.

Thayer WR Jr, Denucci T: Miscellaneous diseases of the large bowel and anal canal. Chap 25, Part 9. Collagenous colitis, in Kirsner JB, Shorter RG (eds): *Diseases of the Colon, Rectum, and Anal Canal.* Baltimore, Williams and Wilkins, 1988, 574–576.

Thayer WR Jr, Denucci T: Miscellaneous diseases of the large bowel and anal canal. Chap 25, Part 14. Radiation colitis, in Kirsner JB, Shorter RG (eds): *Diseases of the Colon, Rectum, and Anal Canal.* Baltimore, Williams and Wilkins, 1988, 583–585.

Thayer WR Jr, Denucci T: Miscellaneous diseases of the large bowel and anal canal. Chap 25, Part 20. Drug-induced colitis, in Kirsner JB, Shorter RG (eds): *Diseases of the Colon, Rectum, and Anal Canal.* Baltimore, Williams and Wilkins 1988, 593–594.

Colon—General

Earnest DL, Schneiderman DJ: Other diseases of the colon and rectum, in Sleisenger MH, Fordtran JS (eds): *Gastrointestinal Disease: Pathophysiology, Diagnosis, Management,* 4th ed. Philadelphia, Saunders, 1989, 1592–1631.

Goldberg SM, Nivatvongs S, Rothenberger DA: Colon, rectum, and anus, in Schwartz SI, Shires GT, Spencer FC (eds): *Principles of Surgery,* 5th ed. New York, McGraw-Hill, 1989, 1225–1314.

Thayer WR Jr, Denucci T: Miscellaneous diseases of the large bowel and anal canal, Chap 25, Part 11. Cathartic colon, in Kirsner JB, Shorter RG (eds): *Diseases of the Colon, Rectum, and Anal Canal.* Baltimore, Williams and Wilkins, 1988, 578–579.

Colorectal Carcinoma

Bolin S, Franzen L, Nilsson E, et al: Carcinoma of the colon and rectum. Tumors missed by radiologic examination in 61 patients. *Cancer* 61:1999–2008, 1988.

Corman ML: Carcinoma of the colon, in Corman ML: *Colon and Rectal Surgery.* Philadelphia, Lippincott, 1984, pp 267–328.

Corman ML: Diverticular disease, in Corman, ML: *Colon and Rectal Surgery.* Philadelphia, Lippincott, 1984, pp 487–526.

Iijima T: Angiographic diagnosis of the degree of serosal invarion of carcinoma of the colon. *Dis Colon Rectum* 31:46–49, 1988.

Iijima T: Pharmacoangiographic diagnosis of venous invasion of carcinoma of the colon with reference to liver metastases. *Dis Colon Rectum* 31:718–722, 1988.

Naitove A, Almy TP: Diverticular disease of the colon, in Sleisenger MH, Fordtran JS (eds): *Gastrointestinal Disease: Pathophysiology, Diagnosis, Management,* 4th ed. Philadelphia, Saunders, 1989, pp 1419–1434.

Diarrhea

Krejs GJ: Diarrhea, in Wyngaarden JB, Smith LH Jr (eds): *Cecil Textbook of Medicine,* 18th ed. Philadelphia, Saunders, 1988, pp 725–732.

Parsonnet J, Trock SC, Bopp CA, et al: Chronic diarrhea associated with drinking untreated water. *Ann Intern Med* 110:985–991, 1989.

Diverticulitis—Cecal and Transverse Colon

Chappuis CW, Cohn I Jr: Acute colonic diverticulitis. *Surg Clin North Am* 68(2):301–313, 1988.

Crist DW, Fishman EK, Scatarige JC, et al: Acute diverticulitis of the cecum and ascending colon diagnosed by computed tomography. *Surg Gynecol Obstet* 166(2):99–102, 1988.

Graham SM, Ballantyne GH: Cecal diverticulitis. A review of the American experience. *Dis Colon Rectum* 30:821–826, 1987.

Scatarige JC, Fishman EK, Crist DW, et al: Diverticulitis of the right colon: CT observations. *AJR* 148:737–739, 1987.

Shperber Y, Halevy A, Oland J, et al: Perforated diverticulitis of the transverse colon. *Dis Colon Rectum* 29:466–468, 1986.

Wyble EJ, Lee WC: Cecal diverticulitis: Changing trends in management. *South Med J* 81(3):313–316, 1988.

Case 33-1987, Case records of the Massachusetts General Hospital. *N Engl J Med* 317(7):432–441, 1987.

Diverticulitis—Sigmoid

Chappuis CW, Cohn I Jr: Acute colonic diverticulitis. *Surg Clin North Am* 68(2):301–313, 1988.

Freischlag J, Bennion RS, Thompson JE Jr: Complications of diverticular disease of the colon in young people. *Dis Colon Rectum* 29:639–643, 1986.

Johnson CD, Baker ME, Rice RP, et al: Diagnosis of acute colonic diverticulitis: Comparison of barium enema and CT. *AJR* 148:541–546, 1987.

Klein S, Mayer L, Present DH, et al: Extraintestinal manifestations in patients with diverticulitis. *Ann Intern Med* 108:700–702, 1988.

Lubat E, Balthazar EJ: The current role of computerized tomography in inflammatory disease of the bowel. *Am J Gastroenterol* 83(2):107–113, 1988.

Pohlman T: Diverticulitis. *Gastroenterol Clin North Am* 17(2):357–385, 1988.

Diverticulitis—Small Bowel

Geroulakos G: Surgical problems of jejunal diverticulosis. *Ann R Coll Surg Engl* 69:266–268, 1987.

Greenstein S, Jones B, Fishman EK, et al: Small-bowel diverticulitis: CT findings. *AJR* 147:271–274, 1986.

Endometriosis

Adamson GD, Lu J, Subak LL: Laparoscopic CO_2 laser vaporization of endometriosis compared with traditional treatments. *Fertil Steril* 50:704–710, 1988.

Badawy SZA, Freedman L, Numann P, et al: Diagnosis and management of intestinal endometriosis. A report of five cases. *J Reprod Med* 33(10):851–855, 1988.

Barbieri R, Kistner RW: Endometriosis, in Kistner RW (ed): *Gynecology Principles and Practice,* 4th ed. Chicago, Year Book, 1986, pp 393–414.

Davis GD, Brooks RA: Excision of pelvic endometriosis with the carbon dioxide laser laparoscope. *Obstet Gynecol* 72:816–819, 1988.

Fedele L, Arcaini L, Vercellini P, et al: Serum CA 125 measurements in the diagnosis of endometriosis recurrence. *Obstet Gynecol* 72:19–22, 1988.

Graham B, Mazier WP: Diagnosis and management of endometriosis of the colon and rectum. *Dis Colon Rectum* 31:952–956, 1988.

Jones HW Jr, Jones GS: Endometriosis, in Jones HW Jr, Jones GS (eds): *Novak's Textbook of Gynecology,* 10th ed. Baltimore, Williams and Wilkins, 1981, pp 609–635.

Lucero SP, Wise HA, Kirsh G, et al: Ureteric obstruction secondary to endometriosis. Report of three cases with a review of the literature. *Br J Urol* 61:201–204, 1988.

Martin DC, Hubert GD, Vander Zwaag R, et al: Laparoscopic appearances of peritoneal endometriosis. *Fertil Steril* 51(1):63–67, 1989.

Merrill JA: Endometriosis, in Danforth DN (ed): *Obstetrics and Gynecology,* 4th ed. Philadelphia, Harper and Row, 1982, 1004–1014.

Pittaway DE, Fayez JA: The use of CA-125 in the diagnosis and management of endometriosis. *Fertil Steril* 46(5):790–795, 1986.

Pittaway DE, Douglas JW: Serum CA-125 in women with endometriosis and chronic pelvic pain. *Fertil Steril* 51(1):68–70, 1989.

Prystowsky GB, Stryker SJ, Ujiki GT, et al: Gastrointestinal endometriosis. *Arch Surg* 123:855–858, 1988.

Stripling MC, Martin DC, Chatman DL, et al: Subtle appearance of pelvic endometriosis. *Fertil Steril* 49:427–431, 1988.

Thayer WR Jr, Denucci T: Miscellaneous diseases of the large bowel and anal canal. Chap 25, Part 1. Endometriosis, in Kirsner JB,

Shorter RG (eds): *Diseases of the Colon, Rectum, and Anal Canal.* Baltimore, Williams and Wilkins, 1988, 561–562.

Fallopian Tube Carcinoma

Peters WA III, Andersen WA, Hopkins MP, et al: Prognostic features of carcinoma of the fallopian tube. *Obstet Gynecol* 71:757–762, 1988.

Fallopian Tubes—General

Kistner RW: The oviduct, in Kistner RW (ed): *Gynecology Principles and Practice,* 4th ed. Chicago, Year Book, 1986, pp 249–287.

Merrill JA: Lesions of the fallopian tubes, in Danforth DN (ed): *Obstetrics and Gynecology,* 4th ed. Philadelphia, Harper and Row, 1982, pp 1105–1113.

Fitz-Hugh–Curtis Syndrome

Katzman DK, Friedman IM, McDonald CA, et al: *Chlamydia trachomatis* Fitz-Hugh–Curtis syndrome without salpingitis in female adolescents. *AJDC* 142:996–998, 1988.

Gynecologic Infections

Jones HW Jr, Jones GS: Genital tuberculosis, in Jones HW Jr, Jones GS (eds): *Novak's Textbook of Gynecology,* 10th ed. Baltimore, Williams and Wilkins, 1981, pp 484–495.

Kirby P, Corey L: Genital human papillomavirus infections. *Infect Dis Clin North Am* 1(1):123–143, 1987.

Lande IM, Hill MC, Cosco FE, et al: Adnexal and cul-de-sac abnormalities: Transvaginal sonography. *Radiology* 166:325–332, 1988.

Paavonen J, Stamm WE: Lower genital tract infections in women. *Infect Dis Clin North Am* 1(1):179–198, 1987.

Tuomala RE: Gynecologic infections, in Kistner RW (ed): *Gynecology Principles and Practice,* 4th ed. Chicago, Year Book, 1986, pp 667–695.

Infectious Diarrhea

Black RE, Slome S: *Yersinia enterocolitica. Infect Dis Clin North Am* 2(3):625–641, 1988.

Cornick NA, Gorbach SL: Campylobacter. *Infect Dis Clin North Am* 2(3):643–654, 1988.

DuPont HL: Shigella. *Infect Dis Clin North Am* 2(3):599–605, 1988.

Goldberg MB, Rubin RH: The spectrum of Salmonella infection. *Infect Dis Clin North Am* 2(3):571–598, 1988.

Gorbach SL: Infectious diarrhea, in Sleisenger MH, Fordtran JS (eds): *Gastrointestinal Disease: Pathophysiology, Diagnosis, Management,* 4th ed. Philadelphia, Saunders, 1989, pp 1191–1232.

Holmberg SD: Vibrios and Aeromonas. *Infect Dis Clin North Am* 2(3):655–676, 1988.

Panosian CB: Parasitic diarrhea. *Infect Dis Clin North Am* 2(3):685–703, 1988.

Thorne GM: Diagnosis of infectious diarrheal diseases. *Infect Dis Clin North Am* 2(3):747–774, 1988.

Inflammatory Bowel Disease

Condie JD Jr, Leslie KO, Smiley DF: Surgical treatment for inflammatory bowel disease in the older patient. *Surg Gynecol Obstet* 165:135–142, 1987.

Corman ML: Nonspecific inflammatory bowel disease; in Corman ML: *Colon and Rectal Surgery.* Philadelphia, Lippincott, 1984, pp 527–636.

Donaldson RM Jr: Crohn's disease, in Sleisenger MH, Fordtran JS (eds): *Gastrointestinal Disease: Pathophysiology, Diagnosis, Management,* 4th ed. Philadelphia, Saunders, 1989, pp 1327–1358.

Kirsner JB, Shorter RG: Idiopathic inflammatory bowel disease of the large bowel and anal canal, in Kirsner JB, Shorter RG (eds): *Diseases of the Colon, Rectum, and Anal Canal.* Baltimore, Williams and Wilkins, 1988, pp 261–294.

Sackier JM, Wood CB: Ulcerative colitis and polyposis coli. Surgical options. *Surg Clin North Am* 68(6):1319–1338, 1988.

Intestinal Obstruction

Thayer WR Jr, Benucci T: Miscellaneous diseases of the large bowel and anal canal. Part 2. Colonic volvulus, in Kirsner JB, Shorter RG

(eds): *Diseases of the Colon, Rectum, and Anal Canal.* Baltimore, Williams and Wilkins, 1988, pp 563–565.

Intraabdominal Abscess

Walker AP, Condon RE: Peritonitis and intraabdominal abscesses, in Schwartz SI, Shires GT, Spencer FC (eds): *Principles of Surgery,* 5th ed. New York, McGraw-Hill, 1989, pp 1459–1489.

Intraabdominal Testis—Torsion

Elder JS: The undescended testis. Hormonal and surgical management. *Surg Clin North Am* 68(5):983–1005, 1988.

Riegler HC: Torsion of intraabdominal testis. An unusual problem in diagnosis of the acute surgical abdomen. *Surg Clin North Am* 52(2):371–374, 1972.

Irritable Bowel Syndrome

Schuster MM: Irritable bowel syndrome, in Sleisenger MH, Fordtran JS (eds): *Gastrointestinal Disease: Pathophysiology, Diagnosis, Management,* 4th ed. Philadelphia, Saunders, 1989, pp 1402–1418.

Whitehead WE, Schuster MM: The irritable bowel, stress, and the colon, in Kirsner JB, Shorter RG (eds): *Diseases of the Colon, Rectum, and Anal Canal.* Baltimore, Williams and Wilkins, 1988, pp 507–517.

Ischemic Bowel Disease

Glick SN, Teplick SK, Whiteman MS, et al: Small intestine ischemia simulating primary colonic disease. *Radiology* 164:43–46, 1987.

Welling RE, Roedersheimer R, Arbaugh JJ, et al: Ischemic colitis following repair of ruptured abdominal aortic aneurysm. *Arch Surg* 120:1368–1370, 1985.

Large Bowel—Diseases

Bynum TE, Jacobson ED: Vascular disorders of the large bowel, in Kirsner JB, Shorter RG (eds): *Diseases of the Colon, Rectum, and Anal Canal.* Baltimore, Williams and Wilkins, 1988, pp 537–548.

Glick SN, Laufer I: Radiographic methods in the diagnosis of colorectal disease, in Kirsner JB, Shorter RG (eds): *Diseases of the Colon, Rectum, and Anal Canal.* Baltimore, Williams and Wilkins, 1988, pp 183–224.

Grendell JH, Ockner RK: Vascular diseases of the bowel, in Sleisenger MH, Fordtran JS (eds): *Gastrointestinal Disease: Pathophysiology, Diagnosis, Management,* 4th ed. Philadelphia, Saunders, 1989, pp 1903–1932.

Quinn TC, Schuffler MD: The clinical aspects of specific infections of the large bowel and anal canal, including the "Gay Bowel Syndrome." In Kirsner JB, Shorter RG (eds): *Diseases of the Colon, Rectum, and Anal Canal.* Baltimore, Williams and Wilkins, 1988, pp 439–481.

Rogers BHG: Endoscopy in diseases of the large bowel and anal canal, in Kirsner JB, Shorter RG (eds): *Diseases of the Colon, Rectum, and Anal Canal.* Baltimore, Williams and Wilkins, 1988, pp 225–259.

Schwartz JT, Graham DY: Diverticular disease of the large intestine, in Kirsner JB, Shorter RG (eds): *Diseases of the Colon, Rectum, and Anal Canal.* Baltimore, Williams and Wilkins, 1988, pp 519–536.

Zaiman H, Frierson JG, Shorter RG: Clinical aspects of certain parasitic infections affecting the large bowel in humans, in Kirsner JB, Shorter RG (eds): *Diseases of the Colon, Rectum, and Anal Canal.* Baltimore, Williams and Wilkins, 1988, pp 483–506.

Liver Abscess

Crass JR: Liver abscess as a complication of regional enteritis: Interventional considerations. *AJR* 78(11):747–749, 1983.

Musculoskeletal Disorders

Jacobson HG: Musculoskeletal applications of magnetic resonance imaging. *JAMA* 262:2420–2427, 1989.

Modic MT, Pflanze W, Feiglin DHI, et al: Magnetic resonance imaging of musculoskeletal infections. *Radiol Clin North Am* 24(2):247–258, 1986.

Neuropathic Pain—Chronic
Sellman MS, Mayer RF: Thoracoabdominal radiculopathy. *South Med J* 81(2):199–201, 1988.

Obturator Hernia
Bjork KJ, Mucha P Jr, Cahill DR: Obturator hernia. *Surg Gynecol Obstet* 167:217–222, 1988.

Omentum Infarction
Baxter NS, Storey DJ, Airan MC: Infarction of the greater omentum. Elusive cause of acute abdominal pain. *Postgrad Med* 79(5): 141–146, 1986.

Quinn AD, Jothi RK: Idiopathic segmental infarction of the greater omentum. *Postgrad Med* 79(5):133–140, 1986.

Osteomyelitis of the Ilium
Ang JGP, Gelfand MJ: Decreased gallium uptake in acute hematogenous osteomyelitis. *Clin Nucl Med* 8(7):301–303, 1983.

Beaupré A, Carroll N: The three syndromes of iliac osteomyelitis in children. *J Bone Joint Surg Am* 61A(7):1087–1092, 1979.

Chung SMK, Borns P: Acute osteomyelitis adjacent to the sacro-iliac joint in children. *J Bone Joint Surg (Am)* 55(3):630–634, 1973.

Edwards MS, Baker CJ, Granberry WM, et al: Pelvic osteomyelitis in children. *Pediatrics* 61:62–67, 1978.

Ghahremani GG: Osteomyelitis of the ilium in patients with Crohn's disease. *Am J Roentgenol Radium Ther Nucl Med* 118(2):364–370, 1973.

Landy MD, Katz JF: Osteomyelitis of the ilium: Presentation as an abdominal syndrome (letter to the editor). *J Nucl Med* 23(12):1144–1145, 1982.

Morgan A, Yates AK: The diagnosis of acute osteomyelitis of the pelvis. *Postgrad Med J* 42:74–78, 1966.

Sant GR, O'Rourke SK, Dias E: Case Report: Acute osteomyelitis of the ilium. *Ir J Med Sci* 145(12):409–412, 1976.

Vest BT, Rich MM, Gilula LA: Roentgen Rounds #94. *Orthop Rev* 17(5):511–515, 1988.

Weld PW: Osteomyelitis of the ilium. Masquerading as acute appendicitis. *JAMA* 173(6):634–636, 1960.

Yamaguchi H, Nojima T, Yagi T, et al: High-grade surface osteosarcoma of the left ilium. A case report and review of the literature. *Acta Pathol Jpn* 38(2):235–240, 1988.

Ovarian Carcinoma
Bast RC, Hunter V, Knapp RC: Pros and cons of gynecologic tumor markers. *Cancer* 60:1984–1992, 1987.

Flam F, Einhorn N, Sjovall K: Symptomatology of ovarian cancer. *Eur J Obstet Gynecol Reprod Biol* 27:53–57, 1988.

Killackey MA, Neuwirth RS: Evaluation and management of the pelvic mass: A review of 540 cases. *Obstet Gynecol* 71:319–322, 1988.

Krebs H-B, Goplerud DR: Mechanical intestinal obstruction in patients with gynecologic disease: A review of 368 patients. *Am J Obstet Gynecol* 157:577–583, 1987.

Yabushita H, Masuda T, Ogawa A, et al: Combination assay of CA125, TPA, IAP, CEA and ferritin in serum for ovarian cancer. *Gynecol Oncol* 29:66–75, 1988.

Ovarian Hemorrhage
Peters WA III, Thiagarajah S, Thornton WN Jr: Ovarian hemorrhage in patients receiving anticoagulant therapy. *J Reprod Med* 22:82–86, 1979.

Ovarian Remnant or Residual Syndrome
Bukovsky I, Lifshitz Y, Langer R, et al: Ovarian residual syndrome. *Surg Gynecol Obstet* 167:132–134, 1988.

Goldstein SR, Subramanyam B, Snyder JR, et al: The postmenopausal cystic adnexal mass: The potential role of ultrasound in conservative management. *Obstet Gynecol* 73:8–10, 1989.

Pettit PD, Lee RA: Ovarian remnant syndrome: Diagnostic dilemma and surgical challenge. *Obstet Gynecol* 71:580–583, 1988.

Case 6-1988, Case records of the Massachusetts General Hospital (Scully RE, Mark EJ, McNeely WF and McNeely BU, eds). *N Engl J Med* 318(6):366–372, 1988.

Ovarian Torsion
Bowen A: Ovarian torsion diagnosed by ultrasonography. *South Med J* 78(11):1376–1378, 1985.

Graif M, Itzchak Y: Sonographic evaluation of ovarian torsion in childhood and adolescence. *AJR* 150:647–649, 1988.

Ovary—General
Griffiths CT, Berkowitz R: The ovary, in Kistner RW (ed): *Gynecology Principles and Practice,* 4th ed. Chicago, Year Book, 1986, pp 289–377.

Jones HW Jr, Jones GS: Epithelial tumors of the ovary, in Jones HW Jr, Jones GS (eds): *Novak's Textbook of Gynecology,* 10th ed. Baltimore, Williams and Wilkins, 1981, pp 507–558.

Parasitic Diseases
Owen RL: Parasitic diseases, in Sleisenger MH, Fordtran JS (eds): *Gastrointestinal Disease: Pathophysiology, Diagnosis, Management,* 4th ed. Philadelphia, Saunders, 1989, pp 1153–1191.

Pelvic Inflammatory Diseases—Etiology and Therapy
Blanchard AC, Pastorek JG II, Weeks T: Pelvic inflammatory disease during pregnancy. *South Med J* 80(11):1363–1365, 1987.

Brihmer C, Kallings I, Nord C-E, et al: Salpingitis; aspects of diagnosis and etiology: A 4-year study from a Swedish capital hospital. *Eur J Obstet Gynecol Reprod Biol* 24:211–220, 1987.

Burchell HJ, Schoon MG: The value of laparoscopy in the diagnosis of acute pelvic inflammatory disease. *S Afr Med J* 72:197–198, 1987.

Burnakis TG, Hildebrandt NB: Pelvic inflammatory disease: A review with emphasis on antimicrobial therapy. *Rev Infect Dis* 8(1):86–116, 1986.

Burnett LS: Gynecologic causes of the acute abdomen. *Surg Clin North Am* 68(2):385–398, 1988.

Dodson MG, Faro S, Gentry LO: Treatment of acute pelvic inflammatory disease with aztreonam, a new monocyclic beta-lactam antibiotic, and clindamycin. *Obstet Gynecol* 67:657–662, 1986.

Eschenbach DA: Pelvic Infections, in Danforth DN (ed): *Obstetrics and Gynecology,* 4th ed. Philadelphia, Harper and Row, 1982, pp 981–1003.

Fraiz J, Jones RB: Chlamydial infections. *Annu Rev Med* 39:357–370, 1988.

Golden N, Neuhoff S, Cohen H: Pelvic inflammatory disease in adolescents. *J Pediatr* 114:138–143, 1989.

Jones HW Jr, Jones GS: Pelvic inflammatory disease, in Jones HW Jr, Jones GS (eds): *Novak's Textbook of Gynecology,* 10th ed. Baltimore, Williams and Wilkins, 1981. Pelvic Inflammatory Disease. pp 462–483.

Kinghorn GR, Duerden BI, Hafiz S: Clinical and microbiological investigation of women with acute salpingitis and their consorts. *Br J Obstet Gynecol* 93:869–880, 1986.

Kiviat NB, Wølner-Hanssen P, Peterson M, et al: Localization of *Chlamydia trachomatis* infection by direct immunofluorescence and culture in pelvic inflammatory disease. *Am J Obstet Gynecol* 154:865–873, 1986.

Phillips RS, Hanff PA, Wertheimer A, et al: Gonorrhea in women seen for routine gynecologic care: Criteria for testing. *Am J Med* 85:177–182, 1988.

Raggio ML, Bostrom SG, Harden EA: Hodgkin's lymphoma of the uterus presenting as refractory pelvic inflammatory disease. A case report. *J Reprod Med* 33(10):827–830, 1988.

Sweet RL, Blankfort-Doyle M, Robbie MO, et al: The occurrence of chlamydial and gonococcal salpingitis during the menstrual cycle. *JAMA* 255(15):2062–2064, 1986.

Teisala K, Heinonen PK, Aine R, et al: Second laparoscopy after treatment of acute pelvic inflammatory disease. *Obstet Gynecol* 69:343–346, 1987.

Trachtenberg AI, Washington AE, Halldorson S: A cost-based decision analysis for chlamydia screening in California family planning clinics. *Obstet Gynecol* 71:101–108, 1988.

Wasserheit JN, Bell TA, Kiviat NB, et al: Microbial causes of proven pelvic inflammatory disease and efficacy of clindamycin and tobramycin. *Ann Intern Med* 104:187–193, 1986.

Wølner-Hanssen P: Oral contraceptive use modifies the manifestations of pelvic inflammatory disease. *Br J Obstet Gynaecol* 93:619–624, 1986.

Wølner-Hanssen P, Paavonen J, Kiviat N, et al: Outpatient treatment of pelvic inflammatory disease with cefoxitin and doxycycline. *Obstet Gynecol* 71:595–600, 1988.

Pelvic Inflammatory Disease—Tuboovarian Abscess

Collins CG, Jansen FW: Treatment of pelvic abscess. *Clin Obstet Gynecol* 2:513–522, 1959.

Landers DV, Sweet RL: Current trends in the diagnosis and treatment of tuboovarian abscess. *Am J Obstet Gynecol* 151:1098–1110, 1985.

Landers DV, Sweet RL: Tubo-ovarian abscess: Contemporary approach to management. *Rev Infect Dis* 5(5):876–884, 1983.

O'Connor KF, Bagg MN, Croley MR, et al: Pelvic actinomycosis associated with intrauterine devices. *Radiology* 170:559–560, 1989.

Reich H, McGlynn F: Laparoscopic treatment of tuboovarian and pelvic abscess. *J Reprod Med* 32(10):747–752, 1987.

Rivlin ME, Hunt JA: Ruptured tuboovarian abscess. Is hysterectomy necessary? *Obstet Gynecol* 50:518–522, 1977.

Rivlin ME: Clinical outcome following vaginal drainage of pelvic abscess. *Obstet Gynecol* 61:169–173, 1983.

Schmidt E, Nehra P: Tubo-ovarian abscess: A study of 17 patients. *Am Fam Physician* 37(4):181–185, 1988.

Pelvic Pain—Chronic

Avant RF: Dysmenorrhea. *Prim Care* 15(3):549–559, 1988.

Bahary CM, Gorodeski IG: The diagnostic value of laparoscopy in women with chronic pelvic pain. *Am Surg* 53(11):672–674, 1987.

Beard RW, Reginald PW, Wadsworth J: Clinical features of women with chronic lower abdominal pain and pelvic congestion. *Br J Obstet Gynaecol* 95:153–161, 1988.

Gaul JN: Evaluation of chronic pelvic pain. *Minn Med* 71:546–548, 1988.

Harrop-Griffiths J, Katon W, Walker E, et al: The association between chronic pelvic pain, psychiatric diagnoses, and childhood sexual abuse. *Obstet Gynecol* 71:589–594, 1988.

Miró J, García-Moncó C, Leno C, et al: Pelvic pain: an undescribed paroxysmal manifestation of multiple sclerosis. *Pain* 32:73–75, 1988.

Quan M: Chronic pelvic pain. *J Fam Pract* 25(3):283–288, 1987.

Risser WL, Pokorny SF, Maklad NF: Ultrasound examination of adolescent females with lower abdominal pain. *J Adolesc Health Care* 9:407–410, 1988.

Slocumb JC, Kellner R, Rosenfeld, et al: Anxiety and depression in patients with the abdominal pelvic pain syndrome. *Gen Hosp Psychiatry* 11:48–53, 1989.

Pregnancy—Tubal

Brenner PF, Benedetti T, Mishell DR: Ectopic pregnancy following tubal sterilization surgery. *Obstet Gynecol* 49(3):323–324, 1977.

Buck RH, Joubert SM, Norman RJ: Serum progesterone in the diagnosis of ectopic pregnancy: A valuable diagnostic test? *Fertil Steril* 50:752–755, 1988.

Cartwright PS, Vaughn B, Tuttle D: Culdocentesis and ectopic pregnancy. *J Reprod Med* 29:88–91, 1984.

Cartwright PS, Herbert CM III, Maxson WS: Operative laparoscopy for the management of tubal pregnancy. *J Reprod Med* 31:589–591, 1986.

Cartwright PS, Victory DF, Moore RA, et al: Performance of a new enzyme-linked immunoassay urine pregnancy test for the detection of ectopic gestation. *Ann Emerg Med* 15:1198–1199, 1986.

Dashefsky SM, Lyons EA, Levi CS, et al: Suspected ectopic pregnancy: Endovaginal and transvesical US. *Radiology* 169:181–184, 1988.

Droegemueller W: Ectopic pregnancy, in Danforth DN (ed): *Obstetrics and Gynecology,* 4th ed. Philadelphia, Harper and Row, 1982, pp 407–422.

Dubuisson JB, Aubriot FX, Cardone V: Laparoscopic salpingectomy for tubal pregnancy. *Fertil Steril* 47(2):225–228, 1987.

Fernandez H, Rainhorn JD, Papiernik E, et al: Spontaneous resolution of ectopic pregnancy. *Obstet Gynecol* 71:171–174, 1988.

Hutton JD, Narayan R: Is ectopic pregnancy too often diagnosed too late? *N Z Med J* 99:3–5, 1986.

Jain KA, Hamper UM, Sanders RC: Comparison of transvaginal and transabdominal sonography in the detection of early pregnancy and its complications. *AJR* 151:1139–1143, 1988.

Jones HW Jr, Jones GS: Ectopic pregnancy, in Jones HW Jr, Jones GS (ed): *Novak's Textbook of Gynecology,* 10th ed. Baltimore, Williams and Wilkins, 1981, pp 636–658.

Leeton J, Davison G: Nonsurgical management of unruptured tubal pregnancy with intra-amniotic methotrexate: Preliminary report of two cases. *Fertil Steril* 50(1):167–169, 1988.

Kim DS, Chung SR, Park MI, et al: Comparative review of diagnostic accuracy in tubal pregnancy: A 14-year survey of 1040 cases. *Obstet Gynecol* 70:547–554, 1987.

O'Connor DM, Kurman RJ: Intermediate trophoblast in uterine curettings in the diagnosis of ectopic pregnancy. *Obstet Gynecol* 72:665–670, 1988.

Rempen A: Vaginal sonography in ectopic pregnancy. A prospective evaluation. *J Ultrasound Med* 7:381–387, 1988.

Shapiro BS, Cullen M, Taylor KJW, et al: Transvaginal ultrasonography for the diagnosis of ectopic pregnancy. *Fertil Steril* 50:425–429, 1988.

Taylor RB, Padula C, Goldsmith PC: Pitfall in the diagnosis of ectopic pregnancy: Immunocytochemical evaluation in a patient with false-negative serum beta-hCG levels. *Obstet Gynecol* 71:1035–1038, 1988.

Tuomivaara L, Kauppila A, Puolakka J: Ectopic pregnancy—an analysis of the etiology, diagnosis and treatment in 552 cases. *Arch Gynecol Obstet* 237:135–147, 1986.

Weinstein L, Morris MB, Dotters D, et al: Ectopic pregnancy—a new surgical epidemic. *Obstet Gynecol* 61:698–701, 1983.

Zeiderman AM, Wiles PJ, Espino DV: Ectopic pregnancy: Six atypical cases. *Postgrad Med* 83(4):297–306, 1988.

Prostatic Pain

Meares EM: Acute and chronic prostatitis: Diagnosis and treatment. *Infect Dis Clin North Am* 1(4):855–873, 1987.

Miller HC: Stress prostatitis. *Urology* 22(6):507–510, 1988.

Schellhammer PF, Whitmore RB III, Kuban DA, et al: Morbidity and mortality of local failure after definitive therapy for prostate cancer. *J Urol* 141:567–571, 1989.

Shortliffe LMD: Prostatitis. *Prim Care* 12(4):787–794, 1985.

Pseudoobstruction

Freilich HS, Chopra S, Gilliam JI: Acute colonic pseudo-obstruction or Ogilvie's syndrome. *J Clin Gastroenterol* 8(4):457–460, 1986.

Thayer WR Jr, Denucci T: Miscellaneous diseases of the large bowel and anal canal. Part 3. Pseudoobstruction of the colon, in Kirsner JB, Shorter RG (eds): *Diseases of the Colon, Rectum, and Anal Canal.* Baltimore, Williams and Wilkins, 1988, pp 566–567.

Psoas Abscess

Leu S-Y, Leonard MB, Beart RW Jr, et al: Psoas abscess: Changing patterns of diagnosis and etiology. *Dis Colon Rectum* 29:694–698, 1986.

Renal Stones

Blute ML, Segura JW, Patterson DE: Ureteroscopy. *J Urol* 139:510–512, 1988.

Brown RD, Preminger GM: Changing surgical aspects of urinary stone disease. *Surg Clin North Am* 68(5):1085–1104, 1988.

Coury TA, Sonda LP, Lingeman JE, et al: Treatment of painful caliceal stones. *Urology* 22(2):119–123, 1988.

Jagjivan B, Moore DJ, Naik DR: Relative merits of ultrasound and intravenous urography in the investigation of the urinary tract. *Br J Surg* 75:246–248, 1988.

Nelson C-E, Nylander C, Olsson AM, et al: Rectal v. intravenous administration of indomethacin in the treatment of renal colic. *Acta Chir Scand* 154:253–255, 1988.

Stewart C: Nephrolithiasis. *Emerg Med Clin North Am* 6(3):617–630, 1988.

Renal and Perirenal Infection

Ahlering TE, Boyd SD, Hamilton CL, et al: Emphysematous pyelonephritis: A 5-year experience with 13 patients. *J Urol* 134:1086–1088, 1985.

Fallon B, Gershon C: Renal carbuncle: Diagnosis and management. *Urology* 17(4):303–309, 1981.

Johnson JR, Stamm WE: Diagnosis and treatment of acute urinary tract infections. *Infect Dis Clin North Am* 1(4):773–791, 1987.

Kaplan GW, Keiller DL: Ureteral obstruction after appendectomy. *J Pediatr Surg* 9(4):559–560, 1974.

Koch MO, McDougal WS: Urologic causes of the acute abdomen. *Surg Clin North Am* 68(2):399–413, 1988.

Lipsky BA: Urinary tract infections in men. Epidemiology, pathophysiology, diagnosis, and treatment. *Ann Intern Med* 110(2):138–149, 1989.

Makker SP, Tucker AS, Izant RJ Jr, et al: Nonobstructive hydronephrosis and hydroureter associated with peritonitis. *N Engl J Med* 287(11):535–537, 1972.

Malgieri JJ, Kursh ED, Persky L: The changing clinicopathological pattern of abscesses in or adjacent to the kidney. *J Urol* 118:230–232, 1977.

Mendez G Jr, Isikoff MB, Morillo G: The role of computed tomography in the diagnosis of renal and perirenal abscesses. *J Urol* 122:582–586, 1979.

Moore CA, Gangai MP: Renal cortical abscess. *J Urol* 98:303–306, 1967.

Patterson JE, Andriole VT: Renal and perirenal abscesses. *Infect Dis Clin North Am* 1(4):907–926, 1987.

Piccirillo M, Rigsby C, Rosenfield AT: Contemporary imaging of renal inflammatory disease. *Infect Dis Clin North Am* 1(4):927–964, 1987.

Thorley JD, Jones SR, Sanford JP: Perinephric abscess. *Medicine* (Baltimore) 53(6):441–451, 1974.

Vehmas T, Paivansalo M, Taavitsainen M, et al: Ultrasound in renal pyogenic infection. *Acta Radiol* 29:675–678, 1988.

Tumors

Wilkins RM, Pritchard DJ, Burgert EO, et al: Ewing's sarcoma of bone. Experience with 140 patients. *Cancer* 58:2551–2555, 1986.

Winawer SJ: Neoplasms of the large and small intestine, in Wyngaarden JB, Smith LH Jr (eds): *Cecil Textbook of Medicine,* 18th ed. Philadelphia, Saunders, 1988, pp 766–774.

Case 43-1987, Case records of the Massachusetts General Hospital. *N Engl J Med* 317(17):1076–1083, 1987.

Case 3-1989, Case records of the Massachusetts General Hospital. *N Engl J Med* 320(3):171–178, 1989.

Uterus and Fallopian Tubes—Diseases

Jones JW Jr, Jones GS: *Novak's Textbook of Gynecology,* 10th ed. Baltimore, Williams and Wilkins, 1981. Adenomyosis of the uterus, pp 443–451; Tumors of the tube, paraovarium, and uterine ligaments, pp 496–506; Infertility, recurrent and spontaneous abortion, pp 694–732.

Merrill JA, Gusberg SB, Deppe G: Lesions of the corpus uteri, in Danforth DN (ed): *Obstetrics and Gynecology,* 4th ed. Philadelphia, Harper and Row, 1982, pp 1076–1104.

Yersiniosis and Mesenteric Adenitis

Aleksic S, Bockemuhl J: Diagnostic importance of H-antigens in *Yersinia enterocolitica* and other *Yersinia* species. *Contrib Microbiol Immunol* 9:279–284, 1987.

Hoogkamp-Korstanje JAA, de Koning J, Samsom JP: Incidence of human infection with *Yersinia enterocolitica* serotypes 03, 08, and 09 and the use of indirect immunofluorescence in diagnosis. *J Infect Dis* 153(1):138–141, 1986.

Leino R, Granfors K, Havia T, et al: Yersiniosis as a gastrointestinal disease. *Scand J Infect Dis* 19:63–68, 1987.

Puylaert JBCM: Mesenteric adenitis and acute terminal ileitis: US evaluation using graded compression. *Radiology* 161:691–695, 1986.

GENERALIZED ABDOMINAL PAIN REFERENCES
(Chapters 27 and 28)

Acute Abdomen—AIDS

Nylander WA Jr: The acute abdomen in the immunocompromised host. *Surg Clin North Am* 68(2):457–470, 1988.

Acute Abdomen—Children

Neblett W, Pietsch JB, Holcomb, GW JR: Acute abdominal conditions in children and adolescents. *Surg Clin North Am* 68(2):415–430, 1988.

Acute Abdomen—Diagnosis

Shaff MI, Tarr RW, Partain CL, et al: Computed tomography and magnetic reasonance imaging of the acute abdomen. *Surg Clin North Am* 68(2):233–254, 1988.

Acute Abdomen—General

Hickey MS, Kiernan GI, Weaver KE: Evaluation of abdominal pain. *Emerg Med Clin North Am* 7(3):437–452, 1989.

Neblett WW III, Pietsch JB, Holcomb GW Jr: Acute abdominal conditions in children and adolescents. *Surg Clin North Am* 68(2):415–430, 1988.

Poole SR: Recurrent abdominal pain in childhood and adolescence. *Am Fam Physician* 30(2):131–137, 1984.

Purcell TB: Nonsurgical and extraperitoneal causes of abdominal pain. *Emerg Med Clin North Am* 7(3):721–740, 1989.

Shaff MI, Tarr RW, Partain CL, et al: Computed tomography and magnetic resonance imaging of the acute abdomen. *Surg Clin North Am* 68(2):233–254, 1988.

Silen W: *Cope's early diagnosis of the acute abdomen,* 17th ed. New York, Oxford, 1987, pp 107–127 pp 153–208.

Diseases of the Mesentery, Omentum, and Peritoneum

Bender MD: Diseases of the peritoneum, and Diseases of the mesentery and omentum, in Wyngaarden JB, Smith LH Jr (eds): *Cecil*

Textbook of Medicine, 18th ed. Philadelphia, Saunders 1988, pp 790–795, pp 795–796.

Isselbacher KJ, LaMont JT: Diseases of the peritoneum and mesentery, in Braunwald E, Isselbacher KJ, Petersdorf RG, et al. (eds): *Harrison's Principles of Internal Medicine,* 11th ed. New York, McGraw-Hill, 1987, pp 1306–1307.

Mast WH: Splenic flexure traction syndrome: Role of the greater omentum. *Int Surg* 53:363–367, 1970.

Williams LF Jr: Mesenteric ischemia. *Surg Clin North Am* 68(2):331–353, 1988.

Diverticulitis/Diverticulosis

Geroulakos G. Surgical problems of jejunal diverticulosis. *Ann R Coll Surg Engl* 69:266–268, 1987.

Greenstein S, Jones B, Fishman EK, et al: Small-bowel diverticulitis: CT findings. *AJR* 147:271–274, 1986.

Food Poisoning

Altman DF: Food poisoning, in Wyngaarden JB, Smith LH Jr (eds): *Cecil Textbook of Medicine,* 18th ed. Philadelphia, Saunders, 1988, pp 784–787.

Infectious Diarrhea

Black RE, Slome S: *Yersinia enterocolitica. Infect Dis Clin North Am* 2(3):625–641, 1988.

Cornick NA, Gorbach SL: *Campylobacter. Infect Dis Clin North Am* 2(3):643–654, 1988.

DuPont HL: *Shigella. Infect Dis Clin North Am* 2(3):599–605, 1988.

Fairchild PG, Blacklow NR: Viral diarrhea. *Infect Dis Clin North Am* 2(3):677–684, 1988.

Goldberg MB, Rubin RH: The spectrum of *Salmonella* infection. *Infect Dis Clin North Am* 2(3):571–598, 1988.

Holmberg SD: *Vibrios* and *Aeromonas. Infect Dis Clin North Am* 2(3):655–676, 1988.

Panosian CB: Parasitic diarrhea. *Infect Dis Clin North Am* 2(3):685–703, 1988.

Thorne GM: Diagnosis of infectious diarrheal diseases. *Infect Dis Clin North Am* 2(3):747–774, 1988.

Intestinal Obstruction

Case 7-1987, Case records of the Massachusetts General Hospital. *N Engl J Med* 316(7):394–403, 1987.

Levine MS, Drooz AT, Herlinger H: Annular malignancies of the small bowel. *Gastrointest Radiol* 12:53–58, 1987.

Martin RG: Malignant tumors of the small intestine. *Surg Clin North Am* 66(4):779–785, 1986.

Richards WO, Williams LF Jr: Obstruction of the large and small intestine. *Surg Clin North Am* 68(2):355–376, 1988.

Silen W: Acute intestinal obstruction, in Braunwald E, Isselbacher KJ, Petersdorf RG, et al. (eds): *Harrison's Principles of Internal Medicine,* 11th ed. New York, McGraw-Hill, 1987, pp 1302–1304.

Lymphoma

Shepherd NA, Hall PA, Coates PJ, et al: Primary malignant lymphoma of the colon and rectum: A histopathological and immunohistochemical analysis of 45 cases with clinicopathological correlations. *Histopathology* 12:235–252, 1988.

Slater DN, Bleehen SS, Beck S: Gastrointestinal complications of mycosis fungoides. J R Soc Med 77:1149, 1984.

Tabbane F, Mourali N, Cammoun M, et al: Results of laparotomy in immunoproliferative small intestinal diseases. *Cancer* 61:1699–1706, 1988.

Metabolic Causes of Abdominal Pain

Adams PC, Halliday JW, Powell LW: Early diagnosis and treatment of hemochromatosis. *Adv Intern Med* 34:111–126, 1989.

Barrett EJ, Sherwin RS: Gastrointestinal manifestations of diabetic ketoacidosis. *Yale J Biol Med* 56:175–178, 1983.

Berger GMB: An incomplete form of familial lipoprotein lipase deficiency presenting with type I hyperlipoproteinemia. *Am J Clin Pathol* 88:369–373, 1987.

Bissell DM: Porphyria, in Wyngaarden JB, Smith LH Jr (eds): *Cecil*

Textbook of Medicine, 18th ed. Philadelphia, Saunders, 1988, pp 1182–1187.

Collen MJ, Lewis JH, Deschner WK, et al: Abdominal pain in hereditary angioedema: The role of acid hypersecretion. *Am J Gastroenterol* 84(8):873–877, 1989.

Duffens K, Marx JA: Alcoholic ketoacidosis: A review. *J Emerg Med* 5:399–406, 1987.

Gardner EC, Hersh T: Primary hyperparathyroidism and the gastrointestinal tract. *South Med J* 74(2):197–199, 1981.

Hift RJ, Meissner PN: Acute intermittent porphyria: An underdiagnosed cause of abdominal pain. *S Afr Med J* 76:44–45, 1989.

Holman JR, Green JB: Acute intermittent porphyria: More than just abdominal pain. *Postgrad Med* 86(5):295–298, 1989.

Karcz A, Farkas PS: Acute porphyria in the emergency department. *J Emerg Med* 7:279–285, 1989.

Kelly TR, Zarconi J: Primary hyperparathyroidism: Hyperparathyroid crisis. *Am J Surg* 142:539–542, 1981.

Laiwah ACY, McColl KEL: Management of attacks of acute porphyria. *Drugs* 34:604–616, 1987.

Moore GP, Hurley WT, Pace SA, et al: Hereditary angioedema. *Ann Emerg Med* 17:1082–1086, 1988.

Palmer JP: Alcoholic ketoacidosis: Clinical and laboratory presentation, pathophysiology and treatment. *Clin Endocrinol Metabol* 12(2): 381–389, 1983.

Poole GV, Albertson DA, Myers RT: Causes of the failed cervical exploration for primary hyperparathyroidism. *Am Surg* 54:553–557, 1988.

Weinstock LB, Kothari T, Sharma R, et al: Recurrent abdominal pain as the sole manifestation of hereditary angioedema in multiple family members. *Gastroenterol* 93:1116–1118, 1987.

Miscellaneous Inflammatory Diseases of the Intestine

Sleisenger MH: Miscellaneous inflammatory diseases of the intestine, in Wyngaarden JB, Smith LH Jr (eds): *Cecil Textbook of Medicine,* 18th ed. Philadelphia, Saunders, 1988, pp 800–807.

Neutropenic Enterocolitis

Keidan RD, Fanning J, Gatenby RA, et al: Recurrent typhlitis: A disease resulting from aggressive chemotherapy. *Dis Colon Rectum* 32:206–209, 1989.

Koea JB, Shaw JHF: Surgical management of neutropenic enterocolitis. *Br J Surg* 76:821–824, 1989.

Peritonitis—Iatrogenic

Arbuck SG, Trave F, Douglass HO Jr, et al: Phase I and pharmacologic studies of intraperitoneal leucovorin and 5-fluorouracil in patients with advanced cancer. *J Clin Oncol* 4:1510–1517, 1986.

Caruana RJ, Wolfman NT, Karstaedt N, et al: Pancreatitis: An important cause of abdominal symptoms in patients on peritoneal dialysis. *Am J Kidney Dis* 7(2):135–140, 1986.

Ekberg O: Complications after herniography in adults. *AJR* 140:491–495, 1983.

Johnson RJ, Ramsey PG, Gallagher N, et al: Fungal peritonitis in patients on peritoneal dialysis: Incidence, clinical features and prognosis. *Am J Nephrol* 5:169–175, 1985.

Kaplan RA, Markman M, Lucas WE, et al: Infectious peritonitis in patients receiving intraperitoneal chemotherapy. *Am J Med* 78:49–53, 1985.

Linton IM, Leahy SI, Thomas GW: *Mycobacterium gastri* peritonitis in a patient undergoing continuous ambulatory peritoneal dialysis. *Aust N Z J Med* 16:224–225, 1986.

Reynolds M, Sherman JO, McIone DG: Ventriculoperitoneal shunt infection masquerading as an acute surgical abdomen. *J Pediatr Surg* 18(6):951–954, 1983.

Shohat J, Shapira Z, Shmueli D, et al: Intestinal incarceration in occult abdominal wall herniae in continuous ambulatory peritoneal dialysis. *Isr J Med Sci* 21:985–987, 1985.

Peritonitis—Secondary

DeRiso AJ II, Kemeny M, Torres RA, et al: Multiple jejunal perforations secondary to cytomegalovirus in a patient with acquired immune deficiency syndrome: Case report and review. *Dig Dis Sci* 34(4):623–629, 1989.

Greenstein AJ, Barth JA, Sachar DB, et al: Free colonic perforation without dilatation in ulcerative colitis. *Am J Surg* 152:272–275, 1986.

Marbet UA, Stalder GA, Vogtlin J, et al: Diffuse peritonitis and chronic ascites due to infection with *Chlamydia trachomatis* in patients without liver disease: New presentation of the Fitz-Hugh–Curtis syndrome. *Br Med J* 293:5–6, 1986.

Torosian MH, Turnbull ADM: Emergency laparotomy for spontaneous intestinal and colonic perforations in cancer patients receiving corticosteroids and chemotherapy. *J Clin Oncol* 6:291–296, 1988.

Walter N, Krishnaswami H: Granulomatous peritonitis caused by *Ascaris* eggs: A report of three cases. *J Trop Med Hyg* 92:17–19, 1989.

Peritonitis—Spontaneous

Ajao OG, Ajao AO: "Idiopathic" intra-abdominal abscess. *Trans R Soc Trop Med Hyg* 76(1):75–76, 1982.

Caralis PV, Sprung CL, Schiff ER: Secondary bacterial peritonitis in cirrhotic patients with ascites. *South Med J* 77(5):579–583, 1984.

Conn HO: Spontaneous bacterial peritonitis: Variant syndromes. *South Med J* 80(11):1343–1346, 1987.

DiPiro JT, Mansberger JA, Davis JB Jr: Current concepts in clinical therapeutics: Intra-abdominal infections. *Clin Pharm* 5:34–50, 1986.

Freij BJ, Votteler TP, McCracken GH Jr: Primary peritonitis in previously healthy children. *AJDC* 138:1058–1061, 1984.

Ing TS, Daugirdas JT, Gandhi VC: Peritoneal sclerosis in peritoneal dialysis patients. *Am J Nephrol* 4:173–176, 1984.

Liebowitz D, Valentino LA: Exogenous peritonitis. *J Clin Gastroenterol* 6:45–49, 1984.

Maddaus MA, Ahrenholz D, Simmons RL: The biology of peritonitis and implications for treatment. *Surg Clin North Am* 68(2):431–443, 1988.

Pusateri R, Ross R, Marshall R, et al: Sclerosing encapsulating peritonitis: Report of a case with small bowel obstruction managed by long-term home parenteral hyperalimentation, and a review of the literature. *Am J Kidney Dis* 8(1):56–60, 1986.

Shaked Y, Samra Y: Primary pneumococcal peritonitis in patients with cardiac ascites: Report of two cases. *Cardiology* 75:372–374, 1988.

Wilcox CM, Dismukes WE: Spontaneous bacterial peritonitis: A review of pathogenesis, diagnosis, and treatment. *Medicine* 66(6):447–456, 1987.

Wongpaitoon V, Sathapatayavongs B, Prachaktam R, et al: Spontaneous *Vibrio vulnificus* peritonitis and primary sepsis in two patients with alcoholic cirrhosis. *Am J Gastroenterol* 80(9):706–708, 1985.

Peritonitis—Tuberculous

Addison NV: Abdominal tuberculosis: A disease revived. *Ann Ry Coll Surg Engl* 65:105–111, 1983.

Palmer KR, Patil DH, Basran GS, et al: Abdominal tuberculosis in urban Britain: A common disease. *Gut* 26:1296–1305, 1985

Yampolski I, Wolloch Y, Dintsman M: Tuberculous peritonitis. *Isr J Med Sci* 20:1064–1067, 1984.

Pregnancy-Related Pain

Goplerud CP: Bleeding in late pregnancy, in Danforth DN (ed): *Obstetrics and Gynecology.* Philadelphia, Harper & Row, 1982, pp 443–454.

Pritchard JA, MacDonald PC: *Williams Obstetrics,* 16th ed. New York, Appleton-Century-Crofts, 1980, pp 375–382, pp 495–503, pp 859–876.

Ruptured Abdominal Aneurysm

Mannick JA, Whittemore AD: Management of ruptured or symptomatic abdominal aortic aneurysms. *Surg Clin North Am* 68(2):377–384, 1988.

Toxicologic Causes of Acute Abdominal Disorders

Mueller PD, Benowitz NL: Toxicologic causes of acute abdominal disorders. *Emerg Med Clin North Am* 7(3):667–682, 1989.

Vascular Diseases

Agha FP, Nostrant TT, Keren DF: Leucocytoclastic vasculitis (hypersensitivity angiitis) of the small bowel presenting with severe gastrointestinal hemorrhage. *Am J Gastroenterol* 81(3):195–198, 1986.

Anger BR, Seifried E, Scheppach J, et al: Budd-Chiari syndrome and thrombosis of other abdominal vessels in the chronic myeloproliferative diseases. *Klin Wochenschr* 67:818–825, 1989.

Belman AL, Leicher CR, Moshe SL, et al: Neurologic manifestations of Schöenlein-Henoch purpura: Report of three cases and review of the literature. *Pediatrics* 75:687–692, 1985.

Coglin WK, Elliott BM, Deppe SA: Nifedipine-induced hypotension and mesenteric ischemia. *South Med J* 82(2):274–275, 1989.

Grendell JH: Vascular diseases of the intestine, in Wyngaarden JB, Smith LH Jr (eds): *Cecil Textbook of Medicine,* 18th ed. Philadelphia, Saunders, 1988, pp 760–765.

Jacobsen SEH, Petersen P, Jensen P: Acute abdomen in rheumatoid arthritis due to mesenteric arteritis. *Dan Med Bull* 32:191–193, 1985.

Keshavarzian A, Saverymuttu SH, Chadwick VS, et al: Noninvasive investigation of the gastrointestinal tract in collagen-vascular disease. *Am J Gastroenterol* 79(11):873–877, 1984.

Maung R, Kelly JK, Schneider MP, et al: Mesenteric venous thrombosis due to antithrombin III deficiency. *Arch Pathol Lab Med* 112:37–39, 1988.

Shepherd HA, Patel C, Bamforth J, et al: Upper gastrointestinal endoscopy in systemic vasculitis presenting as an acute abdomen. *Endoscopy* 15:307–311, 1983.

Toffelmire EB, Clark WF, Cordy PE, et al: Plasma exchange in thrombotic thrombocytopenic purpura. *Can Med Assoc J* 131:1371–1376, 1984.

Vesole DH: Diffuse large-cell lymphoma in an adult with Schönlein-Henoch purpura. *Arch Intern Med* 147:2026–2027, 1987.

Vogelzang RL, Gore RM, Anschuetz SL, et al: Thrombosis of the splanchnic veins: CT diagnosis. *AJR* 150:93–96, 1988.

Wongrowei D, Pollak A, Okon E, et al: Collagenous colitis and rheumatoid arthritis with response to sulfasalazine: A case report and review of the literature. *J Clin Gastroenterol* 9(4):456–460, 1987.

PART SIX
Acute Back and Buttock Pain

Acute Interscapular and Scapular Pain

☐ **SUMMARY**

Acute myocardial infarction may cause dull, aching, interscapular pain, either alone or in association with anterior chest, neck, or jaw pain. There may be associated lightheadedness, palpitations, sweating, nausea, and vomiting. The electrocardiogram (ECG) and serum cardiac isozymes will confirm the diagnosis. The chest radiograph will usually be normal, or show pulmonary vascular congestion and early evidence of pulmonary edema.

A *dissecting aortic aneurysm* causes excruciating, severe anterior chest, neck, and jaw pain that may extend into the interscapular and lower thoracic regions of the back. The pain has been described as "tearing" or "ripping" in up to 50 percent of cases. Syncope, dyspnea, aphasia, and hemiparesis may occur. The chest radiograph usually demonstrates a widened upper mediastinum. If retrograde dissection occurs, a new murmur of aortic insufficiency may appear (50 percent of cases), and a myocardial infarction may occur (16 percent).

The diagnosis can be confirmed by a CT scan or by an aortogram.

A *common bile duct stone* may cause epigastric, subxiphoid, and right upper abdominal pain. It may also refer pain to the left interscapular area. Other symptoms include dark urine, jaundice, chills, and fever. The diagnosis can be confirmed by endoscopic retrograde cholangiography. Surgical or endoscopic removal of one or more common bile duct stones may be necessary to prevent suppurative cholangitis and sepsis, or biliary obstruction.

Acute pyelonephritis may cause lumbar and interscapular pain and tenderness; fever; rigors; and irritative bladder symptoms. The urine contains leukocytes and bacteria, and symptoms resolve promptly with antibiotic therapy.

Acute pleuritis (manifested by pleuritic posterior lower chest and interscapular pain) may occur with *bacterial pneumonia* (i.e., cough, purulent sputum, fever, and rigors), *pulmonary embolism* (i.e., dyspnea, hemoptysis, positive V/Q scan or angiogram), *serositis in collagen vascular disease* (e.g., lupus or rheumatoid arthritis), or *viral pleuritis* (i.e., fever and a negative perfusion lung scan).

Myofascial pain causes a mild to severe ache in the interscapular region. This pain is seldom affected by jarring or general movement, but may be made more intense by specific movements of the muscles of the upper back and paraspinal region (e.g., turning to one side or extending the upper back). There may be one or more local trigger points in the muscles along the spine and between the scapulae. Such pain may be relieved immediately by an anesthetic injection of the causative trigger point.

Pathologic fracture of the spine can result from osteoporosis or malignancy. Such fractures cause the sudden onset of moderate to severe, sharp, midline pain. Jarring and generalized movement intensify the pain. Plain films and computed tomography (CT) scans will demonstrate the fracture and abnormal lytic bone associated with it.

Herpes zoster causes burning or aching back and anterolateral chest pain, in association with a rash composed of grouped, tiny, red-based vesicles and crusted ulcers, which appears in the painful region.

Transverse myelitis causes local midline interscapular pain and tenderness. Lancinating, sharp and diffuse aching or burning anterolateral chest pain may accompany the midline interscapular pain. Within hours of onset of the pain, leg weakness and anesthesia develop and progress rapidly. Bowel and urinary function may be impaired. CT and MRI do not reveal any evidence of a mass (e.g., abscess, disc, tumor, or hematoma) affecting the spinal cord. The cerebrospinal fluid may show an elevated protein concentration and an increased leukocyte count. There is usually no history of prior or concurrent neurologic defects. Optic neuritis may accompany a small number of cases of transverse myelitis. A similar syndrome has been described with multiple sclerosis, sarcoid, and systemic lupus erythematosus.

An *acute epidural abscess* may present with similar back and radicular pain, but the temperature is higher and there is a complete or partial block seen on the myelogram. An abscess will be identified by a CT scan or magnetic resonance imaging (MRI), and neurologic impairment may be reversed by prompt surgical drainage, under cover of intravenous antibiotics.

Trauma can cause fractures and/or subluxations, with back pain, tenderness, muscle spasm, and soft tissue injury, with local pain made worse by movement. Plain thoracic spine radiographs will demonstrate fractures and subluxations.

Osteomyelitis of the spine may cause back pain, spasm, and tenderness of the spine and adjacent muscles. Fever may occur, but is reported in only 50 percent of cases. During the first 2 weeks, plain radiographs and CT scans of the spine may be negative, but a bone scan may identify the affected vertebral segment. This disorder responds to intravenous antibiotic therapy.

The sudden onset of posterior lower neck, interscapular, and/or scapular pain may be caused by herniation of a C5–C6 or C6–C7 disc. Neck rotation to the painful side may initiate or exacerbate pain in the arm, hand, or fingers. Coughing or straining at stool has the same effect. Weakness of specific

TABLE OF DISEASE INCIDENCE

INCIDENCE PER 100,000 (APPROXIMATE)

Common (>100)	Uncommon (>5–100)	Rate(>0–5)
Myofascial pain	Acute myocardial infarction	Transverse myelitis
Pathologic fracture due to osteoporosis	Dissecting aortic aneurysm	Acute epidural abscess
Trauma	Common bile duct stone	Acute pyelonephritis
	Pathologic spine fracture due to tumor or myeloma	Acute pleuritis
	Herpes zoster	
	Osteomyelitis of the spine	
	Cervical radiculopathy due to disc herniation	

arm and hand muscles, hypesthesia of specific fingers, and loss of reflexes are of localizing value. Scapular pain and tenderness is nonlocalizing, and may be associated with C6, C7, or C8 radiculopathies. The herniated disc may be visualized by myelography, with or without CT scan augmentation. Surgical decompression of the affected root leads to recovery.

☐ DESCRIPTION OF LISTED DISEASES

1. ACUTE MYOCARDIAL INFARCTION

Interscapular pain, alone or associated with substernal and/or anterior chest pain, can be caused by coronary artery spasm or occlusion due to thrombus. The pain may be severe or mild, but it is constant, and continues for hours. It may be described as a pressure, a squeezing, or a "weight on the chest." Breathing, bodily movements, and changes of position have no effect on the intensity of the pain. Sweating, nausea, vomiting, dyspnea, and light-headedness may occur in association with the pain.

Examination reveals decreased intensity of the first heart sound and a gallop rhythm in 40 to 60 percent of patients. The electrocardiogram may show Q waves and ST-segment elevation and T-wave inversion in leads with Q waves. In 20 percent of cases, the ECG may be normal, but serum isozyme studies usually reveal elevated levels of CPK-MB and LDH_1. If the diagnosis of severe myocardial ischemia and infarction is made during the first 4 h after the onset of the pain, thrombolytic therapy and angioplasty can be utilized to restore coronary patency and myocardial perfusion.

Tissue plasminogen activator or streptokinase can be given intravenously or by direct coronary artery perfusion.

Thrombolytic activity will restore patency in 60 to 70 percent of cases within 1 to 2 h. Direct use of angioplasty without thrombolytic agents can restore coronary patency and perfusion within 1 h or less.

If the patient arrives more than 4 h after the onset of pain, admission to a coronary care unit and supportive therapy is given to control arrhythmias, hypotension, and congestive heart failure. Warfarin may be used to prevent formation of mural thrombi and embolization.

2. DISSECTING AORTIC ANEURYSM

Severe tearing or ripping pain occurs initially in the substernal area, and may radiate to the neck, lower jaw, and teeth. With extension of the dissection to the aortic arch and descending aorta, a sharp, tearing pain may be felt in the interscapular area and thoracolumbar area. There may be weakness, dizziness, and shortness of breath. The pain can be so severe that the patient writhes in bed, despite large doses of morphine.

Sometimes the pain may be accentuated by each heartbeat. Loss of consciousness, aphasia and/or hemiparesis, paraplegia, and loss of limb or carotid pulses may occur. The chest and back pain may persist for hours, or may be very transient.

A diastolic murmur of aortic insufficiency may appear for the first time (50 percent of cases). Hoarseness, Horner's syndrome, and/or dyspnea may occur. A myocardial infarction with electrocardiographic changes can follow retrograde dissection (16 percent of cases). In some patients, neck vein distension occurs because of superior vena cava compression or cardiac tamponade resulting from bleeding of the aneurysm into the pericardium.

A chest radiograph usually demonstrates a widened mediastinum. Aortography or CT scanning with contrast medium will confirm the diagnosis and define the extent of the dissection and the location of the initial intimal tear.

This disorder may be treated with intravenous nitroprusside to lower the systolic blood pressure to the 100–120 mmHg range. Intravenous propranolol should also be used to reduce the rate of aortic pressure increase with time.

Aortic arch lesions (types I and II) can dissect proximally, leading to severe aortic insufficiency or myocardial infarction. Dissecting aneurysms may rupture into the pleural cavity, causing exsanguination, or into the pericardial sac, causing tamponade with hypotension and distended neck veins. Involvement of aortic branches can cause stroke (innominate or left carotid artery), severe abdominal pain, distension and fever (superior mesenteric artery), and paraplegia (lumbar arteries to the spinal cord). Type I and type II lesions require surgical intervention

with replacement of the arch, aortic root, and valve. Type III lesions begin at the left subclavian artery and dissect down the aorta. These cases require surgery for impending rupture, progressive aneurysmal enlargement, or slow leakage.

Most patients with dissecting aortic aneurysms have one or more of the following predisposing disorders:

1. Severe hypertension.
2. Marfan's syndrome. This is a genetic disorder that is dominantly inherited. Musculoskeletal abnormalities include a tall stature with an upper segment (top of head to pubic symphysis)–to–lower segment (symphysis to floor) ratio of less than 0.75, arachnodactyly, scoliosis, and pectus excavatum or carinatum. Cardiovascular lesions include mitral valve prolapse and regurgitation, aortic insufficiency, aortic dilatation, and dissecting aneurysm. Eye problems include lens dislocation and myopia. Most patients with Marfan's syndrome who suffer dissecting aneurysm have normal blood pressure.
3. Pregnancy.
4. Bicuspid aortic valves.
5. Coarctation of the aorta.
6. Ehlers-Danlos syndrome.
7. Relapsing polychondritis.
8. Trauma.

3. COMMON BILE DUCT STONE

Pain occurs in the epigastrium and right upper abdomen. It can also be felt beneath the xiphoid process and in the upper back. The pain is constant and severe; it may be relieved by meperidine, or by spontaneous passage of the stone into the duodenum. Ascending infection is associated with biliary pain, jaundice, chills, and fever. Tenderness is usually localized to the right upper abdomen.

If ductal obstruction occurs, a suppurative cholangitis may develop. The ductal contents become purulent. Delirium and shock, due to gram-negative sepsis, may soon follow. Multiple small hepatic abscesses can occur, and can lead to death. In addition, common duct stones may obstruct the pancreatic duct and cause epigastric and left upper abdominal pain due to pancreatitis.

Serum bilirubin and alkaline phosphatase levels are high; transaminase levels may be only 2 to 3 times normal. Very high transaminase levels may occur with severe cholangitis, due to hepatic microabscess formation and liver necrosis.

The leukocyte count usually exceeds 12,000 per mm^3 and blood cultures are frequently positive. Rapid biliary decompression, using endoscopic retrograde drainage and intravenous antibiotics, will salvage patients who otherwise would succumb to suppurative cholangitis. Stones can be identified with a sensitivity of 90 to 95 percent, using endoscopic retrograde cholangiography. After stabilization, laparoscopic or open cholecystectomy and endoscopic or open exploration of the common duct are required. All common duct stones should be identified and removed. Despite open surgical exploration and T-tube drainage of the common duct, 2 to 10 percent of patients still retain common duct stones. Common duct stones can be removed by endoscopic techniques.

4. ACUTE PYELONEPHRITIS

Renal infection may cause unilateral or bilateral lumbar ache and fever. Aching pain and muscle tenderness may extend cephalad to the interscapular region. Fever, chills, and irritative bladder symptoms (e.g., frequency, urgency, dysuria) are commonly present. Costovertebral angle tenderness on one or both sides, and sometimes anterior abdominal tenderness, is present. The urine is grossly cloudy and often foul-smelling. It contains red cells and leukocytes—singly, in clumps, and in casts. Bacteria are present in large numbers, and fever and pain resolve with appropriate antibiotic therapy.

5. ACUTE PLEURITIS

A. Bacterial Pneumonia　Cough, chills or rigors, and fever are associated with posterior chest and interscapular pain. The pain is sharp and stabbing, and is intensified by a deep inspiration. It may be referred to the ipsilateral shoulder. The sputum has a purulent, rusty or currant-jelly appearance. Gram stain and culture of sputum, or of a transtracheal aspirate, may aid in identifying the causative infectious agent. Pain and fever resolve with antibiotic therapy.

B. Pulmonary Embolism　Pleuritic lower posterior chest and interscapular pain, hemoptysis, and dyspnea may result from an acute pulmonary infarction due to embolism. A V/Q scan and a Doppler sonographic study of the thigh veins may support the diagnosis. Pulmonary angiography may be required if the V/Q scan is not high probability and the Doppler study is negative. Symptoms resolve on anticoagulant therapy.

C. Serositis in Collagen Vascular Disease　Systemic lupus erythematosus or rheumatoid arthritis may be associated with attacks of pleuritic pain, with or without fever. The pain may be localized to the lower posterior chest and interscapular area. Radiographs may be negative or may show a small pleural effusion. The diagnosis depends on associated clinical findings, and can be supported by laboratory studies (e.g., ANA and LE preparation for lupus, and rheumatoid factor for rheumatoid arthritis). Pleural effusions associated with these disorders are exudates. In systemic lupus erythematosus the pleural fluid may contain LE cells and an ANA titer greater than that of the patient's serum. Patients with systemic lupus usually have pleural fluid titers of 1:160 or greater. Fluid ANA titers in patients with other causes of pleural effusion are not significantly elevated. Rheumatoid pleural effusions have a low glucose (<50 mg/dL) and a pH below 7.3. Rheumatoid factor is present in the fluid, and complement levels are reduced.

D. Viral Pleuritis　Fever and pleuritic pain similar to that described can be caused by a viral agent. Lack of risk factors for thromboembolism, together with a negative perfusion lung scan, distinguishes these patients from those with embolism.

6. MYOFASCIAL PAIN

Pain begins abruptly as an ache or as a sharp, sticking, interscapular pain. Movement of the scapulae and spine may intensify the pain. For example, moving the vertebral borders of the scapulas together may worsen the pain on account of a painful tender area in the rhomboids. Spine extension may aggravate pain originating in paraspinal muscles. Trigger points (localized, fingertip-sized, tender areas in the muscles) may or may not be present. Trigger-point pain sites can be treated with local injection of lidocaine and methylprednisolone, with dramatic relief of pain.

Not all trigger points are primary in the muscle. Some are secondary to spine and nerve-root disease. For example, extramedullary spinal cord tumors may produce secondary trigger points in the paraspinal muscles, on one or both sides.

Trapezius muscle pain may also occur in the interscapular area. This may be intensified by rotation of the head to the side of the pain, and/or by neck extension. Jarring, walking, or moving about has little or no effect on myofascial pain. Plain radiographs, CT scans, sedimentation rates, and serum calcium and alkaline phosphatase levels usually are all normal.

7. PATHOLOGIC FRACTURE OF THE SPINE

Severe, sharp, midline interscapular spinal pain may be caused by a nontraumatic fracture of one or more vertebral bodies in the interscapular region. These fractures may occur from such minimal efforts as lifting a package or opening a window. This type of pain is intensified by spine movement, jarring, stair climbing, and walking.

There is localized tenderness over the spine. If the fracture compresses the spinal cord, one or both legs may become clumsy, weak, or paralyzed. Variable sensory losses may also occur, with partial or complete loss of pinprick sensitivity as well as position, vibration, and touch sensations below a given level in the upper abdomen or chest. Bowel and urinary function may be impaired.

Metastatic cancer can cause vertebral destruction; this may first manifest itself as a sharp, stabbing pain caused by vertebral collapse. In most cases there is a prior history of a diagnosed cancer and surgical or radiation therapy. Plain radiographs will show vertebral destruction and collapse; a CT scan will demonstrate destructive lesions in greater detail. A skeletal survey or bone scan may demonstrate asymptomatic lesions in other areas of the skeleton. The serum calcium and alkaline phosphatase levels may be elevated or normal. Tumors that frequently metastasize to the spine include primary tumors arising in the lung, breast, kidney, prostate, thyroid, colon, ovary, and uterus. Surgical resection of localized vertebral metastatic disease and reconstruction of the spine may be used to treat radioresistant, renal, and other carcinomas. Local palliative radiotherapy may be used with radiosensitive tumors, because of the limited life expectancy of patients with such disease. Multiple myeloma may arise as a bone marrow tumor that can erode a vertebral body. Such lesions are associated with a monoclonal electrophoretic spike in the serum or urine. A normochromic, normocytic anemia is commonly present. Myeloma can be treated with local radiotherapy and with melphalan and prednisone.

Osteoporosis of the postmenopausal type causes trabecular absorption in the vertebral bodies. Affected vertebrae appear, on plain radiographs, to have prominent end plates and vertical trabeculae, or appear as ''empty'' rectangular boxes without trabecular bone. Such vertebrae will crush with minor trauma, giving rise to sharp, and then aching, midline back pain. In advanced cases of osteoporosis, one or two thoracic or lumbar vertebrae may fracture each year. Women beyond their mid-sixties are prone to this disorder. Estrogen progesterone cyclic therapy and oral calcium supplements may prevent this disorder, if begun at age 50 and continued for life.

8. HERPES ZOSTER

Herpes zoster may cause an interscapular aching or burning pain that radiates in a band around one side of the upper back and anterior chest. Within 2 or 3 days of the onset of pain, small, red-based, tender vesicles and pustules erupt, in groups of 3 to 8, on the skin of the paraspinal area and the lateral and anterior chest. There is associated surrounding skin redness. These vesicles soon rupture and become covered with reddish-brown crusts. Acyclovir, taken orally, may decrease viral shedding, but its effect on pain duration and intensity is minimal.

9. TRANSVERSE MYELITIS AND ACUTE EPIDURAL ABSCESS

A. Transverse Myelitis This disorder begins abruptly with localized, midline, interscapular pain that may, or may not, radiate anterolaterally around the chest on one side. This radiating component may be a dull ache or a burning pain. Sharp, lancinating jabs may also occur. Low-grade fever may be present (50 percent of cases), and there is usually local spine tenderness. Within a few hours to 3 days, there is progressive loss of muscle power and sensation in the lower extremities, leading to profound paraplegia and to partial or complete loss of sensation below a transverse level in the upper abdomen or lower chest.

A myelogram should be done to rule out spinal cord compression by disc, abscess, hematoma, or tumor. Plain radiographs taken with the myelogram may show vertebral destruction if the cord syndrome is due to tumor or infection; with idiopathic transverse myelitis they are usually normal. A CT scan or MRI may show localized swelling of the spinal cord at the site of the myelitis, but no cord compression. Spinal fluid shows a slightly elevated protein level and increased numbers of neutrophiles. Counts as high as 1000 cells per mm^3 have been recorded, but this is unusual.

There is no specific therapy for idiopathic transverse myelitis. Corticosteroids have been used with questionable efficacy. One-third of patients may recover completely, and one-third partially; one-third sustain permanent, severe damage.

Transverse myelitis may occur in association with optic or retrobulbar neuritis as a symptom of multiple sclerosis, or as an isolated illness with no subsequent neurologic symptoms or signs. A similar syndrome has been described, rarely, in patients with sarcoidosis and systemic lupus erythematosus.

B. Acute Epidural Abscess An acute epidural abscess caused by hematogenous dissemination of bacteria from an infected heart valve, or from a skin infection, may begin abruptly with severe aching interscapular pain and tenderness, and a high fever. Within hours the patient may develop leg weakness, numbness, and paresthesias, as well as loss of bowel, urinary, and sexual function. Root involvement may develop, causing anterolateral chest or upper abdominal pain of an aching and/or lancinating, sharp quality. A myelogram will show a partial or complete block, and a CT scan or MRI will demonstrate the abscess. Lumbar puncture reveals an elevated protein level, and neutrophils up to 150 per mm³; manometry shows evidence of a block caused by the abscess. Weakness will often progress to complete paralysis within 36 h, so immediate surgical drainage of the abscess should be performed under cover of intravenous antibiotics, to prevent permanent damage.

10. TRAUMA

Rapid deceleration, as in an automobile crash, can cause spinal fractures and dislocations as well as muscle and ligament injuries. If the upper thoracic spine is injured, there is severe muscle spasm and pain, which is intensified by movement. Local spine and muscle tenderness is usually present. Plain radiographs of the cervical and thoracic spine may show fractures, subluxations, or dislocations. Minor fractures missed on plain radiographs may be detected by a CT scan. Severe injuries with loss of posterior elements and spinal instability may cause spinal cord injury and resultant paraplegia. Nonfracture injuries of this region of the back may cause recurrent aching back pain over a period of many years. Even injuries that are apparently minor, and that improve spontaneously within 1 week, may be the source of recurrent attacks of pain. It is important to obtain a careful, complete history to exclude prior injury to the same region of the back, since old trauma may explain current spontaneous back pain.

11. OSTEOMYELITIS OF THE SPINE

Acute mild to severe pain in one or two vertebral bodies may be due to acute osteomyelitis of the spine. *Staphylococcus aureus* and certain gram-negative bacteria are the most common causes. In most cases the pain is mild and low-grade, but it may be a severe and disabling ache that is made more intense by walking or jarring. Fever and chills may occur, as well as radicular pain that spreads anterolaterally around one side of the chest, simulating lung or heart disease. Most often the pain is localized over the spine. Plain radiographs and CT scans taken during the first 2 weeks of such an illness may be normal. The sedimentation rate and white blood cell count are often elevated. A radionuclide bone scan will usually be positive, identifying a bone-related disorder. MRI may be as sensitive as, or more sensitive than, a radionuclide scan in early osteomyelitis of the spine. Needle biopsy and culture will confirm the diagnosis of osteomyelitis. Parenteral antibiotic therapy should be continued for 4 to 8 weeks.

12. CERVICAL RADICULOPATHY DUE TO DISC HERNIATION

Herniation of soft disc material at the C5–C6 (C6 root) or C6–C7 (C7 root) disc level may cause posterior aching neck, interscapular pain, and/or scapular pain on the affected side. Neck rotation toward the painful side may increase the pain and initiate radiation of lancinating severe pain down the posterolateral arm (C7 root) into the hand (index and middle fingers). C6-related pain may radiate down the anterior, medial, and/or lateral upper arm into the lateral forearm and thumb and, sometimes, the adjacent index finger.

The interscapular and/or scapular area may ache continuously. Arm abduction does not intensify the scapular, shoulder, and arm pain; but coughing, sneezing, or straining at stool may cause electric-like pain to radiate into the scapular, arm, hand, and fingers. Spurling's test, performed by compression on the head with the neck rotated to the side contralateral to the pain and laterally flexed to the ipsilateral side, will be positive. This maneuver sends pain and paresthesia down the arm into the hand and fingers (i.e., thumb [C6] or index and middle finger [C7]). C8 radiculopathy may also cause neck and scapular pain, with pain and paresthesia radiating into the ring and little fingers. The Spurling test should not be used until cervical spine disease (fracture, subluxation, and destructive bone disease) has been excluded by radiographic studies.

Clinical localization of the affected root can be achieved by testing for motor weakness and sensory and reflex losses. C6 root compression causes biceps and brachialis muscle weakness, hypesthesia of the thumb and index finger, and loss or diminution of the biceps reflex. A C7 root lesion may cause weakness of the triceps, pectoralis major, flexor carpi ulnaris and radialis, and pronator teres, and sometimes of the serratus anterior (e.g., causing scapular winging, with demonstration by pushing forward against a wall at shoulder or waist level). Hypesthesia of the index and middle finger may be present, and the triceps reflex is diminished or absent. Since there may be tenderness in the interscapular area or along the medial scapular border, a herniated disc may be confused with myofascial syndromes, or with the scapulocostal syndrome prior to radiologic studies.

The abnormal disc can be demonstrated by a myelogram or CT-augmented myelogram. Many cases respond to rest, use of a cervical collar, or analgesics, but discectomy may be required for persistent pain or neurologic loss. Disc removal usually leads to a resolution of symptoms and recovery of neurologic function.

30

Acute Midline Thoracolumbar Pain

☐ DIAGNOSTIC LIST

1. Pathologic vertebral fracture
   A. Metastatic carcinoma
   B. Multiple myeloma
   C. Osteoporosis
   D. Pyogenic or tuberculous osteomyelitis
2. Acute epidural abscess

3. Acute transverse myelitis
4. Herpes zoster
5. Myofascial pain
6. Acute pancreatitis
7. Duodenal ulcer with penetration into the pancreas
8. Fractures and soft tissue injuries

☐ SUMMARY

A *pathologic vertebral fracture* may be asymptomatic, or may begin with severe sharp midline pain or a dull ache that is increased by movement or jarring. Sneezing, coughing, or straining at stool may intensify the pain. Radicular pain may spread around one loin from the back into the abdomen. This may be a dull aching or burning discomfort, accompanied by jabs of sharp lancinating pain.

Metastatic carcinoma may cause isolated vertebral fractures without eroding intervertebral discs. There is often a history, or current physical evidence, of a cancer of the lung, prostate, breast, kidney, thyroid, colon, or uterus. *Multiple myeloma* is associated with weakness, anemia, and back pain. Usually there is a monoclonal spike on a urine or serum electrophoretic pattern and the sedimentation rate is elevated. A needle biopsy of the affected vertebral body will confirm the diagnosis of carcinoma or myeloma.

Osteoporosis may cause anterior wedge or crush fractures of one or more vertebral bodies, but it spares the intervertebral discs. Most vertebral bodies show a marked loss of bone density, and prominent vertebral body end plates, as well as vertical trabeculae; or inwardly ballooned vertebral end plates

(''codfish'' vertebrae); or total loss of all trabeculae (''empty box'' vertebral bodies). Osteoporosis attacks women between age 55 and age 70, and both sexes after age 70.

If *osteomyelitis* is the cause of vertebral fracture, there may be a low-grade fever, a paravertebral abscess, and lytic destruction of the vertebral body and adjacent disc. Needle biopsy and culture of the affected vertebrae will usually identify a pyogenic organism or *Mycobacterium tuberculosis*.

The symptoms of an *epidural abscess* begin with a high fever, chills, severe back pain and tenderness, and rapid loss of motor strength and sensation in the legs. A myelogram will show a block, and a computed tomography (CT) scan or magnetic resonance imaging (MRI) will demonstrate the epidural abscess.

Acute transverse myelitis begins with acute back pain and, sometimes, radicular pain radiating into the abdomen along a 2- to 3-inch wide band from the midline of the back. This is followed, in minutes or hours, by loss of motor strength and sensation and of bladder and bowel control. The myelogram and CT scan of the spine usually show no evidence of a tumor, herinated disc, epidural abscess, or hematoma. There is no block on the myelogram in 90 percent of cases.

Herpes zoster causes back and dermatomal pain on one side

TABLE OF DISEASE INCIDENCE

INCIDENCE PER 100,000 (APPROXIMATE)

Common (>100)	Uncommon (>5–100)	Rare (>0–5)
Pathologic vertebral fracture due to osteoporosis	Pathologic vertebral fracture due to metastatic carcinoma or multiple myeloma	Pathologic vertebral fracture due to osteomyelitis
Myofascial pain	Herpes zoster	Epidural abscess
Acute pancreatitis	Duodenal ulcer with penetration into the pancreas	Transverse myelitis
Fractures and soft tissue injuries		

of the trunk with an erythematous vesicular rash in the painful region. It may mimic a surgical abdominal disorder.

Myofascial pain produces aching, dull discomfort partially relieved by a change in posture or by general exercise. Jarring, coughing, and sneezing have little effect on the pain. Sitting for prolonged periods may intensify it. There may be local trigger points in the muscles. Pressure over a trigger point may reproduce the characteristic pain and its radiation. Radiographs and bone scans are negative in patients with myofascial pain.

Acute pancreatitis begins with constant upper anterior abdominal pain and midline back pain (50 percent of cases), nausea, vomiting, dizziness, and fever. The serum amylase level is usually elevated (80 percent). There may be upper abdominal direct and rebound tenderness, and guarding. Usually the patient has gallstones or is an alcoholic. The back pain is improved by sitting up with the spine flexed, and made worse by extending the back or lying supine.

A *duodenal ulcer with penetration into the pancreas* causes midline back pain that may be temporarily relieved by food and antacids, or H_2-blocking drugs. The pain may be associated with an elevated serum amylase level. The diagnosis can be confirmed by a double contrast upper gastrointestinal series or by endoscopy.

Trauma can cause *fractures* and dislocations of the bony spine, visible on radiographs; or *soft tissue injury* of muscles and ligaments, with associated local tenderness and spasm. The pain and tenderness begin with, or shortly after, the injury, and are related to it.

☐ DESCRIPTION OF LISTED DISEASES

1. PATHOLOGIC VERTEBRAL FRACTURE

Pathologic vertebral fracture is associated with the abrupt onset of moderate to severe midline back pain. This pain may be initially sharp and then become a severe, constant,

boring ache. Jarring (e.g., during walking, running, or descending stairs), coughing, sneezing, or straining at stool may intensify the pain. Sitting or standing may make the pain worse, while lying supine or on a side may lessen it. Pain, and sometimes paresthesias, may radiate around one loin to the mid- or lower abdomen. In some cases this may simulate the severe pain of an acute (surgical) abdomen and lead to an operation. Such pain suggests associated nerve root compression by the vertebral fracture and collapse. Local tenderness is usually present over the fracture site.

The possible causes of pathologic vertebral fracture include:

A. Metastatic Cancer   Tumors of the lung, breast, prostate, kidney, female genital tract, colon, and lymphatic system may metastasize to the spine. Such tumors grow in one or more vertebral bodies, and destroy and replace trabecular bone. Metastases may be asymptomatic until a vertebral fracture occurs, or they may cause low-grade back pain that comes and goes. Plain spine radiographs may reveal vertebral osteolysis and collapse. Lesions causing wedge fractures of the posterior superior aspect of the vertebral body are suspect. Intervertebral discs are rarely involved. A CT scan will provide fine cross-sectional detail of the destructive process. A needle biopsy will confirm the diagnosis. Such patients may benefit from palliative radiation. In some centers, radioresistant tumors, such as renal cell carcinomas, are being operated on to resect the tumor in the spine; the vertebral body is then reconstructed using methyl methacrylate. Superior symptomatic improvement and prolonged survival have been claimed for this type of operative intervention. Radiosensitive tumors can be treated with radiation and/or chemotherapy.

B. Multiple Myeloma   Patients with this disorder may present with the sudden onset of severe back pain due to a vertebral fracture. Small oval-to-round lytic lesions or a washed-out osteoporotic appearance of the vertebrae may be seen on plain radiographs. The diagnosis can be confirmed by finding a monoclonal globulin spike on a urine or serum electrophoresis, or by detecting sheets of abnormal plasma cells on needle biopsy of an osteolytic lesion or other region of the bone marrow. This disorder can be treated with melphalan, with or without prednisone, with remission of bone pain and hematologic abnormalities.

C. Osteoporosis   Back pain due to fracture begins to increase in frequency in women after age 55, and in men after age 70. Plain radiographs show loss of vertebral body density and accentuation of vertical trabeculae and vertebral end plates. Anterior wedge fractures and crush fractures occur. The former type tends to occur in women between 55 and 70 and is the more painful of the two. A CT scan of vertebral bone can be quantitated to establish the diagnosis of osteoporosis. Intervertebral discs are not affected.

The use of cyclic estrogen therapy and supplemental calcium may prevent progression of osteoporosis, but such a regimen will not increase bone strength and density. Fluoride will improve density but it can also cause side effects, such as lower extremity pain in the knees and ankles; it may also increase the frequency of fractures. Epigastric pain and nausea are other common side effects.

It is important to rule out potentially treatable secondary causes of diffuse osteoporosis, such as hyperthyroidism, male hypogonadism, Cushing's disease, parathyroid tumor, steroid therapy, and multiple myeloma.

D. Pyogenic or Tuberculous Osteomyelitis Patients with pyogenic osteomyelitis may have prior low-grade localized thoracolumbar pain and tenderness. Their sedimentation rates are usually elevated, but white blood cell counts and temperatures may be in the normal range in up to 50 percent of cases. The intervertebral discs may be narrowed or destroyed by pyogenic or *Myobacterium tuberculosis* infections. Pathologic fracture produces sharp, constant, severe pain that may be intensified by jarring, straining, sneezing, or coughing. Radicular pain and muscle guarding may occur in the abdomen on one side, simulating an acute abdomen. This pain originates in the midline of the back and radiates to the front. CT scans provide a detailed display of the destructive process.

Needle biopsy of the affected vertebral body and biopsy culture will usually identify a pyogenic organism or *M. tuberculosis*. Pyogenic osteomyelitis follows urinary tract infections, skin infections, bacterial endocarditis, and respiratory infections. Intravenous drug abusers are also at risk. In the United States, tuberculosis of the spine occurs mainly in the elderly and in recently arrived Asian immigrants.

Pyogenic osteomyelitis requires treatment with 4 to 8 weeks of intravenous antibiotic therapy. Surgery is reserved for patients with spinal cord compression secondary to epidural abscess formation or vertebral collapse.

M. tuberculosis infection of the spine can usually be treated with 2 or 3 drugs. These include isoniazid, rifampin, ethambutol, streptomycin, and pyrazinamide. Since up to 25 percent of cases of bone tuberculosis worldwide are caused by isoniazid-resistant organisms, it may be necessary to replace isoniazid with pyrazinamide in a triple drug regimen. Surgery is currently used to decompress the spinal cord and nerve roots, and correct bony deformities secondary to spinal fractures. Medical therapy is highly effective without surgery if cord compression is not present.

2. ACUTE EPIDURAL ABSCESS

An acute epidural abscess may result from a prior pyogenic osteomyelitis, or from direct hematogenous seeding of the epidural space by bacteria metastatic from a different site. High fever, chills, and the abrupt onset of severe back pain and tenderness signal the onset of this disorder. Within hours, leg weakness, paresthesias, and numbness occur. Loss of urinary, bowel, and sexual functions may soon follow. Such patients may appear to be in a toxic condition, or may appear to be relatively normal except for the severity of their back pain. Root involvement may cause pain that radiates into the abdomen, groin, or thigh on one side. A myelogram will show a complete or partial block in 90 to 100 percent of cases. A CT scan or MRI will demonstrate the abscess. The cerebrospinal fluid (CSF) protein concentration is usually elevated, the glucose level normal, and the cell count increased up to 150 per/mm^3. Most of these cells are polymorphonuclear leukocytes. Weakness may progress to irreversible, complete paralysis and sensory loss within 24 h, so surgical intervention should be initiated promptly under cover of intravenous antibiotic therapy.

3. ACUTE TRANSVERSE MYELITIS

This syndrome begins suddenly with sharp, severe, localized midline thoracolumbar pain. Radicular pain may radiate around the lumbar area into the abdomen on one side. This pain may be a constant, dull ache with superimposed jabs of lancinating sharp pain. Local spine tenderness and a low-grade fever may occur (50 percent of cases). Within 72 h there is a progressive loss of motor power and sensation in the legs, which may progress to complete paraplegia and sensory loss with a transverse sensory level on the lower trunk. With idiopathic transverse myelitis, plain radiographs and CT scans will show no evidence of extrinsic spinal cord compression or destructive bone lesions. The sudden onset of paralysis and sensory loss over a period of minutes suggests that occlusion of the arterial supply to a region of the spinal cord is the cause and not myelitis.

A myelogram, a CT scan or MRI should be done to rule out spinal cord compression by a tumor, herniated disc, epidural abscess, or hematoma. A CT scan will also exclude aortic aneurysm as a cause of occlusion of the arterial supply to the thoracolumbar region of the spinal cord. Other causes of spinal artery occlusion, such as disseminated arteritis or the small vessel disease associated with systemic lupus erythematosus, can be diagnosed by the associated clinical picture of the underlying multisystem disease.

Patients with motor weakness and partial or complete sensory loss in the legs, with or without a transverse sensory level and a negative CT scan or MRI, most likely have idiopathic transverse myelitis. This may occur in association with optic neuritis (Devic's disease). Multiple sclerosis is the usual cause of Devic's disease in adults. Transverse myelitis may be treated with corticosteroids.

The prognosis is guarded. One-third of patients recover completely, and one-third partially; the remainder do not improve.

4. HERPES ZOSTER

This illness begins with aching and/or burning pain in the back and abdomen that radiates from back to front in a bandlike dermatomal pattern on one side of the trunk. Itching, tenderness, and paresthesias may also occur in the same region.

Within a few days a rash erupts in the painful zone. This consists of tiny grouped vesicles, clustered in groups of 3 to 8, on erythematous, slightly swollen skin. These lesions may be tender, but often are not. The vesicles may form pustules within 3 days. Shortly thereafter the vesicles and pustules rupture, dry, and form crusts. The skin in the painful zone may be hyperesthetic and tender; because of this, intraabdominal disease may be simulated.

5. MYOFASCIAL PAIN

This may present as a diffuse ache in the thoracolumbar area, with local tenderness over the paraspinal muscles and spine. There may be marked variation of pain intensity from day to day. Some postures and movements may intensify the pain. Exercise may alleviate the pain, or may make it more intense. Jarring by walking or running, coughing, sneezing, or straining at stool does not usually intensify the pain, but at times it may. The pain may spread from the thoracolumbar region to the interscapular region.

Some patients have localized painful trigger points that can be detected by fingertip pressure near the spinous processes in the midline region. Palpation of these trigger points may cause diffuse pain radiation to the flank and up or down the paraspinal region. Injection of these points with lidocaine will usually relieve the pain and tenderness, but such relief may be only transient.

In most patients with pain caused by myofascial disorders, radionuclide bone scans and spine radiographs are negative; the sedimentation rate and white blood cell count are normal; and there are no systemic symptoms such as fever, weakness, weight loss, fatigue, or malaise.

6. ACUTE PANCREATITIS

This disorder begins with a steady pain in the epigastrium and left upper abdomen. The pain begins gradually and achieves peak intensity over a period of 15 to 20 min. It radiates directly through to the midline of the thoracolumbar region in up to 50 percent of patients. The back pain is usually increased by lying supine or extending the back, and eased by flexing the spine. Patients may be found curled up in a "fetal" position, or sitting hunched over in a chair or on the side of the bed. Nausea, vomiting, and fevers up to 101°F occur. Dizziness and weakness are common, and there is usually an accompanying orthostatic or supine hy-

potension. Abdominal distension due to ileus may occur. There is often upper abdominal direct and rebound tenderness and guarding, and evidence of hypovolemia.

Cholelithiasis and alcoholism account for more than 80 percent of cases of acute pancreatitis. Hydrochlorothiazide or estrogen therapy may cause pancreatitis, as may elevated serum levels of triglycerides or calcium.

The diagnosis can be established by measuring the serum amylase and amylase isozyme levels.

Treatment of pancreatitis usually requires narcotics for pain, and intravenous fluids; sometimes nasogastric intubation and suction are required. Attacks of pain and tenderness may persist continuously for 5 to 15 days. Recurrence is common.

7. DUODENAL ULCER WITH PENETRATION INTO THE PANCREAS

A duodenal ulcer penetrating into the pancreas may cause midline thoracolumbar back pain in addition to, or in the absence of, midepigastric pain. The back pain is constant and boring and may be relieved by food and antacids, or by H_2 blockers. The diagnosis can be confirmed by an upper gastrointestinal tract series or by endoscopy.

Therapy with antacids or H_2 blockers, or both, will usually relieve symptoms and lead to the ulcer's healing. An ulcer that fails to heal in 6 to 8 weeks may require surgical intervention for pain relief or to prevent gastrointestinal bleeding.

An ulcer penetrating into the pancreas may also elevate the serum amylase level. Despite the elevated amylase level, the clinical picture of acute pancreatitis—with constant upper abdominal pain and tenderness and guarding—usually is not simulated. Pancreatic pain does not respond to antacids and H_2 blocking drugs, unlike the pain of a penetrating duodenal ulcer.

8. FRACTURES AND SOFT TISSUE INJURIES

Back trauma may result from (1) a deceleration injury—e.g., a fall from a height or an automobile collision with a stationary or moving object; or (2) an acceleration injury—e.g., a blow, or a moving car striking a stationary victim.

Midline thoracolumbar pain may be felt immediately, or may not begin until the next day. There is usually local tenderness. Paresthesias and pains extending into the legs suggest nerve root or spinal cord trauma. Local paraspinal muscle tenderness and spasm may occur. Moving about may be painful; bending over may be impossible. Radiographs may be normal, or may show vertebral body fractures or subluxations due to fractures of posterior articular processes and the disruption of ligaments. A CT scan is more sensitive than plain radiographs for vertebral fractures, and for nerve root compression by a fracture or sub-luxation.

Severe and persistent soft tissue (i.e., muscle and ligament) injuries may occur, which may take months or years to resolve. Radiologic studies in patients with soft tissue injuries are usually normal. Pain, muscle spasm and stiffness, and exacerbation of pain by changes of position are common complaints. These injuries can be treated by rest and administration of analgesics, muscle relaxants, and nonsteroidal anti-inflammatory drugs.

Acute Lumbosacral Pain

☐ **DIAGNOSTIC LIST**

1. Lumbosacral sprain and strain
2. Disc disruption without herniation or protrusion
3. Disc degeneration with herniation and sciatica
4. Disc degeneration with central herniation and acute cauda equina syndrome
5. Infarction of the conus medullaris
6. Nerve root compression in the lateral recess or spinal canal
   A. Lateral recess stenosis
   B. Anomalous conjoined nerve roots
   C. Intraspinal synovial cysts
7. Epidural abscess and epidural hematoma
   A. Acute epidural abscess
   B. Acute nontraumatic epidural hematoma
8. Facet syndrome (posterior joint syndrome)
9. Acute sacroiliitis
   A. *Yersinia enterocolitica* infection
   B. Acute brucellosis
   C. Reiter's syndrome
   D. Pyogenic infection
10. Spondylolysis and spondylolisthesis
11. Pathologic vertebral fractures
    A. Metastatic carcinoma
    B. Local primary bone tumors
    C. Multiple myeloma
    D. Metabolic bone disease
       1. Osteoporosis
       2. Paget's disease
12. Trauma
    A. "Sprung back"
    B. Fractures and subluxations
    C. Hyperextension injury
13. Trochanteric bursitis
14. Maigne's syndrome
15. Myofascial syndromes
    A. Gluteus maximus syndrome
    B. Quadratus lumborum syndrome
    C. Piriformis syndrome
16. Referred pain from intraabdominal structures
    A. Erosive aortic or iliac aneurysm
    B. Diverticulitis of the colon
    C. Acute pelvic inflammatory disease
    D. Acute prostatitis

☐ SUMMARY

Acute nonspecific lumbosacral pain may begin spontaneously, or after ''overuse'' of the back, or after minor trauma. Usually, pain due to *lumbosacral sprain or strain* is constantly present for the first 2 or 3 days, and is made worse by sitting in a chair. Lying curled in bed, on one side, is often the most comfortable posture. Attempts to walk any distance, dress, tie shoelaces, or engage in sexual intercourse usually intensify the pain. Carrying weights as light as 10 or 15 lb may make the pain worse. In addition to this lumbosacral ache, acute paroxysms of low back pain may occur, which ''freeze the victim in his tracks'' until they subside. These painful spasms usually cease after 2 or 3 days of bed rest. Referred pain may occur in the buttock and upper posterior thigh on one or both sides. There may be local tenderness over the spines of L4 and L5 in the midline, and over the gluteal region on one or both sides. Straight leg raising is normal, but elevation above 30° to 45° may cause back pain. Sciatic lancinating pain does not usually occur, although referred sclerotome pain down one leg may mistakenly be attributed to sciatic neuropathy. Muscle strains and ligament sprains, disc degeneration without herniation, facet inflammation or subluxation, or facet joint capsular injury may be the cause of some of these episodes of acute pain. Since the discomfort resolves, in 80 to 90 percent of cases, after 2 to 10 days of rest, most acute attacks of lumbosacral pain without sciatica go undiagnosed as to their specific cause. Patients with more prolonged and troublesome pain (i.e., pain showing no sign of improvement after 20 to 60 days of conservative therapy) are likely to have more extensive diagnostic testing done.

Persistent lumbosacral pain, with sacral and buttock aching, may result from *disc disruption without herniation*. Discograpy will usually reproduce or intensify the patient's pain, and a postdiscography CT scan will show asymmetrical penetration of dye into the disc anulus. Injection of lidocaine into such a disc will ameliorate the pain. Lumbar pain with *sciatica* is most commonly due to *disc degeneration with herniation*, of a nucleus pulposus at the L4–L5 or L5–S1 level. A metrizamide-enhanced CT scan will demonstrate the protruding or extruded disc, and demonstrate its relationship to the adjacent L5 or S1 nerve root. The patient's aching or sharp posterior thigh, calf, and foot pain (i.e., sciatica) is intensified or precipitated by coughing, sneezing, or straining at stool. Conservative treatment usually brings resolution of both lumbosacral and sciatic pain; if such pain persists for 3 to 6 months, it can usually be relieved by laminectomy and discectomy.

Acute lumbosacral pain associated with unilateral or bilateral sciatica, leg heaviness and weakness, paresthesias and patchy anesthesia of the legs and saddle area, and, sometimes, urinary and/or fecal incontinence requires an emergency myelogram followed by a CT scan. This acute *cauda equina syndrome* is usually caused by a large *central disc herniation* at the L5–S1 or L4–L5 level. Emergency discectomy is required to prevent permanent neurologic damage.

The sudden onset of severe lumbosacral, buttock, and leg pain, with paresthesias, patchy anesthesia, leg weakness, and incontinence of urine and feces, may be caused by *infarction of the conus medullaris*. In this form of cauda equina region involvement, the myelogram and CT fail to reveal any mass lesion compressing a nerve root (e.g., disc, abscess, tumor, or hematoma). Such patients usually achieve partial recovery after 3 to 6 months, but seldom recover completely.

Various forms of *nerve root compression* can cause pain in the lumbosacral area. These include *lateral recess stenosis*, which causes lumbosacral pain and sciatica. The stenosis should be apparent on a CT scan or MRI. It may result from severe narrowing of the adjacent disc space, which allows cephalad movement of the superior articular process of the inferior vertebrae. This encroaches on the lateral recess. The recess and foramen can also be compromised by a high-grade spondylolisthesis. Stenosis of a lateral recess or foramen may mimic the symptoms of a protruding or extruded disc. *Anomalous conjoined nerve roots* may cause sciatica, since they are prone to compression by mild degrees of disc protrusion or lateral recess stenosis. *Intraspinal synovial cysts* can also cause nerve root compression and sciatic pain. Both abnormalities can be identified by a contrast-enhanced CT scan.

An *acute epidural abscess* in the lumbosacral area causes midline ache and tenderness, sciatic pain on one or both sides, and leg weakness and numbness, and may cause urinary and fecal incontinence. Associated fever, chills, rigors, prostration, and leukocytosis suggest the diagnosis, which can be confirmed by a CT scan or MRI or a myelogram. Surgical drainage and parenteral antibiotic therapy will usually lead to resolution of all complaints.

Severe localized lumbar pain may occur suddenly in a patient who is on warfarin or who has severe liver disease. In as little as 6 h leg weakness and numbness occur, and bladder and bowel dysfunction may begin. A myelogram usually reveals a lumbar block, and a CT scan or MRI will demonstrate an *acute nontraumatic epidural hematoma* in the lumbar region. Administration of fresh frozen plasma and vitamin K will partly correct the clotting defect. Surgery is required to remove the hematoma.

Patients with a *facet syndrome* (facet joint dysfunction or inflammation) have difficulty sitting for prolonged periods. Rotation and extension of the lumbosacral area will often intensify the pain. Manipulation therapy and lidocaine injection into one or more facet joints may transiently relieve it. A CT scan may reveal facet joint abnormalities. Some patients find relief in standing and in walking or other exercise.

Lumbosacral and buttock pain occur frequently with acute facet joint disease, but thigh pain is uncommon.

Lumbosacral and medial buttock pain may be due to *acute sacroiliitis*. This can follow a diarrheal illness caused by *Yersinia enterocolitica*. This organism may also cause right lower abdominal pain and tenderness, as it involves the ileum and mesenteric nodes. Acute *brucellosis* causes fever, sacroiliitis, and lumbar and thoracic spine aching due to spondylitis. Blood cultures and/or serologic studies will establish the diagnosis. Sacroiliitis related to *Reiter's syndrome* is associated with an attack of dysentery or urethritis. Sacroiliitis and asymmetrical peripheral arthritis occur with conjunctivitis and/or anterior uveitis. This diagnosis depends on the presence of the clinical triad of urethritis, conjunctivitis, and arthritis. Such mucocutaneous lesions as keratoderma blennorrhagicum, balanitis circinata, and painless oral ulcers support the suspected diagnosis when they are present. *Pyogenic infection* (septic arthritis) *of the sacroiliac joint* causes high fever, chills, medial buttock pain and tenderness on one side, and leukocytosis. This disorder responds to parenteral antibiotic therapy.

Low back pain, tenderness, and muscle spasm occurring in adolescents and young adults engaged in athletics (e.g., gymnastics and football) may be due to *spondylolysis* at L5 and, sometimes, at L2 to L4. This pain is caused by a fatigue fracture of the pars interarticularis on one or both sides of L5. Immobilization in a body cast or corset usually leads to healing in 6 to 8 weeks and to the disappearance of symptoms. About 50 percent of patients with untreated fatigue fractures develop *spondylolisthesis*. Severe trauma rarely causes pars interarticularis fractures; usually any spondylolisthesis following such an injury is mild. Congenital spondylolisthesis may begin before age 6 and progress to cause severe lumbosacral pain. An elongated pars interarticularis allows the development of a high grade of spondylolisthesis.

A *pathologic vertebral fracture* may cause severe acute lumbar or lumbosacral pain. Local muscle spasm and tenderness occur at, and near, the fracture site. Spine radiographs will reveal osteolytic lesions and the fracture. A CT scan provides better resolution of the lytic lesions and the relationship of the pathologic fracture to adjacent nerve roots. Cauda equina involvement with unilateral or bilateral sciatic pain may occur. Most patients with *metastatic carcinoma* to the spine have a history of a recently diagnosed cancer; breast, lung, prostate, thyroid, liver, kidney, and bowel are the most common primary sites. Rarely, a pathologic spine fracture is caused by a *local primary bone tumor*.

Multiple myeloma may cause pathologic spine fractures. This diagnosis can be confirmed by serum or urine electrophoresis and a bone marrow examination. Symptoms improve with administration of melphalan.

Metabolic bone disease, such as *osteoporosis* or *Paget's disease,* may cause acute lower back pain because of a pathologic fracture. Bone biopsy may be required for diagnosis; but very often, radiographic changes in adjacent bones establish the nature of the disorder.

Trauma can cause soft tissue injury. A severe flexion injury may tear the supraspinous ligament. This painful ligamentous disruption is associated with increased pain on spine flexion, and with relief on hyperextension. This injury is called a *sprung back*. There is local tenderness and a depression at the site of the injured ligament. By contrast, facet joint injuries result in low back pain made worse by back extension or rotation; partial relief occurs with back flexion. Manipulation of the spine may aid in the relief of painful *subluxation* of facet joints.

Low back pain and tenderness due to *fractures* can be de-

TABLE OF DISEASE INCIDENCE

INCIDENCE PER 100,000 (APPROXIMATE)

Common (>100)	Uncommon (>5–100)	Rare (0–5)
Lumbosacral strain and sprain	Acute sacroiliitis due to Reiter's syndrome	Cauda equina syndrome due to central disc herniation.
Disc degeneration (with or without herniation)	Pathologic fracture due to carcinoma or myeloma	Conus medullaris infarction
Lateral recess stenosis	Paget's disease	Acute epidural abscess
Spondylolysis and spondylolisthesis	Traumatic "sprung back"	Acute nontraumatic epidural hematoma
Facet syndrome	Hyperextension injury of the spine	Acute sacroiliitis due to *Yersinia enterocolitica,* brucellosis, or pyogenic infection
Traumatic fractures and subluxations	Maigne's syndrome	
Osteoporosis with fractures	Erosive aortic or iliac aneurysm	
Trochanteric bursitis	Acute prostatitis	Pathologic vertebral fracture due to a local primary bone tumor
Myofascial syndromes	Lateral recess stenosis associated with anomalous nerve roots	
Diverticulitis of the colon	Intraspinal synovial cyst	
Acute pelvic inflammatory disease		

tected on plain spine radiographs. *Hyperextension injury* may damage one or more facet joints. Lumbosacral pain intensified by rotation or hyperextension occurs. Pain relief may follow anesthetic injection of the injured facet joint.

Trochanteric bursitis causes trochanteric pain that radiates into the low back and down the lateral thigh. A lidocaine injection of the tender trochanteric bursa immediately relieves the pain.

Maigne's syndrome causes posterior iliac crest pain and tenderness on one or both sides. Thoracolumbar facet joint anesthetic injection or manipulation will relieve the pain.

Myofascial syndromes are associated with trigger points in specific muscles. Low back and buttock pain occur together. *Gluteus maximus* trigger points cause low back, buttock, and posterior thigh pain on one side. *Quadratus lumborum* involvement causes ipsilateral groin and anterior thigh pain, and posterior iliac crest and buttock pain. Pain related to the *piriformis* muscle usually involves the buttock and the posterior region of the ipsilateral leg. Injection of lidocaine into a tender trigger point gives immediate relief of the local and referred pain. In many cases, muscle stretching after the anesthetic injection permanently relieves the pain.

Referred pain to the lumbosacral region may arise in the retroperitoneum or from the colon, prostate gland, or fallopian tubes. An *erosive aortic or iliac aneurysm* causing vertebral erosion can cause low back pain. It can be diagnosed by an abdominal sonographic or CT scan. *Diverticulitis of the colon* can cause left lumbar and left lower abdominal pain, fever, localized direct tenderness, rebound tenderness, and guarding in the left lower quadrant. A mass may develop because of a pericolic abscess. A CT scan and/or a barium enema will establish the diagnosis. Acute *pelvic inflammatory disease* causes bilateral or unilateral abdominal and lower back pain. There may be fever and vaginal discharge. Pelvic exam reveals tenderness of one or both fallopian tubes. Antibiotic therapy is usually curative. *Acute prostatitis* causes high fever, chills, dysuria, frequency and urgency, and suprapubic, perineal, penile, and low back pain. In acute prostatitis the urinalysis may reveal many leukocytes, singly and in clumps, and bacteria. There is a good response to antibiotic therapy. Jarring or walking may intensify the pain associated with pelvic inflammatory disease and diverticulitis.

☐ DESCRIPTION OF
LISTED DISEASES

1. LUMBOSACRAL SPRAIN AND STRAIN

Nonspecific aching lower back pain of varying severity may begin gradually and build in severity until it is disabling. In some cases it may start abruptly after a fall, while lifting a heavy object, or while bending over. Such pain is aggravated by sitting for even brief periods of time. It may be improved, or made worse, by standing. Lying in bed usually relieves the pain, but certain positions, such as lying supine, may be associated with a sustained aching lumbar pain. It may be made transiently more severe when walking or jogging is attempted. Rising from the bed to go to the bathroom may cause more intense lumbosacral pain. It may be felt in the midline of the low back, or in the right or left paravertebral region, or bilaterally.

Dressing and tying shoelaces may become impossible without help from a family member. Slight bending, into either flexion or extension, may precipitate excruciating muscle spasms in the low back that make the patient ''freeze in his tracks'' until the pain decreases. Each step or movement may precipitate another spasm that may last for a few seconds or several minutes. Walking with the support of a 4-foot pole, rather than a cane, may allow movement without precipitating spasms. Coughing, sneezing, and straining at stool may cause a mild increase in low back pain without causing lancinating leg pain (negative Dejerine's sign).

There is no sciatic pain, though there may be a dull ache in one or both buttocks and upper posterior thighs; and there are no associated symptoms. Physical examination reveals marked limitation of forward bending and extension and a loss of the normal lumbar lordosis. Straight leg raising may cause an increase in back pain, but there is no pain radiation down the leg. In most cases the leg can be raised above 45°. The knee and ankle jerks are normal. Local tenderness is often present over the lower lumbar spinous processes, or over the upper gluteal region on one or both sides. Plain radiographs usually reveal no specific abnormalities. Routine blood counts, blood biochemical analyses, and the sedimentation rate are within normal limits.

Patients with acute lower back pain should be placed on bed rest for 2 to 4 days and should be given analgesics, such as aspirin, acetaminophen, ibuprofen, or diflunisal. Manipulation therapy may provide dramatic relief in some patients. Muscle relaxants (e.g., cyclobenzaprine) may prevent back spasms. Local application of heat may provide some symptomatic benefit.

Spine radiographs have a low diagnostic yield in patients under age 50 with acute low back pain. They are useful only for the diagnosis of serious disorders, such as vertebral osteomyelitis, metastatic carcinoma, epidural abscess, and vertebral fracture. Spinal radiographs have a higher likelihood of providing new diagnostic information in patients who have the following risk factors for serious disease:

1. Age over 50.
2. Severe trauma.
3. History of a recent malignancy, or evidence on physical examination or by radiography of cancer at another site.
4. Continuous pain while at bed rest for over 1 week.
5. Unexplained weight loss.
6. Drug or alcohol abuse.
7. Recent or current therapy with corticosteroids.
8. A temperature above 38°C, or an elevated sedimentation rate or white blood cell count.
9. Historical evidence compatible with a diagnosis of ankylosing spondylitis.

As many as 80 percent of attacks of low back pain as described above go without specific diagnosis, and are attributed to lumbar strain or sprain. Most patients with such pain recover with bed rest and analgesics. But there is a subset of patients with similar complaints who continue to have persistent pain, stiffness, and disability. These patients have disc disease, facet disorders, lateral recess stenosis, central canal stenosis, spondylolisthesis, sacroiliitis, myofascial syndromes, serious infections, and neoplastic involvement of the spine. These disorders are described below.

2. DISC DISRUPTION WITHOUT HERNIATION OR PROTRUSION

Patients suffering from this disorder have aching lumbosacral pain that is increased by sitting for prolonged periods. This ache may spread to one or both buttocks and upper posterior thighs. There is no lancinating or aching sciatic pain. The region over the spinous processes of L5 and S1 and the upper gluteal area may be locally or diffusely tender. There is marked limitation of back flexion and extension. Straight leg raising and lower extremity reflexes are normal. Plain radiographs of the spine may show disc space narrowing or may be normal. A CT scan may show a bulging disc, or gas in the disc, or it may be normal. A discogram injection will usually reproduce or exacerbate the patient's pain. This has been interpreted as evidence that the degenerated disc itself is the source of the pain. A CT scan done after dye injection into the abnormal disc may show abnormalities of disc structure, such as asymmetrical migration of contrast material into the peripheral anulus. Some surgeons have done anterior interbody fusions to treat this cause of persistent low back pain, with good results. Use of discography and interbody fusion is controversial.

3. DISC DEGENERATION WITH HERNIATION AND SCIATICA

Patients with this condition have lumbosacral pain and tenderness that are made worse by sitting for prolonged periods, walking, jogging, bending forward, dressing, and lifting. Pain may be eased by standing or lying down. The protruding nuclear material may compress one or more nerve roots, causing a sciatic syndrome. Radicular pain radiates down the posterior aspect of the thigh from the lower back. It usually extends into the calf and foot. Disc herniations are most common at the L4–L5 and L5–S1 interspaces. An L4–L5 herniation impinges on the L5 root, so that pain radiates down the posterolateral thigh and lateral calf into the big toe. There may be weakness of big toe and foot dorsiflexion, and normal knee and ankle reflexes. An L5–S1 herniation causes posterior thigh and calf pain, as well as heel and lateral foot pain. Eversion of the foot is weakened, and the ankle jerk may be absent or decreased. Big toe pain has been considered localizing for an L5 root lesion, and heel pain for an S1 root compression.

Typical pain with localizing features for L5 and S1 root compression is usually present in only 25 percent to 38 percent of cases. S1 root compression is most frequent. Some patients have an L3–L4 disc with L4 root compression. This results in anterior thigh, knee, and medial calf pain, weakness of foot inversion, and a diminished knee jerk.

Sciatic pain may occur as a persistent, dull ache or may be felt as jabs or trains of electric-like pain that radiate from the low back down the thigh into the calf and foot. Both types of pain may occur in the same patient at different times.

Jabs of this electricity-like pain may be precipitated by

a cough, a sneeze (positive Dejerine's sign), or straining at stool—or voluntarily, by the Valsalva maneuver. This finding may be present in 48 to 84 percent of patients with nerve root compression. In the past, neurologists have used the presence of this sign as an indication for myelography, and its absence as a reason to delay intervention. Paresthesias and numbness occur in 30 percent of patients, and subjective feelings of ankle and leg weakness in only 6 percent. The straight leg raising test will be positive in 90 to 99 percent, while the crossed sign, which is 98 percent predictive of root compression, is positive in only 15 percent. A positive straight leg raising test should result in reproduction of the sciatic pain—not just back pain—when the leg is raised from 0° to 45°. Hypesthesia of the big toe (L5), or little toe and lateral foot (S1), may also occur.

Sciatic pain must be differentiated from referred "sclerotome" pain, which is felt as a vague, deep, boring ache that spreads from the lower back into the buttock, and often into the posterolateral thigh on one or both sides. Rarely sclerotome pain extends to the calf. It is not associated with paresthesias, numbness, or weakness, and there are no reflex changes. The straight leg raising test causes only back pain, and Dejerine's sign is negative. This type of pain is associated with facet arthritis, sacroiliitis, and myofascial syndromes in the gluteal region. It is not caused by root compression.

Disc herniation can be confirmed by metrizamide myelography. This test has an 80 to 90 percent sensitivity and an 87 percent specificity. It may miss 25 to 30 percent of disc herniations at L5–S1, and may miss small central herniations and larger lateral ones. Specificity is also a problem with the myelogram, since lumbar defects may occur in up to 24 percent of asymptomatic patients. Demonstrable abnormalities in these patients include nerve root sleeve deficits, narrowing of the transverse diameter of the contrast column, and partial and complete obstruction of the subarachnoid space.

A metrizamide-enhanced CT scan shows a clear relationship between nerve roots and adjacent disc herniations; it will also demonstrate nerve root anomalies, postoperative scar tissue, and arachnoiditis. This procedure has a higher sensitivity and specificity than myelography. The role of MRI in the diagnosis of disc herniation is currently being evaluated.

Nonenhanced CT scans of asymptomatic patients may show a 35 percent incidence of abnormality. The most common findings in one series were a herniated nucleus pulposus (15 to 31 percent), spinal stenosis (2 to 9 percent), and facet degeneration (4 to 16 percent). The wide ranges reported were due to interobserver disagreement between the 3 different radiologists reading the same films. These abnormalities have also been detected in the postmortem examinations of patients who had never had sciatic pain. Protruded discs were found in 39 percent.

Because of the poor specificity of radiologic studies, it is essential to do a careful clinical history and physical examination in any case of lumbosacral pain with sciatica. The clinical diagnosis and root localization should correspond to the myelographic and CT findings; if they do not, surgery may be directed at a radiologic defect that is not the cause of the patient's symptoms, in which case the surgery will be a failure and the pain will persist.

Most patients with low back pain and sciatica caused by herniation of a nucleus pulposus will recover on conservative therapy within 3 months. Others may respond to epidural injections of corticosteroids. The use of such injections is controversial; their efficacy has been questioned, and there is a low-frequency risk of causing arachnoiditis. Patients with residual pain and disability may require surgical intervention (5 to 6 percent). In the recent past, many of these patients have been treated with chymopapain injections (chemonucleolysis) to dissolve protruding or extruded disc material. Such therapy is effective in 75 percent of cases. Chemonucleolysis is not without hazard: Anaphylaxis occurs in 0.5 to 1 percent of patients, and at least four deaths have occurred. Subarachnoid bleeding may occur if the injection is into the subarachnoid space. Paraplegia due to transverse myelitis may occur in 1 of 3500 cases; thirty-five cases of this catastrophic complication have already occurred. Persistent muscle spasms may occur in up to 20 percent of patients after chemonucleolysis. Patients who fail to respond to enzyme injection usually have a sequestered disc fragment, lateral recess stenosis, or another underlying problem. While some centers continue to use chemonucleolysis, these complications make surgery a more attractive option.

There are three basic operations for disc removal. *Microdiscectomy* is currently popular because of the minimal surgical trauma to the bony spine. Only the extruded fragment, with a small amount of residual disc material, is removed. Standard *unilateral discectomy* allows for more extensive removal of disc space material. (Total discectomy is not possible.) The recurrence rates for these two procedures approach 15 percent. *Bilateral radical discectomy* allows more effective removal of disc material; the recurrence rate is only 2 percent.

Discectomy is 95 percent effective, but it primarily relieves sciatica; though lumbosacral pain may also be relieved, often it is not. Operations done primarily for lumbosacral pain have a low success rate. Failure of discectomy is due to the missing of a disc fragment, recurrent herniation, periradicular fibrosis, arthritic spurs, or an incorrect initial diagnosis (e.g., missed lateral recess stenosis). Complications include infections, such as discitis; epidural abscess; arachnoiditis; and dural tears with cerebrospinal fluid leaks. Rarely, damage to the aorta or iliac vessels may occur.

Emergency surgery is usually unnecessary unless there is a large midline herniation that produces a cauda equina syndrome (2.5 percent of cases). Most patients should not be operated on until they have had 3 to 6 months of conservative care.

4. DISC DEGENERATION WITH CENTRAL HERNIATION AND ACUTE CAUDA EQUINA SYNDROME

In this condition there is an abrupt or gradual onset of severe lumbosacral and buttock pain. There may be pain radiation down one or both posterior legs into the calves or ankles. Paresthesias and numbness may occur in the same distribution as the pain. Dejerine's sign will be positive, as will the straight leg raising test on one or both sides. Buttock, genital, and thigh (i.e., saddle area) hypesthesia or anesthesia may be present. There may be urinary retention, followed by overflow incontinence, as well as anal sphincter incompetence and incontinence of stool. Leg weakness may be absent, mild, or severe. Hip abduction and extension, knee flexion, and ankle plantar flexion and dorsiflexion are commonly affected. A myelogram or a metrizamide-enhanced CT scan will reveal a midline disc protrusion or extrusion. Bilateral radical discectomy should be done as soon as possible to prevent the development of permanent leg weakness and incontinence.

5. INFARCTION OF THE CONUS MEDULLARIS

In this condition severe lumbosacral, and unilateral or bilateral buttock, and thigh pain occurs abruptly and is followed by the rapid onset of leg weakness, saddle anesthesia, or hypesthesia—with additional sensory loss, in some cases, in the legs and feet. Urinary and stool incontinence develop. The urinary incontinence usually is of the overflow type and follows urinary retention. The anal sphincter is usually patulous. Hip extension and abduction, knee flexion, and ankle dorsiflexion and extension are usually impaired, and lower extremity reflexes may be absent. Aortic surgery, use of an intraaortic balloon catheter, advanced age, smoking, and vascular disease are risk factors for this rare disorder, which can mimic a central disc herniation. There may be prodromal recurrent brief attacks of low back, buttock, and thigh pain, and numbness and lower extremity weakness involving one or both limbs. The myelogram and CT scan are negative for disc herniation. There is no effective therapy, but spontaneous partial recovery may occur over a period of months. This disorder is a form of spinal cord "stroke" involving the conus medullaris. L4 to S5 segments are involved.

6. NERVE ROOT COMPRESSION IN THE LATERAL RECESS OR SPINAL CANAL

A. Lateral Recess Stenosis   Lumbosacral aching pain made worse by sitting and walking may reflect disc degeneration at L4–L5 or L5–S1. Sciatic pain may radiate into one or both buttocks, posterior thighs, and calves. Coughing, sneezing, and straining at stool may precipitate sciatic pain, and the straight leg raising test is positive.

Plain radiographs may show marked disc-space narrowing (e.g., from a normal width of 15–20 mm to 5–10 mm). Enlargement and upward subluxation of the adjacent superior facet joint and hypertrophy and displacement of the ligamentum flavum may cause stenosis of the lateral recess or nerve root foramen, resulting in ipsilateral sciatic pain. Spondylosis and spondylolisthesis can cause lateral recess narrowing. Lateral stenosis can be confirmed by a CT scan. Disc herniation is not usually present. Myelography is usually fairly reliable for the diagnosis of disc disease, but it is not sensitive enough for the detection of lateral stenosis. CT and MRI diagnose this disorder accurately and can confirm the absence of disc protrusion. Decompressive nerve-root-canal laminectomy is necessary to relieve the buttock and leg pain. Some patients with disc degeneration and unilateral sciatica have nerve root compression caused by a fragment of sequestered vertebral end plate cartilage, which requires removal. Lateral recess stenosis should be sought on a CT scan when disc protrusion and extrusion are not present.

A congenital variant that affects spinal canal dimensions and the width of the lateral recess is the narrowed trefoil canal. This too can give rise to lateral recess stenosis.

B. Anomalous Conjoined Nerve Roots   Anomalous conjoined nerve roots may be mistaken for extruded or protruding disc material on CT scans of patients with lumbosacral pain and sciatica. The pain is often, but not always, on the side of the conjoined-nerve-root anomaly. Some surgeons believe that these roots, because of their size, are prone to compression by mild degrees of disc protrusion and lateral recess stenosis. Lateral recess decompression may be required for the relief of symptoms if a herniated disc is not present adjacent to the affected conjoined root. The incidence of this anomaly is 2 percent; most cases are asymptomatic. The discovery of such an anomaly on CT in a patient without symptoms does not warrant further treatment.

C. Intraspinal Synovial Cysts   Intraspinal synovial cysts can cause nerve root compression with lower back and sciatic pain, requiring surgical intervention. They can be detected by a CT scan.

Failure to recognize lateral recess stenosis is a common reason for surgical failure in operations performed to remove herniated nucleus pulposus material.

7. EPIDURAL ABSCESS AND EPIDURAL HEMATOMA

A. Acute Epidural Abscess   A central lumbar spinal ache and exquisite tenderness develop rapidly. High fever, rigors, and/or chills accompany the pain. Root pains radiate into the posterior aspects of one or both legs. There is urinary retention followed by overflow incontinence. Stool incontinence may also be present. There is weakness or heaviness of one or both legs. There is variable sensory loss over the buttocks, genitalia, and lower extremities. The leukocyte count is elevated, and spinal fluid examination reveals an elevated protein level and white blood cell count and a normal cerebrospinal fluid sugar level. A CT scan or MRI will establish the diagnosis. Surgical drainage, under cover of parenteral antibiotics, should be done as soon as possible.

B. Acute Nontraumatic Epidural Hematoma   Most patients who develop this disorder are taking anticoagulants like warfarin or have chronic liver disease. There may be an onset while straining at stool or doing heavy manual work, such as woodcutting. On the other hand, this disorder can begin without any precipitating event or activity. The first symptom is the abrupt onset of severe local midline lumbar pain associated with tenderness. Pain may radiate down the back of one or both legs into the feet. Such pain may be intensified by coughing or straight leg raising. Neurologic dysfunction begins 6 h or more after the onset of the back pain. It consists of patchy sensory loss and leg weakness. Bladder and bowel function may be partly or completely impaired. Fever and chills are not part of the clinical picture. The prothrombin time may be moderately or severely prolonged. A myelogram will show a spindle-shaped lower lumbar block, and a CT scan will accurately locate the hematoma. Vitamin K and fresh frozen plasma should be given, and laminectomy performed to decompress the cauda equina and remove the hematoma. Patients with partial neurologic lesions have a good prognosis for recovery. Those with complete neurologic lesions have a poor prognosis. (Fewer than 50 percent recover.) The longer surgery is delayed, the worse the prognosis becomes. A rapid progression of neurologic signs is ominous; a gradual loss of neurologic function over a period of several days correlates with a smaller hematoma.

8. FACET SYNDROME
(POSTERIOR JOINT SYNDROME)

In this syndrome, lumbosacral ache usually begins abruptly and is aggravated by sitting for prolonged periods. Walking and standing may ease the pain. Rotational movements, flexion, and hyperextension of the spine usually intensify the pain. Referred dull, deep, boring pain may spread to one or both buttocks. There may be localized paravertebral tenderness over the affected facet joints. The buttock and leg pain is usually sclerotome-referred pain and not due to nerve root compression. Local injection of tender facet joints with the long-acting local anesthetic bupivacaine may separate patients with acute lumbosacral pain (i.e., pain present less than 3 months) into responder and nonresponder groups.

In one series, responders (55 percent of patients) usually had an abrupt onset of lumbosacral pain, which was made worse by sitting and was usually not exacerbated by standing. It was often eased by walking. Flexion usually increased pain in the back, as did straight leg raising. Straight leg raising did not usually produce leg pain. Forty-two percent of responders in a small series had permanent relief after an anesthetic injection into a tender facet joint. Posterior thigh pain was uncommon in the responders, who usually had unilateral lumbosacral and buttock pain, midline lumbosacral pain, or bilateral buttock and lumbosacral pain.

If the specificity of pain relief by facet joint anesthetic injections is high, then the above description probably corresponds to a clinical description of facet-related low back pain. Since local anesthetic may diffuse away from the joint injected and affect adjacent structures, the specificity of a facet injection response is still controversial. Hypertonic saline-solution injections (e.g., during clinical research studies) into facet joints have demonstrated that these joints can give rise to low back, buttock, and, sometimes, posterior thigh pain.

Patients who are temporarily relieved of rest- and movement-related back pain by anesthetic and corticosteroid injection of one or more facet joints may be permanently relieved of such pain by radiofrequency denervation of the same joints. Spinal manipulation may also provide pain relief for those with acute pain related to facet joint subluxation. Manipulation may be tried before injection

Facet joint capsules may be stretched and torn by violent movements of the spine into hyperextension. Laxity of the ligamentous capsules of these joints may allow the development of joint subluxation and osteoarthritis.

9. ACUTE SACROILIITIS

Acute sacroiliitis causes unilateral or bilateral sacroiliac, buttock, and posterior thigh pain of an aching nature that is made worse by walking or jarring. There is local fist-percussion tenderness over one or both sacroiliac joints. The pelvic rock test, with the patient supine, and Gaenslen's sign are both positive. (In the pelvic rock test, the examiner places a hand on each iliac crest with thumbs on the anterior-superior iliac spines, and palms on the iliac tubercules. The pelvis is then compressed toward the midline. If the patient complains of pain, the test is positive. In testing for Gaenslen's sign, the patient is asked to draw both legs up with knees and hips flexed. He or she is then moved to the side of the table with one buttock extending over the edge. The unsupported leg is dropped and extended. A positive test occurs when ipsilateral sacroiliac pain is felt on the side of the dangling leg.) The patient is usually HLA-B27-positive.

Acute sacroiliitis may occur with the following disorders:

A. *Yersinia Enterocolitica* Infection   Patients with this disorder develop generalized crampy abdominal pain, fever, and diarrhea. Right lower quadrant pain, guarding, and rebound tenderness may develop, mimicking acute appendicitis. These symptoms are caused by acute mesenteric adenitis; this occurs in children and younger adolescents (ages 5 to 15).

Diarrhea, right lower abdominal pain, and fever, with local tenderness, occur in older adolescents and adults. This disorder may mimic Crohn's disease. Usually it is self-limited and is followed in 1 to 6 weeks by a symmetrical polyarthritis that tends to be migratory. There is sacroiliac pain (20 to 25 percent of cases) and involvement of the knees, ankles, and small joints of the hands and feet. The diagnosis can be confirmed by stool cultures on enriched media, and by measuring agglutination titers to *Yersinia enterocolitica*. Serologic testing is not as reliable as culture, since some strains to not lead to antibody production and because rising titers may fall rapidly. Erythema (multiforme or nodosum), urethritis, and uveitis may accompany the arthritis. Antibiotic therapy is usually not effective in cases with sacroiliitis and arthritis.

B. Acute Brucellosis   Acute brucellosis may cause acute sacroiliitis and spondylitis, with sacroiliac pain and fever, and pain over the upper lumbar and thoracic vertebrae. Peripheral joint involvement may occur in 10 to 15 percent of cases. Blood cultures and agglutinin tests for brucella are useful in establishing a diagnosis. Spine radiographs may remain negative for months, as may serologic tests. Many patients with this disorder are slaughterhouse workers, veterinarians, butchers, farmers, or cattlemen; or have eaten meat, or unpasteurized milk or cheese from an underdeveloped country. Antibiotic therapy with tetracycline and streptomycin is effective.

C. Reiter's Syndrome   In this syndrome sacroiliitis may occur, with additional involvement of knee, shoulder, hip, and other joints in an asymmetrical fashion. There may be only one peripheral joint involved at a time, and the arthritis may be migratory. Spondylitis affecting the lumbar vertebrae may also occur, causing lumbosacral pain extending up to the thoracolumbar area.

The incidence of sacroiliitis in Reiter's syndrome is 20 to 25 percent. Conjunctivitis (30 to 40 percent of cases) may be mild or severe, with a serosanguineous discharge. Anterior uveitis occurs in 50 percent of cases with sacroiliitis. Keratitis and episcleritis may also occur. Urethritis, with a clear mucoid discharge, and dysuria complete the triad of urethritis, conjunctivitis, and arthritis (Reiter's syndrome). Mucocutaneous lesions such as keratoderma blennorrhagicum (macules and pustules on the soles of the feet and palms), balanitis circinata, and painless buccal papules and ulcers may also occur. Fever is usually low-grade, but occasionally the temperature exceeds 102°F. Nonsteroidal anti-inflammatory drugs may be used for treatment.

D. Pyogenic Infection Pyogenic infection may cause acute sacroiliac pain and swelling of the overlying soft tissue. There may be severe localized tenderness. High fever, chills, and severe disability occur. The leukocyte count may be elevated above 15,000 per mm^3. There is a therapeutic response to appropriate antibiotic therapy.

10. SPONDYLOLYSIS AND SPONDYLOLISTHESIS

This disorder causes lumbosacral and right or left paravertebral aching pain, associated with local muscle spasm, in children and young adults. The pain may also be felt in one or both buttocks and upper thighs. Many patients with this disorder are involved in athletics; gymnasts and football players are at greatest risk. (Their risk is 4 times the average.) High-quality lumbosacral oblique spine radiographs should be taken and, if negative, repeated in 3 to 6 weeks. A linear fatigue fracture of the pars interarticularis of L5 is the most common lesion found in this clinical setting. Similar defects may occasionally occur in L2, L3, and L4, but L5 is the most common site. These fatigue fractures may be unilateral or bilateral. Sometimes a particularly violent fall or mishap involving the back precipitates the back pain; in most cases it comes on gradually. Some patients have an elongated pars interarticularis but no fracture. This is believed to be due to prior undetected fractures that have healed, allowing pars elongation. This disorder is the most common cause of spondylolisthesis, occurring between ages 6 and 50 (6 percent prevalence). Most patients with a spondylolytic defect have probably had it since age 6. Usually the radiographic appearance of the fracture is characteristic enough to determine if it is new or old. A radionuclide scan can be done if there is doubt about the age of the fracture. Spondylolisthesis of L5 on S1 develops in about 50 percent of patients with spondylolysis and is usually less than 30 percent in extent. Once detected in a child or young adult, a pars interarticularis fracture should be treated by body cast or corset immobilization for 6 to 8 weeks. Some fractures will heal without treatment. Usually symptoms remit after fracture healing. Such therapy probably prevents progression to spondylolisthesis. This latter process becomes maximal by age 20, and usually does not progress after that.

Dysplastic or congenital spondylolisthesis affects the L5–S1 articulation. Usually spina bifida occulta of the sacrum and L5 is present. The usual defects are in the sacral articular processes. The pars interarticularis of L5 is usually intact. This disorder may cause lumbosacral pain in children and adolescents. Slippage of L5 on S1 may be severe, and can lead to sciatic pain superimposed on the lumbosacral and buttock ache that is the initial complaint.

Many patients with spondylolytic lesions and with varying degrees of spondylolisthesis are asymptomatic. The development of spondylolisthesis is usually gradual after the pars interarticularis defect occurs, and may take many years.

An acute fracture of the pars interarticularis resulting from severe trauma (e.g., a major fall or a pedestrian accident) causes severe lumbosacral back pain and spasm and a mild-to-moderate degree of spondylolisthesis, which may develop at the time of the fracture. These pars fractures usually heal with bed rest and immobilization with an extension brace, and the patients usually become asymptomatic within 3 to 6 months.

11. PATHOLOGIC VERTEBRAL FRACTURES

Lumbosacral pain associated with pathologic spine fractures may be constant and severe; or it may be mild, and troublesome only during certain movements or after prolonged sitting.

A. Metastatic Carcinoma Metastatic carcinoma to the spine may be clinically silent, or may cause only mild intermittent lumbosacral discomfort until a pathologic fracture occurs. Pain then becomes severe and constant, and is intensified by movement and jarring. If there is vertebral displacement in the lumbar region associated with the fracture, there may be compression of lumbar and sacral roots. This can cause sciatic pain on one or both sides, as well as leg weakness and sensory loss. Severe epidural compression may lead to urinary retention or urinary and fecal incontinence.

In most cases there is a history of a recently diagnosed or treated malignancy of the breast, lung, prostate, kidney, thyroid, liver, or large bowel, or of some other site. Lumbosacral muscle spasm and bony tenderness may be present. There may be anemia, elevated serum calcium and alkaline phosphatase levels, and a positive radionuclide bone scan. Plain spine radiographs show the fracture and osteolytic vertebral lesions. A CT scan through the area of the fracture will define the extent of the osteolytic lesions and demonstrate the relationship of the fracture to the nerve roots of the cauda equina. In a small percentage of cases, a pathologic fracture may be the first symptom of metastatic carcinoma. (Tumors of the stomach, pancreas, and rectum may first present as bone metastases.) Most bone metastases are clinically silent. Premenopausal metastatic breast cancer can be treated with oophorectomy, or with tamoxifen. Chemotherapy with 5-fluorouracil, cyclophosphamide, and methotrexate may induce remission of bone pain when endocrine ablation is no longer effective. Prostatic cancer can be treated by orchiectomy or estrogen administration. Renal carcinoma may respond to therapy with interleukin-2-stimulated autologous killer lymphocytes. Metastatic thyroid cancer can be treated with thyroid hormone and with radioiodine. Small cell and other lung tumors can be treated with multiple-agent chemotherapy. If the fracture causes nerve root compression, corticosteroids should be given and surgical decompression should be carried out without delay. During this procedure the involved portion of the vertebral body can be resected and methyl methacrylate reconstruction of the resected region completed. Radiotherapy can be used postoperatively. Excellent palliative results have followed surgical resection, with recovery of leg weakness and sensory disturbances.

B. Local Primary Bone Tumors Local primary bone tumors can produce a pathologic fracture of one vertebrae and may cause nerve root compression with radicular pain. They are rare. Both benign and malignant lesions can cause localized back and root pain. Plain lumbosacral spine radiographs are 99 percent sensitive for detection of symptom-producing lesions. A metrizamide enhanced CT scan is useful for demonstrating the relationship of the tumor to nerve roots. MRI can be used to scan the entire spinal canal. It is more sensitive than CT in detecting skip lesions and metastases.

Malignant tumors include solitary plasmacytoma (a premyeloma lesion), chordoma, chondrosarcoma, lymphoma, Ewing's sarcoma, osteosarcoma, and fibrosarcomas. Surgical extirpation is the recommended treatment, except for solitary plasmacytoma; this more sensitive lesion can be treated with radiation, and carries a good prognosis for long-term survival. Patients with this lesion should be observed for the development of multiple myeloma. Benign lesions include osteoblastoma, osteochondroma, giant cell tumor, and bone cyst.

C. Multiple Myeloma Multiple myeloma causes punched-out, round-to-oval, 0.5- to 2-cm lytic lesions, and/or a radiologic picture of generalized osteoporosis. Pathologic fractures occur, causing local and root pain

and dysfunction. This lesion is radiosensitive, but radicular compression requires surgical intervention. The diagnosis can be confirmed by local bone biopsy, serum and urine electrophoresis, and bone marrow aspiration. Therapy with melphalan and prednisone may produce remission.

D. Metabolic Bone Disease

1. Osteoporosis Osteoporosis may cause a pathologic fracture of one or more vertebral bodies. These bones usually have a hypodense radiographic appearance on x-ray and may show prominent vertical trabeculae and vertebral end plates, or an "empty box" appearance with no trabeculae. Women between ages 55 and 70, and both men and women after age 70, are at risk. Rarely osteoporosis is secondary to another disorder, such as hyperthyroidism, Cushing's syndrome, male hypogonadism, or hyperparathyroidism.

2. Paget's Disease Other metabolic disorders, such as Paget's disease, may cause pathologic fractures of anterior or posterior spinal elements, resulting in low back and nerve root pain.

12. TRAUMA

A. "Sprung Back" This injury occurs when the lumbar spine is overflexed (e.g., in a motor vehicle accident where the victim is unrestrained or wearing only a lap belt; while carrying a heavy object with another person where the latter suddenly drops the load; or following a fall while moving at high speed on a motorcycle, a bicycle, or skis).

There is a sudden onset of sharp midline pain at the L4–L5 and/or L5–S1 interspaces. This pain is intensified by flexion, and relieved by extension, of the lower back. (Extension might be, for example, sitting straight with a pillow in the lumbar area.) It may spread as a dull ache to one or both anterior or lateral thighs and buttocks. The straight leg raising test is negative, and the knee and ankle reflexes are normal. Localized tenderness is present over the L4–L5 and/or L5–S1 interspaces. A palpable depression of the tender zone is due to interruption of the supraspinous ligament resulting from the injury. Local anesthetic injection into the affected supra- and interspinous ligaments provides immediate pain relief. The use of an extension back brace or corset allows the torn ligaments to heal in 6 to 8 weeks. There is a tendency toward recurrence.

B. Fractures and Subluxations A vertebral fracture caused by hyperflexion or axial loading of the spine may cause acute lumbosacral pain that can spread to the buttocks and/or thighs. Plain radiographs will identify the fracture, which can be treated by bed rest or by surgical intervention. Root compression causing radicular pain may require surgical intervention. Severe hyperflexion may cause a tear in the posterior longitudinal ligament and disc herniation. If the disc compresses nerve roots then a typical cauda equina syndrome may develop, with bladder and rectal incontinence. Alternatively, the disc herniation may produce only back pain and sciatica; in most cases of this type, surgery is unnecessary.

Fractures of the pars interarticularis of L5 or L4 may lead to acute lower back pain and spondylolisthesis with sciatic-type pain on one or both sides, secondary to nerve root compression. Such fractures are uncommon, and the degree of spondylolisthesis produced does not usually require surgical intervention. Acute slippage, causing severe low back, buttock, and leg pain, with hamstring muscle spasm, may require surgical intervention.

C. Hyperextension Injury   Forceful hyperextension of the low back causes this injury. It may result from falling backward with the lumbar area striking a low wall or the back or armrest of a low chair, a fall from a height, or a motor vehicle collision in which the victim is unrestrained. There is tearing and stretching of the ligamentous capsule about one or more facet joints. These joints become hypermobile and may develop traumatic arthritis.

There is localized low back pain, exacerbated by rotation or hyperextension of the back. Flexion is less painful, but often is not entirely pain-free. Referred aching deep pain may be present in one or both buttocks and thighs, posterolaterally. Sleeping prone, sitting erect, rising from a chair, or holding and lifting a weight at arm's length with the back straight may intensify the pain.

The back pain may be accompanied by local tenderness over one or more facet joints. If this pain persists despite rest and analgesics, bupivacaine injections of one or more facet joints may be given for diagnostic and therapeutic purposes. Recurrent injuries of this type may cause segmental instability and lead to progression of facet joint disease, producing lateral recess stenosis and sciatica. This progression may take many years.

In many cases of hyperflexion or hyperextension injury, the affected ligamentous structures heal and the back pain and referred pain disappear. In such a case, however, the back may be functionally insufficient, and pain may recur with minimal flexion or hyperextension stress.

13.   TROCHANTERIC BURSITIS

Trochanteric bursitis may occur spontaneously in elderly women and may develop in young adults who are active in athletics (e.g., tennis, jogging, cycling). Pain is felt over the greater trochanter and radiates upward into the buttock and low back, and downward to the lateral thigh and knee. Local tenderness is present in a half-dollar-sized area over the greater trochanter. Patients often report that they are unable to lie on the affected side because of the pain produced by pressure against the mattress. Walking and jogging intensify or precipitate the pain. An injection of lidocaine and methylprednisolone into the tender trochanteric area may temporarily or permanently relieve the pain. Plain radiographs of the hip should be done for patients over age 50, since metastatic cancer may sometimes mimic trochanteric bursitis. Calcium deposits may or may not be present in the bursa, but otherwise such radiographs are usually negative.

14.   MAIGNE'S SYNDROME

In Maigne's syndrome pain occurs over one or both posterior iliac crests. There may be skin hyperesthesia in the posterior iliac crest region. The source of the pain is facet joint dysfunction at the T12–L1 level. Rest and analgesics may ameliorate this disorder. Manipulation of the thoracolumbar facet joints usually provides rapid relief and should be tried before facet joint injection.

15.   MYOFASCIAL SYNDROMES

In these syndromes, aching myofascial pain occurs in lumbosacral muscle groups; the pain is related to one or several trigger points. Pressure on these points may cause wide referral of pain, and will often reproduce the primary and referred pain arising in a particular muscle. These disorders usually cause unilateral discomfort. There is often an area of muscle induration or spasm, which feels ropy to palpation beneath, or adjacent to, the trigger point. Passive or active stretching of such muscles causes pain. Cough- and sneeze-related jabs of pain do not occur, and the straight leg raising, Gaenslen, and pelvic rock tests are negative. Pain in these sites is immediately relieved by lidocaine injection into the trigger point, followed by active muscle stretching. Coolant spraying, followed by passive full-length muscle stretching, can be used for treatment with somewhat less efficacy than an anesthetic injection.

Bending, walking, and jogging usually worsen the pain, but active stretching, even in the presence of discomfort, may produce pain relief.

Repeat injections may be required if relapse occurs, but 92 percent cure rates may occur with injection, or with spray-and-stretch techniques. These disorders may mimic the facet syndrome, sacroiliitis, a herniated disc, or lateral recess stenosis.

The common myofascial syndromes causing lumbosacral and buttock pain, and sometimes thigh pain, are listed below:

A. Gluteus Maximus Syndrome   Trigger points are found in the buttock on the ipsilateral side. Pain is felt in the low back, buttock, and upper posterior thigh.

B. Quadratus Lumborum Syndrome   Pain is felt in the groin, upper anterior thigh, posterior iliac crest, and buttock region on one side. An active trigger point is present between the posterior iliac crest and the last rib.

C. Piriformis Syndrome   Pain occurs in the low back, buttock, posterior thigh, calf, and foot on one side. The trigger point is usually in the buttock.

16. REFERRED PAIN FROM INTRAABDOMINAL STRUCTURES

Referred pain to the lumbosacral area may arise from retroperitoneal structures (e.g., aorta, common iliac artery) or from the colon, female reproductive organs, or prostate gland.

A. Erosive Aortic or Iliac Aneurysm   An enlarging aneurysm may cause lumbosacral pain secondary to pressure on, and erosion of, a vertebral body. Aneurysms can arise in the lower aorta and in the proximal common iliac artery. Leakage may also occur, causing a tender, pulsatile lower abdominal mass (i.e., hematoma). A sonographic study will identify the aneurysm. A CT scan will also demonstrate the aneurysm, adjacent eroded vertebrae, and a hematoma if partial rupture has occurred. Immediate surgical resection of the aneurysm, with graft replacement, is required.

B. Diverticulitis of the Colon   Diverticulitis of the left colon may begin with fever, chills, and left lumbosacral pain. Within 1 or 2 days, left lower abdominal pain and tenderness develop. There may be left lower abdominal guarding and rebound tenderness, and a palpable mass due to a pericolic abscess may appear. The leukocyte count is usually elevated. Involvement of the left ureter by an inflammatory mass can cause acute hydronephrosis and left flank pain. A plain radiograph of the abdomen may show an accumulation of gas and fluid in the left lower quadrant, or free air beneath the diaphragm. A CT scan may demonstrate inflamed pericolic fat, bowel wall thickening, and the involved diverticulum. If a barium enema is done after 1 or 2 weeks of parenteral antibiotics there may be barium leakage from the involved diverticulum, fistula formation, and a pericolic abscess.

The left kidney should be studied by ultrasonography to rule out ureteral obstruction in the presence of an abscess. Patients with this condition require hospitalization, a clear liquid diet, and parenteral antibiotics. Up to 50 percent of complicated cases require surgical drainage and resection of the involved colonic segment.

C. Acute Pelvic Inflammatory Disease   Acute pelvic inflammatory disease causes unilateral or bilateral lower abdominal pain that may be intensified by walking, jarring, or sexual intercourse. Pain and tenderness may also be present on one or both sides of the lumbosacral region. It is usually made worse by walking and jarring, and often by bending or extending the back. Fever, vaginal discharge, nausea, and vomiting may or may not be present. There is usually direct lower abdominal tenderness, and sometimes guarding and rebound tenderness. Pelvic examination reveals tender, and sometimes enlarged, fallopian tubes and ovaries and cervical motion provoked lower abdominal and back pain. This disorder usually resolves with administration of parenteral antibiotics. Oral therapy may be effective in milder cases.

D. Acute Prostatitis   Patients with acute prostatitis have high fever, chills, and suprapubic and perineal pain. There is often dysuria, frequency, a sensation of incomplete bladder emptying, and clear or cloudy urine. Lumbosacral backache may occur, and in some cases may be the most prominent painful symptom. The suprapubic pain may temporarily improve or disappear after voiding, only to recur 1 or 2 h later. If a three-glass test is done, the first and third glasses may show leukocytes. Oral and/or parenteral antibiotics will usually lead to symptom resolution. Urine cultures will frequently grow the causative organism. Diagnostic prostatic massage to express secretions should not be done until 2 or 3 weeks after resolution of the infection.

The lumbosacral pain is relieved by antibiotic therapy and is not intensified by bending, walking, sitting, or jarring.

CHAPTER
32

Acute Unilateral Buttock Pain

☐ DIAGNOSTIC LIST

1. Furuncle of the buttock skin
2. Anorectal Abscess
   A. Ischiorectal abscess
   B. Supralevator abscess
   C. Deep posterior anal abscess
3. Sacroiliitis
   A. *Yersinia enterocolitica*
   B. Acute brucellosis
   C. Reiter's syndrome
   D. Pyogenic infection
4. Facet syndrome (posterior joint syndrome)
5. Spondylolisthesis
6. Degenerative disc disruption
7. Ischial bursitis
8. Myofascial syndromes
9. Hamstring strain or tear
10. Nodular fasciitis (episacroiliac lipomas)
11. Trochanteric bursitis
12. Nonspecific low back pain
13. Epidural abscess
14. Sacral neuralgia due to primary genital herpes

☐ SUMMARY

A *furuncle* causes localized buttock pain associated with skin redness and with fluctuance or induration. Such lesions may be single or multiple. They usually resolve after spontaneous or surgical drainage. An *injection-related abscess* usually occurs in the upper outer quadrant of the buttock and causes fluctuance or induration deep in the buttock. Bowel movements do not intensify the pain associated with this lesion.

An *anorectal abscess* may cause deep medial buttock pain that is intensified by sitting, walking, and defecation. Rectal digital and proctoscopic examinations are extremely painful, but the latter may identify pus coming from an internal opening of the abscess in the base of an anal crypt. Fever, rigors, and chills occur in some cases, and a tender fluctuant mass may be present in the painful region. Incision and drainage of the abscess will usually relieve the pain.

Sacroiliitis causes upper medial buttock pain that is increased by jarring or walking, but not by coughing or defecation. There is localized percussion tenderness over the sacroiliac joint. Gaenslen's test and the pelvic rock test are positive. In some patients, activity relieves the pain, while prolonged sitting and rest in bed worsen it.

Some cases of sacroiliitis occur after a febrile diarrheal illness associated with right lower quadrant pain and tenderness. *Yersinia enterocolitica* may be cultured from the stool, or there may be a rise in serum antibody to this organism. *Brucellosis* occurs in slaughterhouse workers, butchers, ranchers, farmers, and veterinarians. These patients may have fever, as well as lumbar and thoracic spine pain and tenderness and sacroiliitis. The diagnosis requires a positive blood culture or a fourfold rise in the brucella agglutinin titer. *Reiter's syndrome* causes sacroiliac and, usually, asymmetrical peripheral joint involvement, with swelling and pain most often affecting the larger joints of the lower extremities. Urethritis, conjunctivitis, balanitis circinata, and keratoderma blennorrhagicum are other findings that, when present, support this diagnosis. *Pyogenic infection* can cause *sacroiliitis*, resulting in fever and chills, local skin swelling, redness, and tenderness. There is usually a good response to intravenous antibiotic therapy.

Facet syndrome (facet joint inflammation or subluxation) causes lumbar and/or lumbosacral and buttock pain, which is made more intense by prolonged sitting and by back rotation and extension. Activity decreases the pain in some cases, but not in all. Standing may be more comfortable than sitting. Spinal manipulation or bupivacaine injection into a tender facet joint may dramatically relieve the pain. Maigne's syndrome results from facet joint subluxation at T12–L1. It causes pain referred to the posterior iliac crest or upper buttock, and is relieved by manipulation or injection.

Spondylolisthesis may develop acutely, causing low back, buttock, and posterior thigh pain. There is usually an underlying spondylolysis of L5. There may be marked hamstring spasm and a painful abnormal gait.

Disc disruption causes low back and buttock pain. The back pain may be midline and/or paraspinal. It is relieved by bed rest and worsened by prolonged sitting, carrying a load, and pushing heavy objects. Discography precipitates or intensifies the pain, whereas disc injection with bupivacaine relieves it. A computed tomography (CT) study done after discography shows disc degeneration.

Ischial bursitis causes pain and tenderness over the ischial tuberosity, intensified by walking, running, and prolonged sitting on a hard chair. Local injection of methylprednisolone and avoidance of pressure on the bursal area lead to resolution. Ischial bursitis occurs in novice cyclists, people who sit for prolonged periods resting on their buttocks (i.e., weaver's bottom), and adolescent runners doing speed training.

Myofascial syndromes cause buttock pain associated with painful trigger points. Pressure over these points reproduces or intensifies the patient's pain. Injection of these tender spots with lidocaine, followed by muscle stretching, relieves the pain. Trigger points may occur in the gluteus maximus, piriformis, and quadratus lumborum muscles. A *hamstring strain or tear* may mimic ischial bursitis. A tear of the hamstring at its origin causes deep pain and tenderness over the ischial tuberosity. Surgical repair may be required. The injury usually occurs suddenly, during running or jumping.

Nodular fasciitis causes upper buttock pain associated with tender, mobile subcutaneous nodules. This pain can be relieved by local injection of lidocaine and methylprednisolone into a tender nodule. *Trochanteric bursitis* causes pain and tenderness over the greater trochanter of the femur. Pain may radiate to the buttock and down the lateral thigh. Local injection of lidocaine and methylprednisolone into the bursa relieves the pain and tenderness immediately, and often permanently.

Nonspecific low back pain may cause a lumbosacral ache and buttock pain. Painful low back muscle spasms may accompany certain movements or attempts at ambulation. Prolonged sitting, walking, carrying a load, or pushing a heavy

TABLE OF DISEASE INCIDENCE

INCIDENCE PER 100,000 (APPROXIMATE)

Common (>100)	Uncommon (>5–100)	Rare (>0–5)
Furuncle	Sacroiliitis due to Reiter's syndrome	Sacroiliitis due to brucellosis
Facet syndrome	Sacroiliitis due to *Yersinia enterocolitica*	Sacroiliitis due to pyogenic infection
Spondylolisthesis		
Disc degeneration		
Myofascial syndromes (gluteus maximus, quadratus lumborum)	Ischial bursitis	Epidural abscess
	Hamstring strain or tear	
	Acute anorectal abscess	
Nodular fasciitis	Myofascial syndrome (piriformis)	
Trochanteric bursitis		
Nonspecific low back pain	Injection-related abscess	
Sacral neuralgia due to genital herpes		

object intensifies the pain. Most patients respond well to bed rest and analgesics, and recover in 2 to 7 days. More resistant cases may be caused by disc degeneration, facet disease, or torn supraspinous and/or interspinous ligaments. The cause of nonspecific low back pain, by definition, goes undetermined, since there is rapid spontaneous symptom resolution. In most cases, a muscular strain or a ligamentous sprain is probably causative. Small numbers of cases may be due to disc degeneration without herniation, or to facet joint disease.

An *acute epidural abscess* causes severe low back and buttock pain, and sometimes upper and lower leg pain, associated with marked tenderness over the lower lumbar spine. Fever, rigors, and/or chills occur, and the leukocyte count is elevated. Leg weakness, buttock and leg sensory loss, and urinary and fecal incontinence may follow the onset of pain and fever. The diagnosis can be confirmed by CT, magnetic resonance imaging (MRI), or myelography. Symptoms resolve after surgical drainage of the abscess and decompression of the cauda equina. In *sacral neuralgia due to genital herpes,* there are painful tender vesicular or ulcerative lesions of the labia or penis, and of adjacent skin, associated with aching or burning buttock and thigh pain.

☐ DESCRIPTION OF LISTED DISEASES

1. FURUNCLE OF THE BUTTOCK SKIN

Initially, an area of skin the size of a quarter becomes painful, tender, and red. Within 24 to 36 h this lesion enlarges and becomes more intensely erythematous and indurated. Within 2 to 3 days the indurated region becomes fluctuant. Sitting on, or placing pressure over, the reddened area intensifies the pain, while coughing and defecation usually do not affect it. Such lesions may resolve without drainage, or they may form a pustular head and begin to discharge small amounts of yellow-green pus. Staphylococci are the main cause of such abscesses. Fluctuant lesions should be drained surgically. Antistaphylococcal oral antibiotics may be used to ensure resolution of the infection.

Anal cultures and nares cultures may grow *Staphylococcus aureus*. Careful disinfection of clothing and bed linens (e.g., using chlorine bleach in the wash), frequent showers, use of bacitracin ointment in the nares, and oral administration of dicloxacillin may prevent further attacks of ''boils'' in patients who suffer from recurrent lesions on the buttocks and at other sites.

Injection-Related Abscess   Injections of antibiotics and other drugs into the upper outer quadrant of the buttock can cause pain, swelling, local tenderness, and fluctuance. Such an abscess may be sterile or infected. It may drain spontaneously, or require drainage; or it may resolve, after many weeks, into a small, hard nodule. Defecation does not itensify the pain produced by such a lesion.

2. ANORECTAL ABSCESS

An anorectal abscess is usually connected to an anal crypt by a fistulous tract. It may be classified by its location in relation to the rectum, and the sphincter and levator muscles.

A. Ischiorectal Abscess   This type of abscess usually develops from infection of an anal gland. It causes severe aching and sometimes throbbing medial buttock pain, made worse by sitting, walking, coughing, and defecation. There is exquisite tenderness of the medial buttock, which may be swollen and either indurated or fluctuant. Rectal examination may be so painful that the patient refuses to allow completion of the examination. The presence of an internal fistulous opening can be confirmed, and the site identified, by passing an anoscope and compressing the abscess. Pus may exude from the orifice of the fistulous tract at the base of one of the anal crypts. Fever, chills, and sweats often accompany the buttock pain.

A medial incision into the mass will drain 30 to 300 ml of foul-smelling pus, with prompt improvement of all symptoms. The abscess should be irrigated and the cavity loosely packed with iodoform gauze. Intravenous antibiotics should be used for 48 to 72 h. The iodoform gauze wick can be removed at 24 to 48 h, and the fistulous tract can be excised surgically 10 to 14 days after the abscess is drained.

B. Supralevator Abscess   This type of abscess causes deep buttock, sacral, and perianal pain. It is severe, continuous, and aching, and may become throbbing. In some cases the abscess arises from an intraabdominal site (e.g., diseased colon from Crohn's disease, diverticulitis, appendicitis, or salpingitis); in others the abscess is connected by a fistulous tract to the anal canal.

The pain is made worse by sitting, walking, coughing, defecation, and rectal digital examination. Fever, chills, sweats, and leukocytosis are commonly present.

Supralevator abscesses arising from intraabdominal disease that are not connected by a fistulous tract to the rectum should be drained into the rectum.

A supralevator abscess secondary to extension of an intersphincteric abscess should also be drained into the rectum. A supralevator abscess secondary to an ischiorectal abscess should be drained through the ischiorectal fossa. Intravenous antibiotics should be used for 2 or 3 days. With adequate abscess drainage, fever and pain rapidly subside.

C. Deep Posterior Anal Abscess   There is deep posterior rectal pain, made worse by bowel movements and digital examination. Fever, chills, and leukocytosis occur. The pain is aching and continuous and may be throbbing. It radiates to the buttock and sacrum. Physical examination may reveal only posterior rectal tenderness. Needle aspiration of pus from the abscess, located between the rectum and coccyx in the midline, will usually establish the diagnosis. This pus may invade the ischiorectal fossa(e) on one or both sides (horseshoe abscess). Surgical drainage and irrigation should be carried out.

3. SACROILIITIS

Acute sacroiliitis may cause medial buttock and, sometimes, posterior thigh pain of an aching nature, that is intensified by walking and jarring but not by coughing or defecation. There is local fist percussion tenderness over the sacroiliac joint on the painful side. The pelvic rock test, Gaenslen's test, and fabere sign are usually positive. Many patients are seropositive for HLA-B27 antigen.

The causes of acute sacroiliitis include:

A. *Yersinia enterocolitica*   Diarrhea, right lower abdominal pain, fever, and chills occur. There is localized direct, and sometimes rebound, abdominal tenderness in the same region. This disorder may mimic acute appendicitis or an acute episode of Crohn's disease. It is due to a localized inflammation of the ileum and the adjacent mesenteric nodes.

Within 1 to 6 weeks after the onset of abdominal symptoms, small numbers of patients develop a migratory symmetrical arthritis that may mimic acute rheumatic fever. Twenty-five percent of patients with polyarthritis develop sacroiliitis. The diagnosis of yersiniosis can be confirmed by culture of stool or a surgically excised mesenteric lymph node, or by serologic testing for an antibody rise. Erythema multiforme, erythema nodosum, urethritis, or anterior uveitis may occur in association with the arthritis. Antibiotic therapy with doxycycline and other drugs usually fails to control the joint-related symptoms.

B. Acute Brucellosis This disorder causes medial buttock aching secondary to sacroiliitis, and lumbar and thoracic aching from spondylitis. There may be local sacroiliac and spine tenderness. Spine radiographs may remain negative for months. A radionuclide bone scan will usually show sacroiliac and spinal uptake even when radiographs are negative. Peripheral joint symptoms and splenomegaly occur in fewer than 15 percent of cases. The diagnosis can be confirmed by blood or bone biopsy cultures, or by serologic tests for brucella agglutinins. Most cases in the United States occur in slaughterhouse workers, veterinarians, cattlemen, farmers, butchers, and persons ingesting unpasteurized milk or cheese.

C. Reiter's Syndrome Pain in one buttock and over the sacroiliac area may occur in association with a migratory arthritis of the large weight-bearing joints (i.e., hips, knees, and ankles). The peripheral joint involvement is often asymmetrical. Sacroiliitis occurs in 25 percent of cases. Conjunctivitis (30 to 40 percent of cases) and urethritis are the other components of the diagnostic triad.

Mucocutaneous lesions, such as keratoderma blenorrhagicum, balanitis circinata, painless oral papules and ulcers, and a low-grade fever may occur in some cases. Most symptoms respond to nonsteroidal anti-inflammatory drugs.

D. Pyogenic Infection Pyogenic infection may cause sacroiliac pain, with soft tissue swelling, redness, and tenderness over the joint. High fever, chills, and severe disability may occur. Leukocytosis is common. This disorder usually responds to intravenous antibiotic therapy.

4. FACET SYNDROME (POSTERIOR JOINT SYNDROME)

Buttock pain of an aching quality, and of mild to moderate severity, may be caused by facet joint inflammation or subluxation. Lumbar or lumbosacral joints are usually involved. The pain may be precipitated by lifting, snow-shoveling, or prolonged sitting. It may begin abruptly after bending or twisting the back. Rotation and extension of the spine intensify the pain; standing and moving about may alleviate it. Spinal manipulation may result in dramatic relief. An injection of bupivacaine into a tender facet joint may also alleviate the discomfort. After either procedure, however, the pain may recur.

A CT scan may show hypertrophic articular processes and irregular facet joint spaces. Careful correlation of symptoms and radiographic findings is necessary, since many asymptomatic patients have abnormal facet joints on their spinal CT scans.

Maigne's syndrome is caused by a disorder of the facet joint between T12 and L1. Pain is felt over the posterior iliac crest and upper buttock. The ipsilateral T12–L1 facet joint is tender. Manipulation or joint injection relieves the pain. This disorder usually arises from degenerative changes in the facet joints and intervertebral discs. Bilateral involvement may occur.

5. SPONDYLOLISTHESIS

A patient with spondylolysis of the pars interarticularis of L5 may suddenly develop severe sharp buttock pain, which may radiate into the upper posterior thighs. Spine radiographs may show slippage of L5 on S1. The pain may lead to hamstring spasm and an abnormal gait. Symptoms are worse when the patient is standing. Such acute episodes are very uncommon. Rest in bed, analgesics, and muscle relaxants usually provide relief, but severe cases may require surgical decompression and spinal fusion to prevent recurrence.

6. DEGENERATIVE DISC DISRUPTION

Lumbosacral and buttock pain of an aching quality occur. The intensity is moderate to severe. Sitting for a prolonged period intensifies the pain; lying down alleviates it. Injection of contrast dye into the suspected disc reproduces and intensifies the buttock pain, whereas injection of lidocaine into the disc abolishes it. A CT study done after discography shows that the contrast dye has penetrated through the anulus in an asymmetrical fashion, indicating disc degeneration. Most patients recover with conservative treatment. A small percentage may require anterior interbody fusion for permanent pain relief. Careful assessment of the subjective response to disc injection is necessary, because many patients with asymptomatic discs may have abnormal CT discography. The use of discography is not accepted by all authorities.

7. ISCHIAL BURSITIS

Ischial bursitis occurs over the bony prominence of the buttock. The area over the ischial spine is tender and painful. Pressure from prolonged sitting on a hard surface is a common cause. The pain may be intensified by sitting on a hard chair or bench. Avoidance of sitting on uncushioned surfaces, combined with local injection of methylprednisolone and lidocaine into the bursa, usually provides relief. This disorder has been called *weaver's bottom,* since it occurred in weavers during the nineteenth century. It occurs frequently in novice cyclists and in young runners doing speed work.

8. MYOFASCIAL SYNDROMES

Buttock pain may be caused by a myofascial syndrome. Walking may intensify the pain, while rest relieves it. There may be well-localized tender trigger points in the buttock. Pressure over these points with the examiner's fingertip may increase the pain. Local trigger-point injection with lidocaine, and muscle stretching exercises relieve the pain. Relief may also occur after spraying the trigger point with a coolant and then stretching the painful buttock muscle. Common myofascial syndromes include:

Gluteus maximus syndrome, in which there is aching pain in one buttock and posterior thigh. The trigger point is in the buttock.

Piriformis syndrome, in which buttock and posterior thigh pain may occur. The trigger point is in the buttock near the sciatic notch.

Quadratus lumborum syndrome, in which pain of an aching nature occurs in the buttock, groin, and anterior upper thigh. The trigger point is located in the deep musculature midway between the twelfth rib and the posterior iliac crest, 2 or 3 in. from the midline of the back. Trunk movements intensify the pain.

9. HAMSTRING STRAIN OR TEAR

Hamstring-related pain (strain) may be intensified by walking. The pain may begin after several hundred meters of walking and continue until the patient rests. There may be minimal local tenderness over the ischial tuberosity. Stretching exercises relieve the pain, which may mimic ischial bursitis except for the minimal amount of local tenderness present. An acute tear of a hamstring muscle at its origin from the ischial tuberosity causes severe buttock pain and local tenderness. This injury usually happens abruptly during running or jumping. Rest, followed by gentle stretching exercises, will help mild injuries. Severe hamstring tears require surgical repair.

10. NODULAR FASCIITIS (EPISACROILIAC LIPOMAS)

Aching pain occurs in the upper buttock; it may be intensified by bending forward. There are one or more tender mobile subcutaneous firm nodules that measure 2 to 4 cm in size. They are soft to firm in consistency. They may represent herniations of fat through the deep fascia. Local injection of these lesions with lidocaine and methylpred-

nisolone relieves the pain. Alternatively, repeated puncturing of the tender nodule with a large-bore needle will fragment the lesion and lead to pain relief.

11. TROCHANTERIC BURSITIS

Pain occurs over the greater trochanter and radiates down the lateral thigh and into the buttock. It is intensified by lying on the affected side, walking, and running. There is localized tenderness over the greater trochanter. Injection of lidocaine and methylprednisolone into the bursa immediately relieves the pain. One or two injections usually suffice to provide prolonged pain relief. In fewer than 5 percent of cases, surgical excision of the bursa may be required because of a failure to respond to injection therapy.

12. NONSPECIFIC LOW BACK PAIN

Aching lumbosacral and buttock pain begins insidiously during, or shortly after, some unaccustomed activity such as lifting, pushing a heavy object, or shoveling snow.

The pain is intensified by flexion, prolonged sitting, and trunk rotation. It is relieved by lying in bed. Sometimes, lying on the side, with the thighs flexed on the trunk, is the least painful position. Attacks of severe low back spasm may limit ambulation.

These acute episodes usually respond to 2 to 7 days of bed rest; warm, moist heat; analgesics; nonsteroidal anti-inflammatory drugs; and muscle relaxants. The patient's bed should have a firm, nonsagging mattress, and a back support should be used during driving.

The cause of nonspecific low back pain usually is not investigated unless the pain persists. Some cases are due to a muscle strain or ligament sprain, while others are caused by disc disruption, facet joint inflammation, vertebral subluxation, or segmental instability.

13. EPIDURAL ABSCESS

Severe pain occurs in the lower lumbar area, buttock, and upper thigh. There is severe midline spinal pain and tenderness. Chills, fever, and leukocytosis occur. Weakness of one or both legs may occur, as well as patchy lower extremity and buttock sensory loss. Urinary and stool incontinence may follow. Cerebrospinal fluid (CSF) examination may demonstrate an elevated or normal leukocyte count, an increased CSF protein level, and a normal sugar level. The caudad extent of the abscess can be determined by a myelogram or a contrast-enhanced CT scan. Abscess drainage under cover of intravenous antibiotic therapy will usually lead to full recovery if surgical intervention is not delayed beyond 36 h after the onset of neurologic symptoms. Delay beyond 48 h is frequently associated with irreversible neurologic damage.

14. SACRAL NEURALGIA DUE TO PRIMARY GENITAL HERPES

Aching unilateral buttock pain and posterior and medial thigh pain may be present for 2 or 3 days before a tender group of vesicles and small ulcers develops on the labia and perineal skin in women, or on the penis and adjacent areas in men. Fever, chills, generalized myalgias, and anorexia may accompany these other complaints. Typical grouped, paired, or single vesicles and crusted ulcerations are present on the genital skin. Local tenderness may be so severe as to lead to temporary sexual abstinence, or so mild as to go unnoticed. Some patients have pruritus, rather than local pain and tenderness.

Other complaints include dysuria, urinary frequency, and sometimes urinary retention. Neurologic symptoms (e.g., headache, stiff neck, and photophobia) may occur in up to 10 percent of cases. Severe cases of genital herpes, with extensive systemic and local symptoms, can be treated with intravenous acyclovir; milder cases can be treated with oral acyclovir.

33 Acute Bilateral Buttock Pain

☐ **DIAGNOSTIC LIST**

1. Anorectal abscess
2. Furuncules
3. Sacroiliitis
   A. *Yersinia enterocolitica*
   B. Brucellosis
   C. Reiter's syndrome
4. Facet syndrome
5. Spondylolisthesis
6. Disc disruption
   A. Disc disruption without herniation
   B. Disc disruption with herniation
7. Ischial bursitis
8. Epidural abscess
9. Infarction of the conus medullaris
10. Nontraumatic epidural hematoma
11. Buttock trauma
12. Sacral neuralgia due to primary genital herpes

☐ **SUMMARY**

A *horseshoe abscess* causes severe bilateral buttock pain and fever, made worse by defecation and by proctoscopic examination. It responds to surgical drainage of the postero-anorectal and ischiorectal spaces. *Furuncles* appear as red, tender, fluctuant lesions on the buttock skin. They respond to drainage and the use of dicloxacillin. *Sacroiliitis* causes medial buttock pain on both sides, made worse by jarring, bending, and thigh extension on the hip. There is localized sacroiliac fist percussion tenderness. The pelvic rock test and Gaenslen's test are positive. This disorder may occur suddenly after a febrile diarrheal illness caused by *Yersinia enterocolitica;* after a flulike illness produced by a species of *Brucella;* or as part of a migratory arthritis, associated with urethritis and conjunctivitis (*Reiter's syndrome*). *Bilateral facet joint synovitis or subluxation* (*facet syndrome*) causes low back pain and bilateral buttock pain that is made worse by prolonged sitting, back rota-

tion, or hyperextension. It is dramatically improved by spine manipulation or by facet joint injection. A CT scan may confirm facet joint abnormalities. *Spondylolisthesis* of L5 on S1, developing acutely, can cause bilateral buttock pain. The diagnosis can be confirmed by a standing lateral radiograph of the lumbosacral spine.

Disc disruption without herniation can cause low back pain and bilateral aching buttock pain that is intensified by prolonged sitting or by lifting a load. Discography should precipitate or intensify the characteristic pain (i.e., as the contrast medium is injected). Injection of lidocaine into the same disc relieves it. *Disc herniation* may cause sciatica in addition to low back and buttock pain. Midline herniation may cause a cauda equina syndrome with leg weakness, sensory symptoms, and incontinence. A computed tomography (CT) scan will demonstrate the herniated disc.

Ischial bursitis causes local pain and tenderness over the ischial tuberosities. This pain can be relieved by cushioning

TABLE OF DISEASE INCIDENCE

INCIDENCE PER 100,000 (APPROXIMATE)

Common (>100)	Uncommon (>5–100)	Rare (>0–5)
Furuncles	Anorectal abscess (horseshoe abscess)	Sacroiliitis due to a Brucella species
Sacroiliitis due to Reiter's syndrome	Sacroiliitis due to *Yersinia enterocolitica*	Epidural abscess
Facet syndrome		Conus medullaris infarction
Disc disruption	Spondylolisthesis	Epidural hematoma
Buttock trauma	Ischial bursitis	
Primary genital herpes and sacral neuralgia		

hard surfaces used for prolonged sitting, and by the injection of lidocaine and methylprednisolone into one or both of the bursae.

An *epidural abscess* usually begins with low back and buttock pain, fever, chills, and a toxic appearance. This is soon followed by a rapidly progressive cauda equina syndrome. *Infarction of the conus medullaris* begins suddenly with buttock, thigh, and perineal pain. Leg weakness, sensory loss, paresthesias, and incontinence occur. CT and myelographic studies reveal no evidence of a mass lesion. Recovery occurs gradually over a period of months. An epidural abscess will resolve only with surgical drainage and antibiotic therapy. A *nontraumatic epidural hematoma* occurs in patients who have severe liver disease, or a prolonged prothrombin time from anticoagulant therapy. There is an abrupt onset of low back and buttock pain, followed within hours by cauda equina symptoms. The diagnosis can be confirmed by a myelogram and a CT study. Symptoms respond to laminectomy and removal of the hematoma. Buttock *trauma* may cause local pain, swelling, tenderness, bony crepitus, and blue-black cutaneous discoloration. *Primary genital herpes* can cause genital ulcerations; there may also be bilateral buttock aching and sometimes paresthesias, which precede the onset of the local lesions by 2 or 3 days.

☐ DESCRIPTION OF LISTED DISEASES

1. ANORECTAL ABSCESS

Fever, chills, sweats, and deep anorectal pain are the initial complaints. Initially, the pain is a mild ache that is intensified during and after bowel movements. Pus collects posterior to the rectum. Within a 1- or 2-day period the pain becomes severe and throbbing. It spreads to involve one, then both, medial buttocks. Needle aspiration will obtain pus from the region posterior to the anus. The

infection may spread to involve both ischiorectal fossae (*horseshoe abscess*). Drainage of both the ischiorectal and deep postanal spaces will relieve symptoms. Intravenous antibiotics are useful for the first 3 days after surgical drainage, to eradicate infection in the soft tissue surrounding the abscess cavity.

2. FURUNCLES

Painful, red, tender, 3- to 10-cm furuncles may occur simultaneously on both buttocks. These may resolve spontaneously, or drain, or require surgical incision and drainage. Antistaphylococcal antibiotics are useful in the management of this disorder.

3. SACROILIITIS

Pain occurs in the low back and medial buttock region bilaterally. It is felt over the sacroiliac joints. Walking, jogging, bending forward, rising from a chair, or sitting down will transiently increase the intensity of the pain. Discomfort may radiate down one or both posterior thighs. The pelvic rock test, Gaenslen's test, and the fabere sign are positive bilaterally. Straight leg raising may cause buttock and low back pain, but not leg and foot pain. There is fist percussion tenderness over both sacroiliac joints. Morning stiffness usually accompanies the low back and buttock pain. Acute bilateral sacroiliitis may be caused by the following disorders:

A. *Yersinia enterocolitica* This microorganism causes fever, diarrhea, and right lower abdominal pain and tenderness, because of inflammation of the ileum and mesenteric lymph nodes. The clinical findings mimic acute appendicitis or regional ileitis. Between 1 and 6 weeks after the onset of gastrointestinal symptoms some patients develop a symmetrical migratory polyarthritis. Up to 25 percent of patients with polyarthritis develop sacroiliitis. Sacroiliac involvement may also occur without peripheral joint symptoms. Erythema multiforme, erythema nodosum, urethritis, and iritis may accompany the joint symptoms in some cases. Most patients recover spontaneously after 2 to 3 months. A small number may experience recurrent symptoms. Diagnosis depends on the isolation of *Yersinia enterocolitica* from the stool or mesenteric lymph nodes, or on the demonstration of a rise in antibody titer to the organism.

B. Brucellosis This disorder may begin with flulike complaints, fever, and bilateral buttock, lumbar, and thoracic paraspinal pain. Spine and sacroiliac radiographs may be normal for months, but radionuclide bone scans usually show increased radioisotope uptake in the lumbar and sacroiliac regions. Low back and buttock pain may be so severe that the patient is wheelchair-bound despite negative radiographic studies. In time there develop lytic and sclerotic lesions of one or more vertebral bodies or intervertebral discs. Sacroiliac joint-margin blurring, irregularity, and para-articular sclerosis usually develop. The diagnosis can be made by blood or bone culture, or by demonstration of a rise in the brucella agglutinin titer. Most patients with this disorder in the United States are slaughterhouse workers, farmers, ranchers, butchers, and veterinarians. In addition, ingestion of raw milk or other unpasteurized milk products may lead to infection. There is a good response to therapy with doxycycline and streptomycin.

C. Reiter's Syndrome   Sacroiliitis is usually accompanied by conjunctivitis (30–40 percent of cases), urethritis, and peripheral arthritis. Fever occurs in some cases. Mucocutaneous lesions are commonly present. Painless oral ulcers and papules, balanitis circinata, and keratoderma blennorrhagicum occur. Nonsteroidal anti-inflammatory drugs control the fever and joint complaints. Up to one-third of patients develop persistent or recurrent peripheral joint and sacroiliac complaints.

4. FACET SYNDROME

Lumbar and bilateral buttock ache may occur without thigh or calf pain. The pain is made worse by prolonged sitting, bending forward, or back rotation or extension. In some patients the pain is lessened by standing and by activity. Spine manipulation or facet joint injection with bupivacaine usually relieves the pain. Joints for injection are selected on the basis of localized tenderness. CT scans of affected joints may show irregularity or joint space narrowing. Hypertrophic changes of the articular processes and joint subluxation may also occur. CT scans may also show similar changes in asymptomatic patients, so a careful correlation of clinical and radiologic findings should be made.

5. SPONDYLOLISTHESIS

A patient who has had low back pain due to spondylolysis for many months or years may abruptly develop acute bilateral buttock and upper posterior thigh pain. Severe hamstring spasm may occur, resulting in an abnormal shuffling or "waddle" gait. A standing lateral radiograph of the lumbosacral spine reveals marked slippage of L5 on S1. If bed rest and analgesics fail to resolve symptoms, surgical decompression and spinal fusion may be required to allow the patient to become ambulatory and capable of working.

6. DISC DISRUPTION

A. Disc Disruption without Herniation   Aching pain occurs in the lumbosacral area and in both buttocks. The pain is intensified by flexion, extension, prolonged sitting, walking, and load carrying, and is relieved by bed rest. The injection of contrast medium into the abnormal disc space during discography usually precipitates or exacerbates the pain; injection of lidocaine abolishes it. A CT scan done immediately after disc injection shows asymmetrical penetration of contast medium into the anulus of the disc. Again, careful clinical-radiographic correlation is necessary, since many patients have disc disruption visible on discography but have no symptoms. This disorder usually responds to bed rest, analgesics, and avoidance of lifting and prolonged sitting.

B. Disc Disruption with Herniation   This disorder causes low back and buttock pain. Unilateral or bilateral sciatica may occur with positive straight leg raising and Dejerine signs. There may be weakness of one or both legs and patchy lower extremity and/or saddle area sensory loss. Midline disc herniations may cause fecal and urinary incontinence. The diagnosis can be confirmed by a contrast-enhanced CT scan or myelogram. This disorder may resolve on bed rest, or may require laminectomy and removal of the herniated disc.

7. ISCHIAL BURSITIS (TAILOR'S OR WEAVER'S BOTTOM)

Prolonged sitting on a hard surface can cause bilateral buttock pain with associated tenderness over the ischial tuberosities. Novice cyclists and adolescent runners doing speed work may also acquire this disorder. Avoidance of pressure over the ischial tuberosities, through the padding or cushioning of hard seats, and injection of lidocaine and methylprednisolone into the tender site, on one or both sides, bring about symptom resolution.

8. EPIDURAL ABSCESS

Severe pain and tenderness develop abruptly over the lumbar spine or lumbosacral area. The pain radiates into both buttocks and is intensified by jarring or movements of the lower spine. Sciatica may occur in one or both legs. Fever, chills, and sweats accompany the back and buttock pain. Leg weakness on one or both sides, paresthesias and sensory loss, and urinary and fecal incontinence soon follow. The diagnosis can be confirmed by a myelogram, which shows a complete block in the lumbar region. The extent of the lesion can be determined by magnetic resonance imaging (MRI), which can demonstrate the cephalocaudal dimensions of the abscess. Laminectomy and drainage of the abscess will bring about a reduction in pain and recovery of neurologic function. Failure to operate within 48 h after the onset of neurologic symptoms can lead to irreversible damage. Parenteral antibiotics should also be used to aid in the prompt resolution of this disorder.

9. INFARCTION OF THE CONUS MEDULLARIS

Sudden, severe low back and buttock pain occurs. Perineal and thigh pain may also be present. This is followed by the rapid onset of leg weakness, saddle paresthesias, and hypesthesia. Patchy sensory loss and paresthesias may also affect the thighs, lower legs, and feet. Fecal and urinary incontinence often occur. The anal sphincter is usually patulous. Hip extension and abduction, knee flexion, and ankle movements are weak or paralyzed. Lower extremity reflexes may be absent.

Risk factors for this disorder include aortic surgery; use of an intraaortic balloon to treat shock; smoking; and generalized atherosclerosis. The disorder can mimic central disc herniation. In some cases repeated brief attacks of saddle area pain and hypesthesia, leg weakness, and numbness may precede the major attack. Myelography and CT studies for a mass lesion are negative. Fever and chills, common associated symptoms in patients with an epidural abscess, are not present. There is no specific therapy.

Neurologic symptoms and signs subside partially over a period of months.

10. NONTRAUMATIC EPIDURAL HEMATOMA

There is sudden onset of midline lumbosacral or lumbar pain, with radiation into the buttocks and down one or both legs. Most patients who develop this disorder are taking oral anticoagulants or have severe chronic liver disease with clotting abnormalities. Neurologic dysfunction begins within a few hours of the onset of the pain. Leg weakness, paresthesias and hypesthesia, and incontinence soon follow. Fever and chills are not part of the clinical picture. The prothrombin time is usually prolonged. A myelogram will confirm the presence of a mass lesion. The extent of the hematoma can be determined by MRI of the lumbar spine. Vitamin K and fresh frozen plasma should be given, and laminectomy performed to decompress the cauda equina. Partial neurologic lesions respond well to decompression. Complete lesions have a poor prognosis, which grows worse the longer surgery is

delayed. Rapid progression of neurologic signs is ominous; gradual loss of neurologic function, over a period of several days, correlates with a smaller hematoma.

11. BUTTOCK TRAUMA

Falls and motorcycle and automobile accidents can cause severe pain in both buttocks, beginning at the time of injury. There may be local swelling, tenderness, bony crepitus, and blue-black discoloration of the skin. Induration of the soft tissues may occur because of bleeding. Radiographs may show one or more pelvic fractures. Severe pelvic fractures may cause enough blood loss to produce hypotension and tachycardia. Blood loss usually responds to fluid and blood replacement; but uncontrolled pelvic bleeding may require iliac artery arteriography and the use of clot embolization to control continuing hemorrhage.

12. SACRAL NEURALGIA DUE TO PRIMARY GENITAL HERPES

A primary episode of genital herpes may begin with lumbosacral aching pain that spreads to both buttocks and to the posterior and medial thighs. Buttock, perineal, and leg paresthesias and burning may accompany the pain. Fever is commonly present; it may persist for several days. Painful, and sometimes pruritic, genital ulcers and vesicles develop. These are usually tender and may be associated with dysuria, urinary frequency, and, sometimes, urinary retention. In females, vulvar and clitoral lesions are painful, while vaginal and cervical lesions are not. In males, lesions may involve the corona and shaft of the penis, the scrotum, the urethra and perineum, and the anorectal area. Ulcerative bladder lesions may occur. Up to 10 percent of patients may develop headache, nuchal pain and stiffness, vomiting, and photophobia (i.e., aseptic meningitis).

Local vaginal ulceration, vaginal discharge, and tender inguinal adenopathy may develop. Oral acyclovir can effectively treat a primary attack of genital herpes. Severe cases may require intravenous therapy.

Acyclovir therapy decreases pain, viral shedding, and the time needed for lesion healing, but early treatment does not appear to prevent recurrent disease—which becomes a problem in 75 percent of patients with symptomatic infection.

BACK AND BUTTOCK PAIN REFERENCES

Arachnoiditis (Chronic Mycotic Meningitis)

Stein SC, Corrado ML, Friedlander M, et al: Chronic mycotic meningitis with spinal involvement (arachnoiditis): A report of five cases. *Ann Neurol* 11:519–524, 1982.

Autonomic Disorders

McLeod JG, Tuck RR: Disorders of the autonomic nervous system: 1. Pathophysiology and clinical features. *Ann Neurol* 21:419–430, 1987.

Brucellosis/Spondylitis

Goodhart GL, Zaken JF, Collins WC, et al: Brucellosis of the spine. Report of a patient with bilateral paraspinal abscesses. *Spine* 12(4):414–416, 1987.

Norton WL: Brucellosis and rheumatic syndromes in Saudi Arabia. *Ann Rheum Dis* 43:810–815, 1984.

Rajapakse CNA, Al-Aska K, Al-Orainey I, et al: Spinal brucellosis. *Br J Rheumatol* 26:28–31, 1987.

Samra Y, Hertz M, Shaked Y, et al: Brucellosis of the spine. A report of 3 cases. *J Bone Joint Surg* 64B(4):429–431, 1982.

Torres-Rojas J, Taddonio RF, Sanders CV: Spondylitis caused by *Brucella abortus*. *South Med J* 72(9):1166–1169, 1979.

Case Records of the Massachusetts General Hospital. Case 37-1986. *N Engl J Med* 315(12):748–754, 1986.

Computed Tomography—Asymptomatic Patients

Wiesel SW, Tsourmas N, Feffer HL, et al: A study of computer-assisted tomography: 1. The incidence of positive CAT scans in an asymptomatic group of patients. *Spine* 9:549–551, 1984.

Hitselberger WE, Witten RM: Abnormal myelograms in asymptomatic patients. *J Neurosurg* 28:204–206, 1968.

Epidural Hematoma

Mattle H, Sieb JP, Rohner M, et al: Nontraumatic spinal epidural and subdural hematomas. *Neurology* 37:1351–1356, 1987.

Facet Syndrome

Fairbank JCT, Park WM, McCall IW, et al: Apophyseal injection of local anesthetic as a diagnostic aid in primary low-back pain syndromes. *Spine* 6(6):598–605, 1981.

Mooney V, and Robertson J: The facet syndrome. *Clin Orthop* 115:149–156, 1976.

Shields C, Williams PE Jr: Low back pain. *Am Fam Physician* 33:173–182, 1986.

Fibrositis/Fibromyalgia

Bennet RM: Fibromyalgia (editorial). *JAMA* 257(20):2802–2803, 1987.

Bennett RM: Current issues concerning management of the fibrositis/fibromyalgia syndrome. *Am J Med* 81(suppl 3A):15–18, 1986.

Bennett RM: Fibrositis: Evolution of an enigma (editorial). *J Rheumatol* 13:676–678, 1986.

Calabro JJ: Fibromyalgia (fibrositis) in children. *Am J Med* 81(suppl 3A):57–59, 1986.

Campbell SM: Is the tender point concept valid? *Am J Med* 81(suppl 3A):33–37, 1986.

Campbell SM, Bennett RM: Fibrositis. *Dis Mon* 32(1):653–722, 1986.

Carette S, McCain GA, Bell DA, et al: Evaluation of amitriptyline in primary fibrositis. A double-blind, placebo-controlled study. *Arthritis Rheum* 29(5):655–659, 1986.

Caro XJ: Immunofluorescent studies of skin in primary fibrositis syndrome. *Am J Med* 81(suppl 3A):43–49, 1986.

Cathey MA, Wolfe F, Kleinheksel SM, et al: Socioeconomic impact of fibrositis. A study of 81 patients with primary fibrositis. *Am J Med* 81(suppl 3A):78–84, 1986.

Dinerman H, Goldenberg DL, Felson DT: A prospective evaluation of 118 patients with the fibromyalgia syndrome: Prevalence of Raynaud's phenomenon, sicca symptoms, ANA, low complement, and Ig-deposition at the dermal-epidermal junction. *J Rheumatol* 13(2):368–373, 1986.

Gatter RA: Pharmacotherapeutics in fibrositis. *Am J Med* 81(suppl 3A):63–66, 1986.

Goldenberg DL: Fibromyalgia syndrome. An emerging but controversial condition. *JAMA* 257(20):2782–2787, 1987.

Goldenberg DL: Psychologic studies in fibrositis. *Am J Med* 81(suppl 3A):67–70, 1986.

Goldenberg DL, Felson DT, Dinerman H: A randomized, controlled trial of amitriptyline and naproxen in the treatment of patients with fibromyalgia. *Arthritis Rheum* 29(11):1371–1377, 1986.

Gupta MA, Moldofsky H: Dysthymic disorder and rheumatic pain modulation disorder (fibrositis syndrome): A comparison of symptoms and sleep physiology. *Can J Psychiatry* 31:608–616, 1986.

Hadler NM: A critical reappraisal of the fibrositis concept. *Am J Med* 81(suppl 3A):26–30, 1986.

Hartz A, Kirchdoerfer E: Undetected fibrositis in primary care practice. *J Fam Pract* 25(4):365–369, 1987.

Hench PK, Mitler MM: Fibromyalgia: 1. Review of a common rheumatologic syndrome. *Postgrad Med* 80(7):47–56, 1986.

Hench PK, Mitler MM: Fibromyalgia: 2. Management guidelines and research findings. *Postgrad Med* 80(7):57–69, 1986.

Hench PK: Secondary fibrositis. *Am J Med* 81(suppl 3A):60–62, 1986.

McCain GA: Role of physical fitness training in the fibrositis/fibromyalgia syndrome. *Am J Med* 81(suppl 3A):73–77, 1986.

Moldofsky H: Sleep and musculoskeletal pain. *Am J Med* 81(suppl 3A):85–89, 1986.

Molony RR, MacPeek DM, Schiffman PL, et al: Sleep, sleep apnea and the fibromyalgia syndrome. *J Rheumatol* 13:797–800, 1986.

Muller W: The fibrositis syndrome: Diagnosis, differential diagnosis and pathogenesis. *Scand J Rheumatol* (suppl 65):40–53, 1987.

Rice JR: "Fibrositis" syndrome. *Med Clin North Am* 70(2):455–468, 1986.

Russell IJ, Vipraio GA, Morgan WW, et al: Is there a metabolic basis for the fibrositis syndrome? *Am J Med* 81(suppl 3A):50–54, 1986.

Smythe H: Tender points: Evolution of concepts of the fibrositis/fibromyalgia syndrome. *Am J Med* 81(suppl 3A):2–6, 1986.

Smythe H: Referred pain and tender points. *Am J Med* 81(suppl 3A):90–92, 1986.

Wolfe F: The clinical syndrome of fibrositis. *Am J Med* 81(suppl 3A):7–14, 1986.

Wolfe F: Development of criteria for the diagnosis of fibrositis. *Am J Med* 81(suppl 3A):99–104, 1986.

Yunus MB, Kalyan-Raman UP, Kalyan-Raman K, et al: Pathologic changes in muscle in primary fibromyalgia syndrome. *Am J Med* 81(suppl 3A):38–42, 1986.

Idiopathic Skeletal Hyperostosis and Low Back Pain

Forestier J, Rotes-Querol J: Senile ankylosing hyperostosis of the spine. *Am Rheum Dis* 91:321–330, 1950.

Resnick D, Niwayama G: Radiographic and pathologic features of spinal involvement in diffuse idiopathic skeletal hyperostosis (DISH). *Radiology* 119:559–568, 1976.

Resnick D, Shaul SR, Robins JM: Diffuse idiopathic skeletal hyperostosis (DISH): Forestier's disease with extraspinal manifestations. *Radiology* 115:513–524, 1975.

White AA III, McBride ME, Wiltse LL, et al: The management of patients with back pain and idiopathic vertebral sclerosis. *Spine* 11(6):607–616, 1986.

Low Back Pain—CT Studies

Rosa M, Capellini C, Canevari MA, et al: CT in low back and sciatic pain due to lumbar canal osseous changes. *Neuroradiology* 28:237–240, 1986.

Low Back Pain—Diagnosis

Quebec Task Force on Spinal Disorders, Spitzer WO (chairman): Scientific approach to the assessment and management of activity-related spinal disorders: A monograph for clinicians: 1. Approach to the problem. *Spine* 12:S9–11, 1987; 3. Diagnosis of the problem (The problem of diagnosis). *Spine* 12:S16–21, 1987; 4. Treatment of activity-related spinal disorders. *Spine* 12:S22–30, 1987; 5. Management guidelines. *Spine* 12:S31–36, 1987; 6. Conclusions, recommendations, and research priorities. *Spine* 12:S37–39, 1987.

Mooney V: Where is the pain coming from? Presidential Address, International Society for the study of the lumbar spine, Dallas, 1986. *Spine* 12:754–759, 1987.

Low Back Pain—Geriatric

Swezey RL: Low back pain in the elderly: Practical management concerns. *Geriatrics* 43:38–44, 1988.

Low Back Pain—Medical Therapy

Aghababian RV, Volturo GA, Heifetz IN: Comparison of diflunisal and naproxen in the management of acute low back strain. *Clin Ther* 9(suppl C):47–51, 1986.

Bell GR, Rothman RH: The conservative treatment of sciatica. *Spine* 9:54–56, 1984.

Bigos SJ, Battie MC: Acute care to prevent back disability. Ten years of progress. *Clin Orthop* 221:121–130, 1987.

Brown FL Jr, Bodison S, Dixon J, et al: Comparison of diflunisal and acetaminophen with codeine in the treatment of initial or recurrent acute low back strain. *Clin Ther* 9(suppl C):52–58, 1986.

Deyo RA, Diehl AK, Rosenthal M: How many days of bed rest for acute low back pain? A randomized clinical trial. *N Engl J Med* 315:1064–1070, 1986.

Linton SJ, Kamwendo K: Low back schools. A critical review. *Phys Ther* 67:1375–1383, 1987.

Ward NG: Tricyclic antidepressants for chronic low-back pain. Mechanisms of action and predictors of response. *Spine* 11:661–665, 1986.

Low Back Pain—Metabolic/Osteomalacia

Coburn JW, Norris KC, Nebeker HG: Osteomalacia and bone disease arising from aluminum. *Semin Nephrol* 6:68–89, 1986.

Cushner HM, Adams ND: Review: Renal osteodystrophy-pathogenesis and treatment. *Am J Med Sci* 291:264–275, 1986.

Fukumoto S, Tarui S, Tsukiyama K, et al: Tumor-induced vitamin D-resistant hypophosphatemic osteomalacia associated with proximal renal tubular dysfunction and 1,25-dihydroxyvitamin D deficiency. *J Clin Endocrinol Metab* 49:873–878, 1979.

Nebeker HG, Coburn JW: Aluminum and renal osteodystrophy. *Annu Rev Med* 37:79–95, 1986.

Parker MS, Klein I, Haussler MR, et al: Tumor-induced osteomalacia. Evidence of a surgically correctable alteration in vitamin D metabolism. *JAMA* 245:492–493, 1981.

Quarles LD, Gitelman HJ, Drezner MK: Aluminum: culprit or accessory in the genesis of renal osteodystrophy. *Semin Nephrology* 6:90–101, 1986.

Nephrology Forum: Renal osteodystrophy. Coburn JW, principal discussant. *Kidney Int* 17:677–693, 1980.

Low Back Pain—Metabolic/Osteoporosis/Paget's Disease

Crane SM, Hulick MF: Metabolic Bone Disease in Wilson JD, Braunwald E, Isselbacher KJ et al (eds): *Harrison's Principles of Internal Medicine*, 12th ed. New York, McGraw-Hill, 1991, vol 2, pp 1921–1926.

Lane JM, Werntz JR, Healey JH, et al: Metabolic bone disease and Paget's disease in the elderly: I. Metabolic bone disease. *Clin in Rheum Dis* 12:49–70, 1986.

Merkow RL, Lane JM: Metabolic bone disease and Paget's disease in the elderly: II. Paget's disease. *Clin in Rheum Dis* 12:71–96, 1986.

Raisz LG: Local and systemic factors in the pathogenesis of osteoporosis. *N Engl J Med* 318:818–828, 1988.

Low Back Pain—Pregnancy

Berg G, Hammar M, Moller-Nielsen J, et al: Low back pain during pregnancy. *Obstet Gynecol* 71:71–75, 1988.

Fast A, Shapiro D, Ducommun EJ, et al: Low-back pain in pregnancy. *Spine* 12:368–371, 1987.

Low Back Pain—Psychogenic/Malingering

Blumer D, Heilbronn M: Chronic pain as a variant of depressive disease. The pain-prone disorder. *J Nerv Ment Dis* 170:381–406, 1982.

Chapman SL, Brena SF: Learned helplessness and responses to nerve blocks in chronic low back pain patients. *Pain* 14:355–364, 1982.

Folks DG, Freeman AM III: Munchausen's syndrome and other factitious illness. *Psychiatr Clin North Am* 8:263–278, 1985.

Frymoyer JW, Rosen JC, Clements J, et al: Psychologic factors in low-back-pain disability. *Clin Orthop* 195:178–184, 1985.

Keel PJ: Psychosocial criteria for patient selection: Review of studies and concepts for understanding chronic back pain. *Neurosurgery* 15:935–941, 1984.

King BH, Ford CV: Pseudologia fantastica. *Acta Psychiatr Scand* 77:1–6, 1988.

Leavitt F: The value of the MMPI conversion 'V' in the assessment of psychogenic pain. *J Psychosom Res* 29:125–131, 1985.

Leavitt F, Sweet JJ: Characteristics and frequency of malingering among patients with low back pain. *Pain* 25:357–364, 1986.

McCreary C, Turner J, Dawson E: Principal dimensions of the pain experience and psychological disturbance in chronic low back pain patients. *Pain* 11:85–92, 1981.

Mayer TG, Gatchel RJ, Kishino N, et al: Objective assessment of spine function following industrial injury. A prospective study with comparison group and one-year follow-up. *Spine* 10:482–493, 1985.

Prokop CK: Hysteria scale elevations in low back pain patients: A risk factor for misdiagnosis? *J Consult Clin Psychol* 54:558–562, 1986.

Rosen JC, Johnson C, Frymoyer JW: Identification of excessive back disability with the Faschingbauer Abbreviated MMPI. *J Clin Psychol* 39:71–74, 1983.

Shafer N, Shafer R: Factitious diseases including Munchausen's syndrome. *NY State J Med*, March 1980, pp 594–604.

Trief P, Stein N: Pending litigation and rehabilitation outcome of chronic back pain. *Arch Phys Med Rehabil* 66:95–99, 1985.

Turner JA, Herron L, Weiner P: Utility of the MMPI pain assessment index in predicting outcome after lumbar surgery. *J Clin Psychol* 42:764–769, 1986.

Ward NG: Tricyclic antidepressants for chronic low-back pain. *Spine* 11:661–665, 1986.

Low Back Pain—Review Articles and General References

Bernard TN Jr, Kirkaldy-Willis WH: Recognizing specific characteristics of nonspecific low back pain. *Clin Ortho* 217:266–280, 1987.

Frymoyer JW: Back pain and sciatica. *N Engl J Med* 318:291–300, 1988.

Herkowitz HN: Current status of percutaneous discectomy and chemonucleolysis *Orth Clin of NA* 22:327–332, 1991.

Keim HA, Kirkaldy-Willis WH: Low back pain. *Clin Symp* 39:2–29, 1987.

Kuslich SD, Ulstrom CL, Michael CJ: The tissue origin of low back pain and sciatica: A report of pain response to tissue stimulation during operations on the lumbar spine using local anesthesia *Arth Clin of NA* 22:181–187, 1991.

Lipson SJ: Low back pain, in Kelley WN, Harris ED Jr, Ruddy S, et al (eds): *Textbook of Rheumatology*. Philadelphia, Saunders, 1981, pp 451–471.

McCowin PR, Borenstein D, Wiesel SW: The current approach to the medical diagnosis of low back pain. *Orth Clin of NA* 22:315–325, 1991.

Nachemson AL: Advances in low-back pain. *Clin Orthop* 200:266–278, 1985.

Shields C, Williams PE Jr: Low back pain. *Am Fam Physician* 33:173–182, 1986.

Turek SL: *Orthopaedics: Principles and Their Application*, 4th ed. Philadelphia, Lippincott, 1984.

Low Back Pain—Risk Factors

Bongers PM, Boshuizen HC, Hulshof CTJ, et al: Back disorders in crane operators exposed to whole-body vibrations. *Int Arch Occup Environ Health* 60:129–137, 1988.

Bowden T: Back pain in helicopter aircrew: A literature review. *Aviation, Space and Environmental Medicine* 58:461–467, 1987.

Buckle P, Erg M: Epidemiological aspects of back pain within the nursing profession. *Int J Nurs Stud* 24:319–324, 1987.

Damkot DK, Pope MH, Lord J, et al: The relationship between work history, work environment and low-back pain in men. *Spine* 9:395–399, 1984.

Dwyer AP: Backache and its prevention. *Clin Orthop* 222:35–43, 1987.

Kelsey JL, Githens PB, White AA III, et al: An epidemiologic study of lifting and twisting on the job and risk for acute prolapsed lumbar intervertebral disc. *J Orthop Res* 2:61–66, 1984.

Patenaude SS, Sommer MA: Low back pain. Etiology and prevention. *AORN J* 46:472–479, 1987.

Vallfors B: Acute, subacute and chronic low back pain. Clinical symptoms, absenteeism and working environment. *Scand J Rehabil Med Suppl* 11, pp 5–98, 1985.

Lumbar Disc Disease—CT Studies

Burton CV: High resolution CT scanning: The present and future. *Orthop Clin North Am* 14:539–551, 1983.

Gado M, Patel J, Hodges FJ III: High resolution CT of the spine in lumbar disc disease. *Clin Neurosurg* 32:654–676, 1983.

Graves VB, Finney HL, Mailander J: Intradural lumbar disk herniation. *AJNR* 7:495–497, 1986.

Hakelius A, Hundmarsh J: The comparative reliability of preoperative diagnostic methods in lumbar disc surgery. *Acta Orthop Scand* 43:235–238, 1972.

Holtas S, Nordstrom C-H, Larsson E-M, et al: MR imaging of intradural disk herniation. *J Comput Assist Tomogr* 13:353–356, 1987.

Hudgins WR: Computer-aided diagnosis of lumbar disc herniation. *Spine* 8:604–615, 1983.

Kaplan DM, Knapp M, Romm FJ, et al: Low back pain and x-ray films of the lumbar spine: A prospective study in primary care. *South Med J* 79:811–814, 1986.

Kelen GD, Noji EK, Doris PE: Guidelines for use of lumbar spine radiography. *Ann Emerg Med* 15:245–251, 1986.

Peyster RG, Teplick JG, Haskin ME: Computed tomography of lumbosacral conjoined nerve root anomalies. Potential cause of false-positive reading for herniated nucleus pulposus. *Spine* 10:331–337, 1985.

Pyhtinen J, Lahde S, Tanska E-L, et al: Computed tomography after lumbar myelography in lower back and extremity pain syndromes. *Diagn Imag* 52:19–22, 1983.

Simeone FA, Rothman RH: Clinical usefulness of CT scanning in the diagnosis and treatment of lumbar spine disease. *Radiol Clin North Am* 21:197–200, 1983.

Yetkin Z, Chintapalli K, Daniels DL, et al: Gas in spinal articulations. *Neuroradiology* 28:150–153, 1986.

Lumbar Disc Disease—Medical Therapy

Altman R: International experiences with diclofenac in osteoarthritis. *Am J Med* 80(suppl 4B):48–52, 1986.

Benzon HT: Epidural steroid injections for low back pain and lumbosacral radiculopathy. *Pain* 24:277–295, 1986.

Buchanan WW, Kassam YB: European experience with flurbiprofen: A new analgesic/anti-inflammatory agent. *Am J Med* 80(suppl 3A):145–152, 1986.

Chu KH: Collagenase chemonucleolysis via epidural injection. A review of 252 cases. *Clin Orthop* 215:99–104, 1987.

Corrigan AB, Carr G, Tugwell S: Intraspinal corticosteroid injections. *Med J Aust* Mar 6; 1(5):224–225, 1982.

Crawshaw C, Frazer AM, Merriam WF, et al: A comparison of surgery and chemonucleolysis in the treatment of sciatica. A prospective randomized trial. *Spine* 9:195–198, 1984.

Dilke TFW, Burry HC, Grahame R: Extradural corticosteroid injection in management of lumbar nerve root compression. *Br Med J* 2:635–637, 1973.

Konings JG, Williams FJB, Deutman R: The effects of chemonucleolysis as demonstrated by computerised tomography. *J Bone Joint Surg [Br]* 66:417–421, 1984.

Lumbar Disc Disease—Reoperation

Brown BM, Bedell JE, Frank E: Contrast-enhanced computed tomography scanning of the postoperative spine. *Surg Neurol* 25:351–356, 1986.

de Divitiis E, Spaziante R, Cappabianca P, et al: Lumbar disk: Surgical tricks for safeguarding the "root's ecology." *Surg Neurol* 22:73–75, 1984.

Firooznia H, Kricheff II, Rafii M, et al: Lumbar spine after surgery: Examination with intravenous contrast-enhanced CT. *Neuroradiology* 163:221–226, 1987.

Gartland JJ: Judgment in lumbar disc surgery. *Orthop Clin North Am* 2:507–520, 1971.

Goldner JL, Urbaniak JR, McCollum DE: Anterior disc excision and interbody spinal fusion for chronic low back pain. *Orthop Clin North Am* 2:543–568, 1971.

Lewis PJ, Weir BKA, Broad RW, et al: Long-term prospective study of lumbosacral discectomy. *J Neurosurg* 67:49–53, 1987.

Teplick JG, Haskin ME: Intravenous contrast-enhanced CT of the postoperative lumbar spine: Improved identification of recurrent disk herniation, scar, arachnoiditis, and diskitis. *AJR* 143:845–855, 1984.

Lumbar Disc Disease—Surgical Therapy

Day AL, Friedman WA, Indelicato PA: Observations on the treatment of lumbar disk disease in college football players. *Am J Sports Med* 15:72–75, 1987.

Hakelius A: Prognosis in sciatica. A clinical follow-up of surgical and nonsurgical treatment. *Acta Orthop Scand,* suppl 929, pp 6–76, 1970.

Hirsch C, Nachemson A: The reliability of lumbar disk surgery. *Clin Orthop* 29:189–193, 1962.

Hirsch C: Reflections on the use of surgery in lumbar disc disease. *Orthop Clin North Am* 2:493–498, 1971.

Rothman RH: The clinical syndrome of lumbar disc disease. *Orthop Clin North Am* 2:463–475, 1971.

Weber H: Lumbar disc herniation. A controlled, prospective study with ten years of observation. *Spine* 8:131–140, 1983.

Lumbosacral Plexopathy

Evans BA, Stevens JC, Dyck PJ: Lumbosacral plexus neuropathy. *Neurology* 31:1327–1330, 1981.

Foley KM: Pain syndromes in patients with cancer. *Med Clin North Am* 71:169–184, 1987.

Jaeckle KA, Young DF, Foley KM: The natural history of lumbosacral plexopathy in cancer. *Neurology* 35:8–15, 1985.

Thomas JE, Cascino TL, Earle JD: Differential diagnosis between radiation and tumor plexopathy of the pelvis. *Neurology* 35:1–7, 1985.

Young RJ, Zhou YQ, Rodriguez E, et al: Variable relationship between peripheral somatic and autonomic neuropathy in patients with different syndromes of diabetic polyneuropathy. *Diabetes* 35:192–197, 1986.

Musculoskeletal Syndromes and Malignancy

Caldwell DS: Musculoskeletal syndromes associated with malignancy. *Semin Arthritis Rheum* 10(3):198–223, 1981.

McAfee JG: Radionuclide imaging in metabolic and systemic skeletal diseases. *Semin Nucl Med* 17(4):334–339, 1987.

Myofascial Pain

Keefe FJ, Dolan E: Pain behavior and pain coping strategies in low back pain and myofascial pain dysfunction syndrome patients. *Pain* 24:49–56, 1986.

Mance D, McConnell B, Ryan PA, et al: Myofascial pain syndrome. *J Am Podiatr Med Assoc* 76:328–331, 1986.

Osteoarthropathy—Pulmonary

Amin R: Hypertrophic osteoarthropathy in association with pulmonary metastases from carcinoma of bladder. *Urology* 26(6):581–582, 1985.

Booth BW, Van Nostrand D, Graeber GM: Hypertrophic pulmonary osteoarthropathy and breast cancer. *South Med J* 80(3):383–386, 1987.

Cohen AM, Yulish BS, Wasser KB, et al: Evaluation of pulmonary hypertrophic osteoarthropathy in cystic fibrosis. *Am J Dis Child* 140:74–77, 1986.

Dalgleish AG: Hypertrophic pulmonary osteoarthropathy: Response to chemotherapy without documented tumour response. *Aust N Z J Med* 13:513–516, 1983.

Leung FW, Williams AJ, Fan P: Indomethacin therapy for hypertrophic pulmonary osteoarthropathy in patients with bronchogenic carcinoma. *West J Med* 142:345–347, 1985.

Webb JG, Thomas P: Hypertrophic osteoarthropathy and pulmonary tuberculosis. *Tubercle* 67:225–228, 1986.

Osteoporosis—Therapy

Finkelstein JS, Klibanski A, Neer RM, et al: Osteoporosis in men with idiopathic hypogonadotropic hypogonadism. *Ann Intern Med* 106:354–361, 1987.

Hansson T, Roos B: The effect of fluoride and calcium on spinal bone mineral content: A controlled, prospective (3 years) study. *Calcif Tissue Int* 40:315–317, 1987.

Maharaj B, Kalideen JM, Leary WP, et al: Carcinoma of the prostate with multiple osteolytic metastases simulating multiple myeloma. *South Afr Med J* 70:227–228, 1986.

Schnitzler CM, Sweet MBE, Blumenfeld TS, et al: Radiographic features of the spine in fluoride therapy for osteoporosis. *J Bone Joint Surg [Br]* 69(2):190–194, 1987.

Spencer H, Rubio N, Rubio E, et al: Chronic alcoholism. Frequently overlooked cause of osteoporosis in men. *Am J Med* 80:393–397, 1986.

Plexopathy—Brachial

Bateman JE: Neurologic painful conditions affecting the shoulder. *Clin Orthop* 173:44–54, 1983.

Cascino TL, Kori S, Krol G, et al: CT of the brachial plexus in patients with cancer. *Neurology* 33:1553–1557, 1983.

Kori SH, Foley KM, Posner JB: Brachial plexus lesions in patients with cancer: 100 cases. *Neurology* 31:45–50, 1981.

Salner AL, Botnick LE, Herzog AG, et al: Reversible brachial plexopathy following primary radiation therapy for breast cancer. *Cancer Treat Rep* 65:797–802, 1981.

Polymyositis

Adams EM, Hafez GR, Carnes M, et al: The development of polymyositis in a patient with toxoplasmosis: Clinical and pathologic findings and review of literature. *Clin Exp Rheumatol* 2:205–208, 1984.

Behan WMH, Behan PO, Draper IT, et al: Does toxoplasma cause polymyositis? *Acta Neuropathol [Berl]* 61:246–252, 1983.

Dowsett RJ, Wong RL, Robert NJ, et al: Dermatomyositis and Hodgkin's disease. *Am J Med* 80:719–723, 1986.

Edwards RHT, Round JM, Jones DA: Needle biopsy of skeletal muscle: A review of 10 years experience. *Muscle and Nerve* 6:676–683, 1983.

Halla JT, Fallahi S, Koopman WJ: Penicillamine-induced myositis. Observations and unique features in two patients and review of the literature. *Am J Med* 77:719–722, 1984.

Hochberg MC, Feldman D, Stevens MB: Adult onset polymyositis/dermatomyositis: An analysis of clinical and laboratory features and survival in 76 patients with a review of the literature. *Sem Arth Rheum* 15(3):168–178, 1986.

Lakhanpal S, Duffy J, Engel AG: Eosinophilia associated with perimyositis and pneumonitis. *Mayo Clin Proc* 63:37–41, 1988.

Lott JA, Landesman PW: The enzymology of skeletal muscle disorders. *Crit Rev Clin Lab Sci* 20(2):153–190, 1984.

Mastaglia FL, Ojeda VJ: Inflammatory myopathies: 1. *Ann Neurol* 17:215–227, 1985.

Peters WA III, Andersen WA, Thornton WN Jr: Dermatomyositis and coexistent ovarian cancer: A review of the compounding clinical problems. *Gynecol Oncol* 15:440–446, 1983.

Rhoades DW, Pascucci RA: Cardiac involvement in polymyositis: Report of case and review of literature. *J Am Osteopath Assoc* 87(4):310–313, 1987.

Strongwater SL, Annesley T, Schnitzer TJ: Myocardial involvement in polymyositis. *J Rheumatol* 10:459–463, 1983.

Tymms KE, Webb J: Dermatopolymyositis and other connective tissue diseases: A review of 105 cases. *J Rheumatol* 12:1140–1148, 1985.

Whitaker JN, Bertorini TE, Mendell JR: Immunocytochemical studies of cathepsin D in human skeletal muscle. *Ann Neurol* 13:133–142, 1983.

Wolfe SM, Pinals RS, Aelion JA, et al: Myopathy in sarcoidosis: Clinical and pathologic study of four cases and review of the literature. *Semin Arthritis Rheum* 16(4):300–306, 1987.

Psoas Abscess

Leu S-Y, Leonard MB, Beart RW Jr, et al: Psoas abscess: Changing patterns of diagnosis and etiology. *Dis Colon Rectum* 29(11):694–698, 1986.

Rheumatic Disorders—Ankylosing Spondylitis

Calin A, Elswood J: The natural history of juvenile-onset ankylosing spondylitis: A 24-year retrospective case-control study. *Br J Rheumatol* 27:91–93, 1988.

Calin A, Porta J, Fries JF, et al: Clinical history as a screening test for ankylosing spondylitis. *JAMA* 237:2613–2614, 1977.

Jajic I, Jajic Z: The prevalence of osteoarthrosis of the sacroiliac joints in an urban population. *Clin Rheumatol* 6:39–41, 1987.

Roberts WN, Liang MH, Pallozzi LM, et al: Effects of warming up on reliability of anthropometric techniques in ankylosing spondylitis. *Arthritis Rheum* 31(4):549–552, 1988.

Wordsworth BP, Mowat AG: A review of 100 patients with ankylosing spondylitis with particular reference to socio-economic effects. *Br J Rheumatol* 25:175–180, 1986.

Rheumatic Disorders—Polymyalgia Rheumatica

Andersson R, Malmvall B-E, Bengtsson B-A: Long-term survival in giant cell arteritis including temporal arteritis and polymyalgia rheumatica. *Acta Med Scand* 220:361–364, 1986.

Boesen P, Sørensen SF: Giant cell arteritis, temporal arteritis, and polymyalgia rheumatica in a Danish county. *Arthritis Rheum* 30(3):294–299, 1987.

Dasgupta B, Duke O, Kyle V, et al: Antibodies to intermediate filaments in polymyalgia rheumatica and giant cell arteritis: A sequential study. *Ann Rheum Dis* 46:746–749, 1987.

Davison S, Spiera H: Polymyalgia rheumatica. *Clin Orthop* 57:95–99, 1968.

Ehrlich GE: Diagnosis and management of rheumatic diseases in older patients. *J Am Geriatr Soc* 30(11 suppl):S45–S51, 1982.

Ettlinger RE, Hunder GG, Ward LE: Polymyalgia rheumatica and giant cell arteritis. *Annu Rev Med* 29:15–22, 1978.

Golbus J, McCune WJ: Giant cell arteritis and peripheral neuropathy: A report of 2 cases and review of the literature. *J Rheumatol* 14:129–134, 1987.

Jubb RW: Therapeutic progress, review XXV: Osteoarthritis—Are we making progress? *J Clin Pharm Ther* 12:81–90, 1987.

Manolios N, Schrieber L: Polymyalgia rheumatica. *Aust Fam Physician* 15(10):1298–1300, 1986.

Nuessle WF, Miller HE, Norman FC: Polymyalgia rheumatica, giant-cell arteritis and blindness: A review and case report. *J Am Geriatr Soc* 14(6):566–577, 1966.

Smith AJ, Kyle V, Cawston TE, et al: Isolation and analysis of immune complexes from sera of patients with polymyalgia rheumatica and giant cell arteritis. *Ann Rheum Dis* 46:468–474, 1987.

Wilske KR, Healey LA: Polymyalgia rheumatica and giant cell arteritis. The dilemma of therapy. *Postgrad Med* 77(8):243–248, 1985.

Sciatic Pain—Other Causes

Anderson NE, Willoughby EW: Infarction of the conus medullaris. *Ann Neurol* 21:470–474, 1987.

Hadler NM: Regional back pain. *N Engl J Med* 315:1090–1092, 1986.

Holtzman RNN, Dubin R, Yang WC, et al: Bilateral symptomatic intraspinal T12–L1 synovial cysts. *Surg Neur* 28:225–230, 1987.

O'Neil DJ, Harding D: Crohn's disease with pelvic abscess appearing as lumbar disc herniation. *Clin Orthop* 222:174–180, 1987.

Scoliosis

Bradford DS: Adult scoliosis. Current concepts of treatment. *Clin Orthop* 229(4):70–87, 1988.

Weinstein SL: Idiopathic scoliosis. Natural history. *Spine* 11:780–783, 1983.

Segmental Instability

Frymoyer JW, Selby DK: Segmental instability. Rationale for treatment. *Spine* 10:280–286, 1985.

Kirkaldy-Willis WH, Farfan HF: Instability of the lumbar spine. *Clin Orthop* 165:110–123, 1982.

McGill SM, Normal RW: Partitioning of the L4–L5 dynamic moment into disc, ligamentous, and muscular components during lifting. *Spine* 11:666–678, 1986.

Nachemson A: Lumbar spine instability. A critical update and symposium summary. *Spine* 10:290–291, 1985.

Spondylolisthesis

Cope R: Acute traumatic spondylolysis. Report of a case and review of the literature. *Clin Orthop* 230:162–165, 1988.

Frederickson BE, Baker D, McHolick WJ, et al: The natural history of spondylolysis and spondylolisthesis. *J Bone Joint Surg [Am]* 66:699–707, 1984.

Hanley EN Jr: Decompression and distraction-derotation arthrodesis for degenerative spondylolisthesis. *Spine* 11:269–276, 1986.

Kaneda K, Kazama H, Satoh S, et al: Follow-up study of medial facetectomies and posterolateral fusion with instrumentation in unstable degenerative spondylolisthesis. *Clin Orthop* 203:159–167, 1986.

Lee C, Woodring JH, Rogers LF, et al: The radiographic distinction of degenerative slippage (spondylolisthesis and retrolisthesis) from traumatic slippage of the cervical spine. *Skeletal Radiol* 15:439–443, 1986.

Wiltse LL, Widell EH Jr, Jackson DW: Fatigue fracture: The basic lesion in isthmic spondylolisthesis. *J Bone Joint Surg [Am]* 57:17–22, 1975.

Stenosis—Lateral Recess

Arnoldi CC, Brodsky AE, Cauchoix J, et al: Lumbar spinal stenosis and nerve root entrapment syndromes. *Clin Orthop* 115:4–5, 1976.

Crock HV: Isolated lumbar disk resorption as a cause of nerve root canal stenosis. *Clin Orthop* 115:109–115, 1976.

Tuberculosis of the Spine

Adendorff JJ, Boeke EJ, Lazarus C: Pott's paraplegia. *S Afr Med J* 71:427–428, 1987.

Coppola J, Muller NL, Connell DG: Computed tomography of musculoskeletal tuberculosis. *Can Assoc Radiol J* 38:199–203, 1987.

Dawson JW, Daniell SJN: Lumbar abscess resulting from tuberculosis of the spine. *J Roy Soc Med* 77:689–690, 1984.

Hsu LCS, Leong JCY: Tuberculosis of the lower cervical spine (C2 to C7). A report on 40 cases. *J Bone Joint Surg [Br]* 66(1):1–5, 1984.

Humphries MJ, Gabriel SM: Spinal tuberculosis presenting with abdominal symptoms—a report of two cases. *Tubercle* 67:303–307, 1986.

Rajasekaran S, Shanmugasundaram TK: Prediction of the angle of gibbus deformity in tuberculosis of the spine. *J Bone Joint Surg [Am]* 69(4):503–509, 1987.

Thommesen P, Bartholdy N, Bunger E: Histiocytosis X. VIII. Histiocytosis X simulating tuberculosis. *Acta Radiol [Oncol]* 22(4):295–297, 1983.

A controlled trial of six-month and nine-month regimens of chemotherapy in patients undergoing radical surgery for tuberculosis of the spine in Hong Kong. Tenth report of the Medical Research Council Working Party on Tuberculosis of the Spine. *Tubercle* 67:243–259, 1986.

Tumor—Carcinomatous Meningitis

Ito U, Tomita H, Yamazaki S, et al: CT findings of leptomeningeal and periventricular dissemination of tumors. *Clin Neurol Neurosurg* 88:115–120, 1986.

Olson ME, Chernik NL, Posner JB: Infiltration of the leptomeninges by systemic cancer. *Arch Neurol* 30:122–137, 1974.

Wasserstrom WR, Glass JP, Posner JB: Diagnosis and treatment of leptomeningeal metastases from solid tumors: Experience with 90 patients. *Cancer* 49:759–772, 1982.

Tumors—Epidural/Extradural Spinal

Bates DW, Reuler JB: Back pain and epidural spinal cord compression. *J Gen Intern Med* 3:191–197, 1988.

Breuer AC, Kneisley LW, Fischer EG: Treatable extramedullary cord compression. Meningioma as a cause of the Brown-Séquard Syndrome. *Spine* 5(1):19–22, 1980.

Ch'ien LT, Kalwinsky DK, Peterson G, et al: Metastatic epidural tumors in children. *Med Pediatr Oncol* 10:455–462, 1982.

Epstein JA, Marc JA, Hyman RA, et al: Total myelography in the evaluation of lumbar discs. With the presentation of three cases of thoracic neoplasms simulating nerve root lesions. *Spine* 4(2):121–128, 1979.

Giannotta SL, Kindt GW: Metastatic spinal cord tumors. *Clin Neurosurg* 25:495–503, 1978.

Gilbert MR, Grossman SA: Incidence and nature of neurologic problems in patients with solid tumors. *Am J Med* 81:951–954, 1986.

Gilbert RW, Kim J-H, Posner JB: Epidural spinal cord compression from metastatic tumor: Diagnosis and treatment. *Ann Neurol* 3:40–51, 1978.

Hahn YS, McLone DG: Pain in children with spinal cord tumors. *Child's Brain* 11:36–46, 1984.

Kleinman WB, Kiernan HA, Michelsen WJ. Metastatic cancer of the spinal column. *Clin Orthop* 136:166–172, 1978.

Kostuik JP: Anterior spinal cord decompression for lesions of the thoracic and lumbar spine, techniques, new methods of internal fixation results. *Spine* 8(5):512–531, 1983.

Kuban DA, El-Mahdi A, Sigfred SV, et al: Characteristics of spinal cord compression in adenocarcinoma of prostate. *Urology* 28(5):364–369, 1986.

Levy WJ, Bay J, Dohn D: Spinal cord meningioma. *J Neurosurg* 57:804–812, 1982.

Nather A, Bose K: The results of decompression of cord or cauda equina compression from metastatic extradural tumors. *Clin Orthop* 169:103–108, 1982.

Nicholas JJ, Christy WC: Spinal pain made worse by recumbency: A clue to spinal cord tumors. *Arch Phys Med Rehabil* 67:598–600, 1986.

Overby MC, Rothman AS: Anterolateral decompression for metastatic epidural spinal cord tumors. Results of a modified costotransversectomy approach. *J Neurosurg* 62:344–348, 1985.

Posner JB: Back pain and epidural spinal cord compression. *Med Clin North Am* 71:185–205, 1987.

Posner JB, Howieson J, Cvitkovic E: "Disappearing" spinal cord compression: Oncolytic effect of glucocorticoids (and other chemotherapeutic agents) on epidural metastases. *Ann Neurol* 2:409–413, 1977.

Rodriguez M, Dinapoli RP. Spinal cord compression with special reference to metastatic epidural tumors. *Mayo Clin Proc* 55:442–448, 1980.

Schaberg J, Gainor BJ: A profile of metastatic carcinoma of the spine. *Spine* 10(1):19–20, 1985.

Sherman RMP, Waddell JP: Laminectomy for metastatic epidural spinal cord tumors. *Clin Orthop* 207:55–63, 1986.

Stern WE: Localization and diagnosis of spinal cord tumors. *Clin Neurosurg* 25:480–494, 1978.

Vasilakis D, Papaconstantinou C, Aletras H: Dumb-bell intrathoracic and intraspinal neurofibroma. Report of a case. *Scand J Thorac Cardiovasc Surg* 20:171–173, 1986.

Case 52-1985, Case records of the Massachusetts General Hospital. *N Engl J Med* 313:1646–1656, 1985.

Tumors—Epidural/Spinal/Therapy

Kuhlman JE, Fishman EK, Leichner PK, et al: Skeletal metastases from hepatoma: Frequency, distribution, and radiographic features. *Radiology* 160:175–178, 1986.

O'Neil J, Gardner V, Armstrong G: Treatment of tumors of the thoracic and lumbar spinal column. *Clin Orthop* 227:103–112, 1988.

Schulz U, Bamberg M: Relationship between curative radiation therapy of paravertebral tumors and the incidence of radiation myelitis. *Tumori* 64:305–312, 1978.

Siegal T, Siegal T: Surgical decompression of anterior and posterior malignant epidural tumors compressing the spinal cord: A prospective study. *Neurosurgery* 17(3):424–432, 1985.

Sundaresan N, Scher H, DiGiacinto GV, et al: Surgical treatment of spinal cord compression in kidney cancer. *J Clin Oncol* 4:1851–1856, 1986.

Tumors—Imaging

Baleriaux D, Deroover N, Hermanus N, et al: MRI of the spine. *Diagn Imaging Clin Med* 55:66–71, 1986.

Bradley WG, Waluch V, Yadley RA, et al: Comparison of CT and MR in 400 patients with suspected disease of the brain and cervical spinal cord. *Radiology* 152:695–702, 1984.

Chadduck WM, Flanigan S: Intraoperative ultrasound for spinal lesions. *Neurosurgery* 16(4):477–483, 1985.

Di Chiro G, Doppman JL, Dwyer AJ, et al: Tumors and arteriovenous malformations of the spinal cord: Assessment using MR. *Radiology* 156:689–697, 1985.

Kent DL, Larson EB: Magnetic resonance imaging of the brain and spine. *Ann Intern Med* 108:402–424, 1988.

Sherman JL, Barkovich AJ, Citrin CM: The MR appearance of syringomyelia: New observations. *AJR* 148:381–391, 1987.

Sze G, Krol G, Zimmerman RD, et al: Malignant extradural spinal tumors: MR imaging with Gd-DTPA. *Radiology* 167:217–223, 1988.

Tumors—Intradural/Extramedullary Spinal

Divers WA, Hoxsey RJ, Dunnihoo DR: A spinal cord neurolemmoma in pregnancy. *Obstet Gynecol* 52(1)(suppl):47S–50S, 1978.

Onofrio BM: Intradural extramedullary spinal cord tumors. *Clin Neurosurg* 25:540–555, 1978.

Tumors—Intramedullary Spinal

Cooper PR, Epstein F: Radical resection of intramedullary spinal cord tumors in adults. *J Neurosurg* 63:492–499, 1985.

Garrido E, Stein BM: Microsurgical removal of intramedullary spinal cord tumors. *Surg Neurol* 7:215–219, 1977.

Grem JL, Burgess J, Trump DL: Clinical features and natural history of intramedullary spinal cord metastasis. *Cancer* 56:2305–2314, 1985.

Heppner F, Ascher PW, Holzer P, et al: CO_2 laser surgery of intramedullary spinal cord tumors. *Lasers Surg Med* 7:180–183, 1987.

Post MJD, Quencer RM, Green BA, et al: Intramedullary spinal cord metastases, mainly of nonneurogenic origin. *AJR* 148:1015–1022, 1987.

Stein BM: Intramedullary spinal cord tumors. *Clin Neurosurg* 30:717–741, 1983.

Tumors—Primary

Weinstein JN, McLain RF: Primary tumors of the spine. *Spine* 12:843–851, 1987.

Tumors—Retroperitoneal

Braasch JW, Mon AB: Primary retroperitoneal tumors. *Surg Clin North Am* 47:663–678, 1967.

Tumors—Scapula

Malawer MM, Dick HM: Neoplasms affecting the upper extremity, in Dee R, Mango E, Hurst LC (eds): *Principles of Orthopaedic Practice*, New York, McGraw-Hill, 1988, vol 1, pp 751–755.

PART SEVEN

Acute Genital, Perineal, and Anal Pain

Acute Penile Pain

☐ DIAGNOSTIC LIST

1. Ulcerative penile lesions
   A. Primary genital herpes
   B. Chancroid (soft chancre)
   C. Primary syphilis
   D. Trauma
   E. Pyoderma
   F. Chancroid-like ulcers
      1. *Haemophilus ducreyi*–like bacteria
      2. Secondarily infected herpetic and traumatic ulcers
      3. Combined syphilis and chancroid
   G. Balanitis due to fixed drug eruption
   H. Infectious balanoposthitis
      1. Bacterial balanoposthitis
      2. Erosive and gangrenous balanoposthitis
      3. Candidal balanoposthitis
   I. Herpes zoster
2. Urethritis
   A. Gonococcal urethritis
   B. Nongonococcal urethritis
      1. *Chlamydia trachomatis*
      2. *Ureaplasma urealyticum*
      3. *Mycoplasma hominis*
      4. Nongonococcal urethritis of unknown cause
         A. *Mycoplasma genitalium*
         B. *Bacteroides* species
         C. Adenovirus types 19 and 37
         D. *Haemophilus ducreyi*

3. Other causes of urethral pain
   A. Acute bacterial prostatitis
   B. Prostatic abscess
   C. Acute bacterial cystitis
   D. Acute pyelonephritis
   E. Pseudocystitis due to carcinoma in situ
   F. Urethral calculi
   G. Urethral foreign bodies
4. Penile trauma
   A. Penile fracture due to blunt trauma
   B. Gunshot wound
   C. Genital skin loss
      1. Avulsion injuries
   D. Urethral injuries
      1. Anterior (penile) urethra
      2. Posterior urethra
5. Painful erection
   A. Peyronie's disease (idiopathic)
   B. Peyronie's disease and other disorders
   C. Mimics of Peyronie's disease
      1. Thrombophlebitis of the dorsal vein of the penis
      2. Penile sarcoma
      3. Fibrotic plaques from prior surgery or trauma
   D. Priapism
      1. Hematologic disorders
      2. Neoplastic disorders
      3. Behçet's disease
      4. Neurologic disorders
      5. Drug-related priapism
      6. Infectious diseases

7. Renal failure
8. Trauma to the penis and perineum
9. Idiopathic priapism
10. Nonischemic idiopathic priapism
6. Generalized skin disorders with balanitis
   A. Toxic epidermal necrolysis
   B. Stevens-Johnson syndrome
7. Local skin disorders

    A. Contact dermatitis
    B. Neurodermatitis
8. Penile and perineal infections
   A. Periurethral abscess
   B. Necrotizing fasciitis of the scrotum, penis, and perineum
9. Referred pain
   A. Anorectal disorders
   B. Appendicitis
10. Psychogenic pain

☐ SUMMARY

Primary herpes simplex infection of the penis begins with a prodrome (50 percent of cases) of local penile pain, tenderness, and paresthesias—sometimes with dull, aching buttock and posteromedial thigh and calf pain. This is followed within 1 to 2 days by the bilateral (84 percent of cases) eruption of 1- to 3-mm grouped painful and tender papules and vesicles on the penile shaft and coronal sulcus. These lesions may form pustules, or may ulcerate and crust. The surrounding skin may be erythematous and tender. Fever, chills, myalgias, and malaise may occur in severe cases. Dysuria, and even urinary retention, may complicate a primary attack. Viral cultures and direct immunofluorescence of lesion exudate can confirm the diagnosis. Herpes simplex virus type 2 (HSV 2) is responsible for 85 percent of cases of primary genital herpes, and herpes simplex virus type 1 (HSV 1) for 15 percent. There is a therapeutic response to oral or intravenous acyclovir.

Chancroid is caused by *Haemophilus ducreyi*. Lesions may be single or multiple. The initial lesion is a papule that soon ulcerates, forming an irregular, ragged, painful and tender ulcer with an undermined erythematous edge and a purulent base. Secondary ulcers on the thigh and scrotum occur by autoinoculation and, when present, are of diagnostic value. Gram-stained smears of ulcer exudate show parallel chains of gram-negative coccobacilli ("railroad tracks"); cultures on special media may grow the organism. Painful and tender lymphadenitis may occur in one or both inguinal regions. Chancroid is rare in the United States; and male cases have been associated with prostitute contact in large cities like Atlanta, New York, and Boston. There is a good therapeutic response to erythromycin.

Primary syphilis forms a 0.5- to 3-cm erosion on the glans, coronal sulcus, or shaft of the penis. The chancre has a firm, indurated base and edge. The base is usually dry or may exude serous exudate. It is usually not painful, but it may be tender (33 percent). It has a beefy-red or "raw ham" appearance. Dark-field examination of lesion exudate reveals *Treponema pallidum*; a VDRL or RPR test is positive in 70 percent. A single injection of benzathine penicillin leads to resolution of the chancre, and to a fall in the VDRL or RPR titer over a period of months.

Some linear or irregular superficial ulcers are secondary to friction during sexual activity or to bites during fellatio (*traumatic ulcers*). These ulcerations may become secondarily infected, forming a purulent ulcer or a fluctuant pustule (*pyoderma*). The usual causative organisms are *Streptococcus pyogenes* and *Staphylococcus aureus*. *Trichomonas vaginalis* has been isolated from some chancroid-like, foul-smelling penile ulcers.

Painful, tender, ragged *chancroid-like ulcers* may be caused by *H. ducreyi–like bacteria* or by *secondary bacterial infection of herpetic or traumatic ulcers*. In endemic areas, up to 15 percent of patients have *complex chancres* caused by *T. pallidum* and *H. ducreyi*. These lesions usually resemble chancroidal ulcers; but *T. pallidum* can be detected by dark-field examination, and *H. ducreyi* by use of selective culture media. Treatment with benzathine penicillin and erythromycin usually results in resolution. A *fixed drug eruption* due to use of tetracycline or a sulfonamide may cause an acutely painful circumscribed glans erosion or ulcer that appears within 8 h of ingestion of the drug. Discontinuance of the drug usually leads to resolution of symptoms.

Severe edema, redness, pain, and tenderness of the prepuce, in association with a purulent discharge from beneath the foreskin (*balanoposthitis*), is caused by a local *bacterial skin infection* and responds to local cleansing and antibiotic therapy. Repeated episodes may require circumcision. Severe involvement of the foreskin by *spirochetes and vibrios* may lead to gangrene of the prepuce, and sometimes to necrosis of the glans. Extensive ulceration of the glans and shaft may also occur, and precede necrotic changes. The infection can be controlled by a dorsal slit in the foreskin and parenteral antibiotic therapy.

Candidiasis of the foreskin and glans presents with local pain, tenderness, redness, edema, and white, curdlike flecks of exudate on the glans and foreskin. Erosions and ulcerations of the glans and urethral meatus may occur. Microscopic examination of these curds in 10% KOH reveals the pseudohyphae and hyphae of a *Candida* species. *Herpes zoster* begins with burning penile pain and tenderness, followed by the unilateral eruption of clusters of vesicles, pustules, and crusted ulcers. Paresthesias and local areas of penile numbness may occur. Viral cultures will identify varicella-zoster virus as the causative agent.

Urethritis presents with dysuria and/or a urethral discharge, without urinary frequency and urgency. *Gonococcal urethritis* usually causes a purulent or mucopurulent discharge; the Gram stain of the discharge is 95 percent sensitive and 99 percent specific. Culture will usually detect cases missed by Gram stain, and will allow determination of the penicillin resistance of the isolate.

Chlamydia trachomatis causes most cases of postgonococcal urethritis, and 30 to 50 percent of cases of acute *nongonococcal urethritis*. The diagnosis is suggested by an incubation period of 10 to 14 days or more and a mucoid or yellow-white discharge. Culture, a direct immunofluorescent antibody stain, and an ELISA test can be used to confirm the diagnosis of chlamydial infection. *Ureaplasma urealyticum* may cause up to 40 percent of cases of nongonococcal urethritis. *Trichomonas vaginalis*, HSV, and other microorganisms cause only a small percentage of cases of nongonococcal urethritis. Up to 20 percent of cases of urethritis are of unknown etiology.

Dysuria accompanied by frequency, suprapubic and perineal pain, strangury, fever, chills, malaise, myalgias, and an enlarged, boggy, tender prostate is most likely due to an *acute bacterial prostatitis*. There is a good response to antibiotic therapy. A fluctuant, tender, prostatic lobe associated with symptoms of acute prostatitis that fail to respond to antibiotic therapy may be caused by a *prostatic abscess*. This diagnosis can be confirmed by a pelvic CT scan or transrectal ultrasonography. Drainage of the abscess and antibiotic therapy result in symptom resolution.

Acute cystitis presents with frequency, nocturia, urgency, and dysuria, but without chills, rigors, and fever. The urine may be cloudy and foul-smelling, and gross hematuria may occur. Urinalysis reveals leukocytes, singly and in clumps, and large numbers of bacteria. Urine culture reveals more than 10^4 colony-forming units (cfu) per ml. There is usually a prompt response to antibiotic therapy. A 3- to 7-day course of antibiotic therapy is usually sufficient, and the relapse rate is low.

Acute pyelonephritis may present with flank and anterior ipsilateral abdominal pain, chills, and fever. Lower tract irritative symptoms such as dysuria, frequency, and urgency are common. The urine contains leukocytes—singly, in clumps, and sometimes in casts—erythrocytes, albumin, and bacteria. There is a good response to antibiotic therapy, but a short course (1 to 3 days) is commonly followed by a relapse.

Pseudocystitis, with dysuria, frequency, and urgency, may be secondary to carcinoma in situ of the bladder. The urine may contain some leukocytes, erythrocytes, and atypical epithelial cells. Gross hematuria and penile pain may also occur. The diagnosis may be confirmed by urine cytology and/or by cystoscopic biopsy of Brunn's nests (yellow, comedo-like areas of the bladder mucosa).

A *urethral calculus* may cause severe dysuria, dribbling and/ or stuttering urination with local urethral tenderness, and a palpable stone along the course of the urethra. The urine may contain erythrocytes and leukocytes. The diagnosis can be confirmed by a retrograde urethrogram or endoscopy. Urethral stricture, bladder stones, neurogenic bladder, urethral diverticula, and prostate hypertrophy are associated with urethral stones. A *urethral foreign body* may cause similar symptoms. Removal of the stone or foreign body results in symptom relief.

Penile fracture usually results from violent bending of the erect penis during sexual intercourse, but other mechanisms of blunt injury may also be responsible. A popping or cracking noise is accompanied by pain in the penile shaft, detumescence, and rapid swelling and discoloration of the penile shaft, with curvature to the contralateral side and bizarre distortion of the organ. A cavernosogram will determine if the tunica albuginea has been ruptured. Rupture of the tunica requires immediate surgical repair and evacuation of the hematoma to prevent sequelae, such as permanent penile deformity and impotence. *Penetrating, avulsion, and degloving injuries* also occur. Mutilating penectomy has been reported in psychotic patients, with successful reattachment.

Injury to the penis and *rupture of the anterior urethra* with an intact Buck's fascia results in severe, painful swelling and discoloration of the shaft of the penis. An associated rupture of Buck's fascia results in swelling and discoloration of the anterior abdominal wall, perineum, scrotum, and penis. *Posterior urethral rupture* results in blood at the urethral meatus, gross or microscopic hematuria, a floating, high-riding prostate on rectal examination, and inability to void. A retrograde urethrogram will usually localize the site of injury.

Peyronie's disease causes penile curvature and pain associated with an erection. Impotence may develop as this disorder progresses. An indurated fibrous plaque may be present beneath the skin on the dorsum of the shaft of the penis. Excision of the plaque may relieve pain and penile deformity. *Mimics of Peyronie's disease* include *penile thrombophlebitis*, *penile sarcoma*, and *fibrous plaques* resulting *from prior surgery* or *trauma* (i.e., penile fracture).

Priapism is a sustained, painful erection not resulting from sexual stimulation and not relieved by ejaculation or cold showers. The corpora cavernosa are rigid, but the glans and corpus spongiosum remain soft. Most cases are veno-occlusive; in such cases the problem is delayed venous outflow.

Hematologic disorders, such as sickle cell anemia, chronic leukemia, myeloma, polycythemia, macroglobulinemia, and protein C deficiency, may cause priapism. *Penile metastases* may cause penile pain and/or priapism. Painful priapism may occur with *Behçet's disease*, because of a thrombophlebitis of the corpora cavernosa. *Neurologic disorders*, such as Wilson's disease, tuberous sclerosis, cerebral infarction, and central nervous system tumors, have been associated with priapism. *Antidepressant drugs* (trazodone), *antipsychotics*, *antihypertensives* (prazosin), *cocaine, alcohol, testosterone, diazepam*, and *discontinuation of heparin* have been associated with priapism. *Intracavernous injection therapy for impotence* using papaverine/phentolamine also may cause priapism. Rare cases

TABLE OF DISEASE INCIDENCE

PREVALENCE PER 100,000 (APPROXIMATE)

Common (>100)	Uncommon (5>5–100)	Rare (>0–5)
Herpes simplex infection	Primary syphilis	Chancroid
Trauma	Herpes simplex urethritis	Chancroid-like ulcers
Pyoderma	Acute bacterial prostatitis	Fixed drug eruption
Bacterial balanoposthitis	Carcinoma in situ of the bladder	Gangrenous balanoposthitis
Candidal balanoposthitis	Anterior urethral rupture	Herpes zoster
Gonococcal urethritis	Posterior urethral rupture	*Mycoplasma hominis* urethritis
Chlamydial urethritis	Peyronie's disease associated with other disorders	*Bacterioides* urethritis
Ureaplasma urealyticum urethritis	Priapism due to sickle cell anemia	Adenovirus urethritis
Acute bacterial cystitis	Priapism due to drugs	*Trichomonas vaginalis* urethritis
Acute pyelonephritis	Priapism due to intracavernosal injection of	*Haemophilus ducreyi* urethritis
Peyronie's disease	papavarine/phentolamine	*Mycoplasma genitalium* urethritis
	Idiopathic priapism	Prostatic abscess
	Toxic epidermal necrolysis	Urethral calculus
	Stevens-Johnson syndrome	Urethral foreign body
	Periurethral abscess	Penile fracture
	Psychogenic pain	Penile gunshot wound
		Penile avulsion injuries
		Penile thrombophlebitis
		Penile sarcoma
		Posttraumatic penile scarring
		Priapism due to:
		Neoplasms
		Hematologic disorders
		Behçet's disease
		Neurologic disorders
		Infectious diseases
		Renal failure
		Trauma
		Penile contact dermatitis
		Penile neurodermatitis
		Referred penile pain from anorectal disorders and acute appendicitis
		Necrotizing fasciitis
		Nonischemic idiopathic priapism

occur with *systemic infections* and *renal failure*. High-flow painless priapism may result from *trauma* causing disruption of an artery in a cavernous body. Clot embolism of the leaking vessel results in detumescence. Idiopathic cases are frequently associated with *exercise*, *sexual intercourse*, and *masturbation*. Some early cases of idiopathic painful priapism may be due to *high inflow*; these may be relieved by α agonist therapy.

Toxic epidermal necrolysis is a generalized inflammatory skin disorder that causes diffuse blistering and may involve the genitalia. The *Stevens-Johnson syndrome* also may cause cutaneous and penile bullae associated with a generalized macular rash with target lesions. Urticarial plaques may also occur; lip involvement results in hemorrhagic crusting of the vermilion border. *Contact dermatitis* of the penis and/or scrotum causes penile and foreskin redness, edema, vesiculation, ulceration, oozing, and crusting. Poison ivy, local antibiotics or anesthetics, or chemicals from new unwashed underwear may cause this disorder. Use of local or oral corticosteroids leads to resolution within 3 to 10 days. *Neurodermatitis* produces similar findings, but results from chronic scratching.

A *periurethral abscess* causes ventral penile pain and a localized tender swelling. It may be associated with a urethral stricture or acute gonococcal urethritis. Spontaneous rupture of the abscess may result in a draining urethrocutaneous perineal fistula. *Necrotizing fasciitis* causes severe penile, perineal, and scrotal pain, and is associated with local skin erythema, edema, and blackening. The skin becomes indurated and the blackening spreads. Skin crepitus may be present. Sloughing of the skin and surgical debridement of necrotic tissue may leave the penis and testicles partially or completely bare. Fever, chills, rigors, and prostration occur. Survival depends on extensive debridement and antibiotic therapy.

Referred pain to a clinically normal penis may result from *anorectal disease* or *appendicitis*. *Psychogenic pain* occurs in patients with no organic disease of the penis. Some of these patients may have neurologic pain secondary to recurrent HSV 2 infection without skin lesions (i.e., in a prodrome or with clinically insignificant penile lesions), but most have a somatization disorder or a depression; often these patients have abiding fear of a sexually transmitted disease or a malignancy.

☐ DESCRIPTION OF LISTED DISEASES

1. ULCERATIVE PENILE LESIONS

A. Primary Genital Herpes The initial symptoms may be a burning penile discomfort, superficial tenderness, and paresthesias. Aching, deep pain in one or both buttocks and down the posteromedial thigh may also occur as part of the prodrome. Small grouped vesicles and/or pustules appear on one or both sides (84 percent) of the distal shaft of the penis, near the corona. The number of lesions averages 16.3 (nearly 3 times the average number seen in recurrent attacks). These soon ulcerate and crust. Some of the small vesicles or ulcers may coalesce, forming large, irregularly bordered ulcers proximal to the corona. A narrow erythematous rim borders each lesion. Often the lesions are too tender to allow sexual activity. Within 1 week, unilateral or bilateral, painful and/or tender lymphadenopathy develops (80 percent). Urinary frequency, dysuria (44 percent), and, sometimes, urinary retention may occur. Fever, myalgias, headache, and malaise are common associated symptoms (60 percent). Penile lesions heal without scarring in 2 to 6 weeks (mean, 19 days). Viral cultures taken from the lesions may remain positive for 14 to 21 days. Primary infection may be associated with aseptic meningitis (13 percent) or, rarely, encephalitis.

A Tzanck test may be done for immediate confirmation of the clinical diagnosis. The base of a vesicle is scraped, and the cells obtained are smeared on a slide and stained with Wright's, Giemsa, or Papanicolaou's stain. Multinucleated giant cells, intranuclear inclusion bodies, and ballooning degeneration are found in up to 60 percent of cases. The Tzanck test does not differentiate between varicella-zoster, HSV 1, and HSV 2 infections. A direct immunofluorescence stain of lesion exudate is 70 percent as sensitive as viral culture. Cell cultures usually become positive in 1 to 3 days (95 percent of isolates are positive within 5 days); cytopathic effects, while relatively specific, require confirmation by neutralization or immunofluorescence tests. Seroconversion after a primary episode can be documented by complement fixation or microneutralization tests. The initial serum should be obtained at the onset of the infection. HSV 2 causes 75 to 85 percent of primary genital herpes infections, and HSV 1 the remainder. There is a therapeutic response to oral or intravenous acyclovir.

B. Chancroid (Soft Chancre) *Haemophilus ducreyi* may cause painful genital ulcers 4 to 7 days after exposure. These begin as tender papules that soon ulcerate, forming irregular, ragged, soft, tender ulcers covered with a purulent exudate. An erythematous rim borders the ulcer, and the edge may be undermined. Multiple ulcers

occur in up to 75 percent of cases. Ulcerative lesions on the thigh or scrotum may be due to autoinoculation of *H. ducreyi*. The presence of these satellite lesions may be helpful diagnostically.

Unilateral, and sometimes bilateral, painful and tender inguinal lymphadenitis develops within the first week in 33 to 50 percent of cases. Without specific therapy, these nodes may enlarge into fluctuant buboes that may drain spontaneously through the skin. Gram-stained smears of ulcer exudate reveal parallel chains (''railroad tracks'') of gram-negative coccobacilli. These coccobacilli may occur within polymorphonuclear cells, or may be extracellular. A ''school of fish'' pattern of *H. ducreyi* has also been described on smears taken of tissue exudate or solid media colonies.

H. ducreyi is difficult to grow and requires special media containing hemin (e.g., hemoglobin or myoglobin), albumin, selenium, and 1-glutamine for optimum growth. Vancomycin is added to suppress the growth of competing bacteria. *H. ducreyi* will grow on gonococcal agar base augmented with 1% bovine hemoglobin, 1% IsoVitale X, and vancomycin (3 $\mu g/\mu l$). It grows best at 35°C in a 5% CO_2 atmosphere.

The diagnosis is commonly made by exclusion of primary syphilis and herpes simplex infection. Painful ulceration and/or painful tender lymphadenopathy, and a prompt response to erythromycin preceded by no response to penicillin or tetracycline, is also supportive of the diagnosis. Many cases are diagnosed on clinical findings, since culture media are not always available and the sensitivity of culture may be only 60 to 70 percent.

Chancroid is rare in the United States. It may occur in single cases or in localized epidemics (e.g., Florida, New York City, Boston, Texas), in which it is typically spread through prostitution. In these outbreaks, the male:female ratio has varied from 3:1 to 25:1. It is a common sexually transmitted disease in the third world (e.g., Africa, Asia). In the United States this disorder is most likely to occur in black and Hispanic men who patronize prostitutes. Men returning from developing countries, or from endemic regions in the United States (e.g., New York, Texas, California, Florida, Georgia), with painful genital ulcers should also be suspected of having this disease.

C. Primary Syphilis After an incubation period of 14 to 21 days, a red, painless papule appears on the penis; within 1 to 3 days it ulcerates. In one large series (642 men with primary syphilis), the chancres were located on the coronal sulcus (35 percent), the glans (29 percent), the shaft (22 percent), the prepuce (19 percent), the frenulum (10 percent), and the urethral meatus (1 percent). Up to 37 percent of patients had multiple penile chancres.

Chancres are usually round, but may be elongated. The base is usually dry, with a dark ''beefy'' or light-red ''raw ham'' appearance. Some are covered by a thin yellow or gray-white exudate. The ulcer margin, and often the base, are indurated, in contrast to the soft consistency of chancroidal ulcers. Up to 35 percent of these lesions are tender to palpation, but they are seldom spontaneously painful. The lesion is usually sharply outlined, and there is no undermining of the edge as occurs with chancroid. Up to 10 percent of lesions may have a purulent pseudomembrane or irregular undermined edge, mimicking chancroid. Inguinal adenopathy on one or both sides may occur, and may be tender in up to 23 percent of cases. Exudate from all genital ulcerations should be studied by dark-field examination, and a Venereal Disease Research Laboratory (VDRL) or rapid plasma reagin (RPR) test should be performed, even though the false-negative rate in primary syphilis is 30 percent. The fluorescent treponemal antibody absorption (FTA-ABS) test and the microhemagglutination assay (MHA-TP) are positive in 90 percent of cases of primary syphilis. The reagin tests are used as a baseline for follow-up after treatment. The FTA-ABS and MHA-TP remain positive for life, and are seldom useful in the diagnosis and management of primary syphilis. Benzathine penicillin G (2.4×10^6 units IM weekly for 3 doses) is usually curative.

D. Trauma   Friction from vigorous intercourse or masturbation, or human bites during fellatio, may cause penile abrasions and ulcers. Severe lacerations, and sometimes avulsion of the glans, have followed accidents during masturbation using an electric broom or vacuum cleaner for autostimulation. Erosions occurring from rough, unlubricated intercourse or masturbation are more likely to be mistaken for chancroid or herpes since they are painful and tender, and there may be no recollection of a causative traumatic incident.

E. Pyoderma   A traumatic erosion or a herpetic ulcer of the shaft of the penis may become secondarily infected by pyogenic bacteria *(Staphylococcus aureus, Streptococcus pyogenes)*, producing a large ulcer surrounded by erythema and edema, or a pustule. Such lesions are usually painful and tender and, if eroded, are covered by a purulent exudate. Culture and Gram stain of the exudate will identify the causative organism. *Trichomonas vaginalis* has been isolated from some painful penile ulcerations. *T. vaginalis* has been associated with deep, foul-smelling, chancroid-like ulcers that were initiated by herpesvirus-induced ulceration.

F. Chancroid-Like Ulcers

1. Haemophilus ducreyi–Like Bacteria   Chancroid-like, painful, purulent ulcers with undermined edges have been associated with *Haemophilus ducreyi*–like bacteria that differ from *H. ducreyi* in many biochemical characteristics.

2. Secondarily Infected Herpetic and Traumatic Ulcers   Chancroid-like ulcers (purulent, soft, tender,

painful ulcers with a red, friable base) have been associated with positive herpes simplex cultures. These probably represent herpes lesions secondarily infected by pyogenic bacteria. In some cases neither herpes virus nor pyogenic bacteria have been isolated. Some of these may represent false-negative culture results. In some cases, *Haemophilus ducreyi* may also secondarily infect traumatic ulcers.

3. Combined Syphilis and Chancroid   In developing nations, where both syphilis and chancroid are common disorders, up to 15 percent of patients with chancroid may also contract primary syphilis. Secondary infection of one or more chancres by *Haemophilus ducreyi* causes pain, tenderness, preputial redness, and edema, associated with well-circumscribed, indurated ulceration. Granulation tissue and a dirty gray exudate cover the ulcer base. Dark-field study of serous fluid obtained from such an ulcer reveals *Treponema pallidum*. Gram stain of the exudate may reveal gram-negative coccobacilli in parallel chains (''railroad tracks''); cultures for *H. ducreyi* are positive. Treatment with benzathine penicillin G and erythromycin usually leads to ulcer healing.

Careful microbiologic study of 100 penile ulcers seen in Detroit (1973–1975) revealed 15 cases of infection with *T. pallidum*, 34 with HSV 2, and 2 with chancroid. There were 7 traumatic ulcers, and 1 due to fixed drug eruption. Cultures of penile ulcers revealed a polymicrobial flora in 97 percent of cases, with 2 to 10 isolates reported per patient. [These included aerobic (100 percent) and anaerobic (64 percent) bacteria.]

G. Balanitis Due to a Fixed Drug Eruption   Ingestion of tetracycline has been reported to cause severe pain, swelling, erythema, and tenderness of the glans penis. The lesion is a sharply circumscribed red plaque. Eruptions have appeared within 1 to 8 h of ingestion of the drug. The lesion may sometimes progress rapidly to a painful hemorrhagic ulceration. Sulfonamides, phenolphthalein, and barbiturates have also been reported as causes of penile fixed drug eruptions. Discontinuance of the offending drug leads to rapid resolution of pain and erythema.

H. Infectious Balanoposthitis

1. Bacterial Balanoposthitis   Severe edema and redness of the foreskin and glans are accompanied by pain, tenderness, and purulent exudate. Gram stains reveal single or mixed bacterial infections. There is a good response to oral and/or intravenous antibiotics. Severe cases cause so much tenderness and edema of the prepuce that phimosis occurs, but this is usually reversible after treatment of the infection. Cases caused by group B streptococci, group A streptococci, and mixed aerobic/anaerobic bacterial infections have been reported.

Haemophilus ducreyi infection beneath the prepuce may cause diffuse foreskin edema, redness, and phimosis, relieved by erythromycin therapy.

2. Erosive and Gangrenous Balanoposthitis

A severe form of preputial and glans infection with spirochetal and *vibrio* organisms may cause severe pain associated with induration, edema, redness, and tenderness of the prepuce. The foreskin may become black and necrotic, and neglect may lead to necrosis of the glans and the shaft. Extensive ulceration and edema of the glans and shaft may precede necrotic changes. A dorsal foreskin slit, to expose the occluded region to air; cleansing soaks and/or baths; and antibiotic therapy will usually prevent progression and lead to recovery.

3. Candidal Balanoposthitis (Candidiasis of the Prepuce and Glans)

Edema, redness, pain, and tenderness of the prepuce are present. Whitish, curdlike deposits occur on the glans and foreskin; they may be accompanied by shallow, tender ulcerations of the glans, meatus, and foreskin. Microscopic examination of the whitish curds in 10% KOH reveals candidal pseudohyphae and hyphae. Oral therapy with fluconazole is effective. Local therapy with butoconazole or nystatin may also lead to resolution.

I. Herpes Zoster Unilateral penile pain is associated with the eruption of ipsilateral grouped vesicles on a red, edematous base. The lesions soon ulcerate and crust. They remain unilateral, but may be mistaken for herpes simplex infection. Specific fluorescent antibody stains or viral culture can establish the diagnosis if differentiation is required.

2. URETHRITIS

A purulent or mucopurulent urethral discharge is accompanied by severe burning penile and perineal discomfort during urination (dysuria) and for a variable time afterward. Urinary frequency, nocturia, and urgency are not usually present unless the bladder neck is inflamed.

A. Gonococcal Urethritis Urethritis may result from vaginal or rectal intercourse or fellatio. The risk per contact with an infected female with genital tract gonorrhea is 17 percent. The incubation period may be as short as 12 h or as long as 3 months; it is usually 3 to 10 days. In most cases the discharge is yellow (purulent), but it may be whitish-gray (mucoid) or pale yellow (mucopurulent). Urethral cultures obtained with a calcium alginate swab are usually satisfactory. Smears demonstrating polymorphonuclear leukocytes, with intracellular gram-negative diplococci, are 95 percent sensitive and 99 percent specific. Culture of the alginate swab on modified Thayer-Martin or New York City medium is very sensitive and specific. Culture is useful for confirmation, for testing for antibiotic resistance, and to identify infections missed by Gram stain. Serologic and fluorescent antibody tests have been developed, but they have not enhanced diagnostic sensitivity above that resulting from cultures and Gram stains. This disease may respond to therapy with penicillin G, ampicillin, doxycycline, erythromycin, or ofloxacin. Up to 30 percent of patients with gonococcal urethritis are simultaneously infected with *Chlamydia trachomatis* or *Ureaplasma urealyticum* and require additional therapy with doxycycline, erythromycin, or quinolone antibiotics.

B. Nongonococcal Urethritis Dysuria, and/or a mucopurulent or mucoid discharge, and meatal and urethral itching are common complaints. *Chlamydia trachomatis* causes 30 to 50 percent of cases; *Ureaplasma urealyticum* (T-mycoplasma) may cause up to 40 percent of such cases. *Trichomonas vaginalis*, herpes simplex virus, and other microorganisms may cause a small percentage of cases. *C. trachomatis* is the cause of up to 80 percent of cases of postgonococcal urethritis.

1. Chlamydia trachomatis

C. trachomatis infection is usually associated with a spontaneous or a "milked" urethral discharge. Urethral discharge and leukocytosis are most commonly present in the morning, before urination, and are most easily demonstrable at this time. Urethral leukocytosis has been defined as an average of 5 or more polymorphonuclear leukocytes (PMNs) in 5 (1000×) microscopic fields of a Gram-stained urethral smear, or 15 or more PMNs in any of 5 randomly picked (400×) microscopic fields of a centrifuged sediment of a 10-ml sample of first-voided morning urine.

In one large study, cell culture was positive in 80 percent of patients positive for *Chlamydia* antigen by a solid-phase immunoassay. The immunoassay was negative in 14 percent of those positive by cell culture. Up to 90 percent of patients with detected antigen and a negative culture probably had *C. trachomatis* infection, and required treatment with doxycycline or erythromycin.

Fluorescent monoclonal antibodies may also be used to detect chlamydial elementary bodies on a urethral smear. The sensitivity of antigen detection tests varies with the intensity of the inflammatory reaction in the urethra. Male sensitivities for the IDEIA test (Boots Celltech) varied from a low of 68 percent to 83 percent (e.g., in males with more than 20 leukocytes per field in the sediment of the first-voided morning urine). Chlamydial infection responds to 7 days of tetracycline, doxycycline, or erythromycin.

2. Ureaplasma urealyticum

This T-strain mycoplasma may be isolated from the urethra in 50 to 70 percent of asymptomatic sexually active men. Evidence of a role of *U. urealyticum* as a cause of nongonococcal, nonchlamydial urethritis includes the following: (1) *U. urealyticum* is present in large numbers (i.e., more than 10^4 colony-forming units in urethral discharges from men with chlamydia-negative nongonococcal urethritis. (2) Selective therapeutic studies in patients with chlamydia-negative nongonococcal urethritis demonstrate that *U. urealyticum*–positive patients respond to spectinomycin (an antibiotic active against *U. urealyticum*) and not to drugs with low activity against *U. urealyticum* (e.g., rifampin or sulfonamides). Resolution of urethral infections associated with conversion of positive *U. urealyticum* cultures to negative also supports a role for *U. urealyticum*. (3) Urethral inoculation of ureaplasmas into human volunteers has caused urethritis. (4) A serologic response to *U. urealyticum*, with broad serotype specificity, has been detected by an ELISA test in 67 percent of nongonococcal nonchlamydial urethritis patients.

Up to 30 percent of cases of nongonococcal urethritis are associated with *U. urealyticum* infection.

3. Mycoplasma hominis A role for this organism as a cause of nongonococcal urethritis has also been suggested, but the frequency of isolation from cases of nongonococcal urethritis is low. It has been isolated in high concentrations in patients with urethritis and a high titer culture of *Ureaplasma urealyticum*. Its role as a cause of urethritis remains unsettled.

4. *Nongonococcal Urethritis of Unknown Cause* *Chlamydia trachomatis* and *Ureaplasma urealyticum* are not isolated from urethral infections in up to 20 percent of heterosexual men and most homosexual men. The cause of urethritis in these cases is, at present, unknown.

A. mycoplasma genitalium This is a tetracycline-sensitive mycoplasma that has recently been isolated from a small percentage of men with nongonococcal urethritis. It requires a special medium (SP4) for growth.

B. bacteroides species These infections have also been considered as etiologic in a small percentage of cases of nongonococcal urethritis.

C. adenovirus types 19 and 37 These viruses have been isolated from the urethras of men with nongonococcal urethritis in western Australia. The isolation rate was less than 1 percent. Conjunctivitis may be associated with the urethritis. An important role for this virus as a cause of urethritis in the United States is unlikely.

D. haemophilus ducreyi Urethral discharge, dysuria, and a discharge that is culture-positive for *H. ducreyi* may occur in 2 percent of patients with chancroid-positive ulcers. Even in endemic areas, only a small fraction of cases of nongonococcal ure-

thritis are caused by *H. ducreyi*. Asymptomatic urethral carriage of this organism does not usually occur in men with culture-proven chancroidal ulcers.

Up to 20 percent of cases of acute urethritis are of unknown etiology, but may be doxycycline- and/or erythromycin-responsive.

3. OTHER CAUSES OF ACUTE URETHRAL PAIN

A. Acute Bacterial Prostatitis There is an abrupt onset of chills, rigors, and fever associated with low back and perineal pain. Burning urethral pain occurs during and after voiding and may persist for hours. Small, frequent voidings may occur, and severe, sharp suprapubic and penile pain may occur in association with repeatedly interrupted voiding (stuttering urination), because of bladder neck inflammation and spasm. This sharp pain in association with stuttering urination has been called *strangury*.

Rectal examination reveals an enlarged, tender, boggy prostate. In some cases it may be firm and indurated. Prostatic secretions are filled with single and clumped polymorphonuclear leukocytes. Cultures reveal the causative bacteria. There is a good response to parenteral or oral antibiotic therapy.

B. Prostatic Abscess This disorder is usually a complication of acute bacterial prostatitis. Urinary retention or frequency, and burning penile pain during and after urination, occur in up to 49 percent of cases. Fever occurs in only 41 percent. An associated epididymo-orchitis may occur (24 percent), as may rectal pain (14 percent).

Fluctuance of a prostatic lobe, with associated tenderness, is suggestive of an abscess. Another clue is failure of fever and prostatic symptoms to respond to antibiotic therapy. The diagnosis can be confirmed by CT scan or transrectal ultrasonography. The abscess may rupture into the urethra (6 percent). It is preferable to confirm the diagnosis prior to spontaneous rupture, and drain the abscess surgically.

C. Acute Bacterial Cystitis Symptoms include frequency, urgency, suprapubic aching, low back pain, nocturia, and burning penile pain during and after urination. Gross hematuria may occur occasionally, but fever, chills, rigors, and flank pain do not. Tenderness may be present in the suprapubic area. A midstream urine sample contains polymorphonuclear leukocytes, singly and in clumps, but no leukocyte casts. Gram stain reveals the causative bacterium in large numbers. Urine culture reveals more than 10,000 bacteria per ml of urine. There is usually a prompt response to antibiotic therapy; a short course of 3 to 7 days of treatment is usually effective. The relapse rate is minimal.

D. Acute Pyelonephritis This disorder usually presents with high fever, chills, rigors, upper abdominal pain, and flank pain, with radiation of pain into the ipsilateral mid- and lower abdomen. There is usually frequency, urgency, and penile pain on voiding. This may persist for minutes or hours after urination. There is costovertebral angle, abdominal, and, sometimes, suprapubic tenderness. The urine contains polymorphonuclear leukocytes, singly, in clumps, and in leukocyte casts; red blood cells; and bacteria. There is a good response to antibiotic therapy.

E. Pseudocystitis Due to Carcinoma in situ Penile urethral pain of a burning quality occurs on voiding and for minutes or hours afterward. This discomfort is associated with urinary frequency and urgency, mimicking a bacterial cystitis. The urine may contain erythrocytes, some leukocytes, and many atypical epithelial cells. Gram stains of the urinary sediment and urine cultures are usually negative. Urine cytologic studies identify malignant cells. Cystoscopic biopsy of portions of the bladder mucosa containing Brunn's nests (yellow, comedo-like areas of the mucosa) confirms the diagnosis. Localization of in-situ carcinoma to the urethra causes edema of the surrounding connective tissue stroma and is the cause of severe penile pain during and after voiding. This disorder may be mistaken for idiopathic interstitial cystitis, tuberculosis, and schistosomiasis of the bladder.

F. Urethral Calculi Urethral calculi consist of bladder or renal stones that become impacted in the urethra on their way to the outside. Rarely, urethral stones arise at a stricture or in a diverticulum of the urethra.

Symptoms include sudden stoppage of urine flow during voiding, or dribbling or stuttering urination due to partial obstruction. Dysuria may be severe and radiate into the glans penis. A stone localized to the anterior urethra will cause local shaft or glans pain; the patient may sometimes be able to palpate the stone. Palpation of the penis and perineum or prostate by the physician will usually detect the causative stone. The urine may contain erythrocytes and leukocytes. The diagnosis can be confirmed by radiography (i.e., retrograde urethrography) and/or panendoscopy. Stones less than 10 mm in diameter usually pass spontaneously unless a urethral stricture is present. Urethral stones may become lodged in the posterior, bulbous, or penile urethra. Urethral stricture, bladder stones, neurogenic bladder, a urethral diverticulum, and prostatic hypertrophy are frequently associated with urethral stones.

Surgical removal of the impacted urethral stone is required for symptom relief.

G. Urethral Foreign Bodies Foreign bodies are usually introduced into the urethra for erotic purposes during masturbation, or in the course of a drug- or alcohol-induced state of confusion.

Possible symptoms include frequency, dysuria, nocturia, hematuria, urethral bleeding and pain, partially obstructed voiding, and complete urinary obstruction. Foreign bodies found in the urethra have included a rifle bullet, a crystal highball stirrer, needles, surgical instruments, a squirrel tail, a decapitated snake, a fish, a fishhook on a string, pins, paper clips, pencils, pens, metal screws, parts of plastic spoons, a bedspring, and paint chips. Foreign body insertion into the urethra was used by prisoners at a maximum security hospital for the criminally insane, as a form of self-mutilation. Removal of the intraurethral foreign body and initiation of antibiotic therapy is required for relief of symptoms.

4. PENILE TRAUMA

A. Penile Fracture Due to Blunt Trauma This injury occurs only when the penis is erect. There is an abrupt onset, on penile bending during intercourse, of severe penile pain, accompanied by an audible popping or cracking sound. There is immediate detumescence; swelling and blue-black discoloration over one or both corpora cavernosa; and penile distortion.

Other, noncoital, causes include bending of the erect penis when rolling over in bed, kneading when trying to cause detumescence, and falling onto objects from a height.

The penis is deviated to the side opposite the injury; an associated tear in Buck's fascia may result in a large scrotal hematoma. Urethral rupture with urinary extravasation may occur in up to 33 percent of cases. These patients may have blood at the meatus and/or gross hematuria. A periurethral hematoma and angulation of the penis may cause urinary retention. A urethrogram should be done to exclude urethral injury. Cavernosography will detect a tear in the tunica albuginea. Patients without a demonstrable tear can be treated conservatively. Those with a rent require surgical evacuation of the hematoma, repair of the tear in the tunica albuginea, and urethral catheter drainage.

Sequelae may include penile deformity and decreased erectile firmness, leading to difficulty during intercourse. These complications can be prevented by immediate surgical repair.

B. Gunshot Wound A penetrating injury to the penis causes a cylindrical defect in the skin and corpora, and sometimes disrupts the urethra. There is local pain, tenderness, and bleeding. Surgical debridement and repair are required.

C. Genital Skin Loss

1. Avulsion Injuries Avulsion injuries of the penis may result in degloving of the penile shaft, with pain and bleeding. These injuries may occur in motor vehicle and pedestrian accidents and in falls, or by engulfment of the penis by a rotatory machine. Autostimulation with a vacuum cleaner or an electric broom may cause lacerations, avulsion of the glans, edema, ecchymoses, and/or degloving of the skin of the penis. Severe injury can cause a residual urethral stricture and penile deformity. These injuries result from placing the penis in a vacuum cleaner hose or in the body of the vacuum cleaner. Some psychotic patients have performed self-penectomy. Prompt and skilled surgery has resulted in successful reattachment.

D. Urethral Injuries

1. Anterior (Penile) Urethra   Rupture and/or perforation of the urethra below the urogenital diaphragm may result from catheterization or other iatrogenic causes, a gunshot, a fall-astride injury, a direct blow to the perineum, insertion of foreign bodies for erotic stimulation, a human bite during fellatio, or penile fracture during intercourse. If the anterior urethra ruptures and the escaping urine and blood are confined by Buck's fascia, there is severe, painful swelling and discoloration of the shaft of the penis. Rupture through Buck's fascia leads to bleeding and urinary extravasation into the anterior abdominal wall, perineum, and scrotum in addition to penile swelling. A butterfly hematoma (blue-black discoloration of both buttocks inferomedially) and hemorrhagic discoloration, swelling, and fullness of the scrotum may be present. Immediate surgical repair and suprapubic cystotomy are required.

2. Posterior Urethra   Rupture of the urethra superior to the urogenital diaphragm causes blood to appear at the meatus; it also causes difficulty in voiding, or inability to void. Perineal swelling during or after voiding represents urinary extravasation.

Examination may reveal blood at the meatus. Rupture of the urethra may result in inability to void. The glans and shaft of the penis appear normal. Rectal examination may reveal a high-riding or free-floating prostate and/or a diffuse bogginess anterior to the rectum. Urinalysis reveals gross or microscopic hematuria. A retrograde urethrogram will localize the site of urethral injury. Catheterization is to be avoided prior to urethrography, since it can convert a partial rupture into a complete one. Urethral rupture above the urogenital diaphragm frequently occurs in association with pelvic fractures suffered in motor vehicle accidents.

Partial urethral injuries that permit voiding are associated with dysuria and gross or microscopic hematuria.

Complete ruptures of the urethra superior to the urogenital diaphragm may be managed by a suprapubic cystotomy or by drainage of the pelvic hematoma and urethral realignment over a fenestrated catheter held in place by traction.

5. PAINFUL ERECTION

A. Peyronie's Disease (Idiopathic)   Penile pain and curvature occur with an erection. The pain is relieved by detumescence. Erectile impotence may occur, or penile curvature may be so severe that it interferes with entry into the vagina. A firm, circumscribed plaque is palpable on the dorsum of the shaft. The length of the plaque averages 3 cm and the width 1.4 cm. Downward curvature is uncommon (6 percent), while dorsal or dorsolateral deviation occurs in 67 percent of cases. Pain provoked by erection occurs in up to 65 percent. Plaque tenderness may be present. Patients with severe forms of this disorder are unable to have intercourse because of penile curvature or impotence. Erectile impotence has been shown to be due to abnormal drainage of blood from the corpora cavernosa because of insufficient venous closure. Dynamic ^{133}Xe washout from the corpora cavernosa and dynamic infusion cavernosography have demonstrated abnormal drainage of the corpora cavernosa in 87 percent of patients with Peyronie's disease and erectile impotence. The plaque somehow causes failure of venous closure, allowing detumescence.

Ultrasonography of the penis may disclose plaques that are missed by palpation (e.g., at the root of the shaft or in the midline septum). Calcified plaques are detected easily as hyperechoic lesions with clear acoustic shadowing. Sonography can differentiate recently formed lesions from end-stage calcified plaques. The latter are best treated by surgery. Similarly, CT scans of the penis may detect lesions missed by palpation and may differentiate early from advanced lesions. CT may be used to follow lesion progression. Usually, each plaque is seen to be larger on CT than it has appeared on clinical examination.

Surgical excision of plaques that are causing pain and interfering with coitus may provide symptomatic relief. Dermal grafts may have to be used to replace the excised tissue.

B. Peyronie's Disease and Other Disorders   Peyronie's disease has been associated with Dupuytren's contracture (10 percent of cases), Ledderhose's (i.e., thickening of the plantar aponeuroses), and Weber-Christian disease, systemic sclerosis, and rheumatoid arthritis.

C. Mimics of Peyronie's Disease

1. Thrombophlebitis of the Dorsal Vein of the Penis   This disorder may present with a painful and tender bluish linear plaque-like area beneath the skin on the dorsum of the penis. Vigorous sexual intercourse or masturbation may be the cause, but a case has been reported in association with pancreatic carcinoma; in that patient, migratory phlebitis involving the arm was also present. Tumors frequently associated with migratory phlebitis include lung, pancreatic, and gastric carcinomas.

Table 34-1
CAUSES OF PRIAPISM

Hematologic disorders
  Sickle cell disease or trait
  Nonspherocytic hemolytic anemia
  Chronic leukemia
  Myeloma and amyloidosis
  Congenital protein C deficiency
  Polycythemia
  Macroglobulinemia
Neoplastic disorders
  Metastatic carcinoma from bladder, prostate, kidney, or
    colorectum
Behçet's disease
Neurologic disorders
  Spinal cord injury
  Wilson's disease
  Tuberous sclerosis
  Cerebral infarction
  Central nervous system neoplasms
Drug-associated
  Antidepressants (trazodone)
  Antipsychotics (phenothiazines, butyrophenones)
  Antihypertensives (prazosin, hydralazine, guanethidine, labetalol)
  Cocaine
  Alcohol and marijuana
  Testosterone
  Discontinuance of heparin
  Warfarin therapy
  Intracavernous papaverine/phentolamine injections
  Adrenal corticosteroids
  Psychedelic street drugs
  General anesthesia
  Hyperalimentation (fat emulsions)
  Diazepam
Infections
  Rocky Mountain spotted fever
  Tularemia
  Brucellosis
  Rabies
  Mumps orchitis
  Local penile or pelvic abscesses
Renal failure
High flow (arterial priapism) secondary to intracavernosal arterial
    injury caused by:
  Trauma
  Injection therapy for impotence
Idiopathic priapism associated with:
  Excessive sexual activity
  Diabetes mellitus
  Rheumatoid arthritis
  Coagulopathies
  Familial
  Nonischemic high-flow priapism

2. Penile Sarcoma Early lesions may rarely present with subcutaneous induration of the penis mimicking Peyronie's disease. The diagnosis can be confirmed by biopsy.

3. Fibrotic Plaques from Prior Surgery or Trauma A fibrotic plaque on the lateral aspect of the shaft may result from penile fracture caused by blunt trauma. This may cause mild-to-moderate curvature of the penis to the side opposite the plaque. Scarring resulting from penile surgery may have a similar effect.

D. Priapism Priapism is a prolonged and often painful erection not caused by sexual arousal. The most common type is veno-occlusive in origin (i.e., a low-outflow disorder). Both corpora cavernosa are rigid, while the glans is usually soft. The erection does not subside with orgasm or a cold shower. The causes of painful priapism are discussed below and listed in Table 34-1. High-flow, or external, priapism is rare, and usually results from laceration of an intracavernosal artery secondary to trauma.

1. Hematologic Disorders

A. SICKLE CELL DISEASE AND SICKLE CELL TRAIT The venous outflow from the corpora may become obstructed by sticky and viscous blood containing sickle cells. Priapism may occur in short, stuttering episodes lasting 2 to 6 h that resolve with simple measures and do not usually lead to impotence. A major attack of priapism lasting over 24 h causes clotting in the vascular spaces of the corpora and eventual fibrous obliteration of these bodies. Sickle cell trait is less commonly associated with priapism. Treatments that have been effective in patients with sickle cell–related priapism include aspiration of blood from the corpora and irrigation of these bodies with dilute epinephrine and/or exchange transfusion. Failure of these measures requires surgical creation of a cavernosum-spongiosum shunt. Early intervention with an exchange transfusion and/or epinephrine irrigation may preserve potency. Erectile function is frequently lost after prolonged episodes of priapism, despite all therapeutic measures. Nonspherocytic hemolytic anemia has also been associated with priapism.

B. CHRONIC LEUKEMIA Patients with very high leukocyte counts (i.e., greater than 100,000 cells per mm^3.) are at risk. The leukocytes may obstruct venous outflow from the corpora, resulting in priapism.

C. MYELOMA AND AMYLOIDOSIS These disorders have also been associated with priapism.

D. CONGENITAL PROTEIN C DEFICIENCY Patients with protein C deficiency suffer from repeated episodes of venous thrombosis and embolism. Iliofemoral, mesenteric, renal, and intracerebral veins may be involved. Priapism may result from occlusive disease involving the corpora cavernosa.

E. POLYCYTHEMIA This disorder may be associated with priapism secondary to increased blood viscosity.

F. MACROGLOBULINEMIA This disorder has been reported to be associated with priapism.

2. Neoplastic Disorders   Metastatic carcinoma arising in the bladder or prostate can cause severe penile pain and/or painful priapism. (Priapism occurs in 40 percent of cases of penile metastasis.) Induration of the shaft and/or subcutaneous penile nodules may be palpable. Cavernosography or a CT scan of the penis can identify the intracavernous neoplasm, and fine-needle or open biopsy can be used to confirm the diagnosis. In a series of 218 cases of penile metastasis, the primary tumor arose in the bladder in 30 percent, in the prostate in 30 percent, in the kidney in 11 percent, and in the rectosigmoid in 16 percent.

3. Behçet's Disease   This disease may cause recurrent bouts of thrombophlebitis, usually involving the legs. A case of Behçet's syndrome with painful priapism secondary to thrombophlebitis of the corpora cavernosa has been reported. Oral aphthous ulcers; iritis or iridocyclitis; genital ulcers; skin pathergy; and erythema nodosum are other frequent components of this disease.

4. Neurologic Disorders

   A. SPINAL CORD INJURY   Priapism may occur as a symptom of cervical spinal cord injury in association with a myotome-level motor loss, and dermatome-level sensory loss. There may be inability to extend the elbows, with preservation of elbow flexion; generalized muscular flaccidity and areflexia; a patulous anal sphincter; diaphragmatic breathing; and spinal shock. The priapism is not painful, because of sensory interruption above the sacral segments.

   B. WILSON'S DISEASE   Truncal myoclonus and tremors, in association with recurrent priapism and spontaneous seminal ejaculation, have been reported in a patient with Wilson's disease. D-penicillamine therapy caused resolution of all symptoms within 6 months.

   C. OTHER NEUROLOGIC DISORDERS   Priapism has been associated with tuberous sclerosis, cerebral infarction, and central nervous system tumors.

5. Drug-Related Priapism   Drugs with vasodilator activity or with α-adrenergic blocking activity have been reported to produce both painful and nonpainful priapism. These episodes have been reversed pharmacologically using intra-cavernous injections of epinephrine, norepinephrine, metaraminol, or oral terbutaline. Drugs reported to cause priapism include the following:

   A. ANTIDEPRESSANTS   Trazodone has α-adrenergic receptor and serotonin blocking activity. Priapism can be treated by aspiration of blood and irrigation of the corpora with epinephrine or norepinephrine. Shunt surgery may be required for relief; impotence may follow.

   B. ANTIPSYCHOTICS   Phenothiazines, such as thioridazine and chlorpromazine, and butyrophenones have been associated with painful priapism due to their α-adrenergic blocking activity. Terbutaline therapy may alleviate phenothiazine-induced priapism.

   C. ANTIHYPERTENSIVES   Prazosin, hydralazine, guanethidine, and labetalol have been associated with priapism. Prazosin has central and peripheral α-adrenergic blocking activity. Intracorporal injection of epinephrine, metaraminol, or phenylephrine is often effective in relieving priapism due to prazosin. Shunt surgery may be required if pharmacologic intervention is unsuccessful.

   D. COCAINE (TOPICAL APPLICATION OR NASAL INSTILLATION)   Priapism related to the use of cocaine topically on the penis may respond to aspiration of blood from the corpora cavernosa and epinephrine irrigations; but shunting may be required to prevent impotence. Intranasal cocaine abuse has also been associated with painful erection (one reported case); corpora cavernosa-to-spongiosum shunting was required for relief after failure of corporeal irrigation with epinephrine.

   E. ALCOHOL AND MARIJUANA   Alcohol and marijuana abuse may cause priapism.

   F. TESTOSTERONE INJECTIONS   Testosterone injections for delayed male puberty have been associated with painful priapism.

   G. DISCONTINUANCE OF HEPARIN   This may cause priapism because of rebound hypercoagulability.

   H. INTRACAVERNOUS INJECTION OF PAPAVERINE (WITH OR WITHOUT PHENOTOLAMINE)   This treatment for impotence may occasionally cause priapism, requiring the use of α agonists, such as oral terbutaline or intracavernous epinephrine, to achieve pain relief and detumescence. The incidence of drug-induced priapism is 4 to 9 percent; this can be reduced to 1 percent by avoidance of phentolamine mesylate in the first three injections, and the use of gradual increments of papavarine dosages in high-risk patients (i.e., those with a penile-to-brachial blood pressure ratio higher than 0.7 and a good response to visual sexual stimulation). Patients with paraplegia- and multiple sclerosis–related impotence are more prone to develop priapism after therapy.

   I. ADRENAL CORTICOSTEROIDS

   J. PSYCHEDELIC STREET DRUGS

   K. GENERAL ANESTHESIA

   L. HYPERALIMENTATION WITH FAT EMULSIONS

   M. DIAZEPAM

6. Infectious Diseases Rare occurrences of priapism have been reported in Rocky Mountain spotted fever, tularemia, brucellosis, rabies, mumps, and orchitis, and with local penile or pelvic abscess.

7. Renal Failure Renal failure, with or without hemodialysis therapy, may be associated with priapism. The mechanism is unknown.

8. Trauma to the Penis and Perineum (High-Flow Arterial Priapism) Trauma to the perineum (e.g., straddle injury) may cause perineal pain and painless priapism. Doppler studies may reveal strong corporal arterial pulsations. Corporeal aspiration reveals bright red blood. Selective internal pudendal arteriography reveals a cavernosal arterial blush due to laceration of an artery. Clot embolization of this artery relieves the priapism and preserves potency.

A similar type of high-output priapism secondary to intracavernosal arterial laceration may result from injection therapy for impotence; this can be managed by clot embolization. Arterial priapism occurring after injection therapy should be suspected if the erection is painless, there is good blood flow (i.e., the aspirated blood is bright red), and adrenoreceptor irrigation therapy fails. ^{99m}Tc penile scans have also been used to differentiate high- and low-flow priapism, and may be useful, since the presence of arterial pulsation and bright red aspirate do not rule out veno-occlusive priapism. α-Agonist therapy and shunting are not effective in high-flow priapism.

9. Idiopathic Priapism This group includes all patients without any of the above described associations. Some of these patients have engaged in prolonged and vigorous intercourse or masturbation prior to the onset of their painful sustained erection. Other disorders associated with idiopathic priapism include diabetes mellitus, rheumatoid arthritis, and coagulopathies. In some cases, excessive sexual activity may have provoked priapism in patients taking a priapism-associated drug or having a priapism-associated disorder (e.g., sickle cell anemia or leukemia). Idiopathic priapism is usually of the low-flow veno-occlusive type, and may respond to intracavernosal α-agonist therapy or may require shunting. A rare family with idiopathic priapism has been reported.

10. Nonischemic Idiopathic Priapism Some patients with painful idiopathic priapism have good arterial flow to the corpora (seen on duplex sonography and pulsed Doppler study) accompanied by nonischemic oxygen levels in corpora cavernosa blood. This high-flow disorder is not related to arterial injury. It may respond to intracavernosal α-agonist therapy, or may require shunting to preserve potency. Shunts are usually required in cases presenting long after the onset of the painful erection.

6. GENERALIZED SKIN DISORDERS WITH BALANITIS

A. Toxic Epidermal Necrolysis This disorder begins with patches of confluent erythema and edema of the skin that soon develop into flaccid bullae. There is local pain and tenderness. The conjunctiva, mouth, lips, anorectal region, and penis may be involved. The blisters soon rupture, leaving denuded areas on the skin and mucous membranes. The Nikolsky sign is positive in regions of erythema. Fever and leukocytosis are commonly present. Allergy to sulfonamides, other antibiotics, or phenytoin is frequently causative. Cases have also been reported in association with measles, varicella, herpes zoster, herpes simplex, *Escherichia coli* septicemia, pulmonary aspergillosis, lymphomas, and leukemias. Early administration of corticosteroids, fluid and electrolyte therapy, and thorough local care and protection of the skin increase the chances for recovery.

B. Stevens-Johnson Syndrome This bullous erosive form of erythema multiforme begins with a prodrome of fever, malaise, arthralgias, myalgias, cough, sore throat, chest pain, vomiting, and diarrhea. Bullous lesions then appear over the skin, oral mucosa, lips, and bulbar conjunctivae. Genital involvement may cause a painful, tender balanitis. The inner mucosal surface of the lips may be coated by a grayish-white pseudomembrane, and the vermilion border by hemorrhagic crusts. In most cases this disorder is idiopathic; but some cases are related to herpes simplex virus, *Mycoplasma* or other infections, drug allergy, or other hypersensitivity reactions.

7. LOCAL SKIN DISORDERS

A. Contact Dermatitis Contact dermatitis may involve the penis and scrotum. Local swelling, redness, vesiculation, oozing, and crusting may occur, accompanied by pain, tenderness, and pruritus. Topical anesthetics or antibiotics, poison ivy or poison oak, or chemicals in new unwashed underwear may cause this disorder. Use of local or oral corticosteroids usually leads to resolution within 3 to 10 days.

B. Neurodermatitis (Lichen Simplex Chronicus) This disorder may arise from chronic scratching. The resultant dermatitis consists of red, edematous skin, with ulceration and crusting involving the penis and/or scrotum. The clinical appearance is difficult to distinguish from that of contact dermatitis.

8. PENILE AND PERINEAL INFECTIONS

A. Periurethral Abscess This disorder presents with local perineal (posterior urethral) or penile (anterior urethral) pain, tenderness, and fluctuant swelling. Dysuria may be present. Some abscesses occur in the vicinity of a urethral stricture; these are usually located in the perineum. Gonococcal urethritis, with a purulent discharge and dysuria, may precede the onset of a painful fluctuant mass in the ventral portion of the penile shaft (*gonococcal periurethral abscess*). Drainage and antibiotic therapy relieve symptoms. Spontaneous rupture of a periurethral abscess because of delay in treatment may lead to urine leakage through a urethrocutaneous perineal or penile fistula during micturition.

B. Necrotizing Fasciitis of the Scrotum, Penis, and Perineum Penile, perineal, and scrotal pain, erythema, swelling, and diffuse tenderness occur. The edematous skin of the painful region becomes indurated and then blackened, indicating skin necrosis. Subcutaneous crepitus due to gas-producing bacteria may be present adjacent to the area of discoloration. Chills, rigors, fever, and leukocytosis are usually present. Progression of the necrotizing process leads to blackening and induration of the scrotum, perineum, and penis. Sloughing and surgical debridement leave the penis and testicles bare, as though they were dissected-out for an anatomy demonstration. There may be severe-to-excruciating perineal, scrotal, and penile pain. This disease may arise from a perirectal or periurethral abscess, a minor local laceration, anorectal surgery, or a burn. Cultures of the exudate reveal a polymicrobial synergistic infection with *Escherichia coli,* a

Bacteroides species, and streptococci. Extensive debridement and broad-spectrum antibiotic therapy offer the best opportunity for survival.

9. REFERRED PAIN

A. Anorectal Disorders Rarely, anorectal lesions, such as fissures, carcinoma, proctitis, or ulcerations, may cause penile, as well as anorectal, pain. The genital pain is ameliorated by treatment of the anorectal disorder.

B. Acute Appendicitis Epigastric or periumbilical pain, followed by right lower abdominal pain, is a typical presentation. Some cases develop scrotal or penile pain. Nausea, vomiting, and low-grade fever may also occur. All symptoms resolve with appendectomy.

10. PSYCHOGENIC PAIN

Some patients present with penile pain with no visible lesions, no evidence of urethritis, and no abnormality on penile palpation. There is no tenderness. Very often there is fear of sexually transmitted disease because of an extramarital activity, or fear of malignancy. These patients respond to careful examination followed by reassurance. The role of herpes-related neuropathic pain in some of these cases is unclear, since herpetic lesions may be so small as to go unnoticed. Recurrent neuropathic pain may occur in the absence of herpetic lesions.

PENILE PAIN REFERENCES

Balanitis

Alinovi A, Barella PA, Benoldi D: Erosive lichen planus involving the glans penis alone. *Int J Dermatol* 22(1):37–38, 1983.

Baldwin HE, Geronemus RG: The treatment of Zoon's balanitis with the carbon dioxide laser. *J Dermatol Surg Oncol* 15:491–494, 1989.

Bale PM, Lochhead A, Martin HCO, et al: Balanitis xerotica obliterans in children. *Pediatr Pathol* 7:617–627, 1987.

Bargman H: Pseudoepitheliomatous, keratotic, and micaceous balanitis. *Cutis* 35(1):77–79, 1985.

Beljaards RC, Van Dijk E, Hausman R: Is pseudoepitheliomatous, micaceous and keratotic balanitis synonymous with verrucous carcinoma? *Br J Dermatol* 117:641–646, 1987.

Castle WN, Wentzell JM, Schwartz BK, et al: Chronic balanitis owing to pemphigus vegetans. *J Urol* 137(2):289–291, 1987.

Chanda JJ: Extramammary Paget's disease: Prognosis and relationship to internal malignancy. *J Am Acad Dermatol* 13:1009–1014, 1985.

Dodds PR, Chi T-N: Balanitis as a fixed drug eruption to tetracycline. *J Urol* 133(6):1044–1045, 1985.

Escala JM, Rickwood AMK: Balanitis. *Br J Urol* 63:196–197, 1989.

Ferrándiz C, Ribera M: Zoon's balanitis treated by circumcision. *J Dermatol Surg Oncol* 10:622–625, 1984.

Ganti SU, Sayegh N, Addonizio JC: Simple method for reduction of paraphimosis. *Urology* 25(1):77, 1985.

Gray MR, Ansell ID: Pseudo-epitheliomatous hyperkeratotic and micaceous balanitis: Evidence for regarding it as pre-malignant. *Br J Urol* 66(1):103–104, 1990.

Horan DB, Redman JF, Jansen GT: Papulosquamous lesions of glans penis. *Urology* 23(1):1–4, 1984.

Irvine C, Anderson JR, Pye RJ: Micaceous and keratotic pseudoepitheliomatous balanitis and rapidly fatal fibrosarcoma of the penis occurring in the same patient. *Br J Dermatol* 116:719–725, 1987.

Jamieson NV, Bullock KN, Barker THW: Adenosquamous carcinoma of the penis associated with balanitis xerotica obliterans. *Br J Urol* 58(6):730–731, 1986.

Jenkins D Jr, Jakubovic HR: Pseudoepitheliomatous, keratotic, micaceous balanitis. *J Am Acad Dermatol* 18:419–422, 1988.

Kossard S, Shumack S: Lichen aureus of the glans penis as an expression of Zoon's balanitis. *J Am Acad Dermatol* 21(4, part 1):804–806, 1989.

Lucks DA, Venezio FR, Lakin CM: Balanitis caused by group B streptococcus. *J Urol* 135(5):1015, 1986.

Morrissey R, Xavier A, Nguyen N, et al: Invasive candidal balanitis due to a condom catheter in a neutropenic patient. *South Med J* 78(10):1247–1249, 1985.

Murray WJG, Fletcher MS, Yates-Bell AJ, et al: Plasma cell balinitis of Zoon. *Br J Urol* 58:689–691, 1986.

Neuhofer J, Fritsch P: Treatment of localized scleroderma and lichen sclerosus with etretinate. *Acta Derm Venereol (Stockh)* 64:171–174, 1984.

Nishimura M, Matsuda T, Muto M, et al: Balanitis of Zoon. *Int J Dermatol* 29(6):421–423, 1990.

Rosenberg SK: Carbon dioxide laser treatment of external genital lesions. *Urology* 25(6):555–558, 1985.

Tompkins KJ, James WD: Persistent bullae on the penis of an elderly man. *Arch Dermatol* 123(10):1394–1395, 1987.

Zungri E, Chéchile G, Algaba F, et al: Balanitis xerotica obliterans: Surgical treatment. *Eur Urol* 14:160–162, 1988.

Behçet's Syndrome

Fairley C, Wilson JW, Barraclough D: Pulmonary involvement in Behçet's syndrome. *Chest* 96:1428–1429, 1989.

Feagin OT: Behçet's disease: The Ochsner experience, 1979 to 1982. *South Med J* 77(4):442–446, 1984.

Bladder Stones

Ashworth M, Hill SM: Endemic bladder stones in Nepal. *Arch Dis Child* 63(12):1503–1505, 1988.

DiTonno F, Forte M, Guidoni E, et al: A giant bladder stone. *Br J Urol* 62(1):90–91, 1988.

Krawitt DR, Addonizio JC: Ultrasonic aspiration of prostate, bladder tumors, and stones. *Urology* 30(6):579–580, 1987.

Lewi HJE, White A, Abel BJ, et al: Fused vesical calculi. *Urology* 30(3):267–268, 1987.

Lopez JR, Jenkins CE, Millares M: Irrigating solutions in bladder stone dissolution. *Drug Intell Clin Pharm* 21:872–874, 1987.

Schnall RI, Baer HM, Seidmon EJ: Endoscopy for removal of unusual foreign bodies in urethra and bladder. *Urology* 34(1):33–35, 1989.

Srivastava RN, Hussainy MAA, Goel RG, et al: Bladder stone disease in children in Afghanistan. *Br J Urol* 58:374–377, 1986.

Thomas PL: Haematuria, running, bladder stone (letter to editor). *Br J Sports Med* 19(1):49, 1985.

Yip YL, Tin H: Electrohydraulic lithotripsy of bladder stones: A Hong Kong experience. *Br J Urol* 62:148–149, 1988.

Zhaowu Z, Xiwen W, Fenling Z: Experience with electrohydraulic shockwave lithotripsy in the treatment of vesical calculi. *Br J Urol* 61:498–499, 1988.

Carcinoma—Penis

Abdennader S, Lessana-Leibowitch M, Pelisse M: An atypical case of penile carcinoma in situ associated with human papillomavirus DNA type 18. *J Am Acad Dermatol* 20:887–889, 1989.

Bandieramonte G, Lepera P, Marchesini R, et al: Laser microsurgery for superficial lesions of the penis. *J Urol* 138(2):315–319, 1987.

Bandieramonte G, Santoro O, Boracchi P, et al: Total resection of glans penis surface by CO_2 laser microsurgery. *Acta Oncol* 27(5):575–578, 1988.

Bissada NK: Post-circumcision carcinoma of the penis: 2. Surgical management. *J Surg Oncol* 37:80–83, 1988.

Bissada NK, Morcos RR, El-Senoussi M: Post-circumcision carcinoma of the penis: 1. Clinical aspects. *J Urol* 135(2):283–285, 1986.

Blatstein LM, Finkelstein LH: Laser surgery for the treatment of squamous cell carcinoma of the penis. *J Am Osteopath Assoc* 90(4):338–344, 1990.

Fraley EE, Zhang G, Sazama R, et al: Cancer of the penis: Prognosis and treatment plans. *Cancer* 55:1618–1624, 1985.

Goldminz D, Scott G, Klaus S: Penile basal cell carcinoma: Report of a case and review of the literature. *J Am Acad Dermatol* 20:1094–1097, 1989.

Johnson DE, Lo RK, Srigley J, et al: Verrucous carcinoma of the penis. *J Urol* 133(2):261–268, 1985.

Kearsley JH, Roberts SJ, Kynaston B: Curative radiotherapy for stage IV carcinoma of the penis. *Med J Aust* 145(9):474–475, 1986.

Löning T, Riviere A, Henke R-P, et al: Penile/anal condylomas and squamous cell cancer: A HPV DNA hybridization study. *Virchows Arch [A]* 413:491–498, 1988.

McKee PH, Lowe D, Haigh RJ: Penile verrucous carcinoma. *Histopathology* 7:897–906, 1983.

Onuigbo WIB: Carcinoma of skin of penis. *Br J Urol* 57:465–466, 1985.

Persky L, deKernion J: Carcinoma of the penis. *CA* 36(5):258–273, 1986.

Rothenberger KH: Value of the neodymium-YAG laser in the therapy of penile carcinoma. *Eur Urol* 12(suppl 1):34–36, 1986.

Srinivas V, Khan SA: Penile carcinoma. *Hosp Pract* 20(1):154–155, 158–159, 1985.

Stern RS, and members of the photochemotherapy follow-up study: Genital tumors among men with psoriasis exposed to psoralens and ultraviolet A radiation (PUVA) and ultraviolet B radiation. *N Engl J Med* 322(16):1093–1097, 1990.

Sulaiman MZC, Polacarz SV, Partington PE: Basal cell carcinoma of penis: Case report. *Genitourin Med* 64:128–129, 1988.

Ejaculation Pain

Edwards IS, Errey B: Pain on ejaculation after vasectomy. *Br Med J* 284(6330):1710, 1982.

Karamcheti A, Berg G: Seminal vesicle cyst associated with ipsilateral renal agenesis. *Urology* 12(5):572–574, 1978.

Lucon AM, Nahas WC, Wroclawski ER, et al: Congenital cyst of the seminal vesicle. *Eur Urol* 9:362–363, 1983.

Miller HC: Stress prostatitis. *Urology* 32(6):507–510, 1988.

Erectile Pain—Peyronie's Disease

Devine CJ Jr, Horton CE: Peyronie's disease. *Clin Plast Surg* 15(3):405–409, 1988.

Gingell JC, Desai KM: Peyronie's disease. *Br J Urol* 63:223–226, 1989.

Griff LC: Peyronie's disease: The role of radiation therapy and a general review. *Am J Roentgenol Radium Ther Nucl Med* 100(4):916–919, 1967.

Hemal AK, Goswami AK, Sharma SK, et al: Penile venous haemangioma. *Aust N Z J Surg* 59:814–816, 1989.

Hinman F Jr: Etiologic factors in Peyronie's disease. *Urol Int* 35:407–413, 1980.

Horn AS, Pecora A, Chiesa JC, et al: Penile thrombophlebitis as a presenting manifestation of pancreatic carcinoma. *Am J Gastroenterol* 80(6):463–465, 1985.

Horton CE, Devine CJ Jr, McCraw JB, et al: Penile curvatures. *Plast Reconstr Surg* 75(5):752–759, 1985.

Horton CE, Sadove RC, Devine CJ Jr: Peyronie's disease. *Ann Plast Surg* 18(2):122–127, 1987.

Malloy TR, Wein AJ, Carpiniello VL: Advanced Peyronie's disease treated with the inflatable penile prosthesis. *J Urol* 125:327–328, 1981.

Metz P, Ebbehøj J, Uhrenholdt A, et al: Peyronie's disease and erectile failure. *J Urol* 130(6):1103–1104, 1983.

Ordi J, Selva A, Fonollosa V, et al: Peyronie's disease in systemic sclerosis (letter to the editor). *Ann Rheum Dis* 49(2):134–135, 1990.

Rollandi GA, Tentarelli T, Vespier M: Computed tomographic findings in Peyronie's disease. *Urol Radiol* 7:153–156, 1985.

Schiffman ZJ, Gursel EO, Laor E: Use of Dacron patch graft in Peyronie disease. *Urology* 25(1):38–40, 1985.

Strachan JR, Pryor JP: Prostacyclin in the treatment of painful Peyronie's disease. *Br J Urol* 61:516–517, 1988.

Wooldridge WE: Four related fibrosing diseases: When you find one, look for another. *Postgrad Med* 84(2):269–271, 274, 1988.

Erectile Pain—Priapism/Disease-Associated

Douglas L, Fletcher H, Serjeant GR: Penile prostheses in the management of impotence in sickle cell disease. *Br J Urol* 65:533–535, 1990.

Frouws S, Reeders JWAJ, Valcke AAP: Corpus cavernosography. *Diagn Imag* 52:145–153, 1983.

Hashmat AI, Raju S, Singh I, et al: ^{99m}Tc penile scan: An investigative modality in priapism. *Urol Radiol* 11:58–60, 1989.

Lue TF, Hellstrom WJG, McAninch JW, et al: Priapism: A refined approach to diagnosis and treatment. *J Urol* 136(1):104–108, 1986.

Maconochie IK, Scopes JW: Priapism in a 6½-year-old boy with sickle cell disease. *J R Soc Med* 81:606, 1988.

Melissari E, Kakkar VV: Congenital severe protein C deficiency in adults. *Br J Haematol* 72:222–228, 1989.

Moala M, Gabsi M, El Ouakdi M, et al: Behçet disease and priapism. *J Rheumatol* 17(4):570–571, 1990.

Nagler HM, White RdV, Roberts M: Familial idiopathic priapism: A case report. *J Urol* 131(3):542–543, 1984.

Nair KR, Pillai PG: Trunkal myoclonus with spontaneous priapism and seminal ejaculation in Wilson's disease (letter to editor). *J Neurol Neurosurg Psychiatry* 53(2):174, 1990.

Neuwirth H, Frasier B, Cochran ST: Genitourinary imaging and procedures by the emergency physician. *Emerg Med Clin North Am* 7(1):1–28, 1989.

O'Brien WM, O'Connor KP, Lynch JH, et al: Priapism: Current concepts. *Ann Emerg Med* 18:980–983, 1989.

Savion M, Livne PM, Mor C, et al: Mixed carcinoma of the prostate with penile metastases and priapism. *Eur Urol* 13:351–352, 1987.

Sneed RC, Stover SL: Undiagnosed spinal cord injuries in brain-injured children. *Am J Dis Child* 142:965–967, 1988.

Walker TG, Grant PW, Goldstein I, et al: "High-flow" priapism: Treatment with superselective transcatheter embolization. *Radiology* 174:1053–1054, 1990.

Winter CC, McDowell G: Experience with 105 patients with priapism: Update review of all aspects. *J Urol* 140:980–983, 1988.

Witt MA, Goldstein I, Saenz de Tejada I, et al: Traumatic laceration of intracavernosal arteries: The pathophysiology of nonischemic, high flow, arterial priapism. *J Urol* 143:129–132, 1990.

Witters S, Cornelissen M, Vereecken RL: Malignant priapism. *Eur Urol* 11:431–432, 1985.

Erectile Pain—Priapism/Drug-Related

Baños JE, Bosch F: Prazosin-induced priapism (letter to editor). *Br J Urol* 64:205–206, 1989.

Bénard F, Lue TF: Self-administration in the pharmacological treatment of impotence. *Drugs* 39(3):394–398, 1990.

Bilotta JJ, Goldenberg A, Waye JD: Colonoscopic priapism. *Gastrointest Endosc* 35(5):475–476, 1989.

Bullock N: Prazosin-induced priapism. *Br J Urol* 62(5):487–488, 1988.

Burkhalter JL, Morano JU: Partial priapism: The role of CT in its diagnosis. *Radiology* 156:159, 1985.

Carson CC III, Mino RD: Priapism associated with trazodone therapy. *J Urol* 139(2):369–370, 1988.

Fernando IN, Tobias JS: Priapism in patient on tamoxifen (letter to editor). *Lancet* 1(8635):436, 1989.

Fiorelli RL, Manfrey SJ, Belkoff LH, et al: Priapism associated with intranasal cocaine abuse. *J Urol* 143:584–585, 1990.

Fishbain DA: Re: Priapism associated with trazodone therapy (letter to editor). *J Urol* 142(3):831, 1989.

Fouda A, Hassouna M, Beddoe E, et al: Priapism: An avoidable complication of pharmacologically induced erection. *J Urol* 142:995–997, 1989.

Girdley FM, Bruskewitz RC, Feyzi J, et al: Intracavernous self-injection for impotence: A long-term therapeutic option? Experience in 78 patients. *J Urol* 140:972–974, 1988.

Gold DD Jr, Justino JD: "Bicycle kickstand" phenomenon: Prolonged erections associated with antipsychotic agents. *South Med J* 81(6):792–794, 1988.

Halsted DS, Weigel JW, Noble MJ, et al: Re: Papaverine-induced priapism: 2 case reports (letter to editor). *J Urol* 140(2):386, 1988.

Hanno PM, Lopez R, Wein AJ: Trazodone-induced priapism. *Br J Urol* 61:94–100, 1988.

Key LL, Myers MC, Kroovand RL, et al: Priapism following testosterone therapy for delayed puberty. *Am J Dis Child* 143:1001–1002, 1989.

Levine SB, Althof SE, Turner LA, et al: Side effects of self-administration of intracavernous papaverine and phentolamine for the treatment of impotence. *J Urol* 141:54–57, 1989.

Molina L, Bejany D, Lynne CM, et al: Diluted epinephrine solution for the treatment of priapism. *J Urol* 141:1127–1128, 1989.

Mooradian AD, Morley JE, Kaiser FE, et al: Biweekly intracavernous administration of papaverine for erectile dysfunction. *West J Med* 151:515–517, 1989.

Morera A, Estrada AG, Valenciano R: Priapism and neuroleptics: A case report. *Acta Psychiatr Scand* 77:111–112, 1988.

Mouritsen L, Lyngdorf P, Frimodt-Møller C: The intracavernous injection of papaverine as a diagnostic procedure in patients with erectile dysfunction. *Scand J Urol Nephrol* 22:161–163, 1988.

Mueller SC, Lue TF: Evaluation of vasculogenic impotence. *Urol Clin North Am* 15(1):65–76, 1988.

Rodríguez-Blázquez HM, Cardona PE, Rivera-Herrera JL: Priapism associated with the use of topical cocaine. *J Urol* 143:358, 1990.

Ruch W, Jenny P: Priapism following testosterone administration for delayed male puberty (letter to editor). *Am J Med* 86:256, 1989.

Sayer J, Parsons CL: Successful treatment of priapism with intracorporeal epinephrine. *J Urol* 140:827, 1988.

Selby IR, Sugden JC: Priapism and general anaesthesia. *Anaesthesia* 44(12):1016, 1989.

Shantha TR, Finnerty DP, Rodriquez AP: Treatment of persistent penile erection and priapism using terbutaline. *J Urol* 141:1427–1429, 1989.

Siegel S, Streem SB, Steinmuller DR: Prazosin-induced priapism: Pathogenic and therapeutic implications. *Br J Urol* 61:165, 1988.

Simsek U, Ozyurt M: Phenytoin toxicity causing priapism. *Br J Urol* 61:261, 1988.

van Driel MF, Joosten EAHM, Mensink HJA: Intracorporeal self-injection with epinephrine as treatment for idiopathic recurrent priapism. *Eur Urol* 17:95–96, 1990.

Neoplastic Lesions—Metastatic

Dewit L, Ang KK, Van der Schueren E: Acute side effects and late complications after radiotherapy of localized carcinoma of the prostate. *Cancer Treat Rev* 10:79–89, 1983.

Dictor M, Nelson C-E, Uvelius B: Priapism in a patient with endometrioid prostatic carcinoma: A case report. *Urol Int* 43:245–247, 1988.

Finkelstein LH, Manfrey SJ, Arsht DB, et al: Penile metastases from intraductal carcinoma of prostate diagnosed by corpora cavernosa aspiration biopsy. *J Am Osteopath Assoc* 82(8):549–550, 1983.

Gupta NM: Penile metastases from esophageal carcinoma (letter to editor). *Am J Gastroenterol* 84(3):339–340, 1989.

Haddad FS, Kivirand AI: Metastases to the corpora cavernosa from transitional cell carcinoma of the bladder. *J Surg Oncol* 32:19–21, 1986.

Haddad FS, Kovac A, Kivirand A, et al: Cavernosography in diagnosis of penile metastases secondary to bladder cancer. *Urology* 26(6): 585–586, 1985.

Kelleher JP, Ashpole R, Pengelly AW: Penile plaque: A presentation of metastatic renal carcinoma. *Br J Urol* 64:428, 1989.

Mukamel E, Farrer J, Smith RB, et al: Metastatic carcinoma to penis: When is total penectomy indicated? *Urology* 29(1):15–18, 1987.

Powell FC, Venecie PY, Winkelmann RK: Metastatic prostate carcinoma manifesting as penile nodules. *Arch Dermatol* 120:1604–1606, 1984.

Penile Pain—Psychogenic

Schover LR: Psychological factors in men with genital pain. *Cleveland Clin J Med* 57:697–700, 1990.

Penile Pain—Referred

Corder AP. Penile pain and direct inguinal hernia. *Br J Hosp Med* 42(3):238, 1989.

Penile Trauma

Barbagli G, Selli C, Stomaci N, et al: Urethral trauma: Radiological aspects and treatment options. *J Trauma* 27(3):256–261, 1987.

Benson RC Jr: Vacuum cleaner injury to penis: A common urologic problem. *Urology* 25(1):41–44, 1985.

Bertini JE Jr, Corriere JN Jr: The etiology and management of genital injuries. *J Trauma* 28(8):1278–1281, 1988.

Cass AS: Diagnostic studies in bladder rupture: Indications and techniques. *Urol Clin North Am* 16(2):267–273, 1989.

Dierks PR, Hawkins H: Sonography and penile trauma. *J Ultrasound Med* 2:417–419, 1983.

Hricak H, Marotti M, Gilbert TJ, et al: Normal penile anatomy and abnormal penile conditions: Evaluation with MR imaging. *Radiology* 169:683–690, 1988.

Klein FA, Smith MJV, Miller N: Penile fracture: Diagnosis and management. *J Trauma* 25(11):1090–1092, 1985.

McAninch JW, Kahn RI, Jeffrey RB, et al: Major traumatic and septic genital injuries. *J Trauma* 24(4):291–298, 1984.

Sant GR: Rupture of the corpus cavernosum of the penis. *Arch Surg* 116:1176–1178, 1981.

Sonda LP, Wang S: Evaluation of male external genital diseases in the emergency room setting. *Emerg Med Clin North Am* 6(3):473–486, 1988.

Penile Ulcers—Chancroid

Albritton WL: Biology of *Haemophilus ducreyi*. *Microbiol Rev* 53(4):377–389, 1989.

Becker TM, DeWitt W, Van Dusen G: *Haemophilus ducreyi* infection in south Florida: A rare disease on the rise? *South Med J* 80(2):182–184, 1987.

Joyce JP, Waldman PC, Hood AF: Persistent genital ulceration. *Arch Dermatol* 125(4):552, 554–556, 1989.

Mindel A: Chancroid: Epidemics in some developing countries but still rare in Britain. *Br Med J* 298(6666):64–65, 1989.

Ronald AR, Plummer FA: Chancroid and *Haemophilus ducreyi* (editorial). *Ann Intern Med* 102(5):705–707, 1985.

Schalla WO, Sanders LL, Schmid GP, et al: Use of dot-immunobinding and immunofluorescence assays to investigate clinically suspected cases of chancroid. *J Infect Dis* 153(5):879–887, 1986.

Schmid GP: The treatment of chancroid. *JAMA* 255:1757–1762, 1986.

Penile Ulcers—Herpes Simplex

Greenstein A, Matzkin H, Kaver I, et al: Acute urinary retention in herpes genitalis infection: Urodynamic evaluation. *Urology* 31(5):453–456, 1988.

Hassel MH, Lesher JL Jr: Herpes simplex mimicking leukemia cutis. *J Am Acad Dermatol* 21:367–371, 1989.

Kaufman R: Herpes genitalis. *Ala J Med Sci* 23(3):289–292, 1986.

Penile Ulcers—Other Etiologies

Chapel T, Brown WJ, Jeffries C, et al: The microbiological flora of penile ulcerations. *J Infect Dis* 137(1):50–56, 1978.

Penile Ulcers—Syphilis

Al-Egaily S: Gumma of the testis and penis. *Br J Vener Dis* 53:257–259, 1977.

Drusin LM: Syphilis: Clinical manifestations, diagnosis, and treatment. *Urol Clin North Am* 11(1):121–130, 1984.

Fiumara NJ, Exner JH: Primary syphilis following a human bite. *Sex Transm Dis* 8(1):21–22, 1981.

Lundquist CD: A mixed infection of syphilis and chancroid. *J Am Acad Dermatol* 10:354–356, 1984.

Mehta SP: A case of monorecidive syphilitic chancre. *Sex Transm Dis* 8(3):222–223, 1981.

Phimosis

Stenram A, Malmfors G, Okmian L: Circumcision for phimosis: A follow-up study. *Scand J Urol Nephrol* 20:89–92, 1986.

Prostate

Lee F, Torp-Pederson ST, Siders DB: The role of transrectal ultrasound in the early detection of prostate cancer. *CA* 39(6):337–360, 1989.

Recurrent Cystitis

Boon ME, Blomjous CEM, Zwartendijk J, et al: Carcinoma in situ of the urinary bladder: Clinical presentation, cytologic pattern and stromal changes. *Acta Cytol* 30(4):360–366, 1986.

Johnson LW, Heth WL: Infections of the male genitourinary system. *Prim Care* 16(4):929–940, 1989.

Meares EM Jr: Acute and chronic prostatitis: Diagnosis and treatment. *Infect Dis Clin North Am* 1(4):855–873, 1987.

London RL: Diverticulum of the urinary bladder. *Am Fam Physician* 30(4):151–153, 1984.

Stewart C: Prostatitis. *Emerg Med Clin North Am* 6(3):391–402, 1988.

Urethral Lesions

Ahmed S, Morris L: Foreign body urethral calculus 9 years after traumatic perforation of the rectum. *Br J Urol* 57(3):359, 1985.

Ali Khan S, Kaiser CW, Dailey B, et al: Unusual foreign body in the urethra. *Urol Int* 39:184–186, 1984.

Djulepa J, Potempa J: Urethrotomy technique in urethral strictures: 6-year results. *J Urol* 129(5):955–957, 1983.

Frank JD, Pocock RD, Stower MJ: Urethral strictures in childhood. *Br J Urol* 62:590–592, 1988.

Grumet GW: Pathologic masturbation with drastic consequences: Case report. *J Clin Psychiatry* 46:537–539, 1985.

Mahmood SA, Thomas JA: Primary penile urethral carcinoma. *Br J Urol* 58(3):333, 1986.

Palaniswamy R, Bhandari M: Point of focus: Poor genital hygiene and terminal urethral strictures. *Trop Geogr Med* 35:139–143, 1983.

Rada RT, James W: Urethral insertion of foreign bodies: A report of contagious self-mutilation in a maximum-security hospital. *Arch Gen Psychiatry* 39:423–429, 1982.

Ruutu M, Alfthan O, Heikkinen L, et al: Unexpected urethral strictures after short-term catheterization in open-heart surgery. *Scand J Urol Nephrol* 18:9–12, 1984.

Selli C, Barbagli G, Carini M, et al: Treatment of male urethral calculi. *J Urol* 132(1):37–39, 1984.

Urethritis—Gonococcal

Ariyarit C, Panikabutra K, Chitwarakorn A, et al: Efficacy of ofloxacin in uncomplicated gonorrhoea. *Infection* 14(suppl 4):S311–S313, 1986.

Harrison WO: Gonococcal urethritis. *Urol Clin North Am* 11(1):45–53, 1984.

Kim J-H, Choi K-H, Kim Y-T, et al: Treatment of infections due to multiresistant *Neisseria gonorrhoeae* with sulbactam/ampicillin. *Rev Infect Dis* 8(suppl 5):S599–S603, 1986.

Sadof MD, Woods ER, Emans SJ: Dipstick leukocyte esterase activity in first-catch urine specimens: A useful screening test for detecting sexually transmitted disease in the adolescent male. *JAMA* 258:1932–1934, 1987.

Soendjojo A: Gonococcal urethritis due to fellatio. *Sex Transm Dis* 10(1):41–42, 1983.

Tegelberg-Stassen MJAM, van der Hoek JCS, Mooi L, et al: Treatment of uncomplicated gonococcal urethritis in men with two dosages of ciprofloxacin. *Eur J Clin Microbiol* 5(2):244–246, 1986.

Urethritis—Nongonococcal

Charuwichitratrana S, Polnikorn N, Puavilai S, et al: Prevalence of chlamydial infection in patients with gonococcal urethritis. *J Med Assoc Thailand* 72(5):280–283, 1989.

Harnett GB, Phillips PA, Gollow MM: Association of genital adenovirus infection with urethritis in men. *Med J Aust* 141:337–338, 1984.

Holst E, Mårdh P-A, Thelin I: Recovery of anaerobic curved rods and *Gardnerella vaginalis* from the urethra of men, including male heterosexual consorts of female carriers. *Scand J Urol Nephrol Suppl* 86:173–177, 1984.

Ibsen HHW, Møller BR, Halkier-Sørensen L, et al: Treatment of nongonococcal urethritis: Comparison of ofloxacin and erythromycin. *Sex Transm Dis* 16(1):32–35, 1989.

Kaplan JE, Meyer M, Navin J: *Chlamydia trachomatis* infection in a male college student population. *J Am Coll Health* 37(4):159–161, 1989.

Kunimoto DY, Plummer FA, Namaara W, et al: Urethral infection with *Haemophilus ducreyi* in men. *Sex Transm Dis* 15(1):37–39, 1988.

McCormack WM: *Ureaplasma urealyticum*: Ecologic niche and epidermiologic considerations. *Pediatr Infect Dis* 5(6):S232–S233, 1986.

Moi H, Danielsson D: Diagnosis of genital *Chlamydia trachomatis* infection in males by cell culture and antigen detection test. *Eur J Clin Microbiol* 5(5):563–568, 1986.

Taube, OM: *Chlamydia trachomatis* urethritis presenting as hematuria in an adolescent male (letter to editor). *J Adolesc Health Care* 9:505–506, 1988.

Taylor-Robinson D: The male reservoir of *Ureaplasma urealyticum*. *Pediatr Infect Dis* 5(6):S234–S235, 1986.

Taylor-Robinson D: The role of *Mycoplasmas* in non-gonococcal urethritis: A review. *Yale J Biol Med* 56:537–543, 1983.

Taylor-Robinson D, Furr PM, Webster ADB: *Ureaplasma urealyticum* in the immunocompromised host. *Pediatr Infect Dis* 5(6):S236–S238, 1986.

Tjiam KH, van Heijst BYM, van Zuuren A, et al: Evaluation of an enzyme immunoassay for the diagnosis of chlamydial infections in urogenital specimens. *J Clin Microbiol* 23(4):752–754, 1986.

van der Willigen AH, Polak-Vogelzang AA, Habbema L, et al: Clinical efficacy of ciprofloxacin versus doxycycline in the treatment of non-gonococcal urethritis in males. *Eur J Clin Microbiol Infect Dis* 7(5):658–661, 1988.

Veeravahu M, Clay JC: First-catch urine screening for male urethritis. *Lancet* 2(8417–8418):1467, 1984.

CHAPTER

35

Acute Scrotal Pain

☐ **DIAGNOSTIC LIST**

1. Testicular torsion
2. Epididymitis and epididymo-orchitis
   A. Nonspecific bacterial epididymitis
   B. Sexually transmitted epididymitis
      1. *Chlamydia trachomatis*
      2. *Neisseria gonorrhoeae*
3. Rare causes of epididymitis
   A. Tuberculosis
   B. Brucellar epididymitis or epididymo-orchitis
   C. Hematogenous bacterial infections
      1. *Salmonella* enteritidis
      2. *Pseudomonas pseudomallei*
      3. Other bacterial causes
   D. Fungal disease
   E. Parasitic diseases
   F. Drug-related epididymitis (amiodarone)
   G. Behçet's disease
   H. Idiopathic hematoma of the epididymis
   I. Sarcoidosis
4. Torsion of a testicular appendage
5. Orchitis
   A. Viral orchitis
      1. Mumps orchitis
      2. Other viral agents
   B. Acute hematogenous bacterial or rickettsial orchitis

C. Granulomatous orchitis
   1. Idiopathic granulomatous orchitis
   2. Specific granulomatous orchitis
      A. Tuberculous epididymo-orchitis
      B. Lepromatous leprosy
      C. Blastomycosis, histoplasmosis, and coccidioidomycosis
      D. Actinomycosis
      E. Syphilis
      F. Brucellosis
      G. Sarcoidosis
D. Focal orchitis
E. Familial Mediterranean fever orchitis
F. Self-palpation orchitis
G. Drug-related (mazindol) orchitis

6. Orchitis associated with immunosuppression
   A. AIDS
      1. Toxoplasma orchitis
      2. Cytomegalovirus orchitis
   B. Immunosuppression for cardiac transplantation

7. Complications of epididymo-orchitis
   A. Testicular abscess
   B. Testicular infarction

C. Pyocele of the testis
D. Scrotal abscess or draining sinus
8. Testicular neoplasms
   A. Primary solid tumors
   B. Metastatic tumor
   C. Acute lymphocytic leukemia
9. Polyarteritis nodosa
10. Scrotal trauma
    A. Hematocele and testicular rupture
    B. Traumatic testicular torsion
    C. Traumatic scrotal hernia
    D. Bilateral testicular injury due to gunshot
11. Referred testicular pain
    A. Renal colic due to a ureteral stone
    B. Ureteropelvic junction obstruction
    C. Acute appendicitis
    D. Aneurysm of the common iliac artery or aorta
    E. Acute bacterial prostatitis
    F. Seminal vesiculitis
    G. Spinal cord tumor
12. Scrotal infection
    A. Scrotal abscess
    B. Fournier's gangrene
13. Acute bilateral testicular pain

☐ SUMMARY

Testicular torsion usually begins abruptly, with severe unilateral scrotal pain; nausea and vomiting; and no fever or irritative urethral or bladder symptoms. Some cases may have a more gradual onset. There may be a history of one or more similar brief attacks in the past that resolved spontaneously (6 to 63 percent of cases). The painful testis is retracted into the upper scrotum and is swollen and tender, and a palpable twist may be present in the cord. The scrotum may be red and edematous. The cremasteric reflex is absent on the affected side. The epididymis may be normal to palpation during the first hour, but it soon becomes swollen and indurated, and its palpable boundaries become obscured by edema. The urine may contain increased numbers of leukocytes, but a normal urinalysis is the rule in the majority of cases. Both testes may have an abnormal axis if examined in the standing position (i.e., horizontal position of the long axis). Up to 50 percent of cases are typical; and these cases are usually surgically explored without further investigation. The remainder may be studied by radionuclide imaging or by color Doppler ultrasonography. These procedures can document decreased or absent blood flow to the affected testis. Manual detorsion in the emergency room may also be of diagnostic and therapeutic value. If surgery is performed within 2 to 6 h, there is a high testicular salvage rate. Delay in surgical intervention beyond 6 h usually results in orchiectomy, because the testis has infarcted and become necrotic.

Epididymitis begins with a slowly progressive scrotal ache without nausea and vomiting. It may be associated with fever, frequency, dysuria, and/or urethral discharge. The testis is usually normal in size and consistency, and not tender. The epididymis is focally or diffusely swollen and tender. The urine may contain leukocytes and bacteria, or there may be a urethral discharge. A smear of the discharge or urethral exudate (i.e., obtained with an alginate swab) may show gonococci (Gram stain), or chlamydia (fluorescent antibody stain). In cases secondary to urinary tract infection, bacteriuria caused by coliforms, *Pseudomonas*, or *Enterococcus* species is usually present. Epididymitis may be confused, in some cases, with torsion. Radionuclide imaging or color Doppler ultrasonography will demonstrate normal or increased testicular blood flow. There is a good response to antibiotic therapy, with symptom resolution in 1 to 4 days. Cases not receiving prompt antibiotic therapy may progress and develop testicular involvement, with pain, tenderness, and swelling (i.e., *epididymo-orchitis*). Most cases of epididymitis and epididymo-orchitis are secondary to urinary tract infection or are sexually acquired.

Rare causes of epididymo-orchitis include *tuberculosis* and *brucellosis*. The former may be diagnosed by urine culture or biopsy of the testis and/or epididymis, and by detection of tuberculosis of the kidney and renal pelvis. Brucellar infection has a febrile systemic component and produces a painful, tender epididymo-orchitis. The diagnosis is usually confirmed by demonstration of a high agglutination titer, and occasionally by a positive blood culture. Exposure to farm animals, and/or a history of ingestion of raw milk or cheese made from unpasteurized milk, is frequently associated with brucellosis.

Epididymo-orchitis may arise secondarily to *bacteremia*. *Salmonella* species, *Pseudomonas pseudomallei*, *Neisseria meningitidis*, *Haemophilus influenzae*, and *Streptococcus pneumoniae* have been reported as causes of acute epididymal and/or testicular infection. *Fungal disease (blastomycosis)* and parasitic diseases (*filariasis, schistosomiasis, amebiasis*) may also cause epididymo-orchitis. Use of the drug *amiodarone* may cause acute epididymitis. *Behçet's disease* and *sarcoidosis* have been reported to cause epididymo-orchitis. A *hematoma of the epididymis* may mimic acute epididymitis. The latter diagnosis is usually made after epididymectomy.

Torsion of a testicular appendage causes localized testicular pain and tenderness (i.e., at the superior pole of the testis), and a "blue dot" sign (produced by viewing the cyanotic appendage through the thin, pink scrotal skin of the young male). This disorder occurs primarily in those under 14, but occasional cases occur in older boys and men. It can be differentiated from torsion by radionuclide imaging, since the lesion usually demonstrates normal or increased uptake. Surgical intervention is not required unless the pain persists or is very severe.

Viral orchitis is usually caused by *mumps*. The testicular pain, swelling, and tenderness follow the onset of parotitis by 2 to 6 days but, in some cases, may precede parotid involvement or may occur as the sole manifestation of mumps. *Other viral agents*, such as *varicella-zoster, coxsackievirus B,* and *dengue virus,* may cause acute orchitis. *Hematogenous orchitis,* caused by deposition of bacteria (*Corynebacterium diphtheriae, Salmonella* species, *Streptococcus pyogenes*) or *Rickettsia prowazekii* (i.e., epidemic typhus), has been described.

Granulomatous orchitis may be *idiopathic* or may be secondary to *tuberculosis, leprosy, systemic fungal disease, actinomycosis, syphilis, brucellosis,* or *sarcoidosis.*

Focal orchitis presents as a localized form of testicular inflammation secondary to epididymitis. Ultrasonography reveals a peripheral, hypoechoic, intratesticular lesion adjacent to an enlarged epididymis. This localized form of bacterial orchitis usually resolves with antibiotic therapy. *Rare causes of orchitis* include *familial Mediterranean fever,* excessive *self-palpation* of the testis because of cancerophobia, and use of *mazindol,* a drug used to promote weight reduction.

AIDS patients with scrotal pain and tenderness may have a testicular infection caused by *cytomegalovirus, Toxoplasma gondii,* or *Mycobacterium avium-intracellulare.*

Complications of epididymo-orchitis include *testicular abscess, testicular infarction,* and *pyocele.* Real-time ultrasonography may demonstrate an early or mature testicular abscess, a testicular infarction, or a pyocele.

A *scrotal abscess* may arise from drainage of a testicular abscess into the scrotal sac. Needle aspiration of the fluctuant scrotal mass reveals pus and bacteria.

Up to 37 percent of primary *testicular neoplasms* may present with testicular pain, tenderness, and swelling, and may mimic an epididymo-orchitis or torsion. *Teratoma* is commonly associated with pain, but painful masses have been reported with *seminoma* and *embryonal carcinoma.* A torsive testicle may rarely contain a malignant tumor. Tumors may be associated with elevated levels of α-fetoprotein (embryonal carcinoma, endodermal sinus tumor) or human chorionic gonadotropin (embryonal carcinoma, seminoma, choriocarcinoma). Ultrasonography of the testicular lesion reveals areas of decreased echogenicity interspersed with zones of normal echogenicity, or a diffuse region of decreased echogenicity. These findings are nonspecific; orchiectomy is required for a definitive diagnosis.

Painful testicular swelling may rarely be caused by *metastatic tumor.* There is usually a history of a recently treated malignancy. Sonography may reveal a focal sonolucency. The most frequent primary sites that metastasize to the testicle include the prostate (35 percent), lung (17 percent), colon (8 percent), and skin (melanoma) (8 percent).

Only 6 percent of patients presenting with a painful testicular metastatic nodule have this symptom as the initial presentation of an occult, distant primary tumor. *Acute lymphocytic leukemia* in relapse may present with painless or painful testicular swelling. The diagnosis can be confirmed by needle aspiration or wedge biopsy of the testis.

Rare cases of *polyarteritis nodosa* present with severe testicular pain, tenderness, and swelling as the initial presentation of vasculitis. The diagnosis can be confirmed by biopsy of the testicle. Clinical testicular involvement occurs in up to 18 percent. Systemic symptoms, and evidence of renal, intraabdominal, cardiac, and skin involvement, may also occur. Testicular pain and swelling, systemic symptoms, and other symptoms respond to prednisone/cyclophosphamide therapy.

Scrotal trauma can cause a scrotal *hematoma, hematocele, hydrocele,* or *pyocele;* an *epididymal and/or testicular hematoma; posttraumatic epididymitis; acute traumatic torsion of the testis or an appendage;* or *testicular rupture.* Up to 6 percent of cases of testicular torsion follow trauma. An *acute scrotal hernia* may result from lower abdominal blunt trauma. *Bilateral testicular rupture* usually follows gunshot wounds. Suspicion of testicular rupture requires exploration and repair.

Referred testicular pain may result from *ureterolithiasis, ureteropelvic junction obstruction, acute appendicitis,* an *iliac or lower abdominal aortic aneurysm, acute prostatitis and/or seminal vesiculitis,* or a *spinal cord tumor* at the T12–L2 root level.

Scrotal infection may present with a painful and tender scrotal swelling and/or a draining scrotal sinus. Aspiration of the scrotal mass (*abscess*) yields pus. Drainage and antibiotic therapy leads to resolution. *Fournier's gangrene* involves the skin of the perineum, perianal region, scrotum, penis, lower abdomen, and buttock. Acute edema and erythema are followed by skin blackening and induration, and sloughing of necrotic skin. There is severe perineal and scrotal pain and tenderness. The infection is polymicrobial. Extensive debridement and antibiotic therapy are required for survival.

Some of the disorders discussed may also cause bilateral testicular pain; these are listed in Table 35-1.

☐ DESCRIPTION OF LISTED DISEASES

1. TESTICULAR TORSION

There is an abrupt onset of unilateral testicular pain. The pain is usually severe, and may radiate into the inguinal region and lower abdomen. Nausea and vomiting are commonly associated. Up to 35 percent of cases may have

TABLE OF DISEASE INCIDENCE

INCIDENCE PER 100,000 (APPROXIMATE)

Common (>100)
Testicular torsion
Nonspecific bacterial epididymitis
Sexually transmitted epididymitis (*Neisseria gonorrhoeae, Chlamydia trachomatis*)
Mumps orchitis
Testicular trauma (hematocele and/or rupture of testis)
Referred pain due to ureteral stone or prostatitis

Uncommon (>5–100)
Torsion of a testicular appendage
Orchitis due to other viral agents
Idiopathic granulomatous orchitis
Focal orchitis secondary to epididymitis
Testicular abscess
Testicular infarction
Primary testicular neoplasm
Traumatic testicular torsion
Penetrating trauma of the testis

Rare (>0–5)
Tuberculous epididymitis
Brucellar epididymitis
Hematogenous bacterial epididymitis
Fungal epididymitis
Parasitic epididymitis
Amiodarone-related epididymitis
Behçet's disease–associated epididymitis
Idiopathic hematoma of the epididymis
Sarcoid epididymitis
Hematogenous bacterial or rickettsial orchitis
Specific granulomatous orchitis
Epididymo-orchitis secondary to familial Mediterranean fever
Self-palpation orchitis
Mazindol-related orchitis
Toxoplasma orchitis in AIDS
Cytomegalovirus orchitis in AIDS
Nocardia epididymo-orchitis
Pyocele of the testis
Scrotal abscess
Fournier's gangrene
Metastatic tumor involving the testis
Acute lymphocytic leukemia relapse involving the testis
Polyarteritis nodosa
Referred pain due to ureteropelvic junction obstruction; appendicitis; seminal vesiculitis; aneurysm; or spinal cord tumor
Traumatic scrotal hernia

a more gradual onset. There is a history of prior similar episodes that subsided spontaneously in 6 to 63 percent of patients with this disorder. Fever, urethral discharge, dysuria, frequency, and urgency do not usually occur. Torsion occurs most frequently in the under-20 age group (65 percent of cases), but a significant number of cases occur in the 20-to-30 age group (23 to 45 percent of cases). Torsion is quite rare after age 30. Examination reveals scrotal edema and redness on the painful side, but this may not be evident during the first 2 to 3 h after onset. The affected testis is often elevated in the scrotum, and there may be a palpable twist in the spermatic cord. The epididymis may be edematous and indistinguishable from the testis; if it is palpable it will be in an abnormal position. (The normal position is posterolateral.) There may be an abnormal axis of the involved and the contralateral testis (i.e., horizontal position of the long axis) if the patient is examined in the standing position. Severe tenderness and induration due to edema may prevent a useful examination. Some patients may have no tenderness, or tenderness localized only to the epididymis. Prehn's sign (i.e., pain exacerbation in patients with torsion, and relief in patients with epididymitis, by elevating the scrotal contents for 1 h) is unreliable as a diagnostic test. The cremasteric reflex (i.e., retraction of the scrotal

contents after stroking the posteromedial thigh) is rarely, if ever, present in torsion. It is present in up to 50 percent of cases of epididymitis and other causes of the "acute scrotum." The presence of a cremasteric reflex argues against a diagnosis of torsion. A patient with torsion of more than 24 h duration *and* a cremasteric reflex has been reported (i.e., a false-negative case). Leukocytosis and pyuria may occur (up to 30 percent of cases).

Patients who develop torsion usually have a "bell-clapper" deformity (i.e., the testis has a horizontal position in the scrotum, and the spermatic cord and epididymis are superior) or a loose epididymal attachment to the testis. The tunica vaginalis completely surrounds the bell-clapper testis and distal cord, and there is insufficient attachment, or no attachment, to the scrotal sac.

Up to 50 percent of patients have a typical clinical picture; these patients are often taken to surgery without further study. Other cases of the acute scrotum, occurring in those over age 20 and/or with an atypical presentation, should be evaluated further in order to prevent unnecessary surgical exploration. In surgical series where every acute scrotum was explored, the rate of unnecessary surgery ranged from 30 to 50 percent.

Radionuclide scrotal imaging has been a valuable procedure for differentiating torsion from epididymitis and/

or orchitis. Technetium 99m pertechnetate is given intravenously, and the scrotal contents are scanned with a gamma scintillation camera. There is an abrupt cutoff or decreased perfusion in the angiographic phase. In the tissue phase, a round, cold area replaces the affected testis; this cold spot may be outlined by activity in the dartos layer of the scrotum. Uptake in the contralateral testis is normal. A "nubbin sign" has been described that represents a dilated group of spermatic vessels that show an abrupt cutoff (i.e., at the site of the torsion) during the angiographic phase of the scan. False-negatives may occur, because of increased radionuclide uptake in the testis, during the first 1 to 2 h after torsion begins.

The scan in patients with acute epididymitis and/or orchitis is markedly different from that in patients with torsion; it demonstrates increased flow in the affected spermatic cord during the angiographic phase. Increased activity is found superolaterally (i.e., in epididymitis), and in some cases more medially as well (indicating epididymo-orchitis). Radionuclide imaging has a sensitivity of 80 to 100 percent and a specificity of 89 to 100 percent for the diagnosis of testicular torsion, and is 86 to 100 percent accurate. Gray-scale sonography and continuous-wave Doppler ultrasonography are not accurate in differentiating torsion from epididymitis. Continuous-wave Doppler studies may miss torsion in up to 67 percent of cases, because arterial flow in peritesticular vessels is difficult to distinguish from intratesticular flow.

Color Doppler ultrasonography combines gray-scale parenchymal imaging with blood flow measurement in the testicular arteries. Flow can be visualized and mapped with good resolution. Color Doppler imaging may be useful in selected cases that pose diagnostic problems (i.e., without definite clinical findings that differentiate torsion from epididymitis). Patients with torsion have decreased or absent flow, whereas those with epididymitis have normal or increased flow, on color Doppler imaging. In two reported series, color Doppler imaging correctly diagnosed torsion (early and delayed) in 100 percent of 14 cases. It was also accurate in correctly labeling patients with acute or chronic epididymitis. When compared to radionuclide imaging, it appeared to be as accurate. Use of color Doppler imaging, instead of scintigraphy, has been proposed for the initial evaluation of the acute scrotum with equivocal clinical findings. Magnetic resonance imaging (MRI) has also been shown to accurately differentiate torsion from epididymitis. Torsion knot and whirlpool patterns of the spermatic cord can be identified, in patients with torsion, by MRI. These are the most sensitive and specific MRI signs of torsion.

Use of MRI is investigational and, because of the cost and time delay imposed on the diagnostic workup, it is not likely to become a widely used clinical method for the diagnosis of torsion. Successful manual detorsion in the emergency room can be of diagnostic and therapeutic value.

Surgical exploration and detorsion before 6 h results in an 80- to 100-percent rate of testicular salvage. Delayed or missed cases extending beyond 24 h have a salvage rate of only 20 percent. In a surgical series where early exploration was undertaken on clinical grounds, the immediate salvage rate was 90 percent, and the long-term rate 73 percent. Surgical fixation of each testis to the scrotum (orchiopexy) is required, since the predisposing defect is usually bilateral. Infarction with necrosis requires orchiectomy.

2. EPIDIDYMITIS AND EPIDIDYMO–ORCHITIS

There is a gradual onset of pain and tenderness in one side (91 percent), or both sides (9 percent), of the scrotum over a period of 1 to 2 days. Up to 50 percent of patients have a low-grade fever; a similar percentage may have a urethral discharge and/or dysuria. Nausea and vomiting do not usually occur. In some cases the onset of pain may be abrupt, mimicking torsion. This condition is unusual as a cause of acute scrotal pain in the 0- to 16-year age group (4 to 15 percent of cases); but it is the most common cause of such pain after age 20 (80 to 100 percent of cases). Early in the course (i.e., during the first 6 h after pain onset), the epididymis, or a localized segment of it, becomes firm, swollen, and tender, while the testis remains nontender and of normal consistency. Inflammation may extend to the testis (epididymo-orchitis), causing swelling, tenderness, and obliteration of the palpable boundries between testis and epididymis. The latter is due to induration and edema. Scrotal edema and erythema, and a reactive hydrocele, may also occur. Urethral discharge may be spontaneous, or may require stripping of the urethra for its demonstration. Vasitis is usually present; palpation of the vas deferens usually reveals induration and tenderness.

Vasitis, with inguinal and testicular pain, may occur as an equivalent disorder to epididymitis in patients who have had a vasectomy, the latter preventing extension to the epididymis. Such patients may have a tender and indurated vas up to the point of the vasectomy.

Epididymitis has different predominant etiologies in different age groups.

A. Nonspecific Bacterial Epididymitis In children, up to 50 percent of cases of this disorder are associated with an underlying genitourinary lesion such as a meatal stenosis, posterior urethral valves, urethral stricture, an ectopic opening of the ejaculatory duct, or a congenital colovesical fistula. In patients older than age 40 there is an association of epididymitis with prostatitis; prostatic hypertrophy; urethral stricture; renal, vesical, or prostatic stones; chronic bacteriuria; prostatectomy; or the presence of an indwelling urinary catheter. In patients with epididymitis secondary to urinary tract infection, a midstream urine sample contains increased numbers of leukocytes, and urine culture reveals more than 10^4 colony-forming units per ml of a coliform, or *Pseudomonas* species. In some reports, gram-positive organisms, such as enterococci or staphylococci, were also frequently isolated. This type of nonspecific bacterial urinary tract infection is the most frequent cause of epididymitis in men older than 35. However, gonococcal and chlamydial epididymitis occurred in 38 percent of patients older than 35 in one reported series. Coliform epididymitis is predominant in homosexual males and may be sexually transmitted in this group.

B. Sexually Transmitted Epididymitis

1. **Chlamydia trachomatis**   *Chlamydia trachomatis* is a frequent cause of acute epididymitis in sexually active heterosexual males in the 16- to 35-year age group. *C. trachomatis* has been isolated from urethral swabs and epididymal aspirates, and detected by fluorescent antibody–stained smears of urethral discharge. Milking the urethra is often necessary to deliver the scant watery discharge caused by this agent. The median interval from a prior sexual exposure to the onset of epididymitis is 10 days, with some cases occurring as long as 45 days after contact. There is a good response to doxycycline or erythromycin therapy.

2. **Neisseria gonorrhoeae**   Up to 21 percent of cases of acute epididymitis in the 16-to-35 age group are caused by *Neisseria gonorrhoeae*. Many of these patients have no history of urethral discharge. Milking the urethra may detect a discharge in up to 50 percent of cases. Many patients have no recent history of sexual exposure, demonstrating that gonococci may be carried with few, if any, symptoms for long periods before the onset of epididymitis. Gram stain and culture of material obtained from the urethra will establish a diagnosis of gonococcal urethritis. There is a good clinical response to amoxicillin or ceftriaxone. *Ureaplasma urealyticum* has been isolated from the urethra of patients with acute epididymitis, but it has only occasionally been grown from an epididymal aspirate. Its role in the etiology of acute epididymitis is believed to be minor. Up to 20 percent of cases of acute epididymitis have no known cause, and are classified as idiopathic.

The diagnosis of epididymitis and epididymo-orchitis can be supported by radionuclide imaging and color Doppler ultrasonography, as described above.

3. RARE CAUSES OF EPIDIDYMITIS

A. Tuberculosis   Tuberculous epididymitis or epididymo-orchitis causes dull, aching pain in one side of the scrotum that is intensified by jarring, movement, and pal-

pation. There is a tender intrascrotal mass, scrotal skin edema, and sometimes erythema. Examination may reveal a beaded vas deferens and a contracted prostate that feels like a bag of BB shot. A reactive hydrocele is commonly present as a fluctuant mass adjacent to the testis. Sterile pyuria is uncommon (only 15 percent of cases). An epididymal or testicular abscess may be present. There may be a history of active tuberculosis (25 percent) or of exposure to tuberculosis from a family member (15 percent). Irritative bladder symptoms occur in 25 percent of cases. The epididymis is usually enlarged, irregular, hard, and tender, and the testis may also be swollen. A fistula from a scrotal abscess may drain pus through the scrotal surface. The diagnosis can be confirmed by histopathologic examination of a biopsied epididymis or testis, and culture of pus and/or urine for *Mycobacterium tuberculosis*. Up to 50 percent of patients have negative urine cultures. Patients with negative cultures may have evidence of upper tract tuberculosis on an intravenous pyelogram (e.g., renal cavities; dilated, irregular, and sometimes stenotic calices; renal calcification; unilateral absence of renal function; or hydronephrosis). Up to 73 percent of patients may have an abnormal upper urinary tract; bilateral renal disease is not uncommon. Some cases present as a painless testicular mass mimicking tumor. Antituberculous therapy is effective, but orchiectomy may be required if tumor is suspected.

B. Brucellar Epididymitis or Epididymo-Orchitis

This disorder has been reported in the Middle East. Patients have presented with high fever, weakness, fatigue, malaise, and an acute scrotum. The local scrotal pain is accompanied by swelling and tenderness of a testicle. Most cases have combined epididymal and testicular involvement on the painful side, but orchitis or epididymitis may occur as an isolated finding in a small percentage of cases. Dysuria, frequency, and urgency occurred in 64 percent of patients in one report. The diagnosis was made by determination of brucella agglutination titers (a titer equal to, or greater than, 1:160 was considered diagnostic), with confirmation in 14 percent of cases by a positive blood culture. Liver function abnormalities were common (79 percent), and were probably due to granulomatous hepatitis. Current recommended therapy is rifampim, 600 mg/day, and doxycycline, 200 mg/day, for 6 weeks. Clues to the diagnosis of brucellar epididymo-orchitis include a subacute to chronic course, a history of animal contact or ingestion of unpasteurized milk or cheese, and an intermittent febrile course.

C. Hematogenous Bacterial Infections

1. **Salmonella** *Enteritidis*   This invasive organism caused acute epididymo-orchitis beginning 3 weeks after an episode of gastroenteritis. Three other cases of epididymo-orchitis due to *Salmonella* infection have been published. A case of relapsing acute *Salmonella hadar* epididymo-orchitis was successfully treated with ciprofloxacin.

2. Pseudomonas pseudomallei A case of acute epididymo-orchitis, secondary to *Pseudomonas pseudomallei* infection, has been reported in Thailand. Gross hematuria and fever were present. The patient had been immunosuppressed with prednisone.

3. Other Bacterial Causes Cases of epididymitis caused by *Neisseria meningitidis*, *Haemophilus influenzae*, and *Streptococcus pneumoniae* have occurred secondarily to bacteremia.

D. Fungal Disease Blastomycosis is the most common fungal infection associated with epididymitis; other systemic fungal diseases may rarely be causative (histoplasmosis, coccidiodomycosis).

E. Parasitic Diseases Epididymitis has been associated with filariasis, schistosomiasis, and amebiasis.

F. Drug-Related Epididymitis (Amiodarone) Antiarrhythmic therapy with amiodarone has been reported to cause, first, acute unilateral epididymitis, and then (within 3 weeks) bilateral epididymitis, with pain, epididymal swelling, and tenderness, in 11 percent of those taking the drug. This disorder may resolve within 10 weeks, whether or not the drug is discontinued. Dose reduction or cessation of therapy leads to resolution of symptoms within 1 to 2 weeks.

G. Behçet's Disease This disorder causes oral aphthous ulcers, genital ulcers, anterior uveitis, and skin disease (erythema nodosum, superficial thrombophlebitis, pustular lesions, and/or skin pathergy). Thirty-one percent of patients in a series reported in Iraq had acute or recurrent unilateral epididymo-orchitis with swelling, pain, and tenderness. Other reports have recorded a 4- to 9-percent rate of epididymo-orchitis in Behçet's disease.

H. Idiopathic Hematoma of the Epididymis A small series of 3 cases was reported in Spain. This disorder mimicked epididymitis, with pain, local tenderness, and epididymal enlargement. Resection and histopathologic examination of the epididymis revealed an encapsulated hematoma. No associated local or systemic disease was associated, and the cause was unknown.

I. Sarcoidosis This multisystem disorder has also been associated with epididymitis.

4. TORSION OF A TESTICULAR APPENDAGE

Torsion of the appendix testis (92 percent of cases) or of the appendix epididymis (7 percent of cases) may occur at any age, but is most common during adolescence. It may account for up to 35 percent of cases of unilateral scrotal pain in children up to age 15. Scrotal pain may begin abruptly or gradually (88 percent). The pain may be localized to the upper pole of the testis, the groin, or the lower abdomen. Nausea and vomiting and irritative bladder symptoms are rarely present. Examination may reveal a "blue dot" sign (so called because of the cyanotic appendage's appearance through the thin, pink scrotal skin of a young male) and/or localization of tenderness to the upper pole of the testis.

Testicular enlargement, and edema and erythema of the involved half of the scrotum, may occur secondarily to necrosis of the appendage. A secondary hydrocele may form. This disorder can be differentiated from testicular torsion by radionuclide or color Doppler imaging. The radionuclide scan usually demonstrates normal or slightly increased uptake on the painful side. Rarely, torsion of the appendix testis has been misdiagnosed as testicular torsion by scintigraphy, because the small focal area of decreased uptake caused by the torsive appendage was mistaken for testicular torsion. Surgical intervention is not required; pain and swelling will resolve in 2 to 12 days with conservative therapy. Surgical removal of the infarcted appendage may be performed to relieve persistent or severe pain.

5. ORCHITIS

A. Viral Orchitis

1. Mumps Orchitis Orchitis occurs on one or both sides in 9 to 20 percent of postpubertal patients with mumps. Testicular pain and swelling occur 4 to 6 days after the onset of parotitis, but may occur prior to the onset of parotitis (fewer than 10 percent of cases) or as the only localizing symptom of mumps infection. Fever, chills, headache, nausea, and vomiting accompany unilateral testicular pain, swelling, and tenderness. In up to 30 percent of cases, contralateral testicular involvement follows within 1 to 9 days. Examination reveals diffuse testicular and epididymal enlargement and tenderness, and scrotal edema and erythema. The testis may be swollen to 3 or 4 times its normal size. Fever and testicular swelling resolve within 5 to 7 days, but testicular tenderness may persist for longer than 2 weeks in up to 20 percent of patients with gonadal involvement. Testicular atrophy may follow in up to 50 percent, but infertility is uncommon.

2. Other Viral Agents Orchitis has been associated with chicken pox, and coxsackievirus B, and dengue virus infections. Very rare causes of orchitis include Epstein-Barr virus, adenovirus, lymphocytic choriomeningitis virus, echovirus types 6 and 9, and influenza virus. Testalgia, without documentation of actual testicular swelling or tenderness, has been reported in up to 25 percent of postpubertal cases of rubella.

B. Acute Hematogenous Bacterial or Rickettsial Orchitis Metastatic deposition of microorganisms in the testis resulting in acute orchitis has been reported in diphtheria, typhoid fever, typhus, paratyphoid fever, and scarlet fever. High fever, chills, pain, swelling, and tenderness of the involved testicle(s) occurs. Pain may radiate to the inguinal region and/or lower abdomen. Nausea and vomiting may be prominent complaints. The diagnosis is made by attention to the other symptoms and signs of the underlying infectious disease and by appropriate cultures and serologic studies.

C. Granulomatous Orchitis

1. Idiopathic Granulomatous Orchitis Patients with this disorder may present with fever to 103°F, acute unilateral scrotal pain, testicular and epididymal swelling and tenderness, and scrotal erythema and edema. Leukocytosis and an elevated sedimentation rate are usually present. There is no response to antibiotic therapy. Ultrasonography may reveal diffuse hypoechoicity of the involved testicle. The diagnosis can be confirmed by histopathologic study of a testicular biopsy or surgically removed testis. Microscopy reveals replacement of tubules and interstitial tissue by epithelioid cells, lymphocytes, and plasma cells. Multinucleated giant cells occur, but are infrequent. Cultures and special stains for mycobacteria, fungi, and actinomycetes are negative. Orchiectomy is often required, because subacute and chronic cases cannot be differentiated from neoplasm. The cause is unknown, but a reaction to lipids in spermatozoa that have escaped into the interstitium has been suggested as a pathophysiologic mechanism.

2. Specific Granulomatous Orchitis

   A. TUBERCULOUS EPIDIDYMO-ORCHITIS This disorder is discussed above. *Mycobacterium tuberculosis* can usually be cultured from the urine or from the excised testicle.

   B. LEPROMATOUS LEPROSY This disorder may cause painful testicular enlargement persisting for weeks or months. Testicular biopsy or an orchiectomy specimen reveals a dense infiltrate of lymphocytes, eosinophils, histiocytes, and plasma cells. Lepra cells and free lepra bacilli may be present. Skin lesions are usually present, but testicular involvement may be the only manifestation of disease. The testes are uniformly involved in lepromatous leprosy.

   C. BLASTOMYCOSIS, HISTOPLASMOSIS, AND COCCIDIOIDOMYCOSIS Any of these disorders may cause a granulomatous orchitis. Fungi may be detected by histopathologic study or culture of the surgically resected testis.

   D. ACTINOMYCOSIS This disorder may cause granulomatous orchitis with draining scrotal sinuses. Yellow ''sulfur granules'' may occur in the purulent drainage. Fluorescein-labeled antibodies (species-specific) may be used to identify organisms in smears of purulent exudate.

   E. SYPHILIS Syphilis may also cause granulomatous orchitis (syphilitic gumma), but such lesions are usually painless.

   F. BRUCELLOSIS Brucellosis may cause necrotic areas in granulomas. The diagnosis depends on the brucella agglutination titer and on culture of resected tissue or peripheral blood.

   G. SARCOIDOSIS Sarcoidosis may cause testicular involvement. Granulomas are interstitial and not intratubular.

   All forms of chronic granulomatous orchitis may mimic a testicular neoplasm on clinical examination and by ultrasonography. Most cases of idiopathic granulomatous orchitis have been treated by orchiectomy, so as to exclude neoplasm. Some cases have been treated with prednisone, with improvement.

D. Focal Orchitis Testicular inflammation may occur secondarily to epididymitis, as described above. Focal orchitis, in the presence of a thickened epididymis, may present as a peripheral, hypoechogenic, intratesticular lesion on ultrasonography. Such lesions are often adjacent to an enlarged epididymis. These lesions usually clear rapidly with antibiotic therapy. Most cases of orchitis secondary to epididymitis are diffuse.

A strategy of antibiotic treatment of focal orchitis and careful clinical and sonographic follow-up may lead to testicular preservation in the small group of patients with this disorder.

E. Familial Mediterranean Fever Orchitis Attacks of unilateral testicular swelling, pain, and tenderness; scrotal edema and redness; fever; and abdominal pain may occur in familial Mediterranean fever. Leukocytosis and an elevated sedimentation rate usually occur. Edema of the spermatic cord and epididymis may be present. Attacks clear spontaneously within 72 h. Colchicine therapy may prevent recurrent episodes.

F. Self-Palpation Orchitis Some patients practicing self-palpation of the testes for the detection of an early testicular malignancy have been reported to cause persistent testicular pain and tenderness by repeated palpation of a specific site. Avoidance of palpation results in relief of symptoms within 2 weeks.

G. Drug-Related Orchitis   Mazindol, a drug used to promote weight reduction, can cause testicular pain and sexual dysfunction, which resolve when the drug is discontinued.

6. ORCHITIS ASSOCIATED WITH IMMUNOSUPPRESSION

A. AIDS   Occult testicular infections with cytomegalovirus (16 percent), *Mycobacterium avium-intracellulare* (14 percent), and *Toxoplasma gondii* (11 percent) have been detected at autopsy in AIDS patients dying with opportunistic infections.

1. Toxoplasma Orchitis   Clinical orchitis, with pain and/or tenderness and swelling, has been reported in two patients with AIDS. The diagnosis was made histopathologically after orchiectomy. Ultrasonography revealed inhomogeneity of the involved testis, with 1- to 2-cm areas of decreased echogenicity, simulating neoplasia.

2. Cytomegalovirus Orchitis   Cytomegalovirus has been demonstrated to cause antibiotic-resistant epididymitis in a single case report in an AIDS patient. The surgically resected epididymis was found to contain intracytoplasmic and intranuclear inclusions that stained positive for cytomegalovirus by an immunoperoxidase method. This is a rare manifestation of AIDS.

B. Immunosuppression for Cardiac Transplantation
Nocardial infection of the epididymis and testis has been reported after cardiac transplantation.

Three cases of testicular nocardiosis have occurred in men with neoplasms.

7. COMPLICATIONS OF EPIDIDYMO–ORCHITIS

A. Testicular Abscess   Failure of resolution of epididymo-orchitis results in persistent fever, scrotal pain, tenderness, and swelling. Up to 6 percent of cases of epididymo-orchitis may progress to abscess formation. Real-time (10 MHz) high-resolution ultrasonography can identify several stages in the development of suppurative necrosis. Epididymal enlargement, scrotal skin edema, and a reactive hydrocele occur with uncomplicated epididymitis. A peripheral, circular, hypoechoic signal, situated adjacent to the epididymis, occurs with an early focal orchitis. Such a lesion may mimic malignancy. A more

advanced lesion produces a large zone of decreased reflectance surrounded by a capsule of normal-appearing testis. Linear streaks of high reflectance occur in the hypoechoic area. A more advanced abscess demonstrates a fan-shaped pattern of hypoechoic rectangular and triangular spaces separated by echogenic septa. Serial sonographic study of patients with a poor clinical response to antibiotics will identify those cases requiring orchiectomy because of progressive suppuration.

B. Testicular Infarction   This is another complication of epididymo-orchitis that can be recognized by ultrasonography. It produces homogeneous areas of increased reflectance. Abscess formation, infarction, or intractable pain may lead to orchiectomy. A localized abscess may be drained by needle aspiration, facilitating recovery without surgery. Serial real-time ultrasonography is a useful procedure for following the clinical course of severe epididymo-orchitis.

C. Pyocele of the Testis   This may present as a fluctuant, tender scrotal mass that occurs in a patient with slowly resolving epididymo-orchitis. Ultrasonography may demonstrate a fluid collection in the tunica vaginalis. Aspiration will reveal a turbid purulent fluid. Cases associated with rupture of a testicular abscess usually require drainage and orchiectomy.

D. Scrotal Abscess or Draining Sinus   A testicular abscess may also drain directly into the scrotal sac. The scrotum is fluctuant, distended, red, and edematous. Needle aspiration reveals pus. Drainage and orchiectomy are usually required. Some scrotal abscesses drain spontaneously through the scrotal surface.

8. TESTICULAR NEOPLASMS

A. Primary Solid Tumors   Usually, a testicular tumor presents as a slowly enlarging, painless testicular mass. Up to 37 percent of patients may present with testicular pain, swelling, and tenderness; the clinical picture may mimic that of an epididymo-orchitis or testicular torsion. Testicular pain is most common with teratoma, but may occur with seminoma and embryonal carcinoma. Germinal tumors are most prevalent in adults, and include seminoma (40 percent), embryonal carcinoma (20 percent), teratocarcinoma (25 percent), choriocarcinoma (1 percent), and combined tumor types (20 percent).

There have been three case reports of torsion of an intrascrotal testis containing a malignant tumor. There is usually an abrupt onset of testicular pain, tenderness, and swelling, associated with scintigraphic signs of torsion. This is an uncommon type of neoplasia-associated scrotal pain.

α-Fetoprotein serum levels may be elevated in patients with an embryonal carcinoma or endodermal sinus tumor.

Human chorionic gonadotropin serum levels may be elevated in embryonal carcinoma, seminoma, and choriocarcinoma. α-Fetoprotein is never found in pure seminoma. Its presence signifies nonseminomatous elements in the primary tumor or its metastases.

Ultrasonography of neoplastic lesions reveals areas of decreased echogenicity scattered through zones of normal echogenicity, or a diffuse region of decreased echogenicity. Mixed echogenicity may also occur with epididymo-orchitis and other inflammatory lesions (e.g., granulomas).

Sonographic findings are too nonspecific to permit differentiation of benign and malignant lesions; orchiectomy is required for definitive diagnosis.

B. Metastatic Tumor   Pain, swelling, and tenderness of a testis may occur. Sonography may reveal a focal sonolucency. There is no response to antibiotic therapy. Exploration may reveal an epididymal or testicular mass. Histopathologic study reveals metastatic carcinoma. Testicular ultrasonography is useful for differentiating hydroceles and varicoceles from intratesticular metastatic tumor. The common primary tumors that cause testicular metastases are prostate (35 percent), lung (17 percent), colon (8 percent), melanoma (8 percent), and kidney (6 percent). There is usually a history of a recently treated primary malignancy.

Only 6 percent of patients with a testicular metastasis present with a testicular lump as an initial complaint and are then found to have an occult primary tumor. Most patients with testicular metastasis are asymptomatic, or notice a painless swelling of the testis.

C. Acute Lymphocytic Leukemia   Relapse in children and young adults with acute lymphocytic leukemia may cause painless enlargement of one or both testes. Pain or a sensation of heaviness may occur in a minority of cases, because of intratesticular bleeding. Wedge or fine-needle aspiration biopsy of an involved testis will reveal leukemic infiltration. Ultrasonography and MRI of the testis are not sensitive enough to replace biopsy as a screening test for testicular involvement in patients with acute lymphocytic leukemia and clinically normal testes. Ultrasonography of patients with acute lymphocytic leukemia and an enlarged painless, or painful, testis reveals testicular enlargement and focal or diffuse hypoechoic areas that may or may not be homogeneous. These findings are nonspecific and may occur with primary neoplasms, orchitis, testicular torsion, and granulomatous orchitis. Ultrasonography may aid in the selection of a biopsy site. Tes-

ticular relapse, presenting with painless enlargement of a testicle, has been reported in a few long-term survivors of acute nonlymphocytic leukemia.

9. POLYARTERITIS NODOSA

Severe testicular pain, tenderness, and induration is a rare initial presentation of polyarteritis nodosa. The diagnosis can be established by testicular biopsy. Clinical testicular involvement occurs in up to 18 percent of patients with polyarteritis, and histopathologic evidence of testicular vasculitis is present in 60 to 86 percent of autopsied patients with this disorder. The pain and tenderness may be continuous or intermittent, unilateral or bilateral. This disorder has been mistaken for epididymo-orchitis. Only 3 cases of polyarteritis with testicular pain as an initial symptom have been reported. Testicular vasculitis has been reported in Goodpasture's syndrome. The pain may result from testicular infarction. Isolated cases of vasculitis of the testis without systemic vasculitis have been reported; these patients had no testicular symptoms or areas of infarction. Only 20 percent of random biopsies of the testis in a patient with polyarteritis will be positive. Discrete, clinically apparent lesions in the testis increase the diagnostic yield.

Polyarteritis usually presents with systemic symptoms that include fever, anorexia, weakness, weight loss, and malaise. Multisystem involvement occurs as the illness progresses. Renal disease is produced by glomerulitis and polyarteritis. Gross or microscopic hematuria, proteinuria, cellular casts, and renal insufficiency may occur. Hypertension is frequent and is related to the renal involvement. Angiographically demonstrable aneurysms of medium-sized renal vessels occur and are diagnostically useful. Abdominal pain may occur; it is caused by ischemia, ulceration, perforation, or infarction of the bowel produced by inflammatory arterial lesions. Ischemic disease in the appendix and gallbladder may mimic appendicitis or cholecystitis. Hepatomegaly and jaundice may occur, and elevated aminotransferase (ALT, AST) levels reflect hepatic necrosis. Nervous system involvement includes subarachnoid hemorrhage, cerebral infarction, and mononeuritis multiplex. Myalgias and arthralgias reflect ischemia, or are secondary to neuropathy. Pericarditis, myocardial infarction, and congestive heart failure may occur. Skin lesions may appear; they may include purpura, urticaria, ecchymoses, and gangrene of the fingertips and toes. Subcutaneous nodules may develop. Leukocytosis and an elevated sedimentation rate are commonly present. Biopsy of a swollen, tender testicle; a painful muscle; a palpable subcutaneous nodule; the liver; or a kidney may detect arteritis and establish the diagnosis. Testicular and other lesions, and systemic symptoms, respond to combined prednisone and cyclophosphamide therapy.

10. SCROTAL TRAUMA

A. Hematocele and Testicular Rupture Blunt trauma usually affects one testicle. The testicle may be struck by the external object while fixed against the pubic symphysis or thigh. Shortly after the injury there is a unilateral, painful swelling of the scrotum. Severe tenderness and blue-black discoloration of the scrotum may be present. Possible injuries include scrotal hematoma, hematocele (bleeding within the tunica vaginalis), hydrocele, pyocele, epididymal and/or testicular hematoma, posttraumatic epididymitis, acute traumatic torsion of the testis or an appendage, and testicular rupture. Physical examination may not be sensitive enough to detect testicular rupture in the presence of scrotal edema and/or a hematoma or hematocele. In one approach to blunt testicular trauma, immediate exploration is undertaken and the ruptured testis debrided and repaired; this results in a high salvage rate. Ultrasonography has been used to identify a scrotal hematoma (diffuse scrotal thickening with dense echoes), a hematocele (echo-free area between testis and scrotum, with or without low-level internal echoes), and testicular rupture (increased or decreased areas of testicular echogenicity corresponding to areas of hemorrhage or infarction). A discrete fracture plane of the testis or disruption of the tunica albuginea cannot usually be identified.

The sonographic findings of testicular rupture cannot be differentiated from the findings of tumor or abscess, but in a setting of trauma they indicate possible rupture and a need for surgical exploration.

B. Traumatic Testicular Torsion Up to 5 percent of cases of testicular torsion are caused by trauma. Torsion of a testicular appendage may also result from blunt trauma (up to 10 percent of cases). Traumatic torsion is usually associated with sporting events. Acute traumatic torsion is another reason for prompt exploration of an acute scrotum after trauma. Posttraumatic torsion is similar to spontaneous torsion as described above, and is associated with a "bell-clapper" deformity of the testis and spermatic cord.

C. Traumatic Scrotal Hernia An acute, painful, tender scrotal mass appearing soon after lower abdominal blunt trauma may be due to herniation of bowel and omentum into a partially obliterated processus vaginalis. The scrotal mass is firm and tender, and fails to transilluminate. Sonography may demonstrate gas-filled loops of bowel in the scrotal mass. Surgical exploration is required.

D. Bilateral Testicular Injury Due to Gunshot Bilateral injury is rare after blunt trauma (1.5 percent), and more common with penetrating trauma (gunshot) (31 per-

cent). Contusion or testicular rupture may be present. Prompt exploration, debridement, and repair is required.

MRI clearly displays the normal tunica albuginea of the testis, and may be a useful method for detecting the interruption of this layer that occurs with testicular rupture; but too few cases have been studied by this method to warrant any comment on its reliability or potential usefulness.

11. REFERRED TESTICULAR PAIN

A. Renal Colic Due to a Ureteral Stone Unilateral flank and lower abdominal pain of severe-to-excruciating intensity may radiate into the ipsilateral scrotum. The urine may be grossly bloody (20 percent), or microscopic hematuria may be present (70 percent). The testicle and epididymis are structurally normal to examination, and lower abdominal and costovertebral angle tenderness may be present. An intravenous pyelogram may reveal absent filling or delayed filling of a dilated ipsilateral caliceal system and ureter up to the point of the obstructing stone.

B. Ureteropelvic Junction Obstruction A case has been reported of testicular pain caused by ureteropelvic junction obstruction. The pain was provoked by a large fluid intake and by retrograde pyelography. It was permanently relieved by surgical correction of the obstruction.

C. Acute Appendicitis A patient with acute appendicitis usually presents with crampy midline periumbilical or epigastric pain that soon shifts to the right lower abdomen. Referral of pain to the ipsilateral testicle may occur. A rare case of acute appendicitis in the sac of an inguinal hernia, resulting in a painful irreducible scrotal swelling, has been reported; at surgery a scrotal abscess was present.

D. Aneurysm of the Common Iliac Artery or Aorta An iliac artery aneurysm or lower abdominal aortic aneurysm may be associated with unilateral iliac and testicular pain and a pulsatile lower abdominal mass.

E. Acute Bacterial Prostatitis Low back, perineal, and testicular pain are accompanied by fever, chills, urinary frequency, urgency, dysuria, and diminished force and size of the urinary stream. There may be stuttering urination, strangury, a split urinary stream, or complete obstruction. The prostate is enlarged, swollen, and tender. There is usually pyuria due to associated cystitis and urethritis. The testes are normal on examination. There is a good response to antibiotics directed at coliform, *Pseudomonas*, and *Enterococcus* species.

F. Seminal Vesiculitis   This disorder may occur with symptoms like those of acute bacterial prostatitis. Hematospermia and ejaculation pain may also be present. There may be tenderness and fullness superior to the prostate on one or both sides. MRI may demonstrate dilated, cystic, hemorrhagic seminal vesicles on one or both sides, confirming the diagnosis. There is a good response to antibiotic therapy.

G. Spinal Cord Tumor   A spinal cord tumor involving nerve roots from T12 to L2 may cause back, flank, and testicular pain.

12. SCROTAL INFECTION

A. Scrotal Abscess   This lesion may present with a painful, tender scrotal swelling and/or a draining scrotal sinus. It may be firm or fluctuant. Ultrasonography can identify it as extratesticular. Aspiration reveals pus. A scrotal abscess may result from an intraabdominal infection in the presence of a patent processus vaginalis, perforation of a urethral carcinoma, appendicitis in an inguinal hernia, penetrating trauma, or rupture of a pyocele or a testicular or epididymal abscess. Drainage and antibiotic therapy lead to resolution.

B. Fournier's Gangrene   This disorder may begin with perianal or scrotal pain, tenderness, and swelling that initially may simulate a unilateral orchitis or epididymitis. Scrotal edema and erythema soon extend to involve the penis, perineum, buttocks, and lower anterior abdominal wall. Skin blackening, induration, and sloughing occur in the involved areas. Skin crepitus due to gas-forming bacteria may be present. Ultrasonography demonstrates normal testes, scrotal thickening, bilateral peritesticular fluid, and gas in thickened subcutaneous tissue. Subcutaneous gas can also be demonstrated by plain radiography. The pain may be very severe. High fever, rigors, chills, and

marked prostration accompany the local perineal and scrotal findings. Extensive debridement of necrotic tissue is required. The infection is usually polymicrobic; isolates may include *Staphylococcus aureus*, *Bacteroides fragilis*, *Escherichia coli*, and other streptococcal and *Bacteroides* species.

Patients with diabetes, immunosuppression, and severe liver or renal disease are more likely to develop Fournier's gangrene. Other risk factors include periurethral or perianal infection and skin disruption (e.g., from injections or surgery) in the perineal or scrotal region. A CT scan may more clearly delineate the extent of disease prior to surgical intervention. Despite extensive debridement and parenteral antibiotic therapy, the mortality rate may be as high as 33 to 55 percent.

13. ACUTE BILATERAL TESTICULAR PAIN

Disorders causing bilateral pain usually present with unilateral pain, tenderness, and swelling that is followed, after a variable period, by contralateral involvement. The causes of bilateral pain are listed in Table 35-1; all are described above.

Table 35-1
CAUSES OF ACUTE BILATERAL SCROTAL PAIN

Epididymitis (9 percent of cases) due to nonspecific or sexually
  transmitted infection
Epididymitis due to use of amiodarone
Orchitis due to mumps (30 percent of cases) and other viral agents
Polyarteritis nodosa
Penetrating testicular injury due to gunshot wound
Acute bacterial prostatitis
Acute seminal vesiculitis
Fournier's gangrene

SCROTAL PAIN REFERENCES

Abscess—Testis/Scrotum

Desai KM, Gingell JC, Haworth JM: Localised intratesticular abscess complicating epididymo-orchitis: The use of scrotal ultrasonography in diagnosis and management. *Br Med J* 292(6532):1361–1362, 1986.

Mevorach RA, Lerner RM, Dvoretsky PM, et al: Testicular abscess: Diagnosis by ultrasonography. *J Urol* 136:1213–1216, 1986.

See WA, Mack LA, Krieger JN: Scrotal ultrasonography: A predictor

of complicated epididymitis requiring orchiectomy. *J Urol* 139:55–56, 1988.

Slavis SA, Kollin J, Miller JB: Pyocele of scrotum: Consequence of spontaneous rupture of testicular abscess. *Urology* 33(4):313–316, 1989.

Acute Scrotum—Review Articles

Edelsberg JS, Surh YS: The acute scrotum. *Emerg Med Clin North Am* 6(3):521–546, 1988.

Eshghi M, Silver L, Smith AD: Technetium 99m scan in scrotal lesions. *Urology* 30(6):586–593, 1987.

Goulbourne IA, Nixon SJ, Macintyre IMC: Computer aided diagnosis in acute testicular pain. *Br J Surg* 71:528–531, 1984.

Johnson LW, Heth WL: Infections of the male genitourinary system. *Prim Care* 16(4):929–940, 1989.

May DC, Lesh P, Lewis S, et al: Evaluation of acute scrotum pain with testicular scanning. *Ann Emerg Med* 14:696–699, 1985.

Melekos MD, Asbach HW, Markou SA: Etiology of acute scrotum in 100 boys with regard to age distribution. *J Urol* 139:1023–1025, 1988.

Mueller DL, Amundson GM, Rubin SZ, et al: Acute scrotal abnormalities in children: Diagnosis by combined sonography and scintigraphy. *AJR* 150:643–646, 1988.

O'Brien WM, Lynch JH: The acute scrotum. *Am Fam Physician* 37(3):239–247, 1988.

Son KA, Koff SA: Evaluation and management of the acute scrotum. *Prim Care* 12(4):637–646, 1985.

Epididymitis—Amiodarone

Gasparich JP, Mason JT, Greene HL, et al: Amiodarone-associated epididymitis: Drug-related epididymitis in the absence of infection. *J Urol* 133:971–972, 1985.

Ibsen HHW, Frandsen F, Brandrup F, et al: Epididymitis caused by treatment with amiodarone. *Genitourin Med* 65:257–258, 1989.

Epididymitis—Bacterial and Chemical

Berger RE, Alexander ER, Harnisch, JP, et al: Etiology, manifestations and therapy of acute epididymitis: Prospective study of 50 cases. *J Urol* 121:750–754, 1979.

Bruce AW, Reid G: Prostatitis associated with *Chlamydia trachomatis* in 6 patients. *J Urol* 142:1006–1007, 1989.

Bullock KN, Hunt JM: The intravenous urogram in acute epididymo-orchitis. *Br J Urol* 53:47–49, 1981.

Cooke DI, Williams CE, Fowler RC: An evaluation of the role of the intravenous urogram in the management of patients with epididymo-orchitis. *Clin Radiol* 38:255–256, 1987.

Doble A, Taylor-Robinson D, Thomas BJ, et al: Acute epididymitis: A microbiological and ultrasonographic study. *Br J Urol* 63:90–94, 1989.

Epididymo-orchitis (editorial). *Br Med J* [*Clin Res*] 283(6292):627–628, 1981.

Hahn LC, Nadel NS, Gitter MH, et al: Testicular scanning: A new modality for the preoperative diagnosis of testicular torsion. *J Urol* 113:60–62, 1975.

Hawkins DA, Taylor-Robinson D, Thomas BJ, et al: Microbiological survey of acute epididymitis. *Genitourin Med* 62:342–344, 1986.

Kiviat MD, Kiviat NB, Berger RE: *Chlamydia trachomatis* epididymitis diagnosed by fluorescent monoclonal antibody. *Urology* 30(4):395–397, 1987.

Mulcahy FM, Bignell CJ, Rajakumar R, et al: Prevalence of chlamydial infection in acute epididymo-orchitis. *Genitourin Med* 63:16–18, 1987.

Murshidi MS: Intravenous urography as a routine investigation in epididymitis. *Br J Urol* 57:338–340, 1985.

Trambert MA, Mattrey RF, Levine D, et al: Subacute scrotal pain: Evaluation of torsion versus epididymitis with MR imaging. *Radiology* 175:53–56, 1990.

Vordermark JS II: Acute epididymitis: Experience with 123 cases. *Mil Med* 150(1):27–30, 1985.

Epididymo-Orchitis—Brucellosis

Abeles M, Mond CB: Sacroiliitis and brucellosis. *J Rheumatol* 16:136–137, 1989.

Ibrahim AIA, Awad R, Shetty SD, et al: Genito-urinary complications of brucellosis. *Br J Urol* 61:294–298, 1988.

Khan MS, Humayoon MS, Al Manee MS: Epididymo-orchitis and brucellosis. *Br J Urol* 63:87–89, 1989.

Reisman EM, Colquitt LA IV, Childers J, et al: Brucella orchitis: A rare cause of testicular enlargement. *J Urol* 143:821–822, 1990.

Epididymo-Orchitis—Hematogeneous

Jayanetra P, Vorachit M, Indraprasit S: Epididymo-orchitis due to *Pseudomonas pseudomallei*. *J Urol* 130:5576, 1983.

Noble MA, Chan V: Ciprofloxacin treatment of *Salmonella hadar* epididymo-orchitis (letter to editor). *J Antimicrob Chemother* 21(3):383–384, 1988.

Svenungsson B: Suppurative epididymo-orchitis due to *Salmonella enteritidis*. *J Infect* 8:64–66, 1984.

Weinstein ML, Carcillo J, Scott SJ, et al: Paratyphoid orchitis. *Diagn Microbiol Infect Dis* 1:163–164, 1983.

Epididymo-Orchitis Mimics—Behçets Disease

Ardill RH, Manivel JC, Beier-Hanratty S, et al: Epididymitis associated with mullerian duct cyst and calculus: Sonographic diagnosis. *AJR* 155:91–92, 1990.

Nistal M, Martín-López, Paniagua R: Idiopathic hematoma of the epididymis: Presentation of three cases. *Eur Urol* 17:178–180, 1990.

Sharquie KE, Al-Rawi Z: Epididymo-orchitis in Behçets disease (letter to editor). *Br J Rheumatol* 26:468–469, 1987.

Epididymo-Orchitis—Tuberculous

Ferrie BG, Rundle JSH: Tuberculous epididymo-orchitis: A review of 20 cases. *Br J Urol* 55:437–439, 1983.

Heaton ND, Hogan B, Michell M, et al: Tuberculous epididymo-orchitis: Clinical and ultrasound observations. *Br J Urol* 64:305–309, 1989.

Koyama Y, Iigaya T, Saito S: Tuberculous epididymo-orchitis. *Urology* 31(5):419–421, 1988.

Fournier's Gangrene

Begley MG, Shawker TH, Robertson CN, et al: Fournier gangrene: Diagnosis with scrotal US. *Radiology* 169:387–389, 1988.

Leukemia—Testicular

Heancy JA, Klauber GT, Conley GR: Acute leukemia: Diagnosis and management of testicular involvement. *Urology* 21(6):573–577, 1983.

Klein EA, Kay R, Norris DG, et al: Noninvasive testicular screening in childhood leukemia. *J Urol* 136:864–866, 1986.

Lupetin AR, King W III, Rich P, et al: Ultrasound diagnosis of testicular leukemia. *Radiology* 146:171–172, 1983.

Musmanno MC, White JM: Scrotal ultrasonography as adjunct to testis biopsy in leukemia. *Urology* 35(3):239–241, 1990.

Rupp M, Hafiz MA, Hoover L, et al: Fine needle aspiration in the evaluation of testicular leukemic infiltration. *Acta Cytol* 31(1):57–58, 1987.

Shepard BR, Hensle TW, Marboe CC: Testicular biopsy and occult tumor in acute lymphocytic leukemia. *Urology* 22(1):36–38, 1983.

Vukelja SJ, Swanson SJ, Knight RD, et al: Testicular relapse in adult acute lymphocytic leukemia: A case report and literature review. *Med Pediatr Oncol* 17:170–173, 1989.

Wagner VM, Baehner RL: Leukemic infiltration of the testes in acute nonlymphocytic leukemia. *Med Pediatr Oncol* 12:166–168, 1984.

Neoplasms

Cos LR, Peartree RJ, Descalzi M, et al: Torsion of intrascrotal malignant testis tumors. *J Urol* 130:145–147, 1983.

Derksen DJ, Smith AY: Benign conditions of the external genitalia. *Prim Care* 16(4):981–985, 1989.

Fung CY, Garnick MB: Clinical stage I carcinoma of the testis: A review. *J Clin Oncol* 6:734–750, 1988.

Grignon DJ, Shum DT, Hayman WP: Metastatic tumours of the testes. *Can J Surg* 29(5):359–361, 1986.

Kaneti J, Maor E, Lissmer L, et al: Embryonal carcinoma of testis in elderly men. *Int Urol Nephrol* 20(6):641–645, 1988.

Mikhail NE, Tawfic MI, Hadi AA, et al: Schistosomal orchitis simulating malignancy. *J Urol* 140:147–148, 1988.

Moskovitz B, Kerner H, Levin DR: Testicular metastasis from carcinoma of the prostate. *Urol Int* 42:79–80, 1987.

Patel SR, Richardson RL, Kvols L: Metastatic cancer to the testes: A report of 20 cases and review of the literature. *J Urol* 142:1003–1005, 1989.

Vugrin D, Chen A, Feigl P, et al: Embryonal carcinoma of the testis. *Cancer* 61:2348–2352, 1988.

Young RH, Van Patter HT, Scully RE: Hepatocellular carcinoma metastatic to the testis. *Am J Clin Pathol* 87:117–120, 1987.

Neuropathy—Genitofemoral/Ilioinguinal

Ekberg O, Abrahamsson P-A, Kesek P: Inguinal hernia in urological patients: The value of herniography. *J Urol* 139:1253–1255, 1988.

Ekberg O, Persson NH, Abrahamsson P-A, et al: Longstanding groin pain in athletes: A multidisciplinary approach. *Sports Med* 6:56–61, 1988.

Hahn L: Clinical findings and results of operative treatment in ilioinguinal nerve entrapment syndrome. *Br J Obstet Gynaecol* 96:1080–1083, 1989.

Harms BA, DeHaas DR Jr, Starling JR: Diagnosis and management of genitofemoral neuralgia. *Arch Surg* 119:339–341, 1984.

Lichtenstein IL, Shulman AG, Amid PK, et al: Cause and prevention of postherniorrhaphy neuralgia: A proposed protocol for treatment. *Am J Surg* 155(6):786–790, 1988.

Starling JR, Harms BA: Diagnosis and treatment of genitofemoral and ilioinguinal neuralgia. *World J Surg* 13:586–591, 1989.

Starling JR, Harms BA, Schroeder ME, et al: Diagnosis and treatment of genitofemoral and ilioinguinal entrapment neuralgia. *Surgery* 102(4):581–586, 1987.

Orchialgia—Chronic Pain

Davis BE, Noble MJ, Weigel JW, et al: Analysis and management of chronic testicular pain. *J Urol* 143:936–939, 1990.

Sellu DP, Lynn JA: Intermittent torsion of the testis. *J R Coll Surg Edin* 29(2):127–128, 1984.

Weidner W, Schiefer HG, Garbe C: Acute nongonococcal epididymitis: Aetiological and therapeutic aspects. *Drugs* 34(suppl 1):111–117, 1987.

Wiener SL: Testicular pain, in Walker HK, Hall WD, Hurst JW (eds): *Clinical Methods*, 3d ed. Boston, Butterworth, 1990, pp 853–856.

Zvieli S, Vinter L, Herman J: Nonacute scrotal pain in adolescents. *J Fam Pract* 28(2):226–230, 1989.

Orchitis—Granulomatous

Akhtar M, Ali MA, Mackey DM: Lepromatous leprosy presenting as orchitis. *Am J Clin Pathol* 73(5):712–715, 1980.

Heyderman E, O'Donnell PJ, Lloyd-Davies RW: Stony testicle: Case of calcific granulomatous orchitis. *Urology* 31(4):346–348, 1988.

Klein FA, Vick CW III, Schneider V: Bilateral granulomatous orchitis: Manifestation of idiopathic systemic granulomatosis. *J Urol* 134:762–764, 1985.

Librach IM, Regan L: Granulomatous orchitis. *Br J Clin Pract* 37(10):357–358, 1983.

Raju GC, Naraynsingh V: Idiopathic granulomatous orchitis. *Trop Geogr Med* 37(2):188–189, 1985.

Rosi P, Carini M, Gambacorta G, et al: Granulomatous orchitis: Clinical and pathologic aspects. *Eur Urol* 10:130–132, 1984.

Scott RF, Bayliss AP: Ultrasound in the diagnosis of granulomatous orchitis. *Br J Radiol* 58:907–909, 1985.

Sporer A, Seebode JJ: Granulomatous orchitis. *Urology* 19(3):319–321, 1982.

Orchitis—Immunosuppressed/AIDS

Crider SR, Horstman WG, Massey GS: Toxoplasma orchitis: Report of a case and a review of the literature. *Am J Med* 85(3):421–424, 1988.

DePaepe ME, Guerrieri C, Waxman M: Opportunistic infections of the testis in the acquired immunodeficiency syndrome. *Mt Sinai J Med* 57(1):25–29, 1990.

Haskell L, Fusco MJ, Ares L, et al: Case report: Disseminated toxoplasmosis presenting as symptomatic orchitis and nephrotic syndrome. *Am J Med Sci* 298(3):185–190, 1989.

Nistal M, Santana A, Paniaqua R, et al: Testicular toxoplasmosis in two men with the acquired immunodeficiency syndrome (AIDS). *Arch Pathol Lab Med* 110:744–746, 1986.

Randazzo RF, Hulette CM, Gottlieb MS, et al: Cytomegaloviral epididymitis in a patient with the acquired immune deficiency syndrome. *J Urol* 136(5):1095–1097, 1986.

Wheeler JS Jr, Culkin DJ, O'Connell J, et al: Nocardia epididymo-orchitis in an immunosuppressed patient. *J Urol* 136(6):1314–1315, 1986.

Orchitis—Miscellaneous

Eschel G, Zemer D, Bar-Yochai A: Acute orchitis in familial Mediterranean fever. *Ann Intern Med* 109(2):164–165, 1988.

Krieger JN: Epididymitis, orchitis, and related conditions. *Sex Transm Dis* 11(3):173–181, 1989.

Lentini JF, Benson CB, Richie JP: Sonographic features of focal orchitis. *J Ultrasound Med* 8:361–364, 1989.

Schneiderman H, Voytovich A: (Self)-palpation orchitis (letter to editor). *J Gen Intern Med* 3(1):97, 1988.

Orchitis—Viral

Preblud SR, Dobbs HI, Sedmak GV, et al: Testalgia associated with rubella infection. *South Med J* 73(5):594–595, 1980.

Sullivan KM, Halpin TJ, Kim-Farley R, et al: Mumps disease and its health impact: An outbreak-based report. *Pediatrics* 76(4):533–536, 1985.

Turner RB: Orchitis as a complication of chickenpox. *Pediatr Infect Dis J* 6(5):489, 1987.

Referred Pain—Testis/Scrotum

Goldberg SD, Witchell SJ: Right testicular pain: Unusual presentation of obstruction of the ureteropelvic junction. *Can J Surg* 31(4):246–247, 1988.

Møller-Nielsen C, Jensen FS: Urethral cancer presenting with scrotal abscess formation: A differential diagnosis of acute epididymitis. *Urol Int* 43:364–365, 1988.

Ratzan RM, Donaldson MC, Foster JH, et al: The blue scrotum sign of Bryant: A diagnostic clue to ruptured abdominal aortic aneurysm. *J Emerg Med* 5:323–329, 1987.

Read AG, McQuillan TC: Acute appendicitis presenting as a scrotal abscess. *Aust N Z J Surg* 59:425–426, 1989.

Sue DE, Chicola C, Brant-Zawadzki MN, et al: MR imaging in seminal vesiculitis. *J Comput Assist Tomogr* 13(4):662–664, 1989.

Testicular Torsion

Barada JH, Weingarten JL, Cromie WJ: Testicular salvage and age-related delay in the presentation of testicular torsion. *J Urol* 142:746–748, 1989.

Chakraborty J, Hikim APS, Jhunjhunwala J: Torsion of the spermatic cord: A long-term study of the contralateral testis. *Urol Res* 14:257–260, 1986.

Ishizuka E, Noguchi S, Sato K, et al: A classification for intravaginal torsion of the testis. *Eur Urol* 15:108–112, 1988.

Lindsey D, Stanisic TH: Diagnosis and management of testicular torsion: Pitfalls and perils. *Am J Emerg Med* 6:42–46, 1988.

Nagler HM, Deitch AD, deVere White R: Testicular torsion: Temporal considerations. *Fertil Steril* 42(2):257–262, 1984.

Rabinowitz R: The importance of the cremasteric reflex in acute scrotal swelling in children. *J Urol* 132:89–90, 1984.

Smith SP, King LR: Torsion of the testis: Techniques of assessment. *Urol Clin North Am* 6(2):429–443, 1979.

Tonetti JA, Tonetti FW: Testicular torsion or acute epididymitis? Diagnosis and treatment. *J Emerg Nurs* 16(2):96–98, 1990.

Veeraraghavan K, Cass BP, Cass AS: Torsion of the testis and its appendages. *Minn Med* 65(6):337–340, 1982.

Whitaker RH: Diagnoses not to be missed: Torsion of the testis. *Br J Hosp Med* 27(1):66–69, 1982.

Testicular Torsion—MRI

Trambert MA, Mattrey RF, Levine D, et al: Subacute scrotal pain: Evaluation of torsion versus epididymitis with MR imaging. *Radiology* 175:53–56, 1990.

Testicular Torsion—Radionuclide Studies

Chen DCP, Holder LE, Kaplan GN: Correlation of radionuclide imaging and diagnostic ultrasound in scrotal diseases. *J Nucl Med* 27:1774–1781, 1986.

Donoghue GD, Prezio JA, Ricci PE: Early diagnosis of testicular tumor using Tc-99m pertechnetate scrotal imaging. *Clin Nucl Med* 8(12):630–631, 1983.

Dunn EK, Macchia RJ, Chauhan PS, et al: Scintiscan for acute intrascrotal conditions. *Clin Nucl Med* 11(6):381–388, 1986.

Eshghi M, Silver L, Smith AD: Technetium 99m scan in acute scrotal lesions. *Urology* 30(6):586–593, 1987.

Nakielny RA, Thomas WEG, Jackson ER, et al: Radionuclide evaluation of acute scrotal disease. *Clin Radiol* 35:125–129, 1984.

Romics I, Wesscler T, Bach D: Scintigraphy for the diagnosis of testicular torsion and differential diagnosis of acute intrascrotal processes. *Int Urol Nephrol* 20(6):631–639, 1988.

Stage KH, Schoenvogel R, Lewis S: Testicular scanning: Clinical experience with 72 patients. *J Urol* 125:334–337, 1981.

Testicular Torsion—Ultrasonography

Bickerstaff KI, Sethia K, Murie JA: Doppler ultrasonography in the diagnosis of acute scrotal pain. *Br J Surg* 75:238–239, 1988.

Carroll BA, Gross DM: High-frequency scrotal sonography. *AJR* 140:511–515, 1983.

Deeg K-H, Wild F: Colour Doppler imaging: A new method to differentiate torsion of the spermatic cord and epididymo-orchitis. *Eur J Pediatr* 149(4):253–255, 1990.

Gutman H, Golimbu M, Subramanyam BR: Diagnostic ultrasound of scrotum. *Urology* 27(1):72–75, 1986.

Heaton ND, Kadow C, Packham DA: Nodular peri-orchitis. *Br J Urol* 64:546, 1989.

Kratzik C, Hainz A, Kuber W, et al: Sonographic appearance of benign intratesticular lesions. *Eur Urol* 15:196–199, 1988.

Krieger JN, Wang K, Mack L: Preliminary evaluation of color Doppler imaging for investigation of intrascrotal pathology. *J Urol* 144:904–907, 1990.

Levy BJ: The diagnosis of torsion of the testicle using the Doppler ultrasonic stethoscope. *J Urol* 113:63–65, 1975.

Middleton WD, Siegel BA, Melson GL, et al: Acute scrotal disorders: Prospective comparison of color Doppler US and testicular scintigraphy. *Radiology* 177:177–181, 1990.

Pedersen JF, Holm HH, Hald T: Torsion of the testis diagnosed by ultrasound. *J Urol* 113:66–68, 1975.

Pintauro WL, Klein FA, Vick CW III, et al: The use of ultrasound for evaluating subacute unilateral scrotal swelling. *J Urol* 133:799–802, 1985.

Ralls PW, Jensen MC, Lee KP, et al: Color Doppler sonography in acute epididymitis and orchitis. *J Clin Ultrasound* 18:383–386, 1990.

Scott RF, Bayliss AP, Calder JF, et al: Indications for ultrasound in the evaluation of the pathological scrotum. *Br J Urol* 58:178–182, 1986.

Tellier P-P, Hofmann AD, Cohen LH: "Red herrings," adolescents, and testicular tumors. *J Adolesc Health Care* 4(4):282–284, 1983.

Trauma—Testicle/Scrotum

Albert NE: Testicular ultrasound for trauma. *J Urol* 124:558–559, 1980.

Anderson KA, McAninch JW, Jeffrey RB, et al: Ultrasonography for the diagnosis and staging of blunt scrotal trauma. *J Urol* 130:933–935, 1983.

Baker LL, Hajek PC, Burkhard TK, et al: MR imaging of the scrotum: Pathologic conditions. *Radiology* 163:93–98, 1987.

Bertini JE Jr, Corriere JN Jr: The etiology and management of genital injuries. *J Trauma* 28(8):1278–1281, 1988.

Cass AS: Testicular trauma. *J Urol* 129:299–300, 1983.

Cass AS, Ferrara L, Wolpert J, et al: Bilateral testicular injury from external trauma. *J Urol* 140:1435–1436, 1988.

Fournier GR Jr, Laing FC, McAninch JW: Scrotal ultrasonography and the management of testicular trauma. *Urol Clin North Am* 16(2):377–385, 1989.

Jeffrey RB, Laing FC, Hricak H, et al: Sonography of testicular trauma. *AJR* 141:993–995, 1983.

Manson AL: Traumatic testicular torsion: Case report. *J Trauma* 29(3):407–408, 1989.

Mucciolo RL, Godec CJ: Traumatic acute incarcerated scrotal hernia. *J Trauma* 28(5):715–716, 1988.

Schaffer RM: Ultrasonography of scrotal trauma. *Urol Radiol* 7:245–249, 1985.

Stillwell TJ, Reading CC, Leary FJ: Untreated rupture of the tunica albuginea. *Mayo Clin Proc* 61:975–977, 1986.

Vasculitis—Testis/Scrotum

Lee LM, Moloney PJ, Wong HCG, et al: Testicular pain: An unusual presentation of polyarteritis nodosa. *J Urol* 129(6):1243–1244, 1983.

Rosenthal S, Kim Y-D, Wise GJ: Neuropathy and orchialgia in a 40-year-old man. *J Urol* 138(1):114–115, 1987.

Shurbaji MS, Epstein JI: Testicular vasculitis: Implications for systemic disease. *Hum Pathol* 19:186–189, 1988.

Vasectomy

Finkbeiner AE, Bissada NK, Redman JF: Complications of vasectomies. *Am Fam Physician* 15(3):86–89, 1977.

Pfenninger JL: Complications of vasectomy. *Am Fam Physician* 30(5):111–115, 1984.

Schned AR, Selikowitz SM: Epididymitis nodosa: An epididymal lesion analogous to vasitis nodosa. *Arch Pathol Lab Med* 110:61–64, 1986.

Selikowitz SM, Schned AR: A late post-vasectomy syndrome. *J Urol* 134:494–497, 1985.

Temmerman M, Cammu H, Devroey P, et al: Evaluation of one-hundred open-ended vasectomies. *Contraception* 33(6):529–532, 1986.

Vasitis

Balogh K, Travis WD: Benign vascular invasion in vasitis nodosa. *Am J Clin Pathol* 83:426–430, 1985.

Heaton JM, MacLennan KA: Vasitis nodosa: A site of arrest of malignant germ cells. *Histopathology* 10:981–989, 1986.

Hirschowitz L, Rode J, Guillebaud J, et al: Vasitis nodosa and associated clinical findings. *J Clin Pathol* 41:419–423, 1988.

Kiser GC, Fuchs EF, Kessler S: The significance of vasitis nodosa. *J Urol* 136(1):42–44, 1986.

Ryan SP, Harte PJ: Suppurative inflammation of vas deferens: An unusual groin mass. *Urology* 31(3):245–246, 1988.

Taxy JB: Vasitis nodosa: Two cases. *Arch Pathol Lab Med* 102:643–647, 1978.

Warner JJ, Kirchner FK Jr, Wong SW, et al: Vasitis nodosa presenting as a mass of the spermatic cord. *J Urol* 129(2):380–381, 1983.

Zimmerman KG, Johnson PC, Paplanus SH: Nerve invasion by benign proliferating ductules in vasitis nodosa. *Cancer* 51:2066–2069, 1983.

CHAPTER

36

Acute Anorectal/ Perineal Pain

☐ **DIAGNOSTIC LIST**

ANORECTAL PAIN
1. Thrombosed external hemorrhoid
2. Prolapsed strangulated internal hemorrhoids
3. Anal fissure
4. Mimics of idiopathic anal fissure
   A. Perianal herpes simplex infection
   B. Perianal syphilis
      1. Primary syphilis
      2. Secondary syphilis
   C. Chancroid
   D. Anal trauma related to sexual activity
   E. Secondary anal fissures
5. Pruritus ani and perianal dermatitis
6. Anorectal abscess
   A. Intersphincteric and perianal abscesses
   B. Transsphincteric (ischiorectal) abscess
7. Necrotizing perianal and perineal infections
   A. Fournier's gangrene (synergistic necrotizing cellulitis)
   B. Clostridial cellulitis
8. Proctitis
   A. *Chlamydia trachomatis* serovars L1, L2, and L3 (lymphogranuloma venereum)
   B. *Treponema pallidum*
   C. Herpes simplex virus
   D. Colitis and proctitis due to *Shigella* and *Campylobacter* species

   E. *Entamoeba histolytica*
   F. *Clostridium difficile*
   G. *Neisseria gonorrhoeae*
   H. *Chlamydia trachomatis* (non-LGV strains)
9. Foreign body (e.g., animal bone) impaction in the anal canal
10. Proctalgia fugax
11. Mimics of proctalgia fugax
    A. Cauda equina tumors and conus tumors
    B. Familial rectal, ocular, and submandibular pain
    C. Rectal spasm and flatus
12. Rectal trauma
13. Irritant causes of anorectal pain
    A. Arsenic poisoning
    B. Laxative effects
    C. Ectopic pregnancy
PERINEAL PAIN
14. Prostate and seminal vesicles
    A. Acute prostatitis
    B. Prostatic abscess
    C. Seminal vesiculitis
15. Urethral injury
16. Urethral stricture and its complications in the male
    A. Urethral stricture
    B. Periurethral abscess
    C. Carcinoma of the urethra
    D. Urethral perforation and urinary extravasation
17. Perineal muscular pain

☐ SUMMARY

Anorectal Pain

A *thrombosed external hemorrhoid* causes the abrupt onset of aching or burning localized anal pain. A tender lump is palpable. Examination reveals a bluish almond-shaped mass extending outward from the anal canal. Pressure on this lesion intensifies the patient's pain, and excision relieves it. *Prolapsed internal hemorrhoids* present as a painless mass protruding through the anal canal. Acute anal pain, associated with swelling, bleeding, and tenderness of this mass, signals thrombosis and strangulation of the prolapsed mucosa and internal hemorrhoids. Hemorrhoidectomy leads to symptom resolution. *Idiopathic anal fissure* causes painful bleeding with each bowel movement. Examination of the anus reveals a midline linear ulcer at 6 o'clock and, less commonly, at 12 o'clock. Idiopathic anal fissure may be *mimicked* by other disorders. Similar burning pain can be caused by *perianal herpes simplex infection*. Multiple perianal grouped ulcerations occur. These are tender and may bleed after wiping. *Syphilis* may cause a painless chancre in the perianal region. This lesion may become infected with pyogenic bacteria or *Haemophilus ducreyi*, producing a painful, tender, ragged ulcer adjacent to, or straddling, the anal canal. Similarly, *lesions of secondary syphilis*, such as condylomata lata and mucous patches, may become secondarily infected and painful. The diagnosis can be confirmed by dark-field microscopy of lesion exudate or by a VDRL or RPR test. *Chancroid* forms a soft, ragged, irregular ulceration that is painful and tender. The edges are erythematous and undermined. Multiple ulcerations may occur; autoinoculation to the thigh or lower leg may be of diagnostic aid. Gram stain of lesion exudate reveals gram-negative coccobacilli in long parallel chains (''railroad tracks''); culture on selective media is positive in 80 percent of cases. *Trauma* from anal intercourse or manipulation may cause scratches, fissures, and ulcerations. *Secondary anal fissures* are usually multiple or in nonmidline portions of the anal circumference. They are associated with underlying diseases, such as Crohn's disease, leukemia, tuberculosis, lymphoma, and carcinoma.

Pruritus ani causes anal itching and excoriation and, eventually, lichenification. Most cases are idiopathic; specific anorectal lesions causing irritating discharge or excessive secretions (e.g., prolapse, fistula, fissure), dermatologic disorders, and systemic causes of pruritus are responsible for the others.

Anorectal abscess begins with severe aching pain that increases in severity in a crescendolike fashion. Throbbing pain may supervene. Fever, chills, and sweats are common associated symptoms. Local tenderness and a submucosal anal canal mass can be felt on digital examination in those with an intersphincteric abscess. Perianal abscesses present with a localized perianal mass and/or local tenderness. An ischiorectal abscess occurs with severe anal and buttock pain, variable skin erythema, and buttock tenderness. Abscess drainage and antibiotic therapy relieve all symptoms.

Necrotizing perianal and perineal infection (Fournier's gangrene, clostridial cellulitis) begins with a perianal or ischiorectal abscess, a urethral infection, or a cutaneous infection on the scrotum or labia. Most cases involve the scrotum, so this disorder occurs predominantly in men. Diabetes mellitus, immunosuppression, leukopenia, advanced age, vasculitis, and anorectal or urologic surgery place patients at risk for this disorder. Perianal, perineal, scrotal, or labial pain may be the first complaint. Perineal structures soon become swollen, erythematous, and tender. A black spot appears on the scrotum or labium and rapidly enlarges. The involved swollen and erythematous tissues may show evidence of skin crepitus due to production of gas by invading bacteria. Polymicrobial synergism is the usual cause of the necrotizing process. Skin gangrene and debridement result in loss of the scrotum, all or part of the penis, and areas of perineal, thigh, and abdominal wall skin.

Proctitis causes anorectal pain, discharge, hematochezia, tenesmus, frequent bowel movements, anorectal tenderness, and sphincter tightness. Acute *lymphogranuloma venereum proctitis* causes anorectal erythema, ulceration, and friability in the distal 12 cm of the rectum. The diagnosis requires isolation of *Chlamydia trachomatis* serovar L1, L2, or L3. There is a response to doxycycline. *Treponema pallidum* may cause an anal or rectal chancre. Infection with pyogenic bacteria or *Haemophilus ducreyi* may convert the usually indolent chancre into a painful, tender lesion. The diagnosis of rectal syphilis depends on the clinical appearance of the chancre and serologic studies (i.e., VDRL or RPR). Perianal chancres can be examined for *T. pallidum* by dark-field microscopy, but rectal chancres cannot, because of the presence of nonpathogenic morphologically similar spirochetes in the bowel flora. Symptoms respond to benzathine penicillin. Mucosal disease occurs only in the distal rectum.

Herpes simplex virus may cause anorectal burning pain, tenderness, tenesmus, fever, hematochezia, and perianal grouped vesicles and ulcers. Suggestive associated symptoms include aching posterior thigh pain, sacral paresthesias, and difficulty in initiating urination. The diagnosis depends on viral isolation. Acyclovir therapy accelerates recovery. *Shigella and Campylobacter species* may cause colitis and proctitis. Bowel mucosal friability and ulcers extend beyond the reach of the sigmoidoscope. The diagnosis can be established by stool culture. *Entamoeba histolytica* causes proctitis with discrete deep mucosal ulcers and relatively normal intervening mucosa. Lesions may extend to the entire colon. Some cases show coalescing ulcers and friable mucosa, simulating ulcerative colitis. Microscopic examination of ulcer exudate and/or stool will establish the diagnosis.

Clostridium difficile proctitis occurs in patients who have recently taken, or are taking, clindamycin, a synthetic penicillin, a cephalosporin, or other antibiotics. Sigmoidoscopic examination of early cases reveals small, volcano-shaped mucosal ulcers covered with pseudomembranes. The organism can be cultured from the stool, and the toxin can be demonstrated in feces by a cell culture assay or an immunologic method. *Neisseria gonorrhoeae* causes purulent anal discharge, mucosal edema, erythema, and ulceration. The organism can be demonstrated on Gram stains of rectal mucosal exudate, and by culture. *Chlamydia trachomatis* (non-LGV strains) can cause a mild proctitis. The diagnosis can be established by rectal culture and a response to doxycycline therapy.

Impaction of a chicken bone, or other bone, in the anal canal causes severe pain that is relieved immediately by removal of the bone.

Proctalgia fugax causes brief attacks of sharp, aching, cramping, or gnawing anorectal pain that pass spontaneously in seconds or minutes. Recurrent episodes are the rule. There may be associated diaphoresis, nausea, or syncope. Physical examination, endoscopy, and imaging studies are negative. The cause and treatment are unknown. Proctalgia fugax can be *mimicked* by spinal subarachnoid *hemorrhage* (in the cauda equina area) due to an arteriovenous malformation or tumor, or to infarction of a spinal canal tumor. MRI can exclude a cauda equina or conus lesion. *Rectosigmoid gas* and *spasm* may also mimic proctalgia fugax. Severe *rectal trauma* may be associated with male homosexual activity; rectal mucosal laceration, hematoma formation, or perforation may occur from insertion of foreign bodies or "fisting."

Rectal pain or tenesmus may be associated with acute *arsenic poisoning, strong laxatives*, or a *ruptured tubal pregnancy*.

Perineal Pain

Perineal pain may occur with *acute prostatitis*. Irritative bladder symptoms, obstructive complaints, fever, and rectal and low back pain may occur. The prostate is enlarged, firm, and tender. There is a prompt response to antibiotic therapy. Failure of fever and other symptoms to respond to therapy; a rectal ache intensified by sitting; urinary retention; and fluctuance of an area of the prostate suggest abscess formation. Transrectal ultrasonography or a CT scan can confirm the diagnosis of *prostatic abscess*. Surgical drainage and antibiotic therapy lead to recovery. *Seminal vesiculitis* often accompanies acute prostatitis; rarely, it may occur as a separate infection. Symptoms suggestive of seminal vesicle involvement include irritative urinary complaints; hematospermia; painful ejaculation; and rectal, perineal, or scrotal pain. Transrectal ultrasonography or a CT scan may demonstrate cystic swelling of the seminal vesicles and seminal vesicle calculi. There is a good response to antibiotic therapy.

Urethral injury causes suprapubic and/or perineal pain, blood at the urethral meatus, and painful urination. Inability to void suggests urethral rupture. A perineal and/or scrotal hematoma or urinoma may develop. Rectal examination reveals a floating or poorly defined prostate. The diagnosis can be established by a retrograde urethrogram that demonstrates a partial or complete rupture of the urethra.

Urethral stricture causes a urethral discharge with irritative

and obstructive voiding symptoms, and can be demonstrated by retrograde urethrography or voiding cystography. Complications of untreated stricture include *periurethral abscess* and *urethral perforation with subcutaneous extravasation* of infected urine; both of these disorders can cause perineal pain and tenderness. *Carcinoma of the urethra* may occur in patients with stricture. Obstructive urinary symptoms, perineal pain, and urethral induration suggest the diagnosis.

Transient perineal pain occurring with each step during walking or running may be caused by a *muscular strain* resulting from participation in competitive sports. It responds to decreased athletic activity, or more complete rest, within 2 to 14 days.

☐ DESCRIPTION OF LISTED DISEASES

Anorectal Pain

1. THROMBOSED EXTERNAL HEMORRHOID

There is an abrupt onset of severe aching or burning anorectal pain. Bowel movements intensify the discomfort. A tender fingertip-sized lump may be felt by the patient. Examination reveals a tender bluish almond-shaped mass beneath the surface of a narrow sector of the anal region. Excision relieves the severe pain and exquisite tenderness, and complete resolution follows within 3 to 4 days.

Some untreated thrombi may ulcerate, become infected, and drain pus. Local drainage and antibiotic therapy lead to resolution.

2. PROLAPSED STRANGULATED INTERNAL HEMORRHOIDS

There is prolapse of the anal cushions beyond the dentate line on standing or walking. The tissue is palpable by the patient, and may initially respond to manual reduction.

Eventually the prolapsed mucosa protrudes all the time, and resists replacement. Severe pain and local tenderness may occur if the prolapsed hemorrhoids thrombose. These symptoms may be associated with marked edema, redness, and necrotic blackening of the surface of the protuberant mass. Surgical excision (hemorrhoidectomy) is required for complete resolution. Prolapsed internal hemorrhoids may be associated with pregnancy; labor; a family predisposition; a lax anal sphincter mechanism; severe constipation with hard, dry stools; or cancer of the rectum or lower sigmoid colon.

3. ANAL FISSURE

There is sharp, burning anal pain during and after the passage of stool (100 percent of cases). Blood may be

TABLE OF DISEASE INCIDENCE

INCIDENCE PER 100,000 (APPROXIMATE)

Common (>100)	Uncommon (>5–100)	Rare (>0–5)
Thrombosed external hemorrhoid	Perianal syphilis	Chancroid
Prolapsed strangulated internal hemorrhoids	Secondary anal fissures	Fournier's gangrene
Idiopathic anal fissure	*Treponema pallidum* proctitis	Clostridial necrotizing cellulitis
Perianal herpes infection	*Entamoeba histolytica* proctitis	*Chlamydia trachomatis* proctitis (LGV and non-LGV strains)
Anal trauma related to sexual activity	*Clostridium difficile* proctitis	Foreign body (bone) impaction in anus
Pruritus ani and perianal dermatitis	*Neisseria gonorrhoeae* proctitis	Mimics of proctalgia fugax:
Anorectal abscess	Rectal trauma	Spinal subarachnoid hemorrhage due to spinal cord tumor
Herpes simplex virus proctitis	Acute prostatitis	Familial rectal, ocular, and submandibular pain
Shigella colitis and proctitis	Urethral injury	Irritant causes of anorectal pain:
Campylobacter colitis and proctitis	Urethral stricture	Arsenic poisoning
Proctalgia fugax	Periurethral abscess	Laxative effects
Rectal spasm and flatus		Ectopic pregnancy
Perineal muscular pain		Prostatic abscess
		Seminal vesiculitis
		Carcinoma of the urethra
		Urethral perforation and urinary extravasation

visible on the stool surface or on the toilet paper with each bowel movement (80 percent). The pain may persist for minutes or hours. The fear of provoking pain leads to constipation (67 percent). Pruritus ani (33 percent), anal soiling (20 percent), and diarrhea (10 percent) are other, less frequent, complaints. Idiopathic anal fissure may begin as a traumatic linear ulcer caused by overdistension of the anus by a large, hard fecal mass during passage; or it may follow an attack of severe diarrhea. The fissure is located on the anoderm distal to the dentate line in the midposterior position (6 o'clock) in 99 percent of men and in 90 percent of women. In the remainder, it is located in the anterior (midventral) position (12 o'clock). Anterior fissures in the female may result from childbirth. Fissures not situated in the anteroposterior axis of the anal canal, and those extending above the dentate line, require further investigation for a specific etiology. Idiopathic acute fissures usually heal after warm sitz baths and an oral intake of 10 g of unprocessed bran twice a day. Symptom relief and healing occur within 1 to 2 weeks. An edematous sentinel pile may appear distal or proximal to the fissure, and may lead to an erroneous diagnosis of hemorrhoidal disease as a cause of the anal pain.

4. MIMICS OF IDIOPATHIC ANAL FISSURE

A. Perianal Herpes Simplex Infection   Burning anal pain and tenderness may be associated with the eruption of groups of tiny red-rimmed vesicles and crusted ulcers on the perianal skin. These lesions may coalesce into larger ulcers, and similar lesions may occur on the genitalia. The diagnosis can be suspected from the clinical examination, and can be confirmed by isolation of herpes simplex virus (usually type 2; rarely type 1) from an ulcer. Oral acyclovir therapy may accelerate healing and decrease viral shedding.

B. Perianal Syphilis

1. Primary Syphilis   A painful, tender, round-to-ovoid, indurated, smooth-surfaced chancre may be the only finding. Pressure on this slightly elevated erosion may express inflammatory fluid containing *Treponema pallidum*. These organisms can be identified by dark-field microscopy. Reagin tests, such as the VDRL and the RPR, are initially positive in 70 percent of those with a chancre. There is a prompt response to benzathine penicillin therapy.

2. Secondary Syphilis   Condylomata lata are slightly elevated, flat-surfaced, round-to-ovoid, white or pink erosions caused by *Treponema pallidum*. Multiple lesions involving the genitalia and perianal region may occur. Secondary infection by pyogenic bacteria or *Haemophilus ducreyi* can lead to perianal pain and local tenderness. Whitish-gray mucosal erosions (i.e., mucous patches) may also occur. Dark-field microscopy is positive, and the nontreponemal antibody tests (VDRL, RPR) are positive in nearly 100 percent of cases. There is a prompt response to penicillin therapy.

C. Chancroid   Painful, tender, single or multiple perianal and genital ulcers may occur. These ulcers are irregular in shape and have undermined erythematous edges. Their surface is covered with a ragged dirty-gray or purulent exudate. The consistency of these lesions is soft in contrast to the indurated primary lesions of syphilis. Painful and tender unilateral or bilateral inguinal adenopathy may occur and progress to suppuration. Gram stain of ulcer exudate may reveal gram-negative coccobacilli in long parallel chains, resembling "railroad tracks," or in a grouping resembling a "school of fish." Culture on a selective medium grows *Haemophilus ducreyi* with a sensitivity of 80 percent. There is a good therapeutic response to erythromycin therapy.

D. Anal Trauma Related to Sexual Activity   Anal trauma may result from vigorous insertion of the penis, a dildo, a bottle, fingers, or a fist into the anal canal. Linear ulcers may occur, become secondarily infected, and cause painful defecation and bleeding. The diagnosis is based on a history of homo- or heterosexual anal intercourse or manipulation. Abstinence from such activity, combined with sitz baths and ingestion of bran, leads to resolution of symptoms and healing of traumatic anal fissures and ulcerations.

E. Secondary Anal Fissures   Atypical fissures may be multiple and/or non-midline. They occur secondary to other disorders of a chronic nature, such as Crohn's disease, leukemia, tuberculosis, lymphoma, and anal cancer.

5. PRURITUS ANI AND PERIANAL DERMATITIS

Soiling and increased moisture of the perianal region may cause local pruritus, tenderness, and burning pain. Pain may occur transiently after bowel movements and wiping. The perianal skin may become red, raw, and edematous, and tender superficial erosions may occur. These may cause blood to be visible on the toilet tissue after wiping. Most cases are idiopathic, but there may be an association with stress, frequent passage of flatus, prolonged sitting, anal fissures, prolapsing internal hemorrhoids, fistula in ano, condylomata acuminata, carcinoma of the anus, diabetes mellitus, a local dermatologic disorder, diarrhea, leukorrhea, or local perianal infection by *Candida* or *Epidermophyton* species. Lichenification of the perianal skin may result from scratching. Exclusion of possible specific etiologic disorders is necessary before a diagnosis of idiopathic pruritus ani can be made. Improved anal hygiene, bowel habit regulation, and elimination of possible contact irritants or allergens (e.g., toilet paper, detergents or dyes in underclothing, soap) and irritant foods may lead to improvement or complete resolution of the itching. Specific causes of pruritus ani are summarized in Table 36-1. Scratching may result in painful perianal excoriations and erosions.

6. ANORECTAL ABSCESS

A. Intersphincteric and Perianal Abscesses   Aching and/or throbbing pain develops in the anal region and rapidly increases in severity. It is intensified by bowel movements, walking, straining, and coughing. Digital

Table 36-1
CAUSES OF PRURITUS ANI AND PERIANAL DERMATITIS

Local anorectal disorders that may cause a locally irritating discharge or drainage
    Crypt infection
    Mucosal and hemorrhoidal prolapse
    Anal fissures
    Anal fistulas
    Carcinoma or lymphoma of the anus
    Condyloma acuminatum
    Pinworm
Skin diseases
    Lichen sclerosus
    Lichen planus
    Intertrigo
    Seborrheic dermatitis
    Psoriasis
    Candidiasis
    Vulvar intraepithelial neoplasia (carcinoma in situ)
    Extramammary Paget's disease
    Allergic dermatitis or irritant chemical dermatitis (e.g., foods, soap)
Causes of generalized pruritus
    Obstructive jaundice
    Renal failure
    Diabetes mellitus and hyperthyroidism
    Lymphoma and polycythemia vera
    Drug allergy (subclinical)
Idiopathic pruritus ani and perianal dermatitis
Prolonged sitting

finger examination is extremely painful; some patients may refuse to allow it. Fever, malaise, rigors, and/or chills may be associated. Urinary retention and constipation may result from the pain.

These abscesses begin as infections of one or more anorectal glands at the level of the pectinate line. The orifices of these glands open into an anal crypt, and their ducts penetrate the internal sphincter to enter the intersphincteric space (the space between the internal and external sphincters). With infection of these glands, suppuration may occur, leading to abscess formation in the intersphincteric space (i.e., an intersphincteric abscess). Extension of infection distally may produce a tender fluctuant mass in the perianal region (i.e., a perianal abscess). If the suppuration remains confined to the intersphincteric space, the abscess can be detected as a tender submucosal mass by digital examination. Spontaneous local drainage into the rectum leads to the resolution of anorectal pain, fever, chills, and prostration. Many early abscesses do not form a perianal fluctuant tender mass. Perianal tenderness in the presence of a history of crescendo anal pain and fever is suggestive of an anorectal abscess requiring drainage. Such patients require careful digital examination and/or exploration under anesthesia in the operating room.

B. Transsphincteric (Ischiorectal) Abscess   Rupture

of an intersphincteric abscess through the external sphincter into the ischiorectal space may cause buttock pain, tenderness, fluctuance, and erythema of the overlying skin. Bilateral ischiorectal abscesses may occur by spread from the initially affected space through the deep postanal space (i.e., horseshoe abscess). Most abscesses are polymicrobial, containing *Escherichia coli*, *Bacteroides* species, and other coliforms or anaerobic bacteria.

Prompt and complete surgical drainage and use of antibiotics leads to resolution of all symptoms and signs.

7. NECROTIZING PERIANAL AND PERINEAL INFECTIONS

A. Fournier's Gangrene (Synergistic Necrotizing Cellulitis) This disorder usually arises as a complication of a localized infection of the rectum and perirectal area [i.e., ischiorectal or perianal abscess (49 percent of cases)], the urethra [i.e., infection of periurethral glands or stricture (21 percent)], or the skin [folliculitis or balanitis (31 percent)]. This disorder may rarely occur in healthy young adults without an underlying disorder. Increased risk occurs in the presence of diabetes mellitus and following chemotherapy for hematologic malignancy. Others at risk include the elderly, males, and patients with advanced liver or renal disease. Patients with poor personal hygiene, granulocytopenia, leukemia, immunosuppression, or alcoholism are also more susceptible to necrotizing perianal infections. Urethral stricture, chronic use of a Foley catheter, and small-vessel disease (i.e., hypersensitivity vasculitis) may result in an increased incidence of this disorder. Fournier's gangrene has also been associated with a perforated sigmoid diverticulitis, breakdown of a primary colonic anastomosis, anorectal biopsy, digital rectal examination, and hemorrhoidectomy. Urologic procedures associated with this disease have included penile prosthesis surgery, aspiration of hydroceles, and circumcision. Chronic urinary tract infection has also been associated. Most cases occur in males, but females may also develop a similar disorder.

The initial symptoms may reflect the localized infection causing the necrotizing disorder. Severe pain in the perianal area or buttock (abscess) or in the labial or scrotal area (cutaneous infections), or dysuria (urethral infection), may occur. Swelling of the skin of the anogenital area soon follows. Erythema is variable and may occur early or late. Fever occurs in up to 66 percent of cases; it may be associated with severe prostration and shock (18 percent), and with delirium or coma (14 percent). Examination reveals fever; toxicity; local swelling of the genitalia, anal area, and/or perineum; skin crepitus (66 percent); and severe tenderness. A flat, black spot soon develops on the scrotum or labia, and then rapidly enlarges. Blackening at other perineal sites may also occur, and may extend to cover large portions of the anogenital

region, buttocks, and lower anterior abdominal wall. Fissures or ulcerations in the inflamed and necrotic skin may drain a malodorous yellow-brown discharge. Leukocytosis (93 percent), hyponatremia and pseudohyponatremia, hyperglycemia, and an elevated creatinine level are common findings.

Bacterial cultures of the exudate or necrotic skin reveal an average of 4 organisms per patient. Cases arising in an anorectal focus are usually associated with *Escherichia coli* (86 percent), *Peptostreptococcus* species (79 percent), and *Bacteroides* species (100 percent). Urethral foci are associated with coliform and streptococcal isolates and infections of cutaneous origin with group A or B streptococci, *Staphylococcus epidermidis*, *E. coli*, and *Peptostreptococcus* species. It is believed that these mixed infections are synergistic, resulting in severe inflammation, vasculitis, and ischemic necrosis of the skin and fascia.

B. Clostridial Cellulitis In some series of patients with necrotizing anorectal and perineal infection, *Clostridium perfringens* (63 percent) and other *Clostridium* species (19 percent) have been the predominant organisms. Fournier's gangrene, synergistic necrotizing cellulitis, and clostridial cellulitis appear to be clinically very similar, or even to be the same disorder. Cases with predominantly clostridial isolates are examples of clostridial cellulitis.

Some early cases have only acute scrotal pain and tenderness, and no black spots indicating necrosis. Crepitus may be palpable, or gas in the tissues may be detected by ultrasonography or by plain radiographs of the scrotum.

Treatment of necrotizing perineal infection requires extensive surgical debridement of necrotic skin. Resection of the entire scrotum, portions of the penis, and regions of the skin of the perineum, thigh, and abdominal wall may be required. Broad-spectrum multiple-drug antibiotic therapy is also necessary. Some patients may require suprapubic cystotomy and/or a defunctioning colostomy.

8. PROCTITIS

Symptoms of acute anorectal inflammation and ulceration include fever, severe aching or burning anorectal pain, hematochezia, rectal discharge, and frequent bowel movements and/or soft or liquid stools. Tenesmus may occur in severe cases. Lower abdominal cramping, or constant pain, nausea, and vomiting may occur; these are less frequent complaints. Examination reveals fever, left lower abdominal tenderness, anal sphincter tightness, and anal canal tenderness. Sigmoidoscopy reveals evidence of mucosal edema, ulceration, erythema, and exudate. In patients with treponemal, chlamydial, herpetic, or gonococcal proctitis, lesions do not extend above 12 cm from the pectinate line. Proctitis is most commonly seen in homosexual men, or in women, participating in anal intercourse.

A. *Chlamydia trachomatis* **Serovars L1, L2, and L3 (Lymphogranuloma Venereum)** Acute ulcerative proctitis has been reported in homosexual men. Sigmoidoscopy may reveal normal mucosa and/or pus, erythema, a follicular or "cobblestone" appearance of the mucosa, small ulcerations, and friable areas. Mucosal involvement ends 6 to 12 cm proximal to the pectinate line. Painful inguinal lymphadenopathy may occur. The diagnosis can be confirmed by chlamydial cultures and identification of isolates as serovar L1, L2, or L3. Elevated titers may not occur on the LGV complement fixation test. Microimmunofluorescent titers are usually markedly elevated. This test is not specific, since comparable elevations occur in non-LGV *C. trachomatis* proctitis. There is a therapeutic response to doxycycline therapy.

B. *Treponema pallidum* Chancres are usually asymptomatic unless they became secondarily infected. Such lesions may cause anorectal pain, tenesmus, increased stool frequency and urgency, and a mucoid or blood-tinged anal discharge. Cryptitis or small submucosal abscesses may occur. Rectal chancres are firm, sometimes tender, circular lesions, 2 to 3 cm in diameter. Dark-field microscopy is not helpful for rectal lesions, because there are similar, nonpathogenic spirochetes in the bowel flora. Dark-field microscopy has more specificity when spirochetes occur in exudates from anal and perianal lesions. Serologic diagnosis has a false-negative rate of up to 30 percent at the time of onset of symptoms, so the RPR or VDRL test should be repeated at monthly intervals for up to 3 months to exclude syphilis. Some patients with AIDS may fail to develop a positive VDRL test because of abnormal lymphocyte function. One dose of benzathine penicillin G is usually curative for uncomplicated primary syphilis; some authorities recommend three weekly doses to ensure eradication of *T. pallidum.*

C. Herpes Simplex Virus (HSV) Symptoms of herpes simplex proctitis include fever (48 percent), severe anorectal pain (100 percent), tenesmus (100 percent), constipation (78 percent), and tender unilateral or bilateral inguinal adenopathy (57 percent). Associated neurologic symptoms may be helpful diagnostically. These include difficulty in initiating urination (48 percent), sacral paresthesias (13 percent), and posterior thigh pain (25 percent).

Hematochezia (61 percent) and anal pruritus (74 percent) are other common complaints. Perianal or anal grouped vesicles and small ulcers occur in up to 70 percent, and can be detected by direct inspection and anoscopy. Sigmoidoscopy may reveal focal or diffuse mucosal friability, diffuse ulceration of the distal rectum, and small vesiculopustular lesions. Biopsy findings include crypt abscesses, polymorphonuclear leukocytosis in the lamina propria, multinucleated cells with ground-glass nuclei, and intranuclear inclusions. Tzanck preparations taken from an ulcer may be helpful. Direct fluorescent antibody staining is more sensitive and specific than the Tzanck test. Diagnosis depends on viral isolation and identification. Most isolations are HSV 2, but occasional cases caused by HSV 1 have been reported. Extension of the disease process above 10 cm from the pectinate line occurs in fewer than 5 percent of cases. Treatment with acyclovir for 10 days leads to rapid resolution of symptoms and cessation of viral shedding.

D. Colitis and Proctitis Due to *Shigella* **and** *Campylobacter* **Species** These organisms may cause fever and diarrhea. Proctitis, with tenesmus, anorectal pain, and a purulent or hemorrhagic discharge, may also occur. In some cases diarrhea does not occur.

E. *Entamoeba histolytica* Amebic infection can cause a severe proctitis with fever, tenesmus, anorectal pain, abdominal cramps, a mucopurulent anorectal discharge, and hematochezia.

Sigmoidoscopy reveals minimal mucosal erythema, petechial hemorrhages, and small ulcers with hyperemic borders, covered with exudate. The mucosa between the ulcers may be relatively normal or mildly edematous and hyperemic. This endoscopic picture is characteristic of amebiasis or Crohn's disease. Lesions may occur above the 10-cm level (measured from the pectinate line). Fluid aspirated from ulcers may reveal motile amebic trophozoites. Amebic proctitis can also be diagnosed by microscopic examination of stool specimens. Antiamebic antibodies can be detected by an indirect hemagglutination test in 85 percent of patients with invasive intestinal disease. Treatment with metronidazole is effective in relieving symptoms and resolving mucosal lesions. Administration of diiodohydroxyquin is effective against intraluminal cysts.

F. *Clostridium difficile* This infection follows, or occurs during, therapy with clindamycin or broad-spectrum β-lactam antibiotics. Symptoms include watery or mucoid, green, foul-smelling, and sometimes bloody diarrhea; left lower abdominal pain and tenderness; anorectal pain and soreness; tenesmus; passage of bloody mucous; and fever. Sigmoidoscopy in early cases may reveal small volcano-like ulcers covered with pseudomembranes. *C. difficile* can be cultured from the stool on a selective medium [e.g., cycloserine, cefoxitin, fructose agar (CCFA)]. *C. difficile* toxin B can be demonstrated in stool using a cell culture system. An ELISA method for detection of toxin A is under study. Symptoms resolve after treatment with vancomycin or metronidazole.

G. *Neisseria gonorrhoeae* This agent may cause moderate to severe anorectal pain, tenesmus, local tenderness, and a mucopurulent rectal discharge. Fever and chills may occur. The mucosa is hyperemic and edematous, and may be friable. Rectal ulcerations may occur. Gram stain and culture of exudate reveals *N. gonorrhoeae*. Antibiotic therapy leads to rapid resolution of symptoms.

H. *Chlamydia trachomatis* (Non-LGV Strains) Mild anorectal pain and discharge may occur. Sigmoidoscopy reveals mild hyperemia and small erosions or prominent ''follicles,'' and focal friable areas in the distal 10 cm of the rectum. Biopsies reveal mild inflammation of the rectal mucosa and occasional crypt abscesses. The diagnosis requires isolation of *C. trachomatis* from rectal cultures and immunotyping of these isolates. There is a good response to doxycycline therapy.

9. FOREIGN BODY (e.g., ANIMAL BONE) IMPACTION IN THE ANAL CANAL

Acute severe anal pain may occur following a bowel movement. Rectal examination may reveal a hard, bone-like object. Removal of the foreign body (usually a chicken bone or other type of bone) impacted in the anal canal leads to immediate relief. Manual anal dilation, with the help of an anesthetic gel, facilitates manual or forceps removal. Impaction of a swallowed bone is rare in Western nations; it is more common among the Chinese, who chop meat with bones into small pieces before cooking.

10. PROCTALGIA FUGAX

There is an abrupt onset of severe, stabbing, cramping, aching, or gnawing anorectal pain. During the attack, some patients prefer to lie down on one side with their legs drawn up. Cold sweats, priapism, syncope, and nausea have been associated with the pain in small numbers of patients; these symptoms probably represent an autonomic response to the pain. Characteristically, the pain has a brief duration, lasting seconds to minutes (mean time is 3 min). The diagnosis should be questioned if the pain persists for more than 20 min. Attacks have been reported during sleep, while straining at stool, after a bowel movement, and, in males, during coitus. Physicians with this symptom describe a lax anal sphincter and a tender, tense band on one or both sides adjacent to the rectum. Pain attacks have also coincided with forceful sigmoid contractions. Spasm of the levator ani or pubococcygeal muscles has been suggested as an explanation of the pain and the palpable perianal band detected by physicians experiencing this disorder. Functional gastrointestinal disorders (irritable bowel) are commonly associated (52 percent). Examination after an attack reveals no abnormality. All laboratory, endoscopic, and radio-

graphic studies of the anorectal region and pelvis are negative. The diagnosis depends on the history and on exclusion of local disease. Proctalgia fugax is a common disorder, affecting 13 to 19 percent of healthy individuals. Recurrent attacks usually follow the first episode.

11. MIMICS OF PROCTALGIA FUGAX

A. Cauda Equina Tumors and Conus Tumors Cauda equina tumors (schwannomas) and conus tumors (ependymomas) may infarct or bleed into the subarachnoid space, causing severe anorectal pain of a transient or persistent nature. Persistent acute rectal pain with no local disease, the presence of lower extremity motor weakness, pain, and patchy sensory loss, and/or sphincter disturbances are indications for MRI or a CT scan of the lower thoracic and lumbar areas of the spine. Patients with subarachnoid bleeding may subsequently develop headache, photophobia, and a painful stiff neck. Surgical removal of the intraspinal tumor is required.

B. Familial Rectal, Ocular, and Submandibular Pain This triad has been described as a rare familial syndrome. Blanching and erythema of the skin near the areas of pain occurs. There is no effective therapy.

C. Rectal Spasm and Flatus Some patients with considerable amounts of flatus may experience brief (15- to 30-s) attacks of rectal pain. Recurrent pains may occur over a 20-min period. No underlying disorder is present. Some of these patients may be considered to have a form of proctalgia fugax.

12. RECTAL TRAUMA

Anorectal pain, tenesmus, and rectal bleeding may occur within seconds of the traumatic event. Injuries usually result from male homosexual activity. For example, insertion of a fist (''fisting''), a forearm, a baseball bat, or a bottle into the rectum may result in a laceration of the anterior rectal wall, or bowel (anal canal) perforation. Injuries related to penile intercourse are usually mild and superficial, but may be severe. In such cases sigmoidoscopy may reveal a laceration or perforation of the rectosigmoid or, rarely, a large submucosal hematoma. The appearance of anemia or fever indicates a more serious injury. Perforation of the bowel may result in acute peritonitis, with abdominal pain, direct and rebound tenderness, guarding, and fever. Surgical intervention is usually required for perforation and secondary peritonitis, or to evacuate an intramural rectal hematoma. A case of recurrent rectal wall hematoma secondary to male anal rape has been reported.

13. IRRITANT CAUSES OF ANORECTAL PAIN

Tenesmus and/or anorectal pain may be associated with the following:

A. Arsenic Poisoning   Cramping abdominal pain, diarrhea, and rectal pain may occur after arsenic ingestion. Dysphagia, nausea, vomiting, weakness, and a garliclike breath odor may be present. A plain radiograph of the abdomen may show radiopaque material in the stomach and small bowel. Hematuria, epistaxis, polydipsia, periorbital edema, conjunctivitis, skin hyperesthesia, and muscle cramps may occur. Bone marrow depression and a sensorimotor peripheral neuropathy follow if the patient survives beyond the first week after ingestion. The diagnosis can be confirmed by a history of arsenic ingestion and by measurement of arsenic concentrations in blood or urine.

B. Laxative Effects   Castor oil or citrate of magnesia may cause watery diarrhea and painful tenesmus.

C. Ectopic Pregnancy   Rupture of an ectopic pregnancy with bleeding may cause lower abdominal pain, weakness, and pallor. Rectal pain and tenesmus may occur in some cases. The diagnosis can be confirmed by a positive pregnancy test and the absence of an intrauterine pregnancy on ultrasonography. A tubal mass may be imaged in some cases, adding further support to the diagnosis.

Perineal Pain

4. PROSTATE AND SEMINAL VESICLES

A. Acute Prostatitis   This disorder may present with dysuria, frequency, urgency, a thinned or split urinary stream, and aching pain in the rectal and perineal areas. Fever, chills, rigors, low back pain, and generalized myalgias may be present. A sense of incomplete emptying of the bladder may be present, or complete urinary retention may occur. The prostate is swollen and tender. Increased numbers of leukocytes are present in the urine and expressed prostatic secretions. Massage of the prostate to obtain prostatic secretions should be avoided, because of the danger of causing an acute bacteremia. The responsible bacteria are usually *Escherichia coli*, *Pseudomonas*, and *Enterococcus* species. Rare causes include *Salmonella* and *Clostridium* species, *Mycobacterium tuberculosis*, fungi, and *Actinomyces* species. Hospitalization and administration of parenteral antibiotics usually leads to the resolution of symptoms.

B. Prostatic Abscess   This disorder is a complication of acute prostatitis. Symptoms may include suprapubic and perineal pain, persistent fever, tenesmus, rectal aching intensified by sitting, and urinary retention, or frequency, and dysuria. A persistent leukocytosis may be present. Rectal examination may reveal a fluctuant mass in the prostate, or only a firm, tender, enlarged gland. Transrectal ultrasonography and CT scans are superior to physical examination for the detection and delineation of a prostatic abscess. These abscesses may drain spontaneously into the rectum or urethra. This disorder is associated with diabetes mellitus, carcinoma of the prostate (33 percent of cases), immunosuppression, and urologic instrumentation. Common isolates from prostatic abscesses include *Escherichia coli*, *Staphylococcus aureus*, *Proteus* species, *Pseudomonas* species, and *Staphylococcus albus*. A prostatic abscess requires drainage, as well as antibiotic therapy. Drainage can be achieved by needle aspiration with sonographic guidance, by transurethral resection, or by an open approach.

C. Seminal Vesiculitis   This disorder may cause perineal and scrotal pain, rectal pain, hematospermia, and ejaculatory pain. Fever, chills, and irritative and obstructive urinary symptoms may occur as well. Transrectal ultrasonography may demonstrate cystic enlargement of the seminal vesicles, and/or seminal vesicle calculi. Antibiotic therapy usually leads to resolution.

15. URETHRAL INJURY

The urethra may be injured by blunt or penetrating trauma. Up to 11 percent of patients with a pelvic fracture suffer urethral injury. Straddle falls, with direct perineal trauma, commonly cause urethral damage. Suprapubic and perineal pain, blood at the meatus, obstructive symptoms and dysuria, or inability to void, lower abdominal swelling (i.e., from bladder distension), a perineal hematoma or urinoma due to urinary extravasation, or a scrotal hematoma may occur after urethal injury. Urinary extravasation may cause puffy swelling of the perineum, upper thighs, scrotum, and lower anterior abdominal wall. Rectal examination in the male may demonstrate a "high-riding," "floating," or absent prostate, or a poorly defined, boggy fullness in the normal anatomic site of the prostate. Retrograde urethrography will delineate a urethral tear and/or rupture. Such lesions are rare in women, and result from downward extension of bladder lacerations. Suprapubic cystotomy and repair of the urethra result in resolution of symptoms.

16. URETHRAL STRICTURE AND ITS COMPLICATIONS IN THE MALE

A. Urethral Stricture   Urethral stricture follows trauma or infection. Blunt or penetrating trauma may cause urethral tears, and sometimes urethral rupture. Transurethral resection of the prostate, the chronic presence of an indwelling catheter, and soundings may also contribute to stricture formation. Infectious disorders, such as gonococcal or chlamydial urethritis, syphilis, or tuberculosis, may lead to urethral stricture. Strictures are usually localized to one region of the urethra, but up to 11 percent are multiple. The bulbomembranous urethra (70 percent) and the pendulous urethra are the most common sites of postinfectious stricture. Chronic prostatitis and surgical resection of the prostate, with scarring of the urethral wall, may contribute to narrowing of the prostatic urethra.

Common complaints include a chronic urethral discharge (i.e., due to infection in the vicinity of the stricture), dysuria, frequency, and urgency. The obstructive nature of this disorder results in a thin or split urinary stream, and dribbling. Urinary retention may occur. A stricture may interfere with the therapy of chronic prostatitis and may coexist with prostatic hypertrophy, leading to more severe obstructive symptoms. The role of each component in such combined obstructions may be sorted out by observation of the effects on urinary flow of dilation of the stricture, and by endoscopy. Examination may reveal a urethral discharge and localized urethral induration. Stricture may be detected by difficulty in passing a catheter. Stricture severity in the bulbomembranous urethra can be estimated by passage of sounds of varying diameters. Endoscopy and retrograde urethrography will most clearly delineate the site and extent of a stricture. Urethrography may aid in the diagnosis of ulcerative infection, carcinoma, and a urethral diverticulum.

B. Periurethral Abscess This disorder may arise during an attack of gonococcal or chlamydial urethritis, or may be a complication of a chronic stricture. Localized perineal pain and a palpable, tender perineal mass occur proximal to the stricture. Spontaneous rupture of this fluctuant mass may result in a urethrocutaneous fistula, with leakage of urine from the perineum during voiding.

C. Carcinoma of the Urethra This disorder may occur secondarily to obstruction and infection. Increasingly severe obstructive symptoms, local perineal pain, palpable urethral induration, or local metastasis may signal the presence of malignancy. Endoscopic biopsy will confirm the diagnosis.

D. Urethral Perforation and Urinary Extravasation
This complication occurs at, or proximal to, the site of stricture, and is secondary to inflammatory erosion of the urethral wall. Extravasation of infected urine occurs, causing edema, erythema, pain, and tenderness in the perineum and/or scrotum, and in the lower anterior abdominal wall. The penis may become markedly swollen and red. Fever, chills, and malaise may occur. Subcutaneous abscesses may form, with purulent drainage and sloughing of necrotic skin. Urethrocutaneous fistulas may result, with urinary drainage from one or more perineal sites during voiding. Urethral stricture is rare in women; it most commonly results from trauma to the bladder, with urethral extension.

17. PERINEAL MUSCULAR PAIN

Perineal pain provoked with each step during running or walking may be caused by a strained muscle. Rest for 1 to 14 days will usually lead to disappearance of such pain. Precipitants of this disorder include participation in competitive sports that require quick starts and stops, like racquet ball or tennis. Actual recollection of an injury during participation is uncommon; usually the perineal pain begins 1 to 2 days later.

ANAL AND PERINEAL PAIN REFERENCES

Anal Carcinoma

Boey J, Wong J, Ong GB: Epidermoid carcinoma of the anus. *Aust N Z J Surg* 52(5):521–524, 1982.

Brown DK, Oglesby AB, Scott DH, et al: Squamous cell carcinoma of the anus: A twenty-five year retrospective. *Am Surg* 54(6):337–342, 1988.

Cobb JP, Schecter WP, Russell T: Giant malignant tumors of the anus: A strategy for management. *Dis Colon Rectum* 33:135–138, 1990.

Cutuli B, Fenton J, Labib A, et al: Anal margin carcinoma: 21 cases treated at the Institut Curie by exclusive conservative radiotherapy. *Radiother Oncol* 11:1–6, 1988.

Flood HD, Salman AA: Malignant fibrous histiocytoma of the anal canal. *Dis Colon Rectum* 32:256–259, 1989.

Holmes F, Borek D, Owen-Kummer M, et al: Anal cancer in women. *Gastroenterology* 95:107–111, 1988.

Leibach SJ, Kiel K, Brescia RJ: Carcinoma of the anal canal. *Med Pediatr Oncol* 11:367–370, 1983.

Leichman LP, Cummings BJ: Anal carcinoma. *Curr Probl Cancer* 14(3): 117–159, 1990.

Lopez MJ, Bliss DP Jr, Kraybill WG, et al: Carcinoma of the anal region. *Curr Probl Surg* 26(8):525–600, 1989.

Mangiante EC, Dilawari RA, Britt LG: Neoplasia of the extraperitoneal rectum and anus: The perineal dilemma. *Am Surg* 49(2):73–75, 1983.

Shirouzu K, Morodomi T, Isomoto H, et al: Long-term survival case of small (oat) cell carcinoma of the rectum. *Acta Pathol Jpn* 37(1): 111–116, 1987.

Taxy JB, Gupta PK, Gupta JW, et al: Anal cancer: Microscopic condyloma and tissue demonstration of human papillomavirus capsid antigen and viral DNA. *Arch Pathol Lab Med* 113:1127–1131, 1989.

Werdin C, Limas C, Knodell RG: Primary malignant melanoma of the rectum: Evidence for origination from rectal mucosal melanocytes. *Cancer* 61:1364–1370, 1988.

Anal Fissure

Bernard D, Morgan S, Tassé D: Selective surgical management of Crohn's disease of the anus. *Can J Surg* 29(5):318–321, 1986.

Boddie AW Jr, Bines SD: Management of acute rectal problems in leukemic patients. *J Surg Oncol* 33:53–56, 1986.

Corman ML: Anal fissures, in *Colon and Rectal Surgery*. Philadelphia, Lippincott, 1984, pp 73–84.

Farmer G: Perianal infection with group A streptococcus. *Arch Dis Child* 62(11):1169–1170, 1987.

Gibbons CP, Read NW: Anal hypertonia in fissures: Cause or effect? *Br J Surg* 73:443–445, 1986.

Gingold BS: Simple in-office sphincterotomy with partial fissurectomy for chronic anal fissure. *Surg Gynecol Obstet* 165(1):46–48, 1987.

Goldstein SD: Anal fissures and fistulas: Two common but very different maladies. *Postgrad Med* 82(7):86–92, 1987.

Jensen SL: Treatment of first episodes of acute anal fissure: Prospective randomised study of lignocaine ointment versus hydrocortisone ointment or warm sitz baths plus bran. *Br Med J [Clin Res]* 292(6529):1167–1169, 1986.

Notaras MJ: Anal fissure and stenosis. *Surg Clin North Am* 68(6):1427–1440, 1988.

Sweeney JL, Ritchie JK, Nicholls RJ: Anal fissure in Crohn's disease. *Br J Surg* 75:56–57, 1988.

Anal Fistula

Accarpio G, Davini MD, Fazio A, et al: Pilonidal sinus with an anal canal fistula: Report of a case. *Dis Colon Rectum* 31:965–967, 1988.

Beavis RE: Use of hydrogen peroxide to identify internal opening of anal fistula and perianal abscess (letter to editor). *Aust N Z J Surg* 57:137, 1987.

Doberneck RC: Perianal suppuration: Results of treatment. *Am Surg* 53(10):569–572, 1987.

Evaldson GR: Pararectal abscess with pelvic extension simulating gynecological disease. *Acta Obstet Gynecol Scand* 65:803–804, 1986.

Fasth SB, Nordgren S, Hultén L: Clinical course and management of suprasphincteric and extrasphincteric fistula-in-ano. *Acta Chir Scand* 156:397–402, 1990.

Mehta K, Pawel BR: Human immunodeficiency virus-associated large-cell immunoblastic lymphoma presenting as a perianal abscess. *Arch Pathol Lab Med* 113:531–533, 1989.

Radcliffe AG, Ritchie JK, Hawley PR, et al: Anovaginal and rectovaginal fistulas in Crohn's disease. *Dis Colon Rectum* 31:94–99, 1988.

Ross ST: Fistula in ano. *Surg Clin North Am* 68(6):1417–1426, 1988.

Schouten WR, Van Vroonhoven TJMV, Van Berlo CLJ: Primary partial internal sphincterectomy in the treatment of anorectal abscess. *Neth J Surg* 39(2):43–45, 1987.

Shukla HS, Gupta SC, Singh G, et al: Tubercular fistula in ano. *Br J Surg* 75:38–39, 1988.

Tancer ML, Lasser D, Rosenblum N: Rectovaginal fistula or perineal and anal sphincter disruption, or both, after vaginal delivery. *Surg Gynecol Obstet* 171(1):43–46, 1990.

Ward CS, Dunphy EP, Jagoe WS, et al: Crohn's disease limited to the mouth and anus. *J Clin Gastroenterol* 7(6):516–521, 1985.

Anal Lymphoma

Burkes RL, Meyer PR, Gill PS, et al: Rectal lymphoma in homosexual men. *Arch Intern Med* 146:913–915, 1986.

Ioachim HL, Weinstein MA, Robbins RD, et al: Primary anorectal lymphoma: A new manifestation of the acquired immune deficiency syndrome (AIDS). *Cancer* 60:1449–1453, 1987.

Lee MH, Waxman M, Gillooley JF: Primary malignant lymphoma of the anorectum in homosexual men. *Dis Colon Rectum* 29:413–416, 1986.

Anal Trauma

Chen YM, Davis M, Ott DJ: Traumatic rectal hematoma following anal rape. *Ann Emerg Med* 15:850–852, 1986.

Anal Ulcers

Jali HM: Tuberculous anal ulcer. *J R Soc Med* 82(10):629–630, 1989.

Maule WF, Perniciaro C, Ortego TJ: Cavitating ulcers: Pyoderma gangrenosum of the anal canal? *Gastroenterology* 95(4):1158–1159, 1988.

Anorectal Abscess

Corman ML: Anorectal abscess and fistula, in *Colon and Rectal Surgery*. Philadelphia, Lippincott, 1984, pp 85–113.

Anorectal Lesions in AIDS

Carr ND, Mercey D, Slack WW: Non-condylomatous perianal disease in homosexual men. *Br J Surg* 76:1064–1066, 1989.

Miles AJG, Mellor CH, Gazzard B, et al: Surgical management of anorectal disease in HIV-positive homosexuals. *Br J Surg* 77:869–871, 1990.

Colitis—Radiation

Goldberg SM, Nivatvongs S, Rothenberger DA: Colon, rectum, and anus, in Schwartz SI, Shires GT, Spencer FC (eds): *Principles of Surgery*, 5th ed. New York, McGraw-Hill, 1989, pp 1225–1314.

Thayer WR Jr, Denucci T: Miscellaneous diseases of the large bowel and anal canal, in Kirsner JB, Shorter RG (eds): *Diseases of the Colon, Rectum, and Anal Canal*. Baltimore, Williams & Wilkins, 1988, pp 561–594.

Colorectal Carcinoma

Bassett ML, Bennett SA, Goulston KJ: Colorectal cancer: A study of 230 patients. *Med J Aust* 1:589–592, 1979.

Ibrahim NK, Abdul-Karim FW: Colorectal adenocarcinoma in young Lebanese adults: The American University of Beirut-Medical Center experience with 32 patients. *Cancer* 58:816–820, 1986.

Moore PA, Dilawari RA, Fidler WJ: Adenocarcinoma of the colon and rectum in patients less than 40 years of age. *Am Surg* 50(1):10–14,1984.

Pitluk H, Poticha SM: Carcinoma of the colon and rectum in patients less than 40 years of age. *Surg Gynecol Obstet* 157(4):335–337, 1983.

Dermatologic Disorders

Corman ML: Dermatologic anal conditions, in *Colon and Rectal Surgery*. Philadelphia, Lippincott, 1984, pp 177–225.

Diverticulitis—Rectum

Chiu TCT, Bailey HR, Hernandez AJ Jr: Diverticulitis of the midrectum. *Dis Colon Rectum* 26:59–60, 1983.

Foreign Body—Anus

Carr N: Acute anal pain and a chicken bone. *J R Coll Gen Pract* 37:314, 1987.

Fournier's Gangrene

Barkel DC, Villalba MR: A reappraisal of surgical management in necrotizing perineal infections. *Am Surg* 52(7):395–397, 1986.

Baskin LS, Carroll PR, Cattolica EV, et al: Necrotising soft tissue infections of the perineum and genitalia: Bacteriology, treatment and risk assessment. *Br J Urol* 65:524–529, 1990.

Begley MG, Shawker TH, Robertson CN, et al: Fournier gangrene: Diagnosis with scrotal US. *Radiology* 169:387–389, 1988.

Berg A, Armitage JO, Burns CP: Fournier's gangrene complicating aggressive therapy for hematologic malignancy. *Cancer* 57:2291–2294, 1986.

Bubrick MP, Hitchcock CR: Necrotizing anorectal and perineal infections. *Surgery* 86(4):655–662, 1979.

Burpee JF, Edwards P: Fournier's gangrene. *J Urol* 107:812–814, 1972.

DiFalco G, Guccione C, D'Annibale A, et al: Fournier's gangrene following a perianal abscess. *Dis Colon Rectum* 29:582–585, 1986.

Gorbach SL, Bartlett JG: Anaerobic infections: 2. *N Engl J Med* 290(22):1237–1245, 1974.

Pande SK, Mewara PC: Fournier's gangrene: A report of 5 cases. *Br J Surg* 63:479–481, 1976.

Rea WJ, Wyrick WJ Jr: Necrotizing fasciitis. *Ann Surg* 172:957–964, 1970.

Rudolph R, Soloway M, DePalma RG, et al: Fournier's syndrome: Synergistic gangrene of the scrotum. *Am J Surg* 129:591–596, 1975.

Skiles MS, Covert GK, Fletcher HS: Gas-producing clostridial and nonclostridial infections. *Surg Gynecol Obstet* 147:65–67, 1978.

Sohn M, Kistler D, Kindler J, et al: Fournier's gangrene in hypersensitivity vasculitis. *J Urol* 142:823–825, 1989.

Stone HH, Martin JD Jr: Synergistic necrotizing cellulitis. *Ann Surg* 175(5):702–711, 1972.

Hemorrhoids

Asfar SK, Juma TH, Ala-Edeen T: Hemorrhoidectomy and sphincterotomy: A prospective study comparing the effectiveness of anal stretch and sphincterotomy in reducing pain after hemorrhoidectomy. *Dis Colon Rectum* 31:181–185, 1988.

Roe AM, Bartolo DCC, Vellacott KD, et al: Submucosal versus ligation excision haemorrhoidectomy: A comparison of anal sensation, anal sphincter manometry and postoperative pain and function. *Br J Surg* 74:948–951, 1987.

Perineal Pain

Hellendoorn-Smit M, Overweg-van Kints J: Perineal pain: A case report. *Eur J Surg Oncol* 14:197–198, 1988.

Saris SC, Silver JM, Vieira JFS, et al: Sacrococcygeal rhizotomy for perineal pain. *Neurosurgery* 19(5):789–793, 1986.

Temple WJ, Ketcham AS: Surgical palliation for recurrent rectal cancers ulcerating in the perineum. *Cancer* 65:1111–1114, 1990.

Perineal Pain—Delivery-Related

Go PMNYH, Dunselman GAJ: Anatomic and functional results of surgical repair after total perineal rupture at delivery. *Surg Gynecol Obstet* 166(2):121–124, 1988.

Grant A, Sleep J, McIntosh J, et al: Ultrasound and pulsed electromagnetic energy treatment for perineal trauma: A randomized placebo-controlled trial. *Br J Obstet Gynaecol* 96:434–439, 1989.

Haadem K, Dahlstrom JA, Ling L, et al: Anal sphincter function after delivery rupture. *Obstet Gynecol* 70(1):53–56, 1987.

Haadem K, Ohrlander S, Lingman G: Long-term ailments due to anal sphincter rupture caused by delivery: A hidden problem. *Eur J Obstet Gynecol Reprod Biol* 27:27–32, 1988.

Ultrasound/PEME for perineal pain (editorial). *Lancet* 2(8653):22–23, 1989.

Perineal Pain—Neurogenic

Anderson NE, Willoughby EW: Infarction of the conus medullaris. *Ann Neurol* 21:470–474, 1987.

Batta AG, Gundian JC, Myers RP: Neurofibromatosis presenting as perineal pain and urethral burning. *Urology* 33(2):138–140, 1989.

Feldenzer JA, McGauley JL, McGillicuddy JE: Sacral and presacral tumors: Problems in diagnosis and management. *Neurosurgery* 25(6):884–891, 1989.

Launer DP, Miscall BG, Beil AR Jr: Colorectal infarction following resection of abdominal aortic aneurysms. *Dis Colon Rectum* 21(8):613–617, 1978.

Proctalgia Fugax

Altman DF: Chronic rectal pain. *JAMA* 264(8):1043–1044, 1990.

Kornel EE, Vlahakos D: Intraspinal schwannoma presenting solely with rectal pain. *Neurosurgery* 22:417–419, 1988.

Magni G, de Bertolini C, Dodi G, et al: Psychological findings in chronic anal pain. *Psychopathology* 19:170–174, 1986.

Mountifield JA: Proctalgia fugax: A cause of marital dysharmony. *CMAJ* 134:1269–1270, 1986.

Peery WH: Proctalgia fugax: A clinical enigma. *South Med J* 81(5):621–623, 1988.

Scott D: Proctalgia fugax. *Postgrad Med* 72(3):44–45, 1982.

Swain R: Oral clonidine for proctalgia fugax. *Gut* 28:1039–1040, 1987.

Thompson WG: Proctalgia fugax. *Dig Dis Sci* 26(12):1121–1124, 1981.

Thompson WG: Proctalgia fugax in patients with the irritable bowel, peptic ulcer, or inflammatory bowel disease. *Am J Gastroenterol* 79(6):450–452, 1984.

Thompson WG, Heaton KW: Proctalgia fugax. *J R Coll Physicians London* 14(4):247–248, 1980.

Weizman Z, Binsztok M: Proctalgia fugax in teenagers. *J Pediatr* 114(5):813–814, 1989.

Proctitis

Bolan RK, Sands M, Schachter J, et al: Lymphogranuloma venereum and acute ulcerative proctitis. *Am J Med* 72:703–706, 1982.

Cello JP, Schneiderman DH: Ulcerative colitis, in Sleisenger MH, Fordtran JS (eds): *Gastrointestinal Disease: Pathophysiology, Diagnosis, Management*, 4th ed. Philadelphia, Saunders, 1989, pp 1435–1477.

Connolly GM, Shanson D, Hawkins DA, et al: Non-cryptosporidial diarrhoea in human immunodeficiency virus (HIV) infected patients. *Gut* 30:195–200, 1989.

Donaldson RM Jr: Crohn's disease, in Sleisenger MH, Fordtran JS (eds): *Gastrointestinal Disease: Pathophysiology, Diagnosis, Management*, 4th ed. Philadelphia, Saunders, 1989, pp 1327–1358.

Graef JW, Lovejoy FH: Heavy metal poisoning, in Braunwald E, Isselbacher KJ, Petersdorf RG, et al (eds): *Harrison's Principles of Internal Medicine*, 11th ed. New York, McGraw-Hill, 1987, pp 850–855.

Fekety R: Antibiotic-associated colitis, in Mandell GL, Douglas RG Jr, Bennett JE (eds): *Principles and Practice of Infectious Diseases*, 3d ed. New York, Churchill Livingstone, 1990, pp 863–869.

Goodell SE, Quinn TC, Mkrtichian E, et al: Herpes simplex virus proctitis in homosexual men: Clinical, sigmoidoscopic, and histopathological features. *N Engl J Med* 308(15):868–871, 1983.

Kirsner JB, Shorter RG: Idiopathic inflammatory bowel disease of the large bowel and anal canal, in Kirsner JB, Shorter RG (eds): *Diseases of the Colon, Rectum, and Anal Canal*. Baltimore, Williams & Wilkins, 1988, pp 261–277.

Masur H: Infections in homosexual men, in Mandell GL, Douglas RG Jr, Bennett JE (eds): *Principles and Practice of Infectious Diseases*, 3d ed. New York, Churchill Livingstone, 1990, pp 2280–2284.

Mauff AC, Ballard RC, Koornhof HJ: Problems in the diagnosis of lymphogranuloma venereum: A review of 6 cases. *S Afr Med J* 63:55–56, 1983.

Mindel A: Lymphogranuloma venereum of the rectum in a homosexual man: Case report. *Br J Vener Dis* 59:196–197, 1983.

Quinn TC, Goodell SE, Mkrtichian E, et al: *Chlamydia trachomatis* proctitis. *N Engl J Med* 305(4):195–200, 1981.

Ravdin JI, Petri WA Jr: *Entamoeba histolytica* (amebiasis), in Mandell GL, Douglas RG Jr, Bennett JE (eds): *Principles and Practice of Infectious Diseases*, 3d ed. New York, Churchill Livingstone, 1990, pp 2036–2049.

Schachter J, Osoba AO: Lymphogranuloma venereum. *Br Med Bull* 39(2):151–154, 1983.

Sider L, Mintzer RA, Mendelson EB, et al: Radiographic findings of infectious proctitis in homosexual men. *AJR* 139:667–671, 1982.

Thorsteinsson SB: Lymphogranuloma venereum: Review of clinical manifestations, epidemiology, diagnosis, and treatment. *Scand J Infect Dis Suppl* 32:127–131, 1982.

White WB, Hanna M, Stewart JA: Systemic herpes simplex virus type 2 infection: Proctitis, urinary retention, arthralgias, and meningitis in the absence of primary mucocutaneous lesions. *Arch Intern Med* 144:826–827, 1984.

Proctitis—Radiation

Browning GGP, Varma JS, Smith AN, et al: Late results of mucosal proctectomy and colo-anal sleeve anastomosis for chronic irradiation rectal injury. *Br J Surg* 74:31–34, 1987.

Prolapse—Anal Mucosal

Allen-Mersh TG, Henry MM, Nicholls RJ: Natural history of anterior mucosal prolapse. *Br J Surg* 74:679–682, 1987.

Prostatic Abscess

Brawer MK, Stamey TA: Prostatic abscess owing to anaerobic bacteria. *J Urol* 138:1254–1255, 1987.

Chia JK, Longfield RN, Cook DH, et al: Computed axial tomography in the early diagnosis of prostatic abscess. *Am J Med* 81(5):942–944, 1986.

Cytron S, Weinberger M, Pitlik SD, et al: Value of transrectal ultrasonography for diagnosis and treatment of prostatic abscess. *Urology* 32(5):454–458, 1988.

Dennis MA, Donohue RE: Computed tomography of prostatic abscess. *J Comput Assist Tomogr* 9(1):201–202, 1985.

Learmonth DJ, Philp NH: Salmonella prostatic abscess. *Br J Urol* 61(2):163, 1988.

Lee F Jr, Lee F, Solomon MH, et al: Sonographic demonstration of prostatic abscess. *J Ultrasound Med* 5:101–102, 1986.

Lentino JR, Zielinski A, Stachowski M, et al: Prostatic abscess due to *Candida albicans*. *J Infect Dis* 149(2):282, 1984.

Mariani AJ, Jacobs LD, Clapp PR, et al: Emphysematous prostatic abscess: Diagnosis and treatment. *J Urol* 129(2):385–386, 1983.

Morrison RE, Lamb AS, Craig DB, et al: Melioidosis: A reminder. *Am J Med* 84(5):965–967, 1988.

Papanicolaou N, Pfister RC, Stafford SA, et al: Prostatic abscess: Imaging with transrectal sonography and MR. *AJR* 149:981–982, 1987.

Rørvik J, Daehlin L: Prostatic abscess: Imaging with transrectal ultrasound. *Scand J Urol Nephrol* 23:307–308, 1989.

Steinhardt GF: Prostatic suppuration and destruction in patients with myelodysplasia: A newly recognized entity. *J Urol* 140:1002–1006, 1988.

Sugao H, Takiuchi H, Sakurai T: Transrectal longitudinal ultrasonography of prostatic abscess. *J Urol* 136(6):1316–1317, 1986.

Thornhill BA, Morehouse HT, Coleman P, et al: Prostatic abscess: CT and sonographic findings. *AJR* 148:899–900, 1987.

Vaccaro JA, Belville WD, Kiesling VJ Jr, et al: Prostatic abscess: Computerized tomography scanning as an aid to diagnosis and treatment. *J Urol* 136(6):1318–1319, 1986.

Washecka R, Rumancik WM: Prostatic abscess evaluated by serial computed tomography. *Urol Radiol* 7:54–56, 1985.

Weinberger M, Cytron S, Servadio C, et al: Diagnosis of prostatic abscess (letter to editor). *Am J Med* 83(2):379–380, 1987.

Woo ML, Chan PSF, French GL: A case of melioidosis presenting with prostatic abscess in Hong Kong. *J Urol* 137(1):120–121, 1987.

Prostatic Carcinoma

Anzalotta J: Transrectal prostatic ultrasound: Lesions diagnosed. *Bol Asoc Med P R* 81(11):425–426, 1989.

Buonocore E, Hesemann C, Pavlicek W, et al: Clinical and in vitro magnetic resonance imaging of prostatic carcinoma. *AJR* 143:1267–1272, 1984.

Catalona WJ, Scott WW: Carcinoma of the prostate, in Harrison JH, Gittes RF, Perlmutter AD, et al (eds): *Campbell's Urology*. Philadelphia, Saunders, 1979, vol 2, pp 1096–1097.

Dershaw DD, Scher HI, Smart T: Transrectal sonography for serial evaluation of prostatic malignancy. *Urology* 36(2):172–176, 1990.

Moul JW, Davis R, Vaccaro JA, et al: Acute urinary retention associated with prostatic carcinoma. *J Urol* 141:1375–1377, 1989.

Prostatitis/Prostatodynia

Barbalias GA: Prostatodynia or painful male urethral syndrome? *Urology* 36(2):146–153, 1990.

Barbalias GA, Meares EM Jr, Sant GR: Prostatodynia: Clinical and urodynamic characteristics. *J Urol* 130(3):514–517, 1983.

Bruce AW, Reid G: Prostatitis associated with *Chlamydia trachomatis* in 6 patients. *J Urol* 142:1006–1007, 1989.

Brunner H, Weidner W, Schiefer H-G: Quantitative studies on the role of *Ureaplasma urealyticum* in non-gonococcal urethritis and chronic prostatitis. *Yale J Biol Med* 56:545–550, 1983.

de Souza E, Katz DA, Dworzack DL, et al: Actinomycosis of the prostate. *J Urol* 133(2):290–291, 1985.

Di Trapani D, Pavone C, Serretta V, et al: Chronic prostatitis and prostatodynia: Ultrasonographic alterations of the prostate, bladder neck, seminal vesicles and periprostatic venous plexus. *Eur Urol* 15:230–234, 1988.

Drach GW: Prostatitis and prostatodynia. *Urol Clin North Am* 7(1):79–88, 1980.

Gardner WA Jr, Culberson DE, Bennett BD: *Trichomonas vaginalis* in the prostate gland. *Arch Pathol Lab Med* 110:430–432, 1986.

Hanus PM, Danziger LH: Treatment of chronic bacterial prostatitis. *Clin Pharm* 3:49–55, 1984.

Jiménez-Cruz JF, Tormo FB, Gómez JG: Treatment of chronic prostatitis: Intraprostatic antibiotic injections under echography control. *J Urol* 139:967–970, 1988.

Krieger JN: Prostatitis syndromes: Pathophysiology, differential diagnosis, and treatment. *Sex Transm Dis* 11(2):100–112, 1984.

Madsen PO, Jensen KM-E, Iversen P: Chronic bacterial prostatitis: Theoretical and experimental considerations. *Urol Res* 11:1–5, 1983.

Miller HC: Stress prostatitis. *Urology* 32(6):507–510, 1988.

Orland SM, Hanno PM, Wein AJ: Prostatitis, prostatosis, and prostatodynia. *Urology* 25(5):439–459, 1985.

Osborn DE, George NJR, Rao PN, et al: Prostatodynia: Physiological characteristics and rational management with muscle relaxants. *Br J Urol* 53:621–623, 1981.

Paulson DF, Zinner NR, Resnick MI, et al: Treatment of bacterial prostatitis: Comparison of cephalexin and minocycline. *Urology* 27(4):379–387, 1986.

Stewart C: Prostatitis. *Emerg Med Clin North Am* 6(3):391–402, 1988.

Thin RN, Simmons PD: Chronic bacterial and non-bacterial prostatitis. *Br J Urol* 55:513–518, 1983.

Rectal Carcinoma

Corman ML: Carcinoma of the rectum, in *Colon and Rectal Surgery*. Philadelphia, Lippincott, 1984, pp 329–411.

Corman ML: Malignant tumors of the anal canal, in *Colon and Rectal Surgery*. Philadelphia, Lippincott, 1984, pp 413–428.

Faintuch JS, Levin B: Clinical aspects of malignant tumors: Large intestine and anal canal, including therapy, in Kirsner JB, Shorter RG (eds): *Diseases of the Colon, Rectum, and Anal Canal*. Baltimore, Williams & Wilkins, 1988, pp 400–401.

Jones IT, Fazio VW: Anorectal diseases commonly encountered in clinical practice, in Kirsner JB, Shorter RG (eds): *Diseases of the Colon, Rectum, and Anal Canal*. Baltimore, Williams & Wilkins, 1988, pp 687–703.

Rectal Ulcers

Britto E, Borges AM, Swaroop VS, et al: Solitary rectal ulcer syndrome: Twenty cases seen at an oncology center. *Dis Colon Rectum* 30:381–385, 1987.

Eckardt VF, Kanzler G, Remmele W: Anorectal ergotism: Another cause of solitary rectal ulcers. *Gastroenterol* 91:1123–1127, 1986.

Gizzi G, Villani V, Brandi G, et al: Ano-rectal lesions in patients taking suppositories containing non-steroidal anti-inflammatory drugs (NSAID). *Endoscopy* 22:146–148, 1990.

Levine MS, Piccolello ML, Sollenberger LC, et al: Solitary rectal ulcer syndrome: A radiologic diagnosis? *Gastrointest Radiol* 11:187–193, 1986.

Niv Y, Bat L: Solitary rectal ulcer syndrome: Clinical, endoscopic, and histological spectrum. *Am J Gastroenterol* 81(6):486–491, 1986.

Womack NR, Williams NS, Holmfield Mist JH, et al: Anorectal function in the solitary rectal ulcer syndrome. *Dis Colon Rectum* 30:319–323, 1987.

Womack NR, Williams NS, Holmfield JHM, et al: Pressure and prolapse: The cause of solitary rectal ulceration. *Gut* 28:1228–1233, 1987.

Yamagiwa H: Protruded variants in solitary ulcer syndrome of the rectum. *Acta Pathol Jpn* 38(4):471–478, 1988.

Seminal Vesiculitis
Littrup PJ, Lee F, McLeary RD, et al: Transrectal US of the seminal vesicles and ejaculatory ducts: Clinical correlation. *Radiology* 168:625–628, 1988.

Sexually Transmitted Diseases
Burgoyne RA: Lymphogranuloma venereum. *Prim Care* 17(1):153–157, 1990.
Epling S, Reich GA: Report on an outbreak of lymphogranuloma venereum in central Florida. *J Fla Med Assoc* 75(1):29–30, 1988.
Faro S: Lymphogranuloma venereum, chancroid, and granuloma inguinale. *Obstet Gynecol Clin North Am* 16(3):517–530, 1989.
Kalter DC, Rosen T: Sexually transmitted diseases. *Emerg Med Clin North Am* 3(4):693–716, 1985.
Parkash S, Radhakrishna K: Problematic ulcerative lesions in sexually transmitted diseases: Surgical management. *Sex Transm Dis* 13(3):127–133, 1986.

Scieux C, Barnes R, Bianchi A, et al: Lymphogranuloma venereum: 27 cases in Paris. *J Infect Dis* 160(4):662–668, 1989.
Spence MR: The treatment of gonorrhea, syphilis, chancroid, lymphogranuloma venereum, and granuloma inguinale. *Clin Obstet Gynecol* 31(2):453–465, 1988.

Urethral Calculi
Drach GW: Urinary lithiasis, in Harrison JH, Gittes RF, Perlmutter AD, et al (eds): *Campbell's Urology*. Philadelphia, Saunders, 1978, vol 1, pp 859–860.

Urethral Stricture
Nickel WR, Plumb RT: Other infections and inflammations of the external genitalia, in Harrison JH, Gittes RF, Perlmutter AD, et al (eds): *Campbell's Urology*. Philadelphia, Saunders, 1978, vol 1, pp 673–680.

CHAPTER

37

Acute Vulvar and Vaginal Pain

☐ DIAGNOSTIC LIST

1. Vulvar ulceration
   A. Primary herpes simplex virus infection
   B. Primary syphilis
   C. Chancroid
   D. Chancroid-like ulcers
   E. Lymphogranuloma venereum
   F. Granuloma inguinale
2. Vulvovaginitis
   A. Yeast infection
   B. *Trichomonas vaginalis* infection
   C. Bacterial vaginosis
   D. Noninfectious vulvovaginitis
      1. Chemical irritant vulvovaginitis
      2. Contact allergy–related vulvovaginitis
3. Bartholin's gland cyst or abscess
4. Furuncles and carbuncles
   A. Furuncle of labium majus
   B. Carbuncle of labium majus
5. Clitoral abscess
6. Vulvitis
   A. Focal vulvitis
   B. Diffuse vulvitis and acetowhitening
7. Traumatic labial frenum tears
8. Generalized skin disorders
   A. Stevens-Johnson syndrome
   B. Toxic epidermal necrolysis
9. Dysuria syndromes
   A. Internal dysuria
      1. Acute bacterial cystitis
      2. Cystourethritis syndrome
      3. Dysuria and acute pyelonephritis

A. Occult pyelonephritis
B. Acute pyelonephritis and cystitis
C. Idiopathic dysuria
D. Noninfectious disorders (bladder and urethral stones)
   B. External dysuria
      1. Vulvovaginitis
      2. Genital ulcerative disorders
10. Behçet's disease
11. Necrotizing perineal infection
12. Referred pain to the vulva
   A. Renolithiasis
   B. Aortic and common iliac aneurysms
   C. Ilioinguinal or genitofemoral neuralgia
   D. Spine and spinal cord disease
   E. Acute appendicitis
13. Dyspareunia
   A. Superficial dyspareunia
      1. Lack of lubrication
      2. Vaginismus
   B. Deep dyspareunia
      1. Ectopic pregnancy
      2. Acute salpingitis
      3. Endometriosis
      4. Rupture of an ovarian cyst
      5. Torsion of an ovarian cyst
      6. Pelvic abscess due to inflammatory disease of the appendix or sigmoid
      7. Colitis

452

☐ SUMMARY

Vulvar pain may result from a *primary herpes simplex virus infection*. Prodromal aching or burning perineal, buttock, and posteromedial leg pain may occur. Vesicles and ulcers soon appear on the labia and are associated with pain and tenderness. Dysuria and urinary frequency or retention may occur. The diagnosis can be confirmed by a viral culture. There is a clinical response to intravenous acyclovir. *Primary syphilis* causes one or more painless, but often tender, round or oval, indurated, "ham"- or "beef"-colored, relatively clean-looking erosions (chancres). Dark-field examination of exudate expressed from a lesion will reveal *Treponema pallidum*. Alternatively, the diagnosis can be confirmed by a nontreponemal serologic test for syphilis [rapid plasma reagin (RPR)]. *Chancroid* produces one or more painful, irregular, dirty-looking, tender, soft labial ulcers with undermined edges. A Gram's stain of lesion exudate reveals parallel rows of gram-negative coccobacilli (i.e., "railroad track" pattern), and culture of the same material on selective media detects *Haemophilus ducreyi* in 80 percent of cases. *Chancroid-like ulcers* may be caused by superinfection of luetic, herpetic, or traumatic ulcers with pyogenic bacteria. A *ducreyi*-like bacterium has been isolated from chancroid-like ulcers that are culture-negative for *H. ducreyi*. Some cases of chancroid are culture-negative for unknown reasons (false-negative rate of 20 percent). *Lymphogranuloma venereum* (LGV) begins as a labial papule that evolves into an herpetiform ulcer that may be only mildly painful and tender or asymptomatic. Urethral discharge and/or dysuria may also occur. Urethral culture may grow one of the L1, L2, or L3 serovars of *Chlamydia trachomatis* or a significant LGV complement fixation or microimmunofluorescence test titer may be detected in the patient's serum. Unilateral lymphadenopathy occurs in up to 67 percent, and a "groove" sign may occur in 20 percent. Vulval ulceration and pain may occur secondary to *granuloma inguinale*. Donovan bodies can be detected by Giemsa staining of a crush biopsy of an ulcerated granulomatous lesion.

Vulvovaginitis may result in burning vulvar pain, pruritus, and superficial dyspareunia associated with a vaginal discharge, vulvar erythema, and edema. *Candidiasis* occurs in a setting of diabetes mellitus; pregnancy; or administration of estrogen, antibiotics, or corticosteroids. The vaginal discharge is curdlike and resembles cottage cheese. Microscopy of a saline mount of the vaginal discharge reveals leukocytes, squamous cells, pseudohyphae, hyphae, and spores. A KOH preparation confirms the presence of fungal forms. Cultures are more sensitive, but many women with positive cultures are asymptomatic, and there is no valid study confirming the value of treating such patients with antifungal drugs. Symptomatic patients improve rapidly with intravaginal antifungal therapy. *Trichomonas infection* causes a yellow-green discharge containing motile trichomonads and leukocytes. The discharge is malodorous, in contrast to the odorless discharge caused by yeast infection. There is a prompt response of trichomoniasis to metronidazole therapy.

Bacterial vaginosis produces a copious discharge with a fishy amine odor. Mild irritative symptoms occur in only a small percentage of patients. The discharge is homogeneous, thin, and milky ("milk of magnesia" appearance) or grayish-white; releases a fishy odor after addition of a few drops of 10-percent KOH; has a pH greater than 4.5; and, on microscopy, contains clue cells, an abnormal background bacterial flora, and very few leukocytes. *Noninfectious vulvovaginitis* may be caused by a primary *chemical irritant* (e.g., douching agents, vaginal sprays, bubble baths, and antifungal preparations) or a *contact allergy* (e.g., poison ivy or oak and hypersensitivity to semen). Labial erythema, edema, bullae, vesicles, and weeping erosions may occur, causing vulvar burning and dyspareunia.

A *Bartholin's gland cyst or abscess* usually causes pain, swelling, erythema, and tenderness of the affected labium. Aspiration reveals viscid, translucent, sterile mucus if the lesion is a cyst and pus if it is an abscess. Marsupialization and antibiotic therapy lead to resolution of the abscess and preserve the lubricating function of the infected gland.

Furuncles or carbuncles occur on the hair-bearing skin of a labium majus. They cause localized redness, swelling, tenderness, and an aching or throbbing pain that is relieved by surgical or spontaneous drainage and antibiotic therapy. An abscess may involve the clitoris, causing clitoral enlargement, erythema, and severe pain and tenderness.

Focal vulvitis causes severe superficial dyspareunia and vulvar burning pain and pruritus. Focal tenderness and erythema occur at one or more sites in the posterior portion of the vestibule adjacent to the duct openings of the minor vestibular glands and Skene's glands. Acetowhitening of the erythematous foci is usually present, and some patients harbor human papillomavirus DNA in biopsies of erythematous lesions. *Diffuse vulvitis associated with acetowhitening* also occurs. Relief of dyspareunia may require laser or conventional surgical excision of involved areas. *Labial frenum tears* may cause persistent dyspareunia. Careful inspection of this region with a bright light and magnifying lens may be required for their detection.

The *Stevens-Johnson syndrome* causes systemic symptoms, macular and target skin lesions, purulent conjunctivitis, erosive stomatitis, hemorrhagic cheilitis, and bullous lesions and erosions on the labia. *Toxic epidermal necrolysis* causes similar genital and oral lesions and diffuse skin erythema, with the formation of giant, flaccid bullae that soon rupture, producing large, painful erosions.

Dysuria may be internal or external. *Internal dysuria* is felt deep in the vagina and suprapubic region, and it begins before or at the onset of urination. *External dysuria* is felt between the labia as a burning discomfort that begins after the onset of voiding. *Cystitis* causes internal dysuria, urgency, frequency, and cloudy or bloody urine with no systemic symptoms. The urine contains leukocytes and bacteria. Cultures grow *Escherichia coli*, other Enterobacteriaceae, or *Staphylococcus saprophyticus* in concentrations of $\geq 10^2$ colony forming units (CFU)/ml. Such patients respond rapidly to a 1- or 3-day course of oral antibiotics. There is a very low rate of relapse after such therapy. Dysuria may also occur in women with chlamydial, gonococcal, or herpetic infections. Rarely, LGV is the cause of a purulent urethritis. *Trichomonas vaginalis* may cause frequency and dysuria. The trichomonads can be detected by microscopic examination of a catheterized urine specimen.

A "cystitis" syndrome occurs with *occult pyelonephritis.* This infection may mimic simple cystitis without any symptoms or signs related to the upper urinary tract. Clues to the presence of occult pyelonephritis include known urinary tract abnormalities, diabetes mellitus, a urinary tract infection before age 12, pregnancy, an immunocompromising illness, symptoms for more than 7 days, acute pyelonephritis during the prior year, and relapse after a 3-day course of therapy. *Acute pyelonephritis* may present with cystitis-like complaints that are soon followed by fever, chills, flank and abdominal pain, and costovertebral angle tenderness. The urine contains leukocytes singly, in clumps, and sometimes, in casts. Urine colony counts exceed 10^5 CFU/ml. *Idiopathic dysuria* occurs in patients with a normal urinalysis and a negative urine culture. The etiology is unknown. Bladder and urethral stones may cause dysuria, frequency, gross or microscopic hematuria, and obstructive symptoms. External dysuria may be associated with one of the causes of *acute vulvovaginitis* described above or with *genital ulcers. Behçet's disease* causes recurrent oral aphthae, uveitis, vulvar ulcerations and pain, and cutaneous vasculitis. *Necrotizing perineal infections* cause fever, severe systemic symptoms, labial pain, erythema, edema, tenderness, and an enlarging area of vulvar skin-blackening due to gangrene. Progressive infection rapidly involves the perineum, vulva, buttocks, thighs, and abdominal wall. Skin crepitus occurs. Sloughing and debridement of necrotic tissue leave large

areas of the labia and perineum uncovered by skin. These infections are usually caused by clostridial species or mixtures of aerobic and anaerobic bacteria. Referred pain to the vulva may occur secondary to *renal colic,* an enlarging *lower abdominal aneurysm, ilioinguinal or genitofemoral neuralgia, spine or spinal cord disease, acute appendicitis,* and *sigmoid diverticulitis.*

Superficial dyspareunia may result from *failure of vaginal lubrication* due to surgical castration or the menopause or to primary or secondary *vaginismus.* It is also caused by many of the painful disorders described above. Deep dyspareunia, felt deep in the vagina and lower pelvis, may be caused by pelvic inflammatory changes secondary to an *ectopic pregnancy, salpingitis, endometriosis, torsion or rupture of an ovarian cyst, a pelvic abscess resulting from appendicitis or diverticulitis,* or a *colitis* caused by an acute bacterial or amebic infection or inflammatory bowel disease.

☐ DESCRIPTION OF LISTED DISEASES

1. VULVAR ULCERATION

A. Primary Herpes Simplex Virus Infection   Mild burning discomfort and paresthesias in the labial region may be early complaints. Aching, deep pain may be felt in one or both buttocks, with radiation down the back and medial aspect of one or both legs. Systemic symptoms such as fever, chills, myalgias, headache, and malaise may occur (62 percent). Grouped vesicles appear and rapidly break down into small, shallow, painful ulcers. These

TABLE OF DISEASE INCIDENCE

INCIDENCE PER 100,000 (APPROXIMATE)

Common (>100)	Uncommon (>5–100)	Rare (>0–5)
Primary herpes simplex virus infection	Primary syphilis	Chancroid
Vulvovaginitis caused by yeast, *Trichomonas*, or bacterial vaginosis	Chemical irritant vulvovaginitis	Chancroid-like ulcers
	Contact allergy–related vulvovaginitis	Lymphogranuloma venereum
Bartholin's gland cyst or abscess	Carbuncle of the labium majus	Granuloma inguinale
Furuncle of the labium majus	Clitoral abscess	Cystourethritis syndrome due to LGV
Focal vulvitis	Labial frenum tears	Necrotizing perineal infection
Diffuse vulvitis with acetowhitening	Stevens-Johnson syndrome	Referred pain to the vulva due to spinal
Dysuria syndromes (internal)	Toxic epidermal necrolysis	cord disease or acute appendicitis
Acute bacterial cystitis	Idiopathic dysuria	Deep dyspareunia due to pelvic abscess
Cystourethritis syndromes caused by *C.*	Dysuria due to bladder and urethral stones	from appendicitis or sigmoid
trachomatis, N. gonorrhea, herpes simplex	Cystourethritis due to Trichomonas vaginalis	diverticulitis
Acute pyelonephritis and lower tract symptoms	Behçet's disease	
Occult pyelonephritis	Referred pain to the vulva due to renolithiasis,	
Dysuria syndromes (external) due to	aneurysm, or ilioinguinal or genitofemoral	
vulvovaginitis or genital ulcerative disorders	neuralgia	
Superficial dyspareunia due to lack of	Deep dyspareunia due to ectopic pregnancy,	
lubrication, vaginismus or vulvovaginitis	torsion of an ovarian cyst, or colitis	
Deep dyspareunia due to acute salpingitis,		
endometriosis, or rupture of an ovarian cyst		

lesions are usually bilaterally distributed (85 percent), and there may be a unilateral or bilateral tender and painful inguinal adenopathy (80 percent). The ulcerations may coalesce, forming round and ovoid large (0.5–1 cm), shallow, pink ulcers with a narrow, smooth, erythematous margin. Labial edema may occur secondary to the multiple ulcerations. There are local pain, paresthesias, and sometimes hypesthesia. The pain is continuous, aching, and/or burning. External as well as internal dysuria (83 percent) may occur, the latter being caused by an herpetic urethritis. Passage of urine may be so painful that urinary retention requiring catheterization occurs. Retention may also be caused by an associated sacral neuropathy. Herpes simplex virus (HSV) can be isolated from labial lesions (90 percent), the cervical canal (87 percent), and urine (50 percent). Most genital infections are caused by HSV-2 (63–90 percent) and the remainder by HSV-1. Symptoms follow sexual exposure by 3 to 7 days. Many primary infections are subclinical and detected by observing the presence of HSV-2 antibody in patients without a clinical history of genital infection. Acyclovir given intravenously provides effective therapy against a severe primary HSV genital infection, and shortens the course of the attack and duration of viral shedding. Local pain and tenderness may persist for 1 to 2 weeks, while healing of ulcers may require 2 to 4 weeks.

B. Primary Syphilis Primary syphilis causes a chancre on the labia, cervix, anorectal area, fourchette, or skin adjacent to the genital area. Syphilitic chancres begin as single or multiple papules (0.5–1 cm), 2 to 3 weeks after sexual contact. The papules soon ulcerate, forming a flat, usually round, firm lesion with a ''ham''-colored or dark (''beefy'') surface and an indurated, narrow erythematous margin, often with a fine hemorrhagic line at the border of the lesion. Exudate is minimal. These lesions are usually painless, but they may be tender to palpation in up to 33 percent of cases. Bilateral inguinal lymphadenopathy occurs in 70 percent, and in up to 23 percent these nodes may be tender. Up to 10 percent of chancres may have a pseudomembranous purulent surface exudate or undermined edge, mimicking chancroid. The diagnosis of syphilis can be made by darkfield microscopy of lesion exudate or by serial measurement of a nontreponemal test for syphilis [Venereal Disease Research Laboratory (VDRL) test or rapid plasma reagin (RPR) test]. There is a 30 percent false-negative rate for these tests at the time the chancre is present.

Benzathine penicillin therapy leads to rapid resolution of the chancre and cure of the disease. A Jarisch-Herxheimer reaction, consisting of high fever, chills, malaise, and marked exudation of serum from the chancre, may occur in a small percentage of patients within 6 to 8 h of receiving penicillin.

C. Chancroid (Soft Chancre) A tender papule appears on the labia, fourchette, cervix, clitoris, or skin of the thigh 3 to 10 days following a sexual contact. The papule soon breaks down, forming an irregular, purulent, necrotic, painful 0.3- to 2-cm ulcer with an undermined edge. The ulcer is usually soft and tender. Multiple ulcers tend to occur in women (mean number, 4), and secondary ulcers on the thigh or abdomen caused by autoinoculation may provide supportive evidence of the diagnosis. Up to 50 percent of women may be asymptomatic despite the presence of chancroidal ulcers. Tender; unilateral; or, less commonly, bilateral inguinal adenopathy occurs in 33 to 50 percent of patients. Untreated adjacent lesions may coalesce to form giant ulcerations and extensive labial and perineal edema. Labial destruction or perforation may occur. Lymph node suppuration may develop, with sinus formation and spontaneous drainage of pus.

A Gram stain of ulcer exudate demonstrates gram-negative coccobacilli in parallel rows that resemble a ''railroad track'' or ''school of fish'' pattern. A Gram stain of lesion exudate is neither sensitive nor specific. The most sensitive and specific confirming test is culture on special media. *H. ducreyi* can be grown on a gonococcal base agar, with added bovine hemoglobin and fetal calf serum or Mueller-Hinton agar with 5% horse blood and supplementary vitamins. Vancomycin, 3 μg/ml, is added to inhibit other bacteria. Culture of ulcer exudate using both media results in a combined sensitivity of 80-percent for isolation of the organism. *H. ducreyi* is sensitive to erythromycin. Chancroid is most likely to occur in female prostitutes or secondary contacts of men infected by a prostitute.

D. Chancroid-like Ulcers Painful, irregular and/or undermined, soft, friable genital ulcers may fail to grow *H. ducreyi* after culture on selective media. These cases may be caused by (1) true chancroid with false-negative culture results (the false-negative rate approximates 20 percent); (2) HSV infection with secondary infection by pyogenic bacteria; (3) traumatic ulcers secondarily infected by pyogenic bacteria; (4) infection with ducreyi-like bacteria; or (5) ulcers of unknown etiology that are culture negative for *H. ducreyi* and HSV-2 and are dark-field negative. *H. ducreyi* may coinfect with *T. pallidum* or HSV. The resultant ulcers are usually chancroid-like in appearance, and both agents can be detected.

Chancroid-like ulcers should be studied by dark-field microscopy. A Gram stain of the exudate should be examined and cultures for HSV, *H. ducreyi*, and pyogenic bacteria obtained. Nontreponemal serologic tests for syphilis should be done at the time of the appearance of the ulcers and at monthly intervals until positive or for three consecutive months.

E. Lymphogranuloma Venereum LGV begins as labial or fourchette papules or vesicles that ulcerate. The resulting herpetiform ulcer is the commonest primary lesion. It may be mildly painful and tender or completely asymptomatic. Urethral discharge and/or dysuria occur in some cases. Unilateral or bilateral femoral and inguinal adenopathy may occur, causing a "groove sign" due to a depression or cleft between these two anatomic groups of lymph nodes produced by the inguinal ligament (seen in 20 percent). Unilateral inguinal adenopathy may occur in up to 67 percent. The nodes may become large, fluctuant, and painful. One or more nodes may suppurate and drain a purulent exudate from which *C. trachomatis* of the L1, L2, or L3 serotypes may be isolated. The diagnosis can also be supported by showing a fourfold rise in titer on an LGV complement fixation test or a single titer equal to or greater than 1:64 (sensitivity, 80 percent). A microimmunofluorescent test is sensitive and specific. A titer of 1:512 or greater is specific, but false positives may occur with non-LGV serovar infections (e.g., salpingitis or perihepatitis). Doxycycline or erythromycin therapy is effective.

F. Granuloma Inguinale A papule forms on the vulva, fourchette, or cervix or in the vagina. Autoinoculation may result in multiple papules, which soon form painless or painful secondarily infected ulcerations. Adjacent lesions coalesce, forming large granulating ulcerations that are locally destructive.

Donovan's bodies can be detected in histiocytes in scrapings, smears, or crush preparation biopsies stained with Wright's or Giemsa stain. Histopathologic examination of biopsy specimens is less sensitive, and Donovan's bodies are more difficult to find. Electron microscope examination of biopsy specimens will more frequently detect the causative organism (i.e., *Calymmatobacterium granulomatis*) than will routine histologic study. Doxycycline causes the regression of lesions within 7 days.

2. VULVOVAGINITIS

A. Yeast Infection Vulvar pruritus, burning labial discomfort and tenderness, and a "cottage cheese"-like discharge are characteristic complaints. Superficial dyspareunia may occur in those with vulvar and vaginal edema and erythema. The pelvic examination may reveal vulvar edema, redness, and fissuring. Satellite pustules and red nodules may occur on the skin adjacent to the vulvar region. Excoriations secondary to severe pruritus may be present. The vaginal mucosa is usually erythematous, and a nonodorous, white, curdlike discharge may be present. Fewer than 20 percent have mucosal "thrushlike" patches. The incidence of vaginal wall "thrush" rises to 70 percent in pregnant patients. The pH of the discharge is 4.5 or less. Leukocytes are usually increased [>10 per high-power field (HPF)] in a saline preparation of vaginal discharge. Sheets and clumps of squamous epithelial cells are also abundant. Pseudohyphae, hyphae, and spores may be seen on a saline mount or a KOH preparation

(*Candida* species). The presence of only spores suggests infection by *T. glabrata* (responsible for 3–16 percent of yeast infections). Yeast may be cultured on Saboraud's or Nickerson's media. Gram's stain is also sensitive for the detection of hyphal and spore forms. The sensitivity of microscopy (saline and KOH preparation) has been reported to be as low as 36 to 45 percent or as high as 85 percent. The use of culture for diagnosis has been controversial because of a high false-positive rate (i.e., women without symptoms and positive cultures). A slide latex particle test is available that detects *Candida* organisms present in high concentrations in vaginal discharge. This test has a sensitivity of 65 to 81 percent but has not had extensive use. Risk factors for yeast vaginitis include pregnancy, antibiotic administration (penicillins, cephalosporins, tetracyclines, and metronidazole), diabetes mellitus, immunosuppression, tight-fitting clothing, estrogens, orogenital practices, and anal intercourse. Intravaginal instillation of butaconazole nitrate, miconazole, or nystatin leads to the resolution of symptoms and signs.

B. *Trichomonas Vaginalis* Infection Symptoms include a copious, malodorous vaginal discharge (56–67 percent), pruritus (48 percent), dyspareunia, and dysuria (18 to 26 percent). There may be redness of the vulva, the vestibule, and the skin surrounding the introitus. A granular, friable cervix ("strawberry" cervix) is characteristic but occurs in only 2 to 30 percent. The discharge is yellow or yellow-green, and it may be foamy in up to 34 percent of cases. The latter finding is not specific, since it also occurs in bacterial vaginosis. The diagnosis can be confirmed by detecting motile trichomonads on a saline wet mount, a test that has a sensitivity of 50 to 75 percent compared to culture on Feinberg-Wittington or Diamond's medium. *Trichomonas* infection may occur in women without a significant vaginal discharge (44 percent), and leukocytes may be absent from vaginal exudate (19 percent).

Trichomonas infection may produce a vaginal discharge that releases a fishy amine odor when 1 or 2 drops of KOH are added to it. The pH of the discharge in trichomoniasis exceeds 4.5. There is a prompt response to metronidazole therapy. Up to 16 percent of women treated with this drug may develop posttreatment vaginal candidiasis with a curdlike discharge and require antifungal therapy.

C. Bacterial Vaginosis This disorder may cause a malodorous vaginal discharge and only mild symptoms of vulval or vaginal discomfort. The vaginal secretions have an unpleasant fishy odor that is noted by the patient and her sex partner. Vaginal discomfort and dyspareunia occur in less than 15 percent of cases. The discharge is thin, homogeneous, and milky-white or gray and has a pH greater than 4.5. Clue cells [i.e., squamous vaginal epithelial cells coated with coccobacilli (*Gardnerella vaginalis*)] are present in the vaginal discharge, but very few leukocytes are associated. The amine test, which is performed by adding a drop or two of KOH to the vaginal discharge on the speculum, is positive in up to 73 percent of patients. Cultures for *G. vaginalis* are not diagnostically useful, since many women without bacterial vaginosis harbor the organism in small amounts. There is a rapid response of odor, discharge, and irritative symptoms to metronidazole therapy.

The findings in acute vulvovaginitis are tabulated in Table 37-1.

D. Noninfectious Vulvovaginitis This disorder may be caused by a chemical irritant or a contact allergy.

1. Chemical Irritant Vulvovaginitis Burning vulvar pain, pruritus, labial edema, and erythema that may progress to vesicle and bullae formation develop within minutes or hours of contact with the causative agent. Dyspareunia and dysuria result from the inflammatory changes. Causes of irritant vulvovaginitis include douching agents, vaginal sprays, bubble baths, strong detergents used in laundering undergarments, scented toilet tissues, spermicidal jellies or foams, deodorant tampons, and some intravaginally administered antifungal drugs. Gentian violet, intravaginal instillation of 5-fluorouracil, and nitrofurazone may also cause an irritant vulvovaginitis.

2. Contact Allergy-Related Vulvovaginitis Contact allergy causes burning vulvar pain, tenderness, and pruritus beginning days or weeks after initial contact with the provoking substance. Poison oak and poison ivy cause contact reactions with erythema, linear orientation of vesicles, labial edema, pruritus, and excoriation. Transfer of plant oleoresins from the fingers to the genitalia is responsible. Rare cases of an allergy to the male partner's semen that leads to burning pain, vulvar redness, and edema have been reported. Microscopic examination of vaginal discharge may reveal increased numbers of parabasal cells and no evidence of the common vaginal pathogens. The background flora is sparse, and lactobacilli levels are usually decreased. Dysuria and urinary retention may occur in severe cases. Local cleansing, use of dilute Burow's solution compresses, and a corticosteroid cream and/or oral prednisone accelerate recovery.

3. BARTHOLIN'S GLAND CYST OR ABSCESS

This disorder begins as a painful, tender swelling in the posterior third of a labium majus. The pain is usually aching and may be throbbing. Labial swelling and tenderness progress over a period of 1 to 3 days. Sitting for prolonged periods, walking, and contact with tight cloth-

ing intensify the pain. A localized fluctuant or firm, tender labial mass (3–7 cm in diameter) is present. Fever, chills, and leukocytosis may occur. Aspiration of the mass reveals viscous translucent sterile mucus if the lesion is a cyst. Purulent inflammatory fluid with a positive Gram stain is obtained from a Bartholin's gland abscess. Bilateral Bartholin's gland abscesses suggest gonococcal infection. Reported isolates include *Neiserria gonorrhea* (6–61 percent, with 6–10 percent the usual finding), *Haemophilus influenzae* (13 percent), *E. coli* (28 percent), *Bacteroides* species (9 percent), *Streptococcus agalactiae* (9 percent), *Staphylococcus aureus* (9 percent), *C. trachomatis* (2–8 percent), other coliforms, *Pseudomonas* species, and anaerobes. Polymicrobial infection occurs but is infrequent. Surgical incision and drainage or marsupialization of the abscess may be performed under cover of appropriate antibiotics with preservation of glandular function.

4. FURUNCLES AND CARBUNCLES

A. Furuncle of the Labium Majus A painful furuncle may occur at the base of a hair on a labium majus. Within 3 to 5 days, the lesion enlarges, becomes firm and then fluctuant, and drains yellow-green pus containing *S. aureus*. Painful, tender inguinal adenopathy may occur on the ipsilateral side. Local use of warm soaks and oral administration of dicloxacillin usually result in resolution and healing with minimal scaring.

B. Carbuncle of the Labium Majus Multiple furuncles may coalesce to form a complex abscess of the labia, with pain, erythema, edema, and draining sinuses. *S. aureus* is the usual cause. Surgical drainage and parenteral antistaphylococcal drug therapy are required.

5. CLITORAL ABSCESS

Infection of the clitoris can cause marked enlargement (2–4 times normal size), aching and/or throbbing pain, and erythema. Progression to abscess formation results in fluctuance and marked tenderness. Incision and drainage of the abscess under cover of antistaphylococcal antibiotic therapy lead to resolution.

6. VULVITIS

A. Focal Vulvitis (Vulvar Vestibulitis Syndrome) Vulvar burning pain, severe superficial dyspareunia, and pruritus occur. Pain may also be provoked by tampon insertion. The pain is usually sharply localized to one or more sites (up to eleven sites) at the introitus. Pain pro-

TABLE 37-1
ACUTE VULVOVAGINTIS

Type	Symptoms	Signs	Risk Factors	VAGINAL DISCHARGE Gross Appearance of Discharge	pH	Odor	Microscopy	Gram Stain	Response to Therapy with
Yeast: *C. albicans* (84–97 percent); *T. glabrata* (3–16%)	Vulvar burning, pruritus, superficial dyspareunia, cheesy discharge (50–70% are symptomatic)	Vulvar edema and erythema, fissuring, satellite skin pustules and red dermal nodules, curdlike patches adherent to the vaginal mucosa (20%)	Diabetes mellitus, pregnancy, antibiotic therapy, immunosuppression, contraceptive pills, corticosteroids	White, curdlike "cottage cheese"	≤4.5	None	Clumps of epithelial cells, leukocytes in concentrations >10/HPF, hyphae and pseudohyphae and pseudohyphae and spores (*Candida* species), blastospores only (*T. glabrata*)	*Candida* hyphae and pseudohyphae and spores, abundant gram-positive rods (lactobacilli)	Butaconazole, miconazole, nystatin
T. vaginalis	Vulvar burning, pruritus, superficial dyspareunia, copious yellow or yellow-green malodorous discharge, dysuria (50–90% are symptomatic)	Vaginal mucosal erythema; green or yellow-green vaginal discharge that may be foamy (12–24%); "strawberry" cervix with petechial, granular, friable surface lesions (2–30%)	Sexual activity, increased incidence in divorced women and prostitutes	Yellow or yellow-green; foamy, pasty, or watery	>4.5	Fishy odor, especially after addition of 1–2 drops of KOH	Leukocytes in concentrations >10/HPF, parabasal epithelial cells, trichomonads with characteristic "twitching" motility	"Miscellaneous" Gram stain with gram-positive and -negative bacilli and cocci	Metronidazole
Bacterial vaginosis	Scanty or copious malodorous vaginal discharge, vulvovaginal irritation in 16% and superficial dyspareunia in 10% of cases (46% are symptomatic, with one or more of the listed complaints)	Thin white or yellow-white vaginal discharge with a fishy odor. A "milk of magnesia" or "thin flour paste" appearance of the discharge also has been described. A foamy appearance may occur in up to 15%. Mild edema and redness of the vulva (22%)	Sexual activity, intra-uterine device use	Thin, white, gray, or yellow-white	>4.5	Fishy odor with or without addition of KOH (88–96%), which may be more intense after ejaculation or during menses due to increased pH	Clue cells (85–97%) refractile or granular-appearing squamous cells with coccobacilli (*G. vaginalis*) adherent to their edges, few leukocytes (<10/HPF), epithelial cells	Gram-negative or variable coccobacilli; comma-shaped rods, fusiforms, and few gram-positive rods (lactobacilli)	Metronidazole

458

voked by intercourse or tampon insertion may persist as a dull vulvar ache for hours. The pain may be intensified premenstrually or by wearing tight clothing. Examination of the vestibule under bright light with the hymenal ring rolled inward toward the proximal vagina, reveals one to as many as eleven (median number, three) small areas (3–10 mm) of exquisitely tender focal erythema and/or small ulcers. These lesions may represent inflammation of minor vestibular glands and Skene's glands. A "touch test" of these erythematous lesions (performed with the tip of a cotton applicator) reveals severe tenderness. Areas between erythematous lesions are normal in appearance and nontender. Lesions are most commonly located in the region posterior or adjacent to the Bartholin's duct openings (i.e., between 4 and 8 o'clock), although more anterior focal lesions may also occur. In up to 80 percent of cases in one series, the onset of dyspareunia was abrupt during a single episode of intercourse. This acute dyspareunia then became recurrent. Careful search for other causes of vestibular pain such as herpes progenitalis, candidiasis, trichomoniasis, bacterial vaginosis, or a dermatologic disorder yields negative results. Some cases spontaneously improve or resolve, but surgical laser excision of the painful areas may be required for refractory complaints. At colposcopy, the red vestibular areas may show intense acetowhitening.

B. Diffuse Vulvitis with Acetowhitening   Some women with burning vulvar pain, pruritus, and a sensation of rawness intensified by coitus have a normal vestibule on examination. Application of a 5% acetic acid wash prior to colposcopy reveals an intense, diffuse acetowhitening of the mucosa of the vestibule. This whitening may extend to involve the vulvar skin, interlabial sulci, clitoris, and perineum (60 percent), and the labia majora (25 percent). In one report, a subset of patients with vulvodynia and acetowhitening have been shown to harbor human papillomavirus DNA by a Southern blot hybridization technique. Topical 5-fluorouracil therapy may be effective. Laser vulvectomy may be required for relief of vulvar burning and dyspareunia in severe refractory cases.

7. TRAUMATIC LABIAL FRENUM TEARS

A superficial traumatic "split" or tear in the vaginal mucosa at the juncture of the labia minora posteriorly (i.e., labial frenum or fourchette) may occur secondary to sexual activity. These tears may cause superficial dyspareunia. Magnification and a bright light may be required to detect these subtle but troublesome lesions.

8. GENERALIZED SKIN DISORDERS

A. Stevens-Johnson Syndrome   Vulvovaginitis is associated with systemic symptoms (fever, sore throat,

cough, chest pain, headache, malaise, arthralgias, and myalgias) and a generalized skin rash with target and herpes iris lesions, macules, and confluent erythematous patches on extensor surfaces, and over the knees, hips, and soles. Other cutaneous manifestations include polycyclic and arcuate lesions, urticarial plaques, vesicles, and bullae. Bullous and erosive lesions may involve the mouth, lips, and conjunctiva. The mucosa of the lips may become coated with a gray-white pseudomembrane, and hemorrhagic crusts may cover the vermilion portion. Pain associated with oral involvement may be severe enough to prevent eating. A purulent conjunctivitis may occur. Complications such as corneal ulceration, anterior uveitis, and panophthalmitis may develop. The associated vulvovaginitis may become painful secondary to collapse of bullae and formation of mucosal erosions and ulcers. Severe external dysuria may be associated. This disorder is caused by hypersensitivity to a drug or an infectious agent (e.g., HSV and *Mycoplasma*).

B. Toxic Epidermal Necrolysis   There is an acute onset of a diffuse macular rash that rapidly coalesces to form large erythematous patches. Giant flaccid bullae form on these areas of erythematous skin. These rupture, leaving multiple erosions on the trunk and extremities. Nikolsky's sign is positive in erythematous areas. The conjunctiva is injected, and a purulent exudate may be present. The mouth and lips may be painful due to rupture of oral bullae. Vulvar pain may occur, secondary to bullous lesions and their breakdown. Systemic symptoms such as fever, malaise, weakness, anorexia, and severe prostration usually develop.

Etiologic factors include ingestion of drugs (e.g., trimethoprim-sulfamethoxazole, penicillin, tetracycline, phenytoin, and allopurinol), viral infections (e.g., measles, varicella, herpes zoster, and HSV), *E. coli* septicemia, vaccines, lymphomas and leukemias, and tonic water (quinine). Supportive care in an intensive care or burn unit and early administration of high doses of intravenous corticosteroids increase the likelihood of survival.

9. DYSURIA SYNDROMES

A. Internal Dysuria   Felt deep within the vagina and suprapubic region, internal dysuria begins before or with the onset of urination. It is commonly associated with urinary frequency, nocturia, urgency, cloudy and sometimes foul-smelling urine, and/or gross hematuria. The causes include urethral and bladder infections. Some cases of pyelonephritis may cause only lower tract irritative symptoms such as frequency, urgency, and dysuria (occult pyelonephritis), only upper tract complaints such as flank pain, tenderness, and fever, or both.

1. Acute Bacterial Cystitis   Bacterial cystitis causes internal dysuria, frequency, urgency, cloudy urine, gross hematuria, and suprapubic discomfort relieved by voiding. There are usually no systemic symptoms. Tenderness of the urethra, bladder neck, and suprapubic region may be present (10 percent), but the flanks and costovertebral angle are nontender. The urine sediment contains increased numbers of leukocytes singly and in clumps, erythrocytes (40–60 percent of cases), and bacteria (when there are $>10^4$ CFU/ml). Cultures reveal the presence of *E. coli* (80–90 percent of cases) in colony counts of greater than 10^2 CFU/ml. *S. saprophyticus* is also a common cause of cystourethritis in young, sexually active women. Patients with cystitis respond rapidly to a 3-day course of therapy with amoxacillin, trimethoprim-sulfamethoxazole, or doxycycline with a low percentage of relapse unless there is occult upper tract infection. Less common causes of acute cystitis include other Enterobacteriaceae (*Klebsiella* and *Proteus* species) or enterococci. Inclusion of patients with urine colony counts between 10^2 and 10^4 CFU/ml permits an etiologic diagnosis of acute dysuria in up to one-third of women who would have been given a diagnosis of "acute urethral syndrome" of unknown cause if previous cutoff values of greater than or equal to 10^5 CFU/ml were utilized to diagnose infection.

2. Cystourethritis Syndrome   Internal dysuria and frequency may be associated with pyuria and a negative urine culture (i.e., less than 10^2 CFU/ml). Pyuria may be measured by counting unspun urine in a hemacytometer chamber. More than ten polymorphonuclear leukocytes (PMNL) per cubic millimeter of urine is abnormal. Leukocyte excretion rates of more than 400,000 PMNL/h are abnormal. The presence of pyuria can also be established with a leukocyte esterase (LE) dipstick. Patients with pyuria and a negative culture may also have a purulent vaginal discharge and unilateral or bilateral lower abdominal pain and tenderness. Examination may reveal evidence of cervitis as well as cervical motion, and/or adnexal tenderness. Urethral and cervical cultures may grow *C. trachomatis* (20–60 percent of cases), *N. gonorrhea*, or *HSV-2*. Meatal redness, edema, and urethral discharge may occur with *C. trachomatis* and *N. gonorrhea* infections. Dysuria associated with herpes infection is usually associated with labial, vestibular, and cervical vesicles and ulcerations with local pain and tenderness. *LGV* is a rare cause of dysuria and purulent urethral discharge. The appearance of prominent femoral and inguinal lymphadenopathy is useful in establishing the diagnosis. LGV infection can be confirmed by measuring antibody levels (LGV complement fixation) or by culture of the urethra. *T. vaginalis* may cause cystourethritis with dysuria. This can be confirmed by finding the organism in a catheterized urine specimen.

3. Dysuria and Acute Pyelonephritis

A. occult pyelonephritis   Up to 30 percent of women presenting with acute cystitis, characterized by internal dysuria, frequency, urgency, nocturia, and suprapubic discomfort, may have *occult pyelonephritis*. Flank pain and tenderness and fever may be minimal or absent. Historic clues to the presence of occult pyelonephritis include prior urinary structural abnormalities (e.g., renal stones, obstruction, and neurogenic bladder), diabetes mellitus, a urinary tract infection before age 12, an immunocompromising illness, pregnancy, symptoms for more than 7 days, acute pyelonephritis (i.e., flank pain, fever, and chills) during the prior year, and relapse after a 3-day course of antibiotic therapy or failure to respond to 3 days of antibiotic therapy. Localization techniques such as ureteral catheterization, bladder washout, and detection of antibody-coated bacteria are seldom utilized clinically. Failure of response to single-dose therapy or short-course therapy has been used by some physicians as a test for possible occult pyelonephritis. Treatment of women with occult pyelonephritis with oral antibiotics for 2 weeks is usually effective, but for those failing this therapy a 6-week course of therapy is recommended.

B. acute pyelonephritis and cystitis   *Acute pyelonephritis* may begin with irritative bladder symptoms, followed within 2 to 7 days by the onset of fever, rigors, chills, sweats, and severe aching flank and/or abdominal pain and tenderness. Nausea, vomiting, headache, and prostration may occur in severe cases. The urine contains increased numbers of leukocytes singly, in clumps, and sometimes in casts. Urine colony counts usually exceed 10^5 CFU/ml. There is a prompt response to parenteral antibiotic therapy.

C. idiopathic dysuria   Women with *idiopathic dysuria* have internal dysuria, frequency, and urgency but have a normal urinary sediment and negative urine, urethral, and cervical cultures. The etiology is unknown.

D. noninfectious disorders   Renal colic produced by the passage of a *stone* may be associated with flank and lower abdominal pain. After passage of the stone into the bladder, frequency, urgency, and dysuria may occur in association with gross or microscopic hematuria. If the stone becomes impacted in the urethra, dysuria, frequency, and a thin or split urinary stream or urinary retention may occur. A plain radiograph may detect the stone. Cystoscopy may be required to confirm a diagnosis of vesical stones. Symptoms resolve after passage or removal of the calculus. The diagnosis can also be confirmed by straining the urine and recovering the stone.

B. External Dysuria The pain is perceived as coming from the vulvar area, and it begins after the onset of urination and may persist afterward for a brief or longer period of time. Frequency, urgency, and nocturia are not usually present. The causes of external dysuria include vulvovaginitis and genital ulcerative disorders.

1. Vulvovaginitis Vulvovaginitis caused by candidiasis, trichomoniasis, bacterial vaginosis, chemical irritants, or contact allergy may cause burning vulvar pain during and after urination.

2. Genital Ulcerative Disorders HSV-2 infection, chancroid, trauma, and LGV may cause dysuria. A true urethritis, with internal dysuria, may occur with HSV-2, chancroid, and LGV. These disorders and their diagnoses are discussed above.

10. BEHÇET'S DISEASE

Aphthous stomatitis (99 percent), uveitis (66 percent), genital ulcers (80 percent), and cutaneous vasculitis (66 percent) are the four major symptoms associated with this disorder. Cutaneous vasculitis can present as erythema nodosum on the legs, a superficial thrombophlebitis, skin pustules and papules, and skin pathergy. (A cutaneous needle stick results in a pustule at the puncture site.) Vulvar ulcers are painful but usually recur less often than oral ulcers. Vaginal ulcers are usually asymptomatic, unless they cause a vaginal discharge. Synovitis (involving the knees, ankles, and hands), meningoencephalitis, enterocolitis, and venous and/or arterial thrombosis may also occur. Treatment with prednisone and cytotoxic drugs (e.g., chlorambucil) may be effective in controlling this disorder.

11. NECROTIZING PERINEAL INFECTION

There is an abrupt onset of labial pain, edema, tenderness, and subcutaneous crepitation. A black spot appears in the posterior labial region (25 percent) and rapidly enlarges. Sloughing and progressive gangrene of the skin occur. The local edema, redness, and tenderness may spread within hours to the skin of the thighs, anterior abdominal wall, and buttocks. Radiographs or ultrasonography can confirm gas in tissue planes. Fever, severe systemic toxicity, pain, and prostration occur. Cultures reveal *Clostridium perfringens*, *Clostridium septicum*, or other clostridial species. Polymicrobic infection with multiple aerobic and anaerobic bacteria may also be causative. Clostridia may occur in combination with one or more species of streptococci, coliform bacilli, or staphylococci.

Extensive debridement and parenteral antibiotic therapy are required for survival.

12. REFERRED PAIN TO THE VULVA

A. Renolithiasis Renal colic and renolithiasis may cause flank and lower abdominal pain that radiates into the inguinal region and labia. Gross or microscopic hematuria is associated.

B. Aneurysms An enlarging *aortic* or *common iliac aneurysm* may cause unilateral lower abdominal and back pain and referred labial pain. The diagnosis can be suspected from the physical examination and confirmed by abdominal ultrasonography.

C. Ilioinguinal or Genitofemoral Neuralgia Patients may have inguinal and labial aching pain, hyperesthesia, hypesthesia, and/or paresthesias in this region. Selective anesthetic nerve block of one or both of these nerves may be required to determine which is involved. Both may become damaged after lower abdominal surgery (e.g., appendectomy, herniorrhaphy, or a Pfannenstiel incision). Idiopathic varieties of these forms of neuralgia also occur.

D. Spine or Spinal Cord Disease At the level of the T12 to L2 roots, such disorders may cause lower abdominal, inguinal, and labial pain on the ipsilateral side. Spinal cord tumors may cause perineal pain.

E. Acute Appendicitis Patients with acute appendicitis may have pain radiating into the perineum and labia as well as right or mid-lower abdominal pain. Right iliac and rectal tenderness is frequently present.

13. DYSPAREUNIA

A. Superficial Dyspareunia

1. Lack of Lubrication Decreased vaginal secretion prevents adequate lubrication during coitus and may lead to friction-related abrasion of the mucosa of the vagina and vestibule, with persistent burning pain and tenderness. Lack of lubrication may be due to psychologic factors, gonadal dysgenesis, surgical removal of the ovaries, and the menopause. Use of estrogen, vaginal cream, and lubricating jelly may prevent coitus-related vulvar pain and tenderness.

2. Vaginismus Pain occurs at the initial attempt at penetration. There are associated involuntary spasm of the muscles about the introitus and adduction of the thighs. Similar spasm may be observed during the vaginal examination, but this occurs in only a small number of women with this disorder. The causes of vaginismus include fear of pregnancy, aversion to the partner, and fear of provoking a pain similar to that experienced during intercourse in the past. Vaginismus provoked by an organic cause of dyspareunia is called secondary vaginismus. Treatment of the primary cause may relieve this type of vaginismus.

B. Deep Dyspareunia Severe to moderate deep vaginal and lower abdominal pain can be provoked by deep thrusts of the penis. The pain may be felt with each thrust and/or as a dull, continuous ache afterward. Causes of acute deep dyspareunia include ectopic pregnancy, salpingitis, endometriosis, rupture or torsion of an ovarian cyst, and intraperitoneal bleeding from a follicle cyst or ectopic pregnancy. Inflammatory disease of the rectum, acute appendicitis, or sigmoid diverticulitis may also be responsible for deep dyspareunia.

1. Ectopic Pregnancy Patients have unilateral aching or crampy lower abdominal pain, amenorrhea and/or vaginal spotting, a positive pregnancy test, and absence of an intrauterine pregnancy by ultrasonography. In some cases, a tubal mass may be palpated or detected by ultrasonography. The diagnosis may be confirmed by laparoscopy or at laparotomy.

2. Acute Salpingitis Patients may have fever, chills, unilateral or bilateral lower abdominal and back pain, vaginal discharge, and increased pain on cervical motion and palpation of the affected tube and ovary. The diagnosis can be confirmed by laparoscopy. There is a response to antibiotic therapy.

3. Endometriosis This disorder may cause pain in the lower abdomen and deep in the pelvis that begins a day or two prior to the onset of menstrual bleeding and continues through the period. There may be cervical motion and adnexal tenderness. Pea- to walnut-sized nodules may be palpable on pelvic examination. The diagnosis can be confirmed by laparoscopy and biopsy.

4. Rupture of an Ovarian Cyst Acute unilateral or bilateral lower abdominal pain with peritoneal signs may be caused by rupture of an ovarian cyst. The diagnosis of a cyst can be confirmed by ultrasonography and that of rupture with bleeding by laparoscopy.

5. Torsion of an Ovarian Cyst Patients have unilateral abdominal pain and tenderness and a progressively enlarging tender ovarian mass. The diagnosis can be confirmed by ultrasonography and laparoscopy.

6. Pelvic Abscess due to Inflammatory Disease of the Appendix or Sigmoid Inflammatory disease of the appendix or a sigmoid diverticulum may cause lower abdominal pain, tenderness, and a pelvic mass due to abscess formation, which can be responsible for dyspareunia. Patients may have persistent fever, chills, and leukocytosis. The diagnosis can be confirmed by laparoscopy, an abdominal CT scan, or exploratory surgery.

7. Colitis This disorder causes diarrhea, hematochezia, lower abdominal pain, tenesmus, and deep dyspareunia. It may be caused by pathogenic bacteria or Entamoeba histolytica, or it may be secondary to inflammatory bowel disease. The diagnosis can be confirmed by sigmoidoscopy or colonoscopy, stool culture, and microscopy.

Dyspareunia may occur with any of the above-described disorders when the clinical symptoms are not severe enough to preclude sexual activity.

VULVAR AND VAGINAL PAIN REFERENCES

Amebiasis—Genital
Veliath AJ, Bansal R, Sankarian V, et al: Genital amebiasis. *Int J Gynaecol Obstet* 25:249–256, 1987.
Walter A: Diagnosis of amebic vaginitis from cervicovaginal smears (letter to editor). *Acta Cytol* 26(3):378–379, 1982.

Anorectal Infections—Necrotizing
Bubrick MP, Hitchcock CR: Necrotizing anorectal and perineal infections. *Surgery* 86(4):655–662, 1979.

Bartholin's Cysts
Bleker OP, Smalbraak DJC, Schutte MF: Bartholin's abscess: The role of *Chlamydia trachomatis*. *Genitourin Med* 66:24–25, 1990.
Cheetham DR: Bartholin's cyst: Marsupialization or aspiration? *Am J Obstet Gynecol* 152:569–570, 1985.

Downs MC, Randall HW Jr: The ambulatory surgical management of Bartholin duct cysts. *J Emerg Med* 7:623–626, 1989.
Kovar WR, Scott JC Jr: A practical, inexpensive office management of Bartholin's cyst and abscess. *Neb Med J* 68(8):254–255, 1983.
Lashgari M, Keene M: Excision of Bartholin duct cysts using the CO$_2$ laser. *Obstet Gynecol* 67:735–737, 1986.
Quentin R, Pierre F, Dubois M, et al: Frequent isolation of capnophilic bacteria in aspirate from Bartholin's gland abscesses and cysts. *Eur J Clin Microbiol Infect Dis* 9(2):138–141, 1990.

Carcinoma in Situ of the Vulva
Boden E, Rylander E, Evander M, et al: Papillomavirus infection of the vulva. *Acta Obstet Gynecol Scand* 68:179–184, 1989.
Byrne MA, Walker MM, Leonard J, et al: Recognising covert disease

in women with chronic vulval symptoms attending an STD clinic: Value of detailed examination including colposcopy. *Genitourin Med* 65:46–49, 1989.

Hewitt H: Pre-neoplastic lesions of the vulva. *Eur J Gynaec Oncol* 9(5):377–380, 1988.

Husseinzadeh N, Newman NJ, Wesseler TA: Vulvar intraepithelial neoplasia: A clinicopathological study of carcinoma in situ of the vulva. *Gynecol Oncol* 33:157–163, 1989.

Planner RS, Andersen HE, Hobbs JB, et al: Multifocal invasive carcinoma of the vulva in a 25-year-old woman with Bowenoid papulosis. *Aust N Z J Obstet Gynaecol* 27(4):291–295, 1987.

Planner RS, Hobbs JB: Intraepithelial and invasive neoplasis of the vulva in association with human papillomavirus infection. *J Reprod Med* 33(6):503–509, 1988.

Rodke G, Friedrich EG Jr, Wilkinson EJ: Malignant potential of mixed vulvar dystrophy (lichen sclerosus associated with squamous cell hyperplasia). *J Reprod Med* 33(6):545–550, 1988.

Schlaerth JB, Morrow CP, Nalick RH, et al: Anal involvement by carcinoma in situ of the perineum in women. *Obstet Gynecol* 64:406–411, 1984.

Woodruff JD: Carcinoma in situ of the vulva. *Clin Obstet Gynecol* 28(1):230–239, 1985.

Carcinoma of the Female Urethra

Prempree T, Amornmarn R, Patanaphan V: Radiation therapy in primary carcinoma of the female urethra: 2. An update on results. *Cancer* 54:729–733, 1984.

Carcinoma of the Vulva

Berman ML, Soper JT, Creasman WT, et al: Conservative surgical management of superficially invasive stage I vulvar carcinoma. *Gynecol Oncol* 35:352–357, 1989.

Buckley CH, Butler EB, Fox H: Vulvar intraepithelial neoplasia and microinvasive carcinoma of the vulva. *J Clin Pathol* 37:1201–1211, 1984.

Cavanagh D, Roberts WS, Bryson SCP, et al: Changing trends in the surgical treatment of invasive carcinoma of the vulva. *Surg Gynecol Obstet* 162(2):164–168, 1986.

Copeland LJ, Sneige N, Gershenson DM, et al: Bartholin gland carcinoma. *Obstet Gynecol* 67:794–801, 1986.

Eriksson E, Eldh J, Peterson L-E: Surgical treatment of carcinoma of the clitoris. *Gynecol Oncol* 17:291–295, 1984.

Fiorica JV, LaPolla JP, Cavanagh D: Diagnosis and management of vulvar carcinoma. *Comp Ther* 14(5):24–28, 1988.

Hoffman MS, Roberts WS, LaPolla JP, et al: Carcinoma of the vulva involving the perianal or anal skin. *Gynecol Oncol* 35:215–218, 1989.

Hoffman MS, Roberts WS, Ruffolo EH: Basal cell carcinoma of the vulva with inguinal lymph node metastases. *Gynecol Oncol* 29:113–119, 1988.

Kneale BL: Carcinoma of the vulva, Then and now: The 1987 ISSVD Presidential Address. *J Reprod Med* 33(6):496–499, 1988.

Murdoch JB, Torbet TE: Carcinoma of the vulva: A ten year retrospective study in the West of Scotland (1972–1982). *Scott Med J* 31:166–169, 1986.

Siegle RJ, Headington JT, Swanson NA: Early invasive carcinoma of the vulva treated with the Mohs technique of microscopically controlled surgery. *Am J Obstet Gynecol* 147(4):459–461, 1983.

Sutton GP, Stehman FB, Ehrlich CE, et al: Human papillomavirus deoxyribonucleic acid in lesions of the female genital tract: Evidence for type 6/11 in squamous carcinoma of the vulva. *Obstet Gynecol* 70:564–568, 1987.

Thomas RHM, McGibbon DH, Munro DD: Basal cell carcinoma of the vulva in association with vulval lichen sclerosus et atrophicus. *J R Soc Med* 78(suppl 11):16–18, 1985.

Dermatologic Disorders of the Vulva

Bermejo A, Bermejo MD, Román P, et al: Lichen planus with simultaneous involvement of the oral cavity and genitalia. *Oral Surg Oral Med Oral Pathol* 69:209–216, 1990.

Harrington CI: Old and new causes of superficial dyspareunia. *Br Med J* 295(6602):854, 1987.

Soper DE, Patterson JW, Hurt WG, et al: Lichen planus of the vulva. *Obstet Gynecol* 72:74–76, 1988.

Václavínková V, Neumann E: Vaginal involvement in familial benign chronic pemphigus (Morbus Hailey-Hailey). *Acta Derm Venereol* (Stockh) 62(1):80–81, 1982.

Dyspareunia

Boylan P, MacDonald D, Turner M: Vaginal dilation in the treatment of dyspareunia. *Ir Med J* 77(4):104–105, 1984.

Glatt AE, Zinner SH, McCormack WM: The prevalence of dyspareunia. *Obstet Gynecol* 75:433–436, 1990.

Greiss FC Jr: Equestrian dyspareunia. *Am J Obstet Gynecol* 150(2):168, 1984.

Grillo L, Grillo D: Management of dyspareunia secondary to hymenal remnants. *Obstet Gynecol* 56:510–514, 1980.

Huffman JW: Dyspareunia of vulvovaginal origin: Causes and management. *Postgrad Med* 73(2):287–296, 1983.

Lamont JA: Female dyspareunia. *Am J Obstet Gynecol* 136:282–285, 1980.

Riley AJ, Bromwich P: Old and new causes of superficial dyspareunia. *Br Med J [Clin Res]* 295(6597):513–514, 1987.

Sandberg G, Quevillon RP: Dyspareunia: An integrated approach to assessment and diagnosis. *J Fam Pract* 24(1):66–70, 1987.

Setchell ME: Dyspareunia. *Br J Hosp Med* 26(5):538, 540–541, 1981.

Steege JF: Dyspareunia and vaginismus. *Clin Obstet Gynecol* 27(3):750–759, 1984.

Dyspareunia—Focal Vulvitis

Friedrich EG Jr: The vulvar vestibule. *J Reprod Med* 28(11):773–777, 1983.

Growdon WA, Fu YS, Lebherz TB, et al: Pruritic vulvar squamous papillomatosis: Evidence for human papillomavirus etiology. *Obstet Gynecol* 66:564–568, 1985.

Marinoff SC, Turner MLC: Hypersensitivity to vaginal candidiasis or treatment vehicles in the pathogenesis of minor vestibular gland syndrome. *J Reprod Med* 31(9):796–799, 1986.

Miles PA, Reamy K: Flat condyloma of the hymenal ring: An unusual cause of dyspareunia (letter to editor). *Acta Cytologica* 27(2):212–213, 1983.

Oates JK: Focal vulvitis and localised dyspareunia. *Genitourin Med* 66:28–30, 1990.

Peckham BM, Maki DG, Patterson JJ, et al: Focal vulvitis: A characteristic syndrome and cause of dyspareunia. *Am J Obstet Gynecol* 154:855–864, 1986.

Reid R, Greenberg MD, Daoud Y, et al: Colposcopic findings in women with vulvar pain syndromes: A preliminary report. *J Reprod Med* 33(6):523–532, 1988.

Turner MLC, Marinoff SC: Association of human papillomavirus with vulvodynia and the vulvar vestibulitis syndrome. *J Reprod Med* 33(6):533–537, 1988.

Woodruff JD, Friedrich EG Jr: The vestibule. *Clin Obstet Gynecol* 28(1):134–141, 1985.

Woodruff JD, Parmley TH: Infection of the minor vestibular gland. *Obstet Gynecol* 62:609–612, 1983.

Dyspareunia—Obstructive

Friedman M, Gal D, Peretz BA: Management of imperforate hymen with the carbon dioxide laser. *Obstet Gynecol* 74:270–272, 1989.

Heinonen PK: Longitudinal vaginal septum. *Eur J Obstet Gynecol Reprod Biol* 13:253–258, 1982.

Heinonen PK: Uterus didelphys: A report of 26 cases. *Eur J Obstet Gynecol Reprod Biol* 17:345–350, 1984.

Michlewitz H: Laser ablation of hymenal fissures. *J Reprod Med* 31(1):63–64, 1986.

Munsick RA: Introital operations for dyspareunia. *Clin Obstet Gynecol* 23(1):243–271, 1980.

Pinsonneault O, Goldstein DP: Obstructing malformations of the uterus and vagina. *Fertil Steril* 44(2):241–247, 1985.

Woodruff JD, Genadry R, Poliakoff S: Treatment of dyspareunia and vaginal outlet distortions by perineoplasty. *Obstet Gynecol* 57(6): 750–754, 1981.

Wyant GM: Chronic pain syndromes and their treatment: 3. The piriformis syndrome. *Can Anaesth Soc J* 26(4):305–308, 1979.

Dyspareunia Related to Surgery and Radiation Therapy

Adelusi B: Coital function after radiotherapy for carcinoma of the cervix uteri. *Br J Obstet Gynaecol* 87:821–823, 1980.

Grant A: The choice of suture materials and techniques for repair of perineal trauma: An overview of the evidence from controlled trials. *Br J Obstet Gynaecol* 96:1281–1289, 1989.

Grant A, Spencer D: Dyspareunia associated with the use of glycerol-impregnated catgut to repair perineal trauma: Report of a 3-year follow-up study. *Br J Obstet Gynaecol* 96(6):741–743, 1989.

Haadem K, Ohrlander S, Lingman G: Long-term ailments due to anal sphincter rupture caused by delivery: A hidden problem. *Eur J Obstet Gynecol Reprod Biol* 27:27–32, 1988.

Hjortrup A, Kirkegaard P, Friis J, et al: Sexual dysfunction after low anterior resection for midrectal cancer. *Acta Chir Scand* 150:687–688, 1984.

Metcalf AM, Dozois RR, Kelly KA: Sexual function in women after proctocolectomy. *Ann Surg* 204(6):624–627, 1986.

Schover LR, von Eschenbach AC: Sexual function and female radical cystectomy: A case series. *J Urol* 134(3):465–468, 1985.

Spencer JAD, Grant A, Elbourne D, et al: A randomized comparison of glycerol-impregnated chromic catgut with untreated chromic catgut for the repair of perineal trauma. *Br J Obstet Gynaecol* 93:426–430, 1986.

Dysuria

Berg AO, Heidrich FE, Fihn SD, et al: Establishing the cause of genitourinary symptoms in women in a family practice. *JAMA* 251:620–625, 1984.

Berg AO, Soman MP: Lower genitourinary infections in women. *J Fam Pract* 23(1):61–67, 1986.

Bowie WR: Nongonococcal urethritis. *Urol Clin North Am* 11(1):55–64, 1984.

Bowie WR, Jones H: Acute pelvic inflammatory disease in outpatients: Association with *Chlamydia trachomatis* and *Neisseria gonorrhoeae*. *Ann Intern Med* 95:685–688, 1981.

Forland M: Dysuria, in Stein JH (ed): *Internal Medicine*, 2d ed. Boston, Little, Brown, 1987, pp 748–750.

Heller M: Chlamydial infections. *Ann Emerg Med* 13:170–174, 1984.

Iosif CS, Bekassy Z: Prevalence of genito-urinary symptoms in the late menopause. *Acta Obstet Gynecol Scand* 63:257–260, 1984.

Latham RH: Urinary tract infections and the urethral syndrome in adult women: Pathogenesis, diagnosis, and therapy. *Emerg Med Clin North Am* 3(1):75–86, 1985.

Levine DZ: Interstitial cystitis: An overlooked cause of pelvic pain. *Postgrad Med* 88(1):101–102, 107–109, 1990.

Roehrborn CG: Long term follow-up study of the marsupialization technique for urethral diverticula in women. *Surg Gynecol Obstet* 167(3):191–196, 1988.

Wong ES, Stamm WE: Urethral infections in men and women. *Ann Rev Med* 34:337–358, 1983.

Paget's Disease—Vulva

Degefu S, O'Quinn AG, Dhurandhar HN: Paget's disease of the vulva and urogenital malignancies: A case report and review of the literature. *Gynecol Oncol* 25:347–354, 1986.

Dietel M, Bahnsen J, Stegner H-E, et al: Paget's disease of the vulva with underlying apocrine adenocarcinoma and local lymph node invasion. *Pathol Res Pract* 171:353–361, 1981.

Stacy D, Burrell MO, Franklin EW III: Extramammary Paget's disease of the vulva and anus: Use of intraoperative frozen-section margins. *Am J Obstet Gynecol* 155:519–523, 1986.

Tuck SM, Williams A: Paget's disease of the vulva complicated by bladder carcinoma: Case report. *Br J Obstet Gynaecol* 92:416–418, 1985.

Urinary Tuberculosis

Frank IN: Urology, in Schwartz SI (ed): *Principles of Surgery*, 5th ed. New York, McGraw-Hill, 1989, pp 1747–1748.

Teplik JG, Haskin ME: Tuberculosis of the urinary tract, in *Roentgenologic Diagnosis*, 3d ed. Philadelphia, Saunders, 1976, vol 1, pp 206–208.

Vaginismus

Reamy K: The treatment of vaginismus by the gynecologist: An eclectic approach. *Obstet Gynecol* 59:58–62, 1982.

Steege JF, Jelovsek FR: Sexual behavior during pregnancy. *Obstet Gynecol* 60:163–168, 1982.

Vaginitis—Atrophic

Channon LD, Ballinger SE: Some aspects of sexuality and vaginal symptoms during menopause and their relation to anxiety and depression. *Br J Med Psychol* 59:173–180, 1986.

Dennerstein L, Burrows GD, Hyman GJ, et al: Some clinical effects of oestrogen-progestogen therapy in surgically castrated women. *Maturitas* 2:19–28, 1979.

Gambrell RD Jr: The menopause. *Invest Radiol* 21:369–378, 1986.

Michalas S, Papandrikos A, Koutselini E, et al: Local therapy of atrophic vaginal conditions with oestriol suppositories. *J Int Med Res* 8:358–360, 1980.

Osborn M, Hawton K, Gath D: Sexual dysfunction among middle aged women in the community. *Br Med J [Clin Res]* 296(6627):959–962, 1988.

Semmens JP, Tsai CC, Semmens EC, et al: Effects of estrogen therapy on vaginal physiology during menopause. *Obstet Gynecol* 66:15–18, 1985.

Wallis LA: Management of dyspareunia in postmenopausal women. *J Am Med Wom Assoc* 42(3):82–84, 1987.

Vaginitis—Bacterial Vaginosis

Amsel R, Totten PA, Spiegel CA, et al: Nonspecific vaginitis: Diagnostic criteria and microbial and epidemiologic associations. *Am J Med* 74(1):14–22, 1983.

Blackwell AL, Barlow D: Anaerobic vaginosis: Clinical and diagnostic aspects. *Scand J Urol Nephrol Suppl* 86:129–133, 1984.

Dattani IM, Gerken A, Evans BA: Aetiology and management of nonspecific vaginitis. *Br J Vener Dis* 58:32–35, 1982.

Embree J, Caliando JJ, McCormack WM: Nonspecific vaginitis among women attending a sexually transmitted diseases clinic. *Sex Transm Dis* 11(2):81–84, 1984.

Fleury FJ: The clinical signs and symptoms of *Gardnerella*-associated vaginosis. *Scand J Infect Dis Suppl* 40:71–72, 1983.

Gardner HL: "Non-specific" vaginitis: A non-entity. *Scand J Infect Dis Suppl* 40:7–10, 1983.

Høvik P: Nonspecific vaginitis in an outpatient clinic: Comparison of three dosage regimens of metronidazole. *Scand J Infect Dis Suppl* 40:107–110, 1983.

Ison CA, Easmon CSF, Dawson SG, et al: Non-volatile fatty acids in the diagnosis of non-specific vaginitis. *J Clin Pathol* 36:1367–1370, 1983.

Jaramillo D, Allan NK, Raval B: Computed tomography of vaginitis emphysematosa. *J Comput Assist Tomogr* 10(3):521–523, 1986.

Jones BM, Kinghorn GR, Duerden BI: An overview of the diagnosis and treatment of *Gardnerella vaginalis*- and *Bacteroides*-associated vaginitis. *Eur J Clin Microbiol* 1(5):320–325, 1982.

Nelson MS: Clinical diagnosis of bacterial vaginosis. *Am J Emerg Med* 5:488–491, 1987.

Petersen EE, Pelz K: Diagnosis and therapy of nonspecific vaginitis: Correlation between KOH-test, clue cells and microbiology. *Scand J Infect Dis Suppl* 40:97–99, 1983.

Redondo-Lopez V, Meriwether C, Schmitt C, et al: Vulvovaginal candidiasis complicating recurrent bacterial vaginosis. *Sex Transm Dis* 17(1):51–53, 1990.

Spiegel CA, Amsel R, Holmes KK: Diagnosis of bacterial vaginosis by direct Gram stain of vaginal fluid. *J Clin Microbiol* 18(1):170–177, 1983.

van der Meijden WI: Clinical aspects of *Gardnerella vaginalis*-associated vaginitis: A review of the literature. *Scand J Urol Nephrol Suppl* 86:135–141, 1984.

Weaver CH, Mengel MB: Bacterial vaginosis. *J Fam Pract* 27(2):207–215, 1988.

Vaginitis—Candida/Toruplosis

Bergman JJ, Berg AO, Schneeweiss R, et al: Clinical comparison of microscopic and culture techniques in the diagnosis of *Candida* vaginitis. *J Fam Pract* 18(4):549–552, 1984.

Cooper C, Singha HSK: Condylomata acuminata in women: The effect of concomitant genital infection on response to treatment. *Acta Derm Venereol (Stockh)* 65:150–153, 1985.

DeJong AR: Vaginitis due to *Gardnerella vaginalis* and to *Candida albicans* in sexual abuse. *Child Abuse Neglect* 9:27–29, 1985.

Hopwood V: Differential diagnosis of vaginitis (letter to editor). *J Fam Pract* 30(2):230, 232–233, 1990.

Hopwood V, Warnock DW, Milne JD, et al: Evaluation of a new slide latex agglutination test for diagnosis of vaginal candidosis. *Eur J Clin Microbiol* 6(4):392–394, 1987.

Sweet RL: Importance of differential diagnosis in acute vaginitis. *Am J Obstet Gynecol* 152(7):921–923, 1985.

Vaginitis—Desquamative Inflammatory

Jacobson M, Krumholz B, Franks A Jr: Desquamative inflammatory vaginitis: A case report. *J Reprod Med* 34(9):647–650, 1989.

Oates JK, Rowen D: Desquamative inflammatory vaginitis: A review. *Genitourin Med* 66:275–279, 1990.

Vaginitis—Review Articles

Addison LA: The role of the office laboratory in the diagnosis of vaginitis. *Prim Care* 13(4):633–646, 1986.

Bennett EC: Vaginitis: Its diagnosis and treatment. *Health Care Wom Int* 8:65–73, 1987.

Chantigian PDM: Vaginitis: A common malady. *Prim Care* 15(3):517–547, 1988.

Eschenbach DA, Hillier SL: Advances in diagnostic testing for vaginitis and cervicitis. *J Reprod Med* 34(suppl 8):555–565, 1989.

Kaufman RH, Hammill HA: Vaginitis. *Prim Care* 17(1):115–125, 1990.

Lossick JG: Sexually transmitted vaginitis. *Urol Clin North Am* 11(1):141–153, 1984.

Spiegel CA: Vaginitis/vaginosis. *Clin Lab Med* 9(3):525–533, 1989.

van der Meijden WI, Duivenvoorden HJ, Both-Patoir HC, et al: Clinical and laboratory findings in women with bacterial vaginosis and trichomoniasis versus controls. *Eur J Obstet Gynecol Reprod Biol* 28:39–52, 1988.

Vaginitis—Trichomonas

Bennett JR, Barnes WG, Coffman S: The emergency department diagnosis of Trichomonas vaginitis. *Ann Emerg Med* 18:564–566, 1989.

Fouts AC, Kraus SJ: Trichomonas vaginalis: Reevaluation of its clinical presentation and laboratory diagnosis. *J Infect Dis* 141(2):137–143, 1980.

Vulvar Lesions—Review Articles

Arndt KA: Lichen planus, in Fitzpatrick TB, Eisen AZ, Wolff K, et al (eds): *Dermatology in General Medicine*, 2d ed. New York, McGraw-Hill, 1979, pp 655–661.

Bowie WB, Holmes KK: *Chlamydia trachomatis*, in Mandell GL, Douglas RG Jr, Bennett JE (eds): *Principles and Practice of Infectious Diseases*, 3d ed. New York, Churchill Livingstone, 1990, pp 1426–1440.

Bradley JJ, Ridley CM: Historical and psychological considerations: Subjective and traumatic conditions of the vulva, in Ridley CM (ed): *The Vulva*, 2d ed. New York, Churchill Livingstone, 1988, pp 212–227.

Buckley CH, Fox H: Epithelial tumours of the vulva, in Ridley CM (ed): *The Vulva*, 2d ed. New York, Churchill Livingstone, 1988, pp 263–333.

Cohen PR, Young AW Jr, Tovell HMM: Angiokeratoma of the vulva:

Diagnosis and review of the literature. *Obstet Gynecol Surv* 44(5):339–346, 1989.

Edwards JE Jr: *Candida* species, in Mandell GL, Douglas RG Jr, Bennett JE (eds): *Principles and Practice of Infectious Diseases*, 3d ed. New York, Churchill Livingstone, 1990, pp 1943–1958.

Farah FS: Behçet's syndrome, in Fitzpatrick TB, Eisen AZ, Wolff K, et al (eds): *Dermatology in General Medicine*, 2d ed. New York, McGraw-Hill, 1979, pp 907–909.

Faro S: Sexually transmitted diseases, in Kaufman RH, Friederich EG Jr, Gardner HL (eds): *Benign Diseases of the Vulva and Vagina*, 3d ed. Chicago, Year Book Medical, 1989, pp 73–105.

Fox H, Buckley CH: Tumour-like lesions and cysts of the vulva, in Ridley CM (ed): *The Vulva*, 2d ed. New York, Churchill Livingstone, 1988, pp 228–234.

Friedrich EG Jr: Large tumors, in Friedman EA (ed): *Vulvar Disease*, 2d ed. Philadelphia, Saunders, 1983, vol 9, pp 216–236.

Friedrich EG Jr: Red lesions, in Friedman EA (ed): *Vulvar Disease*, 2d ed. Philadelphia, Saunders, 1983, vol 9, pp 108–128.

Friedrich EG Jr: Small tumors, in Friedman EA (ed): *Vulvar Disease*, 2d ed. Philadelphia, Saunders, 1983, vol 9, pp 189–215.

Friedrich EG Jr: Ulcers, in Friedman EA (ed): *Vulvar Disease*, 2d ed. Philadelphia, Saunders, 1983, vol 9, pp 166–187.

Friedrich EG Jr: White lesions, in Friedman EA (ed): *Vulvar Disease*, 2d ed. Philadelphia, Saunders, 1983, vol 9, pp 129–148.

Handfield-Jones SE, Prendiville WJ, Norman S: Vulval lymphangiectasia. *Genitourin Med* 65:335–337, 1989.

Kaufman RH, Friederich EG Jr, Gardner HL: Cystic tumors, in *Benign Diseases of the Vulva and Vagina*, 3d ed. Chicago, Year Book Medical, 1989, pp 237–288.

Kaufman RH, Friederich EG Jr, Gardner HL: Intraepithelial neoplasia of the vulva and vagina, in *Benign Diseases of the Vulva and Vagina*, 3d ed. Chicago, Year Book Medical, 1989, pp 159–193.

Kaufman RH, Friederich EG Jr, Gardner HL: Miscellaneous vulvar disorders, in *Benign Diseases of the Vulva and Vagina*, 3d ed. Chicago, Year Book Medical, 1989, pp 324–360.

Kaufman RH, Friederich EG Jr, Gardner HL: Non-neoplastic epithelial disorders of the vulvar skin and mucosa (vulvar dystrophies), in *Benign Diseases of the Vulva and Vagina*, 3d ed. Chicago, Year Book Medical, 1989, pp 299–323.

Kaufman RH, Friederich EG Jr, Gardner HL: Pyogenic conditions of the vulva, in *Benign Diseases of the Vulva and Vagina*, 3d ed. Chicago, Year Book Medical, 1989, pp 286–298.

Kaufman RH, Friederich EG Jr, Gardner HL: Solid tumors, in *Benign Diseases of the Vulva and Vagina*, 3d ed. Chicago, Year Book Medical, 1989, pp 194–236.

Kohorn EI, Merino MJ, Goldenhersh M: Vulvar pain and dyspareunia due to glomus tumor. *Obstet Gynecol* 67:41S–42S, 1986.

Novick NL: Angiokeratoma vulvae. *J Am Acad Dermatol* 12:561–563, 1985.

Rhatigan RM, Nuss RC: Keratoacanthoma of the vulva. *Gynecol Oncol* 21:118–123, 1985.

Ridley CM: General dermatological conditions and dermatoses of the vulva, in *The Vulva*, 2d ed. New York, Churchill Livingstone, 1988, pp 138–211.

Spiegel CA: *Gardnerella vaginalis*, in Mandell GL, Douglas RG Jr, Bennett JE (eds): *Principles and Practice of Infectious Diseases*, 3d ed. New York, Churchill Livingstone, 1990, pp 1733–1735.

Tramont EC: *Treponema pallidium*, in Mandell GL, Douglas RG Jr, Bennett JE (eds): *Principles and Practice of Infectious Diseases*, 3d ed. New York, Churchill Livingstone, 1990, pp 1794–1808.

Wallace HJ, Hyman AB: Disorders of external genitalia, in Fitzpatrick TB, Eisen AZ, Wolff K, et al (eds): *Dermatology in General Medicine*, 2d ed. New York, McGraw-Hill, 1979, pp 909–920.

Vulvar Ulcerative Lesions

Chancroid (editorial). *Lancet* 2:747–748, 1982.

Daly JA: *Haemophilus ducreyi*. *Infect Control Hosp Epidemiol* 6(5):203–205, 1985.

Diaz-Mitoma F, Benningen G, Slutchuk M, et al: Etiology of non-vesicular genital ulcers in Winnipeg. *Sex Transm Dis* 14(1):33–36, 1987.

Faro S: Lymphogranuloma venereum, chancroid, and granuloma inguinale. *Obstet Gynecol Clin North Am* 16(3):517–530, 1989.

Kaufman RH: Clinical features of herpes genitalis. *J Reprod Med* 31(suppl 5):379–383, 1986.

Lubwama SW: Isolation and identification of *Haemophilus ducreyi* in a clinical laboratory. *J Med Microbiol* 22:175–178, 1986.

Mertz G, Corey L: Genital herpes simplex virus infections in adults. *Urol Clin North Am* 11(1):103–119, 1984.

Mindel A, Tovey SJ, Timmins DJ, et al: Primary and secondary syphilis: 20 years' experience: 2. Clinical features. *Genitourin Med* 65:1–3, 1989.

Ronald AR, Plummer FA: Chancroid and granuloma inguinale. *Clin Lab Med* 9(3):535–543, 1989.

Salzman RS, Kraus SJ, Miller RG, et al: Chancroidal ulcers that are not chancroid: Cause and epidemiology. *Arch Dermatol* 120:636–639, 1984.

Schmid GP, Sanders LL Jr, Blount JH, et al: Chancroid in the United States: Reestablishment of an old disease. *JAMA* 258:3265–3268, 1987.

Scieux C, Barnes R, Bianchi A, et al: Lymphogranuloma venereum: 27 cases in Paris. *J Infect Dis* 160(4):662–668, 1989.

Sturm AW, Stolting GJ, Cormane RH, et al: Clinical and microbiological evaluation of 46 episodes of genital ulceration. *Genitourin Med* 63:98–101, 1987.

PART EIGHT

Acute Shoulder, Arm, and Hand Pain

38

Acute Upper and Lower Arm Pain

☐ DIAGNOSTIC LIST

1. Acute cervical radiculopathy involving one or more nerve roots (C6–T1)
   A. Acute cervical disc herniation
   B. Cervical spondylosis
   C. Cervical osteomyelitis
   D. Cervical epidural abscess
   E. Cervical epidural hematoma
   F. Trauma
      1. Cervical nerve root avulsion from the spinal cord
      2. Herniated nucleus pulposus
      3. Ligamentous injuries
      4. Fracture and/or dislocation of the lower cervical spine
   G. Herpes zoster neuritis
   H. Lyme disease and cervical radiculoneuritis
2. Brachial plexopathy
   A. Acute thoracic outlet syndrome
   B. Acute brachial neuropathy (neuralgic amyotrophy)
   C. Trauma
      1. Blunt trauma
      2. "Burner" syndrome
      3. Penetrating trauma
3. Discogenic syndrome
4. Myofascial pain and brachialgia
5. Vascular pain
   A. Venous
   B. Arterial
6. Infections of the arm
   A. Gas gangrene

B. Anaerobic streptococcal myonecrosis
C. *Aeromonas hydrophila* myonecrosis
D. Synergistic necrotizing cellulitis
E. Necrotizing fasciitis
F. Cellulitis
7. Carpal tunnel syndrome
8. Referred pain to the arm and hand
   A. Acute myocardial infarction or acute coronary insufficiency
   B. Esophageal motor disorder
   C. Chest wall pain
   D. Superior pulmonary sulcus carcinoma
9. Arthritis involving two or more upper extremity joints
   A. Acute gout
   B. Acute rheumatic fever
   C. Gonococcal arthritis
   D. Reiter's syndrome
   E. Yersiniosis
   F. Acute calcium pyrophosphate dihydrate deposition disease
   G. Immune complex arthritis
      1. Hepatitis B
      2. Subacute bacterial endocarditis
   H. Lyme arthritis
   I. Acute rheumatoid arthritis
10. Acute bilateral upper and lower arm pain

☐ SUMMARY

Acute herniation of a cervical intervertebral disc may cause deep, aching posterior neck, medial scapular, and upper arm pain on one side. Sharp jabs of knifelike or electric-like pain may radiate from the neck down the arm and into the hand. Sneezing, coughing, and neck rotation or extension may provoke radiating pain and/or intensify the constant ache. Spurling's maneuver (i.e., head compression with the neck rotated to the contralateral side and laterally flexed) may also intensify or provoke pain. Axial manual traction or shoulder abduction may alleviate neck and arm pain. Clinical identification of the compressed lower cervical root is based on the location of hand and finger hypesthesia and paresthesias, arm and hand weakness, and reflex changes. Radiculopathy secondary to disc herniation usually involves only one root (98 percent of cases). The diagnosis can be confirmed by CT myelography or MRI. A similar syndrome may be caused by lateral recess or foramen compression of a nerve root secondary to *cervical spondylosis.* Cervical CT myelography or MRI will detect lateral nerve root compression in the lateral recess or at the nerve root foramen.

Osteomyelitis of the cervical spine begins with a persistent posterior neck pain that may continue for months before arm and hand pain and paresthesias develop. Fever (50 percent of cases), leukocytosis (50 percent of cases), and an elevated sedimentation rate (95 percent of cases) may occur. Plain spine radiographs may reveal osteolytic lesions of one or more vertebral bodies and destruction of the intervening intervertebral discs. Infectious agents include pyogenic bacteria, fungi, *Mycobacterium tuberculosis,* and *Brucella* species. A CT scan will provide better definition of the destructive bone lesions.

A *cervical epidural abscess* may begin with posterior neck pain and muscle spasm that progress to torticollis. Aching and lancinating arm pain on one or both sides may occur. Accompanying arm weakness, sensory deficits, reflex changes, and pain location indicate multiple root involvement. Neck rotation, coughing, or straining may intensify or provoke neck and arm pain. Fever, chills, sweating, malaise, and leukocytosis are usually present. Leg weakness and sensory loss may occur, and urinary and/or fecal incontinence or inability to void or defecate may follow. The diagnosis can be confirmed by CT myelography or MRI. Symptom resolution follows abscess drainage and antibiotic therapy.

A *cervical epidural hematoma* may cause the abrupt onset of neck pain, torticollis, and radicular pain in one or both arms. Spinal cord compression by the hematoma may cause paresis of one or all four limbs. Fever, chills, and toxicity do not occur. Most cases occur in patients with liver disease or on anticoagulant therapy. The hematoma can be imaged by CT myelography or by MRI. Rapid spinal canal decompression with removal of the hematoma leads to resolution of symptoms.

Cervical nerve root avulsion from the spinal cord may follow a fall from a motorcycle onto one shoulder and the side of the head. The forces at impact widen the angle between the neck and shoulder, stretching the ipsilateral cervical nerve roots. Partial or complete avulsion of one or more roots from the spinal cord may result. Signs of cervical root avulsion include a winged scapula, loss of the ability to adduct or elevate the ipsilateral scapula, and weakness of upper arm abduction. Electromyography may demonstrate paravertebral muscle denervation. Sensory nerve conduction remains intact, but motor conduction is impaired Complete root avulsion causes arm anesthesia and motor loss, while partial root injury may result in persistent aching and lancinating shoulder and arm pain, paresthesias, and upper extremity sensory impairment. CT myelography can directly visualize avulsed roots and detect dye-filled pseudomeningoceles and transverse process fractures. A *herniated disc* secondary to a neck injury causes neck and arm pain and paresthesias. The diagnosis can be confirmed by CT myelography or MRI. *Ligamentous injuries* of the lower cervical spine may cause neck and radiating arm pain. Subluxation of an upper vertebral body over a subjacent body may occur due to ligament disruption and result in root compression. *Fracture* and/or *dislocations* of the cervical spine may cause neck and radicular arm pain. The presence of a cervical spine fracture may be detected by a lateral neck radiograph (80-percent sensitive), a full cervical spine series (85-percent sensitive), or a cervical CT scan (95-percent sensitive).

Herpes zoster may cause unilateral radicular arm pain involving one or two roots. The onset of burning or aching arm and shoulder pain is soon followed by the eruption of grouped vesicles, pustules, and crusted ulcers in the painful dermatomal region. *Lyme disease* initially presents with a characteristic skin lesion (erythema migrans) and an influenza-like illness. Up to 15 percent of untreated patients may develop an aseptic meningitis syndrome and/or shoulder and arm pain secondary to a cervical radiculopathy, plexopathy, or peripheral neuropathy. The diagnosis can be supported by detection of IgM and/or IgG antibody to *Borrelia burgdorferi.* These painful neurologic symptoms may resolve with high-dose intravenous penicillin or ceftriaxone therapy.

Brachial plexopathy may develop acutely, secondary to neck trauma. A "whiplash" injury may cause neck muscle spasm that elevates the first rib and narrows the costoclavicular space, resulting in brachial plexus compression at the thoracic outlet. A trauma-related acute *thoracic outlet syndrome (TOS)* causes neck and head pain and aching shoulder, arm, and hand pain. Pain is usually intensified by arm use, and this exacerbation may persist for several days. Medial forearm and hand pain (fourth and fifth fingers) and paresthesias are most common, but lateral arm and hand pain may also occur with upper plexus involvement. Distal weakness and clumsiness in the use of the affected hand may be reported. Neurologic signs include ulnar hypesthesia and a variable amount of hand and biceps weakness. Arm symptoms may be reproduced by thumb pressure over the brachial plexus in the supraclavicular space or by the 90° abduction external rotation test (Roos test). Surgical decompression of the thoracic outlet by removal of the ipsilateral first rib and resection of tight fibrous bands and scalene muscles attached to the first rib produces symptomatic relief in 79 to 93 percent of cases.

Acute brachial neuropathy (neuralgic amyotrophy) causes persistent shoulder and upper arm pain described as sharp, throbbing, stabbing, or aching. The pain may radiate down the arm into the hand. It is intensified by arm and shoulder movement but not by coughing or sneezing. Severe shoulder and arm pain may persist for 1 to 21 days. Bilateral involvement may occur. As the arm pain begins to subside, weakness of the deltoid, serratus anterior, and spinati muscles may become apparent. Sensory impairment may occur as a small patch of hypesthesia on the shoulder or the lateral aspect of the upper arm. In some cases the brachial plexus localization of this disease may be confirmed by a reduction of the amplitude of peripheral sensory nerve action potentials, a finding not seen in patients with nerve root lesions. This disorder may be precipitated by an infection, trauma, surgery, an immunization, or childbirth.

Shoulder and arm pain may follow a *fall on the shoulder and side of the head* in a motorcycle, motor vehicle, bicycle, or equestrian accident. Paresthesias and dysesthesias may be associated with shoulder, arm, and hand pain. The brachialgia is usually constant, severe, and intensified by use of the arm. Upper plexus injury causes weakness of upper arm abduction and forearm flexion and supination. Middle plexus injury impairs forearm and wrist extension. Lower plexus involvement may cause pareses of the intrinsic muscles of the hand. Sensory losses are usually patchy and mild relative to motor deficits. Brachial plexus lesions are postganglionic. There are preservation of scapula mobility and loss of sensory nerve action potentials (i.e., secondary to proximal detachment of sensory fibers from sensory nerve cell bodies in the dorsal root ganglia).

The *"burner" syndrome* occurs in football players after forceful contact. It is characterized by the abrupt onset, after impact, of a burning pain that originates in the neck or shoulder and radiates into the lateral forearm and hand. Variable degrees of arm weakness may accompany the burning arm pain. In most cases, symptoms resolve within a few minutes, but more severe injuries may cause persistent arm pain and weakness lasting days or weeks. Arm weakness and hypesthesia may continue for months in a small number of cases. A cervical CT scan may be required to exclude a spinal fracture. *Knife and gunshot wounds* may cause plexus injury resulting in arm pain and paresthesias, numbness, and motor weakness.

A *discogenic syndrome* may cause neck and arm pain and arm numbness without neurologic signs. Analgesic discography relieves the neck and arm pain and confirms the diagnosis. More persistent relief follows anterior cervical fusion. The neck and arm pain is secondary to tears in the anulus fibrosus of one or more cervical discs without disc protrusion. *Myofascial pain* may masquerade as a cervical radiculopathy. There are shoulder pain and a local tender trigger point in the trapezius muscle. Pressure on this point provokes radiating arm pain, as do neck rotation and extension. Lidocaine injection of this trigger point transiently relieves provoked arm pain and confirms the diagnosis.

Vascular pain may arise because of a stenosis or occlusion of the axillary or subclavian vein. It may be primary (Paget-Schroetter syndrome) or secondary to a tumor, trauma, heart failure, or estrogen therapy. Rest or exercise-induced arm pain may occur. The pain may be described as aching or bursting, and it is intensified by exercise of the arm. The arm is usually swollen and discolored. Cyanosis or a purplish-red discoloration is most common. Superficial veins are distended, and they usually fail to collapse after arm elevation. In some cases, arm color changes and venous distension appear only after exercise of the arm. Venography will confirm *axillary and/or subclavian vein occlusion or stenosis.* Venous occlusion is an uncommon complication of the thoracic outlet syndrome. *Subclavian or axillary artery occlusion or stenosis* can cause aching arm pain with exercise (claudication) and unilateral Raynaud's phenomenon secondary to microembolization. The blood pressure and pulse pressure in the affected arm may be low relative to the normal contralateral arm. The diagnosis can be confirmed by arteriography.

Severe, rapidly spreading *hand and arm infections* can cause severe upper extremity pain and dysfunction. *Gas gangrene* begins 1 to 3 days after a penetrating arm or hand wound. Severe aching in the wound and generalized arm pain occur. There are diffuse swelling and tenderness of the arm, followed by yellow or brown discoloration of the skin adjacent to the wound. Tense bullae containing dark fluid appear, and areas of green or black skin gangrene develop. Fever, chills, prostration, and malaise soon follow. Skin crepitus may be present, and plain radiographs can detect gas in the fascial spaces and muscles of the arm. A Gram stain of wound exudate reveals large gram-positive bacilli with blunt ends and only a scant number of polymorphonuclear neutrophils. Evidence of myonecrosis is present at surgical exploration. Extensive debridement or upper extremity amputation is required. *Anaerobic streptococcal myonecrosis* also follows a penetrating wound. Local wound redness and swelling are associated with purulent wound drainage. Over a period of 3 to 4 days, the affected arm becomes diffusely swollen, red, painful, and tender. A Gram stain of wound exudate demonstrates streptococci and many polymorphonuclear leukocytes. Severe systemic symptoms occur. Skin crepitus is usually present. This disorder is polymicrobial and is caused by anaerobic streptococci and group A streptococci or *Staphylococcus aureus.*

Aeromonas hydrophilia myonecrosis follows a penetrating wound associated with a freshwater fish or a marine animal. *Synergistic necrotizing cellulitis* begins with small, draining skin ulcerations. Skin gangrene soon appears and may be associated with severe local arm pain, tenderness, and skin crepitus. Fever, chills, and toxicity occur. Cultures of wound pus produce isolates of anaerobic streptococci and/or *Bacteriodes* species and facultative gram-negative bacteria.

Necrotizing fasciitis causes deep, aching arm pain; tenderness; and swelling. The portal of entry is a skin wound. Reddish-purple or black patches appear on the skin, as well as tense bullae containing dark fluid. Severe systemic symptoms occur. Blackened skin areas are anesthetic and can be probed without causing pain to the level of the deep fascia, indicating that a fasciitis, and not a simple cellulitis, is present. Isolates include mixtures of anaerobic and aerobic bacteria.

Cellulitis causes arm and hand pain, tenderness, and diffuse erythema without elevation of the erythematous region above the level of the surrounding normal skin. Fever, chills, and malaise occur. The margin of the erythematous area progresses up the limb and is irregular in outline. Group A streptococci and *S. aureus* are the usual causative agents. There is a prompt response to intravenous nafcillin or vancomycin.

Carpal tunnel syndrome causes hand and finger pain that may radiate proximally as far as the shoulder. Pain, paresthesias, and/or numbness may involve the thumb, index and middle fingers, and the lateral aspect of the fourth finger. Thenar eminence atrophy and hand weakness may occur in advanced cases. Pain and paresthesias may be provoked by tapping on the median nerve at the wrist (Tinel's sign) and by flexion of the wrist for 30 to 90 s with the elbow extended (Phalen's sign). The diagnosis can be confirmed by median nerve conduction studies across the wrist. Surgical decompression of the carpal tunnel relieves symptoms.

Acute myocardial infarction or acute coronary insufficiency may cause left or right arm pain with or without chest pain. The diagnosis of myocardial infarction can be confirmed by electrocardiography and by serum isozyme studies. Coronary insufficiency can be confirmed by observing ST and/or T wave abnormalities on electrocardiograms taken during pain and by coronary arteriography. This test may demonstrate partial coronary occlusion by thrombus, atheroma, or spasm in patients with prolonged or frequent chest pain without infarction.

An *esophageal motor disorder* may cause chest and unilateral or bilateral arm pain. Manometric studies are required to demonstrate diffuse esophageal spasm or a ''nutcracker'' esophagus, esophageal motor disorders associated with chest and arm pain.

Chest wall pain secondary to costochondritis or pectoral myositis may radiate into the axilla and down the arm into the hand. There is local tenderness in the same area as the spontaneous chest wall pain. Various arm and chest movements and maneuvers may provoke pain of a similar quality to that experienced spontaneously.

A *superior pulmonary sulcus carcinoma* (Pancoast's syndrome) may cause shoulder and arm hyperesthesia and pain. Pain and paresthesias may radiate into the ulnar aspect of the forearm and hand. A chest radiograph will demonstrate the tumor at the apex of the ipsilateral lung.

Acute arthritis may affect the shoulder, elbow, wrist, and carpal and finger joints of one or both arms. Joints in the lower extremity may also be involved. *Acute gout* causes severe joint pain, redness, and swelling. Patients have hyperuricemia, and the synovial fluid contains uric acid crystals and polymorphonuclear leukocytes. There is a prompt and dramatic improvement with colchicine therapy.

Acute rheumatic fever causes fever, malaise, and a migratory polyarthritis that may involve the shoulders, elbows, wrists, and fingers. Antibody levels against streptococcal antigens (i.e., streptolysin O, hyaluronidase, and desoxyribonuclease)

are usually elevated, and there is a dramatic response to salicylate therapy.

Acute gonococcal arthritis presents as a migratory polyarthritis. Tenosynovitis involving the wrists and hands is frequent. Characteristic distal extremity skin pustules and hemorrhagic vesicles on an erythematous base occur in some, but not all, cases. Joint fluid may grow *Neisseria gonorrhoeae* in up to 50 percent of cases, or positive cultures may be obtained from the urethra, rectum, cervix, blood, or skin lesions. There is a prompt response to penicillin therapy.

Reiter's syndrome may cause an illness similar to gonococcal arthritis, with migratory arthritis and an associated urethritis and conjunctivitis. There is no response to penicillin therapy.

Yersiniosis may mimic the migratory polyarthritis of acute rheumatic fever. There is a rise in the agglutination titer to *Yersinia enterocolitica,* and this organism may be cultured from the stool.

Acute calcium pyrophosphate dihydrate deposition disease may cause upper extremity arthritis. The diagnosis can be confirmed by finding calcium pyrophosphate dihydrate crystals and polymorphonuclear leukocytes in synovial fluid and by detecting linear calcification (chondrocalcinosis) of articular cartilage in radiographs of the knees, wrists, or shoulders. This disorder may occur in the absence of chondrocalcinosis.

Hepatitis B may have a prodrome consisting of an urticarial or maculopapular pruritic rash and an *immune complex migratory polyarthritis*. Liver function test abnormalities and detection of hepatitis B surface antigen in the serum support the diagnosis. *Subacute bacterial endocarditis* may also present with a migratory polyarthritis secondary to circulating immune complexes. *Lyme arthritis* may affect the joints of the arm, but the most commonly involved joints are the knees and ankles. An enzyme-linked immunosorbent assay (ELISA) for IgG to *B. burgdorferi* is usually positive at the onset of joint symptoms. There is a good response to antibiotic therapy in up to 70 percent of cases. *Acute rheumatoid arthritis* may begin with a symmetrical or asymmetrical polyarthritis involving the arms and hands. Few systemic symptoms may be present. Rheumatoid factor can be detected in the serum in up to 80 percent of cases, but the predictive value of a positive test is only 33 percent because of its nonspecificity. The diagnosis of rheumatoid arthritis may require a long follow-up period before it can be firmly established by additional symptoms, signs, and laboratory findings.

☐ DESCRIPTION OF LISTED DISEASES

1. ACUTE CERVICAL RADICULOPATHY INVOLVING ONE OR MORE NERVE ROOTS (C6–T1)

A. Acute Cervical Disc Herniation Acute cervical disc herniation may cause the abrupt onset of persistent deep

TABLE OF DISEASE INCIDENCE

INCIDENCE PER 100,000 (APPROXIMATE)

Common (>100)	Uncommon (>5–100)	Rare (>0–5)
Acute cervical disc herniation	Trauma: herniated nucleus pulposus and nerve root compression, ligamentous injury and subluxation, and fracture and/or dislocation of lower cervical spine	Cervical osteomyelitis
Cervical spondylosis		Cervical epidural abscess
Acute thoracic outlet syndrome		Cervical epidural hematoma
"Burner" syndrome		Trauma: cervical nerve root avulsion from the spinal cord
Discogenic syndrome	Herpes zoster neuritis	Infections: gas gangrene, anaerobic streptococcal myonecrosis, *A. hydrophila* myonecrosis, synergistic necrotizing cellulitis, and necrotizing fasciitis
Myofascial pain and brachialgia	Lyme disease and cervical radiculoneuritis	
Cellulitis	Acute brachial neuropathy	
Carpal tunnel syndrome	Blunt trauma to the brachial plexus	
Referred brachialgia due to acute myocardial infarction or acute coronary insufficiency	Penetrating trauma to the brachial plexus	Upper extremity arthritis due to acute gout, yersiniosis, acute calcium pyrophosphate dihydrate deposition disease, subacute bacterial endocarditis, or Lyme disease
Chest wall pain	Vascular pain: subclavian and/or axillary vein occlusion or stenosis, and subclavian or axillary artery occlusion or stenosis	
	Referred brachialgia due to esophageal motor disorder or superior pulmonary sulcus carcinoma	
	Upper extremity arthritis due to acute rheumatic fever, gonococcal arthritis, Reiter's syndrome, acute rheumatoid arthritis, or hepatitis B–associated arthritis	

aching pain in the posterior neck, medial scapular region, and upper arm on one side. Pain may also be felt in the forearm and in a localized area of the hand. Proximal pain is more constant and frequent than distal pain. The pain may vary in intensity from moderate to severe. The persistent aching pain may begin spontaneously or may follow neck trauma (e.g., a fall or "whiplash injury"). Pain onset is sometimes preceded by a sensation of a click in the neck during a sudden or forceful neck movement. Lancinating pains may radiate from the neck down the arm. These severe stabbing pains may be superimposed on the deep aching arm discomfort. They may occur spontaneously or follow neck rotation or extension. Sneezing, coughing, or straining at stool may also intensify the aching pain or provoke jabs of pain that radiate down the arm. Axial manual traction by the examiner may alleviate the deep aching neck, shoulder, and arm pain and prevent the sharp jabs of radiating pain. The average age for patients with disc protrusion is 42 ± 8 years. Individuals at increased risk for cervical disc herniation include those who dive, lift heavy objects, and smoke cigarettes. Up to 75 percent of adults with cervical disc disease are male (the male/female ratio is 3:1).

The location of hypesthesia and paresthesias and specific patterns of arm muscle weakness may contribute to the identification of the compressed nerve root and the site of the protruding disc. Reflex changes are also useful for localization. Pain is less specific and, in general, has poor localizing value. Findings useful for identifying the involved cervical root are summarized in Table 38-1.

Acute disc herniation is often accompanied by posterior neck stiffness and muscle tenderness, resulting in limitation of neck mobility.

A number of provocative and pain-alleviating bedside tests have been used to confirm the diagnosis of compression radiculopathy. Provocative tests include the following:

1. *Neck rotation.* Neck rotation to the side of the pain or to the contralateral side may intensify the neck ache or provoke lancinating radicular arm pain and paresthesias.
2. *Coughing or straining (Valsalva's maneuver).* An increase in the intraspinal pressure may provoke lancinating arm pain and paresthesias.
3. *Spurling's head compression test.* The examiner flexes the patient's head laterally and slightly rotates it to the contralateral side and then compresses the head with a downward pressure of approximately 7 kg. Provocation of radicular arm pain or paresthesias in the ipsilateral or contralateral arm and/or hand is considered a positive test result indicative of a cervical intraspinal nerve root lesion. Spurling's original report of 12 patients claimed a sensitivity of 100 percent for the test. Subsequent studies have shown a sensitivity of only 35 percent but a high specificity. This test should not be done until cervical spine radiographs have demonstrated an absence of vertebral destruction by tumor or osteomyelitis.

Pain-alleviating tests include the following:

1. *Axial manual retraction test.* The examiner exerts manual traction (e.g., 10–15 kg) on the patient's head and neck. Complete elimination or easing of radicular arm pain is considered a positive test result. Sensitivity in one study was only 26 percent.

Table 38-1
LOCALIZATION OF THE SITE OF A CERVICAL MONORADICULOPATHY

Involved Nerve Root	Involved Cervical Disc	Pain Location	Hypesthesia/ Paresthesia Location	Motor Impairment	Reflex Diminution or Loss	Percent of Cases
C6	C5–C6	Trapezius ridge Medial scapula Midventral upper arm and forearm, thenar eminence, index finger	Thumb, index finger	Flexion of forearm on upper arm (biceps muscle, brachialis muscle) Abduction of upper arm (deltoid muscle) External rotators	Biceps	20
C7	C6–C7	Medial scapular border Anterior chest and axilla Lateral dorsal upper arm Dorsal forearm, elbow, index finger, middle finger	Index finger, middle finger	Extension of forearm (triceps muscle) Extension of wrist (extensor carpi ulnaris muscle) Pronators, winged scapula (serratus anterior muscle)	Triceps	70
C8	C7–T1	Medial dorsal upper arm, forearm, fourth and fifth fingers	Fifth finger, ulnar half of fourth finger	Intrinsic hand muscles Extension of wrist	None	<10
T1	T1–T2	Medial arm radiating to the medial aspect of the hand Shoulder and axillary pain	Fifth finger, ulnar half of fourth finger Medial arm, axilla to hand Horner's syndrome	Intrinsic hand muscles Extension of wrist	None	<4

2. *Shoulder abduction test.* The seated patient abducts the ipsilateral arm to 90° and places the hand on the top of the head. A decrease or disappearance of radicular arm pain and paresthesias is considered a positive test result. Sensitivity varies from 32 to 68 percent.

These provocative and pain-alleviating tests are useful for establishing a diagnosis of nerve root involvement. The presence of neurologic signs such as hypesthesia, muscle weakness, and diminution of reflexes also supports a diagnosis of radiculopathy. Neurologic signs are essential for the clinical identification of the involved nerve root. Neurologic findings may be present in up to 65 percent of patients with C6, C7, or C8 root lesions. Some patients without neurologic signs may be detected clinically by provocative or alleviating tests. In one large study, neurologic signs and positive provocative or alleviating tests were absent in only 12 percent of cases.

Monoradiculopathy is the rule in patients with acute cervical disc herniation. Multiple root involvement occurs in less than 2 percent of cases. Involvement of two or more roots requires consideration of other etiologies, such as neoplasm, epidural abscess or hematoma, or a specific infectious polyradiculopathy (e.g., Lyme disease).

A herniated cervical disc can be imaged by myelography, CT-enhanced myelography, and MRI. The sensitivity of surface-coil MRI for detection of a herniated cervical nucleus pulposus is 85 percent, and that of CT myelography is 75 percent. Myelography alone may have a sensitivity of only 36 percent. In some centers, MRI is

the initial screening procedure used for the identification of a herniated disc. Both MRI and CT myelography can detect and identify neoplasm, epidural abscess, epidural hematoma, intradural cyst, spondylosis, and syringomyelia. MRI is able to survey the entire cervical spine; its use results in elimination of the neurologic reactions to contrast medium (e.g., confusion, headache, visual loss, and nausea) observed after CT myelography.

Up to 88 percent of patients with a herniated cervical disc respond to conservative therapy with rest, analgesics, cervical traction, and the use of a neck collar. A history of similar prior episodes with spontaneous resolution is also supportive of a benign etiology of the neck and arm pain. Patients with refractory pain or evidence of progressive or disabling neurologic damage require surgical decompression. Such patients usually have a marked improvement in neurologic findings if the surgery is performed within 4 to 6 months of the onset of symptoms.

B. Cervical Spondylosis Bony spurs arising posterolaterally from a facet joint or uncovertebral joint (joint of Luschka or neurocentral joint) may cause acute nerve root compression in the lateral recess or at the foramen. Symptoms may occur abruptly if there is minor or major neck trauma resulting in nerve root injury and swelling. Symptoms include neck, arm, and hand pain. Neck rotation; coughing, sneezing, or straining, and Spurling's test may provoke or intensify pain and paresthesias in the affected arm. The arm abduction test may relieve brachialgia. Axial traction is usually ineffective or may exacerbate symptoms. The involved root can be identified by the characteristic sensory, motor, and reflex changes produced (Table 38-1). Osteophytes may be visualized by plain radiographs of the cervical spine. These radiographs also reveal an absence of a destructive neoplastic or inflammatory process (e.g., pyogenic or tuberculous osteomyelitis). CT myelography and MRI can be used to evaluate the nerve root canals for impingement by bony spurs in the lateral recesses or at the foramina. Lateral decompression (i.e., uncoforaminotomy) usually results in relief of arm pain and resolution of muscle weakness, numbness, and paresthesias.

C. Cervical Osteomyelitis Neck pain of an aching quality, cervical paravertebral muscle spasm, percussion tenderness over the involved vertebrae, and torticollis occur. Fever may be present in up to 50 percent of patients. Shoulder and arm pain may result from nerve root involvement by the inflammatory process. Paresthesias, numbness, and weakness of specific muscles in the arm occur. Plain spine radiographs may be normal for 8 to 12 weeks. After this time interval, destructive changes of the involved vertebral bodies and adjacent disc spaces may be detected. An enlarged prevertebral soft tissue shadow may be apparent. Root compression by epidural granulation tissue may be the cause of radicular arm pain. A radionuclide bone scan or MRI may reveal abnormalities of the cervical spine during the first few weeks after the onset of symptoms. Risk factors for pyogenic cervical osteomyelitis include intravenous drug abuse, septicemia, skin furuncles or carbuncles, and urinary tract infection.

The erythrocyte sedimentation rate is elevated in 95 percent of cases and the white blood cell count in up to 50 percent. Blood cultures may be positive in up to 50 percent of patients with pyogenic osteomyelitis of the spine. Needle biopsy of infected bone or disc tissue or surgical biopsy is necessary to obtain material for culture. Patients with or without radiculopathy may respond to parenteral antibiotic therapy and neck immobilization with cervical tong traction. Patients with clinical and radiologic evidence of spinal cord compression associated with kyphosis (i.e., resulting from vertebral destruction and collapse), epidural pus, or granulation tissue require surgical intervention. Surgical procedures include incision and drainage, debridement, and skeletal stabilization by bone grafting and spinal segment fusion.

D. Cervical Epidural Abscess Neck pain, stiffness, and spasm, sometimes resulting in a painful torticollis, are usually the initial symptoms. Fever and chills are also common and are present in 73 percent of cases. Radicular aching or burning pain, lancinating jabs, or electric-like shocks may be felt in the arms and hands in up to 50 percent of cases. Electric-like shocks may be felt in the feet and legs in some cases. The radicular pain in the arms may be accompanied by paresthesias, numbness, and weakness. Evidence of multiple root involvement on

one side or bilateral pain, sensory changes, and motor loss are commonly present.

Weakness of one or both arms and the legs may follow the onset of neck pain by 2 days to several weeks. A transverse sensory level may develop on the abdomen or upper thorax. Urinary and fecal retention or incontinence may occur.

Physical examination may reveal fever, a toxic appearance, neck stiffness and tenderness, and resistance to movement. One or both arms may display evidence of sensory loss involving two or more nerve roots, and a polyradicular pattern of muscle weakness. Neck rotation, coughing, or straining at stool may provoke or intensify radicular pain. Leukocytosis is commonly present. Cerebrospinal fluid (CSF) analysis may reveal a pleocytosis of up to 150 white blood cells/mm^3 and an elevated CSF protein level. The presence of an epidural abscess can be confirmed by CT myelography or MRI. *S. aureus* is the definitive cause in 67 percent of cases. In some patients, upper airway (e.g., dyspnea, stridor) and pharyngeal symptoms (dysphagia and odynophagia) are associated with a retropharyngeal mass (abscess) due to extension of infection from a vertebral body into the retropharyngeal space.

Most cases of cervical spinal epidural abscess originate in an associated vertebral osteomyelitis. A smaller number of cases arise by a hematogenous route (26 percent) from an upper body cutaneous infection, urinary tract infection, pneumonia, pharyngitis, or dental abscess. *S. aureus* is the most commonly isolated organism (54–100 percent), while gram-negative bacteria may account for up to 20 percent of infections. Radiographic evidence of osteomyelitis may be absent in up to 40 percent of cases of patients with an epidural abscess secondary to vertebral infection. Early spinal cord decompression by surgical drainage of the epidural space and parenteral antibiotic therapy may result in rapid partial or complete resolution of radicular arm pain and other symptoms.

E. Cervical Epidural Hematoma There is an abrupt onset of posterior neck pain, stiffness, tenderness, and/or torticollis, and aching and lancinating pain in one or both arms. Within hours, paraparesis or tetraparesis may develop, but single-limb weakness or asymmetric weakness may also occur. Sensory loss may be patchy, or a transverse sensory level may develop.

Fever and toxicity are not usually associated symptoms as they are with an epidural abscess. An epidural hematoma usually occurs in patients with liver disease or on anticoagulant therapy. Spontaneous epidural hemorrhage may arise from a tumor, epidural hemangioma, or an arteriovenous malformation or may occur during pregnancy or in association with ankylosing spondylitis. The hematoma can be visualized by CT myelography or by MRI. Surgical decompression should be performed as soon as the diagnosis is established to prevent pressure-related cord injury or anterior spinal artery occlusion and spinal cord infarction.

F. Trauma

1. Cervical Nerve Root Avulsion from the Spinal Cord

Avulsion of one or more of the lower cervical roots and Tl most commonly occurs in motorcycle accidents when the cyclist falls on one shoulder and the ipsilateral side of the head. At impact, the angle between the neck and shoulder is widened, placing the nerve root and trunks of the brachial plexus on stretch, resulting in complete or partial disruption of roots and/or components of the plexus.

Neck pain and tenderness and arm weakness, paresthesias, numbness, and burning pain may follow the injury. Nerve root avulsions (preganglionic lesions) may cause a Horner's syndrome (miosis, ptosis, and enophthalmos); a winged scapula (loss of long thoracic nerve function); and paralysis of rhomboid, levator scapula, and deltoid muscles, as well as rotator cuff paralysis. A more distal lesion (postganglionic) involving the brachial plexus leaves serratus anterior, rhomboid, and levator scapula function intact. The presence of intact sensory ganglion cells in patients with root avulsion can be confirmed by demonstrating a skin axon flare response to histamine or cold. Electromyography can confirm root avulsion by demonstrating paravertebral muscle denervation. Sensory nerve conduction preservation associated with loss of motor conduction in the same nerve supports a diagnosis of nerve root avulsion. CT myelography can demonstrate nerve root avulsion by direct imaging of the roots and by detection of dye-filled pseudomeningoceles at sites of meningeal disruption. Fractures of vertebral transverse processes are also frequently present. It is not possible to reattach avulsed roots to the spinal cord. Such arms remain weak and develop muscle atrophy. Severe injuries leave the arm flail and anesthetic. Arm pain and paresthesias are related to partially damaged roots and brachial plexus components, since completely avulsed roots result in anesthesia.

2. Herniated Nucleus Pulposus of the Lower Cervical Spine

Severe neck trauma in a fall or motor vehicle accident can cause acute disc herniation, with severe neck pain, spasm, and tenderness; and aching, burning, and lancinating radicular arm pain. This posttraumatic lesion can be diagnosed by CT myelography or MRI.

3. Ligamentous Injuries of the Lower Cervical Spine

Anterior subluxation of one vertebral body (>2 mm) over the subjacent body may result from disruption of posterior ligaments. Neck pain, muscle spasm, and tenderness are commonly present, and aching and lancinating arm pain and paresthesias may occur secondary to root compression.

4. Fracture and/or Dislocation of the Lower Cervical Spine

Neck pain, muscle spasm, and tenderness or loss of neck mobility are present in almost all cases of cervical spine fracture or dislocation. Rare but important exceptions have been reported. Burst fractures of a vertebral body are most likely to cause nerve root and spinal cord damage with radicular arm pain and paresthesias and evidence of lower extremity motor and sensory loss. Unilateral facet dislocation or bilateral facet dislocations may cause anterior vertebral displacement with radicular pain and/or paresthesias in one or both arms and evidence of spinal cord compression. Plain spine radiographs detect 80 percent of fractures, but significant fractures may be missed unless a CT scan of the cervical spine is performed in patients with persistent neck pain and tenderness.

G. Herpes Zoster Neuritis   Varicella-zoster virus may cause burning and lancinating unilateral arm pain involving one or at most two cervical roots. Skin hyperesthesia may be associated. Within 3 to 4 days, an eruption of grouped vesicles, pustules, and crusted ulcers on a narrow erythematous base appears in the painful dermatomal region and provides evidence supportive of the diagnosis.

H. Lyme Disease   This disorder follows a tick bite. Within 3 to 32 days following the bite, an expanding erythematous skin lesion appears (i.e., erythema migrans) in 48 to 86 percent of cases. This characteristic lesion has a slightly raised or flat, red, ringlike border and a pale, indurated center. Several days after the appearance of the initial skin lesion, up to 50 percent of patients develop smaller, secondary annular lesions. These cutaneous lesions may persist for weeks or may vanish and then reappear (in 5 to 9 percent of cases). Associated symptoms include fever, chills, headache, photophobia, stiff neck, and cutaneous dysesthesias. Migratory joint and muscle pain and deep bone pain may occur. The rash, flulike symptoms, and mild meningeal complaints are characteristic of stage 1 disease. Up to 15 percent of patients develop nervous system involvement 1 to several months after the onset of the rash and fever.

Symptoms of meningitis (headache, stiff neck, and vomiting) and neuritis occur. Cranial neuritis affects the facial nerves, resulting in a unilateral or bilateral Bell's palsy. Nerves III and VI may also be affected, resulting in diplopia. Painful unilateral or bilateral cervical radiculopathy, plexopathy, or peripheral neuropathy may occur. Aching, burning, or lancinating arm pain and motor weakness may be present. Complex mixtures of root, plexus, and peripheral nerve dysfunction may occur. An elevated CSF protein level and a lymphocytic pleocytosis are frequent findings.

The CSF IgM index for *B. burgdorferi* antibody levels is elevated, and oligoclonal bands may be present. Results of an ELISA test for *B. burgdorferi* IgM antibody in serum are usually positive 3 to 6 weeks after the onset of symptoms. Patients with radicular and plexus involvement usually test positive for IgG antibody. False-positive antibody responses to *B. burgdorferi* may occur in patients with syphilis or infectious mononucleosis. Meningoencephalitis and/or painful radiculoneuritis treated with intravenous penicillin (20 million U/day for 10 days) or ceftriaxone (2 gm/day for 14 days) resolves within 2 weeks.

2. BRACHIAL PLEXOPATHY

A. Acute Thoracic Outlet Syndrome   TOS has been reported in 31 percent of patients with a severe cervical strain following a "whiplash" injury in a motor vehicle accident. It may also occur after other types of neck trauma (e.g., falls, sudden pushes or pulls involving heavy loads, or after sustained contraction of neck muscles while completing a task). There are neck pain and stiffness and cephalgia. Pain of an aching or throbbing nature radiates into the arm and hand. The medial forearm, fourth and fifth fingers, and hypothenar eminence are most commonly affected. Coldness of the fingers and paresthesias may be present. Lancinating jabs of neuritic pain are not usually reported. Pain may be provoked by use of the affected arm during hair combing, painting a wall, washing windows, or other activities. This pain exacerbation may be sustained for 2 to 3 days, making the patient fearful of engaging in the same activity again. Rest and avoidance of active use of the arm may minimize discomfort.

Some patients complain of distal weakness in the fingers and forearm, and sensory loss may occur in small areas of the hand and forearm (the ulnar region of the forearm and hand).

The role of neck trauma in provoking brachialgia is related to cervical muscle spasm that elevates the first rib and narrows the costoclavicular outlet.

Examination may reveal mild weakness of the hand and skin hypesthesia in an ulnar distribution. Thumb pressure over the brachial plexus (percussion and thumb pressure test) in the supraclavicular fossa reproduces pain and paresthesias in the symptomatic arm. The most reliable test for evaluating the adequacy of the thoracic outlet is the 90° abduction-external rotation test (AER test, or Roos test).

The upper arm is abducted to a right angle and externally rotated, and the forearm is flexed to 90°. Loss of the radial pulse and the development of forearm and hand pain and paresthesias should be sought. If typical symptoms do not occur, the patient is asked to slowly open and close his or her fists for 3 min. The onset of severe upper extremity heaviness, fatigue, numbness, or aching pain in the forearm and hand are criteria for a positive test result. Patients with TOS are usually unable to keep their arms elevated for 3 min because of the discomfort provoked by this test. Vascular forms of TOS, involving the subclavian artery or vein, are rare and account for only 1 to 5 percent of cases of TOS. Electromyographic and nerve conduction studies are not helpful in documenting brachial plexus compression in the outlet. Nerve conduction studies at the wrist and elbow are helpful in excluding the carpal tunnel syndrome and the cubital tunnel syndrome, respectively. A double-crush syndrome has been described in which 30 percent of TOS patients in one series had a coincident carpal tunnel syndrome or ulnar nerve compression (10 percent of cases) at the elbow. Some authors find that lateral forearm and hand complaints are common with TOS, while others consider the presence of such symptoms evidence against a diagnosis of TOS. There is controversy regarding the criteria used for the diagnosis of TOS and the indications for surgical removal of the ipsilateral first rib.

Patients with TOS secondary to trauma do not usually respond to physical therapy and thoracic outlet exercises. Most patients with posttraumatic TOS are made worse by cervical traction. Removal of the first rib through a transaxillary approach and resection of fibrous bands and scalene muscles will provide complete relief of arm pain, paresthesias, and weakness in 79 percent and partial relief in 14 percent of patients with the clinical symptoms and signs described above.

B. Acute Brachial Neuropathy (Neuralgic Amyotrophy)   There is an abrupt onset of shoulder and upper arm pain. The pain is described as sharp, throbbing, stabbing, or aching. It is persistent and tends to be more severe at night. It may radiate from the shoulder into the neck and down the arm to the hand. It is exacerbated by arm and shoulder movements, but not by neck rotation, coughing, sneezing, or straining. Severe pain may persist for 1 day to 3 weeks, and bilateral symptoms may develop (25–33 percent). The initial intense pain may be replaced during the first 3 weeks by a milder discomfort. Weakness of shoulder and arm muscles becomes apparent during the first 3 weeks as the pain begins to subside. The deltoid, serratus anterior, and the spinati muscles are most frequently affected. Atrophy and sensory loss may be detected on examination. An anesthetic patch on the shoulder and hypesthesia in a radial distribution are the most frequent sensory findings. This disorder is more common in men (the male/female ratio is 1.6:1–10.5:1), and it usually occurs between ages 20 and 70 years. Antecedent events for episodes of this disorder include viral, bacterial, and parasitic infections; trauma and surgery at other sites; immunizations; childbirth; and medical procedures. A similar disorder has been associated with systemic lupus erythematosus, temporal arteritis, and polyarteritis nodosa, and may occur as a familial disease that is inherited in a dominant fashion. Acute brachial neuropathy can be differentiated from a nerve root disorder by a reduction in amplitude of peripheral sensory nerve action potentials and an absence of paraspinal muscle degeneration detectable by electromyography.

Electromyographic studies indicate that acute brachial neuropathy is caused by axonal loss lesions involving the brachial plexus or two or more of the nerves formed from the plexus. Needle electromyography demonstrates fibrillations and/or motor unit potential changes indicative of muscle denervation. Bilateral abnormalities and the anatomic distribution of needle electromyography and sensory nerve action potential abnormalities suggest the diagnosis of acute brachial neuropathy. The location of the primary pathologic changes (e.g., plexus, roots, spinal cord, peripheral nerve) is still not established with certainty.

C. Trauma

1. Blunt Trauma The brachial plexus may be injured in falls that widen the angle between the shoulder and neck at impact, causing stretching, contusion, and sometimes avulsion of the trunks or cords of the brachial plexus. Such falls on the side of the head and shoulder may occur in motorcycle, motor vehicle, bicycle, or equestrian accidents. Sports in which brachial plexus injuries have been reported include skiing, sledding, football, wrestling, gymnastics, and golf.

Shoulder and arm pain, paresthesias, and dysesthesias may occur after the injury in association with specific patterns of arm weakness and muscle atrophy. Skin hyperesthesia or hypesthesia may occur. The brachial pain is usually constant and severe, and arm movements usually intensify it. Upper plexus involvement causes weakness of arm abduction (deltoid and rotator cuff muscles), forearm flexion (biceps and brachialis muscles), and forearm supination (biceps muscle). The rhomboids, levator scapula, and serratus anterior muscles remain intact. Sensory loss is usually mild and may involve the upper, outer region of the arm, thumb, and index finger.

Middle plexus lesions result in paralysis or weakness of forearm and wrist extension.

Lower plexus lesions may result in paralysis or paresis of the forearm flexors and intrinsic muscles of the hand. Sensory loss may involve the medial arm, forearm, and hand. Complete or partial combinations of plexus lesions may occur after trauma, and a plexopathy may occur in association with ipsilateral root and peripheral nerve lesions.

Brachial plexus lesions are postganglionic and are characterized by preservation of scapula mobility (rhomboids, levator scapula, and serratus anterior muscles), loss of sensory nerve action potentials (due to degeneration of sensory fibers after proximal detachment from sensory nerve cell bodies in the dorsal root ganglia), and loss of the axon flare reflex. The non-

dermatomal pattern of sensory loss also places the lesion in the plexus, rather than in the nerve root, region. Somatosensory evoked potentials may sometimes be useful in localizing an injury to the plexus or the spinal roots. Needle electromyography may be used to map the pattern of muscle denervation in the shoulder and arm. Patients with brachial plexus blunt trauma may benefit from surgical exploration of the plexus and the use of external neurolysis; fascicular neurolysis; direct suture repair; placement of autogenous sural nerve grafts; or neurotization procedures using the cervical plexus, intercostal nerves, or spinal accessory nerve for proximal outflow.

2. "Burner" Syndrome This disorder usually occurs in football players after forceful head, neck, or shoulder contact with an opposing player. It may occur in other contact sports. At impact, there is an abrupt onset of a sharp, burning pain that radiates into the lateral side of the forearm and hand. This burning discomfort may be accompanied by weakness of shoulder abduction (deltoid, infraspinatus, and supraspinatus muscle paresis) and elbow flexion (biceps muscle). Pain and weakness usually last for only a few minutes, but in some cases symptoms may persist for 2 weeks or longer. Some patients may have persistent weakness and hypesthesia for weeks or months and sometimes permanently. The exact location of the injury is not known with certainty, but localization to the upper trunk of the plexus has been proposed.

In most cases, there is a reversible block of the axons in the involved region of the plexus (neuropraxia). Axonotmesis probably accounts for more severe and persistent symptoms. Electromyography may detect fibrillation potentials in the biceps, deltoid, and spinati muscles and normal muscle activity in the paraspinal muscles. In some patients, the reverse is true, suggesting cervical nerve root injury. Since similar burning pain may follow a fracture or dislocation of the cervical spine, patients with a "burner" syndrome should have neck immobilization until the stability of the cervical spine can be established by cervical spine radiography or by a CT scan of the neck.

3. Penetrating Trauma The brachial plexus may also be injured by a penetrating knife blade or bullet. Gunshot-related nerve trauma is more focal than a stretch injury and may benefit from direct suture or grafting of the interrupted nerve ends. Good results have been obtained by resection and repair of the C5 and C6 roots, upper trunk, and lateral and posterior cords of the plexus. Less favorable results are reported for repair of the middle and lower trunk. Surgical exploration allows intraoperative electrical testing of injured plexus components and detection of regeneration or failure of regeneration in these elements. Surgery may be delayed after gunshot wounds unless associated vascular injuries or metal impaled in a neural element is present. Knife wounds may benefit by more immediate exploration and primary repair of transected plexus elements.

3. DISCOGENIC SYNDROME

Pain occurs in the scapular region on one side and radiates to the posterolateral neck and head, the shoulder, and arm. Some patients experience arm numbness, but there are no objective neurologic findings. There are local tenderness and spasm of muscles in the medial scapular region and in the posterior neck. Cervical spine radiographs, myelograms, and CT myelograms may be normal or display some evidence of disc degeneration. Pain is caused by tears in the annulus fibrosus of one or more cervical intervertebral discs without disc protrusion.

The involved discs can be identified by analgesic discography (i.e., injecting 1 ml of lidocaine into the center of one or all three lower cervical discs). Injection of a disc responsible for pain results in immediate and complete relief of pain and paresthesias and return of neck mobility. More than one disc may be involved, and additional symptomatic discs can be identified by repeating the procedure.

Patients who test positive by analgesic discography have benefited from surgery. A good-to-excellent response rate (i.e., 81–93 percent) has been reported for anterior cervical fusion with or without discectomy.

4. MYOFASCIAL PAIN

Pain of an aching quality occurs in the posterior shoulder or lower neck on one side. Rotation of the head to the painful side, hyperextension of the head, or a combination of both maneuvers may cause an intensification of posterior neck and shoulder pain and radiation of pain down the arm into the hand. A well-localized, tender trigger point may be identified in the trapezius region below the posterior border of the trapezius ridge. Pressure over this point causes local discomfort and radiating pain into the arm. Injection of 1 percent lidocaine (3 ml) and 40 mg of methylprednisolone into the tender trigger point results in immediate relief of local tenderness and pain. After the injection, neck movements and trigger point pressure fail to provoke arm pain. This response differentiates referred myofascial pain from a cervical radiculopathy, since the latter is not affected by a trigger point injection. Follow-up muscle exercises facilitate symptom resolution and prevent recurrence. A series has been reported of 130 patients with brachialgia and neck pain originating in a myofascial trigger point and treated as described above. Bilateral symptoms occurred in 11 percent. The relapse rate after trigger point injection with lidocaine and methylprednisolone and postinjection exercises was 23 percent;

many of these patients responded to a second course of injection therapy.

5. VASCULAR PAIN

A. Venous Axillary and/or subclavian venous stenosis or thrombosis may be primary (Paget-Schroetter syndrome) or secondary to another disorder. Primary venous thrombosis or stenosis is caused by costoclavicular space compression of the subclavian-axillary vein. Secondary occlusion may be associated with mediastinal or pulmonary tumors or other masses, venous cannulation, estrogen therapy, congestive heart failure, or trauma (clavicular fracture or subluxation of the head of the humerus).

There is an abrupt onset of diffuse, deep, aching arm pain that extends from the shoulder to the hand. Some patients have minimal or no pain until they exercise their arm. The painful arm may be cyanotic or purplish-red in color and swollen. The superficial hand, forearm, and shoulder veins may be full, tense, and distended, failing to collapse when the arm is elevated. Edema, discoloration, and venous distension may be minimal until the arm is exercised.

Venography will reveal the presence of a venous thrombosis or a stenotic, but patent, axillary vein. A chest radiograph is useful to exclude mediastinal or pulmonary mass lesions, cardiomegaly, and fractures of the clavicle.

In patients with venographic evidence of subclavian occlusion, a tender, firm thrombus may be palpable as a cordlike structure in the axilla. Infusion of streptokinase into the thrombosed vein may produce thrombolysis. Recurrence of the clot can be prevented by opening the outlet (e.g., first rib resection) and using transluminal angioplasty to dilate any residual axillary-subclavian vein stenosis. Venous occlusion is an uncommon result of the thoracic outlet syndrome, occurring in less than 4 percent of cases.

Venous thrombosis is more common in women, in young or middle-aged adults, after unusually vigorous or repetitive use of the affected arm, and on the dominant side (right axillary-subclavian vein occlusion occurs in 68–80 percent of cases). Phlegmasia cerulea dolens may progress to limb gangrene in a small number of patients.

B. Arterial Occlusion of the axillary artery by an embolus can cause acute aching pain in the arm and hand, pallor, paresthesias, numbness, and loss of the radial pulse. Gangrene of one or more digits may follow. Raynaud's phenomenon in one hand may represent microembolization.

Claudication may follow subclavian-axillary occlusion or emboli to more distal vessels. The subclavian artery may be compressed at the shoulder by a cervical rib, an elongated C7 transverse process, an abnormal first rib, fibrous bands, or a callus from a clavicular fracture. Subclavian lesions resulting in peripheral embolization include aneurysms, stenotic segments, ulcerated plaques, and occlusive thrombi. The affected arm may be pale and cool, and the radial pulse weak or absent. The blood pressure and pulse pressure may be low relative to the contralateral side. The diagnosis can be confirmed by arteriography. In some cases, it is necessary to position the arm in a manner that provokes symptoms in order to demonstrate arterial obstruction. Arterial reconstruction and decompression of the outlet to prevent recurrence may be required if ischemic symptoms are disabling.

6. INFECTIONS

Generalized arm infections may involve the skin and subcutaneous tissue (cellulitis), extend to the muscle surface (fasciitis), or involve the muscle (myonecrosis). These infections may cause severe extremity pain and systemic toxicity. They are described below and in Table 38-2.

A. Gas Gangrene (Clostridial Myonecrosis) This disorder may follow a penetrating injury of the arm (e.g., a compound fracture, shell fragment, or high-velocity bullet wound) or ischemic necrosis of the limb. Severe aching pain is the initial symptom. It begins 6 to 72 h after injury. The affected arm becomes swollen and tender. A malodorous, serosanguineous discharge drains from the wound. The skin adjacent to the wound becomes tense, swollen, pale, and discolored. This yellow or bronze skin discoloration may spread over the entire upper extremity. Tense bullae containing dark fluid appear on the affected skin, and areas of black and green cutaneous gangrene develop. Skin crepitus may be palpable in the area of discoloration and at the advancing margin of the lesion. Systemic symptoms such as fever, chills, malaise, toxicity, pallor, delirium, or coma usually occur. Jaundice, hypothermia, and hypotension may soon follow. Gram's stain of the wound exudate reveals many large grampositive bacilli with blunt ends and only a few polymorphonuclear leukocytes. Radiographs of the arm show gas in the soft tissues. *Clostridium perfringens* (80–95 percent of cases) and *Clostridium novyi* (10–40 percent of cases) are the usual causative organisms. Treatment includes extensive debridement or arm amputation, intravenous penicillin, and hyperbaric oxygen. The viability of muscle tissue may be evaluated in the operating room. Necrotic muscle has a dull brick-red color, fails to bleed when cut, and does not twitch when stimulated with a forceps.

B. Anaerobic Streptococcal Myonecrosis This disorder may follow an arm or hand wound. At first, there are local edema and copious, seropurulent, sour-smelling wound drainage. The arm becomes red and swollen, and

pain becomes prominent after 3 or 4 days. Crepitus may be palpable, and gas may be seen in the tissues of the arm on a plain radiograph. Gram's stain of the exudate reveals many polymorphonuclear leukocytes and streptococci. On direct inspection in the operating room, affected muscles may show some discoloration, but they usually contract when stimulated. These infections are usually caused by two or more coccal organisms (e.g., anaerobic streptococci with group A streptococci or *S. aureus*). This disorder responds to high doses of intravenous penicillin and surgical debridement. Inadequately treated patients develop fever, rigors, toxicity, and hypotension and may progress to a fatal outcome.

C. *Aeromonas hydrophila* Myonecrosis This disorder follows penetrating arm or hand trauma in fresh water or an injury occurring during contact with fish or other water animals. There is an abrupt onset, over 1 or 2 days, of severe arm and hand pain, swelling of the injured limb, serosanguineous cutaneous blebs, toxicity, skin and deep tissue crepitus, and radiographic evidence of gas in fascial planes. Fever, chills, toxicity, and the condition of the limb mimic the symptoms of clostridial gas gangrene. *A. hydrophila* is a facultative anaerobic gram-negative rod. Debridement and antibiotic therapy will usually control the infection.

D. Synergistic Necrotizing Cellulitis This disorder is a variant of necrotizing fasciitis and occurs in a setting of cardiovascular and renal disease, obesity, or diabetes, or in patients of advanced age. The initial lesions may be small skin ulcers draining foul-smelling, reddish-brown pus ("dishwater" pus). Blue-black gangrene develops in the surrounding skin. Severe local edema, pain, tenderness, and skin crepitus may be present in up to 25 percent of cases. Fever, chills, and toxicity occur. Cultures of wound drainage grow anaerobic streptococci and/or *Bacteroides* species and facultative gram-negative bacteria (*Klebsiella-Enterobacter*, *Escherichia coli*, and *Proteus* species). Surgical debridement and sometimes amputation are required. Antibiotics alone are not effective. This disorder may cause necrosis of the skin, subcutaneous tissue, and fascia as well as some of the underlying muscle.

E. Necrotizing Fasciitis The portal of entry is a skin wound (abrasion, laceration, burn, or insect bite). Severe aching and throbbing arm pain are accompanied by marked swelling and erythema of the arm. The skin becomes shiny, warm, red, tender, and tense. Reddish-purple or black patches appear; skin bullae develop containing serosanguineous or dark fluid, and skin blackening and leathery thickening occur. Subcutaneous gas may be detected by palpation and by radiography. High fever to 40.6°C (105°F), chills, rigors, and toxicity occur. The development of cutaneous anesthesia in the blackened region, with the ability to probe without causing pain to the

Table 38-2
DEEP INFECTIONS OF THE UPPER EXTREMITY

	Initial Injury	Onset	Symptoms	Appearance of Wound and Adjacent Area	Wound Drainage	Gram's Stain and Culture	Laboratory
Gas gangrene Clostridial myonecrosis	Compound fracture Penetrating war wound Arterial insufficiency of the upper extremity	Begins 6–72 h after wounding	Severe local pain Systemic symptoms of shock, renal failure, fever, chills, delirium	Extensive yellow or bronze discoloration of the skin around the wound, which spreads rapidly over the arm Areas of green-black cutaneous necrosis Bullae containing dark fluid Crepitation of skin	Serosanguineous Foul odor Gas bubbles	Gram's stain: gram-positive rods with blunt ends Culture: *Clostridium perfringens* or *Clostridium novyi*	Reduced hematocrit Leukocytosis
Anaerobic streptococcal myonecrosis	Wounding	Begins 3–4 days after injury	Wound edema and copious purulent exudate Onset of pain in 1–3 days Toxemia and shock in untreated cases	Cutaneous erythema and edema that may progress to green-black gangrene	Sour odor Seropurulent discharge	Gram's stain: streptococci and polymorphonuclear leukocytes Culture: anaerobic streptococcus with group A streptococcus or *Staphylococcus aureus*	
Synergistic necrotizing cellulitis (variant of necrotizing fasciitis)	Skin ulcers in patients with diabetes, renal failure, heart failure, or obesity Most cases affect legs and perineum	Acute onset 3–14 days after injury	Small skin ulcers draining foul-smelling, red-brown pus Severe local pain, edema, and tenderness Severe systemic symptoms	Blue-gray gangrene involving the skin around the ulcers Gangrene circumscribed Extensive necrosis of subcutaneous tissue, fascia, and (sometimes) muscle	Red-brown, foul-smelling, "dishwater" pus	Gram's stain: gram-positive cocci and rods and gram-negative rods Culture: anaerobic streptococci or *Bacteroides* species and facultative bacteria (gram-negative rods)	
Aeromonas hydrophila myonecrosis	Penetrating injury in a freshwater environment or in association with marine animals	Abrupt onset in 24–48 h	Severe wound pain Systemic symptoms and toxicity	Serosanguineous bullae Limb edema Local skin crepitus	Serosanguineous	Gram's stain: gram-negative bacteria Culture: *A. hydrophila*	
Necrotizing fasciitis	Laceration, abrasion, burn, or insect bite occurring in a setting of diabetes mellitus, alcohol, or drug abuse	1–4 days after injury	Severe local pain, tenderness, swelling, and skin discoloration due to gangrene High fever, chills, and prostration Necrosis extending to deep fascia from the skin, resulting in skin anesthesia	Initially pain, tenderness, erythema, and edema Progression to gangrene (blue-gray or black patches) of the skin with bullae Skin crepitus prominent	Foul-smelling serosanguineous or seropurulent exudate	Gram's stain: gram-positive cocci and rods and gram-negative rods Culture: *Peptostreptococcus* or *Bacteroides* and facultative anaerobic species of streptococci and one or more of the *Enterobacteriaceae*	Leukocytosis

deep fascia through the necrotic subcutaneous region, indicates that a fasciitis, and not an uncomplicated cellulitis, is present.

Necrotizing fasciitis is usually caused by a mixed infection involving one or more anaerobic species (e.g., *Bacteroides* and *Peptostreptococcus* species) and one or more facultative anaerobic species, such as streptococci (not group A) and gram-negative bacteria (*E. coli* or *Enterobacter, Klebsiella,* or *Proteus* species). Gram-stained smears of wound exudate may show gram-negative bacilli, streptococci, and sometimes gram-positive bacilli.

F. Cellulitis   There are diffuse aching or burning arm and hand pain, diffuse tenderness, and erythema of the skin of the arm with an irregular proximal margin. The erythema may encircle the arm, or it may be localized to the ventral or dorsal region of the extremity. It may begin without an apparent point of origin or may develop secondary to a wound, ulcer, or local abscess. Fever, chills, and malaise occur, and movement of the erythematous and swollen arm intensifies the pain. Painful and tender enlargement of epitrochlear and axillary lymph nodes may occur. Arm involvement by a rapidly spreading cellulitis may occur in women with chronic lymphedema of the arm secondary to mastectomy and axillary node dissection. Group A streptococci and *S. aureus* are responsible for the majority of cases of extremity cellulitis. Streptococci of group G or group C may also be etiologic. Isolation of the responsible agent may be achieved in 25 to 35 percent of cases by injection of sterile saline solution into the center or edge of the erythematous region and aspiration of the injected fluid for culture. Intravenous penicillin, nafcillin, or vancomycin will usually lead to prompt resolution, which is signaled by a decrease in pain and tenderness, fading of cutaneous erythema, and wrinkling of the skin as the subcutaneous edema resolves.

7. CARPAL TUNNEL SYNDROME

Aching pain, paresthesias, and/or numbness may occur on the radial side of the hand. The thumb, the index and middle fingers, and the radial side of the fourth finger are involved. Attacks of pain and tingling paresthesias often begin during the night and are relieved by repositioning the hand or shaking it. Hypesthesia of all or some of the above mentioned fingers may occur, and atrophy and weakness of the thenar muscles may develop. Tinel's sign (tingling paresthesias in the thumb, the index and middle fingers, and sometimes the radial side of the ring finger, produced by tapping the median nerve at the wrist) and Phalen's sign (reproduction of pain and/or paresthesias by flexing the wrist for 30–90 s with the elbow extended) may be positive. Similarly, extension of the wrist with the elbow extended may also provoke wrist and hand pain and paresthesias. Inflation of a blood pressure cuff to a

pressure between the patient's systolic and diastolic pressure for 1 min or more may also intensify or provoke characteristic symptoms. Electrodiagnostic studies reveal slowing of nerve conduction for sensory or motor components of the median nerve across the wrist. Electrodiagnostic studies have a sensitivity of 75 to 90 percent. A frequent cause of carpal tunnel syndrome is an inflammatory process involving the flexor tendons of the hand that share the carpal tunnel with the median nerve. Pain from median nerve compression in the carpal tunnel may sometimes radiate proximally to the forearm and, in some cases, to the shoulder, mimicking the pain of a cervical radiculopathy or a brachial plexus lesion. Surgical decompression of the carpal tunnel results in the relief of generalized arm and/or hand pain and paresthesias. The causes of an acute carpal tunnel syndrome include trauma, nonspecific flexor tenosynovitis, bleeding into the carpal tunnel, and a specific infection of flexor tendon sheaths (e.g., Lyme disease or bacterial infection).

8. REFERRED PAIN TO THE ARM AND HAND

A. Acute Myocardial Infarction or Acute Coronary Insufficiency   Severe aching pain may occur in the chest, neck, back, and one or both arms. In some cases, diffuse aching arm pain, sometimes associated with numbness and paresthesias, occurs alone. A paroxysm of pain beginning in the left wrist, followed in seconds by left elbow and then left shoulder pain, may also occur. The electrocardiogram taken during the pain may show Q waves and/or ST elevation or depression. Progression to infarction is associated with Q waves on the electrocardiogram, vomiting, nausea, diaphoresis, and sometimes hypotension. Lactic acid dehydrogenase type I and creatine kinase-MB isozyme levels rise in the serum of patients with myocardial infarction and remain normal in the presence of coronary insufficiency. A coronary angiogram will reveal coronary occlusion in patients with infarction, and removal of the occlusion by angioplasty or thrombolytic therapy will often dramatically relieve chest and arm pain. Patients with coronary insufficiency may have a severe fixed stenosis, coronary arterial spasm, and/or a partially occluding thrombus. These patients may respond to a calcium channel-blocking drug and afterload reduction, or they may require angioplasty.

B. Esophageal Motor Disorder   Severe crushing chest pain may occur spontaneously or be provoked by swallowing. Pain may radiate into the left or both arms and directly into the midback. Such pain may be associated with diffuse esophageal spasm or a nutcracker esophagus. Acid reflux may also provoke esophageal spasm, with chest and arm pain. Manometric studies, using an intraesophageal balloon, may be used to identify an esophageal motor disorder as a cause of the pain.

C. Chest Wall Pain Spontaneous parasternal, aching or sharp, stabbing pains may occur to the left or right of the sternum. The pain may radiate to the ipsilateral axillae and down the arm to the elbow or hand. There is local tenderness of one or more ipsilateral costal cartilages and/ or costosternal articulations on the affected side. Abduction or adduction of the ipsilateral arm against resistance may reproduce the patient's chest pain. Other tests that may elicit pain in patients with chest wall pain (costochondritis or pectoral myositis) include the "crowing rooster" and the "hug yourself" maneuvers.

D. Superior Pulmonary Sulcus Carcinoma (Pancoast's Syndrome) Pain may begin in the ipsilateral shoulder and medial scapular border and may radiate down the medial side of the arm, down the ulnar side of the forearm, and sometimes into the ring and small finger. The pain is usually severe and constant. The patient may support the elbow of the affected arm with the opposite hand. Severe skin hyperesthesia of the ipsilateral shoulder and upper arm may be present. Weakness and atrophy of the intrinsic muscles of the hand and the triceps muscle may occur. The triceps reflex may be impaired. Horner's syndrome may appear, with involvement of the sympathetic chain and stellate ganglion. A chest radiograph may demonstrate a thin, radiopaque plate at the top of the lung in the area of the superior sulcus or a large apical mass. A CT scan or MRI will demonstrate the size and extent of the tumor. The diagnosis can be confirmed by open or needle biopsy.

9. ACUTE ARTHRITIS INVOLVING TWO OR MORE UPPER EXTREMITY JOINTS

Asymmetrical arthritis of upper extremity joints may occur, giving rise to unilateral arm pain. The affected shoulder, elbow, wrist, or hand joints may be painful only during use, or there may be a persistent ache, requiring analgesics. Warmth, redness, local tenderness, and swelling of the involved joints may occur. One or more joints may be sequentially or simultaneously involved in another extremity, or the arthritic involvement may remain confined to only one arm. The causes of acute upper extremity joint pain include the following.

A. Acute Gout Polyarticular involvement occurs in up to 14 percent of patients. The elbow, wrist, and finger joints may become acutely swollen, red, warm, painful, and tender. An associated painful tenosynovitis may involve the wrist and hand. First metatarsophalangeal joint, ankle, or knee arthritis may precede or follow arm involvement. Fever, leukocytosis, and an elevated sedimentation rate may accompany the joint symptoms. Almost all patients have hyperuricemia (uric acid level >7.5 mg per deciliter), and aspirated synovial fluid contains

monosodium urate crystals in leukocytes, demonstrable by polarized light microscopy (95 percent sensitive). Colchicine therapy usually produces a dramatic therapeutic response.

B. Acute Rheumatic Fever Shoulder, elbow, wrist, and hand pain, and tenderness, accompanied by swelling, warmth, and redness of the overlying skin, may occur. Sequential involvement of these and other joints may occur. In most cases, the pattern of involvement is migratory, and one joint may be improving as the process begins at another site. Fever, leukocytosis, and an elevated sedimentation rate occur. There may be a history of a sore throat or "cold" 2 to 5 weeks prior to the onset of joint complaints. Acute streptococcal antibody levels are increased (antistreptolysin O, antihyaluronidase, and antidesoxyribonuclease), and there is a dramatic response to aspirin therapy.

C. Gonococcal Arthritis There is usually a migratory polyarthritis, and wrist, elbow, and hand involvement may occur. Joint pain, swelling, tenderness, and redness may be severe. A tenosynovitis involving the dorsum of the hands and wrists is frequent. Typical skin manifestations include small pustular lesions and purple hemorrhagic vesicles with a rim of surrounding erythema. These cutaneous lesions occur on the distal portions of the arms and legs. The skin lesions may be tender but usually are culture-negative. Fever, chills, and local symptoms such as urethritis, proctitis, pharyngitis, and a vaginal discharge may occur. Synovial fluid cultures may be negative in 50 percent of cases. A positive culture of *N. gonorrhoeae* from the urethra, cervix, rectum, pharynx, or blood will establish the diagnosis. The sensitivity of mucous membrane cultures is 80 percent. There is a prompt response to parenteral penicillin therapy.

D. Reiter's Syndrome This disorder may mimic gonococcal arthritis. It is not responsive to penicillin therapy and is usually associated with urethritis and conjunctivitis. Constitutional symptoms are less frequent. Shoulder and elbow symptoms occur, but wrist involvement is uncommon. Sacroiliitis, Achilles tendinitis, and knee involvement are common. Complaints may respond to nonsteroidal anti-inflammatory drugs.

E. Yersiniosis *Y. enterocolitica* may mimic the migratory polyarthritis of rheumatic fever. Fever, an elevated sedimentation rate, and a shift of the differential blood count to the left occur. Microscopic hematuria may occur in 33 percent of cases. *Yersinia* agglutination tests become positive in 7 to 14 days after the onset of diarrhea and should be positive at the onset of joint complaints.

F. Acute Calcium Pyrophosphate Dihydrate Deposition Disease This disorder may be polyarticular. The shoulder, elbow, wrist, and hand joints may be involved.

Swelling, redness, heat, pain, and tenderness may occur over one or all painful joints. Chondrocalcinosis may be identified as fine linear calcifications in the cartilage of the knee and the glenohumeral joint and in the triangular disc of the wrist. Chondrocalcinosis is not always present in patients with symptomatic disease. When the shoulder is involved, chondrocalcinosis occurs in only 50 percent of cases. Synovial fluid examination reveals calcium pyophosphate dihydrate crystals (99-percent sensitivity) and an increased number of joint fluid polymorphonuclear leukocytes. Involvement of upper extremity joints may be sequential, with clearing of one joint as one or more additional joints become involved. There is a good therapeutic response to intravenous colchicine.

G. Immune Complex Arthritis

1. Hepatitis B   This disorder may begin with an urticarial or maculopapular skin rash, followed by joint pain. The arthritis may be asymmetrical and migratory, or additive. Abnormal liver function tests caused by hepatitis B virus may be detected at the onset or within the next 10 days. Hepatitis B surface antigen can usually be detected in the serum of patients with acute arthritis. There may be a good response to salicylate therapy.

2. Subacute Bacterial Endocarditis   Patients may have an acute arthritis of two or more upper extremity joints. Fever, a heart murmur, petechiae, splinter hemorrhages in the nails, microscopic hematuria, and blood cultures positive for a bacterial of fungal pathogen are findings that are supportive of the diagnosis.

H. Lyme Arthritis   Several weeks to as long as 2 years after the onset of a characteristic annular erythematous rash, intermittent or persistent arthritis may occur, involving one or both knees and upper extremity joints. In one series, shoulders were involved in 32 percent, elbows in 20 percent, and wrists in 12 percent of cases. Detection of IgM or IgG antibody to *B. burgdorferi* by an ELISA test will support the diagnosis. Antibiotic therapy for 30 days is effective in relieving joint symptoms in up to 70 percent of cases.

I. Acute Rheumatoid Arthritis   Up to 15 percent of cases may present with an acute symmetrical or asymmetrical polyarthritis. At onset, the wrist may be involved in 60 percent, the shoulder in 37 percent, the elbow in 20 percent, the metatarsophalangeal joints in 48 percent, and the proximal interphalangeal joints in 63 percent of cases. Joint swelling, pain, stiffness, warmth, and tenderness are

common, but periarticular erythema is unusual. The presence of rheumatoid factor may be supportive, but not confirmatory, of the diagnosis. The predictive value of a positive test result is only 33 percent. A high-titer rheumatoid factor test may be more specific and of prognostic value. Patients with an acute onset of arthritis may have fever, mild leukocytosis, and an elevated sedimentation rate. Evolution into a chronic phase, with four or more of the following findings, may be required before the diagnosis can be established with certainty: joint stiffness requiring at least 1 h for maximal improvement, involvement of three or more joint areas, hand and/or wrist joint involvement, symmetrical arthritis, subcutaneous nodules, typical radiographic changes of involved joints, and an elevated titer of serum rheumatoid factor.

10. ACUTE BILATERAL UPPER AND LOWER ARM PAIN

Some of the disorders described above may cause bilateral upper and lower arm pain. These are listed in Table 38-3.

Table 38-3
ACUTE BILATERAL UPPER AND LOWER ARM PAIN

1. Cervical radiculopathy
   A. Cervical spondylosis
   B. Cervical osteomyelitis
   C. Cervical epidural abscess
   D. Cervical epidural hematoma
   E. Trauma with cervical fracture and/or dislocation
   F. Lyme disease and radiculoneuritis
2. Brachial plexopathy
   A. Thoracic outlet syndrome
   B. Acute brachial neuropathy (neuralgic amyotrophy)
3. Myofascial pain and brachialgia
4. Carpal tunnel syndrome
5. Referred pain to the arm and hand
   A. Acute myocardial infarction or acute coronary insufficiency
   B. Acute esophageal motor disorder
6. Acute arthritis involving two or more joints in each arm
   A. Acute gout
   B. Acute rheumatic fever
   C. Gonococcal arthritis
   D. Reiter's syndrome
   E. Yersiniosis
   F. Acute calcium pyrophosphate dihydrate deposition disease
   G. Immune complex arthritis (hepatitis B, subacute bacterial endocarditis)
   H. Lyme arthritis
   I. Acute rheumatoid arthritis

UPPER AND LOWER ARM PAIN REFERENCES

Brachial Plexus Disorders

Cascino TL, Kori S, Krol G, et al: CT of the brachial plexus in patients with cancer. *Neurology* 33:1553–1557, 1983.

Devathasan G, Tong HI: Neuralgic amyotrophy: Criteria for diagnosis and a clinical with electromyographic study of 21 cases. *Aust N Z J Med* 10:188–191, 1980.

Kline DG, Hackett ER, Happel LH: Surgery for lesions of the brachial plexus. *Arch Neurol* 43:170–181, 1986.

Kori SH, Foley KM, Posner JB: Brachial plexus lesions in patients with cancer: 100 cases. *Neurology* 31:45–50, 1981.

Sainer AL, Botnick LE, Herzog AG, et al: Reversible brachial plexopathy following primary radiation therapy for breast cancer. *Cancer Treat Rep* 65:797–802, 1981.

Subramony SH: AAEE case report #14: Neuralgic amyotrophy (acute brachial neuropathy). *Muscle Nerve* 11:39–44, 1988.

Urschel HC Jr: Superior pulmonary sulcus carcinoma. *Surg Clin North Am* 68:497–509, 1988.

Cervical Radiculopathy

Dillin W, Booth R, Cuckler J, et al: Cervical radiculopathy: A review. *Spine* 11:988–991, 1986.

Grisoli F, Graziani N, Fabrizi AP, et al: Anterior discectomy without fusion for treatment of cervical lateral soft disc extrusion: A follow-up of 120 cases. *Neurosurgery* 24:853–859, 1989.

Herkowitz HN: A comparison of anterior cervical fusion, cervical laminectomy, and cervical laminoplasty for the surgical management of multiple level spondylotic radiculopathy. *Spine* 13:774–780, 1988.

Mosdal C, Overgaard J: Lateral cervical facetectomy: The surgical pathology of radicular brachialgia. *Acta Neurochir* 70:199–205, 1984.

Quinn SF, Murtagh FR, Chatfield R, et al: CT-guided nerve root block and ablation. *AJR* 151:1213–1216, 1988.

Snyder GM, Bernhardt M: Anterior cervical fractional interspace decompression for treatment of cervical radiculopathy: A review of the first 66 cases. *Clin Orthop* 246:92–99, 1989.

Vassilouthis J, Kalovithouris A, Papandreou A, et al: The symptomatic incompetent cervical intervertebral disc. *Neurosurgery* 25:232–239, 1989.

Cervical Radiculopathy — Clinical Tests

Fast A, Parikh S, Marin EL: The shoulder abduction relief sign in cervical radiculopathy. *Arch Phys Med Rehabil* 70:402–403, 1989.

Makin GJV, Brown WF, Ebers GC: C7 radiculopathy: Importance of scapular winging in clinical diagnosis. *J Neurol Neurosurg Psychiatry* 49:640–644, 1986.

Vikari-Juntura E, Porras M, Laasonen EM: Validity of clinical tests in the diagnosis of root compression in cervical disc disease. *Spine* 14:253–257, 1989.

Cervical Radiculopathy — Disc Disease

Cailliet R: Cervical disc disease as a factor in pain and disability, in *Neck and Arm Pain*. Philadelphia, F.A. Davis, 1981, pp 56–72.

Eriksen EF, Buhl M, Fode K, et al: Treatment of cervical disc disease using Cloward's technique: The prognostic value of clinical preoperative data in 1,106 patients. *Acta Neurochir* 70:181–197, 1984.

Espersen JO, Buhl M, Eriksen EF, et al: Treatment of cervical disc disease using Cloward's technique: 1. General results, effect of different operative methods and complications in 1,106 patients. *Acta Neurochir* 70:97–114, 1984.

Gore DR, Sepic SB: Anterior cervical fusion for degenerated or protruded discs: A review of one hundred forty-six patients. *Spine* 9:667–671, 1984.

Hong C-Z, Lee S, Lum P: Cervical radiculopathy: Clinical, radiographic and EMG findings. *Orthop Rev* 15:433–439, 1986.

Hunt WE, Miller CA: Management of cervical radiculopathy. *Clin Neurosurg* 33:485–502, 1986.

Husag L, Probst C: Microsurgical anterior approach to cervical discs: Review of 60 consecutive cases of discectomy without fusion. *Acta Neurochir* 73:229–242, 1984.

Kelsey JL, Githens PB, Walter SD, et al: An epidemiological study of acute prolapsed cervical intervertebral disc. *J Bone Joint Surg (Am)* 66-A:907–914, 1984.

Mosdal C: Cervical osteochondrosis and disc herniation: Eighteen years' use of interbody fusion by Cloward's technique in 755 cases. *Acta Neurochir* 70:207–225, 1984.

Rainer JK: Cervical disc surgery: A historical review. *J Tenn Med Assoc* 77:12–16, 1984.

Wiesel SW, Feffer HL, Rothman RH: The development of a cervical spine algorithm and its prospective application to industrial patients. *J Occup Med* 27:272–276, 1985.

Wohlert L, Buhl M, Eriksen EF, et al: Treatment of cervical disc disease using Cloward's technique: 3. Evaluation of cervical spondylotic myelopathy in 138 cases. *Acta Neurochir* 71:121–131, 1984.

Cervical Radiculopathy — Spinal Cord Disease Imaging

Brown BM, Schwartz RH, Frank E, et al: Preoperative evaluation of cervical radiculopathy and myelopathy by surface-coil MR imaging. *AJR* 151:1205–1212, 1988.

Elster AD, Jensen KM: Vacuum phenomenon within the cervical spine canal: CT demonstration of a herniated disc. *J Comput Assist Tomogr* 8:533–535, 1984.

Hedberg MC, Drayer BP, Flom RA, et al: Gradient echo (GRASS) MR imaging in cervical radiculopathy. *AJR* 150:683–689, 1988.

Katijki MB, Agrawal R, Kantra TA: The human cervical myotomes: An anatomical correlation between electromyography and CT/myelography. *Muscle Nerve* 11:1070–1073, 1988.

Larsson E-M, Holtas S, Cronqvist S, et al: Comparison of myelography, CT myelography and magnetic resonance imaging in cervical spondylosis and disk herniation. *Acta Radiol* 30(3):233–239, 1989.

Modic MT, Masaryk TJ, Mulopulos GP, et al: Cervical radiculopathy: Prospective evaluation with surface coil MR imaging, CT with metrizamide, and metrizamide myelography. *Radiology* 161:753–759, 1986.

Modic MT, Masaryk TJ, Ross JS, et al: Cervical radiculopathy: Value of oblique MR imaging. *Radiology* 163:227–231, 1987.

Modic MT, Ross JS, Masaryk TJ: Imaging of degenerative disease of the cervical spine. *Clin Orthop* 239:109–120, 1989.

Tsuruda JS, Norman D, Dillon W, et al: Three-dimensional gradient-recalled MR imaging as a screening tool for the diagnosis of cervical radiculopathy. *AJNR* 10:1263–1271, 1989.

Viikari-Juntura E, Raininko R, Videman T, et al: Evaluation of cervical disc degeneration with ultralow field MRI and discography: An experimental study on cadavers. *Spine* 14:616–619, 1989.

Yu YL, duBoulay GH, Stevens JM, et al: Computed tomography in cervical spondylotic myelopathy and radiculopathy: Visualization of structures, myelographic comparison, cord measurements and clinical utility. *Neuroradiology* 28:221–236, 1986.

Cervical Spine — Review

Epstein NE, Epstein JA: Cervical spine stenosis, in Dee R, Mango E, Hurst LC (eds): *Principles of Orthopaedic Practice*. New York, McGraw-Hill, 1989, vol 2, pp 982–990.

Cervical Spine Trauma

Bachulis BL, Long WB, Hynes GD, et al: Clinical indications for cervical spine radiographs in the traumatized patient. *Am J Surg* 153:473–478, 1987.

Balmaseda MT Jr, Wunder JA, Gordon C, et al: Posttraumatic syringomyelia associated with heavy weightlifting exercises: Case report. *Arch Phys Med Rehabil* 69:970–972, 1988.

Barron MM: Cervical spine injury masquerading as a medical emergency. *Am J Emerg Med* 7:54–56, 1989.

Deans GT, Magalliard JN, Kerr M, et al: Neck sprain: A major cause of disability following car accidents. *Injury* 18:10–12, 1987.

Deans GT, Magalliard JN, Rutherford WH: Incidence and duration of neck pain among patients injured in car accidents. *Br Med J* 292:94–95, 1986.

Eckhardt WF, Doyle M, Woodward A, et al: Cervical spine fracture following a motor vehicle accident. *J Emerg Med* 6:179–183, 1988.

Gisbert VL, Hollerman JJ, Ney AL, et al: Incidence and diagnosis of C7–T1 fractures and subluxations in multiple-trauma patients: Evaluation of the advanced trauma life support guidelines. *Surgery* 106:702:709, 1989.

Kim KS, Rogers LF, Regenbogen V: Pitfalls in plain film diagnosis of cervical spine injuries. False positive interpretation. *Surg Neurol* 25:381–392, 1986.

Landells CD, Van Peteghem PK: Fractures of the atlas: Classification, treatment and morbidity. *Spine* 13:450–452, 1988.

Maimaris C, Barnes MR, Allen MJ: "Whiplash injuries" of the neck: A retrospective study. *Injury* 19:393–396, 1988.

McNamara, RM, O'Brien MC, Davidheiser S: Post-traumatic neck pain: A prospective and follow-up study. *Ann Emerg Med* 17:906–911, 1988.

Neifeld GL, Keene JG, Hevesy G, et al: Cervical injury in head trauma. *J Emerg Med* 6:203–207, 1988.

Pavlov H, Torg JS: Roentgen examination of cervical spine injuries in the athlete. *Clin Sports Med* 6:751–766, 1987.

Povisen UJ, Kjaer L, Arlien-Søborg P: Locked-in syndrome following cervical manipulation. *Acta Neurol Scand* 76:486–488, 1987.

Ringenberg BJ, Fisher AK, Urdaneta LF, et al: Rational ordering of cervical spine radiographs following trauma. *Ann Emerg Med* 17:792–796, 1988.

Salomone JA III, Steele MT: An unusual presentation of bilateral facet dislocation of the cervical spine. *Ann Emerg Med* 16:1390–1393, 1987.

Swischuk LE: Neck pain after trauma. *Pediatr Emerg Care* 4:219–221, 1988.

Werthrim SB, Bohlman HH: Occipitocervical fusion: Indications, technique, and long-term results in thirteen patients. *J Bone Joint Surg (Am)* 69-A:833–836, 1987.

Cervical Spondylosis — Radiculopathy and Myelopathy

Bertalanffy H, Eggert H-R: Clinical long-term results of anterior discectomy without fusion for treatment of cervical radiculopathy and myelopathy: A follow-up of 164 cases. *Acta Neurochir (Wien)* 90:127–135, 1988.

Herkowitz HN: The surgical management of cervical spondylotic radiculopathy and myelopathy. *Clin Orthop* 239:94–108, 1989.

Kiwerski J: Treatment of cervical canal stenosis by decompression and anterior fusion. *Arch Orthop Trauma Surg* 107:354–356, 1988.

Mann KS, Khosla VK, Gulati DR: Cervical spondylotic myelopathy treated by single-stage multilevel anterior decompression. *J Neurosurg* 60:81–87, 1984.

Masaryk TJ, Modic MT, Geisinger MA, et al: Cervical myelopathy: A comparison of magnetic resonance and myelography. *J Comput Assist Tomogr* 10:184–194, 1986.

Yu YL, DuBoulay GH, Stevens JM, et al: Computer-assisted myelography in cervical spondylotic myelopathy and radiculopathy. *Brain* 109:259–278, 1986.

Yu YL, Woo E, Huang CY: Cervical spondylotic myelopathy and radiculopathy. *Acta Neurol Scand* 75:367–373, 1987.

Cervical Spondylosis — Review

Bogduk N, Windsor M, Inglis A: The innervation of the cervical intervertebral discs. *Spine* 13:2–8, 1988.

Epstein NE, Zito J: Cervical spondylosis and disc disease, in Dee R, Mango E, Hurst LC (eds): *Principles of Orthopaedic Practice*. New York, McGraw-Hill, 1989, vol 2, pp 969–981.

Lestini WF, Wiesel SW: The pathogenesis of cervical spondylosis. *Clin Orthop* 239:69–93, 1989.

Manabe S, Tateishi A, Ohno T: Anterolateral uncoforaminotomy for cervical spondylotic myeloradiculopathy. *Acta Orthop Scand* 59:669–674, 1988.

Schmidek HH: Cervical spondylosis. *AFP* 33:89–99, 1986.

Uttley D, Monro P: Neurosurgery for cervical spondylosis. *Br J Hosp Med* 42:62–70, 1989.

Discogenic Arm Pain

Osler GE: Cervical analgesic discography: A test for diagnosis of the painful disc syndrome. *S Afr Med J* 71:363, 1987.

Epidural Abscess — Cervical Spine

Baker AS, Ojemann RG, Swartz MN, et al: Spinal epidural abscess. *N Engl J Med* 293:463–468, 1975.

Bouchez B, Arnott G, Delfosse JM: Acute spinal epidural abscess. *J Neurol* 231:343–344, 1985.

Buruma OJS, Craane H, Kunst MW: Vertebral osteomyelitis and epidural abscess due to mucormycosis: A case report. *Clin Neurol Neurosurg* 81:39–44, 1979.

Erntell M, Holtas S, Norlin K, et al: Magnetic resonance imaging in the diagnosis of spinal epidural abscess. *Scand J Infect Dis* 20:323–327, 1988.

Feldenzer JA, Waters DC, Knake JE, et al: Anterior cervical epidural abscess: The use of intraoperative spinal sonography. *Surg Neurol* 25:105–108, 1986.

Lasker BR, Harter DH: Cervical epidural abscess. *Neurology* 37:1747–1753, 1987.

Lownie SP, Ferguson GG: Spinal subdural empyema complicating cervical discography. *Spine* 14:1415–1417, 1989.

McGrath H Jr, McCormick C, Carey ME: Pyogenic cervical osteomyelitis presenting as a massive prevertebral abscess in a patient with rheumatoid arthritis. *Am J Med* 84:363–365, 1988.

Peterson JA, Paris P, Williams AC: Acute epidural abscess. *Am J Emerg Med* 5:287–290, 1987.

Epidural Hematoma — Cervical Spine

Harding JR, McCall IW, Park WM, et al: Fracture of the cervical spine in ankylosing spondylitis. *Br J Radiol* 58:3–7, 1985.

Nagel MA, Taff IP, Cantos EL, et al: Spontaneous spinal epidural hematoma in a 7-year-old girl: Diagnostic value of magnetic resonance imaging. *Clin Neurol Neurosurg* 91:157–160, 1989.

Epidural Metastatic Tumor — Spine

Bates DW, Reuler JB: Back pain and epidural spinal cord compression. *J Gen Intern Med* 3:191–197, 1988.

Ch'ien LT, Kalwinsky DK, Peterson G, et al: Metastatic epidural tumors in children. *Med Pediatr Oncol* 10:455–462, 1982.

Epstein JA, Marc JA, Hyman RA, et al: Total myelography in the evaluation of lumbar discs: With the presentation of three cases of thoracic neoplasms simulating nerve root lesions. *Spine* 4:121–128, 1979.

Giannotta SL, Kindt GW: Metastatic spinal cord tumors. *Clin Neurosurg* 25:495–503, 1978.

Gilbert MR, Grossman SA: Incidence and nature of neurologic problems in patients with solid tumors. *Am J Med* 81:951–954, 1986.

Gilbert RW, Kim J-H, Posner JB: Epidural spinal cord compression from metastatic tumor: Diagnosis and treatment. *Ann Neurol* 3:40–51, 1978.

Kostuik JP: Anterior spinal cord decompression for lesions of the thoracic and lumbar spine, techniques, new methods of internal fixation results. *Spine* 8:512–531, 1983.

Kuban DA, El-Mahdi AM, Sigfred SV, et al: Characteristics of spinal cord compression in adenocarcinoma of prostate. *Urology* 28:364–369, 1986.

Nather A, Bose K: The results of decompression of cord or cauda equina compression from metastatic extradural tumors. *Clin Orthop* 169:103–108, 1982.

Overby MC, Rothman AS: Anterolateral decompression for metastatic epidural spinal cord tumors: Results of a modified costotransversectomy approach. *J Neurosurg* 62:344–348, 1985.

Posner JB: Back pain and epidural spinal cord compression. *Med Clin North Am* 71:185–205, 1987.

Posner JB, Howieson J, Cvitkovic E: "Disappearing" spinal cord compression: Oncolytic effect of glucocorticoids (and other chemotherapeutic agents) on epidural metastases. *Ann Neurol* 2:409:413, 1977.

Rodriguez M, Dinapoli RP: Spinal cord compression: With special reference to metastatic epidural tumors. *Mayo Clin Proc* 55:442–448, 1980.

Sherman RMP, Waddell JP: Laminectomy for metastatic epidural spinal cord tumors: Posterior stabilization, radiotherapy, and preoperative assessment. *Clin Orthop Rel Res* 207:55–63, 1986.

Siegal T, Siegal T: Surgical decompression of anterior and posterior malignant epidural tumors compressing the spinal cord: A prospective study. *Neurosurgery* 17:424–432, 1985.

Sundaresan N, Galicich JH: Treatment of spinal metastases by vertebral body resection. *Cancer Inves* 2:383–397, 1984.

Sundaresan N, Galicich JH, Lane JM, et al: Treatment of neoplastic epidural cord compression by vertebral body resection and stabilization. *J Neurosurg* 63:676–684, 1985.

Sundaresan N, Scher H, DiGiacinto GV, et al: Surgical treatment of spinal cord compression in kidney cancer. *J Clin Oncol* 4:1851–1856, 1986.

Muscle/Tendon Rupture

Grimes HA: Spontaneous rupture of muscles, tendons and insertions of same. *J Ark Med Soc* 75:433–434, 1979.

Myofascial Arm Pain

Baksi DP: Role of fibrositis of supra and periscapular area in aetiology of brachialgia. *J Indian Med Assoc* 82:170–173, 1984.

Simms RW, Goldenberg DL: Symptoms mimicking neurologic disorders in fibromyalgia syndrome. *J Rheumatol* 15:1271–1273, 1988.

Neck and Arm Pain

Goodman BW Jr: Neck pain. *Prim Care* 15:689–708, 1988.

Lipsky PE: Rheumatoid arthritis, in Wilson JD, Braunwald E, Isselbacher RJ, et al (eds): *Harrison's Principles of Internal Medicine,* 12th ed. New York, McGraw-Hill, vol 2, 1991, pp 1437–1443.

Sherk HH, Watters WC III, Zeiger L: Evaluation and treatment of neck pain. *Orthop Clin North Am* 13:439–451, 1982.

Neck and Arm Pain — Review

Gilbert R, Warfield CA: Evaluating and treating the patient with neck pain. *Hosp Pract* 22:223–232, 1987.

Jenkins DG: Clinical features of arm and neck pain. *Physiotherapy* 65:102–105, 1979.

MacRae DL: Head and neck pain in the elderly. *J Otolaryngol* 15:224–227, 1986.

Moskovich R: Neck pain in the elderly: Common causes and management. *Geriatrics* 43:65–92, 1988.

Payne R: Neck pain in the elderly: A management review: 1. *Geriatrics* 42:59–65, 1987.

———: Neck pain in the elderly: A management review: 2. *Geriatrics* 42:71–73, 1987.

Stabile MJ, Warfield CA: Differential diagnosis of arm pain. *Hosp Pract (Off Ed)* 25:55–58, 61, 64, 1990.

Peripheral Nervous System

Fahr LM, Sauser DD: Imaging of peripheral nerve lesions. *Orthop Clin North Am* 19:27–41, 1988.

Pyogenic Osteomyelitis — Cervical

Bartal AD, Schiffer J, Heilbronn YD, et al: Anterior interbody fusion for cervical osteomyelitis: Reversal of quadriplegia after evacuation of epidural spinal abscess. *J Neurol Neurosurg Psychiatry,* 35:133–136, 1972.

Craig JB: Cervical spine osteomyelitis with delayed onset tetraparesis

after penetrating wounds of the neck: A report of 2 cases. *S Afr Med J* 69:197–199, 1986.

Guyer RD, Collier R, Stith WJ, et al: Discitis after discography. *Spine* 13:1352–1354, 1988.

Schwartz JG, Tio FO: Nocardial osteomyelitis: A case report and review of the literature. *Diagn Microbiol Infect Dis* 8:37–46, 1987.

Sinnott JT IV, Multhopp H, Leo J, et al: *Yersinia enterocolitica* causing spinal osteomyelitis and empyema in a nonimmunocompromised host. *South Med J* 82:399–400, 1989.

Stone JL, Cybulski GR, Rodriguez J, et al: Anterior cervical debridement and strut-grafting for osteomyelitis of the cervical spine. *J Neurosurg* 70:879–883, 1989.

Yang EC, Neuwirth MG: *Pseudomonas aeruginosa* as a causative agent of cervical osteomyelitis: Case report and review of the literature. *Clin Orthop Rel Res* 231:229–233, 1988.

Repetition Strain

Sikorski JM, Molan RR, Askin GN: Orthopaedic basis for occupationally related arm and neck pain. *Aust N Z J Surg* 59:471–478, 1989.

Shoulder and Arm Pain — Review

Bateman JE: Neurologic painful conditions affecting the shoulder. *Clin Orthop Rel Res* 173:44–54, 1983.

Spinal Cord and Brain Malformations

Eisenstat DDR, Bernstein M, Fleming JFR, et al: Chiari malformation in adults: A review of 40 cases. *Can J Neurol Sci* 13:221–228, 1986.

El Gammal T, Mark EK, Brooks BS: MR Imaging of Chiari II malformation. *AJR* 150:163–170, 1988.

Herring JA: Klippel-Feil syndrome with neck pain. *J Pediatr Orthop* 9:343–346, 1989.

Hutchins WW, Vogelzang RL, Neiman HL, et al: Differentiation of tumor from syringohydromyelia: Intraoperative neurosonography of the spinal cord. *Radiology* 151:171–174, 1984.

Spinal Cord Diseases — Review

Adams RD, Victor M: Diseases of the spinal cord, in *Principles of Neurology,* 4th ed. New York, McGraw-Hill, 1989, pp 718–754.

Spinal Cord Tumors — Extramedullary/Intradural

Breuer AC, Kneisley LW, Fischer EG: Treatable extramedullary cord compression: Meningioma as a cause of the Brown-Séquard syndrome. *Spine* 5:19–22, 1980.

Ciappetta P, Celli P, Palma L, et al: Intraspinal hemangiopericytomas: Report of two cases and review of the literature. *Spine* 10:27–31, 1985.

Kaufman BA, Kaufman B, Rekate HL: Cervicomedullary junction tumor diagnosed by nuclear magnetic resonance scanning: Case report: *Neurosurgery* 15:878–880, 1984.

Levy WJ Jr, Bay J, Dohn D: Spinal cord meningioma. *J Neurosurg* 57:804–812, 1982.

Schulz U, Bamberg M: Relationship between curative radiation therapy of paravertebral tumors and the incidence of radiation myelitis. *Tumori* 64:305–312, 1978.

Scotti G, Scialfa G, Colombo N, et al: MR imaging of intradural extramedullary tumors of the cervical spine. *J Comput Assist Tomogr* 9:1037–1041, 1985.

Vasilakis D, Papaconstantinou C, Aletras H: Dumb-bell intrathoracic and intraspinal neurofibroma: Report of a case. *Scand J Thorac Cardiovasc Surg* 20:171–173, 1986.

Spinal Cord Tumor — Intramedullary/Metastatic

Grem JL, Burgess J, Trump DL: Clinical features and natural history of intramedullary spinal cord metastasis. *Cancer* 56:2305–2314, 1985.

Post MJD, Quencer RM, Green BA, et al: Intramedullary spinal cord metastases, mainly of nonneurogenic origin. *AJR* 148:1015–1022, 1987.

Spinal Cord Tumor — Intramedullary/Primary

Cooper PR, Epstein F: Radical resection of intramedullary spinal cord tumors in adults: Recent experience in 29 patients. *J Neurosurg* 63:492–499, 1985.

Cybulski GR, Von Roenn KA, Bailey OT: Intramedullary cystic teratoid tumor of the cervical spinal cord in association with a teratoma of the ovary. *Surg Neurol* 22:267–272, 1984.

Garrido E, Stein BM: Microsurgical removal of intramedullary spinal cord tumors. *Surg Neurol* 7:215–219, 1977.

Heppner F, Ascher PW, Holzer P, et al: CO_2 laser surgery of intramedullary spinal cord tumors. *Lasers Surg Med* 7:180–183, 1987.

Rawlings CE III, Giangaspero F, Burger PC, et al: Ependymomas: A clinicopathologic study. *Surg Neurol* 29:271–281, 1988.

Stein BM: Intramedullary spinal cord tumors. *Clin Neurosurg* 30:717–741, 1983. Case 52-1985, Case records of the Massachusetts General Hospital. *N Engl J Med* 313:1646–1656, 1985.

Spinal Cord Tumors—Metastatic

Kleinman WB, Kiernan HA, Michelsen WJ: Metastatic cancer of the spinal column. *Clin Orthop* 136:166–172, 1978.

Kuhlman JE, Fishman EK, Leichner PK, et al: Skeletal metastases from hepatoma: Frequency, distribution, and radiographic features. *Radiology* 160:175–178, 1986.

Schaberg J, Gainor BJ: A profile of metastatic carcinoma of the spine. *Spine* 10:19–20, 1985.

Spinal Cord Tumors—Pain

Copeman MC: Presenting symptoms of neoplastic spinal cord compression. *J Surg Oncol* 37:24–25, 1988.

Nicholas JJ, Christy WC: Spinal pain made worse by recumbency: A clue to spinal cord tumors. *Arch Phys Med Rehabil* 67:598–600, 1986.

Spinal Cord Tumors—Primary

Aprin H: Spinal neoplasms, in Dee R, Mango E, Hurst LC (eds): *Principles of Orthopaedic Practice.* New York, McGraw-Hill, 1989, vol 2, pp 955–969.

Bohlman HH, Sachs BL, Carter JR, et al: Primary neoplasms of the cervical spine: Diagnosis and treatment of twenty-three patients. *J Bone Joint Surg (Am)* 68-A:483–494, 1986.

Grob D, Loehr J: Osteoblastoma of the cervical spine: Case report. *Arch Orthop Trauma Surg* 108:179–181, 1989.

Myles ST, MacRae ME: Benign osteoblastoma of the spine in childhood. *J Neurosurg* 68:884–888, 1988.

O'Neil J, Gardner V, Armstrong G: Treatment of tumors of the thoracic and lumbar spinal column. *Clin Orthop Rel Res* 227:103–112, 1988.

Sherk HH, Nolan JP Jr, Mooar PA: Treatment of tumors of the cervical spine. *Clin Orthop* 233:163–167, 1988.

Spinal Cord Tumors—Review

Hahn YS, McLone DG: Pain in children with spinal cord tumors. *Child Brain* 11:36–46, 1984.

Stern WE: Localization and diagnosis of spinal cord tumors. *Clin Neurosurg* 25:480–494, 1978.

Thoracic Outlet Syndrome—Axillary-Subclavian Venous Thrombosis

Brochner G, Rojas M, Armas AJ, et al: Axillary-subclavian venous thrombosis. *J Cardiovasc Surg* 30:108:111, 1989.

Kunkel JM, Machleder HI: Treatment of Paget-Schroetter syndrome: A staged, multidisciplinary approach. *Arch Surg* 124:1153–1158, 1989.

O'Leary MR, Smith MS, Druy EM: Diagnostic and therapeutic approach to axillary-subclavian vein thrombosis. *Ann Emerg Med* 16:889–893, 1987.

Perler BA, Mitchell SE: Percutaneous transluminal angioplasty and transaxillary first rib resection: A multidisciplinary approach to the thoracic outlet syndrome. *Am Surg* 52:485–488, 1986.

Strange-Vognsen HH, Hauch O, Andersen J, et al: Resection of the first rib, following deep arm vein thrombolysis in patients with thoracic outlet syndrome. *J Cardiovasc Surg* 30:430–433, 1989.

Swenson WM, Rennich D, Capp KA, et al: Axillary vein thrombosis due to thoracic outlet syndrome: Correction via the supraclavicular approach. *AORN J* 46:878–881, 884–886, 1987.

Thoracic Outlet Syndrome—Neurogenic

Baumgartner F, Nelson RJ, Robertson JM: The rudimentary first rib: A cause of thoracic outlet syndrome with arterial compromise. *Arch Surg* 124:1090–1092, 1989.

Bilbey JH, Müller NL, Connell DG, et al: Thoracic outlet syndrome: Evaluation with CT. *Radiology* 171:381–384, 1989.

Brown SCW, Charlesworth D: Results of excision of a cervical rib in patients with the thoracic outlet syndrome. *Br J Surg* 75:431–433, 1988.

Connolly JF, Dehne R: Nonunion of the clavicle and thoracic outlet syndrome. *J Trauma* 29:1127–1133, 1989.

DeSilva M: The costoclavicular syndrome: A "new cause," *Ann Rheum Dis* 45:916–920, 1986.

Kritzer RO, Rose JE: Diffuse idiopathic skeletal hyperostosis presenting with thoracic outlet syndrome and dysphagia. *Neurosurgery* 22:1071–1074, 1988.

Leffert RD, Gumley G: The relationship between dead arm syndrome and thoracic outlet syndrome. *Clin Orthop* 223:20–31, 1987.

Rayan GM: Lower trunk brachial plexus compression neuropathy due to cervical rib in young athletes. *Am J Sports Med* 16:77–79, 1988.

Shields RW Jr, Wilbourn AJ: Headache and the thoracic outlet syndrome (letter to editor). *Headache* 26:209–210, 1986.

Young MC, Richards RR, Hudson AR: Thoracic outlet syndrome with congenital pseudarthrosis of the clavicle: Treatment by brachial plexus decompression, plate fixation and bone grafting. *Can J Surg* 31:131–133, 1988.

Thoracic Outlet Syndrome—Recurrent

Sessions RT: Reoperation for thoracic outlet syndrome. *J Cardiovasc Surg* 30:434–444, 1989.

Urschel HC Jr, Razzuk MA: The failed operation for thoracic outlet syndrome: The difficulty of diagnosis and management. *Ann Thorac Surg* 42:523–528, 1986.

Thoracic Outlet Syndrome—Review

Blair SJ: Avoiding complications of surgery for nerve compression syndromes. *Orthop Clin North Am* 19:125–130, 1988.

Capistrant TD: Thoracic outlet syndrome in cervical strain injury. *Minn Med* 69:13–17, 1986.

Cherington M, Happer I, Machanic B, et al: Surgery for thoracic outlet syndrome may be hazardous to your health. *Muscle Nerve* 9:632–634, 1986.

Cuetter AC, Bartoszek DM: The thoracic outlet syndrome: Controversies, overdiagnosis, overtreatment, and recommendations for management. *Muscle Nerve* 12:410–419, 1989.

Hawkes CD: Neurosurgical considerations in thoracic outlet syndrome. *Clin Orthop* 207:24–28, 1986.

Hurst LC, Paul S: Thoracic outlet syndrome, in Dee R, Mango E, Hurst LC (eds): *Principles of Orthopaedic Practice.* New York, McGraw-Hill, 1988, vol 1, pp 684–686.

Moore M Jr: Thoracic outlet syndrome experience in a metropolitan hospital. *Clin Orthop* 207:29–30, 1986.

Pang D, Wessel HB: Thoracic outlet syndrome. *Neurosurgery* 22:105–121, 1988.

Schlesinger EB: The thoracic outlet syndrome from a neurosurgical point of view. *Clin Orthop Rel Res* 51:49–52, 1967.

Sellke FW, Kelly TR: Thoracic outlet syndrome. *Am J Surg* 156:54–57, 1988.

Stanton PE Jr, Vo NM, Haley T, et al: Thoracic outlet syndrome: A comprehensive evaluation. *Am Surg* 54:129–133, 1988.

Takagi K, Yamaga M, Morisawa K, et al: Management of thoracic outlet syndrome. *Arch Orthop Trauma Surg* 106:78–81, 1987.

Warrens AN, Heaton JM: Thoracic outlet compression syndrome: The lack of reliability of its clinical assessment. *Ann R Coll Surg Engl* 69:203–204, 1987.

Wood VE, Twito R, Verska JM: Thoracic outlet syndrome: The results of first rib resection in 100 patients. *Orthop Clin North Am* 19:131–146, 1988.

Thoracic Outlet Syndrome—Subclavian Artery Occlusion

Al-Hassan HK, Sattar MA, Eklof B: Embolic brain infarction, A rare complication of thoracic outlet syndrome: A report of two cases. *J Cardiovasc Surg* 29:322–325, 1988.

Cormier JM, Amrane M, Ward A, et al: Arterial complications of the thoracic outlet syndrome: Fifty-five operative cases. *J Vasc Surg* 9:778–787, 1989.

Goadsby PJ: A subclavian bruit in the thoracic outlet syndrome (letter to editor). *Ann Intern Med* 110:323, 1989.

Grant DS, Shaw PJ, Adiseshia M: Vascular compression in thoracic outlet syndrome: A potentially missed diagnosis. *J R Soc Med* 81:476–478, 1988.

Riddell DH, Smith BM: Thoracic and vascular aspects of thoracic outlet syndrome: 1986 update. *Clin Orthop* 207:31–36, 1986.

Scher LA, Veith FJ, Samson RH, et al: Vascular complications of thoracic outlet syndrome. *J Vasc Surg* 3:565–568, 1986.

Van Damme H, Fourny J, Zicot M, et al: Giant cell arteritis (Horton's disease) of the axillary artery: Case reports. *Angiology* 40:593–601, 1989.

Tuberculous Osteomyelitis—Cervical Spine

Corea JR, Tamimi TM: Tuberculosis of the arch of the atlas: Case report. *Spine* 12:608–611, 1987.

Neal SL, Kearns MJ, Seelig JM, et al: Manifestations of Pott's disease in the head and neck. *Laryngoscope* 96:494–497, 1986.

Upper and Lower Arm Pain—Review

Aprin H, Dee R: Infections of the spine, in Dee R, Mango E, Hurst LC (eds): *Principles of Orthopaedic Practice*. New York, McGraw-Hill, 1989, vol 2, pp 941–955.

Cailliet R: Differential diagnosis, in *Neck and Arm Pain*. Philadelphia, F.A. Davis, 1981, pp 137–158.

Coyle MP Jr: Nerve entrapment syndromes, in Dee R, Mango E, Hurst LC (eds): *Principles of Orthopaedic Practice*. New York, McGraw-Hill, 1988, vol 1, pp 672–684.

Fauci AS: The vasculitis syndromes, in Wilson JD, Braunwald E, Isselbacher RJ, et al (eds): *Harrison's Principles of Internal Medicine,* 12th ed. New York, McGraw-Hill, 1991, vol 2, pp 1456–1463.

Greenlee JE: Epidural abscess, in Mandell GL, Douglas RG Jr, Bennett JE (eds): *Principles and Practice of Infectious Diseases,* 3d ed. New York, Churchill Livingstone, 1990, pp 791–793.

Hoffman GS: Arthritis due to deposition of calcium crystals, in Wilson JD, Braunwald E, Isselbacher RJ, et al (eds): *Harrison's Principles of Internal Medicine,* 12th ed. New York, McGraw-Hill, 1991, vol 2, pp 1479–1482.

Hurst LC, Badalamente MA, Paul S: Nerve injuries in the upper extremity, in Dee R, Mango E, Hurst LC (eds): *Principles of Orthopaedic Practice*. New York, McGraw-Hill, 1988, vol 1, pp 666–672.

Lipstein-Kresch E, Greenwald R: Crystal deposition and disease, in Dee R, Mango E, Hurst LC (eds): *Principles of Orthopaedic Practice*. New York, McGraw-Hill, 1988, vol 1, pp 220–225.

Swartz MN: Cellulitis and superficial infections, in Mandell GL, Douglas RG Jr, Bennett JE (eds): *Principles and Practice of Infectious Diseases,* 3d ed. New York, Churchill Livingstone, 1990, pp 796–807.

———: Myositis, in Mandell GL, Douglas RG Jr, Bennett JE (eds): *Principles and Practice of Infectious Diseases,* 3d ed. New York, Churchill Livingstone, 1990, pp 812–818.

———: Subcutaneous tissue infections and abscesses, in Mandell GL, Douglas RG Jr, Bennett JE (eds): *Principles and Practice of Infectious Diseases,* 3d ed. New York, Churchill Livingstone, 1990, pp 808–812.

Acute Shoulder, Upper Arm, and Axillary Pain

☐ **DIAGNOSTIC LIST**

SHOULDER AND UPPER
ARM PAIN

1. Calcific tendinitis and subdeltoid bursitis
2. Acute arthritis
   A. Septic arthritis of the glenohumeral joint
   B. Crystal-induced synovitis of the glenohumeral joint
      1. Acute gout
      2. Acute pseudogout
   C. Acute rheumatic fever
   D. Reiter's syndrome
   E. Lyme arthritis
   F. Hepatitis B-associated arthritis
   G. Acute hemarthrosis secondary to hemophilia or anticoagulant therapy
3. Acute osteomyelitis of the shoulder
4. Trauma
   A. Proximal fracture of the humerus
   B. Proximal fracture and dislocation of the humerus
   C. Pathologic fracture of the humerus
   D. Acute dislocation of the glenohumeral joint
      1. Anterior dislocation
      2. Posterior dislocation
   E. Fracture of the humeral shaft
   F. Acromioclavicular separation
   G. Fracture of the clavicle
5. Rupture of the biceps muscle or tendon
6. Tendinitis of the pectoralis major muscle
7. Osteonecrosis of the humeral head
8. Neuralgic amyotrophy
9. Cervical radiculopathy
10. Referred shoulder pain
    A. Cardiac
       1. Acute pericarditis
       2. Acute myocardial infarction
    B. Pleural
       1. Pneumonia
       2. Pulmonary infarction
       3. Primary pleuritis due to systemic lupus erythematosus or other collagen vascular disorders
       4. Tuberculosis
    C. Intraabdominal inflammation
       1. Acute cholecystitis
       2. Duodenal or gastric ulcer perforation and peritonitis
       3. Gastric carcinoma perforation and peritonitis
    D. Hemoperitoneum
       1. Ruptured ectopic pregnancy
       2. Spontaneous rupture of the spleen
       3. Traumatic rupture of the spleen
       4. Hepatic tumor with hemorrhage

5. Abdominal apoplexy
6. Rupture of a splanchnic artery aneurysm
   E. Subphrenic abscess
     1. Right subphrenic abscess
     2. Left subphrenic abscess
   F. Pneumoperitoneum
11. Subclavian-axillary artery aneurysm

AXILLARY PAIN

12. Axillary infection
   A. Cat-scratch disease
   B. Streptococcal axillary lymphadenitis
   C. Staphylococcal axillary lymphadenitis
   D. Axillary skin abscess
   E. Axillary infections in leukemia
   F. Tularemia (ulceroglandular)
   G. Bubonic plague
   H. Bites on the upper extremity
     1. Animal bites
     2. Human bites
   I. Hidradenitis suppurativa

13. Axillary-subclavian venous thrombosis
14. Fracture of the proximal humerus
15. Costochondritis of the anterior chest with axillary pain radiation
16. Axillary myalgic pain
17. Gaseous distension of the stomach
18. Pneumothorax
19. Breast disorders in women (cyst, tumor, and abscess)
20. Pleuropulmonary disease
   A. Carcinoma of the lung or lymphoma
   B. Pyogenic lung abscess
   C. Actinomycosis
21. Radicular pain involving the T1 root
22. Postaxillary dissection pain in patients operated on for breast cancer
23. Bilateral pain
   A. Bilateral acute shoulder and upper arm pain
   B. Bilateral acute axillary pain

☐ SUMMARY

Shoulder and Upper Arm Pain

Calcific tendinitis may cause the sudden onset of severe-to-excruciating unilateral shoulder pain. The pain is localized to the glenohumeral joint and the deltoid region of the upper arm. The arm is held close to the side, and any attempts at movement are resisted. Swelling, increased skin temperature, and exquisite tenderness are present over the region of the greater tuberosity and the deltoid muscle. Plain radiographs reveal calcium deposits in the supraspinatus tendon or, less commonly, in the tendon of one of the other rotator cuff muscles. A secondary *subdeltoid bursitis* may occur and increase the severity of the pain and dysfunction of the shoulder. Needling of the calcific deposit, saline lavage, and local injection of lidocaine provide dramatic and rapid relief of symptoms. *Septic arthritis* may cause a gradual or a sudden onset of severe shoulder pain and limitation of arm motion. The joint effusion may present as an anteromedial fluctuant swelling. Fever and leukocytosis are present in only half the patients. The synovial fluid usually contains more than 10,000 polymorphonuclear leukocytes per cubic millimeter and a reduced glucose concentration. The diagnosis may be established by a positive synovial fluid gram stain (67 percent) and culture (90 percent).

Risk factors for septic glenohumeral arthritis include advanced age, serious medical disorders, prior glenohumeral joint corticosteroid injections, intravenous drug abuse, and recent glenohumeral joint surgery or penetrating trauma. *Acute gout* may rarely present with shoulder pain and dysfunction without prior or associated involvement of other joints. Gouty synovial joint fluid contains an increased number of polymorphonuclear leukocytes and monosodium urate crystals. A similar painful monoarthritis may be caused by *acute pseudogout*; and in this disorder, involvement of the glenohumeral joint occurs more commonly than in gout. Shoulder radiographs may reveal chondrocalcinosis in up to 50 percent of cases. The synovial fluid contains polymorphonuclear leukocytes and calcium pyrophosphate dihydrate crystals. Both gout and pseudogout may respond dramatically to colchicine therapy. *Acute rheumatic fever* causes fever, chills, sweats, generalized aching, weakness, and a migratory arthritis that may involve the shoulders, elbows, wrists, knees, and small joints of the hands and feet. There may be a history of a recent sore throat or upper respiratory infection, and serum levels of antistreptococcal antibodies are elevated. There is a dramatic response to aspirin therapy.

Reiter's syndrome causes an asymmetric polyarthritis that may involve the shoulders, knees, ankles, and sacroiliac joints. Fever and other systemic symptoms may occur. Urethritis, diarrhea, conjunctivitis, and iritis or iridocyclitis are important associated findings. Cutaneous and mucous membrane lesions include keratoderma blennorrhagicum, and balanitis circinata. Enthesopathic features that suggest this disease include insertional tendinitis, periostitis, spurs, peri-insertional osteoporosis, and bony erosions. Foot involvement includes Achilles tendinitis, plantar fasciitis, and subtalar arthritis. Nonsteroidal anti-inflammatory drugs provide symptomatic relief. *Lyme arthritis* begins with an annular, erythematous, slowly enlarging skin lesion at the site of a tick bite. A flulike illness, with symptoms of aseptic meningitis and a mild encephalitis, soon follows the appearance of the rash. Joint pain and swelling may begin 1 month or more after onset. The knees and ankles are usually involved, but shoulders, elbows, and wrists may also be affected. The diagnosis can be confirmed by an enzyme-linked immunosorbent assay (ELISA) for IgM or IgG antibody to *Borrelia burgdorferi*. Joint symptoms respond to therapy with penicillin or ceftriaxone. Infection with *hepatitis B virus* may cause a pruritic skin rash and a migratory or additive polyarthritis that may involve the shoulders (30 percent of cases). A positive serum test for hepatitis B surface antigen and/or abnormal liver function tests support the diagnosis. Joint complaints may respond to aspirin. An acute onset of shoulder pain, swelling, and dysfunction in a patient *with hemophilia or on anticoagulant therapy* suggests an *acute hemarthrosis*. The diagnosis can be confirmed by a CT scan or MRI of the shoulder or by needle aspiration of the glenohumeral joint after correction of the coagulation defect.

Osteomyelitis of the shoulder may involve the humerus, adjacent glenoid, or acromion. There are local pain, swelling, and bone tenderness. An MRI or radionuclide bone scan may demonstrate a bony abnormality within 1 to 2 weeks of the onset of symptoms, while plain radiographs may remain negative for up to 8 weeks. The diagnosis can be confirmed by bone biopsy and culture. There is a therapeutic response to intravenous antibiotic therapy. Most cases in adults are associated with penetrating trauma or reconstructive shoulder surgery.

Proximal humeral fractures are more common in the elderly, and they occur with relatively mild trauma (e.g., fall on an outstretched arm) because of osteoporosis. There is pain and loss of shoulder mobility. The arm is held close to the side, and motion is resisted. The fracture may be palpated beneath the deltoid muscle or in the axilla. Local tenderness and bony crepitus may be present on examination. Plain radiographs of the shoulder will demonstrate the presence or absence of one or more fractures and the extent of fracture displacement. *Fractures* may be *associated with glenohumeral joint dislocation.*

A *pathologic fracture of the humerus* should be suspected if the fracture occurs spontaneously or with minimal trauma. Causes include metastatic or primary bone tumors, osteoporosis, osteomalacia, and Paget's disease. Plain radiographs may identify the associated disease, or superior definition may be achieved with a CT scan or MRI. Bone biopsy will specif-

ically identify the responsible lesion. *Anterior dislocation* of the humerus follows excessive extension, external rotation, and abduction of the arm. Lateral shoulder pain and loss of movement at the glenohumeral joint occur. The arm is held abducted and externally rotated. The patient cannot place the affected arm across the chest and rest the hand on the opposite shoulder. The shoulder profile is squared off below the acromion, and the humerus is absent from the glenohumeral joint. Plain radiographs will confirm the diagnosis. Reduction immediately relieves pain and shoulder dysfunction. *Posterior dislocation* is uncommon (5 percent of cases) and may be caused by an anterior blow or excessive internal rotation, flexion, and adduction of the arm. Posterior dislocation may follow a grand mal seizure or a severe electric shock. The affected shoulder may have a posterior glenohumeral defect or a squared-off appearance and an empty glenohumeral joint space. The humeral head may be palpable posteriorly. Abduction and external rotation of the involved arm are restricted. The arm is held at the side, adducted, and internally rotated. Plain radiographs will confirm the dislocation, although up to 80 percent of cases are initially missed because of failure to read the radiographs correctly. Important confirmatory radiographic signs include the vacant glenoid sign and the 6-mm rim sign. A CT scan may be required to confirm posterior dislocation. Symptoms resolve after closed reduction. *Fracture of the humeral shaft* may cause pain, swelling, tenderness, crepitus, and deformity in the midportion of the upper arm. Arm shortening of 2.5 to 5 cm may occur. The diagnosis can be confirmed by plain radiographs. *Acromioclavicular separation* causes medial shoulder pain that is intensified by abduction of the arm. The diagnosis can be established by palpation of the acromioclavicular joint and by plain radiographs. A *clavicular fracture* causes localized pain, tenderness, and swelling over the clavicle. A bony deformity and crepitus may be palpable. The diagnosis can be confirmed by a plain radiograph. *Rupture of the biceps tendon or muscle* occurs during lifting. There is a sudden pop followed by the appearance of a convex muscle bunch in the profile of the upper arm on attempted forearm flexion. Pain occurs in the shoulder, axilla, and anterior upper arm.

Pectoralis major insertional tendinitis is a rare disorder. Pain and swelling occur in the affected shoulder and upper arm. Soft tissue calcification or a cortical bone defect near the pectoralis insertion may be detected by plain radiographs. Differentiation from parosteal osteosarcoma may require surgical exploration. *Osteonecrosis of the humeral head* may cause glenohumeral joint pain that is intensified by movement. The pain is usually persistent and severe. Plain radiographs may remain normal for months, but early bone abnormalities may be detected within weeks of onset by MRI or a radionuclide bone scan. Most cases follow chronic use of corticosteroids. Diseases such as sickle cell anemia, alcoholism, caisson disease, hyperlipidemia, and systemic lupus erythematosus may also be associated with humeral osteonecrosis. Some cases follow severe shoulder trauma and complex proximal humeral fractures.

Neuralgic amyotrophy begins with severe, persistent aching or burning shoulder and upper arm pain that is intensified by upper arm movement. Within weeks, paresis of shoulder girdle and proximal arm muscles occurs. Bilateral involvement is frequent. Electrodiagnostic studies help in excluding a radicular origin of the pain and weakness. *Cervical radiculopathy* (C5 and C6) may cause neck, shoulder, scapula, and upper arm pain. The pain is aching or burning and is intensified by neck rotation, coughing, or straining. Weakness of arm abduction (C5) and forearm flexion (C5 and C6) may be present. The biceps reflex may be diminished. MRI of the cervical spine will usually demonstrate the causative nerve root compressing lesion. Referred pain to the shoulder arises at a distant site. The pain is dull, aching, and continuous. It may be intensified by a deep inspiration, a change in position, and, less commonly, by neck and shoulder movement. There is no abnormality of the shoulder, the glenohumeral joint, or the upper arm.

Cardiac disorders such as *acute pericarditis* and *acute myocardial infarction* may cause unilateral or bilateral shoulder pain. Central and precordial chest pain may be associated. Pericardial pain involves the trapezius ridge and medial shoulder. It is intensified by lying flat and/or taking a deep breath and relieved by sitting up. The shoulder pain of myocardial infarction is a dull ache or pressure and is unaffected by position or respiration. The diagnosis of pericarditis or myocardial infarction can be supported by serial electrocardiographic studies, echocardiography, and measurement of serum cardiac isozyme levels.

Shoulder pain that is intensified or provoked by a deep breath may be referred from a pleuritic process involving the diaphragm. Causes include *pneumonia*, *pulmonary infarction*, *primary pleuritis due to systemic lupus erythematosus* or *another collagen vascular disorder*, and *tuberculous pleuritis*. The physical examination may reveal evidence of consolidation (e.g., pneumonia or pulmonary infarction) or pleural fluid. Plain chest radiographs may demonstrate infiltrates in patients with pneumonia or pulmonary infarction and a clear lung parenchyma in patients with primary pleuritis or tuberculous pleuritis beginning shortly after primary tuberculous infection. Pneumonias respond to antibiotic therapy, pulmonary infarction to anticoagulant therapy, lupus pleuritis to prednisone, and tuberculous pleuritis to antituberculous drug therapy.

Acute cholecystitis may refer pain to the tip of the right shoulder, and *perforation and leakage of a duodenal ulcer* may also result in right shoulder pain that is intensified by a deep inspiration. *Benign or malignant gastric ulcers* may perforate and cause irritation of the left hemidiaphragm and left shoulder pain. *Hemoperitoneum* may cause aching and sharp unilateral or bilateral shoulder pain. Causes include rupture of a *tubal pregnancy*, *spontaneous or traumatic splenic rupture*, *hemorrhage from a benign or malignant hepatic tumor*, *abdominal apoplexy*, and *spontaneous rupture of a splanchnic artery aneurysm*. A *right or left subphrenic abscess* may cause pleuritic shoulder pain, upper abdominal and lower chest pain,

chills, and high fever. The diagnosis can be confirmed by CT or MRI. *Pneumoperitoneum* may also cause bilateral or unilateral shoulder pain. A *subclavian artery aneurysm* may cause shoulder pain as it expands. The aneurysm is usually palpable in the supraclavicular region or axilla, and/or it can be demonstrated by selective arteriography.

Axillary Pain

Axillary pain may be caused by *infections* that produce a *local cutaneous abscess* (*Staphylococcus aureus*) or *multiple skin abscesses* (*hidradenitis suppurativa*). Painful axillary adenopathy may result from inoculation of an infectious agent into the skin of the hand or forearm. A local papule, vesicle, pustule, or ulcer may form at the inoculation site. *Cat-scratch disease* follows within 2 weeks of one or more upper extremity cat scratches. It may cause axillary node tenderness and enlargement and aching axillary pain. The diagnosis is suggested by a history of a cat scratch and may be supported by the histopathologic findings of a lymph node biopsy.

Streptococcal lymphadenitis causes severe systemic symptoms and painful, tender axillary lymphadenitis associated with extensive chest wall, shoulder, and arm edema. *Staphylococcal lymphadenitis* occurs secondary to a furuncle on the hand. Diffuse hand swelling, redness, and pain and ascending *lymphangitis* are associated with axillary pain and tender adenopathy.

Patients with leukemia undergoing chemotherapy may develop a painful axillary cellulitis, lymphadenitis, and cutaneous ulceration. The causative organism is usually *Pseudomonas aeruginosa*, other gram-negative rods, or *S. aureus*.

Tularemia follows contact with wild rabbit or muskrat tissue or a tick bite. The initial cutaneous lesion occurs on the hand or forearm. Fever, chills, and painful axillary adenopathy follow. The distal site forms a persistent punched-out ulcer. Diagnosis is dependent on the clinical history and the microagglutination test for antibody to *Francisella tularensis*.

A painful, massive axillary nodal swelling may occur in association with fever and systemic symptoms in a patient with *bubonic plague*. Recent residence in an endemic region is suggestive of the diagnosis in a patient with an axillary bubo and fever. Confirmation requires isolation of *Yersinia pestis* from an involved node or the blood. The organism can be rapidly identified by staining a bubo aspirate with Gram's or Wayson's stains.

Animal or human bite wounds of the hand or forearm may cause a local cellulitis; lymphangitis; fever; chills; and painful, tender axillary adenopathy.

Axillary pain due to a phlebitic cord of the axillary vein can occur in a patient with *axillary-subclavian vein thrombosis*. Arm and shoulder pain, reddish-purple arm discoloration and swelling, and distension of shoulder and arm veins may be present at rest or following exercise of the arm (e.g., weightlifting or push-ups). The diagnosis can be confirmed by venography. Axillary pain may result from a *proximal humeral fracture*, from *costochondritis*, from a *muscle strain* involving muscles in the axillary region during use of the arm and shoulder, and from *gaseous distension of the stomach*. An *acute pneumothorax* may cause anterior chest and axillary pleuritic pain and dyspnea. *Breast lesions*, such as a rapidly enlarging cyst, tumor, or abscess, may cause axillary pain. *Pleuropulmonary disease*, such as a *tumor*, *pyogenic abscess*, or *actinomycosis*, may extend from the pleural surface into the upper lateral chest wall (axillary region), and the extent of invasion may be clearly defined by a CT scan. These lesions cause axillary and shoulder pain by direct invasion of the chest wall. Rarely, a T1 *radiculopathy* caused by a T1–T2 disc herniation may cause neck, axillary, shoulder, and medial arm pain. The diagnosis can be confirmed by CT myelography or MRI of the upper thoracic and cervical spine. Persistent axillary pain and hypesthesia of the upper inner arm and axilla may follow *axillary node dissection* in patients undergoing surgery for breast cancer.

☐ DESCRIPTION OF LISTED DISEASES

Shoulder and Upper Arm Pain

1. CALCIFIC TENDINITIS AND SUBDELTOID BURSITIS

There is an abrupt onset of severe-to-excruciating shoulder pain. It is localized over the glenohumeral joint and may radiate distally to the site of the deltoid insertion. The arm is held adducted at the side, and any attempts at movement by the examiner are resisted. Swelling, warmth, and severe localized tenderness are present over the greater tuberosity of the humerus, and there is more diffuse tenderness over the shoulder and upper arm.

Plain radiographs of the shoulder (anteroposterior), taken in a neutral position and in internal and external

TABLE OF DISEASE INCIDENCE

INCIDENCE PER 100,000 (APPROXIMATE)

Common (>100)	Uncommon (>5–100)	Rare (>0–5)
SHOULDER AND UPPER ARM PAIN		
Calcific tendinitis and subdeltoid bursitis	Pseudogout of the glenohumeral joint	Septic glenohumeral arthritis
Proximal humeral fracture	Acute rheumatic fever	Gout of the glenohumeral joint
Anterior glenohumeral dislocation	Reiter's syndrome	Acute hemarthrosis of the glenohumeral joint
Acromioclavicular separation	Lyme arthritis	Acute osteomyelitis of the shoulder
Fracture of the clavicle	Hepatitis B–associated arthritis	Pathologic fracture of the humerus
	Proximal humeral fracture and glenohumeral dislocation	Pectoralis major tendinitis
	Posterior glenohumeral dislocation	Referred shoulder pain due to tuberculous pleuritis; perforation of an ulcer of the duodenum or stomach; perforation of a gastric carcinoma; hemoperitoneum caused by spontaneous splenic rupture, hepatic tumor hemorrhage, abdominal apoplexy, or splanchnic artery aneurysm rupture; subphrenic abscess; and pneumoperitoneum
	Fracture of the humeral shaft	
	Rupture of the biceps muscle or tendon	
	Osteonecrosis of the humeral head	
	Neuralgic amyotrophy	
	Cervical radiculopathy (C5, C6)	
	Referred shoulder pain due to acute pericarditis, acute myocardial infarction, pneumonia and pleuritis, pulmonary infarction and pleuritis, Lupus pleuritis, Acute cholecystitis, and hemoperitoneum caused by ruptured tubal pregnancy or traumatic splenic rupture	Subclavian-axillary artery aneurysm
AXILLARY PAIN		
Cat-scratch disease	Staphylococcal axillary lymphadenitis	Streptococcal axillary lymphadenitis
Axillary skin abscess	Axillary infections in leukemia	Tularemia
Hidradenitis suppurativa	Human bite	Bubonic plague
Animal bite	Pneumothorax	Axillary-subclavian venous thrombosis
Fracture of proximal humerus	Pleuropulmonary disease caused by carcinoma of the lung	Pleuropulmonary disease caused by pyogenic lung abscess, actinomycosis, or lymphoma
Costochondritis with axillary pain radiation	Postaxillary dissection pain	Radicular pain involving the T1 root
Myalgic pain		
Gaseous gastric distension		
Breast disorders in women		

rotation, usually demonstrate calcium in the supraspinatus tendon or in the tendons of the infraspinatus or teres minor muscles. Rupture of a tendinous calcium deposit into the subdeltoid bursa may appear as a thin, radiopaque crescent overlying the tendon calcification that may outline the extent of the bursa. Calcium deposits observed during the acute symptomatic phase of this disorder are often fluffy, cloudlike, and poorly defined and may be barely visible on a plain radiograph.

The adjacent bursa may or may not become inflamed secondary to calcium deposition near or in the bursal sac. Injection of lidocaine into the region of tenderness, followed by needling of the calcific mass and sterile saline lavage, produces dramatic pain relief in 61 to 79 percent of cases. It may be necessary to repeat lidocaine injection two or three times. Addition of corticosteroids to the local anesthestic does not appear to accelerate symptom resolution or provide additional benefit. Surgical removal of a large calcium deposit is reserved for patients who fail to improve after needling of the calcific region in the tendon and injection of lidocaine.

2. ACUTE ARTHRITIS

A. Septic Arthritis of the Glenohumeral Joint

The onset may be acute or more insidious. There is moderate-to-severe aching pain in the affected shoulder. Arm movements intensify the pain, so that range of motion is limited and the arm is usually held extended and at the side. Anteromedial fluctuant glenohumeral swelling and overlying skin erythema and warmth may be present. In some cases, the swelling may be a primary subcutaneous abscess that communicates with the joint.

Diffuse or localized tenderness may be present over the shoulder. In one report, fever occurred in 57 percent, leukocytosis in 50 percent, and an elevated sedimentation rate in 100 percent of cases. The diagnosis may be established by aspiration of synovial fluid. The fluid is usually turbid, and yellow or brown in color. The cell count ranges from 10,000 to over 100,000 leukocytes per cubic millimeter, and the predominant cell is the polymorphonuclear leukocyte. Up to 50 percent of patients with septic arthritis have a joint fluid glucose concentration that is less than 50 percent of the serum level. A Gram stain of synovial fluid will demonstrate the responsible pathogen in 67 percent of cases, while cultures are positive in 90 percent of cases. Blood cultures may be positive in up to 50 percent. Radiographic studies may demonstrate early lytic lesions of osteomyelitis. CT and MRI are more sensitive than plain radiographs for detection of the early changes of osteomyelitis. Septic arthritis of the shoulder joint usually occurs in the elderly (mean age, 65 years) and in patients having one or more serious medical disorders (e.g., diabetes mellitus, rheumatoid arthritis, al-

coholic cirrhosis, malignancy, or a cardiomyopathy). Previous injection or aspiration of the shoulder joint is an important risk factor and, in one series, accounted for up to 44 percent of cases. *S. aureus* is the most common joint pathogen and is even more frequent in cases following joint injection or aspiration. *Neisseria gonorrhoeae* is the most common pathogen in sexually active adults and adolescents. *Streptococcus pyogenes*, *Streptococcus pneumoniae*, group B streptococci, and gram-negative enteric organisms (*Escherichia coli*, *Proteus mirabilis*, and *Salmonella* species) have also been reported to cause septic glenohumeral arthritis. *Pseudomonas aeruginosa* and *Serratia marcescens* are the most likely pathogens to be found in the infected glenohumeral joint of an intravenous drug abuser. Septic arthritis may arise by the hematogenous route or may be secondary to an adjacent osteomyelitis. Direct spread to the glenohumeral joint from a penetrating missile, knife, or surgical wound or a foreign body (e.g., total joint and internal fixation devices) is the most frequent cause of septic arthritis in adults. Despite operative drainage of the glenohumeral joint and the administration of intravenous antibiotics, functional results are usually poor, and up to 50 percent of patients are left without active motion at the glenohumeral joint.

B. Crystal-Induced Synovitis of the Glenohumeral Joint

1. Acute Gout Severe pain, swelling, and redness of the shoulder may occur, and the temperature may reach 39°C (103°F). There is marked limitation of movement of the glenohumeral joint. An initial attack involving the shoulder is rare. Most patients relate a history of one or more episodes of acute arthritis of the first metatarsophalangeal joint (podagra) or one or both ankles, knees, or wrists. Aspirated synovial fluid contains increased numbers of polymorphonuclear leukocytes and monosodium urate crystals. The serum uric acid level is usually elevated. Gout may also cause an acute subacromial bursitis or an acute rotator cuff tendinitis. Glenohumeral arthritis may occur with postoperative gout or in postmenopausal women with polyarticular gout. Colchicine is a specific and effective therapeutic agent in this disorder and usually relieves symptoms within 24 to 48 h.

2. Pseudogout This disorder may present with acute shoulder pain, swelling, tenderness, erythema, and warmth. The arm is held adducted close to the side, and attempts to move it are resisted. Linear, punctate, and stippled calcifications cap the humeral head (i.e., chondrocalcinosis) in up to 50 percent of cases. Synovial fluid contains increased numbers of polymorphonuclear leukocytes and calcium pyrophosphate dihydrate crystals. The knees, wrists, and hips are most frequently involved, but the shoulder may be the first symptomatic joint. Colchicine and nonsteroidal anti-inflammatory drugs are effective. Hyperparathyroidism and hemochromatosis should be excluded in patients with polyarticular pseudogout.

C. Acute Rheumatic Fever   Fever, pain, redness, and swelling of the knees, hips, ankles, elbows, wrists, and shoulders may occur. The involvement is often asymmetrical and migratory, with new joints becoming involved as others begin to improve. Subcutaneous nodules may be felt over the extensor surface of the wrist or elbow region. Shoulder pain and limitation of motion may be severe. There may be a history of a sore throat or ''cold'' 2 to 5 weeks prior to onset (67 percent of cases). Serum levels of antihyaluronidase, antistreptolysin O, and antideoxyribonuclease B are usually elevated. The streptozyme test is a sensitive screening test for detection of a recent group A streptococcal infection. There is an excellent therapeutic response to aspirin therapy. Recurrent attacks of acute arthritis may be prevented by daily oral administration of penicillin.

D. Reiter's Syndrome   Patients present with an asymmetrical polyarthritis (96 percent of cases). Knees, ankles, and hips may be painful and swollen. Shoulder involvement is common and may occur on one or both sides. Urethritis occurs in up to 88 percent of cases, but it is seldom severe (e.g., mild dysuria and scant discharge) and may be overlooked. Conjunctivitis causes mild itching or a foreign body sensation in the eyes and a conjunctival discharge. In some cases, ocular redness is caused by iritis or iridocyclitis. Eye involvement occurs in 59 percent of cases. Keratoderma blennorrhagicum (20 percent of cases) may involve the soles of the feet, glans penis, and toes. Isolated lesions may occur on the scrotum, palms, scalp, and trunk. The skin lesions begin as vesicles and then evolve into hyperkeratotic nodules. A painless circinate balanitis may affect the glans and foreskin (23–50 percent of cases). Back pain occurs in 70 percent and heel pain in 58 percent. The latter is due to Achilles tendinitis, plantar fasciitis, and/or arthritic involvement of the subtalar joints. Enthesopathic features include sausage digits, insertional tendinitis, sacroiliitis, periostitis, spurs, peri-insertional osteoporosis, and erosions. The diagnosis is based on clinical features. Prior to the availability of adequate culture media for *N. gonorrhoeae*, this disorder was frequently confused with acute gonococcal arthritis.

E. Lyme Arthritis   This disease follows a tick bite. The initial manifestation is a flat or slightly elevated erythematous rash. It soon develops central clearing and expands outward as a large annular lesion (erythema migrans). Within 1 to 2 weeks, a febrile disease develops, with myalgias, arthralgias, fever, headache, neck pain, and stiffness. Joint pain and swelling involving the shoulders, elbows, wrists, knees, and ankles may develop during the next 1 to 12 months. The diagnosis can be confirmed by an ELISA test for serum antibody to *B. burgdorferi*. There is a good therapeutic response to intravenous penicillin or ceftriaxone therapy.

F. Hepatitis B-Associated Arthritis   A symmetrical or asymmetrical migratory or additive polyarthritis occurs, lasting several days to as long as 6 months. The fingers are most commonly involved (70 percent), but shoulder joint pain and swelling may occur in 30 percent. Wrists (22 percent), elbows (25 percent), and knees (35 percent) are also frequently involved. A pruritic, urticarial, maculopapular, or petechial rash may occur in up to 50 percent of cases. Abnormal liver function test results and/or a positive serum test result for hepatitis B surface antigen supports the diagnosis. There may be a therapeutic response to salicylates.

G. Acute Hemarthrosis Secondary to Hemophilia or Anticoagulant Therapy   There is an abrupt onset of severe shoulder pain, loss of mobility, and swelling. A CT scan or MRI of the shoulder will reveal intraarticular hemorrhage. An aspirate of the joint contains nonclotting blood. Causes include hemophilia, trauma, and anticoagulant therapy. Secondary bacterial infection and septic arthritis may develop. Hemophilic hemarthrosis can be treated by administration of factor VIII, followed by aspiration and removal of the intraarticular blood.

3. ACUTE OSTEOMYELITIS

Acute hematogenous osteomyelitis is usually a disease of children, but it may be seen in intravenous drug abusers and in adult patients with sickle cell disease. Severe shoulder pain, swelling, and immobility; warmth and redness of the overlying skin; and local bone tenderness may occur. Systemic symptoms such as fever, chills, malaise, and nausea suggest infection. Plain radiographs may remain negative for 2 to 8 weeks after the onset of symptoms. In patients with negative plain radiographs, MRI may demonstrate an irregular area of decreased signal in the humerus or clavicle and evidence of glenohumeral joint fluid. A technetium bone scan may show increased uptake over the affected humerus in up to 90 percent of cases. The diagnosis can be confirmed by a Craig needle bone biopsy. There is a good response to antibiotic therapy. Most cases in adults follow penetrating trauma of the humerus, clavicle, or scapula, or are a complication of reconstructive shoulder surgery. In adults, the humerus is the most frequently involved, but the clavicle is occasionally infected hematogeneously in drug addicts. The scapula may be infected by an intraarticular corticosteroid injection or joint aspiration.

4. TRAUMA

A. Proximal Fractures of the Humerus Local pain, tenderness, and crepitus over the glenohumeral joint and superolateral axilla occur. The pain is aching and persistent and prevents use of the arm. Attempts to flex or abduct the arm intensify the pain and are avoided. The arm is held adducted at the side. Proximal humeral fractures have been classified as minimally displaced (e.g., no segment displaced more than 1 cm or angulated more than 45°) or displaced. Fractures may occur through the anatomic neck (the constricted border of the articular surface), but displacement without separation of the tuberosities seldom occurs. A fracture through the surgical neck (more distal, narrowed region of the shaft below the tuberosities) may be displaced or impacted into the head of the humerus. Open reduction may result in avascular necrosis of the humeral head. Avulsion of the greater tuberosity with upward displacement may occur as an isolated injury or in association with a fracture of the surgical neck. The latter injury may result in posterior rotation of the articular segment. The blood supply to the head of the humerus is usually intact, and aseptic necrosis does not develop. An avulsion fracture of the lesser tuberosity may also occur. With an associated fracture through the surgical neck (three-part injury), the humeral head may be abducted and externally rotated. The articular surface may be rotated anteriorly. If both tuberosities are avulsed (four-part fracture), the blood supply to the head may be lost. Classification of displaced fractures into the categories described requires only plain radiographs of the shoulder.

B. Proximal Fracture and Dislocation of the Humerus Anterior glenohumeral joint dislocation and a proximal humeral fracture result in severe shoulder pain and tenderness. The shoulder has a squared-off contour, and the acromion appears unusually prominent. The absence of the humeral head from the glenoid can be palpated anterolaterally. Comparison with the uninjured side is helpful. Dislocation may be anterior or posterior. The diagnosis can be confirmed by plain radiographs, and relationships can be more clearly defined by a CT scan.

C. Pathologic Fracture Most fractures of the proximal humerus occur in the elderly and follow relatively minor trauma. The incidence is high in this age group because of osteoporosis.

Pathologic fractures may also occur secondary to osteomalacia, Paget's disease, and benign or malignant bone tumors. A history of mild trauma or no trauma preceding the onset of sharp, severe shoulder pain and loss of arm mobility is suggestive of pathologic fracture. Plain radiographs of the shoulder will usually identify metabolic or neoplastic bone disease in the proximal humerus. MRI may identify areas of bone neoplasia not visible on plain radiographs.

D. Acute Dislocation of the Glenohumeral Joint

1. Anterior Dislocation Anterior dislocation is the most common direction of displacement (95 percent of cases). Excessive extension, external rotation, and abduction of the arm constitute the usual cause. Severe pain and immobility occur at the shoulder. The arm is held abducted and in slight external rotation. The patient cannot place the ipsilateral hand across the chest and rest it on the contralateral shoulder. A subcoracoid dislocation may produce a posterior glenohumeral defect and a prominent acromion. The subacromial region may have a squared-off contour, and the humeral head may be absent from the glenoid if the humeral head is dislocated inferiorly. Plain radiographs can confirm the diagnosis. Closed reduction is usually possible and results in immediate relief of pain and immobility.

2. Posterior Dislocation The head of the humerus may be dislocated posteriorly by a direct blow to the anterior shoulder or by a force applied to the arm and shoulder that causes internal rotation, flexion, and adduction of the upper arm. Accidental electric shock or convulsions cause tonic internal rotation of the arms and may result in a posterior dislocation. There is shoulder pain and immobility. The arm is held in adduction and internal rotation. The glenoid is empty, and the bulge of the humeral head can be felt posteriorly. Abduction and external rotation of the involved arm are severely limited. There is an inability to supinate the forearm with the upper arm flexed to 90°. Plain radiographs should include a true anteroposterior view of the shoulder (35–45° oblique to the trunk), a lateral and a physician-assisted axillary view, and a standard anteroposterior view. Dislocation can be confirmed by the vacant glenoid sign and the 6 mm rim sign (seen on a standard anteroposterior view). The vacant glenoid sign is a void observed in the anterior half of the glenoid, and the 6 mm rim sign is present when the distance between the anterior rim of the glenoid and the humeral head exceeds 6 mm. The diagnosis of posterior dislocation is missed in 60 to 80 percent of cases at the initial examination because of an incomplete physical examination and/or radiographic study.

A CT may be helpful in defining the relationship of the humeral head to the glenoid. Closed reduction, using lateral traction, external rotation of the arm, and posterior pressure on the humeral head, will usually relieve shoulder pain and restore a full range of arm motion.

E. Fracture of the Humeral Shaft Pain, swelling, and tenderness occur in the midportion of the upper arm. Crepitus may be present when the proximal and distal fragments are palpated. The arm may be shortened 2 to 5 cm. Deformity of the upper arm may be visible. Fractures of the humeral shaft may be caused by direct blows, arm wrestling, a fall on the hand or elbow, a gunshot wound, or a fall with the arm at the side. Fractures caused by a direct blow are usually transverse or comminuted, while those caused by violent muscular action or a fall on the outstretched arm are spiral. Radial nerve injury may occur, resulting in wrist drop and/or hypesthesia of the dorsum of the hand. Plain radiographs will establish the diagnosis. Fractures occurring in patients older than 65 years are usually associated with osteoporosis.

F. Acromioclavicular Separation   This injury varies in severity. It is usually caused by a direct blow or a fall on the shoulder. Pain occurs over the region of the acromioclavicular joint. The clavicle may be displaced upward or depressed in relation to the acromion. Local swelling and ecchymoses may be present. The diagnosis can be established by palpation and confirmed by plain radiographs.

G. Fractures of the Clavicle   Patients have local pain, tenderness, bony crepitus and deformity, soft tissue swelling, and skin ecchymoses. The bony deformity caused by the fracture may be palpated and confirmed by plain radiography.

5. RUPTURE OF THE BICEPS MUSCLE OR ITS TENDON

The patient usually reports a sudden snap or pop while lifting a heavy object. Pain may occur at the shoulder, in the axilla, and over the upper anterior arm. On attempted flexion of the forearm, the belly of the biceps forms a convex bunch in the distal portion of the upper arm (rupture of the long head of the biceps). A proximal convex bunch and antecubital fossa pain and tenderness occur with rupture of the distal biceps tendon. Rupture usually follows a forceful muscle contraction.

In other patients, biceps rupture is related to repetitive impingement of the biceps tendon and secondary tendinous degeneration.

2. TENDINITIS OF THE PECTORALIS MAJOR MUSCLE

Pain and swelling occur in the shoulder and upper arm. Movement at the shoulder is restricted. A plain radiograph of the humerus may show a soft tissue calcification adjacent to the upper humerus and/or subperiosteal new bone formation at the insertion of the pectoralis major muscle. A lytic cortical bone lesion may also occur. At exploration, the tendon of the pectoralis major muscle shows evidence of degeneration and replacement of ruptured fibers with granulation tissue. The disorder may radiolog-

ically mimic a parosteal osteosarcoma. Differentiation may require surgical exploration.

7. OSTEONECROSIS OF THE HUMERAL HEAD

Severe and persistent pain may occur in the glenohumeral area. The pain is intensified by elevation and abduction of the arm. In some cases, pain only occurs with shoulder movement. Plain radiographs may remain normal for months after the onset of pain. A radionuclide bone scan or MRI may provide evidence of an abnormality of the humeral head long before changes occur on a plain radiograph. Stage 1 (preradiologic disease) may progress but usually resolves. Nontraumatic osteonecrosis is frequently associated with the use of corticosteroids. Disorders associated with osteonecrosis of the head of the humerus are listed in Table 39-1.

8. NEURALGIC AMYOTROPHY (BRACHIAL NEUROPATHY)

There is an abrupt onset of severe, persistent, aching shoulder and upper arm pain. The pain may sometimes be burning or stabbing. It is intensified by arm movement at the shoulder but not by neck rotation, straining, coughing, or sneezing. Severe shoulder and upper arm tenderness may be present. Bilateral pain is frequent. The pain may last for up to 2 weeks or longer. Muscle weakness or paralysis develops as the pain resolves. The deltoid, serratus anterior, and spinati muscles are most frequently involved. Muscle weakness in patients with bilateral disease is often more severe on one side.

Hypesthesia may occur over a small area of the lateral shoulder and upper arm. Sensory loss in the forearm and hand is rarely seen. Electrodiagnostic studies may demonstrate denervation of weakened muscles and other mus-

Table 39-1
DISORDERS ASSOCIATED WITH OSTEONECROSIS OF THE HUMERAL HEAD

Alcoholism
Cirrhosis of the liver
Pancreatitis
Sickle cell anemia (SS or SC disease)
Hyperuricemia and gout
Hyperlipidemia
Gaucher's disease
Lymphoma
Systemic lupus erythematosus
Rheumatoid arthritis
Decompression sickness
Radiation therapy
Corticosteroid therapy (oral, parenteral, or intraarticular)
Trauma

cle groups not clinically paretic. The paraspinal muscles show no evidence of denervation. Sensory nerve action potentials are decreased, since the neural involvement is postganglionic. MRI of the cervical spine is normal. Recovery occurs spontaneously and slowly, and may take 2 or more years. There is no specific therapy.

9. CERVICAL RADICULOPATHY

Compression of roots C5 or C6 may cause shoulder and upper arm pain, as well as scapular pain. The pain is described as a persistent ache or burning discomfort. Lancinating jabs of pain may radiate down the arm to the hand. The biceps reflex may be diminished, and a C6 lesion may cause hypesthesia of the thumb. Weakness of upper arm abduction (C5) or forearm flexion and wrist extension (C6) may be present. Arm movement or use has no effect on the pain, but neck rotation or Spurling's maneuver may intensify constant pain or provoke lancinating radiating arm and hand pain. Actions that increase intraspinal pressure (e.g., sneezing, coughing, or straining at stool) may also intensify or provoke pain. MRI or a CT-enhanced myelogram of the cervical spine can demonstrate nerve root compression by a soft or hard disc, a narrow nerve root canal, an epidural hematoma, an abscess, or a tumor. Surgical intervention may be required to relieve persistent pain or to prevent progressive neurologic damage.

10. REFERRED SHOULDER PAIN

A. Cardiac

1. Pericarditis   Patients with acute pericarditis may present with left shoulder (trapezius ridge) pain or bilateral shoulder pain. There may be associated substernal and precordial pain. The shoulder pain may be aching or stabbing. It is usually intensified by lying flat or on the left side, and relieved by sitting up or standing. A deep breath may also intensify the shoulder and chest pain. Fever, weakness, sweating, and malaise may be associated. A pericardial friction rub may be present. The electrocardiogram may be normal or show generalized ST elevation in the limb and precordial leads. These ST segments become isoelectric within 1 to 2 weeks, and the associated T waves may remain normal, flatten, or become inverted. An echocardiogram may reveal pericardial fluid. Most cases of acute pericarditis are caused by viral infection or an autoimmune process (idiopathic); follow myocardial infarction, cardiac surgery, or trauma; or are associated with a collagen vascular disorder. There is a dramatic response of chest and shoulder pain and fever to prednisone within 1 to 2 days.

2. Myocardial Infarction   Severe aching may occur in the left upper arm and shoulder region. Associated substernal, elbow, forearm, and wrist pain may occur. Sweating, weakness, palpitations, and dizziness may be associated. The electrocardiogram reveals evidence of myocardial infarction. Serum lactic dehydrogenase and creatine kinase isozyme levels become elevated during the first 24 h. Thrombolytic therapy or direct angioplasty may relieve coronary artery obstruction and provide dramatic relief of symptoms. A coronary angiogram will define the causative lesion.

B. Pleural   Pleuritis involving the diaphragmatic pleura may cause aching shoulder pain that is intensified by a deep breath. Breathing becomes shallow and rapid because of the pain. The shoulder and neck may become tender, and after several hours of pain, neck and arm movements may also intensify the pain. This finding may lead to a misdiagnosis of a local musculoskeletal disorder. Lower anterolateral chest pain, intensified by breathing, may also occur. Pleuritic chest and shoulder pain may be associated with the following disorders.

1. Pneumonia   *S. pneumoniae* (25–60 percent of cases), *Hemophilus influenzae* (4–15 percent of cases), *S. aureus* (2–10 percent of cases), gram-negative bacteria, and *Legionella pneumophila* are the commonest causes of community-acquired pneumonia. Aspiration pneumonia caused by aerobic and anaerobic bacteria may also be associated with pleuritic shoulder and anterolateral chest pain.

Pneumonia may cause cough with purulent or rusty sputum, fever, and dyspnea. A chest radiograph may show patchy, segmental, or lobar infiltrates and/or a pleural effusion. There is a good response to antibiotic therapy.

2. Pulmonary Embolism and Infarction   Pulmonary infarction may cause cough, dyspnea, fever, and in some cases hemoptysis. There is no purulent sputum. A chest radiograph may show a patchy infiltrate; a pleural-based, wedge-shaped infiltrate; Kerley's B lines; or segmental opacities. The lung scan will be high-probability, and symptoms may resolve rapidly after initiation of heparin therapy.

3. Primary Pleuritis due to Systemic Lupus Erythematosus or Other Collagen Vascular Disorders   Pleuritis may occur in the absence of pneumonia or pulmonary infarction. A pleural effusion and/or a pleural friction rub may be present. The breath sounds over the affected pleural space are decreased. Patients with pleuritis secondary to systemic lupus may have fever, shoulder and chest pain, dyspnea, and profound weakness. The pleural fluid antinuclear antibody (ANA) titer is at least 1:160 and may be higher than the serum ANA titer. There is no parenchymal infiltrate, and the lung scan is negative or low-probability. There is a dramatic therapeutic response to oral administration of prednisone.

4. Tuberculosis Tuberculous pleuritis may cause fever, cough, and unilateral pleuritic anterolateral chest and shoulder pain. An ipsilateral pleural effusion is usually present. Coexistent pulmonary lesions may be observed in up to 30 percent of cases. The pleural fluid leukocyte count ranges from 500 to 2500 cells/mm³. The differential count reveals over 90 percent lymphocytes in 67 percent of cases. Initial taps may reveal a predominance of polymorphonuclear leukocytes in 12 percent of cases. Culture for *Mycobacterium tuberculosis* is positive in 25 to 33 percent, and pleural needle biopsy reveals granulomas in up to 75 percent of cases. Culture of the biopsy may be positive in the absence of histologic evidence of granulomatous pleuritis. Tuberculin skin test results are positive in over 90 percent of cases, but a negative result does not exclude pleural tuberculosis. Pleural tuberculosis usually occurs in young persons after primary infection but may occur in older patients with active chronic pulmonary tuberculosis. The shoulder and chest pain, fever, and pleural effusion may resolve spontaneously in 2 to 4 months without treatment or more rapidly with isoniazid and rifampin therapy.

C. Intraabdominal Inflammation

1. Acute Cholecystitis Patients may have epigastric, right upper abdominal, and subscapular pain and right shoulder tip pain that are intensified by a deep breath. Fever, chills, sweats, nausea, and vomiting may be associated. There may be right subcostal tenderness and guarding. The diagnosis can be confirmed by ultrasongraphy and a cholescintigraphy with ⁹⁹ᵐTc-diisopropyl iminodiacetic acid.

2. Duodenal or Gastric Ulcer Perforation of a duodenal ulcer or a benign gastric ulcer of the stomach into the subdiaphragmatic region may cause a subphrenic abscess or erosion of the diaphragm, with aching and/or pleuritic right shoulder pain (duodenal ulcer) or left shoulder pain (gastric ulcer).

3. Gastric Carcinoma Perforation of an ulcerative carcinoma of the stomach may cause left shoulder pain that is intensified by respiration. The diagnosis can be confirmed by detection of free air under the diaphragm and by exploration. Some cases develop insidiously and present with shoulder pain secondary to a subphrenic abscess. These cases can be detected by a CT scan or MRI of the abdomen.

D. Hemoperitoneum

Intraperitoneal bleeding may irritate the undersurface of the diaphragm and cause unilateral or bilateral shoulder pain.

1. Ruptured Ectopic Pregnancy Lower abdominal pain on one or both sides, amenorrhea, and/or vaginal spotting or bleeding may precede rupture by several weeks. There is an abrupt onset of generalized abdominal pain and tenderness and shoulder pain that is intensified by a deep breath. Nausea, vomiting, tenesmus, and fainting may also occur. Orthostatic or supine hypotension, tachypnea, and tachycardia result from hypovolemia due to intraabdominal bleeding. Direct and rebound abdominal tenderness and guarding may occur after tubal rupture. Bowel sounds are usually hypoactive or absent. The serum human chorionic gonadotropin (HCG) level is usually elevated. Transvaginal ultrasonography reveals absence of an intrauterine gestation, and this finding, useful for the diagnosis of an ectopic gestation, has a low false-positive rate if the HCG level exceeds 1400 mIU/ml. Transvaginal ultrasonography may allow detection of the adnexal mass produced by the tubal pregnancy. Surgical exploration is required to control bleeding and to excise the ruptured tubal pregnancy.

2. Spontaneous Rupture of the Spleen Rupture of the spleen has been reported with malaria, infectious mononucleosis, polycythemia vera, sarcoidosis, hemolytic anemia, congestive splenomegaly, acute and chronic lymphocytic leukemia, acute and chronic myelocytic leukemia, and Hodgkin's and non-Hodgkin's lymphoma. A normal spleen may also rupture spontaneously, and such cases may result from minor trauma. Splenic enlargement is observed in up to 70 percent of leukemia and lymphoma patients at the time of splenic rupture. Symptoms of rupture include diffuse abdominal pain and tenderness or localized left hypochondriac pain. Pain also occurs in the left shoulder (Kehr's sign). Dizziness on standing is associated with pallor, tachypnea, tachycardia, and hypotension.

Splenic rupture with intraabdominal bleeding can be detected by a CT scan of the abdomen. Intraabdominal hemorrhage can also be demonstrated by ultrasonography.

3. Traumatic Rupture of the Spleen Penetrating or blunt trauma may be responsible. Left lower posterior rib fractures may be associated. Generalized abdominal pain and left shoulder pain occur (Kehr's sign). Placing the patient in the Trendelenburg position may provoke left shoulder pain, if it is not present. Tenderness may be present in the left upper abdomen. Pallor, hypotension, tachycardia, tachypnea, and severe weakness are usually present. A CT scan will identify a subscapular hematoma, disruption of the spleen, and intraabdominal bleeding. Surgical exploration is required. Delayed rupture of the spleen may occur abruptly 1 to 3 weeks after the injury.

4. Hepatic Tumor Necrosis and/or bleeding from a hepatic tumor can cause generalized abdominal and shoulder pain. A CT scan or MRI will demonstrate the tumor and intraperitoneal hemorrhage.

5. Abdominal Apoplexy Diffuse abdominal pain and shoulder pain may follow spontaneous rupture of the splenic, hepatic, or gastroepiploic artery. Surgical exploration is required for diagnosis and treatment.

6. Rupture of a Splanchnic Artery Aneurysm Diffuse abdominal and left shoulder pain is accompanied by hypotension, tachycardia, pallor, and tachypnea. Abdominal tenderness, guarding, and distension and loss of bowel sounds occur. Selective mesenteric arteriography or surgical exploration will establish the diagnosis, and surgical excision of the aneurysm will control symptoms.

E. Subphrenic Abscess

1. Right Subphrenic Abscess A right subphrenic abscess may form secondary to rupture of a hepatic abscess or as a postoperative infection following gastroduodenal surgery. Localized right subphrenic collections may result from generalized peritonitis or from biliary tract surgery or an appendectomy. Pain may occur in the right upper anterior abdomen or right lower chest and in the right shoulder. Fever, chills, weakness, and weight loss are associated. Chest radiographs reveal an elevated right hemidiaphragm, pleural fluid, and atelectasis of a portion of the right lower lobe. The diagnosis can be confirmed by a CT scan or MRI. Drainage through a lateral subcostal incision and intravenous antibiotic therapy lead to resolution.

2. Left Subphrenic Abscess A left subphrenic abscess may be caused by peritonitis, a perforated stomach or colon, or pancreatitis. It may occur after splenectomy. Left upper abdominal and left shoulder pain (Kehr's sign), fever, and chills are commonly present. The diagnosis can be confirmed by a CT scan or MRI. Surgical drainage and antibiotic therapy are required for cure. A perinephric abscess may extend into a subphrenic space and cause back, flank, and/or shoulder pain. The diagnosis of perinephric abscess can be confirmed by ultrasonography or a CT scan.

F. Pneumoperitoneum Bilateral shoulder pain intensified by lying down may result from pneumoperitoneum. This diagnosis can be confirmed by an upright chest radiograph. Painful pneumoperitoneum may result from gastric or bowel perforation, orogenital insufflation during sexual foreplay, douching with an effervescent solution, or extension of a pneumothorax or pneumomediastinum into the peritoneal cavity.

The causes of referred shoulder pain are listed in Table 39-2.

11. SUBCLAVIAN-AXILLARY ARTERY ANEURYSM

There may be an abrupt onset of unilateral shoulder pain secondary to expansion of the aneurysm. The pain may remain localized to the shoulder, or, less commonly, it may radiate into the neck and down the arm. A palpable pulsatile mass is present in the supraclavicular or axillary region in 65 percent of cases. The diagnosis of a true aneurysm or pseudoaneurysm (secondary to trauma) can be confirmed by arteriography. Aneurysms in this region result from atherosclerosis, trauma, and thoracic outlet obstruction.

Axillary Pain

12. AXILLARY INFECTION

A. Cat-Scratch Disease This disorder results from a scratch by a cat. An erythematous papule, vesicle, or pustule develops at the site of the scratch within 1 to 2 weeks. Painful and tender axillary lymph node enlargement (2–4 cm) follows within 1 to 2 weeks. Axillary adenopathy occurs in up to 54 percent of cases. Other sites of nodal enlargement include cervical, preauricular, inguinal, and epitrochlear areas. Low-grade fever, lasting less than a week, occurs in 30 percent of cases, and malaise and fatigue in 25 percent. Single lymph node involvement occurs in 50 percent, while multiple node enlargement at the same site occurs in 20 percent. Adenopathy is usually present for 2 to 4 months, but it may persist for up to 2 years. Suppuration of the involved node may occur in up to 10 percent. Scratches from dogs, rabbits, monkeys, fish bones, and fishhooks have also been reported to cause cat-scratch disease. Lymph node biopsy reveals reticulum hyperplasia, with increased num-

Table 39-2
REFERRED SHOULDER PAIN

Cardiac
    Acute pericarditis
    Acute myocardial infarction
Pleural
    Community-acquired pneumonia
    Aspiration pneumonia
    Pulmonary embolism and infarction
    Primary pleuritis due to systemic lupus erythematosus
    Tuberculous pleuritis
Intraabdominal inflammation
    Acute cholecystitis
    Duodenal or gastric ulcer perforation
    Gastric carcinoma perforation
Hemoperitoneum
    Ruptured ectopic pregnancy
    Spontaneous rupture of the spleen
    Traumatic rupture of the spleen
    Hepatic tumor
    Abdominal apoplexy
    Rupture of a splanchnic artery aneurysm
Subphrenic abscess
Pneumoperitoneum

bers of germinal centers, granulomas, and microabscesses all in the same biopsy. Pleomorphic gram-negative bacilli that stain with a Warthin-Starry silver stain may be found in 87 percent of cases. Use of the Hanger and Rose skin test is not recommended because the antigen is not standardized, it is not a commercially available product, and it poses the risk of transmission of lethal diseases (human immunodeficiency virus and Kreutzfeldt-Jakob disease). There is no effective therapy for cat-scratch disease.

B. Streptococcal Axillary Lymphadenitis   Fever, chills, and severe axillary pain, swelling, and tenderness occur. A distal site of infection may be present on the hand or forearm. The skin of the axillary region is warm and edematous. The arm is held at the side, and flexion and abduction are resisted because of axillary pain. Enlarged, tender axillary nodes may be palpable. Edema of the affected arm and the ipsilateral supraclavicular and pectoral region may be present. A pleural effusion may develop in the adjacent hemithorax, and occlusion of the axillary-subclavian vein has been reported. A CT scan may show soft tissue edema of the axilla and enlarged axillary nodes. The diagnosis has been made by recovery of *Streptococcus pyogenes* from the initial skin site of infection or from a suppurating node. Severe streptococcal axillary lymphadenitis is a rare disorder. There is a response to intravenous penicillin therapy. In the absence of positive cultures, the diagnosis has been established by a rising serum titer on the Streptozyme test.

C. Staphylococcal Axillary Lymphadenitis   A furuncle may form on the dorsum of one of the fingers. The dorsum of the hand may become red, warm, and markedly swollen and painful. Linear erythematous lymphangitic streaks appear on the forearm and upper arm. Aching axillary pain, associated with enlarged, tender axillary lymph nodes, occurs. Fever and chills may be associated. *S. aureus* may be cultured from the finger lesion. There is a gradual response to nafcillin and to spontaneous or surgical drainage of the finger abscess.

D. Axillary Abscess   A cutaneous abscess of the axilla begins with local pain, skin redness, and tenderness. The erythematous area enlarges, becomes convex, and may be firm or fluctuant. A yellow or greenish head may form at the center of the erythematous area within 4 to 7 days. Culture of abscess pus obtained by surgical drainage revealed *S. aureus* in 65 percent and anaerobes in 19 percent of cases, in one reported series.

E. Axillary Infections in Leukemia   Patients undergoing antileukemia chemotherapy may develop axillary pain secondary to cutaneous infection and axillary adenopathy. Cellulitis, fistulas, and shallow or deep, penetrating ulcers may be present. The most frequent causes of axillary infection in these patients are *P. aeruginosa*, other gram-

negative bacteria, or *S. aureus*. There is a response of pain and local inflammation to systemic antibiotic therapy.

F. Tularemia (*Francisella tularensis*)   Within 1 to 14 days of skinning a wild rabbit or muskrat, a skin papule forms on the fingers or hand. This soon evolves into a small ulcer (in 2–4 days). Lymphangitis may occur on the more proximal region of the arm. Epitrochlear and/or axillary lymph nodes become painful, enlarged, and tender. Fever, chills, rigors, and malaise accompany the appearance of the ulcer and painful, regional adenopathy (ulceroglandular tularemia). Axillary nodes become enlarged in 65 to 90 percent of patients with rabbit-associated disease and in 24 percent of patients with tick-borne tularemia. Pneumonia (subsegmental or segmental) may occur in up to 50 percent. There is good clinical response to streptomycin or gentamicin therapy. The diagnosis is usually based on clinical findings and may be confirmed by demonstrating a four-tube rise in agglutination titer after the second week of illness. The sensitivity of this test is 50 to 70 percent at 2 weeks and higher at 4 to 8 weeks.

G. Bubonic Plague (*Yersinia pestis*)   This disease is endemic in the southwestern United States (Arizona, New Mexico, Utah, Colorado, and California). Risk factors include direct contact with rodents or carnivores (e.g., household cat or dog) and flea bites. It is also endemic in parts of Africa, Asia, and South America. There is a sudden onset of fever, rigors, chills, weakness, and headache. Within hours, severe pain develops in one axilla, accompanied by marked tender enlargement of the axillary lymph nodes. Nodal swellings may become as large as 10 cm in diameter. The overlying axillary skin is stretched and may be erythematous, warm, and edematous. The arm may be held splinted in abduction because of the axillary pain. Plague is suggested by the very abrupt onset of fever and nodal enlargement. Distal skin lesions are usually not present (75 percent of cases), as in tularemia, but may occur. Pustules, papules, eschars, or flea bite sites may be present (25 percent of cases) on the hand or forearm. Skin purpura and gangrene may develop. The diagnosis can be confirmed by injection of 1 ml of sterile saline solution into a bubo, aspirating it, and reinjecting it, until the saline solution becomes blood-tinged. Gram's and Wayson's stains of drops of dried aspirate will identify plague bacilli. Culture on blood agar, MacConkey agar, and infusion broth will result in isolation of the organism. Streptomycin or tetracycline therapy will reduce mortality from 50 percent to 5 percent.

This disorder should be considered in patients in, or recently returned from, an endemic area (2–8 days before onset), who present with the sudden onset of fever, chills, prostration, and painful, tender axillary node enlargement.

H. Bites

1. Animal Bite Wounds   Wounds on the fingers, hand, or forearm are likely to become infected if there is a delay of more than 12 h in seeking treatment, the patient is older than 50 years, or the wound is a puncture. Despite prophylactic therapy, up to 28 percent of hand and arm bite wounds may develop infection. Dog bites usually cause infection with *Pasteurella multocida* (20–50 percent), *S. aureus*, *Staphylococcus epidermidis*, and alpha-hemolytic streptococci. Mixed aerobic and anaerobic bite infections are common. *Bacteroides* and *Fusobacterium* species are common anaerobic isolates from dog bite wounds. *P. multocida* is a common cause of infection after a cat bite. Infection of the wound causes localized redness, edema, pain, and tenderness. Fever; tender forearm and upper arm lymphangitis; and painful, tender axillary lymphadenitis may occur in 20 percent of cases. Therapy with amoxicillin and clavulanic acid provides coverage for *S. aureus*, *P. multocida*, and anaerobes. Uninfected wounds are usually contaminated and require therapy.

2. Human Bite Wounds   These wounds may cause local infection, lymphangitis, and lymphadenitis. *Streptococcus viridans*, *S. aureus*, and anaerobic bacteria (e.g., *Bacteroides* species, *Fusobacterium nucleatum*, and *Peptococcus* and *Peptostreptococcus* species) are the usual isolates. Antibiotic therapy (penicillin or amoxicillin/clavulinic acid) will usually lead to resolution of local infection and axillary pain and tenderness.

I. Hidradenitis Suppurativa

This disorder may begin abruptly in one axilla, with pain and subcutaneous induration and tenderness. The overlying skin soon becomes red, warm, and adherent to the involved subcutaneous area. The aching axillary pain is increased by arm movement. The area of induration and tenderness may resolve or increase in size, stretching the overlying skin. An area of softening may occur in the center of the lesion. Drainage of this area leads to the extrusion of only a few drops of viscous pus. Spontaneous resolution of the skin induration then occurs. Multiple small abscesses may form during the first attack or with repeated attacks, and they may drain a foul-smelling discharge. Early surgical drainage and use of metronidazole may lead to complete resolution, but recurrent disease is frequent. Anaerobic bacteria and staphylococci appear to be the principal pathogens in hidradenitis suppurativa.

13. AXILLARY-SUBCLAVIAN VENOUS THROMBOSIS

This disorder may begin abruptly with axillary or more diffuse arm pain. The axillary pain is intensified by abduction or flexion of the arm and is caused by the presence of a tender, phlebitic cord (i.e., the thrombosed vein).

Arm pain and fatigue are intensified or provoked by use of the arm. The upper extremity may be edematous and discolored (cyanotic or purplish-red) at rest, or these changes may only develop after exercise of the arm. Venography will confirm the diagnosis and define the extent of the thrombosis. Veno-obstructive symptoms may respond to thrombolytic therapy and balloon angioplasty (to treat residual venous stenosis). In cases related to thoracic outlet obstruction, surgical decompression of the outlet should be performed to prevent recurrence of venous occlusion.

14. FRACTURE OF THE PROXIMAL HUMERUS

Pain in the shoulder and axillary area may occur after a fall on the outstretched arm. Palpation of the axilla may reveal local tenderness and bony crepitus over the proximal humerus. Plain radiographs will demonstrate the fracture or fractures.

15. COSTOCHONDRITIS OF THE ANTERIOR CHEST

Costochondritis causes parasternal pain and tenderness on one or both sides of the anterior chest. This pain may occur spontaneously and last for seconds, minutes, or hours. It may be provoked by arm movements against resistance or by the ''crowing rooster'' or ''hug yourself'' maneuvers. Pain may radiate from the parasternal region into the axilla and may spread down the arm.

16. AXILLARY MYALGIC PAIN

Axillary aching pain may be associated with recent exercise involving use of the arms (e.g., tennis or racquetball). The pain may be intensified by upper arm movements (e.g., extension and adduction). Local muscular tenderness in the axilla may be present. Spontaneous resolution occurs in 1 to 3 days.

17. GASEOUS DISTENSION OF THE STOMACH

This disorder, associated with a desire to belch and with pyrosis, may cause sticking or aching unilateral or bilateral lateral pectoral or axillary pain. The pain may be relieved by antacids followed by eructation of considerable amounts of trapped gas.

18. PNEUMOTHORAX

There is an abrupt onset of pleuritic-type anterior chest and/or axillary pain. Dyspnea may be associated. Examination reveals decreased expansion of the affected hemithorax, a hyperresonant percussion note, and decreased or absent breath sounds. A chest radiograph will confirm the diagnosis.

19. BREAST DISORDERS IN WOMEN

A rapidly enlarging cyst, a tumor, or an abscess in the axillary extension of the breast in women may cause axillary pain. The diagnosis can be established by physical examination, mammography, or ultrasonography of the breast. Exploration of the lesion and biopsy may be required to exclude malignancy.

20. PLEUROPULMONARY DISEASE

A. Carcinoma of the Lung or Lymphoma   A lung tumor may invade the upper lateral chest wall, causing axillary pain and tenderness. A CT scan will demonstrate chest wall invasion. The diagnosis can be confirmed by a CT-guided needle biopsy.

B. Pyogenic Abscess   An upper lobe abscess may extend into the chest wall in the region of the axilla. Plain radiographs and a thoracic CT scan can demonstrate the abscess and chest wall involvement. Aching and pleuritic axillary pain may occur. The diagnosis can be confirmed by needle aspiration or exploration.

C. Actinomycosis   Aching and pleuritic chest and axillary pain may be caused by pulmonary and chest wall abscesses in the left upper lateral thorax caused by actinomycosis. Abscesses in the upper lobe and soft tissue of the chest wall with air fluid levels may be demonstrated by plain radiographs and a thoracic CT scan. Incision and drainage of pus allows for identification of an *Actinomyces* species by direct microscopy. Intravenous penicillin therapy for 6 weeks leads to resolution.

21. RADICULAR PAIN INVOLVING THE T1 ROOT

A high thoracic disc herniation (T1–T2 interspace) may cause compression of the T1 root. There may be a constant ache in the lower neck, shoulder, and axilla and aching pain in the lower medial arm radiating to the ulnar side of the hand. Hypesthesia may extend down the medial region of the arm to the wrist. No reflex deficits occur. An ipsilateral Horner's syndrome may be present. Motor weakness may be absent or may primarily involve the intrinsic muscles of the hand. CT myelography or MRI of the lower cervical and upper thoracic spine can identify the cause of T1 root compression (e.g., soft or hard disc or tumor).

Axillary pain of radicular origin may be intensified by neck rotation, coughing, sneezing, or straining at stool. Surgical removal of the causative disc or tumor relieves axillary, shoulder, and arm pain.

22. POSTAXILLARY DISSECTION PAIN IN PATIENTS OPERATED ON FOR BREAST CANCER

Persistent aching or burning pain occurs in the axilla and sometimes in the scapular region, shoulder, and inner side of the upper arm. Anesthesia or hypesthesia is present in the axilla and inner side of the upper arm. Less commonly, hyperesthesia and dysesthesia may occur in the same area. Supraclavicular and axillary pain may follow axillary palpation. The onset of pain was 1 to 26 weeks (median, 6 weeks) after axillary lymph node dissection. The cause is an iatrogenic lesion of the intercostobrachial nerve produced during surgical dissection of the axilla.

23. BILATERAL PAIN

A. Bilateral Acute Shoulder and Upper Arm Pain The causes are listed in Table 39-3.

Table 39-3
BILATERAL ACUTE SHOULDER AND UPPER ARM PAIN

Acute rheumatic fever
Reiter's syndrome
Lyme arthritis
Pseudogout
Hepatitis B-associated arthritis
Neuralgic amyotrophy
Referred shoulder pain due to
   Acute pericarditis
   Acute myocardial infarction
   Bilateral pneumonia and pleuritis
   Bilateral pulmonary infarction and pleuritis
   Lupus pleuritis
   Perforation of a gastric or duodenal ulcer
   Hemoperitoneum secondary to
      Ruptured tubal pregnancy
      Splenic rupture
      Hepatic tumor hemorrhage
      Abdominal apoplexy
      Rupture of a splanchnic artery aneurysm
Bilateral subphrenic abscess
Pneumoperitoneum

B. Bilateral Acute Axillary Pain   The causes are listed in Table 39-4.

Table 39-4
BILATERAL ACUTE AXILLARY PAIN

Bubonic plague
Hidradenitis suppurativa
Axillary-subclavian thrombosis
Axillary myalgic pain
Gaseous distension of the stomach
Fibrocystic disease of the breast

SHOULDER, UPPER ARM, AND AXILLARY PAIN REFERENCES

Arthritic Pain—Arm

Klipple GL, Riordan KK: Rare inflammatory and hereditary connective tissue diseases. *Rheum Dis Clin North Am* 15:383–398, 1989.

Arthritis—Shoulder

Ellman MH: Arthritis of the shoulder, in Post M (ed): *The Shoulder: Surgical and Nonsurgical Management,* 2d ed. Philadelphia, Lea & Febiger, 1988, pp 294–315.

Ellman MH, Curran JJ: Causes and management of shoulder arthritis. *Compr Ther* 14:29–35, 1988.

Figgie HE III, Inglis AE, Goldberg VM, et al: An analysis of factors affecting the long-term results of total shoulder arthroplasty in inflammatory arthritis. *J Arthroplasty* 3:123–130, 1988.

Good AE: Enteropathic arthritis, in Kelley WN, Harris ED Jr, Ruddy S (eds): *Textbook of Rheumatology.* Philadelphia, Saunders, 1981, vol 2, pp 1063–1075.

Lecour H, Miranda M, Magro C, et al: Human leptospirosis: A review of 50 cases. *Infection* 17:8–12, 1989.

Leslie BM, Harris JM, Driscoll D: Septic arthritis of the shoulder in adults. *J Bone Joint Surg (AM)* 71-A:1516–1522, 1989.

Lipsky PE: Rheumatoid arthritis, in Wilson JD, Braunwald E, Isselbacher RJ, et al (eds): *Harrison's Principles of Internal Medicine,* 12th ed. New York, McGraw-Hill, 1991, vol 2, pp 1437–1443.

MacDonald PB, Locht RC, Lindsay D, et al: Haemophilic arthropathy of the shoulder. *J Bone Joint Surg (Br)* 72-B:470–471, 1990.

Malawista SE, Steere AC: Viral arthritis, in Kelley WN, Harris ED Jr, Ruddy S (eds): *Textbook of Rheumatology.* Philadelphia, Saunders, 1981, vol 2, pp 1586–1601.

Marantz PR, Linzer M: Diffuse lymphadenopathy as a manifestation of ankylosing spondylitis. *Am J Med* 80:951–953, 1986.

Mills JA: Arthritis of the shoulder, in Rowe CR (ed): *The Shoulder.* New York, Churchill Livingstone, 1988, pp 471–480.

Nesher G, Rosenberg P, Shorer Z, et al: Involvement of the peripheral nervous system in temporal arteritis-polymyalgia rheumatica: Report of 3 cases and review of the literature. *J Rheumatol* 14:358–360, 1987.

Petersson CJ: The acromioclavicular joint in rheumatoid arthritis. *Clin Orthop* 223:86–93, 1987.

————: Painful shoulders in patients with rheumatoid arthritis: Prevalence, clinical and radiologic features. *Scand J Rheumatol* 15:275–279, 1986.

Podgorski MR, Ibels LS, Webb J: Case report 445. *Skeletal Radiol* 16:589 591, 1987.

Schur PH: Psoriatic arthritis and arthritis associated with gastrointestinal disease, in Wilson JD, Braunwald E, Isselbacher KJ, et al (eds): *Harrison's Principles of Internal Medicine,* 12th ed. New York, McGraw-Hill, 1991, vol 2, pp 1482–1484.

Taurog JD, Lipsky PE: Ankylosing spondylitis and reactive arthritis, in Wilson JD, Braunwald E, Isselbacher KJ, et al (eds): *Harrison's Principles of Internal Medicine,* 12th ed. New York, McGraw-Hill, 1991, vol 2, pp 1451–1455.

Wright V: Psoriatic arthritis, in Kelley WN, Harris ED Jr, Ruddy S (eds): *Textbook of Rheumatology.* Philadelphia, Saunders, 1981, vol 2, pp 1047–1062.

Axillary Lymphadenitis

Al-Gindan Y, Kubba R, El-Hassan AM, et al: Dissemination in cutaneous leishmaniasis: 3. Lymph node involvement. *Int J Dermatol* 28:248–254, 1989.

Benjamin DR: Granulomatous lymphadenitis in children. *Arch Pathol Lab Med* 111:750–753, 1987.

Boyce JM: Severe streptococcal axillary lymphadenitis. *N Engl J Med* 323:655–658. 1990.

Fujimori T, Shioda K, Sussman EB, et al: Subacute necrotising lymphadenitis: A clinicopathologic study. *Acta Pathol Jpn* 31:791–797, 1981.

Gerald W, Kostianovsky M, Rosai J: Development of vascular neoplasia in Castleman's disease: Report of seven cases. *Am J Surg Pathol* 14:603–614, 1990.

Gould E, Porto R, Albores-Saavedra J, et al: Dermatopathic lymphadenitis: The spectrum and significance of its morphologic features. *Arch Pathol Lab Med* 112:1145–1150, 1988.

Helmick CG, D'Souza AJ, Goddard N: An outbreak of severe BCG axillary lymphadenitis in Saint Lucia, 1982–83. *West Indian Med J* 35:12–17, 1986.

Oates E, Staudinger K, Gilbertson V: Significance of nodal uptake on indium 111 labeled leukocyte scans. *Clin Nucl Med* 14:282–285, 1989.

Spires JR, Smith RJH: Cat-scratch disease. *Otolaryngol Head Neck Surg* 94:622–627, 1986.

Axillary Pain—Neurogenic

Alberico AM, Sahni KS, Hall JA Jr, et al: High thoracic disc herniation. *Neurosurgery* 19:449–451, 1986.

Axillary Pain—Surgical Complications

Bostwick J, Stevenson TR, Nahai F, et al: Radiation to the breast: Complications amenable to surgical treatment. *Ann Surg* 200:543–553, 1984.

Egan RL: Estimated risk and occurrence of breast cancer in asymptomatic and minimally symptomatic patients. *Cancer* 43:871–877, 1979.

Gutman H, Kersz T, Barzilai T, et al: Achievements of physical therapy in patients after modified radical mastectomy compared with quadrantectomy, axillary dissection, and radiation for carcinoma of the breast. *Arch Surg* 125:389–391, 1990.

Huang TT: Breast and subscapular pain following submuscular placement of breast prostheses. *Plast Reconstr Surg* 86:275–280, 1990.

Janson RA: Implant arm: Axillary compression from breast prostheses. *Plast Reconstr Surg* 75:420–422, 1985.

Narakas AO: Operative treatment for radiation-induced and metastatic brachial plexopathy in 45 cases, 15 having an omentoplasty. *Bull Hosp Joint Dis Orthop Inst* 44:354–375, 1984.

Vecht CJ, Van de Brand HJ, Wajer OJM: Post-axillary dissection pain in breast cancer due to a lesion of the intercostobrachial nerve. *Pain* 38:171–176, 1989.

White GH, Donayre CE, Williams RA, et al: Exertional disruption of axillofemoral graft anastomosis. *Arch Surg* 125:625–627, 1990.

Axillary Subcutaneous Infections

Dreizen S, McCredie KB, Keating MJ, et al: Intertriginous infections in adults receiving antileukemia chemotherapy. *Postgrad Med* 85:223–229, 230, 1989.

Hennessy MJ, Mosher TF: Mucormycosis infection of an upper extremity. *J Hand Surg (Am)* 6:249–252, 1981.

Leach RD, Eykyn SJ, Phillips I, et al: Anaerobic axillary abscess. *Br Med J (Clin Res)* 2:5–7, 1979.

Møller-Jensen B, Kruse-Andersen S, Andersen K: Thoraco-pleural actinomycosis presenting like diffuse pulmonary embolism. *Thorac Cardiovasc Surg* 36:284–286, 1988.

Paletta C, Jurkiewicz MJ: Hidradenitis suppurativa. *Clin Plast Surg* 14:383–390, 1987.

San Joaquin VH, Kimball JB: Subscapular abscess due to *Haemophilus influenzae* type B. *Pediatrics* 65:331–332, 1980.

Yu CC-W, Cook MG: Hidradenitis suppurativa: A disease of follicular epithelium, rather than apocrine glands. *Br J Dermatol* 122:763:769, 1990.

Axillary Tumors

Stewart CA, Glaser AM, Terasaki K: Massive lymphoma of the mediastinum, chest wall, and axilla. *Clin Nucl Med* 14:210–211, 1989.

Axillary Vascular Pain

Aburahama AF, Sadler DL, Robinson PA: Axillary-subclavian vein thrombosis: Changing patterns of etiology, diagnostic, and therapeutic modalities. *Am Surg* 57:101–107, 1991.

Brochner G, Rojas M, Armas AJ, et al: Axillary-subclavian venous thrombosis. *J Cardiovasc Surg* 30:108–111, 1989.

Campbell CB, Chandler JG, Tegtmeyer CJ, et al: Axillary, subclavian, and brachiocephalic vein obstruction. *Surgery* 82:816–826, 1977.

Graham JM, Mattox KL, Feliciano DV, et al: Vascular injuries of the axilla. *Ann Surg* 195:232–238, 1982.

Nemmers DW, Thorpe PE, Knibbe MA, et al: Upper extremity venous thrombosis: Case report and literature review. *Orthop Rev* 19:164–172, 1990.

Pairolero PC, Walls JT, Payne WS, et al: Subclavian-axillary artery aneurysms. *Surgery* 90:757–763, 1981.

Bursitis — Shoulder

LeNoir JL: Subacromial-subdeltoid bursitis of the shoulder. *Orthop Rev* 15:730–732, 1986.

Mena HR: The pain of acute bursitis/tendinitis of the shoulder. *Am J Med* 80(suppl 3A):140, 1986.

Sisto DJ, Jobe FW: The operative treatment of scapulothoracic bursitis in professional pitchers. *Am J Sports Med* 14:192–194, 1986.

Congenital Disorders — Shoulder

Loomer RL: Shoulder girdle dysplasia associated with nail patella syndrome: A case report and literature review. *Clin Orthop* 238:112–116, 1989.

Dislocations — Shoulder

Post M: Dislocations of the shoulder, in Post M (ed): *The Shoulder: Surgical and Nonsurgical Management,* 2d ed. Philadelphia, Lea & Febiger, 1988, pp 518–618.

Rowe CR; Dislocations of the shoulder, in Rowe CR (ed): *The Shoulder*. New York, Churchill Livingstone, 1988, pp 165–291.

Fractures

Post M: Fractures of the proximal humerus, in Post M (ed): *The Shoulder: Surgical and Nonsurgical Management,* 2d ed. Philadelphia, Lea & Febiger, 1988, pp 450–487.

———: Fractures of the shaft of the humerus, in Post M (ed): *The Shoulder: Surgical and Nonsurgical Management,* 2d ed. Philadelphia, Lea & Febiger, 1988, pp 487–517.

Frozen Shoulder

Griffin JW: Hemiplegic shoulder pain. *Phys Ther* 66:1884–1893, 1986.

Moren-Hybbinette I, Moritz U, Schersten B: The clinical picture of the painful diabetic shoulder: Natural history, social consequences and analysis of concomitant hand syndrome. *Acta Med Scand* 221:73–82, 1987.

Murnaghan JP: Frozen shoulder, in Rockwood CA Jr, Matsen FA III (eds): *The Shoulder*. Philadelphia, Saunders, 1990, vol 2, pp 837–862.

Wohlgethan JR: Frozen shoulder in hyperthyroidism. *Arthritis Rheum* 30:936–939, 1987.

Imaging — Shoulder

Bassett LW, Gold RH: Magnetic resonance imaging of the musculoskeletal system: An overview. *Clin Orthop* 244:17–28, 1989.

Bradley WG Jr, Waluch V, Yadley RA, et al: Comparison of CT and MR in 400 patients with suspected disease of the brain and cervical spinal cord. *Radiology* 152:695–702, 1984.

Esdaile J, Rosenthall L: Radionuclide joint imaging. *Comp Ther* 9:54–63, 1983.

Habibian A, Stauffer A, Resnick D, et al: Comparison of conventional and computed arthrotomography with MR imaging in the evaluation of the shoulder. *J Comput Assist Tomogr* 13:968–975, 1989.

Rafii M, Firooznia H, Bonamo JJ, et al: Athlete shoulder injuries: CT arthrographic findings. *Radiology* 162:559–564, 1987.

Impingement — Biceps Tendon

Ahovuo J, Paavolainen P, Slatis P: Diagnostic value of sonography in lesions of the biceps tendon. *Clin Orthop* 202:184–188, 1986.

Burkhead WZ Jr: The biceps tendon, in Rockwood CA Jr, Matsen FA III (eds): *The Shoulder*. Philadelphia, Saunders, 1990, vol 2, pp 791–836.

Gerber C, Terrier F, Ganz R: The role of the coracoid process in the chronic impingement syndrome. *J Bone Joint Surg (Br)* 67:703–708, 1985.

Mariani EM, Cofield RH, Askew LJ, et al: Rupture of the tendon of the long head of the biceps brachii: Surgical *versus* nonsurgical treatment. *Clin Orthop* 228:233–239, 1988.

Neviaser TJ: The role of the biceps tendon in the impingement syndrome. *Orthop Clin North Am* 18:383–386, 1987.

Impingement — Rotator Cuff

Butters KP, Rockwood CA Jr: Office evaluation and management of the shoulder impingement syndrome. *Orthop Clin North Am* 19:755–765, 1988.

Collins RA, Gristina AG, Carter RE, et al: Ultrasonography of the shoulder: Static and dynamic imaging. *Orthop Clin North Am* 18:351–360, 1987.

Crass JR, Craig EV, Feinberg SB: Clinical significance of sonographic findings in the abnormal but intact rotator cuff: A preliminary report. *Clin Ultrasound* 16:625–634, 1988.

Gartsman GM: Arthroscopic acromioplasty for lesions of the rotator cuff. *J Bone Joint Surg (Am)* 72:169–180, 1990.

England S, Farrell AJ, Coppock JS, et al: Low power laser therapy of shoulder tendonitis. *Scand J Rheumatol* 18:427–431, 1989.

Hawkins RJ, Abrams JS: Impingement syndrome in the absence of rotator cuff tear (stages 1 and 2). *Orthop Clin North Am* 18:373–382, 1987.

Hawkins RJ, Brock RM, Abrams JS, et al: Acromioplasty for impingement with an intact rotator cuff. *J Bone Joint Surg (Br)* 70-B:795–797, 1988.

Mann DL, Littke N: Shoulder injuries in archery. *Can J Sport Sci* 14:85–92, 1989.

Matsen FA III, Arntz CT: Subacromial impingement, in Rockwood CA Jr, Matsen FA III (eds): *The Shoulder*. Philadelphia, Saunders, 1990, vol 2, pp 623–646.

Neviaser RJ: Radiologic assessment of the shoulder: Plain and arthrographic. *Orthop Clin North Am* 18:343–349, 1987.

———: Ruptures of the rotator cuff. *Orthop Clin North Am* 18:387–394, 1987.

Injuries — Shoulder

Kristiansen B, Angermann P, Larsen TK: Functional results following fractures of the proximal humerus: A controlled clinical study comparing two periods of immobilization. *Arch Orthop Trauma Surg* 108:339–341, 1989.

Taft TN, Wilson FC, Oglesby JW: Dislocation of the acromioclavicular joint: An end result study. *J Bone joint Surg (Am)* 69:1045–1051, 1987.

Instability — Shoulder

Bigliani LU, Morrison DS: Glenohumeral instability, in Dee R, Mango E, Hurst LC (eds): *Principles of Orthopaedic Practice*. New York, McGraw-Hill, 1988, Vol 1, pp 575–584.

Garth WP Jr, Allman FL Jr, Armstrong WS: Occult anterior subluxations of the shoulder in noncontact sports. *Am J Sports Med* 15:579–585, 1987.

Nobuhara K, Ikeda H: Rotator interval lesion. *Clin Orthop* 223:44–50, 1987.

O'Brien SJ, Warren RF, Schwartz E: Anterior shoulder instability. *Orthop Clin North Am* 18:395–408, 1987.

Rowe CR: Recurrent anterior transient subluxation of the shoulder: The "dead arm" syndrome. *Orthop Clin North Am* 19:767–772, 1988.

Schwartz E, Warren RF, O'Brien SJ, et al: Posterior shoulder instability. *Orthop Clin North Am* 18:409–419, 1987.

Skyhar MJ, Warren RF, Altchek DW: Instability of the shoulder, in Nicholas JA, Hershman EB, Posner MA (eds): *The Upper Extremity in Sports Medicine*. St. Louis, Mosby, 1990, pp 181–212.

Myofascial Pain—Shoulder

Grosshandler SL, Stratas NE, Toomey TC, et al: Chronic neck and shoulder pain. Focusing on myofascial origins. *Postgrad Med* 77:149–151, 154–158, 1985.

Percy EC, Birbrager D, Pitt MJ: Snapping scapula: A review of the literature and presentation of 14 patients. *Can J Surg* 31:248–250, 1988.

Weed ND: When shoulder pain isn't bursitis: The myofascial pain syndrome. *Postgrad Med* 74:97–98, 101–102, 104, 1983.

Neurogenic Pain—Shoulder

Bateman JE: Neurologic painful conditions affecting the shoulder. *Clin Orthop* 173:44–54, 1983.

Brown C: Compressive, invasive referred pain to the shoulder. *Clin Orthop* 173:55–62, 1983.

Cormier PJ, Matalon TAS, Wolin PM: Quadrilateral space syndrome: A rare cause of shoulder pain. *Radiology* 167:797–798, 1988.

McKowen HC, Voorhies RM: Axillary nerve entrapment in the quadrilateral space: Case report. *J Neurosurg* 66:932–934, 1987.

Peterson GW, Will AD: Newer electrodiagnostic techniques in peripheral nerve injuries. *Orthop Clin North Am* 19:13–25, 1988.

Post M, Mayer J: Suprascapular nerve entrapment: Diagnosis and treatment. *Clin Orthop* 223:126–136, 1987.

Polymyalgia Rheumatica

Cohen MD, Ginsburg WW: Polymyalgia rheumatica. *Rheum Dis Clin North Am* 16:325–339, 1990.

Referred Shoulder Pain

Bauer TW, Haskins GE, Armitage JO: Splenic rupture in patients with hematologic malignancies. *Cancer* 48:2729–2733, 1981.

Berger JP, Buclin T, Haller E, et al: Right arm involvement and pain extension can help to differentiate coronary diseases from chest pain of other origin: A prospective emergency ward study of 278 consecutive patients admitted for chest pain. *J Intern Med* 227:165–172, 1990.

Hockaday JM, Whitty CWM: Patterns of referred pain in the normal subject. *Brain* 90:481–496, 1967.

Khoury GF, Stein C, Ramming KP: Neck and shoulder pain associated with hepatic arterial chemotherapy using an implantable infusion pump. *Pain* 32:275–277, 1988.

Leach RE, Ory SJ: Management of ectopic pregnancy. *Am Fam Physician* 41:1215–1222, 1990.

Rotolo JE: Spontaneous splenic rupture in infectious mononucleosis. *Am J Emerg Med* 5:383–385, 1987.

Smally AJ: Referred shoulder pain in a sexually active woman. *Hosp Pract* 24:62–64, 1989.

Valenzuela GA, Mittal RK, Shaffer HA Jr, et al: Shoulder pain: An unusual presentation of gastric ulcer. *South Med J* 82:1446–1447, 1989.

Reflex Sympathetic Dystrophy (Shoulder-Hand Syndrome)

Buell TR, Karlin JM, Scurran BL, et al: Reflex sympathetic dystrophy syndrome: Review with podiatric case studies. *J Am Podiatr Med Assoc* 77:533–538, 1987.

Escobar PL: Reflex sympathetic dystrophy. *Orthop Rev* 15:646–651, 1986.

Markoff M, Farole A: Reflex sympathetic dystrophy syndrome: Case report with a review of the literature. *Oral Surg Oral Med Oral Pathol* 61:23–28, 1986.

Roig-Escofet D, Rodriguez-Moreno J, Martin JMR: Concept and limits of the reflex sympathetic dystrophy. *Clin Rheumatol* 8(suppl 2):104–108, 1989.

Shih W-J, Pulmano C: Hand and forearm Tc-99m HMDP bone image findings of reflex sympathetic dystrophy similar to those of radiopharmaceutical arterial administration in the arm. *Clin Nucl Med* 14:298–300, 1989.

Review—Shoulder Pain

Bergfeld JA: Acromioclavicular complex, in Nicholas JA, Hershman EB, Posner MA (eds): *The Upper Extremity in Sports Medicine*. St. Louis, Mosby, 1990, pp 169–180.

Bigliani LU, Morrison DS: Miscellaneous degenerative disorders of the shoulder, in Dee R, Mango E, Hurst LC (eds): *Principles of Orthopaedic Practice*. New York, McGraw-Hill, 1989, vol 1, pp 621–634.

Bonafede RP, Bennett RM: Shoulder pain: Guidelines to diagnosis and management. *Postgrad Med* 82:185–189, 192–193, 1987.

Boyce JM: *Francisella tularensis* (tularemia), in Mandell GL, Douglas RG Jr, Bennett JE (eds): *Principles and Practice of Infectious Diseases*. New York, Churchill Livingstone, 1990, pp 1742–1746.

Brems JJ: Degenerative joint disease in the shoulder, in Nicholas JA, Hershman EB, Posner MA (eds): *The Upper Extremity in Sports Medicine*. St. Louis, Mosby, 1990, pp. 235–250.

Butler T: Yersinia species (including plague), in Mandell GL, Douglas RG Jr, Bennett JE (eds): *Principles and Practice of Infectious Diseases*. New York: Churchill Livingstone, 1990, pp 1748–1756.

Calin A: Ankylosing spondylitis, in Kelley WN, Harris ED Jr, Ruddy S (eds): *Textbook of Rheumatology*. Philadelphia, Saunders, 1981, vol 2 pp 1017–1030.

———: Reiter's syndrome, in Kelley WN, Harris ED Jr, Ruddy S (eds): *Textbook of Rheumatology*. Philadelphia, Saunders, 1981, vol 2, pp 1033–1046.

Cofield RH: Degenerative and arthritic problems of the glenohumeral joint, in Rockwood CA Jr, Matsen FA III (eds): *The Shoulder*. Philadelphia, Saunders, 1990, vol 2, pp 678–749.

Fischer GW: The agent of cat-scratch disease, in Mandell GL, Douglas RG Jr, Bennett JE (eds): *Principles and Practice of Infectious Diseases*. New York, Churchill Livingstone, 1990, pp 1874–1877.

Goldstein EJ: Bites, in Mandell GL, Douglas RG Jr, Bennett JE (eds): *Principles and Practice of Infectious Diseases*. New York, Churchill Livingstone, 1990, pp 834–837.

Gristina AG, Kammire G, Voytek A, et al: Sepsis of the shoulder: Molecular mechanisms and pathogenesis, in Rockwood CA Jr, Matsen FA III (eds): *The Shoulder*. Philadelphia, Saunders, 1990, vol 2, pp 920–939.

Jobe FW, Ling B: The shoulder in sports, in Post M (ed): *The Shoulder: Surgical and Nonsurgical Management,* 2d ed. Philadelphia, Lea & Febiger, 1988, pp 619–643.

Jobe FW, Tibone JE, Jobe CM, et al: The shoulder in sports, in Rockwood CA Jr, Matsen FA III (eds): *The Shoulder*. Philadelphia, Saunders, 1990, vol 2, pp 961–990.

Leffert RD: Neurological problems, in Rockwood CA Jr, Matsen FA III (eds): *The Shoulder*. Philadelphia, Saunders, 1990, vol 2, pp 750–773.

Luck JV Jr, Andersson GBJ: Occupational shoulder disorders, in Rockwood CA Jr, Matsen FA III (eds): *The Shoulder*. Philadelphia, Saunders, 1990, vol 2, pp 1088–1108.

Malawer MM, Shmookler BM, Feffer S: Principles of orthopaedic oncology, in Dee R, Mango E, Hurst LC (eds): *Principles of Orthopaedic Practice*. New York, McGraw-Hill, 1989, vol 1, pp 317–361.

Matsen FA III, Kirby RM: Office evaluation and management of shoulder pain. *Orthop Clin North Am* 13:453–475, 1982.

Neviaser TJ: Arthroscopy of the shoulder. *Orthop Clin North Am* 18:361–372, 1987.

Norris TR: History and physical examination of the shoulder, in Nicholas JA, Hershman EB, Posner MA (eds): *The Upper Extremity in Sports Medicine*. St. Louis, Mosby, 1990, pp 41–90.

Ogilvie-Harris DJ, Wiley AM: Arthroscopic surgery of the shoulder: A general appraisal. *J Bone Joint Surg (Br)* 68:201–207, 1986.

Ordway C, Dee R, Mango E: Fractures and dislocations of the elbow, arm, and shoulder girdle of adults, in Dee R, Mango E, Hurst LC (eds): *Principles of Orthopaedic Practice.* New York, McGraw-Hill, 1988, vol 1, pp 560–575.

Perry J, Glousman, R: Biomechanics of throwing, in Nicholas JA, Hershman EB, Posner MA (eds): *The Upper Extremity in Sports Medicine.* St. Louis, Mosby, 1990, pp 725–750.

Polisson RP: Sports medicine for the internist. *Med Clin North Am* 70:469–489, 1986.

Post M: Miscellaneous painful shoulder conditions, in Post M (ed): *The Shoulder: Surgical and Nonsurgical Management,* 2d ed. Philadelphia, Lea & Febiger, 1988, pp 322–363.

———: Orthopaedic management of shoulder infections, in Post M (ed): *The Shoulder: Surgical and Nonsurgical Management,* 2d ed. Philadelphia, Lea & Febiger, 1988, pp 139–153.

Priest JD: The shoulder of the tennis player. *Clin Sports Med* 7:387–402, 1988.

Rogers LF, Hendrix RW: The painful shoulder. *Radiol Clin North Am* 26:1359–1371, 1988.

Uhthoff HK, Sarkar K: Calcifying tendinitis, in Rockwood CA Jr, Matsen FA III (eds): *The Shoulder.* Philadelphia, Saunders, 1990, vol 2, pp 774–790.

Rotator Cuff Tendinitis

Chard MD, Hazleman BL: Shoulder disorders in the elderly: A hospital study. *Ann Rheum Dis* 46:684–687, 1987.

Chard MD, Sattelle LM, Hazleman BL: The long-term outcome of rotator cuff tendinitis: A review study. *Br J Rheumatol* 27:385–389, 1988.

Shoulder Pain—Chronic Tendinitis

Chadwick CJ: Tendinitis of the pectoralis major insertion with humeral lesions: A report of two cases. *J Bone Joint Surg (Br)* 71-B:816–818, 1989.

Tumors—Shoulder

Barbera C, Lewis MM: Office evaluation of bone tumors. *Orthop Clin North Am* 19:821–838, 1988.

Conrad EV III: Tumors and related conditions, in Rockwood CA Jr, Matsen FA III (eds): *The Shoulder.* Philadelphia, Saunders, 1990, vol 2, 874–919.

Craig EV, Thompson RC: Management of tumors of the shoulder girdle. *Clin Orthop* 223:94–112, 1987.

Enzinger FM, Zhang R: Plexiform fibrohistiocytic tumor presenting in children and young adults: An analysis of 65 cases. *Am J Surg Pathol* 12:818–826, 1988.

Hankin FM, Braunstein EM, Orringer MB: Timely evaluation of shoulder pain in a teenager. *Am Fam Physician* 33:177–180, 1986.

Huvos AG, Marcove RC: Chondrosarcoma in the young: A clinicopathologic analysis of 79 patients younger than 21 years of age. *Am J Surg Pathol* 11:930–942, 1987.

Keeney GL, Unni KK, Beabout JW, et al: Adamantinoma of long bones: A clinicopathologic study of 85 cases. *Cancer* 64:730–737, 1989.

Lancaster JM, Koman LA, Gristina AG, et al: Pathologic fractures of the humerus. *South Med J* 81:52–55, 1988.

Leung PC, Hung LK: Bone reconstruction after giant-cell tumor resection at the proximal end of the humerus with vascularized iliac crest graft: A report of three cases. *Clin Orthop* 247:101–105, 1989.

Malawer MM, Dick HM: Neoplasms affecting the upper extremity, in Dee R, Mango E, Hurst LC (eds): *Principles of Orthopaedic Practice.* New York, McGraw-Hill, 1989, vol 1, pp 751–774.

Miser JS, Kinsella TJ, Triche TJ, et al: Preliminary results of treatment of Ewing's sarcoma of bone in children and young adults: Six months of intensive combined modality therapy without maintenance. *J Clin Oncol* 6:484–490, 1988.

Pongracz N, Zimmerman R, Kotz R: Orthopaedic management of bony metastases of renal cancer. *Sem Surg Oncol* 4:139–142, 1988.

Rousselin B, Vanel D, Terrier-Lacombe MJ, et al: Clinical and radiologic analysis of 13 cases of primary neuroectodermal tumors of bone. *Skeletal Radiol* 18:115–120, 1989.

Takagishi K, Shinohara N: Prosthetic replacement due to giant-cell tumor in the proximal humerus: A case report. *Clin Orthop* 247:106–110, 1989.

Yamaguchi H, Isu K, Ubayama Y, et al: Clear cell chondrosarcoma: A report of two cases and review of literature. *Acta Pathol Jpn* 36:1577–1585, 1986.

Acute Elbow and Forearm Pain

☐ **DIAGNOSTIC LIST**

1. Fractures
   A. Olecranon fracture
   B. Radial head fractures
   C. Supracondylar fracture of the humerus
   D. Transcondylar fracture of the humerus
   E. Medial epicondylar fracture of the humerus
   F. Intercondylar fracture of the humerus
   G. Monteggia's fracture-dislocation
   H. Radial head fracture with acute distal radioulnar dislocation
2. Simple dislocation of the elbow
3. Anterior elbow pain
   A. Brachialis muscle tear
   B. Rupture of the distal biceps muscle tendon
   C. Biceps muscle tear
   D. Anterior capsular tear
   E. Disruption of the annular ligament and anterior radial head dislocation
   F. Acute thrombophlebitis
      1. Nonsuppurative
      2. Suppurative
4. Medial elbow pain
   A. Rupture of the flexor forearm muscle mass
   B. Rupture or injury of the medial collateral ligament
   C. Little League elbow
   D. Medial epicondylar fracture

   E. Acute ulnar neuropathy
   F. Medial epicondylitis
   G. Epitrochlear lymphadenitis
5. Lateral elbow pain
   A. Rupture of the lateral extensor muscle origin
   B. Disruption of the annular ligament and anterior radial head dislocation
   C. Entrapment of the musculocutaneous or lateral antebrachial cutaneous nerve
   D. Lateral epicondylitis
   E. Osteochondral fracture of the radial head-capitellum articulation
6. Posterior elbow pain
   A. Triceps tendinitis
   B. Triceps rupture
   C. Valgus extension overload syndrome
   D. Stress fracture of the olecranon
   E. Olecranon bursitis
      1. Septic bursitis
      2. Gouty bursitis
      3. Traumatic bursitis
7. Acute monoarticular arthritis
   A. Septic arthritis
   B. Disseminated gonococcal infection (arthritis-dermatitis syndrome)
   C. Gout
   D. Pseudogout
   E. Hemophilic hemarthrosis

8. Acute polyarthritis with elbow
   involvement
   A. Acute rheumatic fever
   B. Acute hepatitis B arthritis
   C. Reiter's syndrome
   D. Lyme disease arthritis
   E. Rubella arthritis
   F. Rubella vaccine-induced
      arthritis
9. Referred pain
   Coronary heart disease
   1. Acute myocardial
      infarction
   2. Coronary insufficiency

10. Acute C8 radiculopathy
11. Vascular disorders
    A. Acute axillary or brachial
       artery occlusion
    B. Impending Volkmann's
       ischemic contracture (anterior
       compartment syndrome of the
       forearm)
    C. Mycotic aneurysm of the arm
12. Grade I muscle strain of the
    forearm
13. Acute bilateral elbow or forearm
    pain

☐ SUMMARY

Most *fractures* at the elbow result from a fall on the outstretched hand or direct trauma to the elbow. An *olecranon fracture* causes posterior elbow pain, swelling, and tenderness. Elbow extension is impaired, and a gap in the olecranon may be palpable before swelling develops. A *radial head fracture* causes anterolateral elbow pain and tenderness. Supination and pronation may be impaired because of pain. Selective injection of the fracture site with lidocaine to relieve movement-related pain allows assessment of mechanical factors that may interfere with supination and pronation. A *supracondylar fracture of the humerus* produces swelling, a Z- or S-shaped deformity, tenderness, and ecchymoses of the distal portion of the upper arm. The brachial artery may be compressed by the fracture fragments, resulting in ischemic peripheral symptoms and a decrease in pulses. Symptoms of radial, median, or ulnar nerve injury may also occur. A *transcondylar fracture* causes pain, swelling, and tenderness in the elbow joint. A *fracture of the medial epicondyle* causes medial elbow pain, swelling, ecchymoses, and limitation of elbow and wrist movement. Valgus instability of the elbow may result from this fracture. *Intercondylar fractures of the humerus* cause diffuse elbow swelling, crepitus, pain, tenderness, and immobility. The diagnosis can be confirmed by plain radiography. Stiffness and loss of range of motion are common sequelae of this type of fracture. A *Monteggia's fracture-dislocation* consists of a fracture of the proximal third of the ulnar and anterior dislocation of the radial head. Medial and lateral elbow pain, tenderness, and swelling occur. The diagnosis can be confirmed by plain radiography.

A *radial head fracture may be associated with an acute distal radioulnar dislocation.* Proximal migration of the radius may occur, resulting in wrist pain and loss of supination. The radial head fracture may cause anterolateral elbow pain, tenderness, swelling, and crepitus.

Simple dislocation of the elbow results from severe elbow hyperextension during a fall on the outstretched arm. The anterior joint capsule and the medial and lateral collateral ligaments are torn. Severe elbow pain, accompanied by prominence of the olecranon, diffuse elbow swelling, tenderness, and joint immobility occur. The elbow is held stiffly in flexion. The diagnosis can be confirmed by plain radiography. Closed reduction results in good return of elbow mobility if postreduction immobilization is limited to 2 weeks. Injury to the brachial artery, ulnar, and median nerves may be associated with dislocation.

Acute anterior elbow pain may be secondary to a *tear in the brachialis muscle.* This injury causes anterior tenderness and swelling over the distal humerus. *Rupture of the distal biceps tendon* occurs with an audible snap. The tendon is no longer palpable in the midantecubital fossa, and the biceps muscle forms a bunch in the proximal portion of the upper arm when forearm flexion is attempted. A *biceps muscle tear* causes distal upper arm pain, swelling, extensive ecchymoses, tenderness, and a palpable muscle defect. Forearm flexion and supination are impaired. It is seen most frequently in military parachutists. An *anterior capsular tear* results from a hyperextension injury. Local anterior elbow pain, swelling, tenderness, and ecchymoses are usually present. Extension at the elbow intensifies the pain. *Disruption of the annular ligament* causes anterolateral elbow pain and tenderness. The *anteriorly dislocated radial head* may be palpable in the antecubital fossa. The diagnosis of radial head dislocation can be confirmed by plain radiography. *Thrombophlebitis* may cause a painful, tender, red cord in the antecubital fossa. Some cases are associated with a tender cord without skin erythema. *Nonsuppurative and suppurative forms* of thrombophlebitis may occur. Suppurative phlebitis occurs in debilitated or burned patients.

Medial elbow pain may result from a *strain of the flexor-pronator forearm muscle mass.* A grade I (stretched muscle fibers) to a grade III strain (tear of muscle and investing fascia) may be present. *Rupture of the medial collateral ligament* occurs with a valgus force applied to the extended elbow. Medial elbow pain, tenderness, swelling, and instability may be present. Medial instability can be demonstrated by a valgus stress radiograph.

Little League elbow occurs in the 8- to 13-year age group. Medial elbow pain and tenderness are associated with loss of the ability to throw hard. Radiographs demonstrate accelerated growth, partial separation, or fragmentation of the medial epiphysis of the distal humerus ("epiphysitis"). A *medial epicondylar fracture* causes medial pain, swelling, tenderness, and medial instability. The avulsed medial epicondyle and attached medial collateral ligament may be displaced into the joint space, resulting in painful locking. A radiographic gravity valgus stress test can be used to demonstrate medial instability. *Acute neuropathy of the ulnar nerve* at the elbow may follow a direct blow, a supracondylar fracture, dislocation of the elbow, or prolonged direct pressure on the nerve. Pain occurs in the medial elbow, forearm, and medial side of the hand. Hypesthesia and paresthesias of the ring and small finger, and weakness of the intrinsic hand muscles may be present. Elbow flexion with wrist extension may provoke or intensify pain and paresthesias. A Tinel's sign and nerve tenderness may be present at the elbow. *Medial epicondylitis* causes medial epicondylar pain and tenderness. The pain may be intensified by flexion of the wrist against resistance or passive extension of the wrist with the elbow extended.

Acute *epitrochlear lymphadenitis* may cause medial elbow pain and epitrochlear lymph node enlargement and tenderness. Most cases are secondary to a hand or forearm cellulitis or abscess. Tularemia and cat-scratch disease may also cause tender and sometimes painful epitrochlear lymphadenitis.

Lateral elbow pain may result from *avulsion of the lateral extensor muscle mass* from its origin on the lateral epicondyle. An audible pop, accompanied by lateral elbow pain, followed by lateral elbow swelling, tenderness, and a skin ecchymoses, occurs. *Disruption of the annular ligament* is *associated with anterior dislocation of the radial head*. *Entrapment of the musculocutaneous or the lateral antebrachial cutaneous nerve* may cause lateral elbow and proximal lateral forearm pain and burning. Hypesthesia and paresthesias extend down the lateral border of the forearm. Elbow and forearm pain is intensified by pronating the forearm with the elbow extended. *Lateral epicondylitis* causes lateral epicondylar pain and tenderness that are intensified by wrist extension against resistance. *Osteochondral fracture of the radial head or capitellum* may result from medial collateral ligament weakness and incompetence and valgus stress on the elbow. Loose bodies may result, and they may cause painful locking. Posterior elbow pain may result from a *triceps insertional tendinitis or rupture* of the triceps muscle. Rupture results in a tender triceps defect and loss of extension power at the elbow. A *valgus extension overload syndrome* results from olecranon impingement in the olecranon fossa. Loose joint bodies may form, and cause pain and locking. A *stress fracture of the olecranon* may cause olecranon pain and tenderness. Plain radiographs may be falsely negative. A radionuclide bone scan is a very sensitive test for the detection of an undisplaced stress fracture and will

usually demonstrate linear uptake of technetium-99m (^{99m}TC) along the fracture line. *Bursitis* causes a cystic swelling, skin redness and warmth, pain, and tenderness over the olecranon posteriorly. *Gout, infection, and trauma* are the major causes of acute bursitis. Bursal fluid aspiration and analysis may be required to exclude infection and gout.

Acute monoarticular arthritis may involve the elbow. The joint is swollen (paraolecranon grooves are full), painful, and tender; and warmth and erythema of the overlying skin may be present. Joint range of motion is moderately to severely limited. *Septic arthritis* is associated with a high synovial fluid (SF) leukocyte count; a polymorphonuclear leukocyte predominance; a low SF glucose level; and a positive Gram's stain and bacterial culture. Common isolates from synovial fluid include *Staphylococcus aureus*, streptococcal species, and gram-negative bacilli. *Neisseria gonorrhoeae* is the most frequent cause of septic arthritis in sexually active patients under age 30. *Disseminated gonococcal infection (arthritis-dermatitis syndrome)* causes a polyarthralgia that localizes to one or two joints. These joints are painful and may be swollen, tender, and warm, but skin erythema is uncommon. A tenosynovitis may affect the fingers, hands, and wrists or the feet and ankles. Pustules and hemorrhagic vesicles on a 1 to 1.5 cm erythematous base may occur on the extremities. Synovial fluid cultures for *N. gonorrhoeae* may be negative in 50 percent of cases, but mucous membrane cultures have a sensitivity of 80 percent. Arthritis, dermatitis, and tenosynovitis respond to parenteral ceftriaxone therapy. *Gout or pseudogout* may cause an acutely painful, swollen, red, tender, warm elbow. Synovial fluid will contain monosodium urate crystals in gout, and calcium pyrophosphate dihydrate crystals in pseudogout. Acute elbow pain in a patient with hemophilia is usually caused by an acute *hemarthrosis*. Evacuation of the blood relieves pain and prevents loss of elbow function. Some forms of *additive or migratory polyarthritis* can involve the elbow, producing an acute arthritis. These include *acute rheumatic fever*, diagnosed by the presence of elevated antistreptococcal antibodies, subcutaneous nodules, and a dramatic response to salicylates; *hepatitis B-associated arthritis*, which may be identified by the presence of abnormal liver function tests and hepatitis B surface antigen in the serum; *Reiter's syndrome*, which causes an asymmetric arthritis that is associated with urethritis, conjunctivitis, or anterior uveitis and/or diarrhea; *Lyme disease arthritis*, identified by the characteristic initial rash (erythema migrans) and a serum enzyme-linked immunosorbent assay (ELISA) for *Borrelia burgdorferi* antibodies; and *rubella* or *rubella vaccine–induced* generalized joint pain and stiffness in women.

Referred elbow and forearm pain may occur with *acute myocardial infarction* or *coronary insufficiency*. A C8 radiculopathy may cause neck, elbow, medial forearm and hand pain and paresthesia that are intensified by neck movement, coughing, or straining.

Acute arterial occlusion in the arm may occur secondary to an embolus, direct trauma to the artery with thrombosis or transection of the vessel, or vasculitis. Pain, paralysis, paresthesia, skin pallor, and an absent radial pulse characterize the distal arm in patients with acute brachial artery occlusion.

Impending Volkmann's ischemic contracture may cause aching forearm pain, muscle firmness and tenderness, and skin erythema. The causes include direct trauma, forearm compression, brachial artery occlusion secondary to injury, or a hematoma in the anterior compartment of the forearm. Symptoms of a compartment syndrome include pain on finger stretch, paresthesias in the hands, and muscle pareses. If the brachial artery is not occluded, pulses remain intact for many hours, and finger color remains normal. If the artery is obstructed, finger pallor and absent pulses may be observed. Some cases develop under a cast used for fixation of a supracondylar or forearm fracture or an elbow dislocation. The cast should be immediately removed and the arm explored. Wick catheter compartment pressures should be recorded. Arm salvage and prevention of ischemic contracture may be achieved by fasciotomy, epimysiotomy, and decompression of the median and ulnar nerves.

A pulsatile, erythematous, tender, focal lesion on the arm in a patient with bacterial endocarditis may be a *mycotic aneurysm* of an intramuscular artery. Aching forearm pain and tenderness after unaccustomed use of the forearms at work or in athletics are usually due to a *grade I muscle strain* in the forearm. Use of the muscles provokes or intensifies the pain for 1 to 3 days after onset.

☐ DESCRIPTION OF LISTED DISEASES

1. FRACTURES

A. Olecranon Fracture Direct impact with the point of the elbow or a strong contraction of the triceps at the time of a fall on the extended arm can cause a fracture of the olecranon. There are posterior elbow pain, swelling, tenderness, ecchymoses, and crepitus. A gap in the olecranon may be palpable before the swelling occurs if the fracture fragments are displaced. The ability to extend the arm may be limited or absent. A displaced olecranon fracture requires open reduction and internal fixation. Articular fractures may be treated with tension band wiring or excision of the olecranon fragment, followed by reattachment of the triceps tendon to the ulna.

TABLE OF DISEASE INCIDENCE

INCIDENCE PER 100,000 (APPROXIMATE)

Common (>100)	Uncommon (>5–100)	Rare (>0–5)
Supracondylar fractures of the humerus (common in children)	Olecranon fracture	Radial head fracture with acute distal radioulnar dislocation
Simple dislocation of the elbow	Radial head fracture	Brachialis muscle tear
Medial epicondylitis	Supracondylar fracture in adults	Rupture of the distal biceps tendon
Lateral epicondylitis	Transcondylar fracture	Biceps muscle tear
Rubella arthritis	Intercondylar fracture of the humerus	Rupture of the flexor forearm muscle mass
Rubella vaccine-induced arthritis	Monteggia's fracture-dislocation	Epitrochlear lymphadenitis
Referred pain from acute myocardial infarction or coronary insufficiency	Anterior capsular tear	Rupture of the lateral extensor muscle origin
Grade I muscle strain of the forearm	Disruption of the annular ligament and anterior radial head dislocation	Entrapment of the musculocutaneous or lateral antebrachial cutaneous nerve
	Acute thrombophlebitis in the antecubital fossa	Triceps rupture
	Rupture or injury to the medial collateral ligament	Valgus extension overload syndrome
	Little League elbow	Stress fracture of the olecranon
	Medial epicondylar fracture	Septic olecranon bursitis
	Acute ulnar neuropathy	Impending Volkmann's ischemic contracture
	Osteochondral fracture of the radial head-capitellum articulation	Mycotic aneurysm of the arm
	Triceps tendinitis	
	Olecranon bursitis caused by gout or trauma	
	Septic arthritis	
	Disseminated gonococcal infection	
	Gout	
	Pseudogout	
	Acute rheumatic fever	
	Acute hepatitis B arthritis	
	Reiter's syndrome	
	Lyme disease arthritis	
	Hemophilic arthropathy	
	Acute C8 radiculopathy	
	Acute brachial artery occlusion	
	Acute bilateral elbow pain	
	Acute bilateral forearm pain	

B. Radial Head Fractures These fractures usually follow a fall on the outstretched hand. Pain, swelling, and tenderness occur over the radial head on the lateral side of the elbow. Type I fractures are not displaced. A type II radial head fracture shows minimal displacement of the fragments, and a type III fracture is comminuted and involves the entire head. After selective injection of lidocaine into the fracture site, the range of pronation and supination may be tested. Inability to obtain the full range of these forearm movements requires open reduction. Radial head fractures may also be associated with dislocation of the elbow (type IV fracture) or with severe elbow instability due to medial collateral ligament disruption.

C. Supracondylar Fracture of the Humerus This type of humeral fracture is most frequent in the first decade of life. There is a fall on the outstretched hand with the elbow extended. The distal humeral fragment is displaced posteriorly. A small percentage of these fractures occur with the elbow in flexion. This leads to anterior angulation of the distal humeral fragment. Pain, tenderness, swelling, crepitus, ecchymoses, and deformity occur over the elbow and distal region of the upper arm. If the distal fragment is displaced posteriorly, an S-shaped deformity is present over the lower humerus. The visible and palpable anterior prominence is the lower end of the humeral shaft. An antecubital ecchymoses or wound may be associated with this fragment (i.e., open fracture). Differentiation from an elbow dislocation is required. The olecranon and the epicondyles form an equilateral triangle posteriorly, and this relationship is preserved with a supracondylar fracture, but not with an elbow dislocation.

Supracondylar fractures may result in injury to the stretched brachial artery and to the radial, median, or ulnar nerves. Symptoms related to these injuries may occur during a delay in treatment or following closed reduction and casting (i.e., impending Volkmann's ischemic contracture). These neurovascular complications of a supracondylar fracture of the humerus and other forearm trauma are discussed below.

D. Transcondylar (Dicondylar) Fracture of the Humerus This fracture follows a fall on the extended outstretched hand or a fall on the flexed elbow. Pain, swelling, and tenderness occur at the elbow. This type of fracture is more commonly seen in the elderly, osteoporotic patient. The diagnosis of an intraarticular fracture can be confirmed by plain radiographs, and the injury may be treated by closed reduction and casting.

E. Medial Epicondylar Fracture of the Humerus This injury may follow a direct blow to the elbow or a fall on the outstretched hand. In the latter case, dislocation of the elbow may be associated. There are local medial elbow pain, swelling, tenderness, ecchymoses, and limitation of elbow and wrist movement. Ulnar nerve injury

may be associated, causing hypesthesia and paresthesias of the ring and small fingers, and hand weakness. Plain radiographs will confirm the fracture. The epicondylar fracture fragment may be trapped in the joint and cause painful limitation of elbow motion. Ulnar neuropathy may develop months or years after the fracture has healed. Elbow instability may result from this fracture.

F. Intercondylar Fracture of the Humerus This intraarticular fracture may follow a fall on the outstretched hand or a direct blow to the elbow. The coronoid process of the ulnar is forcefully wedged into the intercondylar region of the humerus, resulting in a T- or Y-shaped fracture pattern. The diagnosis can be confirmed by plain radiography. Undisplaced or displaced fractures without rotational deformity can be treated by closed reduction. Type III and IV fractures usually require open reduction and internal fixation, or external fixation and skeletal traction. Elbow stiffness, loss of functional range of motion, and ulnar neuropathy after surgery are sequelae of this type of fracture.

G. Monteggia's Fracture-Dislocation There is a fracture of the proximal third of the ulna, with anterior dislocation of the radial head. This fracture may follow a fall on the outstretched hand or a direct injury to the ulna. There are medial elbow pain, swelling, and tenderness. Swelling and tenderness may be present over the lateral elbow region, and the dislocated radial head may be palpable anteriorly. Supination and pronation are impaired. Radial nerve injury may occur in 20 percent of cases. The diagnosis can be made by plain radiography, but the radial dislocation is frequently missed.

H. Radial Head Fracture with Acute Distal Radioulnar Dislocation (Essex-Lopresti's Fracture-Dislocation) This rare type of fracture follows a fall on the outstretched hand that drives the radial head into the capitellum. Disruption of the distal radioulnar joint and interosseous membrane occurs as a result of the same indirect force. There is proximal migration of the radius (5–10 mm), associated with wrist pain and loss of supination. A displaced radial head fracture associated with wrist pain requires careful clinical and radiographic evaluation of the distal radioulnar joint. The radial head fracture causes anterolateral elbow pain and tenderness.

2. SIMPLE DISLOCATION OF THE ELBOW

This injury usually follows a fall on the outstretched arm. Severe hyperextension occurs, which ruptures the anterior capsule of the joint, the anterior oblique ligament, other portions of the medial collateral ligament, and in some cases the lateral collateral ligament. The ulna and radius are displaced posteriorly or posterolaterally in relation to the distal humerus. The dislocated joint is held stiffly, in partial flexion. There are severe elbow pain, diffuse swelling, and local tenderness. Plain elbow radiographs will confirm the diagnosis. The posteriorly displaced olecranon may appear unusually prominent. Closed reduction under general anesthesia is usually successful. The joint is then placed in 90° of flexion in a posterior splint, with the forearm in neutral position. Good functional results, without troublesome pain, require limitation of the period of immobilization to less than 13 days. Early mobilization does not usually result in redislocation. Injury to the brachial artery and ulnar and median nerves may occur. The median nerve may be entrapped during the reduction procedure.

3. ACUTE ANTERIOR ELBOW PAIN

A. Brachialis Muscle Tear   During hyperextension of the elbow, the brachialis muscle may rupture, causing anterior elbow pain, tenderness, and swelling.

B. Rupture of the Distal Biceps Muscle Tendon   During flexion of the elbow against resistance (e.g., while lifting a heavy weight), a severe pain and a tearing sensation or snap is felt in the antecubital fossa. Weakness of forearm flexion and supination become immediately apparent. The antecubital space is tender, but swelling is relatively mild. The biceps tendon is no longer palpable in the midportion of the antecubital fossa. With attempted flexion, the biceps muscle forms a bunch in the proximal upper arm. In proximal rupture of the biceps tendon, the bunch is in the lower arm, the pain is at the shoulder, and only supination is impaired.

C. Biceps Muscle Tear   There is a tearing or popping sensation just above the anterior elbow, followed by severe pain, swelling, and weakness. The pain is felt in the distal upper arm or in the anterior elbow. A palpable defect may be found in the distal biceps, or the tear may be filled by hematoma. If a defect is present, the humerus may be palpable through it. There is ecchymoses over the region of the tear and distal to it. This injury has been most frequently reported in military parachutists.

D. Anterior Capsular Tear   Extreme elbow hyperextension in a fall can tear the anterior capsule of the elbow. Local pain, swelling, tenderness, and ecchymoses may be present. Pain in the antecubital fossa is increased with elbow extension. Immobilization in flexion for a few days, ice, and analgesics lead to relief of pain and full functional use of the arm in 1 to 3 weeks.

E. Disruption of the Annular Ligament   This injury may follow forced flexion against resistance, a fall on the outstretched hand with the forearm pronated, or a direct blow to the elbow. There is anterolateral elbow pain.

Pronation and supination may be painful and impaired. The dislocated radial head may be palpated in the antecubital fossa. Lateral swelling, tenderness, and ecchymoses may be present. The diagnosis of radial head dislocation, secondary to rupture of the annular ligament, can be confirmed by plain radiography of the elbow. A line through the radial shaft should intersect the capitellum. If it does not, a dislocation of the radial head is likely. An associated fracture of the proximal ulna may be present and go undetected, unless a follow-up radiograph is done 2 weeks after the injury. Reduction can be achieved by arm traction and forearm supination, followed by immobilization of the arm in flexion.

F. Thrombophlebitis

1. Acute Nonsuppurative Thrombophlebitis of the Cephalic or Basilic Veins   Aching anterior forearm and/or antecubital pain may be associated with a palpable, tender, subcutaneous cord. Erythema of the skin overlying the cord may be present. This disorder usually follows introduction of a needle or catheter into a peripheral vein.

2. Suppurative Thrombophlebitis   Severe pain, fever, and prostration may be associated with suppurative thrombophlebitis. Blood cultures may isolate *S. aureus*. Exploration of the suspected vein and other veins recently cannulated is required to establish the diagnosis. Suppurative phlebitis occurs in the presence of extensive burns or a severe debilitating medical illness.

4. MEDIAL ELBOW PAIN

A. Rupture of the Flexor Forearm Muscle Mass   Medial elbow pain may result from a strain of the flexor forearm mass (pronator teres, flexor carpi radialis, palmaris longus, and flexor carpi ulnaris). A grade I strain involves stretching of the muscle fibers but no disruption. A partial tear of the involved muscle, with intact overlying fascia, describes a grade II strain. There are local tenderness, swelling, muscle spasm, and a hematoma. Stretch causes pain, and muscle use is limited. Grade III tears involve a complete disruption of the muscle and its investing fascia, resulting in a complete loss of muscle function. Local tenderness, a palpable defect in the muscle, diffuse swelling, and ecchymoses in the overlying skin support the diagnosis of a grade III tear.

Grades I and II strains can be treated conservatively, but grade III strains require operative repair.

B. Rupture of the Medial Collateral Ligament   The ligament is avulsed from the epicondyle (70 percent of cases) or from the ulna (20 percent of cases). Ligament rupture may follow a valgus force on the extended arm. This injury usually occurs after falling on the outstretched hand with an abduction component applied against the medial side of the elbow. Tears may be associated with pitching and javelin throwing. A medial ligament tear occurring during pitching may be heard as a pop by the athlete. After ligament rupture, there are valgus stress instability and severe medial elbow pain and tenderness. Arthrography will demonstrate extravasation of contrast media into the soft tissue on the medial side of the elbow. A valgus stress radiograph can also be used to demonstrate medial elbow instability.

C. Little League Elbow   This disorder occurs in adolescents and young children involved in throwing sports. There are localized pain and tenderness and sometimes swelling over the medial epicondyle. Limitation of elbow motion occurs, and there is a loss of the ability to throw with the velocity achieved prior to the onset of symptoms. Symptoms are exacerbated by throwing curve balls. Radiographs may demonstrate accelerated growth and/or partial separation or fragmentation of the medial epiphysis of the distal humerus (''epiphysitis''). Flexion contracture and an increased valgus carrying angle may occur in severe cases. Compression stress on the lateral radiohumeral joint may result in osteochondritis dissecans involving the radial head and capitellum. Treatment includes rest, ice, nonsteroidal anti-inflammatory drugs, and immobilization.

D. Medial Epicondylar Fracture   This fracture type is discussed above. Medial epicondyle pain and tenderness are associated with valgus instability of the elbow. The avulsed medial epicondyle and attached medial collateral ligament may sometimes be displaced into the elbow joint and interfere with elbow function. A gravity valgus stress radiograph can demonstrate medial instability. Patients with medial instability require operative repair of the fracture and medial ligament. Surgical repair is also recommended for adolescents desiring to return to active competition in throwing sports.

E. Ulnar Neuropathy   Acute ulnar neuropathy may result from a traumatic elbow dislocation, a supracondylar fracture of the humerus, a direct blow to the nerve, or direct pressure on the nerve at the elbow over a period of several hours (e.g., leaning on the elbow while working, in a patient with a drug overdose, or arm board compression in the operating room). Aching pain may occur in the medial elbow and forearm and the ring and small fingers. Paresthesias and hypesthesia may involve the same fingers. Symptoms can be provoked or intensified by elbow flexion combined with wrist extension for up to 3 min (elbow flexion test). A positive Tinel's sign may be present over the ulnar nerve at the elbow, and nerve tenderness may also be present. Severe cases of acute ulnar neuropathy may demonstrate weakness of the intrinsic hand muscles. Electromyographic and nerve con-

duction velocity studies may confirm the clinical diagnosis, but a negative result does not exclude the diagnosis. Conservative management of acute ulnar compression neuropathy usually results in a decrease in medial elbow and forearm pain and resolution of neurologic symptoms. Acute ulnar neuropathy secondary to severe trauma may require operative intervention.

F. Medial Epicondylitis   Pain develops over the medial elbow and is intensified by throwing or by hitting a forehand shot or serve in tennis. Tenderness of the medial epicondyle is present. Flexion of the wrist against resistance or passive extension of the wrist with the elbow extended intensifies the medial elbow pain. Acute symptoms respond to rest and nonsteroidal anti-inflammatory drugs.

G. Epitrochlear Lymphadenitis   Medial elbow pain intensified by movement is associated with enlarged, tender epitrochlear lymph nodes. These nodes drain the medial side of the forearm and hand, and the middle, ring, and small fingers. A bacterial infection of the arm or hand may cause cellulitis or a localized abscess, ascending lymphangitis, and epitrochlear and axillary lymphadenitis. Fever and leukocytosis may be associated. There may be a discrete, palpable, enlarged group of epitrochlear nodes or diffuse medial elbow swelling and tenderness. Group A streptococci and *S. aureus* are the usual pathogens.

Up to 8 percent of patients with ulceroglandular tularemia may develop tender, painful epitrochlear lymphadenitis and sometimes axillary lymphadenitis. The initial skin lesion appears 1 to 14 days after contact with the carcass of a wild rabbit or muskrat as a papule on the hand or forearm. Within 2 to 4 days, this papule ulcerates, and fever, chills, and malaise occur. The diagnosis is suggested by a history of animal contact and the clinical findings, and may be confirmed by a positive blood or sputum culture and/or a fourfold or greater rise in the tularemia tube agglutination or microagglutination titer. Most cases are diagnosed on clinical and serologic evidence.

Epitrochlear lymphadenitis may also occur in cat-scratch disease in association with a low-grade fever (32–60 percent of cases), malaise, and fatigue (25 percent of cases). Single node enlargement and tenderness occur in 50 percent, and multiple node enlargement at a single site occurs in 20 percent. Up to 33 percent of patients have adenopathy at multiple sites (e.g., axilla and inguinal). A primary papule or pustule may form at the site of the cat scratch. Lymph node biopsy is supportive of the diagnosis.

Secondary syphilis may cause fever, malaise, a rash, generalized lymphadenopathy, and bilateral, nonpainful epitrochlear adenopathy. The diagnosis can be confirmed on clinical evidence and by a positive reagin test result for syphilis.

5. LATERAL ELBOW PAIN

A. Acute Rupture of the Lateral Extensor Muscle Origin Involving the brachioradialis, extensor carpi radialis longus, and extensor carpi radialis brevis, this injury occurs with sharp, severe pain and an audible snap. Local tenderness of the lateral epicondyle, loss of extensor function, swelling, and skin ecchymoses occur. Surgical repair is recommended for competitive athletes.

B. Disruption of the Annular Ligament and Anterior Radial Head Dislocation Patients experience a popping sensation and anterolateral pain with varus elbow stress. Forceful supination or flexion may also cause anterior radial head dislocation. Dislocation can be documented by a varus stress radiograph.

C. Entrapment of the Musculocutaneous Nerve or the Lateral Antebrachial Cutaneous Nerve Acute entrapment of the musculocutaneous nerve may follow vigorous use of the arm (e.g., building a wall or weight lifting) or a fracture of the distal humerus. The entrapment may result in paresis of the coracobrachialis, brachialis, and biceps muscles. Lateral elbow and forearm aching may be associated with weakness of forearm flexion. The lateral antebrachial cutaneous nerve may be entrapped by the distal biceps tendon. Pain and burning occur in the lateral elbow and proximal forearm with compression of the nerves. Hypesthesia and paresthesias may extend down the lateral border of the forearm. Elbow pain is intensified by pronating the forearm with the elbow extended.

D. Lateral Epicondylitis Pain and local tenderness occur over the lateral epicondyle and are usually provoked or intensified by use of the arm. Passive flexion of the wrist with the elbow extended increases lateral elbow pain. Extension of the wrist against resistance also intensifies epicondylar pain. Most acute cases respond to splinting, avoidance of the provoking activity, and use of nonsteroidal anti-inflammatory drugs.

E. Osteochondral Fracture of the Radial Head-Capitellum Articulation Compression forces on the capitellum may occur secondary to medial collateral ligament weakness and incompetence. Valgus stress may cause osteochondral fracture of the capitellum or radial head. Such a fracture may result in the formation of loose joint bodies that cause lateral elbow pain and locking. These may be removed and intact osteochondral fractures repaired by arthroscopic surgery.

6. POSTERIOR ELBOW PAIN

A. Triceps Tendinitis Pain and tenderness occur posteriorly over the olecranon. Mild edema may be noted overlying the triceps insertion. Extension of the elbow against resistance intensifies the pain. Radiographs of the elbow are negative. Rest and nonsteroidal anti-inflammatory drugs lead to resolution of symptoms.

B. Triceps Rupture Severe local pain, swelling, tenderness, and skin ecchymoses; a palpable triceps muscle defect above the elbow; and loss of extension power occur. Operative repair is required.

C. Valgus Extension Overload Syndrome Posterior elbow pain follows impingement of the olecranon in the olecranon fossa. Loose bodies may form, resulting in painful locking. Osteophytes may develop on the olecranon tip.

D. Stress Fracture of the Olecranon Extensor overload may cause a painful stress fracture of the olecranon. Plain radiographs may remain negative for weeks or months, despite posterior elbow pain and tenderness. A radionuclide bone scan will demonstrate a linear pattern of increased uptake over the fracture site. Immobilization in extension will usually lead to healing of nondisplaced stress fractures.

E. Olecranon Bursitis Pain and a tender cystic swelling occur over the olecranon posteriorly. Adjacent skin erythema and tenderness are frequently present. The elbow is held in partial flexion. The range of motion is normal, and there is no joint effusion. The causes include the following.

1. Septic Bursitis Skin redness and swelling may be present over the bursal sac and may extend to the surrounding skin. A skin wound of entry is usually present, or there is a history of a recent operation or injection of the bursa. The fluid contains a high concentration of polymorphonuclear leukocytes. Gram's stain is 65- to 90-percent sensitive, and culture has similar sensitivity. The most frequent causative organism is *S. aureus* (80 percent of cases). Group A streptococci account for 10 percent of cases, while *Hemophilus influenzae*, anaerobic bacteria, and gram-negative rods account for the remaining 10 percent of cases. There is a good response to antibiotic therapy and repeated needle aspiration of the bursa.

2. Gouty Bursitis Acute gout may cause local pain, bursal swelling, tenderness, skin erythema, and warmth. The bursal fluid contains a relatively low concentration of polymorphonuclear leukocytes (<6600 cells/mm^3) and monosodium urate crystals. Leukocyte counts in synovial fluid in gout are usually much higher. The reason for the low cell count in gouty bursitis is unknown. There is a response to colchicine.

3. Traumatic Bursitis Patients experience local pain, tenderness, and swelling. Small nodules are palpable within the bursa. There may be a history of injury to the elbow or chronic pressure on the elbow during work. Effusions may be hemorrhagic, and the leukocyte count is usually less than 1500 cells/mm³. The results of culture and examination for crystals are negative.

7. ACUTE MONOARTICULAR ARTHRITIS

A. Septic Arthritis   Severe aching or throbbing pain occurs in the affected elbow. The paraolecranon grooves are full and fluctuant. The elbow is held stiffly, and movement is resisted. The overlying skin is warm and may be erythematous. The entire joint is tender. Fever may reach 38.3°C (101°F) but is frequently low-grade. Blood cultures may be positive in up to 75 percent of cases. Synovial fluid cell counts range from as low as 5000 to over 100,000 cells/mm³, with a polymorphonuclear leukocyte predominance. The joint fluid glucose level may be low (>40 mg/dl below the simultaneously drawn blood glucose) in up to 50 percent of cases. Low synovial glucose concentrations are nonspecific and have also been reported in rheumatoid arthritis and tuberculous arthritis. Synovial cultures for bacteria may be positive in 90 percent of cases. The common isolates in nongonococcal suppurative arthritis include *S. aureus* (70 percent); *Streptococcus* species (*Streptococcus pneumoniae*, groups A and B streptococci, *Streptococcus viridans* and microaerophilic and anaerobic streptococci) (17 percent); and gram-negative bacilli (8 percent).

N. gonorrhoeae infection is the predominant cause of septic arthritis in adults under 30 years of age. It may occur clinically as a monoarthritis with no or few skin manifestations or as a disseminated infection (i.e., dermatitis-arthritis syndrome) with polyarticular symptoms.

Risk factors present in patients with nongonococcal bacterial arthritis include oral corticosteroid therapy (33 percent of cases); preexisting arthritis, such as rheumatoid arthritis, gout, osteoarthritis, or hemophilic arthropathy (24 percent of cases); a recent intra-articular injection (24 percent of cases); other active infections (22 percent of cases); diabetes mellitus (13 percent of cases), joint trauma (12 percent of cases); and splenectomy (< 1 percent).

B. Disseminated Gonococcal Infection (Arthritis-Dermatitis Syndrome)   This illness usually begins 1 to 4 weeks after mucous membrane infection, with additive and/or migratory polyarthralgias involving the knees, elbows, wrists, and hands. Physical examination shows evidence of arthritis or tenosynovitis (periarthritis) in relation to two or more joints. Only a few joints are usually affected by a definite arthritis or periarthritic process (tenosynovitis). This pattern of involvement of only a few joints serves to differentiate this disorder from an immune complex-mediated arthropathy, which usually causes a symmetrical polyarthritis. A characteristic skin eruption occurs in association with the joint complaints in 75 percent of cases. Small pustules and hemorrhagic vesicles on a 1- to 1.5-cm erythematous base occur on the extremities. The number of cutaneous lesions seldom exceeds 40, and as few as 3 to 5 may be present. Without treatment, the arthritis resolves in most sites but tends to persist in one or two joints (e.g., knee, ankle, elbow, and wrist).

Involved joints are painful at rest, tender, swollen, and warm. Synovial fluid cell counts exceed 50,000 cells/mm³, and synovial fluid cultures may be positive. Only 50 percent of patients with this syndrome have positive blood or joint fluid cultures. *N. gonorrhoeae* can be cultured from the urethra, endocervix, anorectum, or throat in 80 percent of cases or from a sexual contact. Gram-stained or immunofluorescent-stained smears and cultures of skin lesion fluid should be obtained. Stains may be positive when cultures are negative.

Finger, hand, and wrist pain and swelling and foot and heel pain may be caused by gonococcal tenosynovitis, and these complaints are supportive of the diagnosis. Administration of ceftriaxone intravenously or intramuscularly for 10 days will usually lead to prompt resolution of all complaints.

C. Gout   Acute pain, swelling, redness, and tenderness of the elbow joint may be caused by gout. The serum uric acid level is usually elevated, and the synovial fluid contains increased numbers of polymorphonuclear leukocytes and monosodium urate crystals.

D. Pseudogout   A goutlike clinical picture of elbow joint arthritis and a synovial fluid containing an increased concentration of polymorphonuclear leukocytes and calcium pyrophosphate dihydrate crystals are present. Chondrocalcinosis of knee, shoulder, and wrist joints may be identified on plain radiographs.

E. Hemophilic hemarthrosis   Acute elbow pain, swelling, tenderness, and warmth are usually due to intra-articular bleeding in a patient with hemophilia. Administration of factor VIII and aspiration of blood from the elbow relieve pain and prevent ankylosis.

8. ACUTE POLYARTHRITIS WITH ELBOW INVOLVEMENT

A. Acute Rheumatic Fever   A migratory polyarthritis associated with fever and subcutaneous nodules is a common presentation. Unilateral elbow involvement is more frequent than bilateral. There may be elbow swelling, redness, pain, tenderness, and limitation of motion. There is usually a history of a sore throat and/or respiratory infection within 2 to 5 weeks prior to the onset of fever and joint symptoms. Serum antibodies to streptococcal antigens are elevated (Streptozyme test). There is a dramatic response to salicylate therapy.

B. Hepatitis B-Associated Arthritis Type B hepatitis causes a pruritic rash (urticarial or, less commonly, a macular, papular, or petechial rash) and a migratory or additive polyarthritis prior to the onset of clinical hepatitis. The elbow may be involved in up to 25 percent of cases. Serum contains hepatitis B surface antigen (HBsAg), and liver function test results are frequently abnormal or soon become so. Symptoms respond to salicylate therapy.

C. Reiter's Syndrome This disorder causes an asymmetrical polyarthritis that may involve the elbows, shoulders, knees, hips, and ankles. Urethritis, diarrhea, and conjunctivitis or anterior uveitis occurs. Skin manifestations include balanitis circinata and keratoderma blennorrhagicum.

D. Lyme Disease Arthritis This disorder begins with an annular erythematous rash. Smaller, satellite, red rings may appear in adjacent skin areas. An acute febrile illness follows the appearance of the rash by 1 to 3 weeks. The illness may be characterized by aseptic meningitis and mild encephalitis. Facial nerve palsy on one or both sides may follow, or a painful radiculoneuritis involving the arms, trunk, or legs may occur. Joint swelling, pain, and tenderness may develop 1 to 6 months after the onset of the illness. The knees (75 percent), ankles (10 percent), shoulders (30 percent), elbows (18 percent), and wrists (12 percent) may be involved. The diagnosis can be supported by measuring IgG antibody to *B. burgdorferi* by an ELISA method. Confirmation by Western blot may also be performed to increase specificity. There is a good response of the joint complaints to high-dose intravenous penicillin or ceftriaxone.

E. Rubella An acute polyarthritis involving the fingers (90 percent), wrists (70 percent), elbows (25 percent), knees (70 percent), and ankles (40 percent) occurs in 15 to 60 percent of women with rubella. Stiffness and pain are the most frequent complaints. Objective signs of joint inflammation are usually absent. Symptoms resolve spontaneously after 5 to 30 days. The rash may precede the arthritis by several days, or it may follow it by as much as a week. Tenosynovitis, carpal tunnel syndrome, and brachial neuritis may occur. This disorder occurs primarily in women and is rare in children and men.

F. Rubella Vaccine-Induced Arthritis This syndrome follows vaccination by 2 to 4 weeks. There is more frequent involvement of only the knees and an increased incidence of carpal tunnel involvement in the vaccine-induced illness. Arthralgias and joint stiffness last for up to 7 weeks. Up to 33 percent with knee involvement may have recurrent attacks of joint pain over several years. Rash, low-grade fever, malaise, painful posterior cervical adenopathy, and sore throat may be associated with the acute joint symptoms.

9. REFERRED PAIN

Coronary Heart Disease

1. Acute Myocardial Infarction Patients may experience left elbow, forearm, and hand pain, numbness, and paresthesias. More proximal pain in the upper arm, shoulder, precordium, substernal region, neck, and scapular region may be present at onset or appear minutes or hours later. The electrocardiogram will demonstrate evidence of myocardial infarction. Abnormal serum levels of creatine kinase and lactate dehydrogenase cardiac isozymes will be detectable during the first 48 h. Thrombolytic therapy and/or direct angioplasty may dramatically relieve pain as the occluding coronary thrombus is lysed.

2. Coronary Insufficiency This syndrome may cause prolonged elbow and forearm pain similar to that seen in myocardial infarction. There is no evidence of myocardial infarction by electrocardiographic studies or by measurement of serum cardiac isozymes. Symptoms may respond to the use of calcium channel-blocking drugs, thrombolytic agents, angioplasty, or bypass surgery.

10. ACUTE C8 RADICULOPATHY

Pain may radiate from the neck into the medial upper arm, elbow, and small and ring fingers. It may take the form of a dull ache, with superimposed lancinating jabs that travel down the arm. Neck rotation, Spurling's maneuver, coughing, sneezing, or straining at stool provoke or intensify the pain. MRI of the cervical and upper thoracic spine will usually identify the cause of the radiculopathy (e.g., acute disc herniation, epidural abscess, epidural hematoma, or tumor). Symptoms may be confused with an acute ulnar neuropathy.

11. VASCULAR DISORDERS

A. Acute Axillary or Brachial Artery Occlusion The five P's describe the symptoms and signs of this acute emergency: pain, paralysis, paresthesias, pallor, and absent pulses. Pain is severe, constant, and persistent and usually involves the fingers, hand, and forearm. Paresthesias and muscle paralysis indicate severe ischemia of the arm. A paralyzed anesthetic arm may begin to develop gangrene 6 h after the onset of symptoms. Pallor occurs because of lack of blood flow and cutaneous vasoconstriction. A line of demarcation may be present between cool, white, ischemic skin and proximal warm, perfused skin. The absence of pulses confirms occlusion and may help in localizing the site of obstruction. Use of a Doppler device and arteriography provides more accurate localization of the site of occlusion. The causes of acute arterial occlusion include emboli from the heart (mural thrombus, valve vegetation, or intraatrial or ventricular tumor) or from an atheromatous plaque or aneurysm of the innominate or subclavian-axillary arteries. Trauma to the chest, shoulder, or upper arm may also cause acute arterial occlusion. Less commonly, a vasculitis, such as giant cell arteritis, Takayasu's arteritis, or Buerger's disease, may cause an acute brachial artery occlusion. Use of the brachial artery for monitoring, for arteriography, or for cardiac catheterization can cause acute thrombotic occlusion. Symptoms resolve if the arterial obstruction is relieved within 6 h and the patency of the occluded vessel is ensured by arterial reconstruction and/or the use of anticoagulants.

B. Impending Volkmann's Ischemic Contracture (Anterior Compartment Syndrome of the Forearm) This disorder may occur several hours after a supracondylar fracture of the humerus or a severe contusion or crush injury of the forearm. Other causes of an acute forearm compartment syndrome include forearm fractures, brachial artery puncture, subfascial intravenous infiltration, an intracompartmental hematoma secondary to a coagulopathy (hemophilia), drug overdose with prolonged arm compression, a gunshot wound, and open fracture of the arm. The initial symptom is deep, aching forearm pain. The volar aspect of the forearm is tender over muscle bellies and red, warm, and swollen; the underlying muscles have a tense, firm consistency. The fingers are flexed, and attempts to passively extend them intensify forearm pain (i.e., stretch pain). The radial and ulnar pulses may be normal, diminished, or absent. Hypesthesia to pinprick and/or touch may be present in the median nerve and/or ulnar nerve sensory areas of the hand. Active finger flexion is weak and usually provokes forearm pain. Major arterial injury due to a humeral fracture may result in arterial occlusion and/or severe spasm. Occlusion of the brachial artery may be associated with aching forearm and hand pain, pain on passive finger extension, paresthesias, pallor of the fingers (poor capillary refill), pulselessness, and paralysis of the forearm muscles and hand.

If the compartment syndrome is due to intracompartmental swelling secondary to a hematoma or direct muscle trauma or to external compression by a tight cast, the five P's may include pulses intact; pink finger color (good capillary refill); palpable forearm muscle induration, tenderness, and swelling; pain on passive extension of the fingers; and paresthesias and hypesthesia in the distribution of the median and ulnar nerves. Unless the brachial artery is occluded, the radial pulse remains palpable, since the radial artery does not pass through the affected anterior compartment.

Impending Volkmann's ischemic contracture is a surgical emergency. If a supracondylar fracture has already been reduced and the arm casted, the cast should be removed. Whatever the cause, exploration is required to confirm the diagnosis and prevent ischemic damage. Intracompartmental pressures in the forearm should be measured for confirmation. The clinical findings alone may be sufficient to warrant fasciotomy, epimysiotomy of individual muscles, debridement of necrotic muscle, and decompression of median and ulnar nerves. The brachial artery should be located, and any injuries identified and repaired, an occluding thrombus removed, and spasm treated to restore the peripheral circulation.

C. Mycotic Aneurysm Secondary to Endocarditis Forearm or distal upper arm pain, redness, tenderness, and a localized pulsation beneath the erythematous region may be secondary to a mycotic aneurysm. The patient will usually have a heart murmur, fever, petechiae, and positive blood cultures, providing evidence of bacterial endocarditis.

12. GRADE I MUSCLE STRAIN OF THE FOREARM

Aching pain in the flexor-pronator or extensor-suppinator forearm muscle groups may follow unaccustomed use of the arms in work or athletics (i.e., weekend softball or bowling). The forearm pain may be intensified or provoked by lifting or other use of the forearm. Local tenderness may be present. Symptoms resolve in 1 to 3 days with rest.

13. ACUTE BILATERAL ELBOW AND FOREARM PAIN

The causes are listed in Table 40-1.

Table 40-1
ACUTE BILATERAL ELBOW AND FOREARM PAIN

Elbow
  Disseminated gonococcal infection
  Polyarticular gout
  Polyarticular pseudogout
  Acute rheumatic fever
  Acute hepatitis B arthritis
  Reiter's syndrome
  Lyme disease arthritis
  Rubella arthritis
  Rubella vaccine-induced arthritis
  Acute coronary insufficiency or myocardial infarction
Forearm
  Grade I muscle strain
  Forearm fractures

ELBOW AND FOREARM PAIN REFERENCES

Arthritis

Canoso JJ, Yood RA: Acute gouty bursitis: Report of 15 cases. *Ann Rheum Dis* 38:326–328, 1979.

Dee R: Rheumatologic and degenerative disorders of the elbow, in Dee R, Mango E, Hurst LC (eds): *Principles of Orthopaedic Practice.* New York, McGraw-Hill, 1989, vol 1, pp 635–645.

Figgie MP, Inglis AE, Mow CS, et al: Total elbow arthroplasty for complete ankylosis of the elbow. *J Bone Joint Surg (Am)* 71:513–520, 1989.

————: Salvage of non-union of supracondylar fracture of the humerus by total elbow arthroplasty. *J Bone Joint Surg (Am)* 71:1058–1065, 1989.

Kudo H, Iwano K: Total elbow arthroplasty with a non-constrained surface-replacement prosthesis in patients who have rheumatoid arthritis. *J Bone Joint Surg (Am)* 72:355–362, 1990.

Leber C, Melone CP Jr: Total elbow replacement. *Orthop Rev* 17:857–863, 1988.

Summers GD, Taylor AR, Webley M: Elbow synovectomy and excision of the radial head in rheumatoid arthritis: A short-term palliative procedure. *J Rheumatol* 15:566–569, 1988.

Elbow Fracture/Dislocation

Ackerman G, Jupiter JB: Non-union of fractures of the distal end of the humerus. *J Bone Joint Surg (Am)* 70:75–83, 1988.

DeLee JC, Green DP, Wilkins KE: Fractures and dislocations of the elbow, in Rockwood CA Jr, Green DP (eds): *Fractures in Adults,* 2d ed. Philadelphia, Lippincott, 1984, vol 2, pp 559–652.

Edwards GS Jr, Jupiter JB: Radial head fractures with acute distal radioulnar dislocation: Essex-Lopresti revisited. *Clin Orthop* 234:61–69, 1988.

Hurley JA: Complicated elbow fractures in athletes. *Clin Sports Med* 9:39–57, 1990.

Letsch R, Schmit-Neuerburg KP, Stürmer KM, et al: Intraarticular fractures of the distal humerus: Surgical treatment and results. *Clin Orthop* 241:238–244, 1989.

Mehlhoff TL, Noble PC, Bennett JB, et al: Simple dislocation of the elbow in the adult: Results after closed treatment. *J Bone Joint Surg (Am)* 70:244–249, 1988.

Ordway C, Dee R, Mango E: Fractures and dislocations of the elbow, arm, and shoulder girdle of adults, in Dee R, Mango E, Hurst LC (eds): *Principles of Orthopaedic Practice.* New York, McGraw-Hill, 1989, vol 1, pp 560–575.

Watson JT: Fractures of the forearm and elbow. *Clin Sports Med* 9:59–83, 1990.

Elbow Pain—Review

Andrews JR, Craven WM: Lesions of the posterior compartment of the elbow. *Clin Sports Med* 10:637–652, 1991.

Turek SL: The elbow, in Turek SL (ed): *Orthopaedics Principles and Their Application,* 4th ed. Philadelphia, Lippincott, 1984, vol 2, pp 967–984.

Watrous BG, Ho G Jr: Elbow pain. *Prim Care* 15:725–735, 1988.

Entrapment Neuropathies

Buehler MJ, Thayer DT: The elbow flexion test: A clinical test for the cubital tunnel syndrome. *Clin Orthop* 233:213–216, 1988.

Campbell WW: AAEE case report #18: Ulnar neuropathy in the distal forearm. *Muscle Nerve* 12:347–352, 1989.

Coyle MP Jr: Nerve entrapment syndromes in the upper extremity, in Dee R, Mango E, Hurst LC (eds): *Principles of Orthopaedic Practice.* New York, McGraw-Hill, 1989, vol 1, pp 672–684.

Glousman RE: Ulnar nerve problems in the athlete's elbow. *Clin Sports Med* 9:365–377, 1990.

Goldberg BJ, Light TR, Blair SJ: Ulnar neuropathy at the elbow: Results of medial epicondylectomy. *J Hand Surg (Am)* 14A:182–188, 1989.

Jones JA: Pitfalls in the management of cubital tunnel syndrome. *Orthop Rev* 18:36–44, 1989.

Kleinman WB, Bishop AT: Anterior intramuscular transposition of the ulnar nerve. *J Hand Surg (Am)* 14A:972–979, 1989.

Posner MA: Compressive neuropathies of the median and radial nerves at the elbow. *Clin Sports Med* 9:343–363, 1990.

Richards RR, Regan WD: Medial epicondylitis caused by injury to the medial antebrachial cutaneous nerve: A case report. *Can J Surg* 32:366–367, 369, 1989.

Epicondylitis

Chop WM Jr: Tennis elbow. *Postgrad Med* 86:301–304, 307–308, 1989.

————: Tennis elbow and life-style factors (reply). *Postgrad Med* 87:32, 34, 1990.

Kamien M: A rational management of tennis elbow. *Sports Med* 9:173–191, 1990.

Kapp R: Tennis elbow and life-style factors (comment). *Postgrad Med* 87:32, 1990.

Ligament Injuries

Garroway RY, McCue FCV III: Ligament injuries of the wrist, hand, and elbow, in Dee R, Mango E, Hurst LC (eds): *Principles of Orthopaedic Practice.* New York, McGraw-Hill, 1989, vol 1, pp 553–560.

Osteochondrosis

Roch DS, Poehling GG: Arthroscopic treatment of Panner's disease. *Clin Sports Med 10:629–636, 1991.*

Trauma

Andrews JR, Schemmel SP, Whiteside JA: Evaluation, treatment and prevention of elbow injuries in throwing athletes, in Nicholas JA, Hershman EG (eds): *The Upper Extremity in Sports Medicine.* St. Louis, Mosby, 1990, pp 781–826.

Bennett JB, Tullos HS: Acute injuries to the elbow, in Nicholas JA, Hershman EB (eds): *The Upper Extremity in Sports Medicine.* St. Louis, Mosby, 1990, pp 319–334.

Nirschl RR: Tennis injuries, in Nicholas JA, Hershman EB (eds): *The Upper Extremity in Sports Medicine.* St. Louis, Mosby, 1990, pp 827–842.

Parkes JC: Overuse injuries of the elbow, in Nicholas JA, Hershman EB (eds): *The Upper Extremity in Sports Medicine.* St. Louis, Mosby, 1990, pp 335–346.

Acute Wrist, Hand, and Finger Pain

☐ **DIAGNOSTIC LIST**

WRIST PAIN

1. Radial wrist pain
   A. Fractures
      1. Distal radius
         a. Colles' fracture
         b. Smith's fracture
         c. Articular margin fracture of the distal radius and carpal dislocation
      2. Scaphoid fracture
      3. Trapezium fracture
   B. Sprains and dislocations
      1. Scapholunate sprain
         a. Disruption of the scapholunate interosseous ligament
         b. Dynamic scapholunate instability
         c. Static rotatory subluxation of the scaphoid
      2. Radial collateral ligament (RCL) sprain
   C. Tenosynovitis (noninfectious)
      1. de Quervain's disease
      2. Tenosynovitis of the extensor pollicis longus
      3. Flexor carpi radialis (FCR) tendinitis
      4. Intersection syndrome
      5. Extensor indicis proprius syndrome
   D. Tenosynovitis (infectious)
      1. Suppurative flexor pollicis longus tenosynovitis
      2. Gonococcal tenosynovitis
      3. Other causes of infectious tenosynovitis
2. Mid-dorsal wrist pain
   A. Fractures
      1. Capitate fracture
      2. Lunate fracture and Kienböck's disease
   B. Sprains and dislocations
      1. Perilunate instability
         a. Dorsal perilunate dislocation
         b. Perilunate fracture-dislocation
         c. Volar Lunate dislocation
         d. Intermediate injury stage (perilunate or lunate dislocation)
3. Acute ulnar wrist pain
   A. Distal radioulnar joint (DRUJ) disorders
      1. Fracture of the distal ulna or radial sigmoid fossa
      2. Fracture of the triquetrum or lunate
      3. Triquetrum avulsion fracture
      4. Dislocation of the distal ulna

5. Dislocation of the lunate or triquetrum
6. Triangular fibrocartilage complex (TFCC) injury
7. Extensor carpi ulnaris (ECU) subluxation and/or tendinitis
8. Extensor digiti minimi tendinitis
   B. Triquetrolunate instability
   1. Triquetrolunate sprain
   2. Triquetrolunate dissociation
   C. Fractures of the ulnar carpal bones
   1. Fracture of the hamate
   2. Fracture of the pisiform
   D. Tendinitis
   1. Flexor carpi ulnaris (FCU) tendinitis
   2. Digital flexor tendinitis
   E. Pisotriquetral arthritis
   F. Midcarpal instability
4. Wrist instability radiographic patterns
   A. Volar intercalated segment instability (VISI)
   B. Dorsal intercalated segment instability (DISI)
5. Diffuse wrist pain
   A. Traumatic ulnar translocation of the carpus
   B. Acute arthritis of the wrist
   1. Septic arthritis
   2. Pseudogout
   3. Gout
   4. Kienböck's disease
   5. Hemophilic arthropathy
   6. Idiopathic arthritis
6. Neurogenic wrist pain
   A. Acute carpal tunnel syndrome
   B. Acute ulnar tunnel syndrome

HAND AND FINGER PAIN

7. Carpometacarpal and metacarpophalangeal (MP) areas
   A. Carpometacarpal dislocation
   B. Metacarpal shaft fractures
   C. MP joint dislocation and ligament injuries
   1. Volar plate disruption
   2. Collateral ligament sprain
   3. Dorsal capsule injuries
   4. Fractures of the metacarpal neck and head
      a. Metacarpal neck fractures

      b. Intraarticular fractures of the metacarpal head
8. Proximal phalanx and proximal interphalangeal (PIP) joint area injuries
   A. Fractures of the proximal phalanx
   1. Base of the proximal phalanx
   2. Shaft of the proximal phalanx
   3. Neck and head of the proximal phalanx
   B. PIP joint area
   1. Ligament sprains
   2. Volar plate injuries
   3. Intraarticular fracture-dislocation
   4. Collateral ligament tears
   5. Volar dislocations
   6. PIP joint deformities
      a. Boutonnière deformity
      b. Pseudoboutonnière deformity
9. Middle phalanx area fractures
10. Distal interphalangeal (DIP) joint area
    A. Extensor tendon disruption (mallet finger)
    B. Flexor tendon disruption from distal phalanx
    C. Fracture of the distal phalanx
    D. Subungual hematoma
    E. Dislocation of the DIP Joint
11. Finger infections
    A. Paronychia and eponychia
    1. Superficial type
    2. Deep type
    B. Eponychia
    C. Runaround infection
    D. Subungual abscess
    E. Pulp space infections
    1. Felon (distal pulp space infection)
    2. Middle and proximal pulp space infection
    F. Web space infections
    G. Tendon sheath infections
    H. Herpetic whitlow
    I. Mimics of acute finger infections
    1. Gouty arthritis and tenosynovitis
    2. Acute calcific tendinitis
    3. Malignant melanoma

involving the nail fold and
   nail bed
   4. Sarcoidosis with acute
      tenosynovitis
12. Hand infections
    A. Bursal infections
       1. Radial bursal infection
       2. Ulnar bursal infection
    B. Space infections
       1. Midpalmar space infection
       2. Thenar space infection
13. Animal and human bites of the
    hand and fingers
    A. Dog bites
    B. Cat bites
    C. Human bites
       1. Paronychia
       2. Occlusive bites
       3. Clenched-fist injuries
    D. Snake bites
    E. Necrotic arachnidism
    F. Rat bites (rat bite fever due to
       Streptobaccilus moniliformis)
14. Diffuse infections of the hand and
    forearm
    A. Acute bacterial cellulitis
    B. Palmar subaponeurotic
       infection
    C. Gas gangrene (clostridial
       myonecrosis)
    D. Clostridial anaerobic cellulitis
    E. Nonclostridial anaerobic
       cellulitis
    F. Anaerobic streptococcal
       myonecrosis
    G. *Aeromonas hydrophila*
       myonecrosis
    H. Streptococcal gangrene
15. Acute polyarthritis with wrist and
    hand involved
    A. Hepatitis B arthritis
    B. Rubella-associated arthritis
    C. Rubella immunization–
       associated arthritis
    D. Acute rheumatoid arthritis
    E. Systemic lupus erythematosus
       arthritis
    F. Acute rheumatic fever
    G. Acute traumatic arthritis
    H. Arthritis-dermatitis syndrome
       due to *Neisseria gonorrhoeae*
    I. Yersiniosis
    J. Acute gout
    K. Arthritis associated with
       inflammatory bowel disease
    L. Psoriatic arthritis

M. Calcium pyrophosphate
   dihydrate deposition
   disease
N. Septic arthritis
16. Vascular hand and finger pain
    A. Acute arterial embolism
       1. Brachial artery
       2. Ulnar artery
       3. Radial artery
    B. Arterial trauma
    C. Secondary Raynaud's
       phenomenon
       1. Acute arterial occlusive
          disease
       2. Drug therapy
17. Entrapment neuropathies
    A. Carpal tunnel syndrome
    B. Ulnar tunnel syndrome
    C. Proximal causes of
       neuropathic hand and finger
       pain
    D. Double-crush syndrome
18. Reflex sympathetic dystrophy
    (RSD)
19. Mononeuritis multiplex
20. Cutaneous disorders of the hand
    A. Dyshidrotic eczematous
       dermatitis
    B. Palmoplantar pustulosis
       1. Pustulosis palmaris et
          plantaris
       2. Pustular psoriasis of
          Barber
    C. Pustular bacterid of the hands
       and feet (Andrew's disease)
    D. Acrodermatitis continua
    E. *Trichophyton rubrum*
       dermatitis
    F. *Staphylococcus aureus*
       cutaneous infection
    G. Erysipeloid
    H. Osler's nodes
    I. Splinter hemorrhages
    J. Frostbite
    K. Photosensitivity secondary to
       drugs
THUMB PAIN
21. Trapeziometacarpal area
    A. Tendinitis
    B. Fractures
       1. Bennett's fracture
       2. Rolando's fracture
    C. Dislocations
22. MP joint of the thumb
    A. Volar plate injury
    B. Collateral ligament injury

☐ SUMMARY

Wrist Pain

A *Colles' fracture* follows a fall on the outstretched hand. Members of either sex and any adult age group may sustain this injury, but it is most frequently seen in postmenopausal women. There are pain, tenderness, swelling, and ecchymoses over the radial aspect of the wrist. The radial styloid is palpated proximal to the ulna styloid and dorsal angulation, and displacement of the distal fragment produces a "dinner fork" deformity. Intraarticular fractures may result in posttraumatic arthritis. An associated fracture of the ulna styloid is usually present. A reverse Colles' fracture, or *Smith's fracture*, occurs after a fall on the dorsum of the hand. Volar displacement of the distal fragment occurs. Plain radiographs and examination findings will differentiate these two common types of radial fractures. *Articular margin fractures of the distal radius* (dorsal lip fractures) can result in dorsal displacement of the carpus and a "dinner fork" deformity of the wrist and hand. Swelling, pain, tenderness, crepitus, and ecchymoses are usually present over the radial aspect of the wrist. *Scaphoid fractures* follow a fall on the extended hand. Pain, swelling, and tenderness occur over the "snuffbox" region, and wrist stiffness becomes severe within 24 h of the injury. Plain radiographs detect 80 to 98 percent of such fractures if four views are taken. Addition of 25° pronation and supination views increases diagnostic sensitivity to 100 percent. At most centers, a negative four-view series is repeated after 2 weeks of wrist immobilization to detect scaphoid fractures not visible on the initial films. Whether the six-view approach will be adapted more widely is at present unknown. Patients with "snuffbox" pain, swelling, and tenderness and no evidence of a fracture or instability of the scapholunate articulation probably have a *partial disruption of the scapholunate intraosseous ligament* and require wrist immobilization for 3 to 4 weeks. *Trapezium ridge fractures* cause pain, swelling, and tenderness over the base of the thumb and thenar eminence. Carpal tunnel radiographs may be necessary to demonstrate the fracture. Excision of the ununited fracture fragment is usually required to relieve pain and tenderness.

Dynamic scapholunate instability is associated with "snuffbox" pain, tenderness, and swelling. Watson's scaphoid test can be used to detect dynamic instability of the scapholunate articulation. An anteroposterior radiograph of the wrist with the forearm and wrist supinated will demonstrate a scapholunate gap greater than 2 mm (Terry-Thomas sign). *Static rotatory subluxation of the scaphoid* may cause similar dorsoradial findings and a painful click as the wrist is moved from ulnar deviation into a neutral position. This click may be reproduced by the examiner by dorsally directed pressure on the scaphoid as the wrist is ulnar-deviated.

In patients with static rotatory subluxation of the scaphoid, radiographs of the wrist will demonstrate a widened scapholunate interval, a "ring sign" of the scaphoid caused by its foreshortened vertical position, and a scapholunate angle greater than 70°. Trapezial area pain and tenderness may be caused by a *radial collateral ligament (RCL) tear*. Radiographs for a fracture of the trapezium are negative, and relief of pain and tenderness by a diagnostic lidocaine injection of the RCL confirms the site of the injury.

De Quervain's disease causes radial styloid pain, swelling, and tenderness of the tendons of the first dorsal compartment on the lateral aspect of the anatomic "snuffbox" and a positive Finkelstein's test (i.e., after the patient grasps the adducted, flexed thumb within his or her fist, the examiner ulnar-deviates the wrist, causing radial styloid pain). Overuse of the involved tendons in job tasks or in athletics is the usual cause. *Extensor pollicis longus tenosynovitis* causes "snuffbox" pain, tenderness, and swelling. Overuse, a distal radial fracture, and rheumatoid arthritis are the common causes of involvement of this tendon. *Flexor carpi radialis (FCR) tendinitis* causes pain and tenderness over the volar aspect of the wrist. Pain is increased by resisted wrist flexion or sudden passive extension of the wrist. A pain-relieving lidocaine injection into the flexor carpi radialis tendon sheath is of diagnostic value. The *intersection syndrome* is caused by friction between the more superficial extensor pollicis brevis and abductor pollicis longus muscle bellies and the radial wrist extensors. Dorsal pain, tenderness, swelling, and a squeaky-type crepitus occur 5 cm proximal to Lister's tubercle. Friction results in a local peritendinitis or an adventitious bursitis. The *extensor indicis proprius syndrome* may cause pain over the mid-dorsum of the wrist. Passive wrist flexion and resisted extension of the index finger intensify or provoke pain.

Infectious tenosynovitis of the flexor pollicis longus can follow a penetrating thumb wound. The thumb, thenar eminence, and first web space are usually swollen and tender, and the thumb is held flexed and adducted. Pain is usually severe and throbbing. Tenderness occurs over the affected tendon, and passive extension of the interphalangeal joint of the thumb provokes pain. *Gonococcal tenosynovitis* may involve extensor or flexor tendons and may be associated with the gonococcal dermatitis-arthritis syndrome. Microbial causes of hand and wrist tenosynovitis other than *N. gonorrhoeae* include *S. aureus* and streptococcal, and *Pseudomonas* species. Rare infections with *Moraxella* species, *Sporothrix schenckii*, or atypical mycobacteria may also occur.

A *capitate fracture* may cause mid-dorsal wrist pain, swelling, and tenderness distal to the lunate. Initial radiographs will usually detect a fracture, but missed fractures may occur. Follow-up radiographs taken 2 weeks after the injury will usually demonstrate an existing fracture. *Lunate fractures* are infrequent and may occur as a cause or result of osteonecrosis. The earliest specific findings of *osteonecrosis of the lunate (Kienböck's disease)* occur on MRI, where there is loss of the lunate marrow signal on a T_1-weighted image.

A *dorsal perilunate dislocation* causes mid-dorsal wrist pain, tenderness, swelling, and a "mini-dinner fork" deformity. Palpation may reveal a capitate edge elevated above the lunate and radius. Plain lateral radiographs reveal that the longitudinal axis of the capitate is dorsal to that of the radius and that the proximal scaphoid is rotated dorsally. *Perilunate fracture-dislocations* cause similar signs and symptoms and require radiographic detection of carpal fractures for diagnosis. *Volar lunate dislocation* causes swelling, pain, and tenderness of the volar aspect of the wrist. Compression of the median nerve by the lunate may cause an acute carpal tunnel syndrome. Plain radiographs will reveal that the lunate is displaced in a volar direction with its concave surface tilted forward or complete volar displacement of the lunate. *Intermediate forms of perilunate or lunate dislocation* provide clinical and radiographic findings that are intermediate between a perilunate and a lunate dislocation.

Radioulnar joint disease may be suspected when passive pronation and supination of the wrist cause distal radioulnar joint (DRUJ) pain. Local tenderness over the DRUJ may also be present. The causes of DRUJ area pain include *fractures of the ulna, radius, triquetrum or lunate; dislocation of the DRUJ, lunate, or triquetrum; and injury to the triangular fibrocartilage complex (TFCC)* of the wrist. *Extensor carpi ulnaris (ECU) subluxation and tenosynovitis* may cause ulnar wrist pain that is difficult to differentiate from an internal disorder of the DRUJ. An *extensor digiti minimi tendinitis* may cause pain and tenderness near the DRUJ. Acute ulnar wrist pain may result from a *triquetrolunate sprain with or without dissociation*. Ballottement of the triquetrum can confirm instability. A painful wrist click may occur when the wrist is moved into ulnar or radial deviation. A carpal instability series will demonstrate overlapping of the lunate and triquetrum with the wrist in ulnar deviation. The lunotriquetral angle (measured on a lateral view) becomes less than 0°. An arthrogram will usually demonstrate disruption of the triquetrolunate ligament. A *fracture of the hook of the hamate or the pisiform* will cause pain, tenderness, and edema over the hypothenar eminence. These fractures may require a carpal tunnel radiograph or a CT scan for diagnosis.

Flexor carpi ulnaris (FCU) *tenosynovitis* causes local pain and tenderness over the tendon and the pisiform bone. This pain may be provoked or intensified by wrist flexion against resistance. *Digital flexor tendinitis* causes midvolar wrist and forearm pain. Swelling and tenderness occur proximal to the wrist flexor creases. *Pisotriquetral arthritis* causes local tenderness and crepitus over the joint. Plain radiographs confirm the diagnosis. *Midcarpal instability* may follow a fall on the outstretched hand or a rotational injury, but it most commonly occurs in the absence of an injury. A painful clunk can be felt in the ulnodorsal aspect of the wrist when the joint is pronated and ulnar-deviated. A prominent volar sag may be visible at the level of the midcarpal joint. This sag disappears with the occurrence of a painful clunk as the midcarpal joint is reduced. Cineradiography is diagnostic and demonstrates an abrupt transition of the proximal carpal row from palmar flexion to dorsiflexion as the hand is ulnar-deviated. *VISI and DISI* can be demonstrated on a lateral radiograph of the wrist. VISI is often associated with triquetrolunate and midcarpal instability and DISI with unstable scaphoid fractures and scapholunate dissociation. *Traumatic ulnar translocation of the carpus* causes massive wrist edema, pain, and tenderness and lateral instability of the carpus. Dislocation of the carpus in an ulnar direction can be demonstrated by clinical examination and plain radiography.

Diffuse wrist pain may be caused by *septic arthritis*. Local swelling, tenderness, and sometimes skin redness also occur. *N. gonorrhoeae* is a common cause of this disorder in young adults. Pyogenic infection with *S. aureus*, streptococcal species, and gram-negative organisms may also occur. The synovial fluid contains increased numbers of polymorphonuclear leukocytes, and cultures are positive in 50 to 90 percent of cases.

Pseudogout or *gout* may cause pain, swelling, and tenderness of the wrist and redness of the overlying skin. Patients with gout usually have an elevated serum uric acid level, and those with pseudogout often have radiologic evidence of chondrocalcinosis. Synovial fluid contains increased numbers of polymorphonuclear leukocytes in both disorders, but gouty joint fluid contains sodium urate crystals, and pseudogout fluid contains calcium pyrophosphate dihydrate crystals. *Kienböck's disease* may cause a localized or a diffuse acute arthritis of the wrist. MRI will confirm the diagnosis in early cases. *Hemorrhage into a wrist* may mimic acute arthritis *in patients with hemophilia*. *Idiopathic wrist arthritis* may also occur and clear spontaneously before a diagnosis can be established.

An *acute carpal tunnel syndrome* may cause wrist and hand pain as well as pain, paresthesias, and hypesthesia in the radial fingers. Phalen's sign and Tinel's sign are frequently positive. The causes of an acute carpal tunnel syndrome include fractures of the radius, volar dislocation of the lunate, a carpal tunnel hematoma, soft tissue infection, septic arthritis of the wrist, and flexor tenosynovitis due to overuse, Lyme disease, or other infectious agents. The *ulnar tunnel syndrome* causes pain, paresthesias, and hypesthesia over the volar aspect of the ulnar fingers, hand, and wrist. Dorsal sensory symptoms and signs occur only with a more proximal ulnar nerve lesion. Sustained pressure over the hypothenar region, repetitive injury of this region, or, rarely, ulnar artery thrombosis in Guyon's canal may cause an acute ulnar tunnel syndrome.

Hand and Finger Pain

Ligament-disrupting flexion or extension forces following a fall may cause *carpometacarpal dislocation*. Dorsal hand deformity and edema are associated with pain and tenderness. Oblique radiographs of the hand are more sensitive than routine views for diagnosis. A missed dislocation may be associated with a bony elevation on the dorsum of the hand, with associated local pain and tenderness.

A *metacarpal oblique or spiral shaft fracture* causes persistent severe aching pain, tenderness, swelling, ecchymoses, and malrotation of the associated finger. Angulation of the involved finger may cause it to overlap an adjacent digit. A transverse *metacarpal fracture* may cause dorsal angulation and metacarpal shortening. *MP joint dislocation* may follow *disruption of the volar plate* of the joint. A bayonet-type dorsal displacement of the proximal phalanx may occur, causing MP joint deformity, pain, and tenderness. The finger may be hyperextended at the MP joint, flexed at the interphalangeal joint, and deviated toward adjacent fingers. The palmar skin volar to the MP joint is often puckered. If the subluxation is partial, the proximal phalanx may hyperextend as much as 90°, and there is no angulation of the finger.

Collateral ligament disruption (sprain) at the MP joint causes local pain, swelling, tenderness, and ulnar (radial collateral ligament tear) or radial (ulnar collateral ligament tear) instability of the flexed joint. Spontaneous deviation of the affected corresponding finger in a radial or ulnar direction may be noted in severe sprains. *Dorsal capsule injuries* cause local pain, tenderness, swelling, and a palpable dorsal capsule defect that may be associated with extensor tendon displacement. These injuries usually occur from direct injury to the closed fist in boxing or karate.

A *fracture of the metacarpal at its neck* may be associated with a painful, bony prominence in the palm due to volar rotation of the distal fragment. There are local pain, tenderness, swelling, and impairment of MP joint extension. *Intraarticular fractures of the metacarpal head* cause loss of joint mobility and swelling, pain, and tenderness of the MP joint. A Brewerton view provides a clear radiographic image of the articular surface of the metacarpal head. *Fractures of the base*

of the proximal phalanx cause local pain, tenderness, swelling, bony deformity, and sometimes volar angulation of the involved phalanx. *Shaft fractures of the proximal phalanx* cause local pain, tenderness, and edema and may extend into the proximal interphalangeal joint, causing stiffness or loss of joint mobility. *Fracture of the neck of the proximal phalanx* may cause volar angulation of the distal fracture surface that may be palpable on the volar side of the finger. A *condylar fracture of the distal end of the proximal phalanx* may cause lateral deviation of the distal portion of the finger to the side of the fracture. Fractures of the proximal phalanx can be imaged by plain radiography. *Proximal interphalangeal (PIP) joint volar plate disruption* follows a severe hyperextension force. There is persistent volar pain, swelling, tenderness, and joint stiffness or immobility. Subluxation of the joint may occur, resulting in hyperextension of the middle phalanx or a bayonet-type dorsal displacement of the middle phalanx. *Intraarticular fractures at the PIP joint* may be associated with joint dislocation. *Collateral ligament tears of the PIP joint* cause local pain, swelling, and tenderness over the region of the disrupted ligament and deviation of the distal portion of the finger to the opposite side. *Volar dislocation of the middle phalanx may* occur as the proximal phalanx ruptures the extensor tendon system after abrupt forced flexion or extreme rotation of the PIP joint.

An acute *boutonnière deformity* results from rupture of the central slip of the extensor tendon from its insertion on the middle phalanx. PIP joint flexion is coupled with extension or hyperextension of the DIP joint. A *pseudoboutonnière deformity* results from PIP volar plate disruption, healing, and fibrotic contracture. DIP joint flexion and extension remain normal. A *middle phalanx fracture* causes local pain, swelling, and tenderness over the fracture line and extension or flexion of the proximal fragment. The direction of proximal fragment displacement is determined by the relationship of the fracture line to the insertion of the extensor and flexor tendons. A *mallet, or "drop," finger* results from *extensor tendon disruption* from the distal phalanx, making active DIP joint extension impossible. Proximal slippage of the detached extensor tendon may cause PIP joint extension, resulting in a "swan neck" deformity of the finger. *Disruption of the flexor tendon from the distal phalanx* renders active DIP joint flexion impossible.

Fracture of the distal phalanx may cause local pain, swelling, and tenderness and can be diagnosed by a plain radiograph. A *subungual hematoma* causes severe throbbing fingertip pain, a blue nail, and severe nail pressure-provoked pain. Dramatic relief occurs after drainage of subungual liquid blood through a small hole in the nail. *DIP joint dislocation* causes local pain, tenderness, swelling, and bony deformity. The deformity is usually transient and disappears after spontaneous or assisted closed reduction.

Paronychia is a pyogenic infection of the nail margin. Local redness, tenderness, pain, and sometimes purulent discharge are present at the edge of the nail and in the adjacent skin. *Eponychia* is a lateral nail fold infection that also involves the eponychium at the base of the nail. A *runaround infection* is a paronychia that begins at one lateral nail fold and spreads around the entire nail. A *subungual abscess* causes severe throbbing pain beneath the nail and a "floating nail" due to underlying pus. Nail removal allows drainage and relieves pain. It may follow as a complication of a paronychia.

Pulp space infections cause swelling, pain, redness, and tenderness of the volar aspect of the finger beneath the distal, middle, or proximal phalanx. An *abscess in the distal pulp space* is called a *felon*. Transillumination of a felon may outline a collection of pus in the distal pulp space of the finger. *Web space infections* cause edema, redness, pain, and tenderness, with splaying of the digits adjacent to the involved web space. The underlying abscess is often an hourglass-shaped collection of pus with a volar and a dorsal component. *Flexor tendon sheath infections* cause uniform swelling of the involved finger, flexion of the involved and other adjacent fingers, tendon sheath swelling, localized tenderness, and marked intensification of pain by passive extension of the involved digit. *Herpetic whitlow* is a localized herpes simplex infection of the skin of a finger or the hand. It causes local pain, tenderness, redness, and vesicular and ulcerative lesions. It may be confused with a paronychia or a localized pyogenic skin infection. Suppurative tenosynovitis of a digit may be mimicked by *acute gouty arthritis* and *tenosynovitis*, *acute calcific tendinitis*, and *sarcoidosis*. Gout may also mimic a septic joint. *Malignant melanama* may mimic a resistant paronychia if it is situated in the nail fold. *Radial bursal infections* are caused by a suppurative tenosynovitis of the thumb. Tenderness along the flexor tendon sheath may extend proximally to the radial volar side of the wrist. The thenar eminence and first web space become swollen, warm, and erythematous, and this appearance may mimic a thenar space infection. Tenosynovitis may develop in the small finger by spread from the infected radial bursa to the *ulnar bursa*. Similarly, an infection of the flexor tendon of the small finger can *infect the ulnar bursa* and, after several days, involve the flexor tendon of the thumb.

A *midpalmar space infection* causes loss of the palmar concavity, swelling of the dorsum of the hand, fever, chills, and malaise. There are redness, tenderness, and pain over the midpalmar space, and passive or active flexion of the fingers increases the pain. *Thenar space infection* is accompanied by swelling, erythema, fluctuance, and tenderness of the thenar eminence. The thumb is held in abduction, and the dorsum of the hand is edematous.

An *infected animal bite* may cause a local cellulitis and sometimes ascending lymphangitis, axillary lymphadenitis, and, in severe cases, sepsis. *Deep bites in the hand by a dog* may cause septic arthritis, tenosynovitis, or osteomyelitis. Isolates from infected dog bites include *Pasteurella multocida*, *S. aureus*, streptococcal species, and anaerobes. *Cat bites* are likely to become infected with *P. multocida* or streptococcal species.

Human bites may cause *paronychia* (biting hangnails) or wound infection and cellulitis due to innoculation of oral flora (*occlusive bites*). *Clenched-fist injury* follows knuckle trauma by an opponent's teeth in a fight. This injury may cause a single or mixed bacterial infection resulting in a cellulitis, tenosynovitis, space infection, or septic arthritis. *Snake bites* by pit vipers or cobras may cause local pain, extensive edema, and tissue necrosis of the hand and fingers. *Necrotic arachnidism* follows a bite by a brown recluse spider. After a latent period of several hours, the bite area becomes pruritic, swollen, and erythematous. The central portion of the lesion becomes pale white or gray, and a large central bulla containing sanguineous fluid may develop. Within several days, extensive central necrosis occurs. A *rat bite* may innoculate the victim with *S. moniliformis*. This organism may cause a bacteremic febrile illness associated with a rash and an asymmetrical polyarthritis or a septic joint. There is usually no local infection of the bite area. The diagnosis can be confirmed by culture of blood or synovial fluid.

Cellulitis may cause diffuse redness, pain, and tenderness of the hand, fingers, and forearm. The area of erythema remains flat. Fever, chills, and malaise may be associated. The usual cause is infection of the skin and subcutaneous area by *S. aureus* or a group A streptococcus. An associated lymphangitis and lymphadenitis may be present. A *subaponeurotic space infection of the palmar aspect of the hand* causes loss of the normal palmar concavity, local pain, erythema, tenderness, and edema. Surgical exploration and drainage of the subaponeurotic collection of pus relieves symptoms.

Gas gangrene follows a compound fracture or bullet wound of the hand that causes muscle injury and contamination. Pain beginning 1 to 2 days after the injury is the initial complaint. There is local malodorous, serosanguineous drainage, sometimes containing bubbles. The wound and adjacent skin become edematous, and the wound margin becomes yellow or bronze in color. Bullae containing dark fluid appear adjacent to the wound, and areas of skin gangrene develop and spread proximally. There may be some skin crepitus, and plain radiographs will demonstrate gas in the skin and underlying muscles and fascial planes. A Gram stain of the wound drainage reveals large gram-positive bacilli. Exploration of the wound confirms myonecrosis. Extensive debridement and sometimes amputation are required.

Clostridial anaerobic cellulitis occurs 3 or more days after a penetrating injury. Local pain is minimal, and a thin malodorous wound discharge and skin crepitus are present. Plain radiographs demonstrate subcutaneous gas, and a Gram stain and culture of wound drainage demonstrate *Clostridium perfringens*. Differentiation from clostridial myonecrosis (gas gangrene) requires surgical exploration and direct testing of the underlying muscle for viability. Local debridement, drainage, and parenteral penicillin lead to resolution. A similar gas-forming disorder, *nonclostridial anaerobic cellulitis*, is caused by a pure anaerobic or a mixed infection with anaerobic and aerobic bacteria. Surgical exploration for muscle viability is required, and Gram stain and culture will differentiate this gas-forming infection from clostridial cellulitis.

Anaerobic streptococcal myonecrosis occurs 3 to 4 days after wounding. There are local wound area swelling, a sour-smelling seropurulent discharge, and diffuse erythema around the wound. Pain develops as the infection spreads and is not a prominent early symptom. Surgical exploration reveals evidence of myonecrosis, and a Gram stain of wound exudate reveals increased numbers of polymorphonuclear leukocytes and large numbers of streptococci. Cultures reveal a mixed infection of anaerobic streptococci and aerobic group A streptococci or *S. aureus*. *Aeromonas hydrophila myonecrosis* occurs after wounding in fresh water or in association with wounds caused by contact with fish or other water animals. Severe local wound pain and edema begin 2 days after the initial injury. Serosanguineous bullae occur near the wound. Systemic complaints and toxicity may be severe. Surgical exploration reveals myonecrosis, and gram-negative bacilli are present in the wound exudate. *Streptococcal gangrene* presents with edema, erythema, tenderness, and pain at a point of hand injury. Bullae containing yellow or reddish-black fluid appear and collapse. Black eschars resembling severe burns replace ruptured bullae. Necrotic sloughing of skin and cutaneous gangrene occur. Group A, C, or G streptococci may be isolated from bullae fluid and blood.

Polyarthritis may involve wrist, hand, and finger joints. The viral causes of acute polyarthritis include *hepatitis B*, *rubella*, and *rubella immunization*. *Acute rheumatoid arthritis*, *systemic lupus erythematosus*, *acute rheumatic fever*, *acute traumatic arthritis of the hands*, the *arthritis-dermatitis syndrome caused by N. gonorrhoeae*, *yersiniosis*, *acute gout*, the *arthritis associated with inflammatory bowel disease*, *psoriatic arthritis*, and *calcium pyrophosphate dihydrate deposition disease* may also involve the wrist and small joints of the hands and fingers.

Involvement of the wrist, MP, PIP, or DIP joints may be due to *septic arthritis* or to gout or pseudogout (calcium pyrophosphate dihydrate deposition disease). Aspiration of a septic joint reveals a high leukocyte count and a positive Gram stain and/or culture.

An *embolus to a brachial artery* may cause aching forearm and hand pain, paresthesias, numbness, pallor, loss of the radial pulse, and paresis of the involved hand. Emboli may arise in the cardiac chambers, valves, or atheromatous lesions near the aortic arch or at the thoracic outlet. *Ulnar artery occlusion* can cause ischemic pain, pallor, paresthesias, and gangrene of the ulnar fingers. *Radial artery occlusion* is usually asymptomatic, but prior ulnar artery occlusion or an incomplete superficial palmar arch may result in digital ischemia and gangrene. *Brachial artery occlusion* may follow blunt or penetrating trauma.

Secondary Raynaud's phenomenon may cause attacks of digital pallor followed by cyanosis and then hyperemic erythema. The color changes and painful hyperemia occur over a 15- to 20-min period. Warming the hands under running water may shorten the duration of an attack. *Acute Raynaud's phenomenon* may be caused by proximal occlusive arterial disease with thrombosis and peripheral embolization as well as by ingestion of beta-adrenergic blocking drugs or ergotamine. Administration of *antitumor drugs* may also provoke Raynaud's phenomenon.

An acute *carpal tunnel syndrome* may cause nocturnal wrist, hand, and radial finger pain and paresthesias. Tinel's sign at the wrist, Phalen's test, or the reverse Phalen's test may be positive. Causes of acute carpal tunnel syndrome include *fractures, volar lunate dislocation, flexor tenosynovitis, direct trauma, midpalmar space abscess, septic arthritis of the wrist*, or a *hematoma*. Electrodiagnostic studies will confirm delayed median nerve conduction across the wrist.

The *ulnar tunnel syndrome* results in ulnar pain in the hand and in the fourth and fifth fingers. Paresthesias and hypesthesia occur in the same area as the pain. Weakness and atrophy of the hand muscles may be associated. Sensory symptoms and losses are usually only volar. Phalen's sign may be positive, provoking medial hand symptoms. Pressure over the hypothenar eminence may cause medial hand and finger discomfort and/or paresthesias (Tinel's sign). This syndrome may be caused by *direct trauma*, a *fracture of the hamate or pisiform bones*, or *ulnar artery thrombosis secondary to repetitive hypothenar trauma*.

Proximal causes of lateral hand, thumb, and index and middle finger pain, paresthesias, and numbness include a *C6 or C7 radiculopathy*, a *thoracic outlet syndrome*, or the *pronator teres syndrome*. *Proximal causes of ulnar nerve-like symptoms* affecting the medial aspect of the hand and the fourth and fifth fingers include a *C8 radiculopathy*, *brachial plexus compression at the thoracic outlet*, or the *cubital tunnel syndrome*. The *double-crush syndrome* is an ulnar or carpal tunnel syndrome occurring simultaneously with a proximal neural compressive lesion. The proximal lesion is believed to predispose the peripheral nerve to symptomatic compression. Peripheral decompression may fail to alleviate symptoms unless the proximal lesion is also corrected.

Reflex sympathetic dystrophy (RSD) follows hand or finger injury and/or corrective surgery for that injury. There is severe hand and finger pain associated with diffuse edema, erythema, warmth, and skin hyperesthesia of the hand. Hyperhidrosis may occur. The joints are painful and stiff. The severity of the pain is out of proportion to the injury or the extent of the corrective surgery. Symptoms are relieved dramatically by a sympathetic nerve block.

Mononeuritis multiplex causes the abrupt onset of severe aching forearm and hand pain, paresthesias, and numbness in a median, ulnar, or radial nerve distribution. Paresis may follow the onset of symptoms by several hours. Pressure over the affected nerve or movement of the arm may provoke shooting, sharp forearm and hand pain and paresthesias. Additional peripheral nerves are usually involved over a period of days or weeks if therapy is not initiated. Ischemia of the involved nerves caused by vasculitis or diabetic vascular disease is the usual cause, although a similar clinical picture has been described in patients with multiple sclerosis.

Painful *cutaneous disorders of the hand* include *dyshidrotic eczematous dermatitis* (multiple, tiny, painful intraepidermal vesicles), *palmoplantar pustulosis*, and the *pustular bacterid of Andrew*. Palmoplantar pustulosis may occur as an isolated disorder and run a brief course, or it may occur in a patient with psoriasis of other areas of the skin and the nails.

Acrodermatitis continua begins about the nail on a single

digit. The skin over the distal phalanx becomes erythematous, fissured, and crusted. Necrosis and sloughing of the skin occurs, and the nail is loosened and floats on an underlying "lake" of pus. This disorder may remain confined to one digit, or it may spread to other fingers on the same or the other hand, and it may progress proximally up the arms. *T. rubrum infection of the hands* may cause weeping, crusting, erosive skin lesions on the palms. Microscopy and cultures of skin scrapings reveal fungal elements. *Furuncles and pustules caused* by *S. aureus* may occur on the dorsum of the proximal phalanx or on other areas of the hand.

Erysipeloid presents as a painful, tender, violaceous skin plaque that may be associated with fever and malaise. It begins at a site of minor trauma in workers handling uncooked fish, poultry, or meat. This disorder is caused by a gram-positive bacillus, *Erysipelothrix rhusiopathiae*, and is responsive to antibiotic therapy. *Osler's nodes* (painful, pink macules on the fingertips) and painful *splinter hemorrhages* in the nail bed may be peripheral manifestations of bacterial endocarditis. Cold exposure of the hands and fingers may cause mild to severe *frostbite*. Pain, erythema, edema, and blistering with superficial gangrene of the skin occur on rewarming of moderately severe cold injuries. After healing, pain, hyperhidrosis, paresthesias, hypesthesia, and cold sensitivity may persist in severe cases. *Drug-related* (e.g., doxycycline) *photosensitivity* may cause bilateral severe, painful redness and blistering of the hands, face, and other exposed areas. Symptoms remit after avoidance of sunlight and cessation of drug ingestion.

Thumb Pain

Tendinitis at the insertion of the abductor pollicis longus tendon on the first metacarpal may cause local pain and tenderness. Similarly, *de Quervain's disease* causes tendon-associated pain and tenderness more proximally between the radial styloid and base of the thumb. *Fractures at the base of the first metacarpal (Bennett's and Rolando's)* cause trapeziometacarpal joint area pain, tenderness, swelling, and loss of joint mobility. *Dislocation of the trapeziometacarpal joint* without a fracture may also occur. These fracture-dislocations and dislocations at the trapeziometacarpal joint can be imaged by plain radiography. *MP joint injuries* include *dislocation* (bayonet-type dorsal dislocation of the proximal phalanx) due to *volar disruption* and *collateral ligament injury*, and *collateral ligament disruptions with radial or ulnar instability of the MP joint*. An *ulnar collateral ligament tear* with instability to a radially directed force has been called "gamekeeper's thumb." This injury is frequently associated with skiing accidents. Violent abduction of the thumb can disrupt the ulnar collateral ligament and cause interposition of the adductor aponeurosis between the avulsed ligament and its detachment site on the proximal phalanx. This interposition (*Stener's lesion*) prevents healing and requires open reduction to prevent chronic instability. *A radial collateral ligament (RCL) injury* allows more than 30° of ulnar deviation of the thumb after application of

an ulnar-directed force to the PIP joint when the MP joint is stabilized in extension. *Bowler's thumb* is a painful pressure neuropathy involving the digital nerve on the ulnar side of the thumb. Paresthesias and hypesthesia of this portion of the thumb may accompany the pain. *Fractures and dislocations of the phalanges of the thumb* cause localized pain, tenderness, swelling, and ecchymoses. *Dislocation of the interphalangeal joint of the thumb* may occur, with local swelling, tenderness, pain, and bony deformity (bayonet type). *Compound dislocation*, with protrusion of the proximal phalanx through the skin, may also occur. A *"drop,"* or mallet, *thumb* may result from *extensor tendon detachment from the distal phalanx*. There are local swelling, pain, tenderness, and ecchymoses over the dorsal surface of the distal phalanx and inability to extend the interphalangeal joint. The causes of bilateral acute wrist, hand, and finger pain are listed in Table 41-1.

☐ DESCRIPTION OF LISTED DISEASES

Wrist Pain

1. RADIAL (LATERAL) WRIST PAIN

A. Fractures

1. Distal Radius

A. COLLES' FRACTURE This fracture usually follows a fall on the extended, outstretched hand. It can occur in either sex and at any adult age, but it is seen most frequently in postmenopausal women because of osteoporosis. The fracture results in local pain, tenderness, swelling, and ecchymoses and dorsal angulation, supination, and radial shortening. Angulation displacement of the distal radial fragment and carpus produces a "dinner fork" deformity. An associated fracture of the ulnar styloid is frequently present. Examination reveals dorsal angulation of the distal radius and carpus with associated tenderness, swelling, and sometimes crepitus. The radial styloid is proximal relative to the ulnar styloid. Plain radiographs taken in anteroposterior, lateral, and oblique views will confirm the clinical findings. Colles' fractures may be extraarticular (12–36 percent) or intraarticular (64–88 percent). The presence of intraarticular disruption may lead to an unsatisfactory result, and it predisposes the patient to posttraumatic arthritis. The majority of distal radius fractures can be treated by closed reduction. The accuracy of reduction can be assessed by measuring the distance between the medial corner of the radius and the ulna head and comparing this distance to the opposite normal wrist, and by measuring radial palmar tilt on a lateral postreduction radiograph (the radial articular

TABLE OF DISEASE INCIDENCE

INCIDENCE PER 100,000 (APPROXIMATE)

Common (>100)	Uncommon (>5–100)	Rare (>0–5)

WRIST PAIN

Common (>100)	Uncommon (>5–100)	Rare (>0–5)
Fracture of the distal radius (Colles' fracture)	Fracture of the distal radius (Smith's fracture)	Other causes of infectious tenosynovitis
Scaphoid fracture	Articular margin fracture of the distal radius	Ulnar dislocation of the carpus
Scapholunate ligament sprain	Trapezium fracture	Hemophilic arthropathy of the wrist
de Quervain's disease	Dynamic scapholunate instability	
Acute carpal tunnel syndrome	Static rotatory subluxation of the scaphoid	
	Radial collateral ligament sprain	
	Tenosynovitis of the extensor pollicis longus	
	Flexor carpi radialis tendinitis	
	Intersection syndrome	
	Extensor indicis proprius syndrome	
	Infectious tenosynovitis: suppurative flexor pollicis longus tenosynovitis, or gonococcal tenosynovitis	
	Capitate fracture	
	Lunate fracture	
	Kienböck's disease	
	Dorsal perilunate dislocation	
	Perilunate fracture-dislocation	
	Volar lunate dislocation	
	Intermediate perilunate or lunate dislocation	
	Distal radioulnar joint disorders due to fracture of the distal ulna or radial sigmoid, fracture of the triquetrum or lunate, triquetrum avulsion fracture, dislocation of the distal ulna, dislocation of the lunate or triquetrum, Triangular fibrocartilage complex injury, extensor carpi ulnaris subluxation, or tendinitis or extensor carpi digiti minimi tendinitis	
	Triquetrolunate sprain or dissociation	
	Fracture of the hamate	
	Fracture of the pisiform	
	Midcarpal instability	
	Flexor carpi ulnaris tendinitis	
	Digital flexor tendinitis	
	Pisotriquetral arthritis	
	Wrist instability patterns: VISI and DISI	
	Acute arthritis of the wrist due to septic arthritis, pseudogout, gout, Kienböck's disease, or idiopathic arthritis	
	Acute ulnar tunnel syndrome	

HAND AND FINGER PAIN

Common (>100)	Uncommon (>5–100)	Rare (>0–5)
Metacarpal fractures	MP joint injuries due to volar plate disruption, collateral ligament injuries, or fracture of the metacarpal head or neck	Carpometacarpal dislocation
Proximal phalanx fracture		MP joint injury due to dorsal capsule disruption
PIP area injuries due to ligament sprain	PIP joint injuries due to volar plate injury, interarticular fracture-dislocation, or collateral ligament tears or extensor tendon, disruption with volar dislocation	Mimics of acute finger infections due to gouty tenosynovitis, acute calcific tendinitis, malignant melanoma, or sarcoidosis
Boutonnière deformity		
Middle phalanx fractures		
Mallet finger (extensor tendon disruption from distal phalanx)	Pseudoboutonnière deformity	Radial bursal infection
Fracture of the distal phalanx	Flexor tendon disruption from the distal phalanx	Ulnar bursal infection
Subungual hematoma	Dislocation of the DIP joint	Midpalmar space infection
Paronychia	Runaround infection	Thenar space infection
Eponychia	Subungal abscess	Rat bite fever
Dog bite	Pulp space infection (felon)	Palmar subaponeurotic infection
Cat bite	Web space infection	Gas gangrene
Human bite	Tendon sheath infection	Clostridial anaerobic cellulitis
Acute bacterial cellulitis	Herpetic whitlow	Nonclostridial anaerobic cellulitis
Polyarthritis due to hepatitis B, rubella, or rubella immunization	Snake bite	Anaerobic streptococcal myonecrosis
Trauma to brachial artery		Aeromonas hydrophila myonecrosis

INCIDENCE PER 100,000 (APPROXIMATE)

Common (>100)	Uncommon (>5–100)	Rare (>0–5)
	HAND AND FINGER PAIN	
Entrapment neuropathies: carpal tunnel syndrome, proximal entrapment syndromes, or double-crush syndrome	Spider bite	Streptococcal gangrene
Dyshidrotic eczematous dermatitis	Polyarthritis due to acute rheumatoid arthritis, systemic lupus erythematosus, acute traumatic arthritis, *N. gonorrhoeae*, gout, inflammatory bowel disease, psoriasis, or calcium pyrophosphate dihydrate deposition disease	Polyarthritis due to acute rheumatic fever or yersiniosis
Staphylococcal cutaneous infection		Septic arthritis
Frostbite		Mononeuritis multiplex
Photosensitivity due to drugs	Acute arterial embolism to brachial artery, radial artery, or ulnar artery	Pustular bacterid of Andrew
	Secondary Raynaud's phenomenon due to acute arterial disease or drugs	Erysipeloid
	Ulnar tunnel syndrome	Osler's nodes
	Reflex sympathetic dystrophy	Splinter hemorrhages
	Palmoplantar pustulosis	
	Acrodermatitis continua	
	Trichophyton rubrum dermatitis	
	THUMB PAIN	
Tendinitis: de Quervain's disease	Abductor pollicis longus tendinitis at its site of insertion	
Bowler's thumb	Fractures: Bennett's fracture or Rolando's fracture	
Fracture of the proximal phalanx	Trapeziometacarpal dislocation	
	MP joint area injury due to volar plate injury, ulnar collateral ligament disruption and Stener's lesion, or radial collateral ligament disruption	
	Interphalangeal joint injury due to dislocation, fracture of the distal phalanx, or mallet thumb (extensor tendon disruption)	

surface usually projects 10–14° palmar relative to the long axis of the shaft). Open reduction may be required for Colles' fractures that have persistent radiographic evidence of displacement after closed reduction. Surgical reduction is also required for a sharp fragment of the proximal radial segment that impinges on a volar nerve or tendon, or to reduce a widely separated or medially rotated fragment of the distal radius.

B. SMITH'S FRACTURE   This fracture results from a fall on the dorsum of the wrist. The fracture collapses into volar flexion, with the radial articular surface displaced in a palmar direction. Local pain, tenderness, and swelling are present over the radial aspect of the wrist. This fracture has been called a reverse Colles' fracture. The displacement of the distal fragment of the radius and carpus is anterior. Extraarticular fractures can usually be treated by closed reduction, but unstable articular fractures require open reduction and internal fixation.

Complications of distal radial fractures include nonunion or malunion, radioulnar joint pain, rupture of the extensor pollicis longus tendon ("drummer boy" palsy), reflex sympathetic dystrophy, carpal tunnel syndrome, degenerative arthritis of the radi-ocarpal joint, a forearm compartment syndrome, and Volkmann's contracture.

C. ARTICULAR MARGIN FRACTURES OF THE DISTAL RADIUS AND CARPAL DISLOCATION.   A dorsal lip fracture of the radius may cause distal radial tenderness, pain, swelling, and a "dinner fork" deformity secondary to carpal dislocation in a dorsal direction. Volar lip fractures may cause anterior carpal displacement. A lateral radiograph will define the site of the fracture and the cause of the deformity.

2. Scaphoid Fracture   This injury follows a fall on the outstretched, extended hand. Immediate pain is felt and persists. Wrist range of motion is initially normal and only mildly painful. Within 24 h, dorsal radial pain and often swelling occur, and wrist stiffness and pain on motion may become severe. Tenderness over the anatomic "snuffbox" (the sulcus distal to the radial styloid between the tendons of the first dorsal compartment [extensor pollicis brevis and abductor pollicis longus] and the extensor pollicis longus) occurs in 100 percent of cases, and "snuffbox" swelling is present in 74 percent. "Snuffbox" region pain can be intensified by supination or pronation against resistance, by longitudinal compression of the thumb metacarpal, and by radial deviation and dorsiflexion of the wrist. A four-view radiographic series of the wrist (neutral postero-anterior, extreme ulnar deviation, radial deviation, and lateral) has a mean sensitivity for the detection of a scaphoid fracture of 83 percent. If the results of a four-view series are negative, performance of two additional views (25° pronation and supination) will increase sensitivity to 100 percent. This sensitivity was confirmed by doing 2-week follow-up radiographs on all patients with negative six-view series results. Additional scaphoid fractures were not detected when the six-view series was negative.

"Snuffbox" tenderness had a specificity of 76 percent and a predictive value positive of 92 percent, and "snuffbox" swelling had a specificity of 72 percent and a predictive value positive of 87 percent in one reported series of 65 fractures.

An alternative diagnostic strategy to the initial six-view series that is currently used is to immobilize the radiographically negative wrist with "snuffbox" tenderness for 2 weeks and then repeat the radiographs. Bone resorption along the fracture line during this interval usually allows identification of any initially missed fractures. Scaphoid fractures can usually be treated by closed reduction and immobilization.

3. Trapezium Fracture   Fracture of the trapezium may result from a fall on the extended, radially deviated hand or a direct blow on the abducted thumb. Localized tenderness is present at the base of the thenar eminence on the volar side of the wrist with a ridge fracture, and pain occurs at the distal end of the "snuffbox" on resisted wrist flexion. An acute carpal tunnel syndrome with thumb, index, and middle finger pain, paresthesias, and hypesthesia may be associated. Demonstration of a ridge fracture requires an oblique view with the ulnar border of the wrist on the cassette and the forearm pronated at 20°. Trapezial ridge fractures are frequently missed with routine radiographic views and may be seen only on a carpal tunnel view. Spontaneous healing of a trapezial ridge fracture is unusual, and persistent complaints may require excision of the ununited fragment.

B. Sprains and Dislocations

1. Scapholunate Sprain

A. DISRUPTION OF THE SCAPHOLUNATE INTEROS-SEOUS LIGAMENT   There is a history of a fall on the outstretched, extended hand. Falling backward on the extended wrist and hand is a frequent cause of this injury. Pain, tenderness, and swelling may be present in the "snuffbox." Routine and stress radiographs of the wrist reveal no evidence of a scapholunate gap.

"Snuffbox" tenderness with negative radiographic results 2 weeks after the injury may be sec-

ondary to this ligamentous injury. Immobilization for 3 to 4 weeks will usually result in symptomatic resolution.

B. DYNAMIC SCAPHOLUNATE INSTABILITY   "Snuff-box" pain, tenderness, and swelling are associated with wrist weakness and loss of mobility. Watson's scaphoid test can be used to demonstrate dynamic instability at the scapholunate articulation. The examiner places four fingers of one hand on the radius and the thumb on the scaphoid tuberosity with the wrist in ulnar deviation (this elongates the scaphoid). Pressure is directed dorsally with the thumb on the scaphoid as the wrist is moved into radial deviation. The pressure on the scaphoid prevents it from becoming vertical and will drive the proximal pole dorsally if the scapholunate ligaments are disrupted. Intensification of pain and/or dorsal movement of the scaphoid are criteria of a positive test result. This injury is also secondary to a fall on the extended wrist and hand. A routine posteroanterior wrist radiograph with the wrist pronated may be normal, but an anteroposterior view with the wrist supinated demonstrates a gap of more than 2 mm between the scaphoid and lunate. This is known as the Terry-Thomas sign. An anteroposterior radiograph of the supinated wrist with the fist clenched (axial loading) may further enhance demonstration of the gap between the scaphoid and lunate. It has been postulated that dynamic instability of this degree requires rupture of the interosseous ligament and rupture or laxity of the dorsal scapholunate or the volar radioscapholunate ligament. Disruption of all three ligaments will give rise to static rotatory subluxation of the scaphoid.

C. STATIC ROTATORY SUBLUXATION OF THE SCAPHOID   Following a fall on the outstretched hand, pain, tenderness, and swelling develop over the "snuffbox." Movement of the wrist from ulnar deviation into a neutral position may give rise to a painful click or clunk. The pain and click may sometimes be reproduced by the following maneuver. The examiner places the thumb and index finger palmar and dorsal to the scaphoid, respectively. Palmar-to-dorsal pressure is exerted as the wrist is ulnar-deviated. A painful click may occur as the scaphoid moves from a palmar flexed position to dorsiflexion in ulnar deviation. A cleft and/or tenderness may be palpated over the scapholunate articulation. A posteroanterior radiograph will demonstrate a "ring sign" due to the vertical and foreshortened position of the scaphoid. The ring represents the cortical rim of the distal pole of the scaphoid. The scapholunate interval exceeds 2 mm on an anteroposterior wrist radiograph with the wrist supinated. On a lateral radiographic view, the lateral scaphoid angle (the angle between longitudinal axes of the scaphoid and lunate) exceeds 70°. Early diagnosis of interosseous ligament disruption can be treated with immobilization for 3 to 5 weeks. More severe degrees of ligamentous injury, with evidence of dynamic or static instability, require open reduction and repair.

2. Radial Collateral Ligament Sprain   Sprain causes pain and tenderness that is intensified by movement over the area of the trapezium in the distal "snuffbox." Results of radiographs for a fracture of the trapezium are negative, and a lidocaine injection of the ligament will transiently relieve the pain.

C. Tenosynovitis (Noninfectious)

1. de Quervain's Tenosynovitis   Pain occurs at the radial styloid (100 percent) and may radiate into the thumb and up the forearm. The pain is related to movement of the first dorsal wrist compartment tendons (abductor pollicis longus and extensor pollicis brevis). It is increased by abduction or extension of the thumb or by grasping, shaking hands, or pouring coffee from a pot. Tenderness over the radial styloid and first compartment tendons occurs in 97 percent of cases. Swelling is present over the affected tendons in 24 percent.

If the patient grasps the adducted flexed thumb within his or her clenched fist and the examiner ulnar-deviates the wrist, pain over the radial styloid is intensified or provoked (Finkelstein's test). This disorder is common in women between ages 30 and 60 and in athletes whose sport requires repetitive ulnar deviation (racquet sports and golf). Direct injury or repetitive hand and wrist activities that involve grasping, twisting, or pinching may provoke an attack. Pregnancy and the postpartum period may be associated with an increased incidence of this disorder. Local injection of lidocaine and dexamethasone into the tendon sheath may be diagnostic and therapeutic. Surgery or immobilization of the wrist in a splint may be required for patients who fail to respond to corticosteroid injection therapy.

2. Tenosynovitis of the Extensor Pollicis Longus   Pain occurs over the radial styloid, and swelling and tenderness of the tendon occur in the "snuffbox" region. This disorder may arise from acute or chronic repetitive trauma. It has been seen acutely in a tennis player repeatedly practicing serves over a period of several hours. Since this tendon has a propensity to rupture when inflamed, injection with dexamethasone should be avoided. Rupture after repetitive use has been called "drummer boy palsy."

3. Flexor Carpi Radialis Tendinitis   Pain occurs over the tendon on the volar aspect of the wrist creases. It is increased by resisted wrist flexion. There are tenderness and swelling over the FCR tendon just ulnar to the radial pulse and adjacent to the trapezium. Women beyond age 60 are most frequently affected. This disorder may be confused with de Quervain's disease, but the pain and tenderness are primarily volar. Pain may be provoked if the relaxed wrist is abruptly moved in a dorsal direction, stretching the flexor tendons. Injection of lidocaine and a corticosteroid into the FCR tendon is of diagnostic and therapeutic value.

4. Intersection Syndrome   The extensor pollicis brevis and abductor pollicis longus muscles cross over the radial wrist extensors 5 cm proximal to Lister's tubercle.

Dorsal radial distal forearm and wrist pain, swelling, tenderness, and squeaky crepitus occur at this site. This disorder is an overuse syndrome and occurs in weight lifters, canoeists, and rowers. Friction of the thumb muscles against the radial extensors produces a peritendinitis or results in the formation of an adventitious bursa. This disorder may easily be confused with de Quervain's disease. There may be a response to rest and a corticosteroid injection, or surgery may be required.

5. Extensor Indicis Proprius Syndrome   Pain occurs over the fourth dorsal compartment located at the mid-dorsum of the wrist (extensor digitorum communis and extensor indicis proprius muscles). Pain may be reproduced by passive wrist flexion and resisted index finger extension. This disorder has been surgically relieved by division of the extensor retinaculum and tenosynovectomy.

D. Tenosynovitis (Infectious)

1. Suppurative Flexor Pollicis Longus Tenosynovitis   Infection can follow a penetrating wound of the thumb or may spread from an adjacent focus (e.g., a felon or paronychia). Splinters, needles, garden thorns, and metal fragments may penetrate the skin and infect the tendon. In a small minority of patients, no apparent entry wound is noted.

The thumb, thenar eminence, and first web space are usually swollen and tender, and the thumb is held in flexion and adduction. The pain is severe and persistent, and may have a throbbing quality. Tenderness is present over the tendon sheath, and passive extension of the interphalangeal joint of the thumb provokes or intensifies the pain. Staphylococcal infection is predominant, but *Pseudomonas* species and *Streptococcus pyogenes* may also be etiologic. Mixed bacterial infections may also occur.

2. Gonococcal Tenosynovitis   Periarthritic symptoms may occur in the dermatitis-arthritis syndrome caused by *N. gonorrhoeae*. Extensor or flexor tendons on the wrists and hands or on the feet may be affected. Involved tendons may be painful, swollen, and tender. Extension of digits or the wrist in the presence of a flexor tendinitis intensifies the pain. A polyarthritis or involvement of only one or two joints may be associated. Skin lesions numbering 5 to 40 are found on the distal extremities. They are usually tender, red-based, small pustules or hemorrhagic, purple vesicles. Fever, chills, and malaise often occur, but systemic symptoms may be mild or absent. Synovial fluid contains more than 10,000 polymorphonuclear leukocytes per cubic millimeter in the majority of cases. Culture results for *N. gonorrhoeae* in synovial fluid are positive in 50 percent of cases, and those from mucous membrane sites (urethra, cervix, and throat) in 80 percent. Typical clinical symptoms and signs, a positive culture result for *N. gonorrhoeae*, and a dramatic response to penicillin or ceftriaxone therapy are useful diagnostic criteria. Tenosynovitis has been reported in up to 68 percent of patients with the arthritis-dermatitis syndrome.

3. *Other Causes of Infectious Tenosynovitis*   Digit and, less commonly, wrist tendon-related pain, swelling, and tenderness may be caused by *S. aureus*, streptococcal species, *Pseudomonas* species, *Moraxella* species, *Sporothrix schenckii*, and atypical mycobacteria.

Operative drainage of the tendon sheath and antibiotic therapy lead to relief of pain and resolution of the inflammatory reaction.

2. MID-DORSAL WRIST PAIN

A. Fractures

1. *Capitate Fracture*   The capitate articulates with the lunate and scaphoid proximally. The lateral surface articulates with the trapezoid distally and the scaphoid proximally. The medial surface articulates with the hamate, and the distal surface with metacarpals 2 to 4. The capitate is present in the mid-dorsal wrist just distal to the lunate and is palpable in a slight depression between the more prominent proximal lunate and the base of the third metacarpal. Tenderness, local swelling, and pain over this region following an injury may be due to a fracture. Direct injury, sudden dorsiflexion, or trauma to the heads of the second and third metacarpals with the wrist palmar flexed may cause a capitate fracture. Nonunion and avascular necrosis of the capitate may occur, as may posttraumatic arthritis. Since capitate, scaphoid, and other carpal fractures may be missed on initial radiographs, follow-up radiographs should be taken of patients with persistent complaints after 10 to 14 days to exclude an initial false-negative result.

2. *Lunate Fracture and Kienböck's Disease*   Local lunate tenderness and pain may be associated with swelling. Radiographs may demonstrate a transverse lunate fracture. Fractures have been documented in patients with Kienböck's disease, but it is not known whether these are the cause or the result of the osteonecrosis. Kienböck's disease may also cause diffuse synovitis with generalized wrist swelling, pain, decreased grip strength, and limitation of motion. Results

of radiographs may be negative in the early symptomatic stages of Kienböck's disease, but MRI will often identify abnormalities of the lunate (loss of the lunate marrow signal on a T_1-weighted image).

B. Sprains and Dislocations

1. *Perilunate Instability*   A fall on the extended wrist and hand results in varying amounts of wrist hyperextension, ulnar deviation, and intercarpal supination. Intercarpal ligamentous injuries begin at the scapholunate articulation and progress clockwise with increased amounts of force. In stage 1 (partial scapholunate joint disruption), the radial collateral, radiocapitate, radioscapholunate, and scapholunate interosseous ligaments rupture. In stage 2, there is complete disruption of the scapholunate and capitolunate joints. In stage 3, the volar radiotriquetral ligaments fail, and there is cumulative disruption of the scapholunate, capitolunate, and triquetolunate joints. In stage 4, the dorsal radiocarpal ligaments are disrupted, resulting in volar dislocation of the lunate or dorsal perilunate dislocation.

A. DORSAL PERILUNATE DISLOCATION   This disorder causes tenderness in the central dorsal wrist, swelling, and a "mini-dinner fork" deformity. The capitate edge may be palpable dorsally. The longitudinal axis of the capitate is dorsal to that of the radius, and the proximal scaphoid is rotated dorsally. In anteroposterior views, the carpus is foreshortened and a scapholunate gap is present.

B. PERILUNATE FRACTURE-DISLOCATION   If the hyperextension force takes a wider arc around the lunate, fracture-dislocations may occur. These greater-arc injuries include a transscaphoid transcapitate perilunate dislocation, transscaphoid transtriquetral perilunate dislocation, and transscaphoid perilunate dislocation. The proximal fracture segments remain attached to the lunate, and the perilunate separation is through the fracture lines. The distal fracture fragments are displaced, attached to the distal carpal row. In transscaphoid perilunate dislocation, there is radial displacement of the distal scaphoid fragment and the attached distal carpus.

C. VOLAR LUNATE DISLOCATION   The longitudinal axis of the capitate is colinear with the radius. The lunate is displaced in a volar direction with its concave surface tilted forward ("spilled teacup" sign). In an anteroposterior radiograph, the lunate has a triangular shape ("piece of cheese" sign). In some cases, the entire lunate may be displaced in a volar proximal direction and come to rest volar to the distal radius. Volar swelling of the wrist due to displacement of the lunate may be noted. An acute carpal tunnel syndrome may occur because of median nerve compression by the lunate.

D. INTERMEDIATE STAGE OF LIGAMENT INJURY (PERILUNATE OR LUNATE DISLOCATION) In some cases, displacement of the lunate and the articulating capitate, scaphoid, and triquetrum is intermediate between a perilunate and lunate dislocation. In this stage, the capitate may be slightly dorsal to the longitudinal axis of the radius, and the lunate may be tipped in a volar direction but not completely dislocated. Distraction radiographs obtained during finger trap traction may reveal the extent of ligament damage and associated fractures in patients with perilunate or lunate dislocations.

Closed reduction of a perilunate dislocation requires regional or general anesthesia and finger trap traction with 10 to 15 lb of weight applied across the upper arm for 5 min, followed by initial dorsiflexion and then gradual palmar flexion and pronation to reduce the dorsally displaced capitate into the articular cup of the lunate.

Volar lunate dislocation may be reduced by stabilizing the lunate while the capitate is brought into palmar flexion, and reduction may be maintained by percutaneously inserted Kirschner wires. The presence of residual scapholunate dissociation or dorsiflexion instability of the lunate after attempted closed reduction requires open reduction and pin fixation.

3. ACUTE ULNAR WRIST PAIN

A. Distal Radioulnar Joint (DRUJ) Disorders Pain occurs on the ulnar side of the wrist, and tenderness may be present over the distal radioulnar joint. Passive forearm motion (pronation or supination) with the elbow flexed and the hand pointed upward causes wrist pain if the DRUJ is involved. Pain-free forearm motion indicates an ulnocarpal origin of the pain.

The causes of acute DRUJ region pain include the following.

1. Fracture of the Distal Ulna or Radial Sigmoid Fossa These fractures cause pain over the ulnar side of the wrist and swelling and tenderness over the DRUJ. They can be diagnosed by plain radiographs or by a CT scan of the DRUJ.

2. Fracture of the Triquetrum or Lunate Pain and local tenderness and swelling occur over the triquetrum or lunate, respectively.

3. Triquetrum Avulsion Fractures There are ulnar wrist pain and tenderness. These fractures follow a hyperextension injury of the wrist with impingement and shearing of a fragment of bone attached to the dorsal radiotriquetral ligament. They can be visualized by a lateral or oblique radiograph of the wrist.

4. Dislocation of the Distal Ulna This disorder causes local pain, swelling, and deformity on the ulnar side of the wrist. A plain radiograph or CT of the DRUJ can define the dislocation.

5. Dislocation of the Lunate or Triquetrum Dislocation of these articulating carpal bones can cause local pain, tenderness, swelling, and deformity. With severe injury of the triquetral ligaments, the triquetrum may be ballotable and dislocation associated with a click.

6. Triangular Fibrocartilage Complex (TFCC) Injury Pain and tenderness are present over the ulnocarpal joint and DRUJ, and a click or snap may be heard during passive forearm motion or wrist flexion. Evaluation by MRI may reveal injury to the TFCC. Arthroscopy is another potentially useful method of evaluating the TFCC and the DRUJ. Arthrography may be used to demonstrate perforation of the TFCC (e.g., by entry of dye into the DRUJ after injection into the radiocarpal joint).

7. Extensor Carpi Ulnaris (ECU) Subluxation and/or Tendinitis This disorder is associated with rupture of the extensor retinaculum. A snap may be heard or felt as the tendon passes palmarly with palmar flexion of the wrist. The subluxating tendon may move dorsally during passive supination of the forearm.

Frictional trauma to the tendon may cause dorsomedial wrist pain, with swelling of the tendon sheath, and local tenderness (tenosynovitis). Resisted wrist extension or passive wrist flexion may intensify the pain. Tenosynovitis of the ECU may occur secondary to overuse without repetitive subluxation.

8. Extensor Digiti Minimi Tenosynovitis Tenosynovitis of the fifth dorsal compartment may cause dorsomedial wrist pain and tenderness that are increased by resisted extension or passive flexion of the small finger. The tendon sheath is usually tender. Excision of the extensor retinaculum may be required to resolve this disorder.

B. Triquetrolunate Instability

1. Triquetrolunate Sprain There are pain on the ulnar side of the wrist and tenderness over the triquetrolunate joint. Some patients complain of wrist stiffness and weakness. The pain usually begins after a fall on the outstretched hand or a twisting injury. Results of static radiographs of the wrist are usually normal. The triquetrolunate interosseous ligament is torn, but the radiotriquetral and the capitotriquetral and ulnotriquetral ligaments remain intact.

2. Triquetrolunate Dissociation Pain occurs on the ulnar side of the wrist, and there is tenderness over the triquetrolunate joint. A painful wrist click may occur when the wrist is moved into ulnar or radial deviation.

The triquetrum can be palpated in the floor of the ulnar ''snuffbox'' on the ulnar side of the wrist. There is a sulcus just beyond the ulnar styloid located between the tendons of the extensor carpi ulnaris (dorsal) and the flexor carpi ulnaris (volar). When the wrist is radially deviated, a rounded bone appears in the ulnar ''snuffbox'' floor. This is the triquetrum. This bone may be tender in the presence of fracture or ligamentous disruption. If the lunate is stabilized by the thumb and index finger of the examiner's hand, the triquetrum can be balloted in the ulnar ''snuffbox'' to displace it dorsally and then by the lunate stabilizing hand to displace it palmarly. This lunotriquetral ballottement (abnormal mobility of the joint) test is helpful in demonstrating triquetrolunate instability. In some cases, a snap or click results from the ballottement test.

A carpal instability radiographic series includes a posteroanterior view in neutral, ulnar, and radial deviation; a clenched-fist (axial loading) anteroposterior view; an oblique view; a 30° off-lateral oblique view to image the pisotriquetral articulation; a lateral view in neutral and in extreme extension and flexion; and a lateral clenched-fist view.

In patients with triquetrolunate dissociation, the triquetrum is displaced proximally and laterally. On ulnar deviation, the lunate and triquetrum may overlap or a gap may be present between them. Lateral radiographs may show dorsiflexion of the triquetrum when compared to the lunate. The lunotriquetral angle measured on a lateral view becomes less than 0 (mean, $-16°$), while it is normally positive. Arthrographic studies will confirm a triquetrolunate ligament tear by demonstrating dye passage from the radiocarpal space to the intercarpal space through the triquetrolunate joint. Arthroscopic studies may also be useful in differentiating a TFCC tear from triquetrolunate dissociation.

C. Fractures of the Ulnar Carpal Bones

1. Fracture of the Hamate   Fracture of the hook of the hamate may result from a fall on the outstretched hand or from a force transmitted through a bat, golf club, or racquet. Persistent pain and localized swelling and tenderness of the proximal hypothenar eminence are the usual clinical findings. Pain may sometimes be felt dorsally.

A carpal tunnel radiographic view or an oblique view, with the forearm in midsupination and the wrist extended and radially deviated, will usually demonstrate a hook fracture. In some cases, trispiral tomography of the carpal tunnel or CT may be necessary. These fractures seldom heal even after open reduction and wire fixation. Relief of hypothenar pain may require operative excision of the ununited fragment. Fractures of the body of the hamate are uncommon. They may result in dorsal dislocation of the fourth and fifth metacarpals. Hamate body fractures may be demonstrated by sagittal CT.

2. Fracture of the Pisiform   Local pain, swelling, and tenderness occur over the proximal ulnar volar region of the wrist over the bony prominence of the pisiform bone. This fracture is usually caused by a fall or a blow to the volar ulnar aspect of the wrist. The fracture can be visualized by a carpal tunnel view or by a 30° supination palm-up view. Pisiform fractures usually heal with 6 weeks of immobilization.

D. Tendinitis

1. Flexor Carpi Ulnaris (FCU) Tendinitis   Pain and tenderness are present over the pisiform and the FCU tendon proximal to the pisiform. Wrist flexion against resistance intensifies the pain. Passive wrist extension has a similar effect. This disorder is usually caused by repetitive trauma (overuse). Symptoms may respond to rest, splinting, and a local corticosteroid injection.

2. Digital Flexor Tendinitis   Midvolar wrist pain and burning occur and radiate into the forearm. An acute carpal tunnel syndrome may be present. Swelling and tenderness occur proximal to the wrist flexor creases.

E. Pisotriquetral Arthritis   There is local tenderness over the area and crepitus. The FCU tendon is not tender. Plain radiographs of the wrist reveal narrowing of the pisotriquetral joint and subchondral sclerosis. Pain may be relieved by pisiform excision.

F. Midcarpal Instability   Symptoms may begin after a fall on the outstretched hand, a rotational injury, or, most commonly, without recalled injury. A painful ulnar click occurs in the midcarpal region when the wrist is ulnar-deviated, pronated, and axially compressed. There is a volar sag of the midcarpal region and localized tenderness over the triquetrohamate articulation. Fullness of the ulnar aspect of the wrist joint may be caused by a secondary synovitis. The click or clunk can be reproduced by moving the hand into ulnar deviation from a neutral position. As ulnar deviation is produced, movement of the proximal carpal row from volar flexion into dorsiflexion occurs abruptly without making a smooth synchronous change. This corrects the volar sag and produces the visible and audible click. Cineradiographic studies confirm the diagnosis as they demonstrate the sudden transition of the proximal carpal row from palmarflexion (VISI) to dorsiflexion as the hand is ulnar-deviated. This abrupt positional change is accompanied by a painful click. With ulnar deviation, the anteriorly subluxated distal row of carpal bones reduces. Results of arthrographic studies are usually normal.

Avoidance of ulnar deviation, pronation, and axial compression of the affected wrist during athletic activities and use of a volar splint may relieve symptoms. Refractory cases with persistent pain may require triquetrohamate arthrodesis.

4. WRIST INSTABILITY RADIOGRAPHIC PATTERNS

A. VISI This instability pattern is diagnosed on a lateral wrist radiograph. It is caused by disruption of the dorsal (dorsal ulnocarpal or ulnoradial ligaments) and/or ulnar stabilizing ligaments of the wrist (lunotriquetral ligament). The lateral radiograph demonstrates a downward tilt of the lunate, a scapholunate axis of 30° or less, and a capitolunate axis angle greater than 30°. VISI is usually associated with the ulnocarpal or midcarpal instabilities described above.

B. DISI This instability pattern is diagnosed by a lateral radiograph of the wrist. The lunate concavity is directed dorsally, and the capitolunate angle exceeds 15°. The scapholunate angle may exceed 60°. DISI is caused by rupture of the scapholunate interosseous ligament and the volar radial scapholunate ligament. The DISI pattern is often associated with unstable scaphoid fractures and scapholunate dissociation.

5. DIFFUSE WRIST PAIN

A. Traumatic Ulnar Translocation of the Carpus There may be a fall on the outstretched hand and pronation of the forearm on the fixed hand. All the palmar radiocarpal ligaments are disrupted. There is massive swelling, pain, and diffuse tenderness of the wrist. Lateral instability of the proximal carpus may be demonstrable by radioulnar pressure on the second metacarpal. Plain wrist radiographs demonstrate carpus dislocation from the radius in an ulnar direction. Less than half the lunate overlaps the radius. The scaphoid-radial styloid distance is increased. Ulnar deviation of the wrist is blocked by the lunate. Primary ligament repair following open reduction is required to relieve pain and instability.

B. Acute Arthritis of the Wrist

1. Septic arthritis N. gonorrhoeae arthritis may begin with fever, chills, malaise, arthralgias, and a migratory polyarthritis. Some patients have only mild systemic symptoms. Localization of the arthritis eventually occurs, with persistent symptoms in one to three joints. N. gonorrhoeae is the most frequent cause of suppurative arthritis in adults under age 30.

Persistent aching wrist pain occurs and may be in-

tensified by slight movement or jarring. The affected wrist is usually warm, diffusely swollen, and tender, and the overlying skin may be erythematous. Synovial fluid usually contains 10,000 to more than 100,000 polymorphonuclear leukocytes per cubic millimeter. Positive synovial fluid cultures for *N. gonorrhoeae* occur in up to 50 percent of cases. A Gram stain demonstrates extracellular and intracellular gram-negative diplococci in a similar percentage of cases. Direct immunofluorescence staining may identify *N. gonorrhoeae* in culture-negative fluids. Cultures of mucous membrane sites will be positive in up to 80 percent of cases. Tenosynovitis of the distal arm or leg may occur in 68 percent of cases. Cutaneous lesions in the form of tender, red-rimmed papules, pustules, or purple vesicles occur most commonly on the forearms, hands, fingers, and feet. There is a prompt response of joint symptoms to antibiotic therapy. Monoarthritis due to *N. gonorrhoeae* is seldom associated with cutaneous lesions.

S. aureus, streptococcal species (*S. pneumoniae*, groups A and B streptococci, viridans group streptococci, and microaerophilic and anaerobic streptococci) and gram-negative bacilli are the major nongonococcal causes of suppurative arthritis in adults. Synovial fluid resulting from infection with these organisms is usually turbid, yellow, and thick or serosanguineous. The leukocyte count may exceed 100,000 cells/mm³ in one-third to one-half the cases, and there is usually a predominance of polymorphonuclear leukocytes. The fluid glucose is often >40 mg/dl lower than the simultaneously drawn blood glucose, and synovial fluid cultures are positive in up to 90 percent of cases. Closed or open drainage and antibiotic therapy result in pain relief and resolution of joint swelling, warmth, and tenderness.

2. Pseudogout Wrist involvement may be unilateral. Pain, swelling, warmth, tenderness, and sometimes redness occur. An attack may be provoked by surgery or by an acute medical illness. The wrist is the second most frequently involved joint after the knee. Joint fluid contains polymorphonuclear leukocytes (mean concentration, 21,350 cells/mm³) and calcium pyrophosphate dihydrate crystals. Chondrocalcinosis of the triangular fibrocartilage in the wrist, articular cartilage in the shoulders, and menisci in the knees occurs. There is a prompt response to intravenous colchicine.

3. Gout Pain, redness, swelling, and tenderness of the wrist joint and sometimes the juxtaarticular flexor and/or extensor tendons occur. The serum uric acid level is usually elevated during an attack, and synovial fluid contains monosodium urate crystals. There is a prompt response to intravenous or oral colchicine.

4. Kienböck's Disease Avascular necrosis of the lunate can cause joint swelling, pain, tenderness, and immobility. An MRI or a bone scan will reveal evidence of avascular necrosis weeks or months before results of plain radiographs become positive.

5. *Hemophilic Arthropathy* An acute hemorrhage into the wrist joint may occur in a patient with known hemophilia. The joint can be aspirated and blood removed after administration of adequate amounts of factor VIII.

6. *Idiopathic Arthritis* Some patients with acute wrist involvement improve spontaneously before a diagnosis is established.

6. NEUROGENIC WRIST PAIN

A. Acute Carpal Tunnel Syndrome An acute carpal tunnel syndrome may cause pain in the wrist and pain, paresthesias, and numbness in the thumb, index, middle finger, and lateral side of the fourth finger. Phalen's sign and Tinel's sign may be positive. Acute carpal tunnel syndrome may be caused by a fracture of the distal radius or a volar dislocation of the lunate, a carpal tunnel hematoma associated with hemophilia or anticoagulant therapy, a thrombosis of a persistent median artery, a soft tissue infection of the hand or forearm, a burn, septic arthritis of the wrist, and Lyme borreliosis. Flexor tenosynovitis due to overuse or pyogenic infection also causes an acute carpal tunnel syndrome. The diagnosis can be confirmed by nerve conduction velocity studies across the wrist. Exploration and decompression of the carpal tunnel is required in rapidly progressing cases.

B. Acute Ulnar Tunnel Syndrome Pain occurs in the medial hand and fourth and fifth fingers (ulnar fingers). Hypesthesia and paresthesias in the volar aspect of the ulnar fingers may be present. Hand weakness and clumsiness may occur. This disorder may follow acute ulnar artery thombosis, repetitive trauma, or sustained pressure over the ulnar region of the hand. Cyclists gripping their handle bars may develop ''handle bar palsy''; other cases develop from the use of crutches or from the use of a paddle in kayaking and from playing handball. A rapidly enlarging ganglion may cause minimal pain and paresthesias while producing significant motor weakness of the involved hand. Palpation by the examiner over Guyon's canal between the hamate and the pisiform bones may elicit tingling paresthesias in the ulnar fingers (positive Tinel's sign). Tinel's sign at the elbow and the elbow flexion test are negative, making a cubital tunnel syndrome unlikely.

The absence of sensory abnormalities on the dorsal aspect of the hand and ulnar fingers is characteristic of a Guyon's canal (ulnar tunnel) lesion. Patients with more proximal ulnar lesions usually have dorsal hand and finger sensory symptoms and signs. Refractory cases of ulnar tunnel compression may require surgical decompression.

Hand and Finger Pain

7. CARPOMETACARPAL AND MP AREAS

A. Carpometacarpal Dislocations Pain, severe swelling, and tenderness occur over the dorsum of the hand several centimeters proximal to the MP joints. Deformity of the dorsal region of the hand may be obscured by edema. Results of routine lateral and anteroposterior radiographs may be normal. Oblique views in one or more projections are likely to profile the injured joints. Dislocation is usually dorsal, but volar displacement of the metacarpal bases may also occur.

Ligament-disrupting extension or flexion forces or a longitudinal force directed at the fifth metacarpal carpal joint following a fall or impact against a hard surface is the usual cause. The second and third carpometacarpal joints are more difficult to disrupt than are the fourth and fifth. A missed dislocation is associated with a localized bony elevation of the dorsum of the hand 3 to 4 cm distal to the wrist, local pain and tenderness, and loss of grasp strength. Fractures of the adjacent carpal bones or the base of the metacarpal may be associated. These injuries are usually treated by closed reduction, percutaneous pin fixation, and casting with the carpometacarpal joints in extension. Dislocations at the trapeziometacarpal joint are discussed below, under ''Thumb Pain.''

B. Metacarpal Shaft Fractures Pain, localized tenderness, and swelling occur over the fractured metacarpal(s). The pain is a dull, constant ache that becomes sharp and severe with passive or active movement. An oblique/spiral fracture may cause malrotation of the associated finger. The malrotation may be observed with the hand open or while making a fist. The involved finger may be directed at a different angle than are the others, and the space between it and an adjacent digit may be widened. The malrotated finger may even overlap another. Anteroposterior, lateral, and sometimes oblique radiographs will identify the metacarpal fracture(s). Oblique/spiral fractures result from a rotational force, and there are frequently overriding of fragments and shortening. Accurate reduction and percutaneous Kirschner pin fixation are usually required. Open reduction and fixation with a small lag screw may also be performed. Transverse fractures may cause dorsal angulation and shortening of the fractured metacarpal.

A test to define metacarpal fractures requiring percutaneous pin fixation has been described. Patients who are able to completely extend the finger associated with the fractured metacarpal without MP joint hyperextension and proximal interphalangeal joint flexion can be treated without wire fixation. This test requires wrist block anesthesia. Clawing of the digits or zigzag collapse due to the effects of the intrinsic hand muscles requires pin fixation.

C. MP Joint Dislocation and Ligament Injuries

1. Volar Plate Disruption   The index and little finger are most frequently involved. Rupture of the volar plate at its membranous attachment to the metacarpal follows sudden forceful hyperextension and leads to dorsal displacement of the proximal phalange so that it may override the metacarpal head. The finger may appear slightly hyperextended at the MP joint and flexed at the interphalangeal joints and may deviate toward or override the adjacent finger. The palmar skin may be puckered in the area of the proximal palmar crease. A defect may be palpated dorsally, proximal to the phalanx due to joint disruption. Radiographs show joint space widening on the anterposterior view and dislocation on the lateral projection. The presence of sesamoid bones, which are usually embedded in the volar plate, within the joint is strong evidence of volar plate disruption and a complex dislocation. Open surgical reduction is required when the volar plate is interposed between the metacarpal head and the base of the proximal phalanx. In a patient with a partial subluxation, the proximal phalanx is positioned directly dorsal to the metacarpal head and may be hyperextended as much as 90°. There is no lateral angulation of the involved digit.

2. Collateral Ligament Sprain   Forced deviation of a finger in an ulnar direction with the MP joint in some degree of flexion is the mechanism of the injury. Pain and sometimes swelling and tenderness occur at the involved MP joint. After swelling and pain have subsided, laxity of the involved MP joint in full flexion can be demonstrated by passive ulnar and radial movements of the corresponding finger. In some cases, the diagnosis may be apparent from deviation of the involved finger to the ulnar side (rupture of radial collateral ligament). Collateral ligament sprain is most common in the ring or little finger but may affect any finger. Surgery is required to correct significant MP joint instability.

3. Dorsal Joint Capsule Injuries   Direct trauma to the knuckle, as occurs in boxing or karate, may cause a contusion or damage to the dorsal hood. Local pain and tenderness occur and persist after use of the affected hand in practice or a match. A tear in the joint capsule may cause extensor tendon displacement (usually to the radial side when the tear is on the ulnar side of the capsule) and a palpable defect over the affected MP joint. Surgical repair of the defect is required.

4. Fractures of the Metacarpal Neck and Head

A. METACARPAL NECK FRACTURES   An injury to the joint with the fist clenched is the usual cause. There are local pain, tenderness, and swelling. Dorsal angulation of a metacarpal neck fracture may cause a painful palm prominence due to the distal fragment, and this may impede grasp. Extension of the MP joint may be mildly impaired, and tendon imbalance may occur. Closed reduction and fixation are usually effective, but instability of this reduction requires surgical fixation.

B. INTRAARTICULAR FRACTURES OF THE METACARPAL HEAD   Pain, tenderness, and swelling occur over the involved MP joint. Loss of joint mobility is usually associated. Lesions include osteochondral joint fragments, comminuted fractures, associated ligament ruptures, and articular surface fractures. The Brewerton radiographic view provides excellent imaging of the articular surface of the metacarpal heads. This radiograph is taken with the dorsum of the hand and fingers on the plate, the MP joints flexed 65°, and the beam angled from 15° on the medial side of the hand. Open reduction and fixation are required.

8. PROXIMAL PHALANX AND PIP JOINT AREA INJURIES

A. Fractures of the Proximal Phalanx

1. Base of the Proximal Phalanx   There are pain, tenderness, swelling, and sometimes deformity involving the base of the proximal phalanx. Rotational deformity of the involved finger may be observed with the hand open or on making a fist. Base fractures are frequently angled in a volar direction because of the pull of the intrinsic hand muscles. These fractures may be demonstrated by lateral or oblique radiographic views. Volar angulation can be detected by palpation. Closed reduction is usually possible.

2. Shaft of the Proximal Phalanx   These fractures may be transverse, oblique/spiral, or comminuted. Local pain, swelling, and tenderness are present over the proximal phalanx. Spiral fractures may extend into the proximal interphalangeal joint and cause limitation of joint flexion if not adequately reduced. A spike fragment in the joint usually requires open reduction to ensure normal joint mobility.

3. Neck and Head of the Proximal Phalanx   Pain, swelling, and tenderness occur at the PIP joint and over the distal portion of the proximal phalanx. The head of the proximal phalanx may be rotated so that the fracture surface is angled in a volar direction and the articular surface is angled dorsally as much as 90°. Surgical reduction and crossed Kirschner pin fixation across the fracture site may be required. Condylar fractures at the distal end of the proximal phalanx may result in lateral deviation of the distal portion of the finger to the side of the condylar fracture. Open reduction and internal fixation are usually required for the displaced condyle.

B. PIP Joint Region

1. Ligament Sprains (First and Second Degree)
Pain, swelling, and tenderness occur at the PIP joint. The joint remains stiff, and there is only limited mobility. Most "jammed" fingers are first- or second-degree sprains, and there is no subluxation or joint instability. Persistent joint swelling, tenderness, and pain may last up to 18 months, and joint size may never return to normal. Pain may be present only at the extremes of joint mobility or with use against resistance.

2. Volar Plate Injuries
These injuries result from a rapid hyperextension of the PIP joint. There are volar pain, tenderness, swelling, and joint stiffness but no joint instability with a type I volar plate rupture. The corner attachments of the volar plate to the middle phalanx remain intact, and only the thin central portion of the plate detaches from the middle phalanx.

Type II volar plate injuries involve the lateral attachments to the middle phalanx. With rupture, hyperextension of the joint or dislocation with dorsal displacement of the middle phalanx occurs. After closed reduction, a dorsal block splint is used to prevent recurrent dislocation.

3. Intraarticular Fracture-Dislocation
At the PIP joint, intraarticular fracture-dislocation may follow a compressive force on the joint or an axial loading force on the partially flexed finger. The volar base of the middle phalanx may then shear against the proximal phalanx, resulting in a fracture-dislocation of the joint that requires open reduction. Instability occurs with middle phalangeal fractures that involve one-third or more of the articular surface.

4. Collateral Ligament Tears
Lateral joint swelling, pain, and tenderness occur over the affected ligament. If the ligament is completely disrupted on one side (usually the radial), there will be deviation of the middle and distal phalanges to the side of the intact collateral ligament with the fingers flexed or extended. Closed reduction and immobilization in slight flexion usually result in a stable joint.

5. Volar Dislocations
These dislocations result from abrupt forced flexion of the middle phalanx or from a severe torsional force on the joint. The head of the proximal phalanx may rupture the extensor tendon system, disrupting the central slip of the extensor tendon. Volar dislocations frequently result in persistent joint stiffness. An irreducible dislocation may occur if the central extensor tendon and one of the lateral extensor bands are entrapped between the joint surfaces or beneath the condyles of the proximal phalanx. A plain lateral radiograph may demonstrate a rotational displacement of the proximal and middle phalanges or a complete dislocation. Closed reduction may be effective, or open reduction may be required.

6. PIP Joint Deformities

A. ACUTE BOUTONNIERE DEFORMITY This deformity (i.e., PIP joint flexion and DIP extension) results from rupture of the central slip of the extensor tendon mechanism. A sudden forceful flexion of the PIP joint can cause this injury. Initially, only pain, tenderness, and swelling occur over the PIP joint. There may be direct tenderness over the site of central tendon insertion on the base of the middle phalanx. The PIP joint becomes flexed as the lateral bands of the extensor mechanism slip volarly. Stabilization of the PIP joint in extension and observation of DIP joint active and passive flexion reveal a decrease in this movement. The PIP joint remains in flexion, and the DIP joint becomes hyperextended or fixed in extension by contracture. Splinting the PIP joint in full extension, with the DIP joint free to move, may lead to resolution of the deformity.

B. PSEUDOBOUTONNIERE DEFORMITY This disorder begins after a hyperextension PIP joint injury. The volar capsule is disrupted, and flexion contracture of the PIP joint follows weeks or months later. There is normal mobility at the DIP joint, including normal passive and active flexion. Surgical release of the flexion contracture at the PIP joint may be required if active and passive PIP joint exercises and dynamic extension splints fail to restore extension.

9. MIDDLE PHALANX AREA FRACTURES

These fractures cause local pain, swelling, tenderness, and deformity with extension or flexion of the proximal fragments. The direction of proximal fragment displacement is determined by the relationship of the fracture line to the insertion of the flexor superficialis tendon and central extensor tendon. If the fracture line is distal to the insertion of the extensor tendon and proximal to the insertion of the flexor tendon, the proximal fragment is extended and the distal fragment flexed. Plain radiographs will define the fracture line.

10. DIP JOINT AREA

A. Extensor Tendon Disruption This disorder occurs in baseball, football, basketball, and volleyball players. A ball strikes the extended finger, forcing the DIP joint into flexion. The extensor tendon is torn or avulsed from the base of the distal phalanx. There are local pain, swelling, tenderness, and inability to extend the distal phalanx. This deformity has been called a mallet, baseball, or drop finger. Slippage of the detached tendon proximally may increase PIP joint extension, resulting in a "swan neck" deformity (i.e., PIP joint extension and DIP joint flexion) of the finger.

B. Flexor Tendon Disruption   Sudden extension of the DIP joint during resisted flexion may cause rupture or avulsion of the flexor profundus tendon from the distal phalanx. There are volar pain, tenderness, swelling, and ecchymoses along the tendon sheath and an inability to flex the DIP joint. In some cases, flexion at the PIP joint may also be limited. A radiograph may show a fragment of bone avulsed from the site of tendon disruption. Surgery is necessary for all acute ruptures of the flexor profundus tendon. This is because the tendon may retract to the level of the PIP joint or even to the palm.

C. Fracture of the Distal Phalanx   These fractures are usually not displaced and heal without complications. There is pain, swelling, and tenderness over the distal phalanx.

D. Subungual Hematoma   A crush injury to the nail bed, with or without fracture of the distal phalanx, may cause excruciating throbbing fingertip pain that is resistant to analgesics. The affected nail is blue secondary to the presence of subungual blood. Drainage of the hematoma by the use of a red-hot paper clip to burn a small hole in the nail will release liquid blood and provide dramatic pain relief. These injuries often follow crushing of the fingertip in a car door.

E. Dislocation of the DIP Joint   Lateral or dorsal dislocation may occur, resulting in pain, tenderness, swelling, and a distal deformity that can usually be reduced by closed manipulation.

11. FINGER INFECTIONS

A. Paronychia and Eponychia

1. Superficial Type   Pain and tenderness are associated with an erythematous, edematous lateral nail margin (paronychia). A small, fluctuant area containing pus may develop adjacent to the lateral nail fold, and this may drain spontaneously or after incision. *S. aureus* is the usual cause.

2. Deep Type   The nail margin and adjacent skin are swollen, erythematous, and tender. Throbbing pain is felt in this area and sometimes beneath the nail. Pressure on the nail may provoke severe localized nail pain. Surgical incision parallel to the nail margin and removal of a quarter of the nail adjacent to the margin will alleviate pain by allowing drainage of subungual pus.

B. Eponychia   Proximal involvement of the nail margin over the nail plate occurs in association with lateral nail fold infection and responds to removal of the proximal third of the nail.

Acute paronychia or eponychia begins after a foreign body lodges between the nail plate and paronychial tissue (e.g., a wood, metal, or glass splinter), from a hangnail

that allows initiation of infection, or after excessive use of nail polish.

C. Runaround Infection   A runaround infection is a paronychia that spreads from one lateral nail fold to the eponychium and then to the opposite lateral nail fold.

D. Subungual Abscess   There is severe aching or throbbing pain beneath the nail. Pressure over the nail elicits pain, and a "floating nail" may be present. Total nail removal allows drainage and pain relief. A subungual abscess may begin with a deep paronychia.

E. Pulp Space Infection   The flexor surfaces of fingers 2 to 5 contain three pulp spaces and the thumb two spaces, bounded by the flexor digit creases. Skin is adherent to the underlying flexor tendon sheath at the flexor creases. Fat in the distal pulp space is divided into compartments by vertical fibrous septa. A direct puncture wound into the pulp space, a neglected paronychia, or a subungual abscess may cause an abscess to develop in the pulp space of a terminal phalanx on the thumb or one of the fingers. This lesion is called a felon.

1. Felon   Severe aching and throbbing pain occurs over the distal pulp space. The distal volar aspect of the affected finger is tensely swollen and exquisitely tender and erythematous. Transillumination of the pulp space beneath the distal phalanx may outline the abscess.

A distal pulp space abscess may drain through a necrotic area of skin, cause an osteomyelitis of the distal phalanx, or cause a septic arthritis of the DIP joint. Radiographs can detect a foreign body in the pulp space or an osteolytic infection of the terminal phalanx. Incision and drainage and use of systemic antibiotics result in relief of pain and tenderness.

2. Middle and Proximal Pulp Space Infection   Local tense swelling, pain, and tenderness with overlying skin warmth and erythema occur over the middle or proximal pulp space. An abscess may form, and infection can spread to the dorsum of the finger or into the adjacent web space.

F. Web Space Infections   Swelling and redness occur in the web space, on the adjacent palm, and over the dorsum of the hand proximal to the involved space. There are severe pain, tenderness, warmth, and erythema of the overlying skin. The digits adjacent to the web space are separated by the underlying abscess and surrounding edema. These abscesses are usually hourglass- or dumbbell-shaped, with dorsal and volar subcutaneous collections of purulent material separated by the palmar fascia and superficial transverse metacarpal ligament. A fissure or puncture in the web space, an infected distal palmar callus, or a subcutaneous abscess volar to the proximal phalanx can cause a web space infection.

Incision and drainage of the dorsal and volar components and systemic antibiotic therapy are required for resolution.

G. Flexor Tendon Sheath Infections   The involved finger is uniformly swollen, and the finger is held in flexion. There are localized tenderness over the involved flexor tendon sheath and pain on passive extension of the involved digit. The index, middle, and ring fingers are most frequently involved. *S. aureus* is the most frequently isolated organism, but gram-negative bacteria have been found to cause up to 20 percent of these infections. Early use of antibiotics alone may relieve finger pain, tenderness, and edema. If there is no improvement within 24 h, incision and drainage and irrigation of the tendon sheath are required for resolution without loss of tendon function. These infections may spread to the deep spaces and bursae of the hand.

H. Herpetic Whitlow   Pain occurs in one finger with associated redness. Small, grouped vesicles or crusted ulcers develop in the area of erythema. Dental and medical personnel are at risk, but this lesion may occur in the absence of occupational exposure. Culture and smears stained with an indirect fluorescent antibody stain to herpes simplex virus will establish the diagnosis. If the infection occurs along the nail margin it can be confused with paronychia, and if it occurs in the distal volar pulp it may be mistaken for a felon. Acyclovir therapy can be used to control recurrent or persistent lesions.

I. Mimics of Acute Infectious Arthritis or Tenosynovitis of a Digit

1. Gout   This disorder may be mistaken for an acute paronychia. It may also cause local redness of the DIP joint, pain, and tenderness. A urate deposit in the skin may drain chalky-white urate crystals and mimic a local cutaneous abscess. Gout may also cause flexor tenosynovitis of a digit.

2. Acute Calcific Tendinitis   Calcium deposition in a tendon or a ligament can cause local finger pain, redness, and tenderness. Calcification may be detected on a plain radiograph at the site of a painful tendon insertion or ligament. Tenderness is usually sharply localized to the area of calcium deposition.

3. Malignant Melanoma Involving the Nail Fold and Bed   A nail fold melanoma may mimic a paronychia that resists therapy. A margin of brownish or black pigmentation provides a clue to the true nature of the lesion. If the lesion is amelanotic, the diagnosis may be missed in 50 percent of cases. A nail bed melanoma with secondary infection may mimic a subungual infection. Identification of the true nature of a persistent nail-associated lesion requires biopsy.

4. Sarcoidosis   This disorder may cause finger swelling, pain, and tenderness secondary to a flexor tenosynovitis. Tender swelling of the flexor tendon may be present. Pain is intensified by finger extension. Extensor tenosynovitis involving the extensor tendons at the wrist is the most frequent form of sarcoid tenosynovitis.

12.   HAND INFECTIONS

A. Bursal Infections   The radial bursa is an extension of the sheath of the flexor pollicis longus tendon that extends into the wrist. The ulnar bursa is a continuation of the flexor sheath of the long flexor of the small finger. This bursa envelops the other flexor tendons in the palm and extends to the volar aspect of the wrist, where it usually communicates with the radial bursa.

1. Radial Bursal Infection   Pain, diffuse swelling, erythema, and flexor tendon tenderness occur in the thumb, and the tenderness extends proximally to the volar aspect of the radial side of the wrist. The thumb is held in flexion, and passive extension of this digit intensifies the pain. The thenar eminence and first web space are swollen, mimicking a thenar space infection. If the radial bursa communicates with the ulnar bursa, pain, swelling, and tenderness can appear in the small finger after a lag period of several days due to secondary spread to the ulnar bursa. This pattern of spread may result in a "horseshoe" abscess and sometimes extension to the distal forearm.

2. Ulnar Bursal Infection   The small finger becomes painful, tender, and diffusely swollen. Passive extension of the flexed finger intensifies the pain. A "horseshoe" abscess may develop after spread to the radial bursa, but this form of infection is uncommon. Bursal infections may result from a puncture wound or from suppurative tenosynovitis of a digit.

B. Space Infections

1. Midpalmar Space   There are diffuse swelling, redness, and tenderness of the midpalm, with loss of the normal palmar concavity. The dorsum of the hand becomes swollen. Fluctuance may develop on the volar side of the hand. Flexion of the fingers intensifies the pain. High fever, chills, weakness, and malaise may occur.

Incision along the distal palmar flexion crease and drainage, accompanied by antibiotic therapy, usually result in cure.

Midpalmar space infections may arise from a direct puncture of the space or by spread of a purulent tenosynovitis (long and ring fingers). The midpalmar space communicates with the second, third, and fourth web spaces through the lumbrical canals.

2. Thenar Space   Swelling, redness, and pain occur over the thenar eminence. The thumb is held in abduction, and the dorsum of the hand is severely swollen. The space is posterior to the muscles of the thenar eminence and anterior to the adductor pollicis. It may become infected by a suppurative tenosynovitis of the flexor tendon of the index finger, by spread from an adjacent space or bursal abscess, or by a direct penetrating wound.

13. ANIMAL AND HUMAN BITES OF THE HAND AND FINGERS

A. Dog Bites   Lacerations, crushing, puncture injuries, or combinations of these forms of tissue trauma occur. Infection of the wound begins with erythema, edema, and tenderness, sometimes accompanied by a purulent and/or malodorous discharge. Fever, usually low-grade; ascending lymphangitis extending up the forearm; and painful axillary adenitis occur in less than 20 percent of cases. Puncture wounds of the hand predispose to abscess formation, while wounds close to the bones and joints may initiate a septic arthritis, tenosynovitis, osteomyelitis, or a space infection. Isolates from infected dog bites include aerobes (e.g., *Pasteurella multocida*, 30–50 percent; *S. aureus*, 30 percent; and streptococcal species) and anaerobes (*Bacteroides* species, 19 percent, and *Fusobacterium* species, 19 percent). Most anaerobic infections are polymicrobial.

B. Cat Bites   These are usually scratches or small puncture wounds. They are likely to become infected. *P. multocida* (80 percent of cases) and streptococcal species are the most frequent isolates.

C. Human Bites

1. Paronychia   This disorder may occur secondary to nail edge biting or thumb sucking. Aerobes or anaerobes are isolated in pure culture (27 percent each) or as a mixed infection (46 percent). The most frequent aerobic isolates in paronychia are viridans streptococci, group A beta-hemolytic streptococci, gamma-hemolytic streptococci, *S. aureus*, and *Eikenella corrodens*. Anaerobic isolates include *Bacteroides* species, *Fusobacterium* species, and anaerobic gram-positive cocci.

2. Occlusive Bites   These bites usually involve the distal phalanx of the long or index finger or both. Viridans streptococci, *S. aureus*, and anaerobes are the usual isolates.

3. Clenched-Fist Injuries   These injuries follow a punch to the opponent's mouth. The target teeth may lacerate or puncture the skin over the flexed MP or PIP joints, inoculating oral bacterial. Local cellulitis with pain, redness, and swelling may begin within 24 to 48 h. Suppurative subcutaneous space or tendon infections may result. Septic arthritis may occur if the joint is punctured. Viridans streptococci, *S. aureus* (30 percent), and *E. corrodens* (25 percent) are common isolates. In addition, anaerobes may be cultured in 55 percent of clenched-fist infections.

D. Snake Bites   Local pain, swelling, and tenderness develop within 15 min of the bite. Two puncture wounds (fang marks) are present, and diffuse edema and pain rapidly spread up the arm. Systemic symptoms in the form of weakness, nausea, vomiting, acroparesthesias, and mucous membrane bleeding may follow. Local necrosis and bullae may develop at the site of the bite, resulting in gangrene of a portion of the hand or a finger. The role of the snake's mouth flora in this necrotizing process is difficult to estimate. Common isolates from the oral cavity of venomous snakes include gram-negative bacilli and anaerobes. Pit viper bites usually cause local necrosis, pain, and edema. Some elapid (cobra) bites may also cause local pain, tenderness, erythema, and necrosis, followed by neurotoxic symptoms.

E. Necrotic Arachnidism (Loxoscelism)   The bite of the brown recluse spider initially causes mild, stinging discomfort. After a latent period of 2 to 8 h, severe local pain occurs at the bite site. This pain is followed within 2 h by pruritus, swelling, and local redness. The central portion of the lesion becomes blue, white, or gray, and a large central bulla containing hemorrhagic fluid may develop. Within 3 to 7 days, a central necrotic ulcer forms.

F. Rat Bites (Rat Bite Fever)   A rat bite in the home or laboratory may be followed within 10 days by an acute febrile illness with chills, headache, myalgias, migratory joint pain, headache, and vomiting. There is usually no local wound infection or regional adenitis in *S. moniliformis* infection (the usual etiologic agent in the United States). The Asian form of this disorder, due to *Spirillum minor* infection, is associated with pain, swelling, and purplish discoloration of the wound and is accompanied by axillary lymphadenitis, a blotchy macular rash, a relapsing febrile course, and a false-positive serologic test for syphilis in 56 percent of cases.

S. moniliformis infection is usually associated with the eruption of a maculopapular or petechial rash on the palms, soles, and extremities. Skin lesions may become confluent and sometimes purpuric. Up to 50 percent develop an asymmetric polyarthritis or septic arthritis. The knees, shoulders, elbows, wrists, ankles, and hips may be involved. Spontaneous resolution of fever and symptoms occurs within 2 weeks. The diagnosis of *S. moniliformis* infection is suggested by a history of a recent rat bite and a febrile illness with rash. A Gram stain of the blood, synovial fluid, or pus demonstrating a gram-negative pleomorphic bacillus (*S. moniliformis*) or positive culture results will confirm the diagnosis. Serodiagnosis by measurement of specific agglutinins may also be confirmatory.

14. DIFFUSE INFECTIONS OF THE HAND AND FOREARM

A. Acute Bacterial Cellulitis Aching pain, redness, and edema involve the hand and extend up the arm. The erythematous margin on the arm is tender but not elevated. Longitudinal, erythematous, tender streaks may occur on the forearm and upper arm due to ascending lymphangitis. The usual cause is skin and subcutaneous infection by a group A streptococcus or *S. aureus*. Tender and painful axillary adenopathy, fever, and chills may occur in some cases. The cause may be an obvious peripheral lesion, such as a furuncle, on the dorsum of a proximal phalanx or a fissuring dermatitis of the hand, or the entry site of the infectious agent may not be apparent. There is a rapid response to intravenous antibiotic therapy.

B. Palmar Subaponeurotic Space Infection Pain, tenderness, erythema, and diffuse edema of the normally concave palm occur, resulting in palmar flattening or convexity. The thumb and fingers are held in flexion, and passive extension causes severe pain. Surgical incision and drainage of pus trapped beneath the palmar aponeurosis and systemic antibiotic therapy lead to rapid resolution.

C. Gas Gangrene (Clostridial Myonecrosis) Muscle injury and contamination by soil or fecal flora is the usual cause. Deep injuries, such as a compound fracture of the hand or a finger or a high-velocity bullet wound, may initiate this disorder. The onset follows within 24 to 72 h of the injury. The initial symptom is severe pain that is out of proportion to the severity of the wound. Systemic symptoms, with fever, diaphoresis, tachycardia, hypotension, pallor, and sometimes jaundice, soon follow. Apathy or apprehension and restlessness may also occur.

The wound becomes edematous and turgid, and local tenderness is present. If the wound is open, edematous muscle may protrude through the wound bed. A serosanguineous malodorous drainage is present, and gas bubbles may be present in the discharge. Careful palpation may reveal crepitus due to subcutaneous gas. Within hours, the pale, edematous skin at the wound margin becomes yellow or bronze in color. Tense bullae containing bloody or dark fluid may occur in the overlying skin, and areas of green-black or black cutaneous gangrene develop. In fulminant cases, progression over the hand and up the arm is rapid, occurring within 4 to 12 h. A Gram stain of the wound exudate reveals large, gram-positive bacilli

and some gram-negative bacteria. Few leukocytes are present. Cultures grow *Clostridium perfringens* (80–95 percent) or *Clostridium novyi* (10–40 percent). Plain radiographs usually reveal gas in muscle, skin, and fascial planes. Wound exploration confirms extensive myonecrosis.

High-dose intravenous penicillin, extensive debridement or amputation, and hyperbaric oxygen therapy may result in partial limb salvage and patient survival.

D. Clostridial Anaerobic Cellulitis Onset follows wounding by 3 to 5 days. Local pain, edema, and systemic symptoms are mild. A thin malodorous drainage occurs, and skin crepitus is prominent locally and may be extensive. Radiographs show subcutaneous gas. A Gram stain and cultures of wound exudate reveal *C. perfringens*. Differentiation from gas gangrene (clostridial myonecrosis) may require operative exploration, with testing of the underlying muscle for twitch, color, and ability to bleed. If necrotic muscle is not found, local debridement, drainage of pus, and high-dose intravenous penicillin therapy will lead to resolution.

E. Nonclostridial Anaerobic Cellulitis This gas-forming disorder is similar clinically to clostridial anaerobic cellulitis. It is usually caused by wound infection with one or more nonspore-forming anaerobes (*Bacterioides* species, peptostreptococci, or peptococci) occurring alone or in a mixed infection with aerobic coliform bacteria (*Escherichia coli* or *Klebsiella*), streptococci, or staphylococci. Surgical exploration of the infected wound site and determination of muscle viability are required. Debridement, drainage, and antibiotic therapy will lead to resolution of the infection and to wound healing.

F. Anaerobic Streptococcal Myonecrosis This disorder begins 3 to 4 days after wounding. There are local edema, a sour-smelling seropurulent discharge from the wound, and diffuse redness around the wound. Gas is present subcutaneously and in muscle and fascial planes. Pain occurs as the infection progresses, and it is not a prominent early complaint, as in gas gangrene. Inadequately treated cases may progress to muscle and cutaneous gangrene, with severe systemic symptoms. The exudate contains streptococci and polymorphonuclear leukocytes in large numbers. Cultures reveal a mixed infection with anaerobic streptococci accompanied by either group A streptococci or *S. aureus*. Exploration reveals muscle discoloration (brick-red color), but muscle twitch may be retained. In patients with limb ischemia, a gram-positive rod, *Bacillus subtilis*, and peptostreptococci may cause a similar infection that, on Gram stain, mimics clostridial gas gangrene. High-dose intravenous penicillin therapy and debridement result in resolution of anaerobic streptococcal myonecrosis.

G. *Aeromonas hydrophila* Myonecrosis This disorder may follow wounding in fresh water or after handling fish or other aquatic animals. The onset is rapid (within 2 days). Local pain is intense, edema is marked, and serosanguineous bullae occur. Systemic symptoms and toxicity may be severe. Radiographs reveal gas in fascial planes. Surgical exploration documents myonecrosis and allows drainage and debridement.

Gram stain of wound exudate reveals gram-negative bacilli. Cultures grow *Aeromonas hydrophila*. There is a response to extensive surgical debridement and antimicrobial therapy.

H. Streptococcal Gangrene This infection usually occurs at a site of injury, but the entry wound may not be apparent. There is an abrupt onset of local pain, redness, edema, and tenderness. Large bullae develop over the next 24 to 72 h. These contain purulent or reddish-black fluid. The bullae collapse into necrotic eschars or ulcers resembling a third-degree burn. Necrotic sloughing of the areas of cutaneous gangrene occurs, and systemic toxicity may be marked. Streptococci can be detected by Gram stain and culture of bulla fluid and the blood. Group A, C, or G streptococci are the usual etiologic agents.

15. ACUTE POLYARTHRITIS WITH WRIST AND HAND INVOLVEMENT

A. Hepatitis B Arthritis A symmetric or asymmetric polyarthritis may occur in 10 to 30 percent of cases of hepatitis B infection prior to the onset of hepatic symptoms. The arthritis may be additive and persistent or migratory. The small joints of the fingers and hands are involved in 80 percent and the wrist in 25 percent of cases. Other joints are involved with a 20 to 40 percent frequency. Tendinitis and bursitis may also occur. In up to 50 percent of cases, an urticarial, macular, or maculopapular pruritic rash appears. The diagnosis can be confirmed by a positive result of a serum test for HB_sAg and abnormal liver function test results.

B. Rubella-Associated Arthritis This disorder causes pain and stiffness in the fingers, wrists, knees, and other joints, often without joint swelling, heat, or redness. There is spontaneous resolution in 1 to 4 weeks. An acute carpal tunnel syndrome, brachial neuritis, or tenosynovitis may occur in a small number of cases. This disorder usually occurs in adult women with rubella infection (in 15–68 percent of rubella infections in women). Rubella-related symptoms include low-grade fever; tender, often painful occipital adenopathy; and a nonpruritic, faint, transient, maculopapular rash. The rash may precede or follow the arthritis.

C. Rubella Immunization Arthritis A similar arthritic illness may follow rubella immunization. In the postvaccination disorder, knee and carpal tunnel involvement have been more frequent. Arthritis is more common in immunized adolescent girls and women than in children. The incidence of arthritis after vaccination is 10 percent.

D. Acute Rheumatoid Arthritis Isolated swelling, tenderness, and movement-provoked pain in one or more PIP joints and/or MP joints may be an early sign of this disorder. Initial involvement may be asymmetric and even monarticular. Involvement of other joints (e.g., knees, wrists, shoulders, elbows, and ankles) soon follows. Results of the serum rheumatoid factor test are positive in 33 to 60 percent of cases at the onset of the disease.

E. Systemic Lupus Erythematosus Arthritis The initial symptom of this disorder may be a symmetric polyarthritis involving the fingers, knees, and other large joints. Results of the serum antinuclear antibody test are positive. Results of the serum test for rheumatoid factor may also be positive, and these patients are often initially diagnosed as having rheumatoid arthritis.

F. Acute Rheumatic Fever This febrile disorder presents as a migratory polyarthritis within 5 weeks of an upper respiratory illness. The joints are red, swollen, painful, and tender. Asymmetric involvement is common. The fingers are less likely to be involved than the knees, wrists, elbows, shoulders, and ankles. The diagnosis can be confirmed by detecting high levels of antistreptolysin O, anti-DNase B, and/or antihyaluronidase in the serum and by a dramatic response to aspirin therapy. Cardiac, cutaneous, and neurologic manifestations (chorea) are uncommon in adults.

G. Acute Traumatic Arthritis Pain, swelling, and stiffness of the PIP joints and MP joints may follow vigorous use of the hands in athletic activities or during performance of work tasks. Results of tests for rheumatoid factor and antinuclear antibodies are negative, and the sedimentation rate is normal. Cessation of the causative activity results in resolution of symptoms in 1 to 3 months.

H. Arthritis-Dermatitis Syndrome *N. gonorrhoeae* dissemination can cause migratory polyarthralgia or polyarthritis. The knees and wrists are frequently affected, while the small joints of the fingers and the ankles are less commonly involved. Associated tenosynovitis may involve the hands, wrists, and feet. Some patients develop 2 to 40 tender skin pustules or hemorrhagic vesicles on an erythematous base that are usually distributed on the distal portions of the limbs. Fever, chills, and systemic signs may be prominent or mild. The diagnosis may be confirmed by mucous membrane cultures (80 percent), culture of the genital region of a sexual partner, blood culture, or joint fluid culture. Results of direct fluorescent antibody stains of joint fluid or skin vesicle or pustule fluid may be positive. There is a rapid response to parenteral antimicrobial therapy.

I. Yersiniosis   Infection with *Yersinia enterocolitica* can result in a migratory polyarthritis that mimics acute rheumatic fever. Sacroiliitis may also occur. The diagnosis can be confirmed by stool culture and by detection of a rise in serum antibody to *Y. enterocolitica*.

J. Gout   Acute gout may involve one or more finger joints or the wrist. The joints are usually red, warm, swollen, painful, and tender. The serum urate level is usually high during an attack, and monosodium urate crystals are present in aspirated synovial fluid. Polyarticular involvement may affect the fingers and large joints.

K. Arthritis Associated with Inflammatory Bowel Disease   Acute arthritis may occur in 9 to 20 percent of patients with inflammatory bowel disease. Patients with large bowel disease and/or complications of the inflammatory bowel disorder are more likely to develop arthritis. It is usually associated with symptomatic bowel disease. The involved joints are red, warm, swollen, and painful. The pattern of involvement is usually asymmetric, polyarticular, and additive, but migratory arthritis may occur in 50 percent of cases. The knees, ankles, elbows, and wrists are more commonly involved than are the small joints of the hands and feet. The clinical picture of ulcerative colitis or Crohn's disease, negative test results for rheumatoid factor and antinuclear antibody, and a response of the arthritis to definitive treatment of the bowel disorder are useful diagnostic criteria.

L. Psoriatic Arthritis   An asymmetric or symmetric arthritis with prominent hand involvement may occur. Sausage-shaped, tender, painful, swollen digits and PIP and DIP arthritis are common, while shoulder, elbow, wrist, knee, and ankle involvement are less frequent. The rash of psoriasis is usually present, and most patients have onychodystrophy (onycholysis, nail pitting and ridging). Symmetric joint involvement may mimic rheumatoid arthritis, but the serum test results for rheumatoid factor are usually negative, nail changes are prominent, and there is increased frequency of HLA-B17 and HLA-B27 antigens in patients with psoriatic arthritis.

M. Calcium Pyrophosphate Dihydrate Deposition Disease   Acute inflammation of the wrist or the second and third MP joints may be manifestations of calcium pyrophosphate dihydrate deposition disease. The knee is the most frequently involved joint. Evidence of chondrocalcinosis may be present in the triangular fibrocartilage complex of the wrist, the articular cartilage of the proximal humerus, and in the articular cartilages and menisci of the knees. Synovial fluid from a swollen, painful, tender joint contains calcium pyrophosphate dihydrate crystals and an elevated concentration of polymorphonuclear leukocytes. There is a good therapeutic response to intravenous colchicine.

N. Septic Arthritis   Involvement of the small joints of the hand is rare, accounting for less than 4 percent of cases of septic arthritis. An involved MP, PIP, or DIP joint is usually swollen, warm, tender, and painful. The synovial fluid leukocyte count is increased to beyond 100,000 cells/mm^3 in 35 to 50 percent of cases, and the fluid culture is positive in 85 percent of cases of nongonococcal septic arthritis. Septic arthritis of the MP or PIP joint may follow a clenched fist injury. Involvement of two or more joints may occur.

16.   VASCULAR HAND AND FINGER PAIN

A. Acute Arterial Embolism

1. Brachial Artery   An embolism to the brachial artery may be asymptomatic or may cause aching, ischemic pain in the hand and fingers, pallor of the digits, paresthesias and/or areas of anesthesia, absence of the brachial and radial pulses, and paresis of the affected hand. Gangrene and painful ulceration of one or more fingertips may occur. The source of the embolism may be the heart, the aortic arch, the right innominate or left subclavian artery in the thorax, or the subclavian artery at the thoracic outlet. Atrial fibrillation, acute myocardial infarction, myocarditis, or mitral stenosis may give rise to clot emboli. A left atrial myxoma or an endocarditis may also embolize to the arm. A subclavian atheroma or aneurysm at the thoracic outlet may also cause a brachial artery embolus. The amount of distal pain and ischemic change is dependent on the collateral circulation around the elbow region.

2. Ulnar Artery   An embolus or trauma to the ulnar artery at the wrist may obstruct the superficial palmar arch, resulting in ischemia, pain and paresthesias, pallor or cyanosis, and sometimes gangrene of the middle, ring, and small fingers. Gangrene is more likely to occur if the superficial palmar arch is incomplete (20 percent of the population) or the radial artery is already occluded by a previous embolus or thrombus.

3. Radial Artery   Traumatic occlusion or an embolus to the radial artery in patients with an incomplete palmar arch may cause severe, painful hand ischemia. An Allen test to evaluate the ability of the radial artery and the ulnar artery to supply the hand and fingers should be done before a radial artery is cannulated or punctured. If the ability of the ulnar artery to supply the hand with the radial artery occluded is inadequate, the radial artery should not be cannulated.

B. Arterial Trauma   Acute traumatic occlusion of the brachial artery may follow blunt and penetrating trauma of the arm. A supracondylar fracture or dislocation of the elbow, an anterior forearm compartment syndrome, brachial artery cannulation or catheterization, and intraarterial injection of illicit drugs may cause brachial artery occlusion. Iatrogenic injury and occlusion of the radial artery may follow arterial puncture or cannulation.

C. Secondary Raynaud's Phenomenon   This disorder may affect one or both hands and the feet, depending on etiology. One or more digits may be affected initially, and in time more digits may become involved. There is a classic triad, after exposure to cold or emotional upset, of digital pallor followed by cyanosis and then rubor, with throbbing pain and/or tingling paresthesias during the hyperemic (rubor) phase.

The entire sequence may last only 15 to 20 min. Warming the hands under running water is frequently helpful and may shorten the attack, which usually resolves spontaneously within a half-hour. Nocturnal attacks of pain and paresthesias are uncommon.

1. Acute Arterial Occlusive Disease   An abrupt onset of Raynaud's phenomenon in one upper extremity may be secondary to arterial occlusive disease due to vasculitis, thrombosis, embolism, or compression at the thoracic outlet. An arteriogram of the involved subclavian artery will usually demonstrate the arterial lesion.

2. Drug Therapy   Administration of beta-adrenergic blocking drugs to treat migraine, angina, or hypertension and ergotamine or methysergide for migraine may occasionally cause bilateral Raynaud's phenomenon. Administration of bleomycin, vinblastine, and cisplatin (e.g., for the treatment of germ cell cancer) has also been reported to precipitate this disorder in up to 44 percent of cases.

17. ENTRAPMENT NEUROPATHIES

A. Carpal Tunnel Syndrome   Acute carpal tunnel syndrome may follow a fracture of the distal radius, volar dislocation of the lunate, an acute suppurative or nonsuppurative flexor tenosynovitis, direct trauma to the palm, a carpal tunnel hematoma secondary to hemophilia or anticoagulation therapy, a midpalmar space abscess, septic arthritis of the wrist, a constricting palmar burn, and Lyme borreliosis. Pain may occur in the wrist, in the volar aspects of the thumb, index finger, and middle finger; and on the radial side of the ring finger. Paresthesias and hypesthesia affect the same digits. Hypesthesia is usually con-

fined to the volar aspect of the affected digits. Symptoms are usually worse at night, often waking the patient with pain and unpleasant paresthesias. Shaking or rubbing the hand and fingers or allowing them to hang over the side of the bed usually relieves symptom intensity and allows return to sleep. Phalen's and the reverse Phalen's sign are often positive, as is Tinel's sign at the wrist. Weakness of the abductor pollicis brevis may occur. The diagnosis can be confirmed by electrodiagnostic studies. Each cause of an acute carpal tunnel syndrome may require a specific surgical and/or medical therapy, as well as surgical decompression of the median nerve.

B. Ulnar Tunnel Syndrome (Guyon's Canal Entrapment of the Ulnar Nerve)   Pain occurs on the medial side of the hand and ring finger and in the little finger. It may be accompanied by paresthesias and hypesthesia of the same volar areas. Weakness and atrophy in the hand reflect motor involvement of the interossei, medial two lumbricals, and adductor pollicis muscles. If hypesthesia is localized to the volar aspect of the medial palm and digits and sensation on the dorsum of the ring and small fingers is normal, it is likely that nerve entrapment is in the region of Guyon's canal, since the dorsoulnar branch that innervates the dorsum of the ring and small fingers leaves the ulnar nerve proximal to Guyon's canal.

Isolated weakness of the intrinsic muscles indicates entrapment of the deep motor branch of the ulnar nerve at or distal to the hook of the hamate. Paresis and atrophy of the hypothenar and intrinsic muscles occur with more proximal entrapment in the canal. There may be local tenderness over the canal and a Tinel's sign at this site. Wrist flexion for 1 to 3 min may intensify symptoms, while results of the elbow flexion test are negative. An acute onset of symptoms may result from direct trauma with fracture of the hamate or pisiform or because of an ulnar artery aneurysm or occlusion.

C. Proximal Causes of Neuropathic Hand and Finger Pain   Cervical radiculopathy of C6 or C7 may cause radial hand and finger pain and hypesthesia. The palmar and dorsal aspects of the thumb and the index and middle fingers are involved. Spurling's maneuver, neck rotation, and/or coughing provoke neck, arm, and hand pain. Thoracic outlet compression of the brachial plexus may cause diffuse hand and forearm pain and weakness, or medial hand pain. The arm abduction external rotation test of Roos, the exaggerated military maneuver, and thumb pressure over the ipsilateral brachial plexus above the clavicle localize entrapment to the plexus. Arm and hand symptoms may become worse after arm and shoulder use, and the increased pain may persist for several days. C8 radiculopathy or compression of the medial cord of the brachial plexus at the thoracic outlet may cause medial arm, forearm, hand, and finger pain and paresthesias. Ulnar nerve compression at the elbow causes medial forearm, wrist, and hand pain and paresthesias. The elbow flexion test is positive, and a Tinel's sign is present at the cubital tunnel with ulnar nerve entrapment at the elbow. Hypesthesia of both the dorsum and palmar aspects of the ring and little fingers may be present. The pronator teres syndrome causes forearm pain and may mimic a carpal tunnel syndrome. However, nocturnal paresthesias and pain do not occur. Phalen's test is negative, and tenderness and Tinel's sign occur in the proximal medial forearm over the pronator teres muscle. Pain and paresthesias in the hand may be provoked by resisted forearm pronation with the elbow extended and by other forearm muscle stress tests.

D. Double-Crush Syndrome   A proximal lesion of the nerves giving rise to the median nerve may predispose that nerve to the carpal tunnel syndrome. A C6 or C7 radiculopathy, brachial plexus compression at the thoracic outlet, or median nerve compression in the region of the pronator teres may facilitate the development of the carpal tunnel syndrome and explain persistent symptoms after carpal tunnel surgery when the proximal site of compression is not treated. Similarly, a C8 radiculopathy, compression of the medial cord of the brachial plexus at the thoracic outlet, or a cubital tunnel syndrome at the elbow may predispose the ulnar nerve to symptomatic compression in the ulnar tunnel.

18. Reflex Sympathetic Dystrophy

This disorder may vary in severity. It may follow minor trauma to the hand, such as a sprain, dislocation, or fracture. It may also follow major wrist and hand injuries or surgery (e.g., major ligamentous disruption, carpal tunnel surgery, displaced or compound fractures, severe dislocations, or crush injuries). There may be a lag period of days or weeks between the injury and the onset of symptoms of RSD.

Severe aching, boring, stinging, or cutting pain that is out of proportion to the existing injury or the corrective surgical procedure occurs. This pain is refractory to most analgesics and is continuous. Severe skin hyperesthesia is associated, and touching the affected hand or fingers causes pain and unpleasant dysesthesias. The hand becomes swollen, warm, and erythematous. In some cases, erythema occurs only over the dorsum of the MP and DIP joints. Hyperhidrosis is often present during the first 2 weeks. Within 3 to 6 weeks the hand and fingers may become cool and pale.

The hand edema is initially pitting and may be decreased by hand elevation. Movement of the finger joints may be resisted because of pain. The extremity may be withdrawn from the examiner during the examination. The wrist is commonly held flexed, the MP joints hyperextended, and the fingers in varying degrees of flexion.

The involved limb may be held and supported by the other hand. This clinical picture may persist for 2 to 3 months unless treatment is begun. Hand and wrist radiographs may show spotty osteoporosis in 30 percent of cases during this stage of the disorder (stage 1), and technetium-99m bone scans may show heavy periarticular uptake over the affected joints. Stellate ganglion or regional nerve blocks can produce a temporary sympathectomy and relieve pain and hyperesthesia. A series of three to seven stellate ganglion blocks, each lasting 1 to 3 days, in conjunction with comprehensive hand physiotherapy to increase mobility and decrease edema, may lead to resolution of this disorder. RSD is more frequent in women (male/female ratio, 2.9 to 1), and its overall frequency is estimated as 0.05 to 5 percent of all trauma cases.

Causalgias due to trauma to a sensory nerve (minor causalgia) or to a major mixed nerve (major causalgia) are forms of RSD and are associated with persistent pain. This is usually burning in quality. Minor causalgia pain is restricted to the distribution of the injured sensory nerve, while the pain of major causalgia may radiate beyond the anatomic distribution of the injured nerve. Sympathetic block relieves causalgic pain and associated skin hyperesthesia and dysesthesia, edema, joint stiffness, and vasomotor skin changes.

19. MONONEURITIS MULTIPLEX

There is an abrupt onset of severe aching or sharp forearm and hand pain, paresthesias, and dysesthesias in the distribution of the median, ulnar, or radial nerves. Skin hyperesthesia or hypesthesia may be present distally. Within hours, motor weakness and further sensory loss may develop in the distribution of the involved peripheral nerve. Palpation of the affected nerve proximally or jarring or movement of the limb may provoke shooting pains and paresthesias that radiate into the hand and fingers. A similar mononeuritis may affect the same or another limb. This disorder usually results from acute ischemia of the involved nerve and is caused by vasculitis (e.g., polyarteritis nodosa, systemic lupus erythematosus, or rheumatoid arthritis), diabetes mellitus, and, rarely, by multiple sclerosis. The initial attack may be confined to a single peripheral nerve, and other attacks of mononeuritis may then follow or may be prevented by therapy. Muscle biopsy that includes nerve twigs in the distribution of the involved nerve may be of use in confirming the clinical diagnosis.

20. CUTANEOUS DISORDERS OF THE HAND

A. Dyshidrotic Eczematous Dermatitis   Slightly painful, small, tender, superficial, clear vesicles appear on the palms and digits without surrounding erythema. Hyperhidrosis may be associated. Persistence of the lesions may lead to scaling, palmar erythema, and painful fissures.

B. Palmoplantar Pustulosis

1. Pustulosis Palmaris et Plantaris   This disorder begins on the palms and soles, with 1 to 2 mm painful and/or pruritic pustules arising on erythematous plaques. The hand lesions first appear over the thenar eminence and then spread to the palm and dorsa of the fingers. The pustules may rupture or dry within 7 to 10 days, leaving a dark crust. These lesions may resolve in 3 weeks without recurrence or sequelae. In the absence of psoriatic lesions at other sites or characteristic psoriatic nail changes, this disorder is called acute pustulosis palmaris et plantaris. It may follow an acute respiratory infection (e.g., sore throat and fever).

2. Pustular Psoriasis of Barber   This disorder is clinically indistinguishable from pustulosis palmaris et plantaris except for the presence of psoriatic lesions at other sites or psoriatic nail changes (pitting, ridging, and onycholysis). Therapy with ultraviolet light may be effective in resolving this dermatitis.

C. Pustular Bacterid of Hands and Feet (Andrew's Disease)

Pustular lesions begin on the midpalm as vesicles that soon become purulent. There is involvement of the web spaces. Local pain and pruritus occur, and the pustules usually dry in situ. Results of cultures of the pustules are usually negative. Microscopic examination shows an intraepidermal pustule. This disorder is often associated with a remote focus of infection, and it frequently clears after effective therapy of that focus (e.g., dental, sinus, or tonsils). Some authorities dispute the role of a focus of infection in the pathogenesis of this disorder.

D. Acrodermatitis Continua

This disorder may begin on a single digit as intraepidermal vesicles and pustules. The site of the initial lesions is usually the distal phalanx surrounding the nail. The skin of the distal phalanx may become diffusely erythematous, fissured, and crusted. Tissue necrosis occurs, causing sloughing and denuded areas. The nails are loosened by underlying "lakes of pus." New pustules form in adjacent inflamed and normal skin. The disease may remain confined to one digit of one hand (dermatitis repens), or it may spread to other digits and may progress proximally. Involvement of other limbs may also occur.

Some cases may evolve into generalized pustular psoriasis. This disorder may be differentiated from pustular psoriasis of Barber and the pustular bacterid of Andrew by its tendency to form "lakes of pus" and large denuded or crusted areas adjacent to the nail margins and the nail bed. The other disorders are usually located on the palms. The presence of spongiform pustules of Kogof on biopsy may aid in establishing the diagnosis.

E. *Trichophyton rubrum* Dermatitis

This disorder may cause a scaling, pruritic dermatitis of the palms and fingers. Weeping, crusting, eczematous, painful palms and finger lesions occur. Small erosions and fissures may occur on the palms. Lesion scrapings examined by direct microscopy and culture will demonstrate fungal elements. Lesions clear with antifungal therapy.

F. *S. aureus* Cutaneous Infection

S. aureus may cause painful, tender, superficial furuncles or a carbuncle on the hand. A Gram stain and culture of pus will reveal the causative organism. The disorder may rarely be confused with cutaneous anthrax (malignant pustule), since the latter is usually painless, and the central pustule or ulcer is surrounded by massive edema.

G. Erysipeloid

This painful, tender, violaceous skin infection occurs at a site of trauma on the hands of workers handling raw fish, poultry, or meat products. The causative organism, *Erysipelothrix rhusiopathiae*, is a grampositive bacillus that is inoculated at the site of minor skin trauma on the hand. Burning pain occurs at the site of injury, and after 2 to 7 days a violaceous plaque appears. Low-grade fever and malaise may occur. The lesion has clearly outlined, raised borders. Arthritis may occur in an adjacent joint. This disorder responds to antibiotic therapy. Biopsy and culture of the lesion margin will allow isolation of the causative organism.

H. Osler's Nodes

These are painful, erythematous 0.5- to 1-cm macules with a slightly elevated, pinhead-size, firm center that occur on the distal volar pads of fingers and toes. They are often mildly painful and tender. Patients describe them as feeling like fingertip papercuts. They are evanescent and vanish within 1 or 2 days. Osler's nodes occur in patients with subacute or acute bacterial endocarditis. The diagnosis can be confirmed by blood culture and by visualization of valvular vegetations by two-dimensional echocardiography.

I. Splinter Hemorrhages

Splinter hemorrhages secondary to bacterial endocarditis may form as brown or black splinterlike lesions in the nail bed. There may be local pain and tenderness to nail bed pressure. These lesions become painless and nontender over a period of 2 to 3 days. Most splinter hemorrhages are painless and nontender.

J. Frostbite

Exposure of the hands and fingers to freezing cold air or to ice may cause burning pain and paresthesias of the fingertips. If exposure continues, the pain decreases, and the part becomes numb and insensitive.

Frostbite has been classified by the degree of severity of tissue injury present after rewarming. First-degree frostbite causes stinging discomfort, hyperemia, and skin edema. Portions of superficial skin may desquamate during the first week after exposure. Pain and paresthesias may occur in the fingers and hands after 3 to 13 days and may not be present in mild cases. Excessive sweating may begin after 2 to 3 weeks and may continue for months or years.

Second-degree frostbite causes finger and hand edema and the formation of vesicles and bullae that collapse into black eschars. Aching finger and hand pain develops after the third day, and hyperhidrosis occurs. After recovery, residual complaints may include cold sensitivity, pain, hyperhidrosis, paresthesias, hypesthesia, and coldness of the hands. Permanent tissue loss does not occur.

Third-degree injuries result in skin gangrene and loss of acral parts.

K. Drug-Related Photosensitivity　Some patients taking photosensitizing drugs, such as doxycycline, may develop severe redness, edema, and burning pain of their hands and face after several hours of sun exposure. Restriction of sunlight exposure, discontinuance of the offending drug, or both will lead to symptom resolution.

Thumb Pain

21. TRAPEZIOMETACARPAL JOINT AREA

A. Tendinitis　Pain occurs at the site of insertion of the abductor pollicis longus tendon at the base of the first metacarpal in the distal corner of the "snuffbox." There may be local tenderness and edema. Adduction of the thumb may intensify the pain. A local injection of lidocaine and a corticosteroid will often relieve the pain and may be of diagnostic value. De Quervain's disease may cause more proximal pain and tenderness between the radial styloid and base of the thumb.

B. Fractures

1. Bennett's Fracture　This injury occurs at the base of the first metacarpal, with local pain, swelling, and tenderness. A small fragment of the first metacarpal remains attached to the second metacarpal and trapezium, while the remainder of the metacarpal is dislocated radially and dorsally by the abductor pollicis longus tendon. Reduction of this fracture-dislocation of the trapeziometacarpal joint by manipulation and fixation of the joint with Kirschner pins will usually provide a satisfactory result.

2. Rolando's Fracture　Pain occurs at the carpometacarpal joint of the thumb, with swelling, ecchymoses, and tenderness. Radiographs reveal a T- or Y-shaped fracture of the metacarpal base. Severe comminution may occur, and posttraumatic arthritis may result.

C. Dislocation of the Trapeziometacarpal Joint　Pain, tenderness, and swelling occur over the distal "snuffbox." Plain radiography will demonstrate the dislocation. Disruption of the volar ligament or the dorsal joint capsule may result from a longitudinal force transmitted down the metacarpal shaft when the carpometacarpal joint is flexed. Surgical fixation may be required if closed reduction and immobilization do not lead to a stable joint.

22. MP JOINT OF THE THUMB

A. Volar Plate Injury　Volar plate disruption follows abrupt, forceful hyperextension of the MP joint. Pain, swelling, and tenderness occur over the volar aspect of the joint. A lateral radiograph will demonstrate dorsal dislocation of the MP joint. A complete dislocation, with the proximal phalanx dorsal and parallel to the metacarpal, requires a complete tear of the collateral ligaments. The metacarpal head may herniate in a volar direction between the flexor pollicis brevis and adductor pollicis muscles. Closed reduction may be successful, but instability requires surgical repair.

B. Collateral Ligament Injuries

1. Ulnar Collateral Ligament Injury　Pain, tenderness, ecchymoses, and marked swelling occur over the ulnar border of the metacarpophalangeal joint. A radially directed force produces 30° or more of instability relative to the unaffected thumb. A rotational supination deformity of the thumb may be present. The effects of radial stress on the MP joint should be checked in extension and at 30° of flexion with the metacarpal stabilized. If the stress test is equivocal, it should be repeated after a radial and median nerve block at the wrist.

Ulnar collateral ligament injuries of the thumb result from forced abduction of the joint. This disorder has been called "gamekeeper's thumb" or "skier's thumb." A frequent cause is skiing accidents in which the strap or grip of the ski pole causes forceful radial deviation of the thumb. Stress testing of the MP joint in full extension is important, since it will distinguish a partial from a complete tear of the ulnar collateral ligament. Angulation of the thumb can be measured with a goniometer placed on the surface of the thumb. Some authors believe that a 20° greater angulation on the affected side is significant. A positive stress test indicates the need for surgical repair of the ligament.

Violent abduction of the thumb may cause interposition of the adductor aponeurosis between the ulnar-avulsed collateral ligament and its insertion site on the proximal phalanx (Stener's lesion). This lesion requires surgical intervention, since the interposed aponeurosis will interfere with healing. Radiographs may also reveal intraarticular condylar or avulsion fractures and volar subluxation of the proximal phalanx. In severe cases, radial angulation of the thumb occurs in the rest position.

2. Radial Collateral Ligament Injury This injury may result after a sudden forced ulnar deviation of the thumb or after a fall in which the thumb is adducted. The ligament may tear at the insertion on the proximal phalanx or on the metacarpal with equal frequency. A pronation ulnar-deviated deformity may be present. Pain, tenderness, swelling, and ecchymoses occur over the radiodorsal joint region. Stress testing is done in extension and at 30° of flexion. Testing with full extension of the MP joint is preferred. An ulnar directed force is applied to the PIP joint with the MP joint stabilized. More than 30° of instability is significant. Complete tears require surgical repair.

23. PROXIMAL PHALANX

A. Neuropathy of the Digital Nerve Local pain, numbness, and paresthesias occur over the ulnar region of the thumb in frequent bowlers ("bowler's thumb"). A tender mass is usually palpable as the digital nerve is rolled back and forth under the palpating finger. Tinel's sign is present over the mass. Mild hypesthesia and impairment of two-point discrimination of the distal thumb may occur. Conservative measures are usually successful, but neurolysis and excision of the thickened epineurium may be required.

B. Fractures Fracture of the proximal phalanx of the thumb may be intraarticular or extraarticular. Local pain, swelling, tenderness, and ecchymoses occur over the proximal phalanx. Transverse fractures are frequently volarly angulated, resulting in deformity of the proximal thumb.

24. INTERPHALANGEAL JOINT AREA

A. Dislocation Dorsal dislocation of the distal phalanx of the thumb occurs with deformity (bayonet type). A compound injury, with protrusion of the proximal phalanx through the skin, may also occur. The dislocation is secondary to disruption of the volar plate of the interphalangeal joint by forced hyperextension.

B. Fracture of the Distal Phalanx Intraarticular fractures may cause interphalangeal joint swelling, pain, and tenderness. Extraarticular fractures cause distal thumb pain, swelling, and diffuse tenderness.

C. Extensor Tendon Disruption (Mallet Thumb) Rupture of the extensor tendon from its insertion on the distal phalanx of the thumb causes local pain, tenderness, swelling, and ecchymoses over the dorsal aspect of the distal phalanx and loss of interphalangeal joint extension. The resultant "drop" or "mallet" thumb will usually be corrected by 6 weeks of extension splinting of the acute injury.

25. BILATERAL ACUTE WRIST, HAND, AND FINGER PAIN

The causes are listed in Table 41-1.

Table 41-1
BILATERAL ACUTE WRIST, HAND, AND FINGER PAIN

Gonococcal tenosynovitis
De Quervain's disease
Acute carpal tunnel syndrome
Kienbock's disease
Polyarthritis due to:
  Hepatitis B
  Rubella
  Rubella immunization
  Acute rheumatoid arthritis
  Systemic lupus erythematosus
  Acute rheumatic fever
  Acute traumatic arthritis (hands)
  Arthritis-dermatitis syndrome due to *N. gonorrhoeae*
  Yersiniosis
  Gout
  Inflammatory bowel disease
  Psoriasis
  Calcium pyrophosphate dihydrate deposition disease
Raynaud's phenomenon due to drugs or without underlying disease
Proximal entrapment syndromes
  Thoracic outlet syndrome
  Cubital tunnel syndrome
Reflex sympathetic dystrophy
Dyshidrotic eczematous dermatitis
Palmoplantar pustulosis
Pustular bacterid of Andrew
Acrodermatitis continua
Osler's nodes
Splinter hemorrhages
Frostbite
Photosensitivity due to drugs

WRIST, HAND, AND FINGER PAIN REFERENCES

Adhesive Capsulitis

Hanson EC, Wood VE, Thiel AE, et al: Adhesive capsulitis of the wrist: Diagnosis and treatment. *Clin Orthop* 234:51–55, 1988.

Maloney MD, Sauser DD, Hanson EC, et al: Adhesive capsulitis of the wrist: Arthrographic diagnosis. *Radiology* 167:187–190, 1988.

Anomolous Muscle

Patel MR, Desai SS, Bassini-Lipson L, et al: Painful extensor digitorum brevis manus muscle. *J Hand Surg (Am)* 14A:674–678, 1989.

Arthritis — General

Ferlic DC: Inflammatory and rheumatoid arthritis, in Lichtman DM (ed): *The Wrist and Its Disorders*. Philadelphia, Saunders, 1988, pp 344–364.

Hooper G: Other arthritic conditions, in Lamb DW, Hooper G, Kuczynski K (eds): *The Practice of Hand Surgery*, 2d ed. Oxford, Blackwell Scientific, 1989, pp 591–595.

Arthritis — Leprosy

Markusse HM, Smelt AHM, Teepe RGC: Unusual arthritis: Be on the alert for leprosy. *Clin Rheumatol* 8:266–268, 1989.

Arthritis — Mycobacterial

Hoppmann RA, Patrone NA, Rumley R, et al: Tuberculous arthritis presenting as tophaceous gout. *J Rheumatol* 16:700–702, 1989.

Jones MW, Wahid IA, Matthews JP: Septic arthritis of the hand due to *Mycobacterium marinum*. *J Hand Surg (Br)* 13-B:333–334, 1988.

Valdazo J-P, Perez-Ruiz F, Albarracin A, et al: Tuberculous arthritis: Report of a case with multiple joint involvement and periarticular tuberculous abscesses. *J Rheumatol* 17:399–401, 1990.

Wendt JR, Lamm RC, Altman DI, et al: An unusually aggressive *Mycobacterium marinum* hand infection. *J Hand Surg (Am)* 11A:753–755, 1986.

Arthritis — Osteoarthritis

Melone CP Jr, Beavers B, Isani A: The basal joint pain syndrome. *Clin Orthop* 220:58–67, 1987.

Pellegrini VD Jr, Burton RI: Osteoarthritis of the proximal interphalangeal joint of the hand: Arthroplasty or fusion? *J Hand Surg (Am)* 15A:194–209, 1990.

Rogers WD, Watson HK: Degenerative arthritis at the triscaphe joint. *J Hand Surg (Am)* 15A:232–235, 1990.

Watson HK, Ryu J: Degenerative disorders of the carpus. *Orthop Clin North Am* 15:337–353, 1984.

Williams WV, Cope R, Gaunt WD, et al: Metacarpophalangeal arthropathy associated with manual labor (Missouri metacarpal syndrome): Clinical, radiographic, and pathologic characteristics of an unusual degenerative process. *Arthritis Rheum* 30:1362–1371, 1987.

Arthritis — Psoriatic

Trail IA, Stanley JK: The hand in psoriasis. *J Hand Surg (Br)* 15-B: 79–83, 1990.

Arthritis — Rheumatoid

Altissimi M, Ciaffoloni E: Surgical treatment of the rheumatoid hand. *Clin Exp Rheumatol* 7(S3):145–148, 1989.

Arnett FC, Edworthy SM, Bloch DA, et al: The American Rheumatism Association 1987 revised criteria for the classification of rheumatoid arthritis. *Arthritis Rheum* 31:315–324, 1988.

Boumpas DT, Wheby MS, Jaffe ES, et al: Synovitis in angioimmunoblastic lymphadenopathy with dysproteinemia simulating rheumatoid arthritis. *Arthritis Rheum* 33:578–582, 1990.

Chalmers TM, Souter WA, Dunkerly DR: Rheumatoid arthritis, in Lamb DW, Hooper G, Kuczynski K (eds): *The Practice of Hand Surgery*, 2d ed. Oxford, Blackwell Scientific, 1989, pp 531–590.

Ellstein JL, Strickland JW: Rheumatoid disorders of the hand and wrist, in Dee R, Mango E, Hurst LC (eds): *Principles of Orthopaedic Practice*. New York, McGraw-Hill, 1989, vol 1, pp 646–665.

Fornage BD: Soft-tissue changes in the hand in rheumatoid arthritis: Evaluation with US. *Radiology* 173:735–737, 1989.

Holbrook JL, Bennett JB: Arthritis of the hand and wrist: Management options for some common arthritic conditions. *Postgrad Med* 87:255–256, 259, 262, 265–266, 271–272, 1990.

Kaye JJ, Fuchs HA, Moseley JW, et al: Problems with the Steinbrocker staging system for radiographic assessment of the rheumatoid hand and wrist. *Invest Radiol* 25:536–544, 1990.

Ngo C, Yaghmai I: The value of immersion hand radiography in soft tissue changes of musculoskeletal disorders. *Skeletal Radiol* 17:259–263, 1988.

Renner WR, Weinstein AS: Early changes of rheumatoid arthritis in the hand and wrist. *Radiol Clin North Am* 26:1185–1193, 1988.

Schmerling RH, Parker JA, Johns WD, et al: Measurement of joint inflammation in rheumatoid arthritis with indium-111 chloride. *Ann Rheum Dis* 49:88–92, 1990.

Stanley D, Norris H: The pathogenesis and treatment of rheumatoid wrist and hand deformities. *Br J Hosp Med* 39:156–160, 1988.

Arthritis — Septic

Gerardi JA, Mack GR, Lutz RB: Acute carpal tunnel syndrome secondary to septic arthritis of the wrist. *J Am Osteopath Assoc* 89:933–934, 1989.

Leslie BM, Harris JM, Driscoll D: Septic arthritis of the shoulder in adults. *J Bone Joint Surg (Am)* 71-A:1516–1522, 1989.

Arthritis — Single Joint

Blocka KLN, Sibley JT: Undiagnosed chronic monarthritis: Clinical and evolutionary profile. *Arthritis Rheum* 30:1357–1361, 1987.

Carpal Tunnel Syndrome

Bloem JJ, Pradjarahardja MCL, Vuursteen PJ: The post-carpal tunnel syndrome: Causes and prevention. *Neth J Surg* 38:52–55, 1986.

Gelberman RH, Rydevik BL, Pess GM, et al: Carpal tunnel syndrome: A scientific basis for clinical care. *Orthop Clin North Am* 19:115–124, 1988.

Halperin JJ, Volkman DJ, Luft BJ, et al: Carpal tunnel syndrome in Lyme borreliosis. *Muscle Nerve* 12:397–400, 1989.

Nkele C: Acute carpal tunnel syndrome resulting from haemorrhage into the carpal tunnel in a patient on warfarin. *J Hand Surg (Br)* 11-B:455–456, 1986.

Nygaard IE, Saltzman CL, Whitehouse MB, et al: Hand problems in pregnancy. *Am Fam Physician* 39:123–126, 1989.

Osterman AL: The double crush syndrome. *Orthop Clin North Am* 19:147–155, 1988.

Urbaniak JR, Roth JH: Office diagnosis and treatment of hand pain. *Orthop Clin North Am* 13:477–495, 1982.

Carpometacarpal Disorders

Gunther SF: The carpometacarpal joints. *Orthop Clin North Am* 15:259–277, 1984.

Mueller JJ: Carpometacarpal dislocations: Report of five cases and review of the literature. *J Hand Surg (Am)* 11A:184–188, 1986.

O'Brien ET: Acute fratures and dislocations of the carpus. *Orthop Clin North Am* 15:237–258, 1984.

Watson HK, Brenner LH: Degenerative disorders of the carpus, in Lichtman DM (ed): *The Wrist and Its Disorders*. Philadelphia, Saunders, 1988, pp 286–292.

Congenital Defects

Fagg PS: Wrist pain in the Madelung's deformity of dyschondrosteosis. *J Hand Surg (Br)* 13-B:11–15, 1988.

De Quervain's Disease
Schned ES: DeQuervain tenosynovitis in pregnant and postpartum women. *Obstet Gynecol* 68:411–414, 1986.

Distal Radioulnar Joint Disease
Palmer AK: The distal radioulnar joint. *Orthop Clin North Am* 15:321–335, 1984.

Foreign Body Granuloma of the Wrist
Goldstein SA, Imbriglia JE: Erosion of the triquetrum and pisiform bones caused by a foreign body granuloma. *J Hand Surg (Am)* 11A:899–901, 1986.

Fracture/Dislocation of the Hand
Steel WM, Belsky MR, Millender LH, et al: Fractures and joint injuries, in Lamb DW, Hooper G, Kuczynski K (eds): *The Practice of Hand Surgery*, 2d ed. Oxford, Blackwell Scientific, 1989, pp 228–290.

Fracture/Dislocation of the Wrist
Melene CP Jr: Unstable fractures of the distal radius, in Lichtman DM (ed): *The Wrist and Its Disorders*. Philadelphia, Saunders, 1988, pp 160–177.
O'Brien ET: Acute fractures and dislocations of the carpus, in Lichtman DM (ed): *The Wrist and Its Disorders*. Philadelphia, Saunders, 1988, pp 129–159.

Hand Pain Review
Hooper G: Miscellaneous conditions, in Lamb DW, Hooper G, Kuczynski K (eds): *The Practice of Hand Surgery*, 2d ed. Oxford, Blackwell Scientific, 1989, pp 649–656.
Mayer VA, McCue FC: Rehabilitation and protection of the hand and wrist, in Nicholas JA Hershman EB, Posner MA (eds): *The Upper Extremity in Sports Medicine*. St. Louis, Mosby, 1990, pp 619–658.
Posner MA: Hand injuries, in Nicholas JA, Hershman EB, Posner MA (eds): *The Upper Extremity in Sports Medicine*. St. Louis, Mosby, 1990, pp 495–594.
Schneider LH: Tendon injuries of the hand, in Nicholas JA, Hershman EB, Posner MA (eds): *The Upper Extremity in Sports Medicine*. St. Louis, Mosby, 1990, pp 595–617.

Infections of the Hand
Glickel SZ: Hand infections in patients with acquired immunodeficiency syndrome. *J Hand Surg (Am)* 13A:770–775, 1988.
Hooper G, Pollen AG: Infections of the hand, in Lamb DW, Hooper G, Kuczynski K (eds): *The Practice of Hand Surgery*, 2d ed. Oxford, Blackwell Scientific, 1989, pp 599–613.
Hurst LC, Nathan J: Infections in the upper extremity, in Dee R, Mango E, Hurst LC (eds): *Principles of Orthopaedic Practice*. New York, McGraw-Hill, 1989, vol 1, pp 741–751.
Siegel DB, Gelberman RH: Infections of the hand. *Orthop Clin North Am* 19:779–789, 1988.

Injuries of the Hand
Isani A: Prevention and treatment of ligamentous sports injuries to the hand. *Sports Med* 9:48–61. 1990.

Injuries of the Wrist
Louis DS, Hankin FM: Arthrodesis of the wrist: Past and present (editorial). *J Hand Surg (Am)* 11A(6):787–789, 1986.
Pin PG, Semenkovich JW, Young VL, et al: Role of radionuclide imaging in the evaluation of wrist pain. *J Hand Surg (Am)* 13A:810–814, 1988.

Kienböck's Disease
Alexander AH, Lichtman DM: Kienböck's disease, in Lichtman DM (ed): *The Wrist and Its Disorders*. Philadelphia, Saunders, 1988, pp 329–343.
Gelberman RH, Szabo RM: Kienböck's disease. *Orthop Clin North Am* 15:355–367, 1984.
Hasselgren G, Jerre R, Ullman M, et al: Liquid silicone as a lunate prosthesis. *J Hand Surg (Br)* 15-B:35–39, 1990.
Jackson MD, Barry DT, Geiringer SR: Magnetic resonance imaging of avascular necrosis of the lunate. *Arch Phys Med Rehabil* 71:510–513, 1990.

Margles SW: Avascular necrosis in the upper extremity, in Dee R, Mango E, Hurst LC (eds): *Principles of Orthopaedic Practice*. New York, McGraw-Hill, 1989, vol 1, pp 781–791.
Nakamura R, Horii E, Imaeda T: Excessive radial shortening in Kienböck's disease. *J Hand Surg (Br)* 15-B:46–48, 1990.
Nakamura R, Imaeda T, Miura T: Radial shortening for Kienböck's disease: Factors affecting the operative result. *J Hand Surg (Br)* 15-B:40–45, 1990.
Sowa DT, Holder LE, Patt PG, et al: Application of magnetic resonance imaging to ischemic necrosis of the lunate. *J Hand Surg (Am)* 14A:1008–1016, 1989.
Viergas SF, Amparo E: Magnetic resonance imaging in the assessment of revascularization in Kienböck's disease: A preliminary report. *Orthop Rev* 18:1285–1288, 1989.

Ligament Injuries—Hand and Wrist
Sampson S, Akelman E, Garroway RJ, et al: Traumatic injury to the upper extremity, in Dee R, Mango E, Hurst LC (eds): *Principles of Orthopaedic Practice*. New York, McGraw-Hill, 1989, vol 1, pp 536–593.

Neuropathies
Chalmers J: Nerve compression syndromes, in Lamb DW, Hooper G, Kuczynski K (eds): *The Practice of Hand Surgery*, 2d ed. Oxford, Blackwell Scientific, 1989, pp 427–447.
Hurst LC, Badalamente MA, Paul S, et al: Peripheral nerve injuries and entrapments, in Dee R, Mango E, Hurst LC (eds): *Principles of Orthopaedic Practice*. New York, McGraw-Hill, 1989, vol 1, pp 666–689.
Massey EW: Hand weakness in elderly patients. *Postgrad Med* 85:59–60, 63–65, 70, 1989.
McCarroll HR Jr: Nerve injuries associated with wrist trauma. *Orthop Clin North Am* 15:279–287, 1984.
————: Nerve injuries associated with wrist trauma, in Lichtman DM (ed): *The Wrist and Its Disorders*. Philadelphia, Saunders, 1988, pp 212–219.

Paget's Disease
Trumble TE, Wu RK, Ruwe PA: Paget's disease in the hand: Correlation of magnetic resonance imaging with histology. *J Hand Surg (Am)* 15A:504–506, 1990.

Reflex Sympathetic Dystrophy—Shoulder-Hand Syndrome
Buell TR, Karlin JM, Scurran BL, et al: Reflex sympathetic dystrophy syndrome: Review with podiatric case studies. *J Am Podiatr Med Assoc* 77:533–538, 1987.
Escobar PL: Reflex sympathetic dystrophy. *Orthop Rev* 15:646–651, 1986.
Markoff M, Farole A: Reflex sympathetic dystrophy syndrome: Case report with a review of the literature. *Oral Surg Oral Med Oral Pathol* 61:23–28, 1986.
Roig-Escofet D, Rodriguez-Moreno J, Martin JMR: Concept and limits of the reflex sympathetic dystrophy. *Clin Rheumatol* 8(suppl 2):104–108, 1989.
Shih W-J, Pulmano C: Hand and forearm Tc-99m HMDP bone image findings of reflex sympathetic dystrophy similar to those of radiopharmaceutical arterial administration in the arm. *Clin Nucl Med* 14:298–300, 1989.

Scaphoid Fracture
DaCruz DJ, Bodiwala GG, Finlay DBL: The suspected fracture of the scaphoid: A rational approach to diagnosis. *Injury* 19:149–152, 1988.
Gumucio CA, Fernando B, Young VL, et al: Management of scaphoid fractures: A review and update. *South Med J* 82:1377–1388, 1989.
Mack GR, Lichtman DM: Scaphoid nonunion, in Lichtman DM (ed): *The Wrist and Its Disorders*. Philadelphia, Saunders, 1988, pp 293–328.
Mehta M, Brautigan MW: Fracture of the carpal navicular: Efficacy of clinical findings and improved diagnosis with six-view radiography. *Ann Emerg Med* 19:255–257, 1990.
Sasaki Y, Sugioka Y: The pronator quadratus sign: Its classification

and diagnostic usefulness for injury and inflammation of the wrist. *J Hand Surg (Br)* 14-B:80–83, 1989.

Skin/Hand Disorders

Burge SM, Ryan TJ: Acute palmoplantar pustulosis. *Br J Dermatol* 113:77–83, 1985.

Epstein E: Hand dermatitis: Practical management and current concepts. *J Am Acad Dermatol* 10:395–424, 1984.

Ferguson CD, Taybos GM: Diagnosis and treatment of pemphigus. *Quintessence Int* 16:473–476, 1985.

Ferlic DC: Pyoderma gangrenosum presenting as an acute suppurative hand infection: A case report. *J Hand Surg (Am)* 8:573–575, 1983.

Goette DK, Morgan AM, Fox BJ, et al: Treatment of palmoplantar pustulosis with intralesional triamcinolone injections. *Arch Dermatol* 120:319–323, 1984.

Hoffmann TJ, Kettler A, Bruce S: Acute acral pustulosis. *Br J Dermatol* 120:107–111, 1989.

Milgraum SS, Friedman DJ, Ellis CN, et al: Pemphigus vulgaris masquerading as dyshidrotic eczema. *Cutis* 35:445–446, 1985.

Rosen MS, Myers AR, Dickey B: Meningococcemia presenting as septic arthritis, pericarditis, and tenosynovitis. *Arth Rheum* 28:576–578, 1985.

Rustin MHA, Robinson TWE, Dowd PM: Toxic pustuloderma: A self-limiting eruption. *Br J Dermatol* 123:119–124, 1990.

Stiff Hand — Posttraumatic

Morey KR, Watson AH: Team approach to treatment of the posttraumatic stiff hand: A case report. *Phys Ther* 66:225–228, 1986.

Tenosynovitis — Acute

Abrahamsson S-O: Gouty tenosynovitis simulating an infection: A case report. *Acta Orthop Scand* 58:282–283, 1987.

Jeffrey RB Jr, Laing FC, Schechter WP, et al: Acute suppurative tenosynovitis of the hand: Diagnosis with US. *Radiology* 162:741–742, 1987.

Zubowicz VN, Raine TR: Sterile flexor tenosynovitis of the hand: A report of three cases. *J Hand Surg (Am)* 11A:140–142, 1986.

Tenosynovitis — Chronic

Lacy JN, Viegas SF, Calhoun J, et al: *Mycobacterium marinum* flexor tenosynovitis. *Clin Orthop* 238:288–293, 1989.

Merle M, Bour C, Foucher G, et al: Sarcoid tenosynovitis in the hand: A case report and literature review. *J Hand Surg (Br)* 11-B:281–286, 1986.

Otto N, Wehbe MA: Steroid injections for tenosynovitis in the hand. *Orthop Rev* 15:290–293, 1986.

Petrini B, Svartengren G, Hoffner SE, et al: Tenosynovitis of the hand caused by *Mycobacterium terrae*. *Eur J Clin Microbiol Infect Dis* 8:722–724, 1989.

Stambaugh JL, Bora FW Jr, DuShuttle RP: Sarcoid flexor tenosynovitis of the finger: A case report. *J Hand Surg (Am)* 11A:436–438, 1986.

Stern PJ: Tendinitis, overuse syndromes, and tendon injuries. *Hand Clin* 6:467–476, 1990.

Stern PJ, Gula DC: *Mycobacterium chelonei* tenosynovitis of the hand: A case report. *J Hand Surg (Am)* 11A:596–599, 1986.

Thorpe AP: Results of surgery for trigger finger. *J Hand Surg (Br)* 13-B:199–201, 1988.

Zachary LS, Clark GL Jr, Kleinert JM, et al: *Mycobacterium chelonei* tenosynovitis. *Am. Plast Surg* 20:360–362, 1988.

Thumb Pain

Gunther SF: The carpometacarpal joint of the thumb: Practical considerations, in Lichtman DM (ed): *The Wrist and Its Disorders.* Philadelphia, Saunders, 1988, pp 187–198.

Tumors — Wrist/Hand — Benign

Bowen CVA, Dzus AK, Hardy DA: Osteoid osteomata of the distal phalanx. *J Hand Surg (Br)* 12-B:387–390, 1987.

DelSignore JL, Torre BA, Miller RJ: Extraskeletal chondroma of the hand: Case report and review of the literature. *Clin Orthop* 254:147–152, 1990.

Mahoney JL: Soft tissue chondromas in the hand. *J Hand Surg (Am)* 12A:317–320, 1987.

Marck KW, Dhar BK, Spauwen PHM: A cryptic cause of monarthritis in the hand: The juxta-articular osteoid osteoma. *J Hand Surg (Br)* 13-B:221–223, 1988.

Sapra S, Prokopetz R, Murray AH: Giant cell tumor of tendon sheath. *Int J Dermatol* 28:587–590, 1989.

Schiffman KL, Harris DCM, Hooper G: Hemangiopericytoma of the median nerve. *J Hand Surg (Am)* 13A:75–78, 1988.

Schütte HE, van der Heul RO: Pseudomalignant, nonneoplastic osseous soft-tissue tumors of the hand and foot. *Radiology* 176:149–153, 1990.

Young L, Bartell T, Logan SE: Ganglions of the hand and wrist. *South Med J* 81:751–760, 1988.

Tumors — Wrist/Hand — General

Bogumill GP: Tumors of the wrist, in Lichtman DM (ed): *The Wrist and Its Disorders.* Philadelphia, Saunders, 1988, pp 373–384.

Chalmers J: Tumours, in Lamb DW, Hooper G, Kuczynski K (eds): *The Practice of Hand Surgery*, 2d ed. Oxford, Blackwell Scientific, 1989, pp 614–634.

Dick H: Tumors of the hand and wrist, in Dee R, Mango E, Hurst LC (eds): *Principles of Orthopaedic Practice.* New York, McGraw-Hill, 1989, vol 1, pp 767–774.

Tumors — Wrist/Hand — Malignant

Cash SL, Habermann ET: Chondrosarcoma of the small bones of the hand: Case report and review of the literature. *Orthop Rev* 17:365–369, 1988.

van der Walt JD, Ryan JF: Parosteal osteogenic sarcoma of the hand. *Histopathology* 16:75–78, 1990.

Zamboni AC, Zamboni WA, Ross DS: Malignant eccrine spiradenoma of the hand. *J Surg Oncol* 43:131–133, 1990.

Vascular Disorders — Hand

Saddler JM, Crosse MM: Ischaemic pain in Buerger's disease. *Anaesthesia* 43:305–306, 1988.

Takeuchi T, Futatsuka M, Imanishi H, et al: Pathological changes observed in the finger biopsy of patients with vibration-induced white finger. *Scand J Work Environ Health* 12:280–283, 1986.

Wigley FM: The differential diagnosis of Raynaud's phenomenon. *Hosp Pract* 261:63–84, 1991.

Wrist Instability

Alexander CE, Lichtman DM: Triquetrolunate and midcarpal instability, in Lichtman DM (ed): *The Wrist and Its Disorders.* Philadelphia, Saunders, 1988, pp 274–292.

———: Ulnar carpal instabilities. *Orthop Clin North Am* 15:307–320, 1984.

Blatt G: Scapholunate instability, in Lichtman DM (ed): *The Wrist and Its Disorders.* Philadelphia, Saunders, 1988, pp 251–273.

Brown DE, Lichtman DM: Physical examination of the wrist, in Lichtman DM (ed): *The Wrist and Its Disorders.* Philadelphia, Saunders, 1988, pp 74–81.

Destouet JM, Gilula LA, Reinus WR: Roentgenographic diagnosis of wrist pain and instability, in Lichtman DM (ed): *The Wrist and Its Disorders.* Philadelphia, Saunders, 1988, pp 82–95.

Gellman H, Schwartz SD, Botte MJ, et al: Late treatment of a dorsal transscaphoid, transtriquetral perilunate wrist dislocation with avascular changes of the lunate. *Clin Orthop* 237:196–203, 1988.

Kleinman WB, Carroll C IV: Scapho-trapezio-trapezoid arthrodesis for treatment of chronic static and dynamic scapho-lunate instability: A 10-year perspective on pitfalls and complications. *J Hand Surg (Am)* 15A:408–414, 1990.

Lichtman DM, Martin RA: Introduction to the carpal instabilities, in Lichtman DM (ed): *The Wrist and Its Disorders.* Philadelphia, Saunders, 1988, pp 244–250.

Mayfield JK: Pathogenesis of wrist ligament instability, in Lichtman DM (ed): *The Wrist and Its Disorders.* Philadelphia, Saunders, 1988, pp 53–73.

————: Wrist ligamentous anatomy and pathogenesis of carpal instability. *Orthop Clin North Am* 15:209–216, 1984.

Rogers WD, Watson HK: Radial styloid impingement after triscaphe arthrodesis. *J Hand Surg (Am)* 14A:297–301, 1989.

Sarrafian SK, Breihan JH: Palmar dislocation of scaphoid and lunate as a unit. *J Hand Surg (Am)* 15A:134–139, 1990.

Wrist Pain — Review

Beckenbaugh RD: Accurate evaluation and management of the painful wrist following injury: An approach to carpal instability. *Orthop Clin North Am* 15:289–306, 1984.

Bogumill GP: Anatomy of the wrist, in Lichtman DM (ed): *The Wrist and Its Disorders*. Philadelphia, Saunders, 1988, pp 14–26.

Braun RM: The trapeziometacarpal joint: Basic principles of surgical treatment, in Lichtman DM (ed): *The Wrist and Its Disorders*. Philadelphia, Saunders, 1988, pp 178–186.

Brown DE, Lichtman DM: The evaluation of chronic wrist pain. *Orthop Clin North Am* 15:183–192, 1984.

Gunther SF: The medial four carpometacarpal joints, in Lichtman DM (ed): *The Wrist and Its Disorders*. Philadelphia, Saunders, 1988, pp 199–211.

Jennings JF, Peimer CA: Ligamentous injuries of the wrist in athletes, in Nicholas JA, Hershman EB, Posner MA (eds): *The Upper Extremity in Sports Medicine*. St. Louis, Mosby, 1990, pp 457–482.

Palmer AK: The distal radioulnar joint, in Lichtman DM (ed): *The Wrist and Its Disorders*. Philadelphia, Saunders, 1988, pp 220–231.

Wilgis EFS, Yates AY Jr: Wrist pain, in Nicholas JA, Hershman EB, Posner MA (eds): *The Upper Extremity in Sports Medicine*. St. Louis, Mosby, 1990, pp 483–494.

PART NINE

Acute Leg and Foot Pain

CHAPTER

42

Acute Unilateral Upper and Lower Leg Pain

☐ **DIAGNOSTIC LIST**

Anterior and anteromedial leg pain
1. Femoral neuropathy (with or without iliacus syndrome)
2. Radiculopathy of L2, L3, or L4 from disc or facet joint disease
3. Lumbar plexopathy (L2–L4)

Posterior and/or posterolateral leg pain
4. Sacral plexopathy (L5–S1)
5. Panplexopathy (L2–S1)
6. Acute sciatic pain
   A. Acute lateral disc herniation
   B. Acute epidural abscess and cauda equina syndrome
   C. Acute epidural hematoma and cauda equina syndrome
   D. Acute cauda equina syndrome due to midline disc herniation

   E. Conus medullaris syndrome due to spinal cord infarction

Lateral leg pain
7. Trochanteric bursitis
8. Meralgia paresthetica

Diffuse or generalized leg pain
9. Myalgic pain
10. Iliofemoral thrombophlebitis
11. Iliofemoral arterial embolism or thrombosis
12. Arthritis in two or more lower extremity joints
13. Sacroiliitis and pseudosciatica
14. Genital herpes

☐ **SUMMARY**

Femoral neuropathy may cause severe aching or pressurelike pain in the anterior and anteromedial thigh and lower leg. This is often associated with weakness of hip flexion and knee extension, and with numbness and tingling of the distal two-thirds of the anterior thigh and lower leg.

A large hematoma in an iliacus muscle may cause an *iliacus syndrome* characterized by severe groin pain and anterior thigh and lower leg pain associated with pain-induced flexion, ab-

duction, and external rotation of the thigh on the hip. Femoral neuropathy related to muscle hemorrhage usually occurs in patients with hemophilia, leukemia, and disseminated intravascular coagulation, and in those on anticoagulants. Vigorous exercise, with sudden flexion or extension of the thigh on the hip, may also precipitate such bleeding. Other possible causes of acute femoral neuropathy include a bleeding aortic aneurysm, and a psoas or appendiceal abscess.

Acute intervertebral disc herniation, causing an *L2, L3, or L4 pressure-related radiculopathy*, can simulate a femoral neuropathy. Patients with this condition usually have low back or buttock pain and tenderness, in addition to anterior thigh and leg pain, and weakness of the hip and knee. A computed tomography (CT) scan will identify a muscle hematoma, an iliac or aortic aneurysm, an abscess, or a herniated disc fragment.

Lumbar plexopathy may cause anteromedial thigh and leg pain, hip and knee weakness, and hypesthesia of the thigh. A CT scan of the pelvis will reveal a hematoma, an abscess, or an aneurysm. In the absence of a pelvic mass lesion on CT, acute inflammatory and vasculitic syndromes involving the lumbar plexus should be considered. Electromyographic evidence of fibrillations in the adductor muscles of the thigh, with absence of fibrillations in the paraspinal muscles, supports a diagnosis of plexopathy. Adductor muscle degeneration requires involvement of more than the femoral nerve, while paraspinal muscle fibrillations are usually seen in patients with radiculopathy.

Patients with unilateral *sacral plexopathy* complain of posterior and posterolateral thigh and leg pain, as well as unilateral buttock and lumbosacral pain. Numbness and tingling paresthesias may occur in the same areas, and may affect the perineum and genitalia as well. Weakness of ankle dorsiflexion and ventral flexion may also occur. Acute involvement of the sacral plexus may be associated with rupture of an aortic or iliac artery aneurysm, trauma, or anticoagulant-related retroperitoneal bleeding. Bleeding associated with these lesions can be detected with a pelvic CT scan. Patients with negative CT scans may have inflammatory or vasculitic involvement of the plexus. *Panplexopathy* may be diagnosed when patients manifest both lumbar (upper) and sacral (lower) plexopathy-associated symptoms and signs.

Sciatic pain with low back pain may begin abruptly after *lateral or central disc herniation* involving the lower two lumbar disc spaces. Central herniation may be associated with a saddle-type hypesthesia and with urinary and fecal incontinence, in addition to sciatic pain. Dejerine's sign and the straight leg raising test are usually positive. A contrast-enhanced CT scan or magnetic resonance imaging (MRI) will identify the herniated disc material. Midline spinal ache and tenderness associated with radiating sciatic pain, chills, rigors, sweats, and fever suggest the possibility of an *acute epidural abscess*. Incontinence of urine and stool may occur. Sensory loss and muscle weakness may develop in the painful area. A contrast-enhanced CT scan or MRI will identify an epidural collection of pus.

Similar complaints to those described for an epidural abscess, but without associated fever, chills, or sweats, suggest the development of an *acute epidural hematoma*. This disorder most commonly occurs in patients who have severe liver disease or are taking anticoagulants. A CT scan or MRI will identify the hematoma.

Leg and low back pain may occur suddenly when there is an *infarction of the conus medullaris*. Mild leg weakness, saddle and thigh hypesthesia, and urinary and fecal incontinence rapidly develop. A CT scan is usually required to eliminate

the possibility of a herniated disc, epidural abscess, or hematoma. Aortic surgery, the use of an intraaortic balloon, smoking, and vascular disease are risk factors that have been associated with conus infarction. Transient prodromal attacks may precede the onset of irreversible symptoms.

Trochanteric bursitis causes lateral hip and thigh pain that may radiate as far as the ankle. This pain is not associated with paresthesias, anesthesia, or limb paresis. Walking, hip abduction, and lying on the affected side intensify the pain. Local injection of 3 ml of lidocaine and methylprednisolone into the painful bursa relieves both local and radiating pain, and confirms the diagnosis. Pressure of a herniated disc, or a subluxated or enlarged facet joint, on the L5 root may cause lateral and posterolateral thigh pain and lower leg pain, paresthesias, and weakness of ankle dorsiflexion. An S1 radiculopathy may cause weakness of plantar flexion and foot eversion. The diagnosis can be confirmed by a contrast-enhanced CT scan or MRI. Pain in the lateral thigh, associated with a circumscribed patch of hypesthesia and a surrounding halo of hyperesthesia, is usually caused by neuropathy of the lateral femoral cutaneous nerve (e.g., *meralgia paresthetica*). Pain from this disorder may sometimes extend into the lateral calf region. *Myalgic pain* is intensified by limb movement, as in walking or climbing stairs, and is not associated with neurologic symptoms or signs. Localized muscle tenderness may or may not be present.

Iliofemoral thrombophlebitis causes a triad of cyanosis of the skin of the leg, generalized leg pain, and swelling. Pedal venous distension and loss or diminution of peripheral arterial pulses may occur. Venous collaterals may develop on the lower abdominal wall. Fever, chills, and nausea may occur. The diagnosis can be confirmed by the use of Doppler ultrasonography, real-time sonography, or impedance plethysmography. In case of doubt, contrast venography can be done.

Iliac or femoral artery emboli or thrombi can cause severe generalized pain in one limb, associated with skin pallor and coldness. Usually all leg pulses are diminished or absent; a line of demarcation may be present. Skin hypesthesia or anesthesia and limb paresis follow the onset of pain. Arteriography will demonstrate a block of the common iliac, external iliac, or femoral artery. *Acute synovitis of the ankle and knee in one leg can* occur in gout, pseudogout, rheumatic fever, Lyme disease, gonorrhea, Reiter's disease, and postinfectious forms of arthritis (e.g., *Shigella*, *Salmonella*, *Campylobacter*, and *Yersinia* species).

Sacroiliitis may occur after an acute diarrheal illness or urethritis (e.g., Reiter's syndrome). *Pseudosciatica* pain may extend from the buttock to the upper calf, and is due to sacroiliac joint involvement. Gaenslen's test and the fist percussion test (i.e., over the sacroiliac joint) are positive, and plain radiographs or scintigraphy confirm the clinical diagnosis of reactive sacroiliitis. *Genital herpes* may cause aching or burning buttock and posteromedial leg pain, fever, and dysuria that precedes—and/or accompanies—an eruption of painful, tender genital papules, vesicles, and crusted ulcers.

☐ DESCRIPTION OF LISTED DISEASES

Anterior and Anteromedial Leg Pain

1. FEMORAL NEUROPATHY

A continuous pain occurs in the inguinal region, and usually radiates down the anterior and medial thigh and into the anteromedial portion of the lower leg and the dorsum of the foot. In some cases the pain may radiate to the lower abdomen and flank on the affected side. The pain is usually continuous, with occasional brief jabs of more severe discomfort.

It is often associated with numbness and tingling paresthesias of the anteromedial thigh. Weakness of hip flexion and knee extension may also occur, and patients may complain of their knees' buckling when they attempt to walk. The knee jerk is diminished, and hypesthesia may occur in the distal two-thirds of the thigh and proximal lower leg.

Femoral neuropathy may be associated with bleeding into the iliacus (iliacus syndrome) or iliopsoas muscles, causing very severe groin pain and resulting in a characteristic appearance of the patient. He or she lies immobile, with the affected leg flexed, abducted, and externally rotated at the hip. Such patients resist any attempts at passive extension of the thigh because of the severe pain produced by even a few degrees of motion. A mass may be palpable in the ipsilateral iliac fossa or in the inguinal region on the affected side. The causative

TABLE OF DISEASE INCIDENCE

INCIDENCE PER 100,000 (APPROXIMATE)

Common (>100)	Uncommon (>5–100)	Rare (>0–5)
Disc herniation (lateral)	Femoral neuropathy	Iliacus syndrome
Trochanteric bursitis	Radiculopathy, L2–L4	Lumbar plexopathy
L5 or S1 radiculopathy due to lateral recess or foramen stenosis	Iliofemoral thrombophlebitis	Sacral plexopathy
	Iliofemoral arterial occlusion	Panplexopathy
	Arthritis in two or more lower extremity joints	Epidural abscess
Meralgia paresthetica		Epidural hematoma
		Midline disc herniation and cauda equina syndrome
Myalgic pain	Sacroiliitis and pseudosciatica	Infarction of the conus medullaris and conus syndrome
Genital herpes		

hematoma may result from hemophilia, leukemia, disseminated intravascular coagulation, or therapeutic anticoagulation. Vigorous exercise, such as judo or gymnastics, may cause an iliopsoas hematoma to develop in a normal (i.e., non-anticoagulated) individual.

An acute onset of the iliacus syndrome may also be associated with rupture and bleeding from an aortic or iliac artery aneurysm. Rarely, pelvic appendicitis with iliopsoas involvement may cause similar complaints. The association of an iliacus syndrome and/or femoral neuropathy with hypotension and a falling hematocrit strongly suggests rupture of an abdominal aneurysm.

Iatrogenic production of a mild femoral neuropathy, with minimal or no pain and predominant findings of limb weakness and hypesthesia, has been reported after such surgical procedures as abdominal hysterectomy and renal transplantation. It has been associated with the use of self-retaining retractors and with assistant-related retractor pressure against the iliopsoas region.

We have known severe anteromedial leg pain to arise from a groin hematoma following coronary angiography, and from an intramuscular injection into the upper anterior thigh. In these cases severe skin hyperesthesia was present, rather than hypesthesia.

The diagnosis of an iliacus or iliopsoas hematoma can be confirmed by abdominal and pelvic CT scanning or ultrasonography. These procedures can also detect the presence of an aneurysm or psoas abscess. Coagulation studies should be done on patients who show evidence of intramuscular bleeding but who have not been engaging in vigorous exercise and have not been treated with heparin or warfarin. Diabetes mellitus may be associated with spontaneous femoral neuropathy.

The pain of femoral neuropathy may respond poorly to narcotic analgesics. Pain associated with hemophilia- or anticoagulant-related hematomas will usually respond promptly to correction of the coagulation disorder and decompressive surgery. Cases of femoral neuropathy without an iliacus syndrome that are related to retractor pressure usually subside, with minimal sequelae, in 2 to 6 months. The literature is controversial regarding the need for decompressive surgery in hemophilia; reports on some series describe excellent recovery after conservative management. Full recovery may take as long as 2 to 3 years.

The pain of femoral neuropathy may be localized to the groin and lower abdomen, or may radiate as far as the knee. It is always anterior and anteromedial in location, and is usually absent in the presence of limb weakness and sensory loss in retractor-related cases.

Weakness of knee extension is due to paresis of the quadriceps muscle. Direct involvement of the nerve by a hematoma in the iliacus muscle may also impair hip flexion by producing iliopsoas muscle paresis. The initial response to intramuscular bleeding is painful iliopsoas and iliacus spasm, with marked hip flexion and abduction; this may be followed by paresis of hip flexion.

2. RADICULOPATHY INVOLVING THE L2, L3, AND/OR L4 NERVE ROOTS

Patients with this condition may complain of the sudden onset of low back and/or buttock pain, associated with pain in the anteromedial thigh and anteromedial lower leg. Quadriceps weakness and atrophy, associated with hypesthesia of the distal two-thirds of the anteromedial thigh and the proximal lower leg, may accompany the pain. In one series herniation or sequestration of a disc, causing the syndrome of low back pain and anterior leg pain, arose in the L2–L3 disc 2 times; in the L3–L4 disc 22 times; and in the L4–L5 disc 21 times. Such syndromes tend to occur at more advanced ages (average age 47) than sciatic syndromes. Radiculopathy may also follow a prior L5–S1 fusion operation. This may result from disc protrusion and/or facet joint arthritis with compression of either the L3 or the L4 nerve root near its foramen. A CT scan or MRI will identify the cause of the problem. Lack of a response to rest may warrant decompressive surgery.

3. LUMBAR PLEXOPATHY

Pain arises from the nerve roots of L2 to L4 in the lumbar plexus. There is pressurelike or aching pain, as well as superimposed jabs of lancinating pain in the anteromedial thigh, the anterior lower leg, and the dorsum of the foot. Localized pain may also occur in the groin and lower abdomen on the involved side. Low back and flank pain may sometimes accompany the leg pain. Weakness of hip flexion and knee extension may begin with, or follow, the onset of the leg pain. In some cases the leg pain does not extend below the knee. Hypesthesia and paresthesias of the painful regions of the leg are commonly associated with the pain.

Acute lumbar plexopathy may follow severe trauma; retroperitoneal bleeding related to injury or clotting disorders; aortic aneurysm with sudden enlargement or bleeding; acute appendicitis with rupture and abscess formation; or inflammatory and vasculitic processes involving the plexus.

A CT study of the lumbosacral area will identify retroperitoneal bleeding, an abscess, or an aneurysm. The CT scan in patients with vasculitis or with inflammatory or idiopathic plexopathies is usually negative.

Electromyographic studies will sometimes, but not always, differentiate femoral neuropathy from lumbar plexopathy. In the latter, adductor muscle fibrillations accompany the same findings in the vastus muscles.

Patients with plexopathy do not usually have fibrilla-

tions in the paraspinal muscles—which are a frequent, but not invariable, finding in patients with L2-to-L4 radiculopathy.

Posterior and/or Posterolateral Leg Pain

4. SACRAL PLEXOPATHY

Aching or pressurelike pain occurs in the low back and/or buttocks, and radiates down the posterior and posterolateral thigh and calf into the big toe (L5) or into the heel and lateral sole (S1). Pain may also occur in the perineum and in the trochanteric region and ankle. Lancinating pain may be superimposed on a more constant pressurelike or aching discomfort. Numbness and paresthesias may develop on the perineum, thigh, and sole, and there may be weakness of foot and big toe dorsiflexion (L5) and foot ventral flexion and eversion (S1). The ankle jerk may be diminished or absent. Acute sacral plexopathy may be associated with a ruptured aneurysm, retroperitoneal bleeding, pelvic fractures, or vasculitic or inflammatory processes involving the plexus. It should be differentiated from a radiculopathy of L5 or S1 caused by a herniated disc or facet disease with lateral recess or foramen stenosis.

Electromyography may sometimes aid in differentiating a cauda equina lesion with multiple radiculopathies, or a high sciatic nerve lesion, from sacral plexopathy. The presence of bilateral findings and/or paraspinal fibrillations favors a diagnosis of multiple radiculopathies (e.g., cauda equina lesion). The presence of fibrillations in plexus-innervated gluteal and tensor fasciae latae muscles favors a diagnosis of sacral plexopathy. In some cases, accurate localization of the lesion by electromyography is impossible. In such cases, CT or MRI studies may identify a lesion and localize it to a specific anatomic region (e.g., root, plexus, peripheral nerve) of the lumbosacral nerves.

5. PANPLEXOPATHY

Both lumbar and sacral plexus involvement may occur, causing pain both in the anterior thigh and lower leg and in the posterior thigh and calf. Pain may also occur in the low abdomen, buttock, perineum, low back, and flank. Weakness may involve knee and hip extension and flexion, and ankle movements. There may be sensory losses on the anterior and posterior aspects of the leg. Such widespread involvement of both components of the plexus is more likely to be associated with retroperitoneal bleeding from a coagulation defect or aneurysmal rupture.

Positive straight leg raising tests and reverse straight

leg tests may occur with both lumbar and sacral plexo-pathies.

Panplexopathy should be suspected in patients without spine pain or paraspinal muscle spasm who have leg pain (i.e., anterior and posterior) with leg weakness and sensory and reflex abnormalities. Abnormal sweating or changes in skin temperature on the leg or foot should also lead to a consideration of plexus involvement. Neurologic examination can detect evidence of involvement of several nerve segments, as well as of the sympathetic trunk. A pelvic CT scan is capable of demonstrating mass lesions in patients in whom plexopathy is suspected. Conversely, it can effectively rule out such lesions, with a high degree of certainty, in patients with other causes of plexopathy.

6. ACUTE SCIATIC PAIN

A. Acute Lateral Herniation of the L4–5 or L5–S1 Disc Pain is felt in the lumbosacral area and radiates down the posterior aspects of the thigh and calf into the foot. The pain is usually intensified by coughing, sneezing, and straining at stool (i.e., positive Dejerine's sign). A positive straight leg raising test is present, and the ankle jerk may be diminished or absent on the affected side. Sensory loss may occur on the affected posterior thigh and calf, and there may be weakness of foot and big toe dorsiflexion (L5) or of plantar flexion and foot eversion (S1). Acute sciatic pain may also be caused by nerve root irritation in a stenotic lateral recess or foramen, or may be secondary to osteoarthritis and disc degeneration or to spondylolisthesis. These disorders can be differentiated from disc herniation by a CT scan or MRI, with careful attention paid to the lateral recesses and foramina. Dynamic CT studies in lateral flexion may disclose root compression not apparent in conventional views. Disc herniation can best be detected by a CT-enhanced myelogram or a CT with contrast injection.

B. Acute Epidural Abscess and Cauda Equina Syndrome Central lumbar ache and tenderness, with cauda equina syndrome, is accompanied by high fever, rigors, and chills. Lancinating pain due to root irritation may radiate down the posterior thigh (L5–S1) or anterior thigh (L2–L4), depending on the level of the abscess. The involvement of the legs may remain unilateral, or may spread to both sides. Urinary retention occurs initially, and is followed by incontinence. Fecal incontinence and a patulous, open anal sphincter may be present. There may be weakness or heaviness of the involved leg, and sensory loss may occur on the buttock, perineum, and leg. The total leukocyte count is usually elevated; the cerebrospinal fluid may show an elevated leukocyte count and protein level, with a normal sugar level. A CT scan

or MRI will establish the diagnosis. Surgical drainage under cover of parenteral antibiotics will relieve the symptoms and lead to resolution of abnormal neurologic findings.

C. Acute Nontraumatic Epidural Hematoma and Cauda Equina Syndrome There is a sudden onset of midline lumbar pain and associated tenderness. Pain in the lumbosacral area and/or buttock radiates into one leg or in some cases, into both. This pain may be increased by straight leg raising or by coughing or straining at stool (i.e., positive Dejerine's sign). Neurologic dysfunction, in the form of patchy sensory loss and leg weakness, usually begins 6 h or more after the onset of the back pain. Bladder and bowel function may be partly or completely impaired. Fever and chills are not present. Most victims of this disorder have severe liver disease, with abnormal coagulation tests, or are taking anticoagulants. A CT scan or MRI will localize and identify the lesion. Administration of vitamin K and fresh frozen plasma will correct the clotting defect if it is due to anticoagulant therapy. Laminectomy should be done to decompress the cauda equina. Partial neurologic lesions have a good prognosis for recovery after removal of the hematoma.

D. Acute Cauda Equina Syndrome Due to a Herniated Midline Disc There is a sudden or rapidly progressive onset of severe lumbosacral and/or buttock pain, with radiation down the back of one thigh to the foot. Paresthesias and numbness may occur in the same distribution as the pain. Dejerine's sign and the straight leg raising test are positive. Buttock, perineal, and posterior-thigh hypesthesia or anesthesia may be present. Evidence of urinary and fecal incontinence may develop. Leg weakness, manifested by decreased ability to abduct or extend the hip, flex the knee, or move the ankle, may occur in severe cases. A CT scan or MRI will confirm the diagnosis by detecting a large herniated midline disc in the lumbar spinal canal.

E. Conus Medullaris Syndrome Due to Spinal Cord Infarction An abrupt, strokelike onset of severe low back and buttock pain occurs, with radiation to the leg. Lower limb weakness, saddle hypesthesia or anesthesia, and thigh hypesthesia rapidly follow. Urinary and fecal incontinence are usually prominent findings. Brief, mild prodromal episodes may occur before a final persistent attack. A CT scan or MRI will reveal no evidence of a space-occupying lesion. Aortic surgery, the use of an intraaortic balloon to treat cardiogenic shock, smoking, and vascular disease are associated with this disorder. There is no specific therapy; partial recovery may occur over a period of several months.

Lateral Leg Pain

7. TROCHANTERIC BURSITIS

Pain and tenderness over the trochanteric region may radiate to the low back and down the lateral side of the leg to the knee, and, in some cases, to the ankle. The pain is intensified by walking and jogging, and by lying on the affected side. When associated with low back pain, it may lead to diagnostic confusion by causing a pseudo-radiculopathy pain syndrome. Pain may be provoked by local palpation, or by abduction or internal rotation of the hip. Local injection, into the painful and tender site, of 3 ml of lidocaine and methylprednisolone immediately relieves all pain and permits pain-free ambulation. Up to 30 percent of patients may require two or more injections.

Relief of pain by the injection of lidocaine into the affected bursa is an important diagnostic test for this disorder, and differentiates it from other causes of lateral thigh pain—such as L5 radiculopathy, meralgia paresthetica, and inflammation of the iliotibial band. A rare case of septic trochanteric bursitis treated with antibiotics and surgical drainage has been reported; this case presented with severe local swelling and heat, findings that do not occur with aseptic trochanteric bursitis.

8. MERALGIA PARESTHETICA

Meralgia paresthetica causes aching pain, associated with a patch of hypesthesia surrounded by a halo of hyperesthesia in the lower third of the lateral thigh. In severe cases, the pain may radiate down the lateral portion of the lower leg. Obesity, pregnancy, diabetes, and iliopsoas hematomas are associated with this disorder. The causative lesion is a neuropathy of the lateral femoral cutaneous nerve.

Diffuse or Generalized Leg Pain

9. MYALGIC PAIN

Pain of an aching quality, intensified by leg movement during walking or stairclimbing, can involve both the calf and the thigh. There may be associated local tenderness. Such pain may be caused by unusual activity involving the affected limb, or by prolonged sitting in a cramped position. Such pain tends to be transient, and often disappears in 1 to 3 days.

10. ILIOFEMORAL THROMBOPHLEBITIS

Generalized leg pain, bluish discoloration, and swelling form a triad of findings in patients with this disorder. The swelling is manifested by an increase in limb circumference, relative to the opposite limb, of 1 cm or more. The skin may feel tense to palpation. Pedal veins stay full despite elevation of the foot above 30°. Collateral vessels may appear on the abdominal wall, with flow away from the affected limb. The pedal pulses may be diminished because of reflex arterial spasm. Inguinal tenderness may be present if the clot extends retrograde to this area.

Iliofemoral thrombophlebitis may sometimes cause acute lower abdominal, groin, and flank pain; fever; chills; and vomiting and ileus. Localized inguinal tenderness may accompany these symptoms.

The diagnosis of iliofemoral vein occlusion can be made more certain by the use of tests such as Doppler ultrasonography (accuracy 82 percent, sensitivity 75 percent, specificity 85 percent); real-time sonography (sensitivity 91–96 percent, specificity 97–100 percent); and impedence plethysmography (IPG) (accuracy 89 percent, sensitivity 71–94 percent, specificity 94–98 percent for femoral and iliac thrombi). IPG can be falsely negative in up to 25 percent of cases. Contrast venography will usually confirm the clinical or laboratory diagnosis of this disorder.

The merits of immediate surgical thrombectomy are not agreed upon. One group obtained excellent results when thrombus removal was completed within 48 h and anticoagulation was continued for 6 months or more. New radionuclide tests, such as indium-111-labeled platelets and technetium-99m-labeled red blood cells, may be used for the diagnosis of deep venous thrombosis, but more thorough evaluation of these radionuclide tests is required before they can be recommended for general use.

11. ILIOFEMORAL ARTERIAL EMBOLISM OR THROMBOSIS

Severe aching pain develops abruptly in the affected limb and may involve the thigh, lower leg, foot, and toes. Skin pallor, or chalky whiteness, and coldness develop rapidly; there may be a line of demarcation. Skin hypesthesia or anesthesia, and limb paresis or paralysis, soon follow. All pulses in the limb are severely diminished or absent. Arteriography will demonstrate the point of obstruction in the iliac or femoral artery. Aortofemoral bypass will usually (60–70 percent of cases) lead to limb salvage. Failure of the graft may result in a cold, pulseless, paralyzed limb. Such cases may require extensive amputation to prevent death.

12. ARTHRITIS IN TWO OR MORE LOWER EXTREMITY JOINTS

Pain in two or more joints of one leg, with radiation proximally and distally, may occur acutely in gout, pseudogout, rheumatic fever, Lyme disease, gonorrhea, Reiter's disease, and other postinfectious forms of arthritis. In gout and pseudogout, the joints are extremely tender and the overlying skin is warm and red. Effusions are present in all of these disorders. Joint aspiration, culture, Gram's stain, and a search for crystals will aid in establishing a diagnosis of gout, pseudogout, or gonorrhea.

Abnormalities in adults with rheumatic fever include joint involvement and, sometimes, cardiac involvement. Erythema marginatum, skin nodules, and chorea are rare. Elevated levels of antistreptococcal enzymes help establish the diagnosis. In patients with Lyme disease, elevated antibody levels to *Borrelia burgdorferi* and the prior or current presence of the characteristic skin rash will confirm the diagnosis. Reactive forms of lower limb arthritis usually follow acute gastrointestinal infection (e.g. *Campylobacter, Shigella, Salmonella,* or *Yersinia* species) or urethritis (e.g., Reiter's disease).

13. SACROILIITIS AND PSEUDOSCIATICA

Sacroiliitis secondary to infections of the gastrointestinal tract (e.g., *Shigella, Salmonella, Campylobacter,* or *Yersinia* species) Reiter's syndrome, brucellosis, or staphylococcal infection of the sacroiliac joint may cause lumbosacral, buttock, and posterior leg pain that extends to the popliteal fossa or upper calf (pseudosciatica). There is local sacroiliac fist percussion tenderness, and a positive Gaenslen's test and fabere sign. Plain radiographs of the pelvis, or scintigraphy, will confirm the diagnosis of sacroiliitis. There is a response to nonsteroidal anti-inflammatory drugs, with resolution of back and leg pain. True sciatic pain with an abnormal straight leg raising test and Dejerine's sign does not develop, and there is no evidence of L5 or S1 compression on a CT scan or MRI. Sacroiliitis secondary to an acute enteric or genitourinary infection clears, in most cases, within 12 months; but a significant percentage of patients may have chronic recurrent or persistent symptoms beyond that time.

14. GENITAL HERPES

An attack of primary genital herpes may begin with a 1- to 3-day prodrome of aching or burning pain, in the buttock and the medial and posterior thigh and lower leg, that precedes the eruption of painful tender grouped papules, vesicles, and crusted ulcers on the penis or labia. The leg pain may cease at the onset of the eruption or continue for several days. Fever, dysuria, urinary frequency, vaginal discharge, and even urinary retention may occur in some cases. Acyclovir given intravenously may reduce the severity of the symptoms and result in more rapid resolution. Recurrent attacks may follow despite use of acyclovir to treat the primary attack.

Acute Bilateral Upper and Lower Leg Pain

☐ DIAGNOSTIC LIST

Anterior and anteromedial leg pain
1. Myalgic pain associated with febrile illness and exercise
2. Lumbar plexopathy

Posterior and posterolateral leg pain
3. Sacral plexopathy
4. Acute bilateral sciatic and low back and/or buttock pain (polyradiculopathy of the cauda equina; acute cauda equina syndrome)
    A. Epidural abscess
    B. Epidural hematoma
    C. Midline disc herniation
5. Infarction of the conus medullaris

Generalized leg pain
6. Acute aortic or bilateral common iliac artery occlusion
7. Polyarthritis of the legs
8. Mononeuritis multiplex
9. Acute spondylolisthesis ("listhetic crisis")
10. Genital herpes

☐ SUMMARY

Myalgic pain is associated with acute febrile disorders, and with leg exercise in untrained or poorly trained persons. Thigh and calf discomfort may be intensified by walking, jogging, or other movements. *Lumbar plexopathy* is associated with anterior and anteromedial leg pain, loss of knee jerks, and weakness of knee extension and hip flexion. Its causes include malignant disease, vasculitis, diabetes, and an inflammatory disorder of unknown etiology.

Sacral plexopathy causes bilateral sciatic pain, sensory loss in a sciatic distribution, and weakness of hip extension, knee flexion, and ankle movements. The causes of sacral plexopathy are similar to those of lumbar plexopathy.

Low back pain and buttock pain with bilateral sciatic pain (and sometimes femoral-nerve-area pain) associated with chills, rigors, and fever occurs with an *acute epidural abscess*. A myelogram, a contrast-enhanced computed tomography (CT) scan, or MRI will detect the abscess, which requires immediate decompression and drainage. Similar symptoms, but without fever or chills, may develop abruptly in patients

who have severe liver disease or are taking anticoagulants. These patients will usually be found to have an *acute epidural hematoma*; this can be confirmed by a CT scan of the lumbar spine. Both epidural abscess and epidural hematoma may be associated with areflexic leg weakness or paralysis, patchy lower extremity sensory loss, and urinary and fecal incontinence (*acute cauda equina syndrome*).

An *acute cauda equina syndrome,* with low back and bilateral leg pain, weakness, sensory loss, and urinary and fecal incontinence, can also arise from a *herniation of a large disc in the midline*. A CT scan will identify the lesion, which requires removal.

Conus medullaris infarction causes perineal and posterior thigh pain. Sensory loss occurs in a saddle distribution. Motor weakness of the legs is minimal initially, but fasciculations may occur. There is early loss of bladder and rectal control, and impotence is a common associated symptom. Usually the onset is sudden, with maximal dysfunction occurring within minutes.

Severe pain radiating into each leg, associated with leg paralysis or paresis, pallor, paresthesias, and then anesthesia, suggests an acute embolic or thrombotic *occlusion of the lower aorta or both common iliac arteries*. Patients may fall suddenly because of leg weakness or paralysis. Embolization is more likely in a setting of relative youth, atrial fibrillation, mitral stenosis, endocarditis, or myocardial infarction.

Involvement of two or more joints in each leg (*polyarthritis*) may cause upper and lower limb pain. Disorders capable of causing lower-extremity arthritis involving multiple joints include rheumatoid arthritis, lupus erythematosus, Lyme disease, Reiter's syndrome, rheumatic fever, and gonococcal arthritis.

Mononeuritis multiplex may cause an acute neuritis of one or more nerves in each leg. The symptoms are often asymmetrical (e.g., the anterior leg may be involved on one side, and the posterior on the other). Paresthesias, numbness, reflex loss, motor weakness, and aching or lancinating pains occur. This type of disorder may occur with polyarteritis nodosa, the vasculitis associated with lupus erythematosus or rheumatoid arthritis, and with diabetes mellitus. In many cases there is no associated disease.

Acute *spondylolisthesis,* with marked slippage, can cause the sudden onset of low back pain and bilateral sciatic pain with severe hamstring spasm, often requiring surgery for relief. *Genital herpes* may cause fever, aching or burning bilateral buttock and posteromedial leg pain, and eruption of painful genital vesicles and crusted ulcers. Dysuria, frequency, and urinary retention may also occur.

TABLE OF DISEASE INCIDENCE

INCIDENCE PER 100,000 (APPROXIMATE)

Common (>100)	Uncommon (>5–100)	Rare (>0–5)
Myalgic pain with febrile illness	Lumbar plexopathy	Epidural abscess
Myalgic pain after exercise	Sacral plexopathy	Epidural hematoma
Polyarthritis of the legs	Midline disc herniation	Infarction of the conus medullaris
Genital herpes	Aortic or bilateral common iliac artery occlusion	Mononeuritis multiplex
		Acute spondylolisthesis

☐ DESCRIPTION OF LISTED DISEASES

Anterior and Anteromedial Leg Pain

1. MYALGIC PAIN

Pain in the hips, thighs, and lower legs may accompany acute febrile disorders, such as influenza and streptococcal pharyngitis. These myalgias may be dramatically relieved by aspirin or acetaminophen. Myalgias may also occur 1 to 2 days after unaccustomed calisthenics; bilateral thigh and lower leg pain has occurred after a "jump squat" calisthenic used to condition soldiers and athletes. In some cases, rhabdomyolysis has accompanied the muscle pain and tenderness.

2. LUMBAR PLEXOPATHY

Bilateral lumbar plexopathy results in anterior and anteromedial thigh and lower limb pain. Usually the pain is accompanied by asymmetrical sensory loss and paresthesias. Variable degrees of weakness of hip flexion and knee extension accompany the sensory loss. Incontinence and impotence are uncommon. Bilateral plexopathy can be caused by cancer, vasculitis, diabetes, or an inflammatory syndrome of unknown etiology. A CT scan of the pelvis and lumbar region will identify neoplasms. The CT will be negative in the presence of the other disorders listed. Plexopathy associated with tumor is frequently associated with a history of a recently treated malignancy, ankle edema, a rectal mass, and a unilateral or bilateral hydronephrosis.

Posterior and Posterolateral Leg Pain

3. SACRAL PLEXOPATHY

Pain may occur as a pressurelike, aching or burning sensation. It may be felt in the buttocks, low back, lower abdomen, flank, and posterolateral aspects of both legs. Skin numbness and paresthesias may occur in the painful leg areas. Weakness of hip extension, knee flexion, ankle dorsiflexion, and ventral flexion may develop. The ankle jerks may be diminished or depressed. In patients with cancer there may be a palpable pelvic mass on rectal examination, and peripheral edema. Sacral plexopathy in cancer patients usually begins as a unilateral syndrome that gradually becomes bilateral. Other processes, such as severe uncontrolled diabetes, vasculitis, inflammatory plexitis with an elevated sedimentation rate, and retroperitoneal bleeding, may have a more acute onset with bilateral findings. A CT scan will be positive in the presence of tumor or hemorrhage, but will show no abnormality in the presence of the other disorders listed.

4. ACUTE BILATERAL SCIATIC AND LOW BACK AND/OR BUTTOCK PAIN (POLYRADICULOPATHY OF THE CAUDA EQUINA; ACUTE CAUDA EQUINA SYNDROME)

A. Epidural Abscess   Fever, neck stiffness, malaise, chills, and sweats are frequent symptoms. Central lumbar ache and tenderness occur with a constant sciatic-type pain in both legs. Anterior thigh pain may also occur on one or both sides. Lancinating jabs of sharp pain radiate from the back to the feet; these pains may be intensified by sneezing, coughing, or straining at stool. Incontinence and leg weakness may develop. Hypesthesia may develop in a saddle distribution and over the posterior thighs and calves. Lumbar puncture usually yields an elevated cerebrospinal fluid leukocyte count and protein level, a normal sugar level, and negative Gram stains and cultures. A myelogram will localize the abscess. It may also be detected by a CT scan or magnetic resonance imaging (MRI). Surgical decompression and abscess drainage under an antibiotic umbrella usually bring about recovery.

B. Epidural Hematoma This disorder occurs in patients with severe liver disease and in patients taking oral anticoagulants. Initially, severe midline lumbar ache and tenderness begin; they are followed by sharp constant pain, radiating into both feet from the buttock region. Dejerine's sign and the straight leg raising test are positive. Leg weakness and numbness begin 6 h or more after the back pain. Urinary retention, and then incontinence, may develop. Fever, chills, and sweats do not occur. The prothrombin time is usually prolonged. A myelogram will demonstrate a spindle-shaped lower lumbar block. CT or MRI will visualize the hematoma. Vitamin K and fresh frozen plasma should be given, and laminectomy performed to decompress the cauda equina.

C. Midline Disc Herniation Severe lumbar or lumbosacral pain and buttock pain occur with bilateral sciatic pain. Paresthesias and numbness may accompany the pain. Straight leg raising, coughing, and straining at stool cause radicular pain. Saddle hypesthesia may occur. Urinary and fecal incontinence may begin within hours. Leg weakness may be absent, mild, or severe. Abduction of the hip, extension and flexion of the knee, and ankle movements may be weakened. A contrast-enhanced CT scan or a myelogram will visualize a midline herniated disc. Bilateral radical discectomy will usually relieve all complaints and prevent neurologic damage.

The above disorders involving the cauda equina tend to produce asymmetrical pain and other symptoms, including asymmetrical sensory and motor changes. Bladder and rectal disfunction usually occur late and are mild to moderate in degree.

5. INFARCTION OF THE CONUS MEDULLARIS

There is an abrupt onset of a severe symmetrical pain in the lumbosacral area, buttocks, and both posterior thighs. The pain is soon followed by mild bilateral leg weakness and saddle hypesthesia or anesthesia. Urinary and fecal incontinence occur early, and are severe relative to the motor loss in the legs. Hip extension and abduction, knee flexion, and ankle movement may be mildly weakened. Prodromal transient attacks of similar symptoms may precede the actual episode of conus infarction. CT studies and myelograms are negative, making hematoma, abscess, tumor, and disc herniation unlikely. Gradual return of neurologic function occurs over a period of many months. Conservative nonsurgical management is indicated. Patients with aortic occlusive disease, or recent aortic surgery or requiring intraaortic balloon use, are at greater risk for conus infarction.

Generalized Leg Pain

6. ACUTE AORTIC OR BILATERAL COMMON ILIAC ARTERY OCCLUSION

There is an abrupt onset of severe aching or sharp pain in the buttocks, thighs, calves, and feet. Tingling paresthesias and numbness develop rapidly, and there is severe weakness, progressing to paralysis, of both lower limbs. The loss of muscle strength may cause the patient to fall and sustain injuries that may confuse the clinical picture. The legs become pale, cool, and sometimes cyanotic. Neither femoral pulse, nor any distal pulse, is palpable. The muscles of the legs are usually soft or doughy shortly after the occlusion. Removal of an occluding embolus, or reconstruction of the thrombosed lower aorta or iliac arteries, should be done before the muscles become firm or hard—changes that indicate myonecrosis.

Embolization is more often present in patients with atrial fibrillation, mitral stenosis, endocarditis, or recent myocardial infarction. Such patients usually give no history of claudication, and often have otherwise normal vessels on arteriography.

Embolectomy, using a Fogarty balloon catheter, will usually remove most emboli or propagating distal thrombi in the iliofemoral vessels; this procedure produces excellent results, with complete remission of symptoms if the procedure is done within 4 to 6 h of the onset of symptoms. Occlusion of the lower aorta by thrombosis in a setting of severe aortoiliac atherosclerosis can be treated by reconstructive techniques, such as endarterectomy or aortofemoral bypass. Balloon angioplasty may be useful in some cases.

7. SYMMETRICAL ARTHRITIS OF TWO OR MORE LOWER EXTREMITY JOINTS (POLYARTHRITIS)

Arthritis of the hip causes groin pain and anterior and medial thigh pain, made worse by walking. Arthritis of the knee causes knee, proximal thigh, and popliteal pain. Involvement of the ankle causes distal extremity pain.

Disorders that may cause bilateral lower-extremity joint involvement include rheumatoid arthritis, rheumatic fever, systemic lupus erythematosus, enteropathic and psoriatic arthritis, Reiter's syndrome, Lyme disease, ankylosing spondylitis, and gonococcal arthritis. Some patients may have persistent arthralgias after a nonspecific febrile illness; the cause of this is seldom determined, since symptoms clear spontaneously.

8. MONONEURITIS MULTIPLEX

A sudden onset of severe aching, burning, or lancinating leg pain, paresthesias, sensory loss, and motor weakness, involving one or more nerves in each leg, usually in an asymmetrical pattern, can be caused by multiple acute mononeuropathies. This disorder may be caused by vasculitis—e.g., polyarteritis nodosa, or the vasculitis associated with lupus erythematosus, rheumatoid arthritis, or mixed connective tissue disease.

This disorder may also occur in patients with severe diabetes, and in those with cryoglobulinemia, sarcoidosis, hypereosinophilic syndromes, amyloidosis, and leprosy. A number of cases are not associated with any underlying disorder. It is believed that the underlying mechanism in most patients is the occlusion of the vasa nervorum, with ischemia and infarction of the affected nerves.

9. ACUTE SPONDYLOLISTHESIS ("LISTHETIC CRISIS")

Acute low back and buttock pain may begin abruptly in the 10- to 15-year age group. Rarely, pain may radiate down both legs to the calves or feet. Such pain is commonly lancinating, and is increased in intensity—or provoked—by coughing, sneezing, or straining at stool (i.e., positive Dejerine sign). This rapid onset is due to a sudden increase in the amount of L5 slippage (i.e., "listhetic crisis"). Physical examination reveals a rigid lumbar spine, scoliosis, flattening of the sacrum, and tightness of the hamstring muscles. The straight leg raising signs are positive bilaterally. Radiographs of the spine reveal marked spondylolisthesis of L5 on S1. Severe sciatic pain related to slippage requires decompressive surgery, arthrodesis, and sometimes the use of Harrington distraction rods to prevent recurrence and stabilize the spine. Symptoms usually resolve after such surgery.

10. GENITAL HERPES

The initial episode may begin with a prodrome of aching or burning pain in the buttocks, posteromedial thighs, and lower legs. Within 1 to 3 days a painful, tender genital eruption of grouped papules, vesicles, and crusted ulcers appears. Fever, dysuria, urinary frequency, and vaginal discharge may also occur. Intravenous acyclovir therapy usually accelerates the resolution of the leg and genital pain and the healing of the vesicular and ulcerative lesions.

UNILATERAL AND BILATERAL UPPER AND LOWER LEG PAIN REFERENCES

Acute Cauda Equina Syndrome

Bahemuka M, Shemena AR, Panayiotopoulos CP, et al: Neurological syndromes of brucellosis. *J Neurol Neurosurg Psychiatry* 51:1017–1021, 1988.

Brodsky AE, Aldama-Lubbert A, Khalil M, et al: Acute cauda equina syndrome secondary to an arteriovenous malformation of the spinal cord: A case report. *Spine* 11:631–632, 1986.

Herb E, Schwachenwald R, Nowak G, et al: Acute bleeding into a filum terminale ependymoma. *Neurosurg Rev* 13:243–245, 1990.

Kardaun JW, White LR, Shaffer WO: Acute complications in patients with surgical treatment of lumbar herniated disc. *J Spinal Disord* 3:30–38, 1990.

Kim SW: The syndrome of acute anterior lumbar spinal cord injury. *Clin Neurol Neurosurg* 92:249–253, 1990.

Kostuik JP, Harrington I, Alexander D, et al: Cauda equina syndrome and lumbar disc herniation. *J Bone Joint Surg (Am)* 68-A:386–391, 1986.

McLaren AC, Bailey SI: Cauda equina syndrome: A complication of lumbar discectomy. *Clin Orthop* 204:143–149, 1986.

Richter RL, Semble EL, Turner RA, et al: An unusual manifestation of Paget's disease of bone: Spinal epidural hematoma presenting as acute cauda equina syndrome. *J Rheumatol* 17:975–978, 1990.

Schuknecht B, Huber P, Buller B, et al: Spinal leptomeningeal neoplastic disease: Evaluation by MR, myelography and CT myelography. *Eur Neurol* 32:11–16, 1992.

Tullberg T, Isacson J: Cauda equina syndrome with normal lumbar myelography. *Acta Orthop Scand* 60:265–267, 1989.

Aortoiliac Stenosis

Baker JD: Hemodynamic assessment of aortoiliac segment. *Surg Clin North Am* 70:31–40, 1990.

Kitslaar PJ, Jorning PJ, Kohlen JP: Assessment of aortoiliac stenosis by femoral artery pressure measurement and Doppler waveform analysis. *Eur J Vasc Surg* 2:35–40, 1988.

Kohler TR, Nance DR, Cramer MM, et al: Duplex scanning for diagnosis of aortoiliac and femoropopliteal disease: A prospective study. *Circulation* 76:1074–1080, 1987.

Piotrowski JJ, Pearce WH, Jones DN, et al: Aortobifemoral bypass: The operation of choice for unilateral iliac occlusion? *J Vasc Surg* 8:211–218, 1988.

van Asten WN, Beijneveld WJ, Pieters BR, et al: Assessment of aortoiliac obstructive disease by Doppler spectrum analysis of blood flow velocities in the common femoral artery at rest and during reactive hyperemia. *Surgery* 109:633–639, 1991.

Aortoiliac Thrombosis

Eldrup-Jorgensen J, Flanigan DP, Brace L, et al: Hypercoagulable states and lower limb ischemia in young adults. *J Vasc Surg* 9:334–341, 1989.

Yuen JC, Riggs OE: Aortoiliac dissection after percutaneous insertion of an intra-aortic balloon pump. *South Med J* 84:1135–1137, 1991.

Conus Medullaris Syndrome

Anderson NE, Willoughby EW: Infarction of the conus medullaris. *Ann Neurol* 21:470–474, 1987.

Ohbu S, Ishimoto A, Honda M, et al: Infarction of the conus medullaris. *Eur Neurol* 30:343–344, 1990.

Overhage, JM Greist A, Brown DR: Conus medullaris syndrome resulting from *Toxoplasma gondii* infection in a patient with the acquired immunodeficiency syndrome. *Am J Med* 89:814–815, 1990.

Scherokman B, Vukelja S: Diabetic neuropathy simulating conus medullaris syndrome. *Arch Intern Med* 148:459–460, 1988.

Epidural Abscess

Arvin MC, Gehring RL, Crecelius JL, et al: Man with progressive lower back pain. *Indiana Med* 84:554–556, 1991.

Goucke CR, Graziotti P: Extradural abscess following local anaesthetic and steroid injection for chronic low back pain. *Br J Anaesth* 65:427–429, 1990.

Mooney RP, Hockberger RS: Spinal epidural abscess: A rapidly progressive disease. *Ann Emerg Med* 16:1168–1170, 1987.

Siao P, Yagnik P: Spinal epidural abscess. *J Emerg Med* 6:391–396, 1988.

Epidural Hematoma

Earman WA, Semba R: Postsurgical epidural hematoma reproducing a lumbar radiculopathy. *Orthop Rev* 17:1201–1204, 1988.

Metzger G, Singbartl G: Spinal epidural hematoma following epidural anesthesia versus spontaneous spinal subdural hematoma: Two case reports. *Acta Anaesthesiol Scand* 35:105–107, 1991.

Mirkovic S, Melany M: A thoracolumbar epidural hematoma simulating a disc syndrome. *J Spinal Disord* 5:112–115, 1992.

Saal JA, Dillingham MF, Gamburd RS, et al: The pseudoradicular syndrome: Lower extremity peripheral nerve entrapment masquerading as lumbar radiculopathy. *Spine* 13:926–930, 1988.

Femoral Neuropathy

Apter S, Hertz M, Rubinstein ZJ, et al: Femoral neuropathy: The role of computed tomography in diagnosis and management in 27 patients. *Clin Radiol* 40:30–34, 1989.

Boontje AH, Haaxma R: Femoral neuropathy as a complication of aortic surgery. *J Cardiovasc Surg* 28:286–289, 1987.

Kumar A, Dalela D, Bhandari M, et al: Femoral neuropathy: An unusual complication of renal transplantation. *Transplantation* 51:1305–1306, 1991.

Mark MD, Kwasnik EM, Wright SC: Combined femoral neuropathy and psoas sign: An unusual presentation of an iliac artery aneurysm. *Am J Med* 88:435–436, 1990.

Meech PR: Femoral neuropathy following renal transplantation. *Aust N Z J Surg* 60:117–119, 1990.

Niakan E, Carbone JE, Adams M, et al: Anticoagulants, iliopsoas hematoma and femoral nerve compression. *Am Fam Physician* 44:2100–2102, 1991.

Olesen LL: Femoral neuropathy secondary to anticoagulation. *J Intern Med* 226:279–280, 1989.

Piazza I, Girardi A, Giunta G, et al: Femoral nerve palsy secondary to anticoagulant induced iliacus hematoma: A case report. *Int Angiol* 9:125–126, 1990.

Puechal X, Liote F, Kuntz D: Bilateral femoral neuropathy caused by iliacus hematomas during anticoagulation after cardiac catheterization. *Am Heart J* 123:262–263, 1992.

Roberts SR, Main D, Pinkerton J: Surgical therapy of femoral artery pseudoaneurysm after angiography. *Am J Surg* 154:676–680, 1987.

Stuart JD, Morgan RF, Persing JA: Nerve compression syndromes of the lower extremity. *Am Fam Physician* 40:101–112, 1989.

Walsh C, Walsh A: Postoperative femoral neuropathy. *Surg Gynecol Obstet* 174:255–263, 1992.

Iliofemoral Venous Thrombosis

Plate G, Einarsson E, Eklof B: Etiologic spectrum in acute iliofemoral venous thrombosis. *Int Angiol* 5:59–64, 1986.

Polak JF, O'Leary DH: Deep venous thrombosis in pregnancy: Noninvasive diagnosis. *Radiology* 166:377–379, 1988.

Qvarfordt P, Eklof B, Ohlin P: Intramuscular pressure in the lower leg in deep vein thrombosis and phlegmasia cerulae dolens. *Ann Surg* 197:450–453, 1983.

Wilson B, Hawkins ML, Mansberger AR Jr: Posttraumatic phlegmasia cerulea dolens: An indication for the Greenfield filter. *South Med J* 82:780–782, 1989.

Lumbar Radiculopathy

Alexander AH, Jones AM, Rosenbaum DH Jr: Nonoperative management of herniated nucleus pulposus: Patient selection by the extension sign, long-term follow-up. *Orthop Rev* 21:181–188, 1992.

Greenspan A, Amparo EG, Gorczyca DP, et al: Is there a role for diskography in the era of magnetic resonance imaging? Prospective correlation and quantitative analysis of computed tomography-diskography, magnetic resonance imaging, and surgical findings. *J Spina Disord* 5:26–31, 1992.

Jinkins JR, Whittemore AR, Bradley WG: The anatomic basis of vertebrogenic pain and the autonomic syndrome associated with lumbar disk extrusion. *AJR* 152:1277–1289, 1989.

Saal JA, Saal JS: Nonoperative treatment of herniated lumbar intervertebral disc with radiculopathy: An outcome study. *Spine* 14:431–437, 1989.

Traycoff RB: "Pseudotrochanteric bursitis": The differential diagnosis of lateral hip pain. *J Rheumatol* 18:1810–1812, 1991.

Lumbosacral Plexopathy

Jaeckle KA: Nerve plexus metastases. *Neurol Clin* 9:857–866, 1991.

Meralgia Paresthetica

Grace DM: Meralgia paresthetica after gastroplasty for morbid obesity. *Can J Surg* 30:64–65, 1987.

Macnicol MF, Thompson WJ: Idiopathic meralgia paresthetica. *Clin Orthop* 254:270–274, 1990.

Streiffer RH: Meralgia paresthetica. *Am Fam Physician* 33:141–144, 1986.

Warfield CA: Meralgia paresthetica: Causes and cures. *Hosp Pract (Off Ed)* 21:40A, 40C, 40I, 1986.

Sciatic Pain

Torkelson SJ, Lee RA, Hildahl DB: Endometriosis of the sciatic nerve: A report of two cases and a review of the literature. *Obstet Gynecol* 71:473–477, 1988.

Trochanteric Bursitis

Collee G, Dijkmans BA, Vandenbroucke JP, et al: Greater trochanteric pain syndrome (trochanteric bursitis) in low back pain. *Scand J Rheumatol* 20:262–266, 1991.

Haller CC, Coleman PA, Estes NC, et al: Traumatic trochanteric bursitis. *Kans Med* 90:17–18, 22, 1989.

Schapira D, Nahir M, Scharf Y: Trochanteric bursitis: A common clinical problem. *Arch Phys Med Rehabil* 67:815–817, 1986.

Acute Inguinal, Trochanteric, Pubic, and Thigh Pain

☐ **DIAGNOSTIC LIST**

INGUINAL AND ANTEROMEDIAL
THIGH PAIN

1. Dislocation and fracture-
   dislocation of the hip
   A. Posterior
   B. Anterior
2. Traumatic fractures of the hip and
   pelvis
   A. Femoral neck fracture
   B. Intertrochanteric fracture
   C. Greater trochanteric fracture
   D. Lesser trochanteric fracture
   E. Subtrochanteric fracture
   F. Central acetabular fracture
      and fracture-dislocation
   G. Fractures at or near the pubic
      symphysis
   H. Impacted fracture of the
      femoral neck
3. Pathologic fracture of the hip
   A. Femoral neck
   B. Intertrochanteric and femoral
      shaft
4. Stress fracture of the hip and
   pelvis
5. Acute arthritis of the hip in adults
   A. Septic arthritis
   B. Acute calcium pyrophosphate
      deposition disease
   C. Acute gout
   D. Acute rheumatic fever
   E. Rheumatoid arthritis
      1. Acute rheumatoid arthritis
         of the hip

2. Chronic rheumatoid
   arthritis with acute
   noninfectious arthritis of
   the hip
   F. Osteoid osteoma
   G. Reiter's syndrome
6. Acute synovitis of the hip in
   children and adolescents
   A. Transient synovitis of the hip
   B. Juvenile rheumatoid arthritis
      of the hip
   C. Legg-Calvé-Perthes disease
   D. Slipped capital femoral
      epiphysis
   E. Pubic osteomyelitis
7. Osteonecrosis of the femoral
   head
8. Iliopsoas muscle disorders
   A. Iliopsoas bursitis
   B. Iliopsoas tendinitis
   C. Iliopsoas abscess
9. Femoral neuropathy
10. Iliofemoral venous thrombosis
11. Inguinal or femoral hernia
    A. Acute inguinal or femoral
       hernia
    B. Incarceration or strangulation
       of an inguinal or femoral
       hernia
12. Inguinal or femoral lymphadenitis
    A. Cellulitis of the leg,
       perineum, or abdominal wall
    B. Pyoderma of the leg,
       perineum, or abdominal wall

C. Specific infections
  1. *Vibrio vulnificus* cellulitis
  2. *Aeromonas hydrophila* cellulitis
  3. Bubonic plague
  4. Ulceroglandular tularemia
  5. Cat-scratch disease
D. Suppurative iliac lymphadenitis
E. Sexually transmitted diseases
  1. Primary genital herpes infection
  2. Chancroid
  3. Lymphogranuloma venereum
  4. Primary syphilis
  5. Gonococcal or nongonococcal urethritis

TROCHANTERIC AND LATERAL THIGH PAIN

13. Hip pointer
14. Avulsion fracture of the iliac crest apophysis
15. Trochanteric bursitis
16. Snapping hip syndrome
17. Meralgia paresthetica
18. Acute arthritis of the hip
19. Osteonecrosis of the hip
20. Fracture of the femoral shaft due to trauma

MEDIAL THIGH PAIN

21. Obturator hernia
22. Greater saphenous vein phlebitis
23. Herpes simplex neuritis
24. Referred pain
  A. Tubo-ovarian lesions
  B. Pubic bone disorders
  C. Ureteral colic
25. Adductor muscle strain
26. Iliopsoas muscle strain or avulsion fracture of the lesser trochanter

PUBIC PAIN

27. Osteitis pubis
28. Osteomyelitis of the pubic bone
29. Pyogenic arthritis of the pubic symphysis
30. Pubic fracture
  A. Pathologic fracture of the pubic bone (disease-associated)
  B. Stress fracture of the pubic bone (athletic activity-associated)
31. Pubic osteolysis
32. Postpartum symphyseal pubic pain

POSTERIOR THIGH PAIN

33. Pyriformis syndrome
34. Hamstring syndrome
35. Hamstring muscle injury
  A. Strain
  B. Ischial apophysis avulsion
36. Ischial bursitis
37. Radicular pain
  A. Disc protrusion
  B. Spinal epidural abscess
  C. Spinal epidural or subdural hematoma
  D. Conus medullaris infarction
38. Posterior femoral cutaneous neuropathy
39. Lumbar facet joint disease
40. Sacroiliitis
  A. Reactive arthritis
  B. Septic arthritis
41. Sacroiliac sprain
42. Myofascial pain
43. Posterior compartment syndrome of the thigh

ANTERIOR THIGH PAIN

44. Bacteremia-associated bilateral anterior thigh pain
45. Femoral neuropathy
46. Radicular pain (L2–L4 spinal roots)
47. Femoral shaft fracture due to trauma
48. Femoral shaft stress fracture in athletes
49. Anterior compartment syndrome of the thigh
50. Sartorius muscle strain
51. Quadriceps muscle strain

GENERALIZED THIGH PAIN

52. Femoral shaft fracture due to trauma
53. Compartment syndromes
54. Sickle cell pain crisis
55. Pathologic fracture due to bone tumor or cyst
56. Pyomyositis
57. Soft tissue sarcoma
58. Retroperitoneal perforation of the colon and thigh infection
59. Retroperitoneal perforation of the colon and lumbosacral plexus involvement
60. Iliofemoral venous thrombosis
61. Stress fracture of the femoral shaft
62. Muscle strain due to overuse
63. Idiopathic dermatomyositis or polymyositis

☐ SUMMARY

Inguinal and Anteromedial Thigh Pain

Posterior dislocation of the hip usually occurs in a motor vehicle or motorcycle accident or a fall. There is severe groin and lateral hip pain, and the leg is shortened and held flexed, adducted, and internally rotated. Plain radiographs or a CT scan will confirm the dislocation and detect associated fractures of the femoral head and acetabulum. *Anterior dislocation* causes groin pain and tenderness. In a superior anterior dislocation, the leg is held extended and externally rotated. In an inferior anterior dislocation, the thigh is abducted, externally rotated, and held in flexion.

Fracture of the proximal femur (e.g., femoral neck, intertrochanteric, or subtrochanteric) usually follows a fall, although some femoral neck fractures occur spontaneously. There are severe groin, anterior thigh, and sometimes trochanteric pain and tenderness. The leg is shortened, held extended at the hip and knee, and externally rotated. Plain radiographs will demonstrate the site and severity of these fractures. *Fracture of the greater trochanter* follows a fall and impact on the trochanter. A forceful abductor muscle contraction may also cause trochanteric pain and tenderness by *avulsing the apophysis of the greater trochanter* in a teenage athlete. *Avulsion of the lesser trochanter* follows a forceful contraction of the iliopsoas muscle. There is medial groin pain, intensified by resisted hip flexion, with fracture of the lesser trochanter. Plain radiographs will identify both types of avulsion fractures. *Acetabular fractures* cause groin and trochanteric pain, and the leg is held immobile. A CT scan may be required to identify and clearly delineate this type of fracture. *Fractures near the pubic symphysis* cause inguinal pain that is intensified by weight bearing and movement. There is local tenderness over the pubic bone. A bone scan or delayed radiographs (2 weeks postinjury) may be required to demonstrate these fractures. Pubic symphysis region fractures usually follow minor trauma in an elderly person with osteoporosis.

An *impacted fracture of the femoral neck* may allow weight bearing with or without mild pain. Because results of plain radiographs may be falsely negative shortly after the onset of pain, diagnostic confirmation may require a radionuclide bone scan or a CT scan. Plain radiographs taken 10 days after the injury often reveal the fracture.

Pathologic fracture of the hip (femoral neck and trochanteric region) may present with acute groin, anteromedial, and sometimes trochanteric and lateral thigh pain and tenderness of gradual or sudden onset. Some patients complain of a sudden painful snap in the hip region or giving way of the leg. Metabolic bone disease, Paget's disease, radiation-related bone injury, and metastatic tumor may cause a pathologic fracture. *Stress fractures of the hip (femoral neck or pubic bone)* cause groin and hip aching that is provoked or intensified by activity or weight bearing. These fractures occur in runners, joggers, and military recruits. The diagnosis can be confirmed by radiographic studies or by a radionuclide bone scan when results of plain radiographs are negative.

Acute septic arthritis of the hip may cause fever, chills, and inguinal, and sometimes trochanteric and anterior thigh pain. The pain is usually persistent, throbbing, or aching and is very severe. Any movement may intensify the discomfort. MRI or ultrasonographic studies may confirm the presence of a joint effusion. Synovial fluid analysis reveals an increased concentration of polymorphonuclear leukocytes; and Gram stain and cultures of the fluid reveal the presence of bacteria. Septic arthritis may be polyarticular or monoarticular. Joint drainage and antibiotic therapy usually result in improvement of systemic and local symptoms in patients with septic arthritis. Gonococcal arthritis rarely involves the hips.

Calcium pyrophosphate deposition disease or gout may involve the hip joint and simulate a septic joint. The joint fluid contains calcium pyrophosphate dihydrate or uric acid crystals, respectively, and culture results are negative. Both forms of crystal-induced arthritis respond to colchicine therapy. *Acute rheumatic fever* may cause a migratory polyarthritis that involves one or both hip joints, fever, and elevated levels of antistreptococcal serum antibodies. There is a dramatic response to aspirin therapy. *Acute rheumatoid arthritis* may present as a monoarthritis of the hip. Rheumatoid factor may be present in the serum in an elevated titer, and subcutaneous nodules may be palpable. *Acute arthritis of one hip may occur in patients with chronic rheumatoid arthritis* and may simulate an acute septic arthritis. Results of synovial fluid cultures are negative, and there is a dramatic response to an intraarticular corticosteroid injection.

A juxtaarticular *osteoid osteoma* may cause an acute synovitis. The diagnosis can be confirmed by plain radiographs or a CT scan. *Reiter's syndrome* causes urethritis, conjunctivitis or uveitis, and an asymmetrical polyarthritis involving the hips, knees, shoulders, and other joints.

Adolescents and younger children may develop unilateral or bilateral groin and trochanteric pain. The causes include *transient synovitis of the hip*. This acute, painful, and sometimes febrile disorder follows a self-limited course and usually spontaneously resolves in 2 to 8 weeks. Plain radiographs reveal no evidence of hip injury. *Juvenile rheumatoid arthritis* may involve the hips in its polyarticular or oligoarticular form. Fever, malaise, anorexia, and a characteristic skin rash may accompany the joint symptoms and signs. *Legg-Calvé-Perthes* disease causes inguinal, anteromedial thigh, and knee pain secondary to unilateral or bilateral osteonecrosis of the head of the femur. A radionuclide bone scan, an MRI, or, later in the course, plain radiographs will demonstrate areas of femoral head osteonecrosis. A *slipped capital femoral epiphysis* may also cause groin and anteromedial thigh pain. The diagnosis can be confirmed by plain radiographs. *Pubic osteomyelitis* may cause pubic, groin, and trochanteric pain and tenderness, and fever. A radionuclide bone scan and a CT scan will demonstrate abnormalities of the pubic bone, and serial radiographs may reveal evidence of bone destruction and reactive sclerosis. A bone biopsy and culture may be necessary for diagnosis.

Osteonecrosis of the femoral head causes groin pain, anteromedial thigh pain, and trochanteric pain that is initially felt during walking, running, and weight bearing. Early confirmation of the diagnosis requires an MRI or a radionuclide bone scan. Plain radiographs may remain normal for months after the onset of hip symptoms. Femoral head osteonecrosis may be posttraumatic or idiopathic. The causes of nontraumatic osteonecrosis include corticosteroid administration, alcohol abuse, sickle cell disease, caisson disease, radiation-induced bone injury, Gaucher's disease, systemic lupus erythematosus, and Legg-Calvé-Perthes disease.

Iliopsoas bursitis may cause pain and sometimes a fluctuant mass in the inguinal region. Tenderness is present 2 cm lateral to the femoral pulse. Walking and passive or active hip extension exacerbate the pain. A local injection of lidocaine and a corticosteroid into the tender inguinal site may relieve the pain and tenderness and confirm the diagnosis. Aspiration of bursal fluid, followed by a lidocaine and corticosteroid injection, will sometimes relieve symptoms in patients with a palpable bursal mass. A similar clinical picture can be produced by a *tendinitis of the iliopsoas tendon* and can be relieved by injecting the painful tendon.

Fever, chills, malaise, and groin pain and in some cases an inguinal mass may be caused by an *iliopsoas abscess*. The ipsilateral leg may be held flexed, abducted, and externally rotated at the hip. A positive psoas sign is usually present, and the patient is frequently unable to fully extend the knee (i.e., place the knee flat on the bed). A CT scan or MRI of the lower abdomen and spine will confirm the diagnosis. Most cases arise from bowel perforation or are secondary to a vertebral osteomyelitis. Drainage of the abscess and antibiotic therapy lead to resolution.

Femoral neuropathy causes groin and anterior thigh pain and may cause anteromedial lower leg pain and paresthesias. Severe cases may cause quadriceps weakness and an impaired patellar reflex. Causes of femoral neuropathy include bleeding into the iliopsoas muscle, lower abdominal abscesses and tumors, surgical procedures on the lower abdomen, sickle cell pain crisis, diabetes mellitus, and arterial damage following catheterization of the femoral artery. *Iliofemoral thrombosis* may cause groin and anteromedial thigh pain, diffuse edema of the involved leg, and aching leg discomfort that is exacerbated or provoked by standing and walking. The diagnosis can be confirmed by Doppler ultrasound, impedence plethysmography, B-mode ultrasonography, or contrast venography.

An *inguinal or femoral hernia* may cause inguinal pain that is intensified by standing and relieved by lying down. When the hernia is not detected by physical examination, it can often be demonstrated by contrast herniography. An *incarcerated or strangulated inguinal or femoral hernia* forms a painful and tender local inguinal or femoral mass, and may be associated with the symptoms and signs of intestinal obstruction (e.g., vomiting, obstipation, distension of the abdomen, constant or colicky abdominal pain, and radiographic evidence of bowel obstruction). Surgical intervention may be required to relieve the intestinal obstruction and repair the hernia.

Inguinal or femoral lymph nodes may become enlarged, tender, and painful secondary to a *cellulitis or pyoderma of the leg, perineum, or abdominal wall*. The usual bacterial pathogens are staphylococcal or streptococcal species.

Vibrio vulnificus infection of the lower leg occurs after an injury occurring in seawater. A severe cellulitis, fasciitis, and myositis may occur. The skin may be reddened and swollen, and hemorrhagic bullae may appear in the erythematous region. The bullae may collapse, forming necrotic ulcers. A painful, tender femoral or inguinal lymphadenitis usually occurs. *Vibrio vulnificus* can be identified on Gram stain and culture of fluid from a bulla. *Aeromonas hydrophila* may cause an acute cellulitis and painful, tender femoral or inguinal lymphadenitis. This infection usually follows trauma in a freshwater lake or river.

Bubonic plague can cause a large unilateral femoral or inguinal mass, fever, and prostration. Aspiration of this painful, tender, inguinal mass, followed by a Gram stain and cultures of the aspirate, will usually establish the diagnosis. History of residence or travel in an endemic area is also an important criterion for diagnosis.

Tick-borne *tularemia* may begin as a unilateral leg ulcer and femoral and/or inguinal lymphadenitis. Fever, malaise, chills, sweats, and pneumonia may follow. The diagnosis may sometimes be established by positive sputum or blood culture results, but most cases are diagnosed on clinical criteria and confirmed within 2 to 3 weeks by serologic tests.

Cat-scratch disease causes femoral or inguinal adenopathy

3 to 10 days after a cat scratch on the foot or leg. Node biopsy histopathologic studies, and the presence of characteristic microorganisms visible on a Warthin-Starry silver stain of an involved node support the diagnosis.

Suppurative iliac lymphadenitis may arise in a cellulitis in the leg, perineum, or lower abdomen. Inguinal node inflammation spreads to the iliac nodes, and suppuration involving the iliacus and iliopsoas muscles may occur. High fever, chills, lower abdominal pain, and prostration follow. The ipsilateral hip is flexed, and the lower abdomen is tender, with spasm of the rectus abdominus muscle. A tender posterolateral pelvic or inguinal mass may be present. A CT scan or MRI can define a collection of purulent fluid adjacent to the iliopsoas and iliacus muscles.

Genital herpes causes painful genital ulcers and vesicles that erupt in small groups and a unilateral or bilateral, painful and tender inguinal lymphadenitis. Culture of the genital ulcers will isolate herpes simplex virus.

Chancroid causes ragged, dirty, irregular, painful, and tender genital ulcers, and painful and tender inguinal lymphadenitis. Culture of the genital ulcer will grow *Haemophilus ducreyi*. There is a good response to quinolone or ceftriaxone therapy.

Lymphogranuloma venereum (LGV) causes painful and tender inguinal adenopathy. A "groove" sign is present in only 15 percent of cases. Nodes may suppurate and drain through the skin. Diagnosis requires isolation and identification of a LGV biovar or serologic testing.

Syphilis may rarely cause tender inguinal adenopathy and a tender or painless genital ulcer. The diagnosis can be confirmed by darkfield microscopic examination of the primary lesion and by serologic tests.

Gonococcal (5 percent of cases) *and nongonococcal urethritis* (1 percent of cases) may cause a painful and tender inguinal lymphadenitis on one or both sides.

Trochanteric and Lateral Thigh Pain

A *hip pointer* results from an injury to the iliac crest in a contact sport or may be secondary to a fall on the side. There are local swelling and tenderness over the iliac crest and spasm of the adjacent muscles. A fluctuant mass (hematoma) may be present over the area. An *avulsion fracture of the iliac crest apophysis* may occur following a sudden, forceful contraction of the abdominal muscles while making a turn during running. There are local pain, tenderness, and swelling over the iliac crest. An oblique radiograph of the involved iliac crest will identify the fracture.

Trochanteric bursitis causes lateral hip, buttock, and lateral thigh pain. The aching pain is provoked or intensified by lying on the inflamed bursa or by crossing the ipsilateral leg over the other. There is local tenderness over one of the trochanteric bursae. An injection of lidocaine and a corticosteroid into the tender bursa provides immediate and sometimes permanent re-

lief of all pain. Such a response is diagnostic. In some cases, the pain radiates to the ankle (pseudoradiculopathy) and may masquerade as lumbosacral disc disease. The *snapping hip syndrome* is caused by painful movement of the iliotibial band over the greater trochanter during flexion and internal rotation of the thigh. This recurrent movement may provoke a painful trochanteric bursitis, resulting in more persistent pain. Surgical release of the iliotibial band may be required to prevent recurrence of pain and trochanteric bursitis. *Meralgia paresthestica* causes pain, hyperesthesia, and hypesthesia of an oval patch of skin in the lower third of the lateral thigh. It is caused by a neuropathy of the lateral femoral cutaneous nerve. Compression of the nerve near the anterior superior spine of the ilium is the usual cause. Pressure or tapping over this area may provoke lower lateral thigh paresthesias and pain (positive Tinel's sign). Lateral thigh and trochanteric pain may occur with *acute arthritis of the hip, osteonecrosis of the femoral head,* and a *traumatic fracture of the shaft of the femur.* The latter disorder follows severe trauma to the knee or thigh and is associated with swelling, tenderness, and deformity of the thigh. A plain radiograph will confirm the fracture.

Medial Thigh Pain

An *obturator hernia* usually occurs in an elderly woman who has suffered a recent weight loss or has severe constipation. Pain and/or paresthesias may occur in the medial ipsilateral thigh or knee. This medial thigh pain is intensified by thigh extension, abduction, and internal rotation (Howship-Romberg sign). Thigh flexion relieves the pain, while coughing provokes or intensifies it. A tender mass (the hernia) may be palpable on rectal examination in the obturator canal anterolateral to the rectum. Vaginal examination may reveal a mass above the inferior ramus of the ischium. Some patients hold the painful leg flexed, adducted, and externally rotated at the hip. Clinical and radiographic evidence of intestinal obstruction is usually present. Surgical exploration for relief of intestinal obstruction and repair of the hernia is required.

Medial thigh pain may be caused by a *thrombophlebitis of the greater saphenous vein.* A palpable, tender cord is present in the usual location of this vein. Fever, leukocytosis, and an elevated sedimentation rate may be present.

Herpes simplex may cause an aching pain in the buttocks, medial thigh, and genitalia prior to the eruption of grouped genital ulcers. Cystic, inflammatory, or neoplastic *lesions of the ovary or tube* may cause lower abdominal and medial thigh pain. *Pubic bone disorders* and *ureteral colic* may also refer pain to the medial thigh.

An *adductor muscle strain* may cause medial thigh and groin pain that is intensified by thigh adduction or abduction. Local tenderness is present over the adductor muscles and their origin on the pubic bone.

An *iliopsoas strain* may cause deep groin and medial thigh pain. Hip flexion against resistance intensifies the pain. The hip is held in flexion. Radiographs may show an *avulsion fracture of the lesser trochanter* in some patients.

Pubic Pain

Osteitis pubis may cause pubic, perineal, medial groin, and thigh pain of an aching or burning nature. There is tenderness of the symphysis and the origins of the adductor muscles, inguinal ligament, and rectus abdominis muscle on the pubic bone. An antalgic or a waddling gait secondary to adductor spasm may occur. Coughing, sneezing, climbing stairs, and resisted abduction or adduction of the thigh intensify the pain. Plain radiographs of the pelvis may show resorption of the medial aspect of the pubic bone, widening of the symphysis pubis, osteopenia of the bones adjacent to the symphysis, erosions and a "moth-eaten" appearance of the pubic bones. This disorder may follow bladder and prostate surgery, pregnancy, or pelvic trauma and may occur in soccer players, runners, and walking racers during training or competition. It may be confused with *pyogenic arthritis of the symphysis pubis* and with pyogenic or tuberculous *osteomyelitis of the pubic bone*. Biopsy and culture of the involved area are often necessary to exclude an infectious process. Some patients with osteitis pubis may have fever and an elevated sedimentation rate, findings usually expected in the presence of infection.

Pathologic fractures of the pubic rami or symphysis may cause local pubic and groin pain. Such fractures occur in elderly women with rheumatoid arthritis and/or osteoporosis. *Stress fractures of the pubic bones* occur in younger women involved in jogging or long-distance running. A pathologic or a stress fracture of a pubic bone may be apparent on a plain radiograph 3 or more weeks after the onset of pain or may be detected only by a radionuclide bone scan. In older patients, a CT scan or a bone biopsy may be required to differentiate a stress fracture from metastatic carcinoma.

Pubic osteolysis may cause groin and lateral hip pain and radiographic evidence of pubic bone osteolysis in elderly women. Because biopsies may be misdiagnosed as a low-grade chondrosarcoma, careful review of biopsy material is necessary before extensive and mutilating surgery is performed.

A small percentage of women may develop disabling *postpartum suprapubic and symphyseal pain* and tenderness. Examination reveals symphyseal separation and tenderness. Walking and weight bearing may be impossible. Symptoms resolve spontaneously over a period of 3 weeks. This disorder may be a mild form of osteitis pubis or a distinct entity (i.e., symptomatic symphyseal separation).

Posterior Thigh Pain

The *pyriformis syndrome* causes unilateral aching upper buttock pain that may radiate down the posterior thigh. This pain is exacerbated by prolonged sitting and is often more severe at night. There is tenderness of the pyriformis muscle on rectal examination. The pain may be intensified by resisted abduction and simultaneous external rotation of the thigh. Forced internal rotation of the extended thigh may also provoke or intensify the pain. Tenderness may be present over the sciatic notch. Injection of the pyriformis muscle with lidocaine and a corticosteroid may relieve symptoms.

The *hamstring syndrome* causes lower gluteal pain and posterior thigh pain that is intensified by sitting and is relieved by standing or another change of position. Stretching exercises, sprinting, hurdling, or kicking a soccer ball provoke the pain. Slow running and lying down are seldom associated with pain. There is local tenderness over the ischial tuberosity. The sciatic nerve is compressed at the ischial tuberosity by fibrous bands and hamstring tendons. Division of the hamstring tendons enough to decompress the sciatic nerve relieves the pain. Patients often have a history of recurrent hamstring "injury," which may be really caused by repeated bouts of sciatic nerve irritation. *Hamstring muscle strain* begins during running or hurdling as a sharp, tearing pain in the lower buttock and/or posterior thigh, sometimes associated with a snapping sound. There are local posterior thigh tenderness and, if the strain is third-degree, a palpable defect in one of the hamstring muscles. Tenderness over the ischial tuberosity on the painful side may be detected. Active flexion of the lower leg against resistance intensifies the pain. A plain radiograph of the thigh and ischial tuberosity should be taken to exclude avulsion of the apophysis of the ischial tuberosity. *Avulsion of the ischial apophysis* usually occurs in running, hurdling, broad jumping, football, dancing, or skating. The age range for this injury is 8 to 24 years, with most cases occurring between 13 and 17 years. *Ischial bursitis* causes pain and tenderness over the ischial tuberosity that is intensified by sitting or by running uphill.

Radicular pain in an L5 or S1 distribution involves the posterolateral and posterior thigh and lower leg. Increases in intraspinal pressure that accompany coughing, sneezing, or straining at stool may provoke or intensify radiating jabs of pain into the thigh, lower leg, and foot. The straight leg-raising test and crossed straight leg-raising test usually provoke thigh and lower leg pain at 30 to 45° of elevation. An S1 root lesion impairs the ankle jerk. Lumbosacral back pain is usually associated with the radicular pain. The common causes include *disc protrusion,* spinal stenosis, and lateral recess stenosis. A *spinal epidural abscess* should be suspected when there are fever, chills, malaise, neck stiffness, midline lumbar ache and tenderness, bilateral or unilateral radiculitis, leg weakness and sensory loss, and symptoms of bowel and bladder dysfunction. Similar findings in an afebrile patient with a history of liver disease or a coagulopathy (e.g., hemophiliacs and anticoagulant users) suggest a *spinal epidural or subdural hematoma*. A disc protrusion, lateral recess stenosis, abscess, hematoma, or tumor can be detected by a CT-enhanced myelogram or MRI. These imaging studies reveal no evidence of a mass lesion in patients with acute bilateral buttock and posterior thigh pain, saddle hypesthesia, and bladder or bowel dysfunction due to *conus medullaris infarction*.

Posterior femoral cutaneous neuropathy causes posterior thigh pain and a patchy hypesthesia of the posterior thigh and/ or scrotum or labium majus. Pressure over the nerve at the ischial tuberosity and direct trauma are possible causes. *Lumbar facet joint disease* may cause buttock and posterior thigh pain on one side. Such pain may be provoked or intensified by extension and rotation of the lumbar area and may be associated with localized lumbar paraspinal tenderness and CT evidence of a facet joint abnormality. A facet joint injection with a local anesthetic and a corticosteroid may provide transient or permanent relief of buttock and posterior thigh pain.

Sacroiliitis causes medial buttock pain associated with morning stiffness. The pain may be unilateral or bilateral and may radiate down one or both posterior thighs to the popliteal region. The pain is often improved by exercise and activity and exacerbated by rest in bed or sitting in a chair. Gaenslen's test and the straight leg-raising test may cause buttock and upper posterior thigh pain. Sacroiliitis may be part of an attack of *reactive arthritis* associated with a diarrheal illness (e.g., caused by *Campylobacter, Shigella, Salmonella, or Yersinia* species) or with urethritis. Many of these patients test positive for HLA-B27. Sacroiliac pain, swelling, and tenderness in association with a spiking fever, chills, sweats, and leukocytosis may be caused by a *septic sacroiliitis. Sacroiliac joint sprain* with pain, local joint tenderness, and a positive Gaenslen's test may occur during athletic activity. The buttock and posterior thigh pain may be intensified by sitting, bending, or running. *Myofascial pain* causes buttock and posterior thigh aching associated with a tender gluteal muscle trigger point. This pain may be relieved by injection of the trigger point with lidocaine and a corticosteroid.

A *posterior compartment syndrome* may follow posterior thigh trauma with or without other injuries. There is excruciating posterior thigh pain that is intensified by active or passive leg movement. The posterior thigh is extremely tender, and there is increased tension in the muscles of the posterior compartment. A measurement of intracompartmental pressure will confirm the diagnosis, and surgical decompression will relieve the thigh pain and distal dysesthesias.

Anterior Thigh Pain

Bilateral anterior thigh muscle pain and tenderness associated with fever and chills may be a manifestation of *bacteremia. Femoral neuropathy* may cause anterior and anteromedial thigh pain and paresthesias. Anteromedial lower leg pain and paresthesias may also occur. Causes include retroperitoneal bleeding, tumors, abscesses, diabetes mellitus, trauma, sickle cell disease, and nerve compression during surgical procedures in the lower abdomen, or as a complication of femoral artery catheterization. *L3 or L4 root compression* may cause similar anterior thigh pain that may be intensified by straight leg-raising, coughing, sneezing, or straining. MRI or a CT-enhanced myelogram will identify a *protruding L2–L3 or L3–L4 disc* or a lateral recess stenosis responsible for the radiculopathy.

Fracture of the femoral shaft may occur secondary to trauma or in association with overuse during running or other athletic activities (i.e., *stress fracture*). Trauma-related fractures can be imaged by a plain radiograph of the thigh, but stress fractures may require a radionuclide bone scan to confirm the diagnosis and identify the fracture site because results of a plain radiograph may be negative or show only nonspecific changes.

An *anterior compartment syndrome* may occur with an injury to the thigh with or without other injuries. There is excruciating anterior thigh pain associated with local tenderness. Palpation of the anterior compartment reveals swelling and increased tension of the underlying muscle mass. Passive stretching of the anterior thigh muscles by flexion of the knee intensifies the pain. The diagnosis can be confirmed by measuring the intracompartmental pressure. Decompression of the anterior compartment before the occurrence of irreversible muscle and nerve damage leads to resolution of pain and weakness.

A *sartorius or quadriceps muscle strain* begins abruptly with sharp anterior thigh pain during athletic activity. Use of the torn muscles or passive stretching provokes or intensifies the pain. There are local muscle tenderness and, in a third-degree strain, a palpable defect in the muscle. In some cases, a hematoma may be palpable in the muscle defect, and skin ecchymoses may appear over the tender area during the first 72 h after the injury.

Generalized Thigh Pain

A high-energy injury to the leg in a motor vehicle accident can cause a *fracture of the femoral shaft* with shortening and lateral or anterior angulation deformity of the thigh with severe pain, swelling, and local tenderness. Plain radiographs confirm the diagnosis. A *complex compartment syndrome* involving the anterior and posterior compartments of the thigh can cause diffuse thigh pain, tenderness, and increased palpable tension in both muscle compartments. The diagnosis can be confirmed by measurement of intracompartmental pressures. *Sickle cell pain crisis* can cause diffuse bilateral or unilateral thigh and sometimes lower leg pain. Skin allodynia and hyperesthesia usually accompany the pain. Knee pain, swelling, and fever may also occur. *Pathologic fracture of the shaft of the femur* may be accompanied by a snapping sound, pain, tenderness, and a sensation of giving way of the leg in the absence of significant trauma. Such fractures occur through cystic, neoplastic, or osteopenic bone. Biopsy may be required for a specific diagnosis.

Pyomyositis may cause fever, chills, malaise, and aching pain in one or several regions of the thigh. It is associated with local swelling, tenderness, induration, and sometimes warmth and redness of the overlying skin. A CT scan of the thigh will demonstrate one or more abscesses in the thigh muscles. Surgical exploration will confirm the diagnosis and allow drainage of pus. This disorder occurs in tropical areas and in patients with poorly controlled diabetes. A *soft tissue sarcoma* may

TABLE OF DISEASE INCIDENCE

INCIDENCE PER 100,000 (APPROXIMATE)

Common (>100)	Uncommon (>5–100)	Rare (>0–5)
	INGUINAL AND ANTEROMEDIAL THIGH PAIN	
Femoral neck fracture	Dislocation of the hip	Pathologic fracture of the intertrochanteric
Intertrochanteric fracture	Greater trochanteric fracture	region or femoral shaft
Transient synovitis of the hip (adolescents)	Lesser trochanteric fracture	Septic arthritis of the hip
Inguinal or femoral hernia	Subtrochanteric fracture	Calcium pyrophosphate deposition disease of
Acute femoral or inguinal lymphadenitis due	Central acetabular fracture and fracture-	the hip
to bacterial cellulitis, bacterial pyoderma,	dislocation	Gouty arthritis of the hip
cat-scratch disease, genital herpes, or	Fractures at or near the pubic symphysis	Acute arthritis of the hip with rheumatoid
gonococcal urethritis	Impacted fracture of the femoral neck	arthritis
	Pathologic fracture of the femoral neck	Juxtaarticular osteoid osteoma
	Stress fracture of the hip and pelvis	Osteomyelitis of the pubic bone
	Acute rheumatic fever	Iliopsoas abscess
	Acute rheumatoid arthritis of the hip	Femoral neuropathy
	Reiter's syndrome	Acute lymphadenitis due to *V. vulnificus*
	Juvenile rheumatoid arthritis of the hip	infection or *A. hydrophila* infection
	(adolescents)	Bubonic plague
	Legg-Calvé-Perthes disease (adolescents)	Tularemia
	Slipped capital femoral epiphysis	Iliac (suppurative) lymphadenitis
	(adolescents)	Chancroid
	Osteonecrosis of the femoral head	LGV
	Iliopsoas bursitis	Primary syphilis
	Iliopsoas tendinitis	
	Iliofemoral venous thrombosis	
	Incarceration or strangulation of inguinal or	
	femoral hernia	
	TROCHANTERIC AND LATERAL THIGH PAIN	
Trochanteric bursitis	Hip pointer	
Snapping hip syndrome	Avulsion fracture of the iliac crest apophysis	
Meralgia paresthetica	Acute arthritis of the hip	
Fracture of the femoral shaft (traumatic)	Osteonecrosis of the hip	
	MEDIAL THIGH PAIN	
Herpes simplex neuritis	Obturator hernia	
Referred pain from tubo-ovarian lesions or	Greater saphenous vein phlebitis	
ureteral colic	Referred pain from pubic bone disorders or	
Adductor muscle strain	iliopsoas avulsion fracture of the lesser	
Iliopsoas muscle strain	trochanter	

cause severe thigh pain, tenderness, and swelling. The diagnosis can be confirmed by a CT scan of the thigh and biopsy. *Retroperitoneal perforation of the colon* secondary to diverticulitis or carcinoma can cause thigh pain, swelling, tenderness, and crepitus associated with fever and chills by spread of infection into the leg. Plain radiographs of the leg will demonstrate gas in the soft tissues. Exploration of the thigh reveals inflammatory fluid and abscesses. Thigh pain may also result from retroperitoneal infection that causes a *lumbosacral plexopathy*. In this situation pain occurs, but no gas is seen in the thigh on plain radiographs.

Iliofemoral venous thrombosis may cause a diffuse thigh ache and swelling of the leg. The pain may be intensified by standing and walking. The skin of the leg may be cool and sometimes pale or cyanotic. Local tenderness medial to the femoral artery may be present. The diagnosis can be confirmed by Doppler ultrasound or impedence plethysmography. *Stress fractures of the femoral shaft* cause diffuse thigh pain and tenderness. They occur in runners or in military trainees.

Muscle strain due to overuse may cause diffuse thigh muscle

aching and tenderness in weekend athletes and in military recruits during the first weeks of basic training. Walking and running intensify the pain, and rest relieves it within 1 to 3 days. Rarely, red-brown urine (myoglobinuria) may accompany the thigh pain and tenderness.

Dermatomyositis or polymyositis may cause diffuse thigh pain, tenderness, and weakness, with or without an accompanying rash. All activities involving the legs may be painful, and the gait may become unsteady and waddling. The diagnosis of polymyositis may be confirmed by measurement of serum creatine kinase and aldolase activities, electromyography, and muscle biopsy. Pain and weakness respond to prednisone therapy. Diagnostic studies to exclude malignancy or an associated connective tissue disorder may sometimes be required. Infectious polymyositis may cause an illness similar to that produced by idiopathic polymyositis. Toxoplasmosis, Lyme disease, and HIV are possible causes of infectious polymyositis.

Rhabdomyolysis causes severe muscle pain and tenderness, and sometimes skin edema and ecchymosis. The creatinine

TABLE OF DISEASE INCIDENCE (*Continued*)

INCIDENCE PER 100,000 (APPROXIMATE)

Common (>100)	Uncommon (>5–100)	Rare (>0–5)
	PUBIC PAIN	
	Osteitis pubis	Osteomyelitis of the pubic bone
	Postpartum symphyseal pain	Pyogenic arthritis of symphysis pubis
	Pathologic fracture of the pubic bone	Stress fracture of the pubic bone
		Pubic osteolysis
	POSTERIOR THIGH PAIN	
Hamstring muscle strain	Pyriformis syndrome	Radicular pain due to epidural abscess,
Myofascial pain	Hamstring syndrome	epidural hematoma, or conus medullaris
Radicular pain due to disc protrusion	Ischial apophysis avulsion	infarction
	Ischial bursitis	Posterior femoral cutaneous neuropathy
	Lumbar facet joint disease	Sacroiliac septic arthritis
	Sacroiliitis due to reactive arthritis or	Posterior compartment syndrome of the
	sacroiliac sprain	thigh
	ANTERIOR THIGH PAIN	
Femoral shaft fracture (traumatic)	Femoral neuropathy	Bacteremia-associated anterior thigh pain
Quadriceps muscle strain	Radicular pain (L2–L4 spinal roots)	Anterior compartment syndrome
	Femoral shaft stress fracture	
	Sartorius muscle strain	
	GENERALIZED THIGH PAIN	
Muscle strain due to overuse	Traumatic fracture of the femur	Pathologic fracture of the femur
Fever-related myalgias	Idiopathic dermatomyositis or polymyositis	Pyomyositis
Sickle cell pain crisis	Iliofemoral venous thrombosis	Soft tissue sarcoma
		Retroperitoneal perforation of the colon and
		thigh infection
		Retroperitoneal perforation of the colon and
		lumbosacral plexitis
		Infectious polymyositis
		Rhabdomyolysis and myoglobinuria
		Combined anterior and posterior
		compartment syndrome
		Stress fracture of the femoral shaft

kinase level is markedly elevated, and *myoglobinuria* is present. Bilateral thigh, lower leg, and sometimes shoulder and arm pain and tenderness may be present. The causes of acute rhabdomyolysis include enzyme, substrate, and electrolyte deficiencies, infectious agents, drugs and toxins, crush injury, and severe myopathies.

Fever may cause diffuse thigh and buttock, and sometimes shoulder girdle and upper arm aching, without local tenderness. This pain responds to aspirin and disappearance of the fever.

☐ DESCRIPTION OF LISTED DISEASES

Inguinal and Anteromedial Thigh Pain

1. DISLOCATION AND FRACTURE-DISLOCATION OF THE HIP

Dislocation of the hip requires a large amount of force. Most cases result from motor vehicle collisions involving unrestrained occupants. Other causes include automobile-

pedestrian or motorcycle accidents, falls, and falls or collisions resulting from football, skiing, and volleyball.

A. Posterior Posterior dislocation is 9 times more frequent than anterior dislocation. Dislocation may occur in a motor vehicle accident when the left knee of the unrestrained driver strikes the dashboard and forces are directed up the thigh toward the hip. When dislocation occurs, groin and lateral hip pain is usually present and is intensified by jarring or attempted movement of the thigh. The leg is shortened and held flexed, adducted, and internally rotated. An associated fracture of the acetabulum, femoral head, or knee may be present. Plain radiographs and a CT scan of the hip will establish the diagnosis and detect other injuries. CT scans are especially useful, since they can detect intraarticular osteochondral fragments and subtle fractures of the femoral head or acetabulum that may be missed on plain radiographs. Sciatic nerve injury with posterior and posterolateral leg pain and paresthesias may occur in up to 19 percent of cases.

B. Anterior Anterior dislocation of the hip may cause similar groin and lateral hip pain and tenderness. If the dislocation is anterosuperior, the leg is held extended and externally rotated, while an anteroinferior displacement of the femoral head results in thigh flexion, abduction, and external rotation. In anterosuperior dislocations, the femoral head may be palpable near the anterosuperior iliac spine (iliac type) or in the groin (pubic type). In the anteroinferior type, the head may be palpable in the obturator foramen. A plain anteroposterior radiograph will demonstrate the dislocation. Assessment of associated femoral head and acetabular fractures and screening for free osteochondral fragments may be accomplished by a CT scan.

2. TRAUMATIC FRACTURES OF THE HIP

A. Femoral Neck Fractures These fractures are more common in women than in men and occur at an average age of 76 years. Most occur after a fall from a standing position to the ground, although a small percentage of femoral neck fractures occur while the patient is standing. The latter group of patients may experience a sudden snap, groin pain, and/or giving way of the limb, resulting in a fall. In one large study ($n = 1449$ fractures), only 3 percent of fractures were unrelated to trauma.

After a fall, severe, constant pain that is intensified by jarring or leg movement occurs in the groin, trochanteric area, and medial thigh. The leg is usually shortened, extended, and externally rotated. Weight bearing and limb movement are extremely painful and are resisted. Edema of the affected leg may occur secondary to immobility and/or venous thrombosis. Plain radiographs and/or a CT scan will define the extent of injury.

B. Intertrochanteric Fractures This extracapsular fracture usually follows a fall from the standing position. The average age of patients with this fracture is 66 to 76 years of age, and the female/male ratio varies from 1.5:1 to 8:1. Extracapsular hip fractures occur with 4 times the frequency of femoral neck fractures.

There is severe groin, trochanteric area, and medial thigh pain that is intensified by jarring or attempted movement of the leg. The leg may be normal in length or, more commonly, shortened. It is extended and may be externally rotated to 90°. The degree of external rotation is often greater than that occurring with femoral neck fractures. Swelling and skin ecchymoses may appear over the hip region during the next 48 h. A true anteroposterior radiograph taken with the limb in internal rotation provides superior visualization of the oblique fracture line. A lateral radiograph is useful in imaging posterior fracture fragments and in determining fracture stability. Intertrochanteric fractures commonly occur through osteoporotic bone, less frequently through osteomalacic bone, and rarely through pagetoid bone.

C. Greater Trochanteric Fracture In adults, a comminuted fracture results from a direct blow to the greater trochanter. In the 7- to 17-year-old age group, an abductor muscle contraction may cause avulsion of the trochanteric apophysis with posterosuperior displacement of the fragment. Lateral hip pain is associated with tenderness of the greater trochanter. The thigh is held in flexion. The diagnosis may be confirmed by a plain radiograph.

D. Lesser Trochanteric Avulsion Fracture This is a fracture of young adults and adolescents. Medial groin pain is associated with femoral triangle tenderness. Pain may be provoked or intensified by hip flexion against resistance. Ludloff's sign (iliopsoas dysfunction) is positive (e.g., the seated patient is unable to lift the affected leg from the ground). This fracture results from a forceful contraction of the ilipsoas muscle, causing avulsion of the apophysis of the lesser trochanter.

E. Subtrochanteric Fracture These fractures involve the region between the lesser trochanter and a transverse line 5 cm distal to it. Direct trauma is the usual cause.

The fracture may be an extension of an intertrochanteric fracture, or it may occur as an independent lesion. It may be seen in an elderly person after a fall or in a young adult after high-energy trauma. The symptoms and signs may mimic those of an intertrochanteric fracture, or more distal fractures may produce a clinical picture usually associated with a femoral shaft fracture. Blood loss into the thigh may exceed 1 liter, resulting in hypovolemia and symptoms and signs of shock. The fracture can be imaged by plain radiography. A plain radiograph of the pelvis should also be obtained to exclude dislocation of the hip or a pelvic fracture.

F. Central Acetabular Fracture and Fracture-Dislocation Central fracture-dislocation may follow a force applied to the lateral aspect of the greater trochanter in a motor vehicle accident or fall, a force applied to the distal femur with the hip in abduction, a spontaneous seizure, or electroconvulsive therapy.

There is severe groin and lateral hip pain that is intensified by attempts to passively move the hip. Slight shortening of the involved leg may be present. Anteroposterior, internal, and external oblique radiographic views and a CT scan will clearly define the extent of these fractures. Sciatic nerve injury is most commonly associated with burst-type fractures, or associated pubic rami, or sacroiliac fractures.

G. Fractures at or near the Pubic Symphysis Severe hip and/or groin pain may follow immediately or several days after minor trauma (e.g., a fall). The pain is intensified by movement, weight bearing, palpation over the pubis, and Patrick's test (fabere sign). Other findings include skin ecchymoses and tenderness over the fracture site on the pubic bone. This injury usually occurs in elderly people in a setting of osteoporosis and/or rheumatoid arthritis. Results of initial plain radiographs and a CT scan of the pelvis may be negative. Radiographs obtained after 10 to 14 days or a technetium-99m bone scan will usually demonstrate fracture of a pubic ramus at or near the symphysis.

Fracture of two rami on the same side may result from a pedestrian-automobile accident, a motor vehicle accident, or a fall. Local tenderness and ecchymoses in the groin and medial thigh may accompany the fracture. The fabere sign will be positive. Plain radiographs will establish the diagnosis.

H. Impacted Fracture of the Femoral Neck A sudden twist of the hip or a minor fall may be followed by groin, medial thigh, and sometimes lateral hip pain that is intensified by walking and weight bearing. Passive range-of-motion testing may cause only minor pain. Percussion over the greater trochanter may be painful. Plain radiography may be falsely negative for a fracture. A radionuclide bone scan, CT scan, or MRI may be required to detect the fracture. Repeated radiographic studies after 10 days of avoidance of weight bearing may also detect an impacted fracture missed on initial radiographic assessment. It is important to avoid weight bearing on such lesions, since displacement of the fracture may occur. Patients with lateral hip pain without evidence of a fracture following trauma probably have a severe contusion of the periosteum and cortical bone.

3. PATHOLOGIC FRACTURE OF THE HIP

There may be abrupt onset of pain in the groin and/or trochanteric area following a sudden twist or a minor fall. Some patients complain of a sudden, painful snap in the hip or giving way of the involved leg. Plain radiographs may demonstrate the fracture and an underlying bone disorder. Weight bearing and ambulation with pain may be possible.

A. Femoral Neck Fracture of the femoral neck may be caused by postmenopausal and senile osteoporosis, osteomalacia, Paget's disease, and renal osteodystrophy or follow radiotherapy to the pelvis for the treatment of carcinoma of the uterus or ovary. Bilateral fractures may occur in up to 40 percent of patients with radiation-related fractures. In patients with postirradiation disease of the femoral neck, pain may precede evidence of a fracture by 1 to 2 months. Activity and weight bearing intensify the pain. Examination may cause pain during rotational movements. Plain radiographs in patients with radiation-related fractures may show a dense transverse line across the femoral neck, a partial fracture line, and/or development of a coxa vara deformity on an anteroposterior radiograph

without any displacement on the lateral view. Metastatic tumor may cause femoral neck fracture with groin and hip pain and loss of the ability to bear weight and walk. The diagnosis can be confirmed at surgery or by an aspiration needle biopsy. Breast and lung carcinomas are the most frequent sources of such metastases, but lymphoma, myeloma, and carcinoma of the kidney, bladder, colon, prostate, and other sites may also metastasize to the hip.

B. Intertrochanteric and Shaft Fracture Pathologic fractures are usually due to metastatic carcinoma (30–50 percent) and rarely to a primary bone tumor (e.g., chondrosarcoma, osteogenic sarcoma, or giant cell tumor). Osteoporosis, sometimes intensified by corticosteroid therapy; osteomalacia; Paget's disease; or Gaucher's disease may also result in pathologic fracture.

4. STRESS FRACTURES OF THE HIP AND PELVIS

Femoral neck or pubic stress fractures have been reported in joggers, runners, and military recruits. Female joggers or runners are more likely to have a stress fracture of a pubic ramus. These injuries are believed to be due to overuse during training. Femoral neck or pubic rami fractures result in groin and hip aching that is intensified by activity and weight bearing. Local inguinal tenderness may be present, and pain may occur at the extremes of passive motion testing at the hip. Results of radiographs taken within a few days of the onset of symptoms may be negative in up to 80 percent of cases. Radiographic abnormalities may never occur if therapy is started early. Symptoms in military recruits begin 2 to 8 weeks after the onset of a physical conditioning program. A radionuclide bone scan will usually establish the diagnosis and localize any fractures.

Radiographic changes occur in stages. Initially, radiographs of the hip and pelvis may appear normal, and only the bone scan results are positive. After several weeks endosteal or periosteal callus (sclerosis) may appear on a radiograph at the site of maximal radionuclide uptake. A cortical crack may then develop, widen, and, if the diagnosis is missed or delayed, fracture displacement may occur. Treatment with bed rest and then partial weight bearing on crutches results in relief of pain and fracture healing in patients with normal radiographs or sclerotic lesions. Patients with more advanced radiographic changes (e.g., widening of the fracture line or fracture of both cortical surfaces) may require surgical intervention.

5. ACUTE ARTHRITIS IN ADULTS

A. Septic Arthritis There is a gradual or abrupt onset of groin, trochanteric, and sometimes anteromedial thigh pain. Referral of pain to the knee is common. Walking, weight bearing, or any movement may provoke or intensify the pain. In some cases, the pain is very severe, throbbing, and persistent at rest, interfering with sleep. Fever and chills may occur but are less common in patients with gonococcal infection. Examination may reveal evidence of toxemia, and, in the case of gonococcal arthritis, there may be red-based pustules and hemorrhagic vesicles on the distal portion of the extremities. The gait is antalgic, or the pain may be too severe to allow weight bearing. In the supine position, the patient may hold the leg flexed, abducted or adducted, and externally rotated. Tenderness and increased skin temperature may be present over the inguinal region. Range of motion is restricted by pain and associated muscle spasm. Radiographic changes may include soft tissue edema in the fat planes around the hip and osteoporosis of the femoral head. Erosive and resorptive changes are late findings and, if present, indicate a process of several months' duration. A radionuclide bone scan may show increased uptake over the hip joint but is nonspecific and cannot differentiate septic arthritis and osteomyelitis. MRI or ultrasonography may confirm the presence of an effusion in the hip joint. Hip arthrocentesis is essential to confirm a diagnosis of septic arthritis. The synovial fluid is often grossly purulent or turbid. The leukocyte count varies from 20,000 to 450,000 cell/mm^3, with a polymorphonuclear leukocyte predominence of 75 percent or greater.

Synovial fluid glucose levels may be decreased (50 percent of cases) and protein concentrations elevated. *Neisseria gonorrhoeae* infection is a frequent cause of septic arthritis in sexually active adults below age 50 but rarely causes monoarthritis of the hip and seldom affects the hip in its polyarthritic form. Septic arthritis of the hip is most frequently caused by *Staphylococcus aureus*. Streptococcal species and *Hemophilus influenzae* are also isolated in some cases. Rare causes of infectious arthritis of the hip include *Pseudomonas* species (e.g., in intravenous drug abusers), *Salmonella* species (e.g., in patients with sickle cell disease), gram-negative bacteria (e.g., in patients with urinary tract infections or intraabdominal sepsis), and *Brucella* species (e.g., in patients ingesting unpasteurized milk or cheese, in visitors from an endemic region, and in workers with an occupational risk for brucellosis). Risk factors for septic arthritis of the hip include preexisting osteoarthritis, rheumatoid arthritis, gout, hemophilic arthropathy, pseudogout, and osteonecrosis of the hip. Chronic disorders such as malignancy, systemic lupus erythematosus, cirrhosis, renal failure, malnutrition, diabetes, and the use of corticosteroids and other immunosuppressive drugs are associated with septic arthritis of the hip and other joints. Some cases may be secondary to an adjacent infection in the femoral head or acetabulum. Needle or surgical drainage of the hip joint and intravenous antibiotic therapy result in gradual resolution of the infection and the return of pain-free, functional use of the hip. Delay in diagnosis may result in permanent hip dysfunction.

B. Acute Calcium Pyrophosphate Deposition Disease
Pain in the groin and trochanteric region and pain on joint motion and weight bearing occur. The synovial fluid contains an increased concentration of polymorphonuclear leukocytes and calcium pyrophosphate dihydrate crystals. Chondrocalcinosis of the knees, wrists, and shoulders may be visible on plain radiographs of these joints.

C. Acute Gout Gouty arthritis of the hip may be indistinguishable from calcium pyrophosphate deposition disease except for an elevated serum uric acid level and the presence of urate crystals in synovial fluid. Both forms of crystal-induced arthritis may respond dramatically to colchicine therapy or nonsteroidal anti-inflammatory drugs.

D. Acute Rheumatic Fever This disorder may present with fever, migratory polyarthritis, subcutaneous nodules, and elevated serum levels of antistreptolysin O, antihyaluronidase, and antideoxyribonuclease B or an elevated and/or rising titer on a Streptozyme test. Leukocytosis and an elevated sedimentation rate are usually present. Shoulder, hip, wrist, knee, ankle, hand, and foot joints may be serially involved. Symptoms respond dramatically to aspirin therapy.

E. Rheumatoid Arthritis

1. Acute Rheumatoid Arthritis Patients may have a monoarthritis of the hip with groin, trochanteric, and sometimes medial thigh pain that is intensified or provoked by walking, weight bearing, and range-of-motion testing. Subcutaneous nodules and positive serum titer results for rheumatoid factor may be present. Within the first 2 years, morning stiffness of the hip and other joints, arthritic involvement of two or more additional joint areas, a symmetrical polyarthritis, involvement of finger and wrist joints, and characteristic radiographic joint changes (e.g., juxtaarticular osteopenia and erosive bone lesions) may also develop.

2. Chronic Rheumatoid Arthritis with Acute Noninfectious Arthritis of the Hip There may be an abrupt onset of pain in one hip severe enough to prevent weight bearing, without fever. Other joints may become painful and swollen. Synovial fluid counts vary from 26,000 to 71,000 cells/mm^3, with a polymorphonuclear predominence, but results of the Gram stain and cultures are negative. There is a dramatic response to intraarticular injection of a corticosteroid into the involved hip.

F. Osteoid Osteoma An osteoid osteoma adjacent to

the hip joint may cause a synovitis with fever, groin and trochanteric pain, decreased range of motion, muscle spasm in the thigh, and pain on walking or running. Night pain, relieved dramatically by aspirin, is characteristic. Plain radiographs may reveal a juxtaarticular, lucent nidus surrounded by sclerotic bone. A CT scan may be required to clearly define the lesion. Surgical excision is necessary.

G. Reiter's Syndrome This disorder may begin with dysuria and discharge from the penis, a conjunctivitis or iridocyclitis, or a diarrheal illness. An asymmetrical arthritis may involve the hip, knees, shoulders, elbows, and wrists. Skin and mucous membrane lesions include balanitis circinata and keratoderma blennorrhagicum. The course may be acute, and symptoms may respond to nonsteroidal anti-inflammatory drugs but not to antibiotics.

6. ACUTE SYNOVITIS OF THE HIP IN CHILDREN AND ADOLESCENTS

Septic arthritis, acute rheumatic fever, monoarticular rheumatoid arthritis, and juxtaarticular osteoid osteoma may also occur in this age range. Disorders usually seen only in patients under age 18 are described in this section.

A. Transient Synovitis of the Hip This disorder occurs in the 3- to 10-year-old age range, but cases in patients as young as 3 months and as old as 15 years have been reported. Male/female ratios vary from 2:1 to 4:1. This disorder is the commonest cause of acute hip pain in children and adolescents. There is a sudden onset of groin and anterior thigh pain, a limp, and fever. The temperature range is 36 to 40.1°C (97 to 104.2°F), with a mean of 37.7°C (99.9°F). The leukocyte count varies from 3300 to 28,000 cells/mm^3 and 88 percent of patients have a count in the normal range. Radiographs may show hip joint distension (25 percent), soft tissue edema (4 percent), or medial joint space widening (3 percent), but in most cases (68 percent) there are no abnormalities. Results of radionuclide scans with technetium 99m were abnormal in only 53 percent of cases in one reported series. Joint fluid is seldom aspirated. In those cases with a successful arthrocentesis, the fluid is serous or serosanguineous, contains few leukocytes, and is culture-negative. Acute symptoms resolve within days or weeks. Severe pain and muscle spasm may require hospitalization, use of Buck's traction, and narcotics. Clinical follow-up is required, since a small minority of patients may differentiate into specific disorders such as juvenile rheumatoid arthritis, osteoid osteoma, or Legg-Calvé-Perthes disease.

B. Juvenile Rheumatoid Arthritis This disorder may present as a polyarthritis (five or more joints involved), an oligoarthritis (four or fewer joints involved), or a febrile, systemic disorder with a rash.

Acute polyarthritis involving one or both hips, knees, ankles, wrists, elbows, and hands may occur. Hip involvement causes groin and trochanteric pain that is intensified or provoked by walking and range-of-motion testing. Neck and back pain and tenderness result from apophyseal joint involvement. Systemic manifestations include a low-grade fever, lymphadenopathy, and hepatosplenomegaly. A characteristic erythematous, morbilliform, macular rash of the trunk and extremities may occur in patients with polyarthritis. Rheumatoid factor is present in only 10 percent, and antinuclear antibody in 40 percent of cases. Oligoarthritis occurs in less than 33 percent, frequently involves the knees, and seldom affects the hips. Systemic symptoms such as malaise, weakness, anorexia, high spiking temperatures, a rash, hepatosplenomegaly, and lymphadenopathy may occur without arthritis in 10 to 15 percent of cases. Skin lesions may be provoked by rubbing the skin (Koebner's phenomenon), a warm bath, or emotional stress. Cutaneous lesions are usually transient and appear in crops. Tenosynovitis of the extensor tendons of the hands and the tendons of the ankle and foot may occur. Subcutaneous nodules may occur in up to 10 percent of cases. The peak age of onset is 1 to 3 years, but cases appear throughout childhood and into adolescence. The diagnosis of juvenile rheumatoid arthritis requires exclusion of other types of arthritis. Other causes of arthritis in this age group include systemic lupus erythematosus and juvenile ankylosing spondylitis.

C. Legg-Calvé-Perthes Disease Inguinal, anteromedial thigh and sometimes knee pain are accompanied by a limp. The gait is antalgic. The pelvis dips on the affected side (gluteal lurch), and the length of stride is shortened. With the patient lying flat, the affected leg may be shortened, and this shortening persists after abducting the legs 20° and bringing them together again. The patient may lie with the thigh flexed, abducted, and externally rotated. Early radiographic changes include bulging of the hip capsule, a round osteopenic lesion on the medial metaphysis of the femoral neck, a small capital epiphysis, and thickening of the cartilaginous surface (widening of the joint space), giving an appearance of hip joint subluxation (Waldenstrom's sign). Increased density of the necrotic region of the femoral head may occur, as may a band of metaphyseal osteopenia. The crescent sign is a lucent line that appears under the articular surface, and it represents a fracture of necrotic subchondral bone. MRI can detect early evidence of bone necrosis in patients with this disorder. Some patients are initially indistinguishable from those with transient synovitis of the hip but can be identified by careful clinical and radiographic follow-up. Other disorders that may be mistaken for unilateral Perthes disease include Gaucher's disease, osteomyelitis, hemophilia, eosinophilic granuloma of the femoral head, and lymphoma.

D. Slipped Capital Femoral Epiphysis   Acute epiphyseal slip causes aching groin pain and anteromedial thigh pain. Walking or weight bearing may provoke or intensify the pain. The involved leg is held externally rotated. Examination of the patient in a supine position by the straight leg-raising test results in external rotation through the hip joint. When the patient is sitting, the thigh is held in adduction and external rotation, and causing the involved leg to cross over the other. Internal rotation and abduction of the hip are limited. Local tenderness may be present in the groin and trochanteric area, and in severe cases, there is loss of all motion at the hip.

Plain radiographs reveal epiphyseal displacement through the physis in a varus and posterior direction. Valgus displacement is less common. Anteroposterior views of the hip and pelvis, with the hips in the frog lateral position (Lowenstein's view), and a true lateral view facilitate diagnosis. In an acute slip, there are no reactive or remodeling changes in the metaphysis. In "acute on chronic" slips, there may be rounding of the metaphysis (anterosuperior region) and new bone formation in the posteroinferior corner. Radiolucency of the metaphysis subjacent to the growth plates also provides evidence of an underlying chronic process. This disorder occurs in the 10- to 16-year-old age group and is more common in males (male/female ratio, 2.5:1). Seventy-five percent of children with this disorder are above the ninetieth percentile for weight relative to their skeletal age. Up to 50 percent are at or above the ninety-seventh percentile for height. Most cases are idiopathic, but some are related to endocrine disorders (e.g., hypopituitarism, hypothyroidism, or hyperparathyroidism), neoplasms, renal osteodystrophy, radiation therapy, or skeletal dysplasias. Many cases begin after a recent growth spurt, and some acute cases are associated with minor trauma.

E. Pubic Osteomyelitis   This disorder may present with fever and trochanteric and/or groin pain. There is usually a good range of passive hip motion without pain, while active movement or jarring may provoke inguinal or lateral hip pain. The sedimentation rate is usually elevated. Sonographic studies show the hip joints to be free of fluid. A radionuclide scan may demonstrate localization to the pubic bone and widening of the symphysis pubis. A bone biopsy and culture may be required to establish a specific diagnosis and guide antibiotic therapy.

7. OSTEONECROSIS OF THE FEMORAL HEAD

Pain may occur in the groin, anteromedial thigh, and/or lateral hip region and may be referred to the knee. Initially, it may occur only during walking, running, and weight bearing. Fever and chills, an elevated sedimentation rate, and leukocytosis do not usually occur. Fist percussion tenderness over the trochanteric area and pain at the extremes of range-of-motion testing may occur. Plain radiographs are usually normal during the first few weeks or months after the onset of symptoms, but MRI and a radionuclide bone scan are usually positive early in the course of this disorder.

The earliest MRI abnormality is a homogeneous band of low signal intensity in the anterosuperior portion of the femoral head on a T_1-weighted image. T_2-weighted images may show a high signal within the low-intensity area due to hypervascular granulation tissue. Low signal intensity on both T_1- and T_2-weighted images occurs with advanced disease in the femoral head (e.g., fibrosis). In some early cases, low signal intensity on the T_1-weighted image is associated with high signal intensity in the same area on a T_2-weighted image (e.g., due to bone marrow edema). Plain radiographs are insensitive to ischemic change and are often normal (stage 1) when an MRI and a radionuclide bone scan demonstrate abnormalities. Stage 2 plain radiographic changes include a lucent area in the femoral head with a sclerotic border, subchondral sclerosis, and sometimes cyst formation. Stage 3 changes include a radiolucent crescent sign that parallels the articular surface and is due to fracture of necrotic subchondral bone. Stage 4 changes include flattening of the femoral head without narrowing of the joint space, and stage 5 is associated with flattening of the femoral head and joint space narrowing and/or acetabular involvement.

Corticosteroid therapy, alcohol abuse, and idiopathic disease account for most patients with this disorder. A list of associated injuries and diseases is presented in Table 44-1. Nontraumatic osteonecrosis may be bilateral in up to 60 percent of cases. Surgical core decompression of the femoral head may relieve pain and prevent progression. Histopathologic examination of the bone core will confirm the diagnosis of osteonecrosis.

8. ILIOPSOAS MUSCLE DISORDERS

A. Iliopsoas (Iliopectineal) Bursitis   Pain occurs in the inguinal region just distal to the inguinal ligament. It may be intensified by walking and by active or passive extension of the hip. A tender mass may be present in the inguinal area. Tenderness is present in patients without a mass and is localized to an area 2 cm lateral to the femoral pulse and just below the inguinal ligament. In patients with a mass lesion, the diagnosis can be confirmed by a CT scan. Aspiration of the mass and injection of lidocaine and a corticosteroid can relieve symptoms. Patients without a mass may be relieved of pain and tenderness by injection of lidocaine and a corticosteroid into the tender area. Some patients with this disorder have radiographic

Table 44-1
OSTEONECROSIS OF THE FEMORAL HEAD: ASSOCIATED CONDITIONS

TRAUMA
    Fracture of the femoral neck
    Fracture or dislocation of the hip
    Hip trauma without fracture
    Hip manipulation and surgery
NONTRAUMATIC DISORDERS
    Corticosteroid administration
    Alcohol abuse
    Sickle cell disease, sickle cell trait, sickle cell-thallasemia disease,
        and sickle cell-hemoglobin C disease
    Caisson disease (e.g., divers and tunnel workers)
    Exposure to high altitude
    Gaucher's disease
    Gout
    Radiation
    Fabry's disease
    Pregnancy
    Cushing's disease
    Tumors in the hip region
    Chronic liver disease
    Pancreatitis
    Systemic lupus erythematosus
    Occlusive vascular disorders (e.g., vasculitis and coagulopathies)
    Psoriasis
    Idiopathic osteonecrosis
NONTRAUMATIC DISORDERS IN CHILDREN AND ADULTS
    Legg-Calvé-Perthes disease
    Slipped capital femoral epiphysis and faulty pin placement or
        forceful surgical manipulation

---

evidence of rheumatoid arthritis, osteoarthritis, or synovial chondromatosis in the hip joint. Besides groin pain and tenderness, other manifestations of iliopsoas bursitis may include ipsilateral pitting (venous compression) or nonpitting edema (lymphatic obstruction); frequency of urination and small urine volumes secondary to intrapelvic extension of the enlarged bursa, producing bladder compression; and simulation of a femoral artery aneurysm by transmission of the arterial pulse through the fluid-filled bursa.

B. Iliopsoas Tendinitis Patients may have groin and anteromedial thigh pain that is intensified by walking and extension of the thigh. Maximal tenderness occurs 2 cm lateral to the femoral pulse and subjacent to the inguinal ligament. Passive external rotation of the extended thigh intensifies the pain. Injection of lidocaine and methylprednisolone into the tender area provides immediate, and sometimes permanent, pain relief.

C. Iliopsoas Abscess Fever, chills, and malaise are accompanied by pain in the groin, in the upper anterior thigh, and sometimes in the iliac fossa. A palpable tender mass may be present in the groin or iliac fossa. The ip-

silateral leg is often held flexed, abducted, and externally rotated. A positive psoas sign may be present, or the patient may refuse to fully extend the thigh and knee. Scoliosis, anemia, and weight loss may be present. A psoas abscess may be primary, resulting from hematogenous dissemination of a distant infection. Most cases are secondary to gastrointestinal disease (e.g., Crohn's disease, appendicitis, carcinoma of the colon, diverticulitis of the colon, bowel perforation, or pancreatic disease). Osteomyelitis of the lumbar vertebrae or T12 (e.g., due to pyogenic organisms or *Mycobacterium tuberculosis*), empyema, a perinephric abscess, ureteral ectopia with obstruction, or an infected retroperitoneal hematoma may also give rise to an iliopsoas abscess. A CT scan will visualize a phlegmon (generalized enlargement of the psoas) or a low-density fluid collection (abscess). Surgical drainage and intravenous antibiotic therapy will lead to resolution.

Complications include ipsilateral leg edema due to iliac vein compression, ipsilateral hydroureter and hydronephrosis, and cutaneous fistula formation in the inguinal region.

9. FEMORAL NEUROPATHY

Femoral nerve compression in the upper thigh causes groin pain that is increased by active or passive thigh extension. Pain, paresthesias, and partial hypesthesia may involve the anterior and anteromedial thigh. Severe cases may cause quadriceps weakness and atrophy. Less commonly, pain, paresthesias, and hypesthesia may involve the anteromedial calf adjacent to the greater saphenous vein. Causes of femoral neuropathy include entrapment in the inguinal region from scarring, a femoral or inguinal hernia, or a pseudoaneurysm of the femoral artery resulting from femoral artery catheterization. An intramuscular injection into the anterior thigh may directly injure the nerve. Neoplastic lesions in the pelvis, a retroperitoneal tumor or hematoma, or compression by a retractor during pelvic surgery may involve the femoral nerve within the abdomen.

Diabetes mellitus is a frequent cause of femoral neuropathy. Some cases follow compression of the femoral nerve by an iliopsoas abscess or a distended iliopsoas bursa. An idiopathic variety also occurs.

10. ILIOFEMORAL VENOUS THROMBOSIS

Pain may occur in the groin, anterior thigh, and sometimes in the ipsilateral iliac fossa. Edema and pallor of the ipsilateral leg, extending from the foot to the groin, is usually present. Superficial venous distension in the inguinal and suprapubic region may occur. There may be tenderness medial to the femoral artery and a palpable cord. This disorder has been called "milk leg" when it occurs in the postpartum period and phlegmasia alba dolens when it appears in obstetrical or other settings. The thrombosis is usually in the iliofemoral and superficial femoral veins.

Progression of this disorder is signaled by cyanosis, coolness of the involved limb, and sloughing of necrotic skin. Hemorrhagic bullae may also occur. This form of iliofemoral thrombosis probably involves all of the major venous channels in the leg, and it is called phlegmasia cerulea dolens.

A quantitative study of the frequency of risk factors, symptoms, and signs in proximal deep vein thrombosis has revealed a significant association with five clinical findings: recent immobilization (41 percent), cancer (20 percent), fever (16 percent), swelling above the knee (50 percent), and swelling below the knee (86 percent). Patients with swelling both above and below the knee had an incidence of proximal deep vein thrombosis of 46 percent. Venography performed on patients with one or more of the five findings missed only 3 percent of cases of proximal deep vein thrombosis. Deep venous thrombosis may be diagnosed by the use of Doppler ultrasound to detect the absence of spontaneous venous flow, the presence of continuous-flow velocity patterns without phasic respiratory variations, and/or diminished augmentation with venous compression. The accuracy of this method (sensitivity, 76–96 percent; specificity, 84–100 percent) is dependent on the skill and experience of the operator.

Impedence plethysmography (IPG) records a decrease in capacitance with thigh-cuff compression (e.g., the usual increase in limb blood volume is limited after thigh cuff inflation because of venous thrombosis) and a decrease in the rate of venous outflow within 3 s of cuff release. Serial IPG studies may be used to confirm the diagnosis of proximal deep vein thrombosis when the initial IPG study is negative or equivocal. IPG is reported to be nearly 100-percent accurate for the diagnosis of proximal venous thrombosis. IPG accuracy is lower in the presence of right-sided heart failure or during ventilator use. Hypervolemia may result in bilateral false-positive results.

B-mode ultrasonography may be used to detect proximal venous thrombi. Venous compressibility indicates patency and the absence of thrombi. Intraluminal thrombus and inability to compress a segment of proximal vein are criteria for the diagnosis of venous thrombosis. Acute and chronic thrombi may also be differentiated by characteristic differences detectable by B-mode ultrasonography. This technique has a reported sensitivity for the diagnosis of popliteal or femoral thrombosis of 100 percent and a specificity of 99 percent. The sensitivity for calf thrombi is only 36 percent. Venography remains the "gold standard" for the diagnosis of proximal and distal venous thrombosis in the leg.

A positive IPG or B-mode sonographic study is suffi-

cient for the initiation of anticoagulant therapy. An equivocal IPG study may be clarified by B-mode ultrasonography or venography. A negative IPG examination in the presence of strong clinical evidence of proximal venous occlusion is an indication for serial IPG studies at 2- to 3-day intervals or for immediate B-mode ultrasonography or venography.

11. INGUINAL OR FEMORAL HERNIA

A. Acute Inguinal or Femoral Hernia   An inguinal hernia may become apparent as a mildly painful and tender bulge following heavy lifting or other strenuous physical activity. The region may remain acutely painful and tender for several days. The pain may be intensified by standing or straining and relieved by lying down. Patients with a femoral hernia usually develop a bulge below the inguinal ligament in the region of the femoral vessels. Many hernias in the inguinal and femoral region may be identified on physical examination in the standing position as a bulge in these areas, in the scrotum, or above the external inguinal ring in the inguinal canal. Some hernias may cause persistent inguinal pain that is often relieved by lying down but may remain undetected on physical examination. Such hernias may be diagnosed by contrast herniography. Surgical repair usually results in the relief of symptoms.

B. Incarceration or Strangulation   Incarceration or strangulation of an inguinal or femoral hernia can cause local pain and a nonreducible, tender mass above (inguinal hernia) or below (femoral hernia) the inguinal ligament. If bowel is trapped in the hernia sac, nausea, vomiting, colicky abdominal pain, and distension of the abdomen secondary to intestinal obstruction may follow. Surgical exploration may be required to prevent bowel necrosis and a lethal peritonitis. Prompt surgical intervention may allow recovery of strangulated bowel and eliminate the need for bowel resection.

At surgery, the hernia sac is opened, the contents are returned to the peritoneal cavity after ensuring their viability, and the hernia is repaired.

12. INGUINAL OR FEMORAL LYMPHADENITIS

A. Cellulitis   The skin of the foot and lower leg becomes painful, tender, red, and warm. The irregular upper margin of the erythematous area spreads proximally. The margin is not elevated above the surrounding skin, but there may be induration and edema of the skin in the erythematous area distally. Pink or red, tender lymphangitic streaks may extend to the thigh, and there may be femoral or inguinal pain associated with tender, enlarged lymph nodes. Occasionally, superficial collections of pus, bullae, and purpura may appear in the center of the erythematous region. Mild-to-moderate temperature elevations may occur. The usual causes are *Streptococcus pyogenes* or *Staphylococcus aureus,* but *Streptococcus sanguis,* gram-negative bacilli, or anaerobic bacteria may be isolated from needle-aspiration cultures obtained from the advancing erythematous margin. This technique has a low sensitivity (5–20 percent) and is not currently recommended for bacteriologic diagnosis. Cellulitis and painful inguinal adenitis will usually respond to intravenous nafcillin or vancomycin within 24 to 72 h. Cellulitis of the abdominal wall or perineum may also cause painful and tender inguinal lymphadenitis.

B. Pyoderma An abscess of the skin of the foot, lower leg, or thigh may cause a surrounding region of erythema and edema, ascending lymphangitis, and painful and tender femoral and/or inguinal lymphadenitis on the ipsilateral side. This disorder responds to antibiotic therapy and drainage of the abscess. An abscess of the lower abdominal wall or perineum may also cause painful unilateral or bilateral femoral and/or inguinal lymphadenitis.

C. Specific Infections

1. **Vibrio vulnificus** *Cellulitis* A leg wound sustained while immersed in seawater or a preexisting wound exposed to contaminated seawater can develop into a cellulitis with an associated fasciitis or myositis. The intense erythematous and edematous cellulitis that occurs may be associated with hemorrhagic bullae and a painful, tender femoral and/or inguinal lymphadenitis. The bullae may collapse, leaving necrotic ulcerations. Aspiration of a bullous lesion may reveal curved, gram-negative bacilli on Gram's stain and *Vibrio vulnificus* on culture. Surgical debridement and doxycycline therapy will usually result in cure of this life-threatening infection.

2. **Aeromonas hydrophila** *Infection* This freshwater organism may cause an acute cellulitis and femoral and/or inguinal lymphadenitis following trauma to the leg sustained in a lake, river, or pond.

3. **Bubonic Plague** **(Yersinia pestis)** There is an abrupt onset of fever, chills, malaise, and prostration. A painful, tender mass of 1 to 10 cm in diameter develops in one or both femoral regions or, less commonly, in the inguinal region. Movement of the leg is resisted because it intensifies the pain. The overlying skin is often red, edematous, and warm. The bubo may appear as a smooth, uniform, ovoid mass or as an irregular cluster of enlarged nodes of varying size. Fever, tachycardia, and low blood pressure are usually present. The liver and spleen may be enlarged and tender. Skin lesions other than flea bites on the lower

leg or abdomen are seldom present, but up to 25 percent of patients may have a pustule, vesicle, papule, or small eschar at the site of a flea bite. Purpura and skin necrosis may occur as the disease progresses. Bubonic plague occurs in New Mexico, Arizona, Colorado, Utah, and California, as well as in South America, Africa, and Southeast Asia. Aspiration of a bubo, followed by Gram's stain and culture of the aspirate, will confirm the diagnosis. Blood culture results may also be positive. Streptomycin therapy will usually lead to rapid resolution of fever and adenopathy.

4. *Ulceroglandular Tularemia* **(Francisella tularensis)** Tick-borne infection most commonly involves the leg. An ulcerated skin lesion occurs on the leg or in the perineal area in more than 50 percent of cases. In cases contracted from contact with a diseased rabbit, perineal and lower-extremity ulcerations are very uncommon. Painful, tender, femoral and/or inguinal lymphadenopathy develops proximal to the skin ulceration. Fever, chills, malaise, and weakness are associated. Pneumonia and pleuritis occur in 10 to 15 percent of ulceroglandular cases, and the onset of these manifestations may be signaled by cough, dyspnea, and pleuritic pain. The diagnosis may rarely be confirmed by Gram's stain and culture of sputum, node aspirates, or ulcer exudate. Almost all cases are usually diagnosed by serologic methods. The tularemia tube agglutination or microagglutination titer exceeds 1:160 in those with acute or past infection. Diagnosis in time to initiate therapy is based on clinical findings, since titers do not rise for 7 to 14 days. Streptomycin or gentamicin therapy will usually result in resolution of symptoms and signs.

5. *Cat-Scratch Disease* There is an inoculation site (cat scratch) present on the foot or leg. A papule or pustule may form in this area 3 to 10 days after the scratch. Low-grade fever, weakness, fatigue, and malaise may occur in up to 25 percent of cases. Inguinal or femoral nodes may enlarge and become painful and tender. A single node enlarges in up to 50 percent of cases, and multiple nodes at the same site occur in 20 percent. Node suppuration occurs in up to 50 percent of cases. Lymph node biopsy demonstrates stellate abscesses with necrotic centers surrounded by epithelioid cells.

Small, pleomorphic, gram-negative bacilli have been seen in endothelial cells and in macrophages lining sinuses in involved nodes. The Warthin-Starry silver impregnation stain will confirm the presence of these organisms. Culture and Gram's stain of aspirated lymph node pus usually reveals no evidence of an etiologic agent. The diagnosis is dependent on the clinical history and signs, the histopathologic findings, and the results of applying the silver impregnation stain to biopsy material. There is no specific therapy.

D. Suppurative Iliac Lymphadenitis   This disorder develops secondary to an infection in the leg, perineum, or lower abdominal wall. Suppuration in the involved iliac nodes spreads to the region of the iliacus and iliopsoas muscles (i.e., to the iliac nodes). Fever, a limp, and low back and hip pain occur. Extension of the thigh causes severe inguinal and iliac pain, but hip abduction and adduction are possible with only mild discomfort. With progression, high fever, chills, lower abdominal pain, prostration, and a marked leukocytosis develop. On examination, the hip is flexed, and there are ipsilateral abdominal muscle (rectus muscle) spasm and a posterolateral pelvic mass or a tender inguinal mass. A CT scan or MRI may define a collection of purulent fluid adjacent to the iliopsoas and iliacus muscles due to abscess formation from iliac node suppuration. *S. aureus* and streptococcal species are the most frequently isolated organisms.

E. Sexually Transmitted Diseases

1. Primary Genital Herpes Infection   Aching perineal, penile, buttock, and thigh pain on one or both sides may precede the appearance of penile or labial grouped vesicles, pustules, or crusted, small ulcers. Inguinal aching pain on one or both sides is followed by the appearance of a slightly enlarged, tender inguinal node. The diagnosis can be confirmed by culture of the penile or labial lesions, by direct immunofluorescent staining of ulcer exudate, or by demonstrating a rise in antibody titer to herpes simplex virus over a period of 2 to 4 weeks. Severe cases may be treated with oral or intravenous acyclovir.

2. Chancroid   Patients with chancroid present with one or more painful genital ulcerations. The ulcers have ragged, irregular, undermined borders, and a soft, tender, purulent base. The incubation period is less than 1 week. Preputial or coronal ulcers cause extensive edema of the distal penis leading to phimosis, which prevents examination and culture of the ulceration(s). Inguinal nodes on one or, less commonly, both sides become enlarged, painful, and tender (65 percent of cases). The overlying skin becomes thin and reddened. Node softening because of suppuration may develop and spontaneous drainage may occur if treatment is not initiated. Autoinoculation ulcerations may occur on the lower leg, thigh, or abdomen, and provide clinical evidence in support of the diagnosis. Genital ulcers accompany the lymphadenitis, and the dark-field examination of ulcer exudate is negative. Isolation of *Haemophilus ducreyi*, the causative organism, requires culture of the ulcer exudate on a serum and vancomycin-containing selective medium. Erythromycin, a quinolone, or ceftriaxone therapy leads to resolution.

3. Lymphogranuloma Venereum   Patients with lymphogranuloma venereum (LGV) present with unilateral or bilateral (33 percent of cases) painful, tender inguinal and/or femoral lymphadenitis. A painless primary lesion consisting of a small papule or ulcer occurs in less than 25 percent of cases and heals in several days without scarring. Both femoral and inguinal nodes may become individually enlarged, painful, and tender. In some cases, the nodes become matted together, and the overlying skin may become indurated and erythematous. Nodes may become fluctuant and drain through the skin. Fever, malaise, fatigue, myalgias, headache, and meningismus may occur prior to or at the onset of the inguinal and/or femoral lymphadenopathy. Femoral and inguinal adenopathies, separated by a furrow caused by the inguinal ligament, give rise to the ''groove sign'' (in up to 15 percent of cases). This sign, while suggestive of LGV, is not pathognomonic and may occur in other infections (e.g., suppurative lymphadenitis) and neoplastic diseases (e.g., lymphoma). Diagnosis requires isolation of the responsible LGV biovar of *Chlamydia trachomatis* from a node aspirate, urethra, rectum, or cervix. Culture, with the capacity to perform biovar analysis, is required for specific diagnosis. Serologic tests, such as the LGV complement fixation test and the microimmunofluorescence antibody test (usually available only in research laboratories), may help support the diagnosis. Tetracycline therapy is effective, but regression of lymphadenopathy is slow after initiation of therapy.

4. Primary Syphilis   This disorder begins with a penile or perineal (women) ulcer that is usually painless, indurated, and nontender. The ulcer has a clean, dry, ''beefy-'' or ''raw ham''-colored surface. Lymph nodes are characteristically enlarged bilaterally (70 percent of cases), painless, and nontender. However, in some cases, the primary lesion and the regional nodes may be tender. The diagnosis can be confirmed by a dark-field microscopic examination of serum exudate from the primary lesion, and it can be supported by a positive result on the rapid plasma reagin (RPR) test.

5. Gonococcal and Nongonococcal Urethritis   Unilateral or bilateral, painful and tender inguinal lymphadenopathy may occur in 5 to 40 percent of patients with acute gonococcal urethritis. Some patients with asymptomatic urethritis may develop tender inguinal adenopathy. The incidence of tender inguinal adenopathy in nongonococcal urethritis is only 1 percent.

Trochanteric and Lateral Thigh Pain

13. HIP POINTER

A fall on the side by a player in a contact sport (e.g., football) may cause a contusion of the iliac crest. There are local pain, tenderness, swelling, and ecchymoses. Severe spasm of adjacent muscles may prevent the patient from standing upright, and gait is usually impaired. Movement of muscles attached to the contused iliac crest does not increase the local pain. A fluctuant mass (hematoma) over the iliac crest may be aspirated to accelerate recovery.

14. AVULSION FRACTION OF THE ILIAC CREST APOPHYSIS

A sudden forceful contraction of the abdominal muscles associated with a directional change during running can cause lateral thigh and iliac crest pain and tenderness (e.g., usually in the 12- to 18-year-old age group). There are local pain, tenderness, and swelling over the iliac crest and discomfort on resisted abduction of the hip. An oblique radiograph of the iliac crest may be required to demonstrate the avulsion fracture.

15. TROCHANTERIC BURSITIS

There are two major bursae (the subgluteus maximus bursa and the subgluteus medius bursa) and one minor bursa (the gluteus minimus bursa) adjacent to the greater trochanter. Inflammation of one or both major bursae may cause aching pain over the lateral hip and thigh that is provoked by walking, squatting, climbing stairs, lying on the affected side, or external rotation or adduction of the thigh. The pain may continue after prolonged activity despite rest. Radiation as far as the knee or, less commonly, down the lateral aspect of the lower leg to the ankle may occur. There is local tenderness over the greater trochanter, and palpation may reproduce the quality, location, and radiation of the pain. Plain radiographs may demonstrate calcification in the supratrochanteric or retrotrochanteric area and should be obtained to exclude bone pathology. Injection of the tender area with lidocaine and methylprednisolone relieves local and radiating pain immediately and sometimes permanently. A dramatic pain-relieving response to lidocaine injection is diagnostic. This disorder has been confused with a L2–L4 radiculopathy (pseudoradiculopathy) and with arthritis of the hip. Predisposing factors include local trauma to the trochanter; inequality of leg length; jogging, especially when the bursitis occurs in women; osteoarthritis of the hip; low back pain that affects the mechanics of walking; jogging on a banked surface, resulting in bursitis in the downside leg; rheumatoid arthritis; abnormal running mechanics (e.g., feet crossing over the midline); and the snapping hip syndrome.

16. SNAPPING HIP SYNDROME

Snapping of the thickened iliotibial band over the greater trochanter may cause an audible and palpable snap and lateral hip pain due to an associated trochanteric bursitis. Snapping can be reproduced by active flexion and internal rotation of the thigh or by running in place. Local bursal pain and tenderness are relieved dramatically by an injection of lidocaine and methylprednisolone.

Cases refractory to conservative therapy may respond to surgical release of the iliotibial band and lengthening or excision of a portion of the iliotibial tract.

In many cases, the snapping hip syndrome is painless, and the development of discomfort requires the development of trochanteric bursitis. Other causes of an audible snap in the region of the hip include stenosing tenosynovitis of the iliopsoas tendon sheath near its insertion on the femur; slipping of the iliopsoas tendon over the iliopectineal eminence of the pelvic bone; slipping of the iliofemoral ligament over the femoral head, or the biceps femoris tendon over the ischial tuberosity; intraarticular loose bodies; and hip subluxation.

17. MERALGIA PARESTHETICA

There is a burning or an aching pain over the lower third of the lateral thigh. Prickling and tingling paresthesias occur in the affected area. Sensory testing reveals a central area of anesthesia surrounded by a rim of hyperesthetic skin. The pain and paresthesias may be provoked or intensified by standing, walking, or extension and adduction of the leg. Sitting or lying prone brings relief. Pressure medial to the anterior superior iliac spine may provoke or intensify the lateral thigh discomfort and paresthesias (positive Tinel's sign). This disorder is frequent in diabetics and may be seen in pregnancy, with obesity, or after a pelvic fracture. It is caused by compression of the lateral femoral cutaneous nerve. L2 or L3 root lesions cause more anteromedial sensory changes, weakness of knee extension and hip flexion, and depression of the knee jerk. Motor impairment and reflex changes do not occur with meralgia paresthetica. Spontaneous improvement is the rule, but corticosteroid injections medial to the anterior superior spine of the ilium may result in temporary improvement.

18. ACUTE ARTHRITIS OF THE HIP

Acute arthritis is discussed above. Pain may occur in the groin, over the trochanter and lateral thigh, and sometimes in the buttock.

19. OSTEONECROSIS OF THE FEMORAL HEAD

Osteonecrosis of the femoral head is discussed above. Pain occurs in the groin and may occur over the trochanter and lateral thigh. It is intensified by weight bearing and walking.

20. FRACTURE OF THE FEMORAL SHAFT

These fractures usually occur in young adults and result from high-energy trauma in motor vehicle or motorcycle accidents or after penetrating wounds (e.g., gunshot injuries). There are severe pain in the thigh, deformity, swelling, and tenderness. The patient is unable to move the hip or knee. Enlargement of the thigh may be secondary to bleeding. Failure of adequate volume replacement may result in hypovolemic shock. The diagnosis can be established by plain radiographs.

Medial Thigh Pain

21. OBTURATOR HERNIA

Medial thigh or groin pain and/or symptoms of intestinal obstruction (e.g., obstipation, colicky abdominal pain, vomiting, and distension) represent the usual presenting symptoms of this disorder. The Howship-Romberg sign may be present in 25 to 50 percent of cases. This sign consists of medial thigh and/or knee pain and/or paresthesias that are exacerbated by thigh extension and abduction or internal rotation. Thigh flexion relieves the pain, while coughing provokes or intensifies it. Hyperesthesia and paresthesias may be present in the painful medial thigh area. Another sign of obturator nerve compression, the Hannington-Kiff sign, may be present in the absence of the Howship-Romberg sign. The former sign is characterized by loss of the adductor reflex and preservation of the patellar reflex on the affected side.

A tender mass may sometimes be palpable on rectal examination in the obturator canal anterolateral to the rectum. Vaginal examination may reveal a mass above the inferior ramus of the ischium. A small mass may be present in the subinguinal area lateral to the adductor longus tendon.

Some patients hold the affected leg flexed, adducted, and externally rotated at the hip. Plain abdominal radiographs may reveal evidence of partial or complete intestinal obstruction. A CT scan may occasionally demonstrate a bowel loop between the pectineal and external obturator muscles or bowel constriction at the hernial orifice. Surgical exploration is required for relief of intestinal obstruction and repair of the hernia. This disorder is more frequent in elderly women (female/male ratio, 9:1) and in older patients with chronic constipation or recent weight loss.

22. GREATER SAPHENOUS VEIN PHLEBITIS

Aching medial thigh pain begins 2 to 4 days after surgery or a delivery. There may be fever, malaise, and a tender cord in the medial thigh without overlying skin redness.

There is no peripheral edema. Leukocytosis and an elevated sedimentation rate may be present.

23. HERPES SIMPLEX NEURITIS

Genital herpes may begin with aching or burning medial thigh and buttock pain. This is followed by the eruption of painful penile or labial vesicles and crusted ulcers. The diagnosis can be confirmed by direct immunofluorescent staining of lesion exudate or by a viral culture.

24. REFERRED PAIN

A. Tubo-ovarian Lesions   Cystic, neoplastic, or inflammatory lesions of the ovary or tube may cause lower abdominal and medial thigh pain.

B. Pubic Bone Disorders   Osteomyelitis, stress fractures of the pubic bone, or osteitis pubis may cause pubic region pain and tenderness and anteromedial thigh pain.

C. Ureteral Colic   A unilateral stone may cause lower abdominal, groin, scrotal, or labial pain. Referral to the medial thigh may occur. The urine contains erythrocytes, and an intravenous pyelogram will demonstrate ureteral dilatation and obstruction.

25. ADDUCTOR MUSCLE STRAIN

Pain occurs in the medial thigh and groin and is intensified by passive abduction of the thigh. The pain is associated with tenderness along the pubic ramus and over the adductor muscles. Squeezing the examiner's fist between the knees may provoke pain due to adductor strain. This injury occurs in hockey and football players. The cause is forced abduction of the thigh while in a split or straddle position. This follows another player's falling on the injured player. Similar adductor injuries occur in bowlers, cricket players, and swimmers who do the breast stroke. The adductor muscles are a common site of muscle strain in professional athletes.

26. ILIOPSOAS STRAIN OR AVULSION FRACTURE OF THE LESSER TROCHANTER

There is an abrupt onset of groin and medial thigh pain during running or after a quick start in running. It results from a sudden, forceful contraction of the iliopsoas muscle with the thigh fixed or a forced hip extension with the leg fixed. Tenderness is present over the lesser trochanter, and hip flexion against resistance intensifies the pain. The hip is usually held in flexion. Radiographs may show an avulsion fracture of the lesser trochanter.

Pubic Pain

27. OSTEITIS PUBIS

This disorder may follow trauma, prostate and bladder surgery, and pregnancy and may also occur in competitive athletes (e.g., runners, race walkers, and soccer players). Burning pain occurs in the pubic region and groin. Pivoting on one leg, kicking a ball, jumping, ascending stairs, or abruptly changing direction during running may intensify the pain. There is severe localized tenderness over the pubic bone and the insertions of the rectus abdominus and adductor muscles. The gait may be antalgic or waddling (due to adductor muscle spasm). Pain in the pubic region and/or groin may occur on flexion of either thigh, on passive hip abduction, and on active abduction or adduction of the thigh against resistance. Plain radiographs of the pelvis may reveal bone resorption of the medial ends of the pubic bones, widening of the symphysis pubis, and loss of density in bone adjacent to the pubic symphysis. Instability of the symphysis pubis may be demonstrated by weight bearing (flamingo) views (35 percent of cases).

A CT scan may show cortical irregularity of the pubic bones. Advanced changes include erosion of the pubic bones, sclerosis of remaining adjacent bone, and widening of the pubic symphysis. The sedimentation rate is sometimes elevated. Application of warm, moist heat; restricted activity; and administration of nonsteroidal anti-inflammatory drugs or prednisone will lead to improvement. Resolution of symptoms and return to athletic activity may take 2 to 3 months.

28. OSTEOMYELITIS OF THE PUBIC BONE

This disorder may cause fever, symphysis pubis, and groin pain that is intensified by walking or jarring. The patient has an antalgic or waddling gait. Radiographs demonstrate widening of the symphysis and "motheaten" rarefaction or extensive destruction of the pubic bones. Pyogenic infection may follow pelvic surgery. *Pseuedomonas, Serratia,* or *Citrobacter* species infections are associated with intravenous drug abuse. Bone biopsy and culture are required for a specific diagnosis. Most cases of osteomyelitis of the pubic bone are due to *S. aureus.* Osteomyelitis responds to intravenous antibiotics.

29. PYOGENIC ARTHRITIS OF THE PUBIC SYMPHYSIS

This disorder may result from osteomyelitis, or it may follow pelvic surgery. It is difficult to differentiate from osteomyelitis of the pubic bone. Fluid aspirated from the symphysis pubis region contains increased numbers of polymorphonuclear leukocytes and contains one or more bacterial species.

30. PUBIC FRACTURES

A. Pathologic Fracture of the Pubic Bone (Disease-Associated)   Elderly women with rheumatoid arthritis or postmenopausal or steroid-induced osteoporosis may develop stress fractures of the pubic bone. There is a gradual or abrupt onset of groin pain. This pain is intensified by weight bearing, walking, or abduction of the thigh. A radionuclide scan will demonstrate a fracture near the symphysis, and after a few days or weeks plain radiographs or a CT scan will demonstrate the fracture. A CT scan will help differentiate a stress fracture from metastatic carcinoma.

B. Stress Fracture of the Pubic Bone (Athletic Activity-Associated)   This disorder begins with groin, trochanteric, and sometimes anterior thigh pain. Inguinal and pubic bone tenderness may be present. Radiographic studies may be negative or demonstrate nonspecific findings. A radionuclide bone scan will demonstrate increased uptake over the pubic bone fracture site. This type of fracture occurs in women joggers or runners and in soccer and football players. Pain may be absent at rest and with weight bearing and may begin only after several miles of running. Rest and avoidance of the causative athletic activity will usually result in healing within 6 to 8 weeks.

31. PUBIC OSTEOLYSIS

Groin and trochanteric pain may begin after a fall or occur spontaneously. There may be local tenderness over an area of the pubic bone. Osteolytic areas are present in the pubic rami or near the symphysis on plain radiographs. Biopsy of the lytic area may show callus, binucleate chondrocytes, increased cellularity, and a myxoid intercellular matrix. Some cases have been incorrectly diagnosed as a low-grade chondrosarcoma and have undergone extensive surgery. Pubic osteolysis follows a more rapid course than chondrosarcoma, and histopathologic examination does not reveal evidence of the nuclear pleomorphism that is present in the latter disorder.

32. POSTPARTUM SYMPHYSEAL PELVIC PAIN

Suprapubic and symphyseal pain and tenderness occur several hours or days after delivery. Pain may radiate to one or both inguinal regions. It may be severe enough to prevent standing or walking. Some patients with this postpartum disorder have some suprapubic discomfort or groin pain during the last trimester. Symphyseal separation is present on physical examination and/or plain radiographs. Some authors consider this transient postpartum disorder (e.g., duration usually less than 3 weeks) a transient form of osteitis pubis, while others consider it a separate entity (i.e., symptomatic symphyseal separation).

Posterior Thigh Pain

33. PYRIFORMIS SYNDROME

Aching pain occurs in the upper buttock and may radiate down the posterior thigh. The pain is often worse at night and after prolonged sitting. A limp may be present on the painful side, or gait may be normal. Palpation of the piriformis muscle during a rectal or vaginal examination reveals localized tenderness. Pain may be provoked or intensified on resisted abduction and simultaneous external rotation of the thigh (Pace's sign). Forced internal rotation of the extended thigh may also provoke or intensify the pain (Freiberg's sign). Dyspareunia may occur in women. There may also be limitation of straight leg-raising on the ipsilateral side. Tenderness may be noted over the sciatic notch. Injection of the piriformis muscle with lidocaine and methylprednisolone results in transient or permanent relief of symptoms.

34. HAMSTRING SYNDROME (GLUTEAL SCIATICA)

Aching pain occurs in the lower gluteal region and radiates down the posterior thigh to the popliteal space. Pain may occur during sitting (e.g., in driving or during a lecture) and remains present until relieved by a change of position or standing. There is often a history of hamstring injury in the past (39 percent of cases). Stretching exercises, sprinting, hurdling, or kicking a soccer ball frequently provoke the pain. Pain is seldom felt while lying down or jogging. There is local tenderness in the region of the ischial tuberosity, but the neurologic examination and the straight leg-raising test are normal. This syndrome results from compression of the sciatic nerve by fibrous bands and tight tendinous origins of the hamstring muscles from the ischial tuberosity. Relief of pain follows division of the taut hamstring tendons and decompression of the sciatic nerve. There is often a history of recurrent hamstring ''injury,'' which may be due to repeated bouts of sciatic nerve irritation.

35. HAMSTRING MUSCLE INJURY

A. Strain There is an abrupt onset of pain and tenderness in the region of ischial tuberosity or in more distal portions of the hamstring muscles. A snapping or popping sound may sometimes be heard at the onset of the pain. A palpable defect in the medial or lateral hamstring muscles may be present. Tears may occur near the ischial tuberosity or in the distal one-third of the hamstring. Hamstring injuries follow a forceful kick, a quick start in running, or stretching to reach a ball.

B. Ischial Apophysis Avulsion Avulsion of the ischial tuberosity causes local ischial pain and tenderness and pain radiation down the posterior thigh. This injury most frequently occurs during running, broad jumping, hurdling, football, and gymnastics. Active flexion of the extended leg intensifies the pain. The diagnosis can be confirmed by a plain radiograph. The peak age range for avulsion of the ischial apophysis is 13 to 17 years, with some cases occurring up to age 24.

36. ISCHIAL BURSITIS

This disorder causes pain and tenderness over the ischial tuberosity. Pain may radiate into the posterior thigh. Prolonged sitting on a hard surface (e.g., ''weaver's'' or ''tailor's bottom''), a direct blow to the tuberosity, or speed work performed by a young runner may cause this disorder. The pain may be intensified by prolonged sitting, wallet pressure, or uphill running. Rest, local heat, and in some cases a local injection of lidocaine and a corticosteroid provide relief.

37. RADICULAR PAIN

A. Disc Protrusion Posterior thigh pain may be associated with lumbosacral, buttock, and calf pain (i.e., sciatica). A dull, aching discomfort may be accompanied by jabs of lancinating pain that radiate from the low back or buttock down the leg.

Radicular pain may be provoked or intensified by sneezing, coughing, or straining at stool. The straight leg-raising test will also provoke buttock and leg pain at 30 to 45° of elevation in patients with root compression or irritation. In 100 cases of proven disc protrusion, ipsilateral straight leg-raising test results were positive in 98 percent, and contralateral (crossed) straight leg-raising test results were positive in 43 percent. In patients with an L5–S1 disc protrusion, the ipsilateral ankle jerk was depressed or absent in 87 percent, while those with an L4–L5 disc protrusion had only a 12-percent incidence of ankle jerk impairment. Muscle atrophy, detected by measuring calf circumference, occurred in 29 percent of patients with disc protrusion, while weakness of ankle dorsiflexion was present in 54 percent. Scoliosis was present in 63 percent. The diagnosis of disc protrusion can be confirmed by myelography, CT-enhanced myelography, or MRI. Posterior thigh and adjacent pain is usually relieved by rest and avoidance of lifting after 4 to 8 weeks. Refractory cases may require surgical removal of the prolapsed disc.

B. Spinal Epidural Abscess Fever, chills, and a midline lumbar ache and tenderness are associated with posterior radicular leg pain, lower limb weakness, and patchy sensory losses in the legs. Retention or incontinence of stool and/or urine may also occur. Reflexes are usually depressed in the presence of a lumbar epidural abscess. Neck stiffness may occur in up to 50 percent of cases, and headache is frequently present. Radiographic evidence of osteomyelitis adjacent to the abscess may occur in only 60 percent of cases. The diagnosis can be confirmed by myelography or MRI. Symptoms resolve with surgical drainage of the abscess and intravenous antibiotic therapy.

C. Spinal Epidural or Subdural Hematoma This disorder occurs in patients with severe liver disease or in those taking anticoagulant drugs. The initial complaint is severe midline low back pain and radiating posterior thigh and calf pain. Within hours or days, motor weakness and sensory loss occur in the legs. Disturbances of bladder and bowel function may soon follow. Coughing, straining, and the straight leg-raising test may provoke lancinating pain in the buttock, posterior thigh, and calf. The diagnosis can be confirmed by myelography, CT scan, or MRI. Removal of the hematoma is required to relieve pain and prevent irreversible neurologic damage.

D. Conus Medullaris Infarction There is an abrupt onset of pain in both buttocks, posterior thighs, and calves. Numbness of the buttocks and heaviness or weakness of the legs may accompany the pain. Saddle hypesthesia (perianal and perineal region) and leg weakness and impairment of the ankle jerks may be present on examination. Retention or incontinence of urine and/or stool are prominent features. A CT scan or MRI will exclude a mass lesion such as a prolapsed disc, abscess, or hematoma. This acute syndrome is most likely due to infarction of the conus medullaris of the spinal cord. There is an association of spinal cord infarction with aortic atherosclerosis, aortic surgery, use of an intraaortic balloon pump, dissecting aneurysm of the aorta, degenerative spine disease, and systemic hypotension combined with stenosis of major segmental arteries. There is no specific therapy, and partial, spontaneous recovery of neurologic function usually occurs.

38. POSTERIOR FEMORAL CUTANEOUS NEUROPATHY

Pain and hypesthesia or hyperpathia involve the posterior thigh. There may be unilateral or bilateral symptoms and signs. Sensory involvement of the labium majus or scro-

tum and the lower buttock may also occur. Direct injury of the posterior femoral cutaneous nerve may occur due to blunt or penetrating trauma. Some cases are caused by compression of the nerve against the ischial tuberosity. An abnormal somatosensory-evoked potential has been demonstrated in one case of isolated posterior femoral neuropathy.

39. LUMBAR FACET JOINT DISEASE

Posterior thigh, low back, and buttock pain on one side are common complaints with a facet joint disorder. Other findings supportive of a diagnosis of facet joint-related pain include localized paraspinal tenderness, provocation of the pain by extension of the back and rotation, and radiographic abnormality (CT scan) of the suspected facet joint. Pain below the knee is unlikely in patients with this syndrome. The presence of three or more of the listed findings predicts a high probability of prolonged pain relief after injection of the tender facet joint with a local anesthetic and a corticosteroid.

40. SACROILIITIS

Acute pain in the medial buttock on one or both sides, with radiation to the posterior thigh(s), may occur in patients with sacroiliitis. There is local sacroiliac joint tenderness, and Gaenslen's sign is positive. Straight leg-raising may cause pain in the buttock(s) and upper thigh(s), but radiating pain does not extend below the knee(s).

A. Reactive Arthritis Sacroiliitis may be part of an attack of acute reactive arthritis (Reiter's syndrome). This disorder may involve knees, hips, shoulders, ankles, and other joints. It occurs in association with acute gastrointestinal infections caused by *Shigella, Salmonella, Campylobacter,* and *Yersinia* species or *Clostridium difficile. C. trachomatis* genitourinary infections may also be associated. Up to 85 percent of patients with reactive arthritis are HLA-B27-positive. Back pain and a predominant involvement of lower-extremity joints are characteristic of reactive arthritis.

Systemic symptoms, such as fever, weight loss, malaise, weakness, and fatigue, may occur. The arthritis is usually asymmetrical and additive. Sacroiliitis is more frequently unilateral or more severe on one side. Dactylitis (sausage digits) occurs and is characteristic of reactive or psoriatic arthritis. Tendinitis and fasciitis may involve the Achilles tendon, the plantar fascia, and the paraspinal region. Peripheral arthritis, conjunctivitis, uveitis, prostatitis, and mucocutaneous lesions (e.g., oral ulcers, keratoderma blennorrhagicum, and balanitis circinata) may be associated with reactive sacroiliitis. Sacroiliac joint films may show blurring of the joint margins, reactive sclerosis of the adjacent bone, joint space narrowing, and irregularity of the margins. Reactive arthritis usually responds to nonsteroidal anti-inflammatory drugs.

B. Septic Arthritis Acute sacroiliitis may result from a joint infection with *S. aureus* or a *Brucella* species. Fever, chills, sweats, leukocytosis, and prostration are associated findings. The diagnosis requires joint fluid aspiration and culture. Tuberculosis may also involve the sacroiliac joint and cause low back, buttock, and posterior thigh pain; fever; and destructive radiographic changes. Specific antimicrobial therapy usually leads to resolution of these infectious disorders.

41. SACROILIAC SPRAIN

Sacroiliac joint pain, with local tenderness, a positive Gaenslen's sign, pain on weight bearing, and limited forward flexion, may result from athletic activities. A sudden hamstring contraction or abdominal muscle tightening can rotate the ilium and sprain the sacroiliac joint. Abrupt rotational motion may also result in a sprain of the sacroiliac joint. Direct trauma to the buttock can cause a similar injury. There may be persistent medial buttock and posterior thigh aching that is intensified by weight bearing, sitting, or bending forward. Rest is required until healing occurs.

42. MYOFASCIAL PAIN

Aching unilateral pain in the lower buttock and upper posterior thigh may be caused by an active myofascial trigger point. Pressure over this localized point may reproduce or intensify buttock and posterior thigh pain, while an injection of lidocaine and a corticosteroid into the trigger point may transiently or permanently relieve the pain.

43. POSTERIOR COMPARTMENT SYNDROME OF THE THIGH

This disorder may follow a closed or open femoral fracture, femoral intramedullary stabilization, blunt trauma, compression of the thigh by body weight during unconsciousness, or vascular injury. The major symptom in alert patients is excruciating posterior thigh pain that is persistent and intensified by movement. Distal limb dysesthesias are associated. Passive stretching of the muscles in the affected compartment intensifies the pain. This can be tested by passively extending the knee with the hip in flexion. Palpation of the posterior compartment reveals swelling, increased tension, and tenderness. The diagnosis can be confirmed by measuring the intracompart-

mental pressure. Measurements exceeding 30 mmHg should be considered abnormal. Serial pressure measurements may be helpful in cases with equivocal initial pressures. Surgical decompression of the involved compartment will relieve pain and prevent extensive ischemic damage to the muscles and nerves within the involved space.

Anterior Thigh Pain

44. BACTEREMIA-ASSOCIATED THIGH PAIN

Bilateral anterior thigh pain and tenderness in a febrile patient may be a manifestation of bacteremia. Leukocytosis, a shift to the left in the differential blood count, and an elevation of the creatine kinase level may be present. Blood culture isolates in patients with anterior thigh pain and tenderness have included *S. aureus*, *N. meningitidis*, *Streptobacillus moniliformis*, *Streptococcus pneumoniae*, *Streptococcus pyogenes*, *Klebsiella pneumoniae*, *Escherichia coli*, and *Pseudomonas aeruginosa*. Leptospirosis and subacute bacterial endocarditis may also cause bilateral anterior thigh pain. Viral and rickettsial disorders may also cause anterior thigh pain and more generalized myalgias. Bilateral anterior thigh pain and tenderness in a febrile patient require exclusion of a bacteremic disorder.

45. FEMORAL NEUROPATHY

Groin and anterior thigh pain occur. Hypesthesia and paresthesias of the anterior and anteromedial thigh may be present. Weakness of knee extension may be apparent and the knee jerk impaired. Walking may be associated with buckling of the affected knee.

Pain and paresthesias may occur in the anteromedial aspect of the lower leg. The pain may be intensified by hip extension or hyperextension. Retroperitoneal bleeding associated with femoral neuropathy may result in a characteristic posture. The knee is flexed and externally rotated, and there may be a palpable iliac mass (e.g., hematoma). A pulsatile mass (e.g., aneurysm) may be palpable in the lower abdomen in a small number of cases of femoral neuropathy. A CT scan will demonstrate a hematoma in the retroperitoneum in cases due to bleeding. An aneurysm adjacent to the hematoma may also be identified. Intraabdominal tumors or lower abdominal abscesses may also be imaged. The causes of acute femoral neuropathy are listed in Table 44-2.

46. RADICULAR PAIN

Groin, anterior, and anteromedial thigh pain with radiation to the knee may be secondary to root compression

Table 44-2
CAUSES OF ACUTE FEMORAL NEUROPATHY

Hemorrhage into the iliopsoas muscle secondary to
  Hemophilia
  Anticoagulant therapy
  Ruptured aortic aneurysm
Mass lesions adjacent to the femoral nerve
  Intraabdominal tumor
  Psoas abscess
  Appendiceal abscess
Iatrogenic causes
  Renal transplantation
  Lithotomy position and spinal anesthesia for hysterectomy
  Retractor pressure during pelvic surgery
  Arterial catheter trauma and femoral artery pseudoaneurysm
Sickle cell pain crisis
Diabetes mellitus
Mononeuritis multiplex
Trauma-related neuropathy (e.g., jumping, judo, and vigorous exercise)

(L2–L4) by a protruding disc or by a hypertrophic facet joint. Protruding discs at the L2–L3 and L3–L4 levels may mimic femoral neuropathy. A protruding lateral L4 disc can produce similar symptoms and signs.

Loss or impairment of the knee jerk may be caused by a disc involving the L3 or L4 root. Weakness of knee extension, quadriceps atrophy, and an impaired knee jerk may be present. Radicular pain may be provoked or intensified by straight leg-raising or by sudden increases in intraspinal pressure (e.g., as in coughing, straining, and sneezing).

High lumbar disc protrusions may be detected by CT-enhanced myelography or MRI. Surgical excision of the responsible prolapsed disc or decompression of the lateral recess or the nerve root foramen may be required to relieve anterior and anteromedial thigh pain.

47. FEMORAL SHAFT FRACTURE DUE TO TRAUMA

A high-speed motor vehicle accident may cause severe pain, swelling, tenderness, and deformity of one of both thighs. The pain may be anterior or diffuse. A plain radiograph will confirm the diagnosis.

48. FEMORAL SHAFT STRESS FRACTURE IN ATHLETES

Pain of an aching nature occurs in the anterior thigh on one side. The pain may be present continuously or only after running or walking. Local tenderness may be present. A plain radiograph will usually demonstrate the fracture. A radionuclide scan may image the fracture be-

fore a plain radiograph. Stress fractures may occur as a linear, oblique radiolucency in the medial cortex of the proximal femur; a spiral oblique fracture of the midfemur; or a transverse fracture of the distal third of the femur. Stress fractures may become displaced. Some stress fractures may be asymptomatic. Femoral shaft stress fractures may occur in soldiers during basic training or in athletes (e.g., runners, baseball players, and basketball players). Rest for 8 to 14 weeks results in recovery. In some cases, use of crutches for 3 to 4 weeks may be required.

49. ANTERIOR COMPARTMENT SYNDROME

Severe pain and tenderness occur in the anterior thigh after an isolated thigh injury or multiple trauma. The thigh is swollen and tense, and passive stretching of the quadriceps muscle (e.g., by flexing the knee with the hip extended) causes excruciating anterior thigh pain. Numbness and dysesthesias in the anteromedial and anterior thigh may occur. Thigh muscle weakness may be present. The diagnosis can be confirmed by measurement of the intracompartmental pressure (saline-injection technique).

An anterior compartment syndrome may be associated with an open or closed femoral fracture, a crush injury or contusion of the thigh, prolonged thigh compression from body weight during prolonged unconsciousness; intracompartmental bleeding from trauma or a coagulopathy, vascular injury and hypotension, and intramedullary stabilization of the femur for a femoral shaft fracture. Early surgical decompression of the compartment will relieve symptoms and preserve neuromuscular function.

50. SARTORIUS MUSCLE STRAIN

A tear of the sartorius muscle may cause anterior thigh pain and tenderness. Avulsion of its origin from the anterior superior iliac spine may occur, with maximum swelling and tenderness at that site.

51. QUADRICEPS MUSCLE STRAIN

Acute pain and tenderness occur in the anterior thigh as the quadriceps contracts forcibly against a fixed lower leg caught in a hole in the ground or fixed by a tackle (e.g., as in football). Forceful contraction of the quadriceps with the hip extended and knee flexed when kicking a ball and encountering unexpected resistance or sudden acceleration while running can also cause a quadriceps strain. There is localized tenderness, and there may be a palpable muscle defect or a hematoma and swelling at the site of injury. Passive and active knee flexion are restricted because of quadriceps spasm and associated anterior thigh pain.

Generalized Thigh Pain

52. FEMORAL SHAFT FRACTURE DUE TO TRAUMA

These fractures are most common in young adults and occur in automobile and motorcycle accidents or as a result of a gunshot wound. Pain begins with the injury and involves the thigh in the region of the fracture. The leg is usually shortened and deformed. Lateral and anterior angulation of the thigh is most common. Pain and muscle spasm prevent voluntary movement at the hip or knee. Marked swelling of the thigh occurs and is caused by traumatic edema and by bleeding at the fracture site. Enough blood volume loss may occur to cause tachycardia and hypotension. Vascular and neurologic impairment distal to the fracture site may occur. Plain radiographs will usually demonstrate the location, type (e.g., oblique, spiral, or transverse), and severity of the fracture (e.g., comminution or segmental fractures with displacement).

53. COMPARTMENT SYNDROME (ANTERIOR AND POSTERIOR)

This disorder is associated with a severe contusion of the thigh, multiple trauma, femoral shaft fractures, intramedullary fixation, thigh compression by body weight, intracompartmental bleeding due to trauma or a coagulopathy, or improper use of military antishock trousers.

Pain may occur in the anterior and posterior thigh in association with marked thigh swelling and increased palpable tension of the anterior and posterior compartments. Passive flexion or extension of the knee intensifies the pain. A measurement of the pressures in both compartments will confirm the diagnosis. Symptoms resolve with decompression of the anterior and posterior compartments of the thigh.

54. SICKLE CELL PAIN CRISIS

Severe unilateral or bilateral thigh pain and paresthesias may occur. There may be superficial burning or deep aching and/or throbbing pain with associated allodynia. MRI may be normal or show one or more bone marrow infarctions. The pain is due to a reversible sensory polyneuropathy (e.g., femoral, lateral femoral cutaneous, and posterior femoral cutaneous nerves), and it resolves spontaneously within 1 to 3 weeks. Some of the provoking causes of a pain crisis include cold, menses, emotional upset, prolonged standing, unusual exertion, and wearing of tight clothing about the upper thighs (e.g., bicycle pants). Pain may migrate to the knees, lower legs, feet, trunk, and upper extremities during the course of an attack.

55. PATHOLOGIC FRACTURE OF A FEMUR

Acute pain in the thigh may occur in association with a snapping sensation or a sudden giving way of the thigh in the absence of significant trauma. Plain radiographs will detect a pathologic fracture of the femur through an associated cystic or neoplastic lesion. Exploration and biopsy will provide a specific diagnosis. Dull, aching pain may sometimes precede the acute, severe pain of the pathologic fracture.

56. PYOMYOSITIS

Pain develops in one region and then spreads to other parts of the thigh. It is accompanied by fever, swelling, local tenderness, induration, and sometimes warmth and erythema of the overlying skin. Local inguinal and generalized adenopathy may occur. The leukocyte count and sedimentation rate are usually elevated. A CT scan of the upper leg will demonstrate one or more abscesses involving the thigh muscles. Surgical drainage reveals purulent and serosanguineous material, and *S. aureus* on culture. The lesion resolves with open drainage and antibiotic therapy. Pyomyositis due to *S. aureus* is most common in tropical and subtropical countries. Cases may occur in temperate climates in recent immigrants or travelers returning from such areas. Poorly controlled diabetics are also susceptible to this rare type of infection.

57. SOFT TISSUE SARCOMA

A soft tissue sarcoma may cause severe thigh pain, swelling, and tenderness and a visible lesion on CT scan. Surgical exploration and biopsy will confirm the diagnosis of malignancy.

58. RETROPERITONEAL PERFORATION OF THE COLON AND THIGH INFECTION

Diverticulitis or a carcinoma of the colon may perforate into the retroperitoneal space. Feces, gas, and bacteria may reach the thigh from the retroperitoneal region by the femoral canal and along the iliopsoas enveloping fascia, the greater and lesser sciatic foramina, and the obturator foramen. Fever, chills, and lower abdominal pain may precede or accompany hip, inguinal, and local or generalized thigh pain. Results of the abdominal examination may be negative or may reveal local tenderness and/or a mass in the ipsilateral iliac region. The painful thigh may be tender and swollen, and crepitus may be palpable. Straight leg-raising may be limited due to tracking of infectious material along the sciatic nerve. Plain radiographs will demonstrate gas in the soft tissues of the leg. Abdominal exploration will reveal a perforated diverticulum or carcinoma of the colon, with local abscess formation and peritonitis. Thigh exploration reveals inflammatory fluid and abscesses. Isolates include aerobic and anaerobic colon bacteria. Survival requires extensive abdominal and thigh drainage, antibiotics, and fecal diversion.

59. RETROPERITONEAL PERFORATION OF THE COLON AND LUMBOSACRAL PLEXUS INVOLVEMENT

Thigh and/or leg pain may also result from infectious involvement of the lumbosacral plexus. Local swelling, crepitus, and tenderness in the leg do not occur, and there is no evidence of gas on a plain radiograph of the thigh. Symptoms resolve after surgical treatment of the intraabdominal infection.

60. ILIOFEMORAL VENOUS THROMBOSIS

Pain occurs in one thigh and/or calf at rest or during exercise of the leg and is associated with edema of the entire leg. An increase in circumference of the calf and thigh of 1.4 cm or more compared with the asymptomatic leg may be present. The skin may be cool and pale or cyanotic. Local tenderness medial to the femoral artery pulse may be present. Doppler ultrasound, impedence plethysmography, or B-mode ultrasonography will confirm the diagnosis. Anticoagulant therapy will decrease the likelihood of pulmonary embolism and prevent thrombus extension.

61. STRESS FRACTURE OF THE FEMORAL SHAFT

Generalized thigh pain may occur at rest or for a variable period of time after running or other activity. There is often diffuse tenderness in the painful region. Stress fractures have been reported in military recruits, runners, baseball and basketball players, skiers, and other athletes. Plain radiographs will identify the fracture. In patients seen within 2 weeks of the onset of pain, the radiographic results may be negative, and a radionuclide bone scan may provide the only evidence of a fracture of the femoral shaft. Stress fractures may occur at any site in the shaft, and they are usually incomplete. Complete fractures with displacement have been reported in military recruits and athletes. Fractures in the middle and distal thirds are more likely to be complete.

62. MUSCLE STRAIN DUE TO OVERUSE

Excessive exercise may result in painful proximal leg muscles. Generalized thigh pain occurs and is increased by passive or active movement of the thigh muscles, and local tenderness and sometimes swelling occur over affected muscle groups in the thigh. Results of a radionuclide bone scan and plain radiographs are negative. This disorder is common in weekend athletes or new military recruits during the first week or two of physical fitness training. Calisthenics involving the thigh muscles may be responsible for crippling thigh muscle pain and weakness and myoglobinemia in a small percentage of participants. Walking, running, and calisthenics intensify the pain, and rest relieves it in 1 to 3 days.

Some runners develop thigh pain during the first 10 min of a 3- to 5-mile run. This myalgic pain improves and disappears as they continue to run. The cause is unknown.

63. IDIOPATHIC DERMATOMYOSITIS OR POLYMYOSITIS

Thigh pain, tenderness, and muscle weakness may occur. Buttock and lower leg pain may be associated. Climbing stairs, running, walking, and rising from a chair may be difficult. The gait may become unsteady and waddling, and frequent falls may occur. Pain and weakness of the arms, shoulders, and neck may follow. Difficulty in chewing and swallowing may be associated. Some patients present with only myalgic pain in the buttocks and thighs, without demonstrable weakness. The diagnosis of myositis can be confirmed by finding evidence of muscle injury by electromyography (e.g., fibrillation potentials, positive sharp waves, decreased amplitude and duration of muscle action potentials, and increased numbers of polyphasic action potentials), an elevated creatine kinase level, and muscle biopsy results. Polymyositis may be idiopathic and may occur with or without a rash (e.g., localized or diffuse erythema, maculopapular eruption, eczematoid dermatitis, or exfoliative dermatitis). A heliotrope (lilac-colored) rash may occur on the eyelids, the bridge of the nose, and the cheeks, as well as around the nails. Some cases of polymyositis or dermatomyositis are associated with a neoplasm (e.g., in the lung, ovary, breast, or gastrointestinal tract) and with myeloproliferative disorders. Others are associated with connective tissue disorders (e.g., scleroderma, rheumatoid arthritis, mixed connective tissue disease, and lupus erythematosus). Diagnostic studies to exclude these associated disorders may be necessary. Pain and weakness respond well to prednisone therapy.

64. INFECTIOUS POLYMYOSITIS

Acute polymyositis may sometimes be associated with toxoplasmosis, Lyme disease, or HIV infection.

65. RHABDOMYOLYSIS AND MYOGLOBINURIA

Severe muscle pain, tenderness, stiffness, weakness, and swelling accompanied by edema and sometimes ecchymoses of the overlying skin occur in association with brownish-red urine (myoglobinuria). The serum creatine kinase level is markedly elevated. There may be severe bilateral thigh and hip girdle aching that is intensified by movement. Renal failure may result from the myoglobinuria. The causes of acute rhabdomyolysis are listed in Table 44-3.

Table 44-3
CAUSES OF RHABDOMYOLYSIS AND MYOGLOBINURIA

Enzyme deficiencies affecting anaerobic glycolysis
  Myophosphorylase
  Phosphofructokinase
  Phosphoglycerate mutase
  Phosphoglycerate kinase
  Lactate dehydrogenase
  Carnitine palmityl transferase
  Myoadenylate deaminase
Substrate deficiencies with increased muscle activity and metabolism
  Malignant hyperthermia
  Neuroleptic malignant syndrome
  Antiparkinsonian drug withdrawal
  Severe exercise in untrained recruits
  Hypoglycemia
  Hypophosphatemia
Electrolyte disorders
  Hypokalemia
  Hypernatremia
  Hyponatremia
  Hypomagnesemia
Infectious disorders
  Influenza A virus
  Epstein-Barr virus
  Herpes simplex virus
  Sepsis
  Coxsackievirus
  Clostridial myonecrosis
Drugs and toxic agents
  Alcohol
  Amphetamines
  Cocaine
  Barbiturates
  Sea snake poison
  Narcotics (heroin)
  Azothioprine
  Amphotericin B
  Clofibrate
  Epsilon amino caproic acid
  Phencyclidine
Ischemic and traumatic causes
  Body-weight pressure on a limb during coma
  Crush injury
  Compartment syndrome
Myopathies
  Acute polymyositis or dermatomyositis
  Systemic lupus erythematosus
  Muscular dystrophies

66. FEVER-RELATED MYALGIAS

Aching bilateral anterior and lateral thigh pain, shoulder pain, and proximal arm pain may be associated with febrile disorders caused by viral, bacterial, and rickettsial organisms. The aching responds to aspirin therapy and to resolution of the infection.

Acute Bilateral Inguinal, Trochanteric, Pubic, and Thigh Pain

Tables 44-4 through 44-10 list the causes of acute bilateral inguinal, trochanteric, pubic, and thigh pain.

Table 44-4
67. BILATERAL INGUINAL AND ANTEROMEDIAL THIGH PAIN

Calcium pyrophosphate deposition disease with hip arthritis
Gout with hip arthritis
Rheumatic fever with hip arthritis
Rheumatoid arthritis with hip arthritis
Reiter's syndrome with hip arthritis
Juvenile rheumatoid arthritis with hip arthritis
Legg-Calvé-Perthes disease
Slipped capital femoral epiphysis
Pubic osteomyelitis
Transient synovitis of the hip
Trauma: bilateral hip fracture and/or dislocation
Osteonecrosis of the femoral head
Iliopsoas bursitis
Femoral neuropathy
Inguinal or femoral hernias
Lymphadenitis (inguinal or femoral)
  Cellulitis of the abdominal wall or perineum
  Bubonic plague
  Genital herpes simplex
  Suppurative iliac lymphadenitis
  Chancroid
  Lymphogranuloma venereum
  Primary syphilis
  Gonococcal urethritis

Table 44-5
68. BILATERAL LATERAL HIP AND THIGH PAIN

Trochanteric bursitis
Meralgia paresthestica
Osteonecrosis of the hip
Arthritis of the hip
Fracture of the femoral shaft due to trauma

Table 44-6
69. BILATERAL MEDIAL THIGH PAIN

Herpes simplex neuritis
Tubo-ovarian disorders (referred pain)
Adductor strain
Pubic bone disorders

Table 44-7
70. BILATERAL PUBIC BONE PAIN

Osteitis pubis
Osteomyelitis of the pubic bone
Pyogenic arthritis of the pubic symphysis
Pubic stress fracture
Pubic osteolysis
Postpartum symphyseal pain

Table 44-8
71. BILATERAL POSTERIOR THIGH PAIN

Ischial bursitis
Disc protrusion and radiculopathy
Epidural abscess and radiculopathy
Epidural or subdural hemorrhage and radiculopathy
Conus medullaris infarction
Sacroiliitis
Sacroiliac sprain
Myofascial pain

Table 44-9
72. BILATERAL ANTERIOR THIGH PAIN

Bacteremia-associated anterior thigh pain
Femoral neuropathy
Radicular pain due to L2, L3, or L4 disc protrusion
Femoral shaft fractures

Table 44-10
73. BILATERAL GENERALIZED THIGH PAIN

Femoral shaft fractures
Sickle cell pain crisis
Muscle strain due to overuse
Dermatomyositis or polymyositis
Infectious polymyositis
Rhabdomyolysis and myoglobinuria
Fever-related myalgias

INGUINAL, TROCHANTERIC, PUBIC, AND THIGH PAIN REFERENCES

Buttock and Upper Thigh Pain
Turek SL. Tuberculosis of the sacroiliac joint, in Turek SL: *Orthopaedics Principles and Their Applications,* 4th ed. Philadelphia, Lippincott, 1984, vol 2, pp 1663–1665.

Coccygodynia
Albrektsson B: Sacral rhizotomy in cases of ano-coccygeal pain: A follow-up of 24 cases. *Acta Orthop Scand* 52:187–190, 1981.
Bayne O, Bateman JE, Cameron HU: The influence of etiology on the results of coccygectomy. *Clin Orthop* 190:266–272, 1984.
Duncan L, Halverson J, De-Schryver-Kecskemeti K: Glomus tumor of the coccyx: A curable cause of coccygodynia. *Arch Pathol Lab Med* 115:78–80, 1991.
Hellberg S, Strange-Vognsen HH: Coccygodynia treated by resection of the coccyx. *Acta Orthop Scand* 61:463–465, 1990.

Maroy B: Spontaneous and evoked coccygeal pain in depression. *Dis Colon Rectum* 31:210–215, 1988.
Thiele GH: Coccygodynia: Cause and treatment. *Dis Colon Rectum* 6:422–436, 1963.
Turek SL: Coccygodynia, in Turek SL: *Orthopaedics Principles and Their Application,* 4th ed. Philadelphia, Lippincott, 1984 vol 2, pp 1658–1661.
Ziegler DK, Batnitzky S: Coccygodynia caused by perineural cyst. *Neurology* 34:829–830, 1984.

Hip Pain—Review
Brady LP: Hip pain: Don't throw away the cane. *Postgrad Med* 83:89–90, 95–97, 1988.
Dee R, Stillwell WT, Mango E: Rheumatologic and degenerative disorders of the hip joint, in Dee R, Mango E, Hurst LC (eds): *Prin-*

ciples of Orthopaedic Practice. New York, McGraw-Hill, 1989, vol 2, pp 1331–1370.

Drummond DS: Congenital and development deformities of the hip, in Steinberg ME (ed): *The Hip and Its Disorders*. Philadelphia, Saunders, 1991, pp 372–389.

Goodman SB, Schurman DJ: Miscellaneous disorders, in Steinberg ME (ed): *The Hip and Its Disorders*. Philadelphia, Saunders, 1991, pp 683–704.

Johnson EW: Location of hip pain (letter to editor). *JAMA* 242:1849, 1979.

Mosca VS: Pitfalls in diagnosis: The hip. *Pediatr Ann* 18:12–14, 16–18, 23, 1989.

Roberts WN, Williams RB: Hip pain. *Prim Care* 15:783–793, 1988.

Schon L, Zuckerman JD: Hip pain in the elderly: Evaluation and diagnosis. *Geriatrics* 43:48–62, 1988.

Turek SL: The hip, in Turek SL (ed): *Orthopaedics Principles and Their Application,* 4th ed. Philadelphia, Lippincott, 1984, vol 2, pp 1109–1268.

Hip Trauma

Canale ST: Intracapsular fractures, in Steinberg ME (ed): *The Hip and Its Disorders*. Philadelphia, Saunders, 1991, pp 144–159.

Kane WJ: Fractures of the pelvis, in Rockwood CA Jr, Green DP (eds): *Fractures in Adults,* 2d ed. Philadelphia, Lippincott, 1984, vol 2, pp 1093–1209.

Kling TF Jr: Pelvic and acetabular fractures, in Steinberg ME (ed): *The Hip and Its Disorders*. Philadelphia, Saunders, 1991, pp 173–197.

Kyle RF: Intertrochanteric fractures, in Steinberg ME (ed): *The Hip and Its Disorders*. Philadelphia, Saunders, 1991, pp 280–291.

Levin PE, Browner BD: Dislocations and fracture-dislocations of the hip, in Steinberg ME (ed): *The Hip and Its Disorders*. Philadelphia, Saunders, 1991, pp 222–246.

Ordway C, Levin PE, Dee R: Fractures of the pelvis and leg, in Dee R, Mango E, Hurst LC (eds): *Principles of Orthopaedic Practice,* New York, McGraw-Hill, 1989, vol 1, pp 1209–1260.

Roberts JM: Extracapsular fractures, in Steinberg ME (ed): *The Hip and Its Disorders*. Philadelphia, Saunders, 1991, pp 160–172.

Tile M: Fractures of the acetabulum, in Steinberg ME (ed): *The Hip and Its Disorders*. Philadelphia, Saunders, 1991, pp 201–221.

Tronzo RG: Femoral neck fractures, in Steinberg ME (ed): *The Hip and Its Disorders*. Philadelphia, Saunders, 1991, pp 247–279.

Wedge JH: Dislocation and epiphyseal separation, in Steinberg ME (ed): *The Hip and Its Disorders*. Philadelphia, Saunders, 1991, pp 129–143.

Zickel RE: Subtrochanteric fractures, in Steinberg ME (ed): *The Hip and Its Disorders*. Philadelphia, Saunders, 1991, pp 292–309.

Inguinal Pain — Adolescents and Adults

Alani WO, Bartal E: Osteoid osteoma of the femoral neck simulating an inflammatory synovitis. *Clin Orthop* 223:308–312, 1987.

Bleck EE: Idiopathic chondrolysis of the hip. *J Bone Joint Surg (Am)* 65-A:1266–1275, 1983.

Bowen JR: Legg-Calvé-Perthes disease, in Dee R, Mango E, Hurst LC (eds): *Principles of Orthopaedic Practice*. New York, McGraw-Hill, 1989, vol 2, pp 1110–1128.

Catterall A: Perthes' disease, in Steinberg ME (ed): *The Hip and Its Disorders,* Philadelphia, Saunders, 1991, pp 419–439.

Cotler JM: Office management in Legg-Calvé-Perthes syndrome. *Orthop Clin North Am* 13:619–627, 1982.

Grogan DP, Sackett JR, Ogden JA: Infection of the hip, in Steinberg ME (ed): *The Hip and Its Disorders*. Philadelphia, Saunders, 1991, pp 354–371.

Haueisen DC, Weiner DS, Weiner SD: The characterization of "transient synovitis of the hip" in children. *J Pediatr Orthop* 6:11–17, 1986.

Hughes RA, Tempos K, Ansell BM: A review of the diagnoses of hip pain presentation in the adolescent. *Br J Rheumatol* 27:450–453, 1988.

Lehman WB: Slipped capital femoral epiphysis, in Dee R, Mango E,

Hurst LC (eds): *Principles of Orthopaedic Practice*. New York, McGraw-Hill, 1989, vol 2, pp 1101–1109.

Speer DP: Slipped capital femoral epiphysis, in Steinberg ME (ed): *The Hip and Its Disorders*. Philadelphia, Saunders, 1991, pp 390–418.

Staheli LT: Acetabular dysplasia: Treatment by pelvic osteotomy, in Steinberg ME (ed): *The Hip and Its Disorders*. Philadelphia, Saunders, 1991, pp 335–353.

Inguinal Pain — Ankylosing Spondylitis and Reactive Arthritis

Finsterbush A, Amir D, Vatashki E, et al: Joint surgery in severe ankylosing spondylitis. *Acta Orthop Scand* 59:491–496, 1988.

García-Morteo O, Maldonado-Cocco JA, Suárez-Almazor ME, et al: Ankylosing spondylitis of juvenile onset: Comparison with adult onset disease. *Scand J Rheumatol* 12:247–248, 1983.

Gordon TP, Sage MR, Bertouch JV, et al: Computed tomography of paraspinal musculature in ankylosing spondylitis. *J Rheumatol* 11:794–797, 1984.

Marks JS, Holt PJL: The natural history of Reiter's disease: 21 years of observations. *Q J Med* 60:685–697, 1986.

Marks SH, Barnett M, Calin A: Ankylosing spondylitis in women and men: A case-control study. *J Rheumatol* 10:624–628, 1983.

Taurog JD, Lipsky PE: Ankylosing spondylitis and reactive arthritis, in Wilson JD, Braunwald E, Isselbacher KJ, et al (eds): *Harrison's Principles of Internal Medicine,* 12th ed. New York, McGraw-Hill, 1991, vol 2, pp 1451–1455.

Thompson GH, Khan MA, Bilenker RM: Spontaneous atlantoaxial subluxation as a presenting manifestation of juvenile ankylosing spondylitis: A case report. *Spine* 7:78–79, 1982.

Vinje O, Dale K, Møller P: Radiographic evaluation of patients with Bechterew's syndrome (ankylosing spondylitis): Findings in peripheral joints, tendon insertions and the pubic symphysis and relations to non-radiographic findings. *Scand J Rheumatol* 14:279–288, 1985.

Inguinal Pain — Arthritis

Altman RD: Criteria for the classification of osteoarthritis of the knee and hip. *Scand J Rheumatol* 16(suppl 65):31–39, 1987.

Altman RD, Fries JF, Bloch DA, et al: Radiographic assessment of progression in osteoarthritis. *Arth Rheum* 30:1214–1225, 1987.

Amstutz HC, Thomas BJ, Jinnah R, et al: Treatment of primary osteoarthritis of the hip: A comparison of total joint and surface replacement arthroplasty. *J Bone Joint Surg (Am)* 66-A:228–241, 1984.

Bennett JC: Rheumatoid arthritis, in Wyngaarden JB, Smith LH Jr (eds): *Cecil Textbook of Medicine,* 18th ed. Philadelphia, Saunders, 1988, vol 2, pp 1998–2004.

Bland JH: The reversibility of osteoarthritis: A review. *Am J Med* 74:16–26, 1983.

Blane CE, Ragsdale CG, Hensinger RN: Late effects of JRA on the hip. *J Pediatr Orthop* 7:677–680, 1987.

Calin A: Ankylosing spondylitis, in Kelley WN, Harris ED Jr, Ruddy S, et al (eds): *Textbook of Rheumatology*. Philadelphia, Saunders, 1981, vol 2, pp 1017–1032.

———: The spondylarthropathies, in Wyngaarden JB, Smith LH Jr (eds): *Cecil Textbook of Medicine,* 18th ed. Philadelphia, Saunders, 1988, vol 2, pp 2004–2009.

Colville J, Raunio P: Total hip replacement in juvenile rheumatoid arthritis: Analysis of 59 hips. *Acta Orthop Scand* 50:197–203, 1979.

Gilliland BC: Relapsing polychondritis and miscellaneous arthritides, in Wilson JD, Braunwald E, Isselbacher KJ, et al (eds): *Harrison's Principles of Internal Medicine,* 12th ed. New York, McGraw-Hill, 1991, vol 2, pp 1484–1490.

Gitelis S, Heligman D, Quill G, et al: The use of large allografts for tumor reconstruction and salvage of the failed total hip arthroplasty. *Clin Orthop* 231:62–70, 1988.

Good AE: Enteropathic arthritis, in Kelley WN, Harris Ed Jr, Ruddy S, et al (eds): *Textbook of Rheumatology*. Philadelphia, Saunders, 1981, vol 2, pp 1063–1075.

Halla JT, Hardin JG: Acute non-infectious arthritis of the hip in patients with rheumatoid arthritis. *Ann Rheum Dis* 46:475–476, 1987.

Harris ED Jr: Rheumatoid arthritis: The clinical spectrum, in Kelley WN, Harris ED Jr, Ruddy S, et al (eds): *Textbook of Rheumatology.* Philadelphia, Saunders, 1981, vol 2, pp 928–963.

Harris WH: Etiology of osteoarthritis of the hip. *Clin Orthop* 213:20–33, 1986.

Howell DS: Osteoarthritis (degenerative joint disease), in Wyngaarden JB, Smith LH Jr (eds): *Cecil Textbook of Medicine,* 18th ed. Philadelphia, Saunders, 1988, vol 2, pp 2039–2041.

Koski JM: Ultrasonographic evidence of hip synovitis in patients with rheumatoid arthritis. *Scand J Rheumatol* 18:127–131, 1989.

Lachiewicz PF, McCaskill B, Inglis A, et al: Total hip arthroplasty in juvenile rheumatoid arthritis: Two- to eleven-year results. *J Bone Joint Surg (Am)* 68-A:502–508, 1986.

Lehtimäki MY, Kaarela K, Hämäläinen MMJ: Incidence of hip involvement and need for total hip replacement in rheumatoid arthritis: An eight-year follow-up study. *Scand J Rheumatol* 15:387–391, 1986.

Lipsky PE: Rheumatoid arthritis, in Wilson JD, Braunwald E, Isselbacher KJ, et al (eds): *Harrison's Principles of Internal Medicine,* 12th ed. New York, McGraw-Hill, 1991, vol 2, pp 1437–1443.

Malawista SE: Infectious arthritis, in Wyngaarden JB, Smith LH Jr (eds): *Cecil Textbook of Medicine,* 18th ed. Philadelphia, Saunders, 1988, vol 2, pp 2009–2011.

Norman A, Abdelwahab IF, Sayon J, et al: Osteoid osteoma of the hip stimulating an early onset of osteoarthritis. *Radiology* 158:417–420, 1986.

O'Brien TM, Moran R, McGoldrick F: The aetiology of degenerative disease of the hip: A review of 400 cases. *Ir J Med Sci* 158:63–66, 1989.

Poss R, Maloney JP, Ewald FC, et al: Six- to 11-year results of total hip arthroplasty in rheumatoid arthritis. *Clin Orthop* 182:109–116, 1984.

Ranawat CS, Atkinson RE, Salvati EA, et al: Conventional total hip arthroplasty for degenerative joint disease in patients between ages of forty and sixty years. *J Bone Joint Surg (Am)* 66-A(5):745–752, 1984.

Reigstad A, Grønmark T: Osteoarthritis of the hip treated by intertrochanteric osteotomy. *J Bone Joint Surg (Am)* 66-A:1–6, 1984.

Saito S, Saito M, Nishina T, et al: Long-term results of total hip arthroplasty for osteonecrosis of the femoral head: A comparison with osteoarthritis. *Clin Orthop* 244:198–207, 1989.

Schur PH: Psoriatic arthritis and arthritis associated with gastrointestinal diseases, in Wilson JD, Braunwald E, Isselbacher KJ, et al (eds): *Harrison's Principles of Internal Medicine,* 12th ed. New York, McGraw-Hill, 1991, vol 2, pp 1482–1484.

Scott RD, Sarokhan AJ, Dalziel R: Total hip and total knee arthroplasty in juvenile rheumatoid arthritis. *Clin Orthop* 182:90–98, 1984.

Steinberg AD: Systemic lupus erythematosus, in Wyngaarden JB, Smith LH Jr (eds): *Cecil Textbook of Medicine,* 18th ed. Philadelphia, Saunders, 1988, vol 2, pp 2011–2018.

White TK, Incavo SJ, Moreland MS: Giant synovial cyst of the hip joint. *Orthop Rev* 17:609–612, 1988.

Wright V: Psoriatic arthritis, in Kelley WN, Harris ED Jr, Ruddy S, et al (eds): *Textbook of Rheumatology.* Philadelphia, Saunders, 1981, vol 2, pp 1047–1062.

Inguinal Pain—Calcium Pyrophosphate Deposition Disease

Sokoloff L, Varma AA: Chondrocalcinosis in surgically resected joints. *Arthritis Rheum* 31:750–756, 1988.

Inguinal Pain—Chronic

Ekberg O, Persson NH, Abrahamsson P-A, et al: Longstanding groin pain in athletes: A multidisciplinary approach. *Sports Med* 6:56–61, 1988.

Wiltz O, Schoetz DJ Jr, Murray JJ, et al: Perianal hidradenitis suppurativa: The Lahey Clinic experience. *Dis Colon Rectum* 33:731–734, 1990.

Inguinal Pain—Hip Replacement

Bierbaum BE, Pomeroy DL, Berklacich FM: Late complications of hip replacement, in Steinberg ME (ed): *The Hip and Its Disorders.* Philadelphia, Saunders, 1991, pp 1061–1096.

Ranawat CS, Figgie MP: Early complications of total hip replacement, in Steinberg ME (ed): *The Hip and Its Disorders.* Philadelphia, Saunders, 1991, pp 1042–1060.

Inguinal Pain—Iliofemoral Thrombosis

Hobson RW II, Mintz BL, Jamil Z, et al: Diagnosis of acute deep venous thrombosis. *Surg Clin North Am* 70:143–157, 1990.

Landefeld CS, McGuire E, Cohen AM: Clinical findings associated with acute proximal deep vein thrombosis: A basis for quantifying clinical judgment. *Am J Med* 88:382–388, 1990.

Inguinal Pain—Iliopsoas Syndrome

Cohen JM, Hodges SC, Weinreb JC, et al: MR imaging of iliopsoas bursitis and concurrent avascular necrosis of the femoral head. *J Comput Assist Tomogr* 9:969–971, 1985.

Fritz P, Mariette X, Clerc D, et al: Rectus femoris sheath: A new localization of hip synovial cyst. *J Rheumatol* 16:1575–1578, 1989.

Grindulis KA: Rheumatoid iliopsoas bursitis (letter to editor). *J Rheumatol* 13:988, 1986.

Hockley NM, Steidle CP, West KW, et al: Ectopic ureter presenting as a psoas abscess. *J Urol* 143:767–769, 1990.

Lotke PA: Soft tissue afflictions, in Steinberg ME (ed): *The Hip and Its Disorders.* Philadelphia, Saunders, 1991, pp 669–682.

Pellman E: Rheumatoid iliopsoas bursitis (reply). *J Rheumatol* 13:988, 1986.

Pellman E, Kumari S, Greenwald R: Rheumatoid iliopsoas bursitis presenting as unilateral leg edema. *J Rheumatol* 13:197–200, 1986.

Sartoris DJ, Danzig L, Gilula L, et al: Synovial cysts of the hip joint and iliopsoas bursitis: A spectrum of imaging abnormalities. *Skeletal Radiol* 14:85–94, 1985.

Underwood PL, McLeod RA, Ginsburg WW: The varied clinical manifestations of iliopsoas bursitis. *J Rheumatol* 15:1683–1685, 1988.

Weinreb JC, Cohen JM, Maravilla KR: Iliopsoas muscles: MR study of normal anatomy and disease. *Radiology* 156:435–440, 1985.

Inguinal Pain—Infections of the Hip

Berquist TH, Bender CE, Maus TP, et al: Pseudobursae: A useful finding in patients with painful hip arthroplasty. *AJR* 148:103–106, 1987.

Bowie WR, Holmes KK: *Chlamydia trachomatis* (trachoma, perinatal infections, lymphogranuloma venereum and other genital infections), in Mandell GL, Douglas RG Jr, Bennett JE (eds): *Principles and Practice of Infectious Diseases.* New York, Churchill Livingstone, 1990, pp 1426–1440.

Boyce JM: *Francisella tularensis* (tularemia), in Mandell GL, Douglas RG Jr, Bennett JE (eds): *Principles and Practice of Infectious Diseases.* New York, Churchill Livingstone, 1990, pp 1742–1746.

Butler T: *Yersinia* species (including plague), in Mandell GL, Douglas RG Jr, Bennett JE (eds): *Principles and Practice of Infectious Diseases.* New York, Churchill Livingstone, 1990, pp 1748–1756.

Collins DN, Nelson CL: Infections of the hip, in Steinberg ME (ed): *The Hip and Its Disorders.* Philadelphia, Saunders, 1991, pp 648–668.

Fischer GW: The agent of cat-scratch disease, in Mandell GL, Douglas RG Jr, Bennett JE (eds): *Principles and Practice of Infectious Diseases.* New York, Churchill Livingstone, 1990, pp 1874–1877.

Flatman JG: Hip disease with referred pain to the knee. *JAMA* 234:967–968, 1975.

Hand WL: *Haemophilus* species, in Mandell GL, Douglas RG Jr, Bennett JE (eds): *Principles and Practice of Infectious Diseases.* New York, Churchill Livingstone, 1990, pp 1729–1733.

Hirsch MS: Herpes simplex virus, in Mandell GL, Douglas RG Jr, Bennett JE (eds): *Principles and Practice of Infectious Diseases.* New York, Churchill Livingstone, 1990, pp 1144–1153.

Kraft SM, Panush RS, Longley S: Unrecognized staphylococcal pyarthrosis with rheumatoid arthritis. *Semin Arthritis Rheum* 14:196–201, 1985.

Phillips FM, Pottenger LA: Acute septic arthritis in chronic osteonecrosis of the hip. *J Rheumatol* 15:1713–1716, 1988.

Rein MF: Inguinal adenopathy, in Mandell GL, Douglas RG Jr, Bennett JE (eds): *Principles and Practice of Infectious Diseases.* New York, Churchill Livingstone, 1990, pp 938–942.

Swartz MN: Cellulitis and superficial infections, in Mandell GL, Douglas RG Jr, Bennett JE (eds): *Principles and Practice of Infectious Diseases.* New York, Churchill Livingstone, 1990, pp 796–807.

———: Subcutaneous tissue infections and abscesses, in Mandell GL, Douglas RG Jr, Bennett JE (eds): *Principles and Practice of Infectious Diseases.* New York, Churchill Livingstone, 1990, pp 808–812.

Tramont EC: *Treponema pallidum* (syphilis), in Mandell GL, Douglas RG Jr, Bennett JE (eds): *Principles and Practice of Infectious Diseases.* New York, Churchill Livingstone, 1990, pp 1794–1808.

Inguinal Pain—Lymphadenitis/Cellulitis

Greenfield LJ: Venous and lymphatic disease, in Schwartz SI (ed): *Principles of Surgery,* 5th ed. New York, McGraw-Hill, 1989, pp 1011–1040.

Hill MK, Sanders CV: Localized and systemic infection due to *Vibrio* species. *Infect Dis Clinic North Am* 1:687–707, 1987.

Krockta WP, Barnes RC: Genital ulceration with regional adenopathy. *Infect Dis Clin North Am* 1:217–233, 1987.

Sachs MK: The optimum use of needle aspiration in the bacteriologic diagnosis of cellulitis in adults. *Arch Intern Med* 150:1907–1912, 1990.

Swartz MN: Lymphadenitis and lymphangitis, in Mandell GL, Douglas RG Jr, Bennett JE (eds): *Principles and Practice of Infectious Diseases.* New York, Churchill Livingstone, 1990, pp 818–825.

Inguinal Pain—Neoplastic

Jeffery CC: Spontaneous fractures of the femoral neck. *Orthop Clin North Am* 5:713–727, 1974.

Meals RA, Hungerford DS, Stevens MB: Malignant disease mimicking arthritis of the hip. *JAMA* 239:1070–1071, 1978.

Murray JA, Parrish FF: Surgical management of secondary neoplastic fractures about the hip. *Orthop Clin North Am* 5:887–901, 1974.

Inguinal Pain—Neuralgia

Smith SE, DeLee JC, Ramamurthy S: Ilioinguinal neuralgia following iliac bone-grafting: Report of two cases and review of the literature. *J Bone Joint Surg (Am)* 66-A:1306–1308, 1984.

Inguinal Pain—Osteonecrosis of the Hip

Bonnarens F, Hernandez A, D'Ambrosia R: Bone scintigraphic changes in osteonecrosis of the femoral head. *Orthop Clin North Am* 16:697–703, 1985.

Hanker GJ, Amstutz HC: Osteonecrosis of the hip in the sickle-cell diseases. Treatment and complications. *J Bone Joint Surg (Am)* 70-A(4):499–506, 1988.

Hickman JG, Tindall JP, McCollum DE: Aseptic (avascular) necrosis of the femoral head in psoriasis. *South Med J* 72:121–126, 1979.

Hungerford DS, Lennox DW: The importance of increased intraosseous pressure in the development of osteonecrosis of the femoral head: Implications for treatment. *Orthop Clin North Am* 16:635–654, 1985.

Jergesen HE, Heller M, Genant HK: Magnetic resonance imaging in osteonecrosis of the femoral head. *Orthop Clin North Am* 16:705–716, 1985.

Maistrelli G, Fusco U, Avai A, et al: Osteonecrosis of the hip treated by intertrochanteric osteotomy: A four- to 15-year follow-up. *J Bone Joint Surg (Br)* 70-B:761–766, 1988.

Mango E: Ischemic necrosis of the femoral head, in Dee R, Mango E, Hurst LC (eds): *Principles of Orthopaedic Practice.* New York: McGraw-Hill, 1989, vol 2, pp 1357–1370.

Meyers MH: Osteonecrosis of the femoral head: Pathogenesis and long-term results of treatment. *Clin Orthop* 231:51–61, 1988.

Myllynen P, Mäkelä A, Kontula K: Aseptic necrosis of the femoral head during pregnancy. *Obstet Gynecol* 71:495–498, 1988.

Saito S, Ohzono K, Ono K: Minimal osteonecrosis as a segmental infarct within the femoral head. *Clin Orthop* 231:35–50, 1988.

Seiler JG III, Christie MJ, Homra L: Correlation of the findings of magnetic resonance imaging with those of bone biopsy in patients who have stage I or II ischemic necrosis of the femoral head. *J Bone Joint Surg (Am)* 71-A:28–32, 1989.

Shupak R, Bernier V, Rabinovich S, et al: Avascular necrosis of bone with rheumatoid vasculitis. *J Rheumatol* 10:261–266, 1983.

Solomon L: Mechanisms of idiopathic osteonecrosis. *Orthop Clin North Am* 16:655–667, 1985.

Steinberg ME, Steinberg DR: Avascular necrosis of the femoral head, in Steinberg ME (ed): *The Hip and Its Disorders.* Philadelphia, Saunders, 1991, pp 623–647.

Stulberg BN, Bauer TW, Belhobek GH, et al: A diagnostic algorithm for osteonecrosis of the femoral head. *Clin Orthop* 249:176–182, 1989.

Sugioka Y: Transtrochanteric rotational osteotomy in the treatment of idiopathic and steroid-induced femoral head necrosis, Perthes' disease, slipped capital femoral epiphysis, and osteoarthritis of the hip: Indications and results. *Clin Orthop* 184:12–23, 1984.

Vakil N, Sparberg M: Steroid-related osteonecrosis in inflammatory bowel disease. *Gastroenterology* 96:62–67, 1989.

Williams IA, Mitchell AD, Rothman W, et al: Survey of the long-term incidence of osteonecrosis of the hip and adverse medical events in rheumatoid arthritis after high-dose intravenous methylprednisolone. *Ann Rheum Dis* 47:930–933, 1988.

Inguinal Pain—Paget's Disease

Goldman AB, Bullough P, Kammerman S, et al: Osteitis deformans of the hip joint. *Am J Roentgenol* 128:601–606, 1977.

Winfield J, Stamp TCB: Bone and joint symptoms in Paget's disease. *Ann Rheum Dis* 43:769–773, 1984.

Inguinal Pain—Pigmented Villonodular Synovitis

Abrahams TG, Pavlov H, Bansal M, et al: Concentric joint space narrowing of the hip associated with hemosiderotic synovitis (HS) including pigmented villonodular synovitis (PVNS). *Skeletal Radiol* 17:37–45, 1988.

Friedman B, Caspi I, Nerubay J, et al: Synovial chondromatosis of the hip joint. *Orthop Rev* 17:994–998, 1988.

Goldberg RP, Weissman BN, Naimark A, et al: Femoral neck erosions: Sign of hip joint synovial disease. *AJR* 141:107–111, 1983.

Janssens X, Veys EM, Cuvelier C: Pigmented villonodular synovitis of the hip: Association with osteochondromatosis. *Clin Exp Rheumatol* 5:329–334, 1987.

Inguinal Pain—Posttraumatic Arthritis

Altenberg AR: Acetabular labrum tears: A cause of hip pain and degenerative arthritis. *South Med J* 70:174–175, 1977.

Inguinal Pain—Review

Bomalaski JS, Schumacher HR Jr: Arthritis and allied conditions, in Steinberg ME (ed): *The Hip and Its Disorders.* Philadelphia, Saunders, 1991, pp 501–526.

Gilliland BC: Relapsing polychondritis and miscellaneous arthritides, in Wilson JD, Braunwald E, Isselbacher KJ, et al (eds): *Harrison's Principles of Internal Medicine,* 12th ed. New York, McGraw-Hill, 1991, vol 2, pp 1484–1490.

Hahn BH: Systemic lupus erythematosus, in Wilson JD, Braunwald E, Isselbacher RJ, et al (eds): *Harrison's Principles of Internal Medicine,* 12th ed. New York, McGraw-Hill, 1991, vol 2, pp 1432–1437.

Hurley HJ Jr: Apocrine glands (hidradenitis suppurativa), in Fitzpatrick TB, Eisen AZ, Wolff K (eds): *Dermatology in Medicine,* 2d ed. New York, McGraw-Hill, 1979, pp 473–484.

Lange TA: Tumors and tumorous conditions, in Steinberg ME (ed): *The Hip and Its Disorders.* Philadelphia, Saunders, 1991, pp 527–588.

Inguinal Pain—Transient Osteoporosis

Gaucher A, Colomb J-N, Naoun AR, et al: The diagnostic value of

99m Tc-diphosphonate bone imaging in transient osteoporosis of the hip. *J Rheumatol* 6:574–583, 1979.

Inguinal Pain — Trauma

DeLee JC: Fractures and dislocations of the hip, in Rockwood CA Jr, Green DP (eds): *Fractures in Adults,* 2d ed. Philadelphia, Lippincott, 1984, vol 2, pp 1211–1356.

Mooney V, Claudi BF: Fractures of the shaft of the femur, in Rockwood CA Jr, Green DP (eds): *Fractures in Adults,* 2d ed. Philadelphia, Lippincott, 1984, vol 2, pp 1357–1427.

Sim FH, Scott SG: Injuries to the pelvis and hip in athletes: Anatomy and function, in Nicholas JA, Hershman EB, (eds): *The Lower Extremity and Spine in Sports Medicine*. St. Louis, Mosby, 1986, vol 2, pp 1119–1169.

Pubic Pain

Gamble JG, Simmons SC, Freedman M: The symphysis pubis: Anatomic and pathologic considerations. *Clin Orthop* 203:261–272, 1986.

Kubitz RL, Goodlin RC: Symptomatic separation of the pubic symphysis. *South Med J* 79:578–580, 1986.

McCarthy B, Dorfman HD: Pubic osteolysis: A benign lesion of the pelvis closely mimicking a malignant neoplasm. *Clin Orthop* 251:300–307, 1990.

Nicholas JJ, Haidet E, Helfrich D, et al: Groin and hip pain due to fractures at or near the pubic symphysis. *Arch Phys Med Rehabil* 70:696–698, 1989.

Tauber C, Geltner D, Noff M, et al: Disruption of the symphysis pubis and fatigue fractures of the pelvis in a patient with rheumatoid arthritis: A case report. *Clin Orthop* 215:105–108, 1987.

Thorne DA, Datz FL: Pelvic stress fracture in female runners. *Clin Nucl Med* 11:828–829, 1986.

Turek SL: Osteitis pubis, in Turek SL: *Orthopaedics Principles and Their Application,* 4th ed. Philadelphia, Lippincott, 1984, vol 2, pp 1661–1662.

Waxman J: Localized rheumatologic diseases: Common diagnostic challenges. *Postgrad Med* 73:189–194, 196, 1983.

Weinberg JR, Berman L, Dootson G, et al: Pubic osteomyelitis presenting as irritable hip. *Postgrad Med J* 63:301–302, 1987.

Wiley JJ: Traumatic osteitis pubis: The gracilis syndrome. *Am J Sports Med* 1:360–363, 1983.

Thigh Pain (Anterior) — Neuropathic/Myopathic

Albert-Ryöppy A, Juntunen J, Salmi T: Femoral neuropathy following anticoagulant therapy for "economy class syndrome" in a young woman: A case report. *Acta Chir Scand* 151:643–645, 1985.

Brozin IH, Martfel J, Goldberg I, et al: Traumatic closed femoral nerve neuropathy. *J Trauma* 22:158–160, 1982.

Fletcher HS, Frankel J: Ruptured abdominal aneurysms presenting with unilateral peripheral neuropathy. *Surgery* 79:120–121, 1976.

Goldman JA, Feldberg D, Dicker D, et al: Femoral neuropathy subsequent to abdominal hysterectomy: A comparative study. *Eur J Obstet Gynecol Reprod Biol* 20:385–392, 1985.

Hallett JW Jr, Wolk SW, Cherry KJ Jr, et al: The femoral neuralgia syndrome after arterial catheter trauma. *J Vasc Surg* 11:702–706, 1990.

Hazlett JW: Low back pain with femoral neuritis. *Clin Orthop* 108:19–26, 1975.

King RB, Bechtold DL: Warfarin-induced iliopsoas hemorrhage with subsequent femoral nerve palsy. *Ann Emerg Med* 14:362–364, 1985.

Louria DB, Sen P, Kapila R, et al: Anterior thigh pain or tenderness: A diagnostically useful manifestation of bacteremia. *Arch Intern Med* 145:657–658, 1985.

Misoul C: Nerve injuries and entrapment syndromes of the lower extremity, in Dee R, Mango E, Hurst LC (eds): *Principles of Orthopaedic Practice*. New York, McGraw-Hill, 1989, vol 2, pp 1420–1430.

Nobel W, Marks SC, Kubik S: The anatomical basis for femoral nerve palsy following iliacus hematoma. *J Neurosurg* 52:533–540, 1980.

Owens ML: Psoas weakness and femoral neuropathy: Neglected signs of retroperitoneal hemorrhage from ruptured aneurysm. *Surgery* 91:363–366, 1982.

Probst A, Harder F, Hofer H, et al: Femoral nerve lesion subsequent to renal transplantation. *Eur Urol* 8:314–316, 1982.

Sisto D, Chiu WS, Geelhoed GW, et al: Femoral neuropathy after renal transplantation. *South Med J* 73(11):1464–1466, 1980.

Sreenivas VI, Pelliccia O Jr, Job G, et al: Femoral neuropathy secondary to anticoagulant therapy. *Int Surg* 65:279–281, 1980.

Tondare AS, Nadkarni AV, Sathe CH, et al: Femoral neuropathy: A complication of lithotomy position under spinal anaesthesia: Report of three cases. *Can Anaesth Soc J* 30:84–86, 1983.

Vaziri ND, Barton CH, Ravikumar GR, et al: Femoral neuropathy: A complication of renal transplantation. *Nephron* 28:30–31, 1981.

Willbanks OL, Willbanks SE: Femoral neuropathy due to retroperitoneal bleeding: A red herring in medicine complicates anticoagulant therapy and influences the Russian communist revolution. *Am J Surg* 145:193–198, 1983.

Yazbeck S, Larbrisseau A, O'Regan S: Femoral neuropathy after renal transplantation. *J Urol* 134:720–721, 1985.

Thigh Pain (Anterior or Posterior) — Lumbosacral Plexopathy

Evans BA, Stevens JC, Dyck PJ: Lumbosacral plexus neuropathy. *Neurology* 31:1327–1330, 1981.

Jaeckle KA, Young DF, Foley KM: The natural history of lumbosacral plexopathy in cancer. *Neurology* 35:8–15, 1985.

Thomas JE, Cascino TL, Earle JD: Differential diagnosis between radiation and tumor plexopathy of the pelvis. *Neurology* 35:1–7, 1985.

Young RJ, Zhou YQ, Rodriguez E, et al: Variable relationship between peripheral somatic and autonomic neuropathy in patients with different syndromes of diabetic polyneuropathy. *Diabetes* 35: 192–197, 1986.

Thigh Pain due to Infections

Aprin H, Dee R: Bone and joint infections, in Dee R, Mango E, Hurst LC (eds): *Principles of Orthopaedic Practice*. New York, McGraw-Hill, 1989, vol 1, pp 294–316.

Thigh Pain due to Intraabdominal Disease

Haiart DC, Stevenson P, Hartley RC: Leg pain: An uncommon presentation of perforated diverticular disease. *J R Coll Surg Edinburgh* 34:17–20, 1989.

Thigh Pain — General

Healey LA: Polymyalgia rheumatica and giant cell arteritis, in Wyngaarden JB, Smith LH Jr (eds): *Cecil Textbook of Medicine,* 18th ed. Philadelphia, Saunders, 1988, vol 2, pp 2033–2034.

Hunder GG, Hazleman BL: Giant cell arteritis and polymyalgia rheumatica, in Kelley WN, Harris ED Jr, Ruddy S, et al (eds): *Textbook of Rheumatology*. Philadelphia, Saunders, 1981, vol 2, pp 1189–1196.

Imparato AM, Riles TS: Peripheral arterial disease, in Schwartz SI (ed): *Principles of Surgery,* 5th ed. New York, McGraw-Hill, 1989, pp 933–1010.

Thigh Pain — General — Compartment Syndromes

Foster RD, Albright JA: Acute compartment syndrome of the thigh: Case report. *J Trauma* 30:108–110, 1990.

Hershman EB, Lombardo J, Bergfeld JA: Femoral shaft stress fractures in athletes. *Clin Sports Med* 9:111–119, 1990.

Schwartz JT, Brumback RJ, Lakatos R, et al: Acute compartment syndrome of the thigh: A spectrum of injury. *J Bone Joint Surg (Am)* 71-A:392–400, 1989.

Singson RD, Feldman F, Staron R, et al: MRI of postamputation neuromas. *Skeletal Radiol* 19:259–262, 1990.

Thigh Pain — General — Neoplasms

Cerroni L, Soyer HP, Smolle J, et al: Cutaneous metastases of a giant cell tumor of bone: Case report. *J Cutan Pathol* 17:59–63, 1990.

Deruyter L, DeBoeck H, Goossens A, et al: An unexpected cause of pathologic hip fracture: Malignant fibrous histiocytoma. *Arch Orthop Trauma Surg* 108:261–263, 1989.

Ding J, Hashimoto H, Tsuneyoshi M, et al: Clear cell chondrosarcoma: A case report with topographic analysis. *Acta Pathol Jpn* 39:533–538, 1989.

Fanning CV, Sneige NS, Carrasco CH, et al: Fine needle aspiration cytology of chondroblastoma of bone. *Cancer* 65:1847–1863, 1990.

Feffer S, Westring D: Other malignancies affecting bone, in Dee R, Mango E, Hurst LC (eds): *Principles of Orthopaedic Practice*. New York, McGraw-Hill, 1989, vol 1, pp 353–361.

Howat AJ, Dickens RV, Boldt DW, et al: Bilateral metachronous periosteal osteosarcoma. *Cancer* 58:1139–1143, 1986.

Klein MJ, Kenan S, Lewis MM: Osteosarcoma: Clinical and pathological considerations. *Orthop Clin North Am* 20:327–345, 1989.

Malawar MM: Neoplasms affecting the lower extremity, in Dee R, Mango E, Hurst LC (eds): *Principles of Orthopaedic Practice*. New York, McGraw-Hill, 1989, vol 2, pp 1395–1419.

Malawar MM, Shmookler BM: Musculoskeletal oncology, in Dee R, Mango E, Hurst LC (eds): *Principles of Orthopaedic Practice*. New York, McGraw-Hill, 1989, vol 1, pp 317–353.

Noel ER, Tebib JG, Dumontet C, et al: Synovial lipoma arborescens of the hip. *Clin Rheumatol* 6:92–96, 1987.

Okada K, Masuda H, Shozawa T, et al: A small aneurysmal bone cyst restricted to the cortical bone of the femur resembling so-called subperiosteal giant cell tumor or subperiosteal osteoclasia. *Acta Pathol Jpn* 39:539–544, 1989.

van Oven MW, Molenaar WM, Freling NJM, et al: Dedifferentiated parosteal osteosarcoma of the femur with aneuploidy and lung metastases. *Cancer* 63:807–811, 1989.

Veth RPH, Nielsen HKL, Oldhoff J, et al: Megaprostheses in the treatment of primary malignant and metastatic tumors in the hip region. *J Surg Oncol* 40:214–218, 1989.

Yoshida H, Yumoto T, Adachi H, et al: Osteosarcoma with prominent epithelioid features. *Acta Pathol Jpn* 39:439–445, 1989.

Thigh Pain (Lateral) — Trochanteric Bursitis

Schapira D, Nahir M, Scharf Y: Trochanteric bursitis: A common clinical problem. *Arch Phys Med Rehabil* 67:815–817, 1986.

Swezey RL: Pseudo-radiculopathy in subacute trochanteric bursitis of the subgluteus maximus bursa. *Arch Phys Med Rehabil* 57:387–390, 1976.

Zoltan DJ, Clancy WG Jr, Keene JS: A new operative approach to snapping hip and refractory trochanteric bursitis in athletes. *Am J Sports Med* 14:201–204, 1986.

Thigh Pain (Medial) — Obturator Hernia

Bjork KJ, Mucha P Jr, Cahill DR: Obturator hernia. *Surg Gynecol Obstet* 167:217–222, 1988.

Carriquiry LA, Piñeyro A: Pre-operative diagnosis of non-strangulated obturator hernia: The contribution of herniography. *Br J Surg* 75:785, 1988.

Glicklich M, Eliasoph J: Incarcerated obturator hernia: Case diagnosed at barium enema fluoroscopy. *Radiology* 172:51–52, 1989.

Kimura I, Ayyar DR, McVeety JC: Saphenous nerve conduction in healthy subjects. *Tohoku J Exp Med* 140:67–71, 1983.

McDonald A, Fletcher PR, Rao AB, et al: Incarcerated obturator hernia. *West Indian Med J* 37:110–113, 1988.

Redwine DB, Sharpe DR: Endometriosis of the obturator nerve: A case report. *J Reprod Med* 35:434–435, 1990.

Rizk TA, Deshmukh N: Obturator hernia: A difficult diagnosis. *South Med J* 83:709–712, 1990.

Siliski JM, Scott RD: Obturator-nerve palsy resulting from intrapelvic extrusion of cement during total hip replacement. *J Bone Joint Surg (Am)* 67-A(8):1225–1228, 1985.

Young A, Hudson DA, Krige JEJ: Strangulated obturator hernia: Can mortality be reduced? *South Med J* 81:1117–1120, 1988.

Thigh Pain (Medial) — Thrombophlebitis

Wilensky RL, Nashel DJ: Case report: Iliofemoral thrombophlebitis presenting as an acute abdomen: Report and literature review. *Am J Med Sci* 295:548–553, 1988.

Thigh Pain — Metabolic Myopathies

Engel AG: Metabolic myopathies, in Wyngaarden JB, Smith LH Jr (eds): *Cecil Textbook of Medicine*, 18th ed. Philadelphia, Saunders, 1988, vol 2, pp 2277–2283.

Thigh Pain — Posterior

Anderson NE, Willoughby EW: Infarction of the conus medullaris. *Ann Neurol* 21:470–474, 1987.

Arnoldussen WJ, Korten JJ: Pressure neuropathy of the posterior femoral cutaneous nerve. *Clin Neurol Neurosurg* 82:57–60, 1980.

Auld AW: Prompt re-exploration for persistent leg pain following disc surgery: A surgical viewpoint. *Mil Med* 142:876–879, 1977.

Barker ME: Pain in the back and leg: A general practice survey: *Rheum Rehabil* 16:37–45, 1977.

Benzel EC, Morris DM, Fowler MR: Nerve sheath tumors of the sciatic nerve and sacral plexus. *J Surg Oncol* 39:8–16, 1988.

Burton CV: Lumbosacral arachnoiditis. *Spine* 3:24–30, 1978.

Dumitru D, Marquis S: Posterior femoral cutaneous nerve neuropathy and somatosensory evoked potentials. *Arch Phys Med Rehabil* 69:44–45, 1988.

Helbig T, Lee CK: The lumbar facet syndrome. *Spine* 13:61–64, 1988.

Hodgson KJ, Sumner DS: Buttock claudication from isolated bilateral internal iliac arterial stenoses. *J Vasc Surg* 7:446–448, 1988.

Julsrud ME: Piriformis syndrome. *J Am Pod Med Assoc* 79:128–131, 1989.

Kerr RSC, Cadoux-Hudson TA, Adams CBT: The value of accurate clinical assessment in the surgical management of the lumbar disc protrusion. *J Neurol Neurosurg Psychiatry* 51:169–173, 1988.

LaBan MM, Meerschaert JR, Taylor RS: Electromyographic evidence of inferior gluteal nerve compromise: An early representation of recurrent colorectal carcinoma. *Arch Phys Med Rehabil* 63:33–35, 1982.

Mattle H, Sieb JP, Rohner M, et al: Nontraumatic spinal epidural and subdural hematomas. *Neurology* 37:1351–1356, 1987.

Puranen J, Orava S: The hamstring syndrome: A new diagnosis of gluteal sciatic pain. *Am J Sports Med* 16:517–521, 1988.

Verner EF, Musher DM: Spinal epidural absess. *Med Clin North Am* 69:375–384, 1985.

Wyant GM: Chronic pain syndromes and their treatment: 3. The piriformis syndrome. *Can Anaesth Soc J* 26:305–308, 1979.

Thigh Pain — Pyomyositis

Meletis J, Yataganas X, Vayopoulos G, et al: Tropical pyomyositis in a Greek adult. *Scand J Infect Dis* 21:343–344, 1989.

Thigh Pain — Trauma

Brody DM: Running injuries, in Nicholas JA, Hershman EB (eds): *The Lower Extremity and Spine in Sports Medicine*. St. Louis, Mosby, 1986, vol 2, pp 1534–1579.

Fox JM: Injuries to the thigh, in Nicholas JA, Hershman EB (eds): *The Lower Extremity and Spine in Sports Medicine*. St. Louis, Mosby, 1986, vol 2, pp 1087–1117.

Nicholas JA: Football injuries, in Nicholas JA, Hershman EB (eds): *The Lower Extremity and Spine in Sports Medicine*. St. Louis, Mosby, 1986, vol 2, pp 1467–1533.

Xethalis JL, Bolardo RA: Soccer injuries, in Nicholas JA, Hershman EB (eds): *The Lower Extremity and Spine in Sports Medicine*. St. Louis, Mosby, 1986, vol 2, pp 1580–1667.

Thigh Pain — Tumors

Ghelman B: Radiology of bone tumors. *Orthop Clin North Am* 20:287–312, 1989.

Greenspan A: Tumors of cartilage origin. *Orthop Clin North Am* 20:347–366, 1989.

Acute Knee and Popliteal Fossa Pain

☐ **DIAGNOSTIC LIST**

GENERALIZED KNEE PAIN

1. Traumatic
   A. Fractures about the knee
      1. Supracondylar fractures of the femur
      2. Patellar fractures
      3. Fractures of the proximal tibia
      4. Fractures of the tibial spines or intercondylar eminence
   B. Acute dislocation of the knee
      1. Anterior dislocation
      2. Posterior dislocation
      3. Medial or lateral dislocation
   C. Acute dislocation of the patella
   D. Intraarticular ligament injury
      1. Anterior cruciate ligament tear
      2. Posterior cruciate ligament tear
      3. Multiple ligament and meniscus injuries
   E. "Dashboard knee"
2. Acute monarthritis of the knee
   A. Septic arthritis
      1. *Neisseria gonorrhoeae* arthritis-dermatitis syndrome
      2. *N. gonorrhoeae* monarthritis
      3. Nongonococcal septic arthritis
   B. Mimics of septic arthritis
      1. Acute pseudogout
      2. Acute gout
      3. Acute leukemic arthritis
      4. Traumatic synovitis
      5. Foreign body synovitis ("cactus thorn synovitis")
      6. Acute hemarthrosis due to coagulopathy
      7. Juvenile rheumatoid arthritis
      8. Acute rheumatic fever
      9. Monarthritis of unknown etiology (idiopathic)
      10. Acute Lyme arthritis
      11. Acute rheumatoid arthritis of the knee
3. Acute polyarthritis involving the knee
   A. Septic arthritis involving the knee
      1. Gonococcal septic polyarthritis
      2. Nongonococcal septic polyarthritis
         a. *Neisseria meningitidis* polyarthritis
         b. Septic polyarthritis due to other bacteria
   B. Reactive arthritis

C. Acute rheumatic fever
D. Crystal-induced polyarthritis
E. Hepatitis B–associated arthritis
F. Acute Lyme arthritis
G. Acute rheumatoid arthritis
H. Gonococcal arthritis (aseptic)
I. Serum sickness response to penicillin
J. Viral arthritis
   1. Rubella arthritis
   2. Rubella vaccine arthritis
   3. Varicella arthritis
K. Still's disease
   1. Acute juvenile-onset rheumatoid arthritis (JRA)
   2. Adult-onset Still's disease
4. Reflex sympathetic dystrophy of the knee
5. Referred pain to the knee

MEDIAL KNEE PAIN
6. Medial meniscus tear
   A. Traumatic
   B. Degenerative
7. Tibial collateral ligament bursitis
8. Tibial collateral ligament injury
   A. Sprain
   B. Rupture
9. Extraarticular displacement of the medial meniscus
10. Osteonecrosis of the medial femoral condyle
11. Hoffa's disease
12. Pes anserine bursitis
13. Pes anserine–gastrocnemius-related tendinitis
14. Semimembranosus tendinitis
15. Osteonecrosis of the proximal tibia

LATERAL KNEE PAIN
16. Iliotibial band friction syndrome
17. Popliteus tenosynovitis
18. Popliteus tendon rupture
19. Lateral meniscus tear
20. Lateral (fibular) collateral ligament injury
21. Tibiofibular joint disorder
22. Biceps femoris tendinitis
23. Osteochondral fracture of the lateral femoral condyle

ANTERIOR KNEE PAIN
24. Patellar tendon injury
25. Patellar tendinitis
26. Prepatellar bursitis
27. Cellulitis of the skin over the knee
28. Retropatellar bursitis
29. Infrapatellar fat pad injury
30. Hoffa's disease
31. Osteochondritis dissecans of the patella
32. Quadriceps tendon rupture
33. Osteochondral fracture of the patella

POSTERIOR KNEE PAIN
34. Gastrocnemius muscle strain
35. Plantaris muscle strain or rupture
36. Hamstring muscle and tendon disorders
   A. Hamstring muscle strain
   B. Hamstring muscle tendinitis
37. Popliteal lymphadenitis
38. Rupture of a popliteal artery aneurysm
39. Muscle spasms (cramps)
40. Posterior cruciate ligament and/or posterior capsule tear

BILATERAL KNEE PAIN

☐ SUMMARY

Generalized Knee Pain

A fall from a height or a high-velocity motor vehicle accident may result in a *supracondylar fracture of the femur*. Pain, edema, tenderness, deformity, ecchymosis, and bony crepitus occur in the supracondylar region. Plain radiographs demonstrate the fracture. Oblique views may be required to image a fracture involving the articular surface of the distal femur. Extension of the fracture into the knee may cause knee pain, stiffness, tenderness, and swelling due to hemarthrosis.

A *patellar fracture* may result from direct impact or from forceful contraction of the quadriceps muscle with the knee in flexion. Pain occurs over the anterior aspect of the knee and is accompanied by diffuse swelling, tenderness, crepitus, and a palpable patellar defect. Hemarthrosis may occur and cause extensive swelling and loss of knee mobility. Routine radiographs are sufficient for the demonstration of transverse and stellate patellar fractures, but a skyline or tangential axial view may be required to exclude a vertical fracture.

Fractures of the proximal tibia may result from a bumper or fender injury to a pedestrian, high-velocity motor vehicle dashboard trauma to the knee, or a fall. Pain and tenderness involve one or both sides of the injured knee. Diffuse swelling due to subcutaneous edema and ecchymoses and intraarticular hemorrhage may occur. Plain radiographs will identify the location and extent of the fracture. *Fractures of the tibial spines or intercondylar eminence* may result from twisting, abducting or adducting, or hyperextension knee injuries. There are a hemarthrosis and severe pain and tenderness that are intensified by knee movement. Plain radiographs will usually demonstrate the fracture. MRI should be performed to exclude associated cruciate or collateral ligament injuries.

Acute anterior dislocation of the knee joint produces severe pain, deformity, swelling, and tenderness; and the tibia and patella are displaced and palpable anterior to the distal femur. Peripheral ischemia may occur secondary to dislocation-related vascular occlusion. *Posterior dislocation* causes acute knee pain, swelling, tenderness, deformity, and extensive ecchymoses. The tibia is displaced posteriorly. The femoral condyles are prominent and easily palpable. A knee effusion or hemarthrosis seldom occurs in patients with dislocation, since the joint capsule is usually torn, allowing intraarticular fluid or blood to escape into the periarticular tissues. *Medial and lateral dislocation* are rare.

Patellar dislocation causes generalized anterior knee pain, swelling, tenderness, and deformity. The patella may be displaced laterally, projecting outward beyond the lateral femoral condyle. Compression of the reduced patella posteriorly against the femoral condyle may cause pain, while pushing the patella laterally makes the patient grab at the examiner's hand (apprehension sign). Plain radiographs of the patella will demonstrate an unreduced dislocation and sometimes an associated osteochondral femoral fracture. A longitudinal axial view of the patella may demonstrate a partial dislocation of the patella.

A *tear of the anterior cruciate ligament (ACL)* usually (78 percent) results from sudden deceleration and a change in direction at the level of the knee. Hyperextension or hyperflexion injuries may also rupture the anterior cruciate ligament. At the time of rupture, a popping sensation occurs in 36 percent of cases and moderate-to-severe anterior knee pain in 70 percent. The painful knee swells in 1 to 2 h secondary to intraarticular hemorrhage. Osteochondral and chondral fractures of the femoral condyles and meniscus tears may accompany ACL rupture.

Positive results of the Lachman test, the flexion-rotation-drawer test, and the Losee test may be demonstrated after aspiration of intraarticular blood that limits knee mobility. Examination under anesthesia is more sensitive for detection of an ACL tear. The Lachman test, the anterior drawer test, and the pivot shift test have sensitivities in the 90 to 100 percent range when performed on an anesthetized patient. Physical examination is less sensitive for partial ACL tears (0–23 percent). ACL disruption can be confirmed by MRI or arthroscopy.

A *posterior cruciate ligament (PCL) tear* frequently results from a posteriorly directed force applied to the proximal tibia with the knee flexed (e.g., a dashboard injury). Severe pain and swelling occur after impact, and range of motion becomes limited by pain and intraarticular bleeding. Results of the posterior Lachman test and the posterior drawer test performed after knee aspiration with the patient anesthetized and/or the

abduction stress test may be positive. MRI has a sensitivity close to 100 percent for PCL disruption. ACL or PCL injuries may be *associated with meniscus tears, patellar dislocation, and collateral ligament tears.*

"Dashboard knee" results when the rider in the passenger side of the front seat of an automobile strikes the dashboard with a flexed knee during a motor vehicle collision. Injuries may include contusion and sprain of the patellar ligament, contusion of the infrapatellar fat pad, damage to the anterior horns of the menisci, chondral or osteochondral fracture of the femoral condyles, and patellar fracture or dislocation. Symptoms include diffuse knee pain and moderate swelling. Sequelae may include chronic recurrent pain and/or limitation of knee rotation and extension.

Acute septic arthritis usually causes severe joint pain of an aching and/or throbbing quality. The pain is constant and is intensified by jarring, palpation, or movement of the knee. Swelling, joint tenderness, skin erythema, and warmth may accompany the pain. *Gonococcal arthritis* occurs in sexually active persons. This disorder may begin as a migratory or additive polyarthritis with pustular skin lesions (*arthritis-dermatitis syndrome*). Most joints gradually improve, but infection may localize to the knee, producing an *acute septic monarthritis*. A reactive oligoarthritis may also cause knee pain, warmth, and swelling and may follow gonococcal urethritis.

Nongonococcal septic arthritis of the knee may present as acute monarthritis with aching or throbbing pain, swelling, redness, tenderness, and warmth. Fever, chills, weakness, diaphoresis, and malaise are usually, but not always, present (68–90 percent of patients have systemic symptoms). The commonest etiologic agents include *Staphylococcus aureus*, streptococcal species, or gram-negative enteric bacteria. The majority of patients developing septic arthritis of the knee are immunosuppressed or have preexisting joint disease, a local or distant site of infection, or a history of recent joint surgery or an intraarticular injection.

Because some cases of septic arthritis are caused by unusual organisms, all suspected cases of joint infection require synovial fluid culture for aerobic and anaerobic organisms, including the bacteria listed in Table 45-3 (e.g., *Hemophilus influenzae*, *Eikenella corrodens*, and *Listeria monocytogenes*). Synovial fluid white blood cell counts may be classified as noninflammatory (200–2000 cells/mm^3), inflammatory (>2000–50,000 cells/mm^3), and infectious (>50,000 WBC cells/mm^3). Up to 50 percent of patients with septic arthritis may have white blood cell counts in the inflammatory range, and up to 30 percent may have negative culture results. Differential counts reveal a predominance of polymorphonuclear leukocytes in patients with infectious and inflammatory joint fluids. The sedimentation rate and the peripheral blood leukocyte count may be elevated or normal, and the synovial fluid glucose level may be decreased or normal in patients with septic arthritis. Septic arthritis may respond dramatically to antibiotic therapy and drainage. A similar response to antibiotics does not occur with other forms of acute monarthritis.

Table 45-1
ETIOLOGIC AGENTS OF NONGONOCOCCAL SEPTIC ARTHRITIS IN ADULTS

Organism	Percent of Cases of Septic Arthritis	Predisposing Factors	Synovial Fluid Leukocyte Counts
Staphylococcus aureus	50–76	Cellulitis, pyoderma, trauma, intraarticular injection or surgery, diabetes mellitus, preexisting joint disease (e.g., osteoarthritis or rheumatoid arthritis)	20,000–250,000
Gram-negative bacteria	14–26	Osteoarthritis (27%), diabetes (23%), rheumatoid arthritis (9%),	11,000–131,000
	9–17	renal failure (9%), steroid use (32%), trauma (18%), urinary tract infection (27–50%), intraarticular injection (9%)	Mean, 54,000
Beta-hemolytic streptococci	11–28		250,000–352,000
	13–17		Mean, 60,000
Group A			
Group G		Extraarticular infection (cellulitis and endocarditis, 61%); major underlying disease (61%)	
Group C			
Group B		Diabetes mellitus	

Table 45-2
NONGONOCOCCAL SEPTIC ARTHRITIS IN ELDERLY PERSONS (AGE 60–87)

Organism	Percent
Gram-positive cocci	
Staphylococcus aureus	54.5
Staphylococcus epidermidis	22.7
Group A beta-hemolytic streptococci	13.6
Group D streptococci	13.6
Streptococcus pneumoniae	4.5
Gram-negative bacteria	
Escherichia coli	9
Pseudomonas species	9
Klebsiella species	4.5
Enterobacter species	4.5
Proteus morganii	4.5
Anaerobes	
Bacteroides fragilis	4.5
Clostridium perfringens	4.5

Mimics of acute septic arthritis of the knee cause moderate-to-severe aching knee pain that is intensified by weight bearing, jarring, and attempted ambulation. The joint is tender, swollen, and warm, and skin erythema may be present.

Pseudogout or gout may be mistaken for joint sepsis. Plain radiographs may reveal chondrocalcinosis of the menisci and articular cartilage in pseudogout. Synovial fluid is shown to contain calcium pyrophosphate dihydrate crystals (pseudogout) or monosodium urate crystals (gout) when viewed by polarized light microscopy. The serum uric acid level is usually, but not always, elevated in gout. Both disorders may respond to colchicine or indomethacin. *Acute leukemia* may present with an acute monarthritis of the knee or as a bilateral migratory or additive arthritis involving the knees and ankles. Synovial tissue and/or fluid, peripheral blood, and bone marrow contain blast cells. *Knee trauma* may cause a reactive knee effusion with warmth and tenderness. Cultures of synovial fluid are negative. A cactus thorn or other sharp *foreign body* may penetrate the skin and enter the knee joint, causing an acute or subacute synovitis. CT visualization of a thorn is possible. The synovial fluid is inflammatory, but cultures are negative. Arthroscopic or open knee surgery may be required to locate and remove the foreign body. *Hemophilia* may cause one or more attacks of knee pain and swelling due to intraarticular bleeding. *Juvenile rheumatoid arthritis (JRA)* may initially involve only one knee. Spiking fevers, sweating, and chills are common associated symptoms, but the evanescent maculopapular rash seen with polyarticular JRA rarely occurs in patients with a monarthritis. JRA occurs in the age group below 16 years. An adult form (adult-onset Still's disease) produces similar symptoms and signs and occurs predominantly in women.

Acute rheumatic fever may involve one or both knees. The knee joint is painful, swollen, tender, warm, and sometimes erythematous. A history of a recent upper respiratory illness is common. The levels of antistreptococcal antibodies, the sedimentation rate, and the leukocyte count are usually elevated. Systemic symptoms include fever, sweats, malaise, and anorexia. Other joints may become involved in a migratory or additive pattern. Chorea, carditis, subcutaneous nodules, and erythema marginatum are rare in adults. There is a dramatic response of symptoms and signs to aspirin therapy.

Monarthritis of the knee may go undiagnosed despite careful clinical and laboratory evaluation. Such cases usually resolve spontaneously without sequelae. *Acute Lyme arthritis* follows erythema migrans and an acute febrile illness. Knees and ankles may become painful and swollen. The enzyme-linked immunosorbent assay (ELISA) for antibody to *Borrelia burgdorferi* reveals an elevated titer.

Rheumatoid arthritis may present as an acute or subacute arthritis of one knee. Pain, swelling, tenderness, and warmth occur, but erythema is unusual. Rheumatoid factor may be present in only 33 percent of cases. Disease progression, with involvement of other joints, provides enough findings to establish the diagnosis.

Knee pain, tenderness, and swelling may occur as a com-

Table 45-3
RARE CAUSES OF SEPTIC ARTHRITIS

Organism	Associations
Hemophilus influenzae	Polyarticular in 48% of cases, extraarticular site of infection (e.g., meninges, lung, throat, sinus, conjunctiva, or skin) in 66%, some form of increased susceptibility to infection or preexisting joint damage (e.g., alcohol abuse, trauma, diabetes mellitus, gout, rheumatoid arthritis, systemic lupus erythematosus, multiple myeloma, lymphoma, splenectomy, or acquired variable hypogammaglobulinemia) in 76%
Eikenella corrodens	Recurrent hemarthrosis of the knee, dental manipulation
Streptococcus faecalis	Preexisting arthritis, prosthetic joint, trauma, alcohol abuse, corticosteroid therapy
Streptococcus pneumoniae	Multiple myeloma (two reported cases), chronic rheumatoid arthritis, recent pulmonary infection (three reported cases)
Salmonella species	Prosthetic joint surgery, trauma, systemic lupus erythematosus, sickle cell disease, malignancy, corticosteroid therapy, diarrhea
Polymicrobial infection with unusual infectious agents (e.g., diphtheroids, *S. viridans, Candida* species)	Factitious disease (needle marks over knee area), penetrating injury to the joint, malignancy
Borrelia burgdorferei	Erythema chronicum migrans and tick exposure in an endemic area
Neisseria meningitidis	Meningococcemia with fever, maculopapular rash, upper respiratory illness
Listeria monocytogenes	Prosthetic joint or chronic rheumatoid arthritis or osteoarthritis, immunosuppression
Pseudomonas aeruginosa	Intravenous drug abuse, primary *Pseudomonas* osteomyelitis adjacent to the joint, infected intravenous line, penetrating local trauma to the femur and knee joint, open fracture, prosthetic joint, internal fixation device
Clostridial species	Penetrating local trauma, arthroscopy, intraarticular injection, immunosuppression
Bacteroides species	Rheumatoid arthritis, prosthetic joint, oral or intraarticular steroid therapy
Streptococcus anginosis	Rheumatoid arthritis, gout, osteoarthritis, steroid therapy
Mycoplasma hominis, Ureaplasma urealyticum	Renal transplantation and hypogammaglobulinemia
Group G streptococcus	Underlying joint disease (e.g., rheumatoid arthritis, prosthetic joint, or osteoarthritis), immunosuppression (e.g., corticosteroid therapy, alcohol abuse, malignancy, or diabetes mellitus), current infection at another site (skin ulcerations, endocarditis)
Nocardia asteroides	Liver transplantation and immunosuppression

ponent of an *acute polyarthritis*. Septic arthritis involving the knee may be *polyarticular*. Multiple joint involvement may occur with *Neisseria gonorrhoeae* (arthritis-dermatitis syndrome), with *Neisseria meningitidis* infection, and in association with infections produced by *S. aureus, streptococcal species, or gram-negative bacteria.*

Reactive arthritis may follow a diarrheal illness or dysuria and urethral discharge resulting from urethritis. Causes include *Salmonella, Shigella, Campylobacter,* and *Yersinia* species and *Clostridium difficile.* These organisms may be cultured from the stool. Arthritis may follow urethral infection with *Chlamydia trachomatis, Ureaplasma urealyticum,* and *N. gonorrhoeae.* Lower-extremity joints (knees, ankles, and hips) are more commonly affected. They may become painful, swollen, warm, and tender. The joint fluid is inflammatory, and culture results are negative. Conjunctivitis, iritis, and urethritis may accompany the joint inflammation. Sexually acquired reactive arthritis (SARA) and *Shigella* species-associated arthritis are more common in men (male/female ratio, 10:1), while other forms of reactive arthritis have a male/female ratio of 1:1.6. Urethritis may occur with postdysenteric reactive arthritis. Musculoskeletal lesions may include enthesopathies (e.g., Achilles tendons and buttock region) and tenosynovitis of the hands or feet, resulting in "sausage" digits.

Reiter's syndrome consists of reactive arthritis, conjuncti-

vitis, and urethritis. Most cases (80 percent) present as an incomplete syndrome with conjunctivitis or urethritis and arthritis, or conjunctivitis and urethritis without arthritis.

Acute rheumatic fever and hepatitis B may cause a migratory and/or additive arthritis involving the knees and other joints. High fever is more common with rheumatic fever. The involved joints become painful, warm, tender, and swollen. Walking may be difficult or impossible because of knee, ankle, or foot pain. Streptococcal antibody levels are elevated in acute rheumatic fever, and there is a dramatic response to aspirin therapy. Hepatitis B-associated arthritis involves the small joints of the fingers in 70 percent of cases and the knees in 35 percent. Up to 50 percent of patients develop urticaria or a pruritic maculopapular or petechial rash that precedes the onset of arthritis. Hepatitis B antigen occurs in the serum, and complement levels are decreased. Liver function test abnormalities may be present.

Lyme arthritis may cause a polyarthritis with knee involvement. There is a history of erythema chronicum migrans followed by a systemic illness with fever, myalgias, arthralgias, aseptic meningitis, and a mild encephalitis. Antibodies to *B. burgdorferi* are present in an elevated titer. *Crystal-induced polyarthritis* may affect the knees and other joints in a symmetrical or asymmetrical fashion. Chondrocalcinosis may be detected in the knees, wrists, hips, or shoulders in calcium pyrophosphate dihydrate deposition disease. Polarized light microscopy of the synovial fluid will reveal either calcium pyrophosphate dihydrate (calcium pyrophosphate deposition disease) or uric acid crystals (gout).

Rheumatoid arthritis may present as an acute arthritis in 15 percent of cases. The knees, as well as the small joints of the hands and wrists, may be involved. Morning stiffness lasting at least 1 h, involvement of three or more joints, symmetrical distribution of joint involvement, subcutaneous nodules, seropositivity for rheumatoid factor, and radiographic evidence of juxtaarticular erosions and osteopenia of the bones of the hands and wrists are other findings supporting a diagnosis of rheumatoid arthritis. *Gonococcal arthritis* may cause an aseptic polyarthritis with skin pustules and vesicles (arthritis-dermatitis syndrome), or a reactive arthritis. The arthritis-dermatitis syndrome responds to ceftriaxone therapy, while reactive arthritis does not respond to treatment of the initiating infection.

Polyarthritis, fever, urticaria, pruritus, and myalgias occurring after penicillin or other drug therapy are suggestive of *serum sickness*. Discontinuance of the responsible drug leads to resolution.

Rubella may cause a symmetrical polyarthralgia and joint stiffness. A similar disorder may occur following *rubella immunization*. Polyarthritis involving one or both knees may rarely occur in children with *varicella*.

JRA may present as an acute polyarthritis or as an oligoarthritis. High, spiking temperatures; joint stiffness; and an evanescent truncal and proximal extremity rash often accompany the polyarthritis. Patients with oligoarthritis seldom develop a rash. Rheumatoid factor may be present in up to 20 percent of patients with this disorder but is rarely present in adults or in children under age 7 with this disease.

Patients with *adult-onset Still's disease* may have fever, chills, malaise, anorexia, and a polyarthritis. Hepatosplenomegaly, lymphadenopathy, and a truncal rash may be present. Neck pain, due to cervical spine arthritis; pericarditis; pleuritis; and abdominal pain may also occur.

Reflex sympathetic dystrophy of the knee may follow knee surgery and major or minor knee trauma. The aching or burning pain caused by this disorder is disproportionately severe for the amount of trauma or the extent of surgery. The knee region may initially become warm and erythematous. After 2 to 6 weeks, the skin over the knee becomes cool, pale, shiny, and taut. Mottling and bluish discoloration occur. Hyperesthesia and allodynia of the skin over the knee may be present, and pain and dysesthesias may radiate distally into the lower leg and foot. Plain radiographs of the knee region reveal early juxtaarticular osteoporosis. A three-phase radionuclide bone scan will demonstrate an increase in blood velocity, blood pool, and early and delayed hyperfixation. A lumbar sympathetic block dramatically relieves most of the disabling symptoms.

Hip disease, such as acute synovitis, may *refer pain to the knee*. Painful limitation of motion occurs at the hip and not in the knee. Medial thigh and knee pain may be caused by an obturator hernia or by another cause of *obturator nerve*

compression. A *lumbosacral plexopathy* or *intraspinal disease* may sometimes *refer pain to the knee*. These disorders can be better defined by a CT scan or MRI of the pelvis and/or lumbosacral spine.

Medial Knee Pain

A *traumatic tear of the medial meniscus* may follow a twisting injury of the flexed knee. A tearing pain, an audible pop, and hemarthrosis may occur. Traumatic synovitis may develop during the first 24 h, resulting in a serosanguineous knee effusion. Tenderness, swelling, and warmth may be localized to the medial joint line. Locking and giving way are other common complaints. A tear may be suggested by a positive McMurray or Apley grind test performed after resorption or aspiration of the joint fluid. MRI has a sensitivity of 77 to 100 percent for the diagnosis of a ''bucket handle'' tear.

Degenerative medial meniscus tears follow minor knee trauma or occur spontaneously. There is medial joint line pain with weight bearing, walking, and running and localized joint line tenderness. For the first 1 to 2 months after onset, swelling and skin warmth may occur over the medial joint line. McMurray's test and the Apley grind test may be positive. The diagnosis of a horizontal degenerative tear of the posterior horn can be confirmed by MRI or arthroscopy.

Mimics of a medial meniscus tear include *tibial collateral ligament bursitis* (*Voshell's bursitis*) or a *sprain or rupture of the tibial collateral ligament*. In patients with Voshell's bursitis, there is local tenderness of the tibial collateral ligament at the joint line. An injection of lidocaine and a corticosteroid into the bursa relieves the pain and tenderness. MRI reveals a normal medial meniscus in 77 percent of cases. A sprain of the tibial collateral ligament causes pain and tenderness over the site of ligamentous insertion into the medial femoral condyle or over other portions of the ligament. Complete rupture of the ligament causes local pain and tenderness and widening of the medial joint space.

Extraarticular displacement of the medial meniscus causes medial knee pain on weight bearing and/or joint movement. Swelling and tenderness occur over the tibial collateral ligament, and the pain may be intensified by external rotation of the lower leg. The diagnosis can be confirmed by MRI or arthroscopy.

Osteonecrosis of the medial femoral condyle causes severe medial knee pain and tenderness that are intensified by weight bearing or walking. Diffuse swelling of the knee, stiffness, and an intraarticular effusion may occur. MRI will define the extent of the osteonecrosis.

Hoffa's disease produces pain, tenderness, and swelling of the patellar fat pad. The pain may be caused by impingement of the joint synovium between articulating surfaces. This disorder may respond to a local injection of lidocaine and corticosteroid into the tender fat pad.

Pes anserine bursitis causes proximal medial pretibial pain, tenderness, and warmth. Inflammatory edema may occur in the painful region. *Pes anserine–gastrocnemius-related tendinitis* causes similar pain, but the tenderness is localized to the region posterior to the pes anserine tendons and adjacent to the gastrocnemius muscle.

Semimembranous tendinitis causes posteromedial knee pain and tenderness. The tenderness is localized to the semimembranous tendon and is just inferior to the joint line.

Osteonecrosis of the proximal tibia causes medial proximal tibial pain and tenderness. MRI will confirm the diagnosis.

Lateral Knee Pain

The *iliotibial band friction syndrome* occurs in long-distance runners. Pain occurs over the lateral aspect of the knee and may be intensified by downhill running. Results of Ober's test may be positive. A creaking sound may occur on flexion and extension of the knee. As the knee is extended from 90° of flexion, thumb pressure over the lateral epicondyle may provoke pain (Noble's test) as the iliotibial band moves beneath the compressing thumb.

Popliteus tenosynovitis causes lateral knee pain during weight bearing with the knee flexed to between 15 and 30°. Downhill walking or running provokes pain. Tenderness is localized to the tendinous portion of the popliteus muscle just anterior to the insertion of the fibular (lateral) collateral ligament on the lateral femoral condyle. *Rupture of the popliteus tendon* rarely occurs as an isolated injury. A sudden external rotation of the tibia with the knee flexed may rupture the tendon. A sudden pop occurs at the time of rupture and is associated with the abrupt onset of lateral knee pain, tenderness, and swelling. The ability to bear weight or walk may be lost because of the severity of the pain. The diagnosis of popliteus tendon rupture may be confirmed by arthroscopy.

A *lateral meniscus tear* occurs with a twisting injury of the flexed knee. Lateral joint line pain and tenderness are present. Locking, "giving way," and a small joint effusion may occur. The diagnosis may be confirmed by MRI or arthroscopy.

A *lateral (fibular) collateral ligament injury* may occur after a fall forward with the lower leg internally rotated when a varus stress is applied to the knee. Pain felt over the lateral side of the knee and tenderness are localized to the ligament. Opening of the lateral joint space occurs with complete rupture of the ligament. This widening of the joint space may be demonstrated by application of an adduction stress at 30° of flexion.

Tibiofibular joint disorders include joint instability and posttraumatic arthritis. Pain and tenderness are localized to the joint. Pain can be provoked by moving the fibular head or placing stress on the joint. Arthritic pain may be immediately relieved by an intraarticular injection of lidocaine.

Biceps femoris tendinitis causes posterolateral knee pain and tenderness of the tendon. The underlying bursa may also be inflamed.

An *osteochondral fracture of the lateral femoral condyle*

may occur after a forceful twist of the flexed knee. Anterolateral knee pain, tenderness, and swelling occur. MRI and arthroscopy will confirm the diagnosis.

Anterior Knee Pain

Direct *trauma to the patella tendon* (dashboard injury) or *patellar tendinitis* (jumper's knee) causes local pain and patellar tendon tenderness. Resisted extension and passive knee flexion may provoke pain. Complete rupture of the tendon is signaled by local pain and tenderness, elevation of the patella, and loss of the ability to actively extend the knee. A gap may be palpable between the tibial tubercle and lower pole of the patella.

Prepatellar bursitis causes pain, tenderness, and swelling over the patella. Direct trauma or direct pressure on the knees from kneeling may cause this disorder.

Fissures of the prepatellar skin or a *cellulitis* may result in a septic *prepatellar bursitis*.

A *retropatellar bursitis* causes local pain, tenderness, and swelling behind and adjacent to the patellar tendon.

Infrapatellar fat pad injury causes local swelling, pain, and tenderness of the fat pad. A recurrent or persistent joint effusion may occur. Extension of the knee against resistance increases the pain.

Hoffa's disease causes aching anterior knee pain that is provoked by exercise and relieved by rest. Pain, tenderness, swelling, and warmth occur over the infrapatellar fat pad. Nontraumatic causes of fat pad inflammation and/or hypertrophy include premenstrual water retention, a space-occupying joint lesion, and a recurvatum deformity of the knee. *Osteochondritis dissecans* of the patella may follow a minor injury, or it may be idiopathic. There are anterior knee pain and localized tenderness of the affected area of the patella. This lesion can be demonstrated by plain radiography, MRI, or arthroscopy.

Rupture of the quadriceps tendon may be preceded by aching pain and soreness over the proximal patella. Rupture may cause local suprapatellar pain and tenderness, and a gap may be palpable above the patella. The ability to actively extend the knee is lost. An *osteochondral fracture of the patella* presents with the sudden onset of tearing anterior knee pain, a breaking sound arising in the knee, localized patellar tenderness, and swelling due to intraarticular bleeding. Such fractures may be caused by an impact force or a twisting force applied to the knee during active extension. The diagnosis can be confirmed by plain radiography, MRI, or arthroscopy.

Posterior Knee Pain

A *gastrocnemius muscle strain* may cause posterior knee pain, which may occur after a sudden start or turn. Tenderness and swelling are localized to the upper portion of the gastrocnemius muscle. There is disagreement as to whether a *disorder (e.g.,*

TABLE OF DISEASE INCIDENCE

INCIDENCE PER 100,000 (APPROXIMATE)

Common (>100)	Uncommon (>5–100)	Rare (>0–5)
	GENERALIZED KNEE PAIN	
Fractures of the proximal tibia	Fractures of the supracondylar femur	Anterior dislocation of the knee
"Dashboard knee"	Fractures of the patella	Posterior dislocation of the knee
Mimics of acute septic monarthritis: acute pseudogout, acute gout, and traumatic synovitis	Fractures of the tibial spines or intercondylar eminence	Medial or lateral dislocation of the knee
	Acute dislocation of the patella	Monarthritis due to unusual organisms
Polyarthritis with knee arthritis: reactive arthritis, crystal-induced polyarthritis, gonococcal arthritis (aseptic), rubella arthritis, and rubella vaccine arthritis	ACL tear	Mimics of acute septic monarthritis: acute leukemic arthritis, foreign body synovitis, and acute hemarthrosis due to coagulopathy
	PCL tear	
	Multiple ligament and meniscus injuries	Polyarthritis with knee arthritis: septic polyarthritis due to *N. meningitidis* or other bacteria
	Arthritis-dermatitis syndrome due to *N. gonorrhoeae*	
	Monarthritis due to *N. gonorrhoeae*	Varicella arthritis
	Monarthritis due to *S. aureus*, streptococcal species, or gram-negative bacteria	Adult-onset Still's disease
	Mimics of acute septic monoarthritis: juvenile rheumatoid arthritis, acute rheumatic fever, idiopathic, Lyme arthritis, and acute rheumatoid arthritis	Reflex sympathetic dystrophy of the knee
	Polyarthritis with knee arthritis: septic polyarthritis due to *N. gonorrhoeae*, acute rheumatic fever, hepatitis B-associated arthritis, Lyme arthritis, acute rheumatoid arthritis, serum sickness response to penicillin, and acute JRA	
	Referred pain to the knee	
	MEDIAL KNEE PAIN	
Medial meniscus tear (traumatic)	Tibial collateral ligament bursitis	Extraarticular displacement of the medial meniscus
Medial meniscus tear (degenerative)	Tibial collateral ligament injury	
Pes anserine bursitis	Osteonecrosis of the medial femoral condyle	Osteonecrosis of the proximal tibia
	Hoffa's disease	
	Pes anserine–gastrocnemius-related tendinitis	
	Semimembranosus tendinitis	
	LATERAL KNEE PAIN	
Iliotibial band friction syndrome	Popliteus tenosynovitis	Popliteus tendon rupture
Lateral meniscus tear	Lateral collateral ligament injury	
Biceps femoris tendinitis	Tibiofibular joint disorder	
	Osteochondral fracture of the lateral femoral condyle	
	ANTERIOR KNEE PAIN	
	Patellar tendon injury	Quadriceps rupture
	Patellar tendinitis	
	Prepatellar bursitis	
	Cellulitis of the skin over the knee	
	Retropatellar bursitis	
	Infrapatellar fat pad injury	
	Hoffa's disease	
	Osteochondritis dissecans of the patella	
	Osteochondral fracture of the patella	
	POSTERIOR KNEE PAIN	
Gastrocnemius muscle strain	Posterior cruciate ligament and/or posterior capsule tear	Plantaris muscle strain or rupture
Hamstring strain or tendinitis		Popliteal lymphadenitis
Muscle spasms (cramps)		Rupture of a popliteal artery aneurysm

strain or rupture) of the plantaris muscle may cause upper calf and popliteal pain and tenderness.

Other causes of posterior knee pain include a *hamstring muscle strain* or *tendinitis*. There is local tenderness over the distal bellies or tendons of the semimembranosus or biceps femoris muscles.

Popliteal lymphadenitis results in a painful, tender, enlarged lymph node in the popliteal fossa. A source of infection is present in the lower leg or foot.

A *popliteal artery aneurysm* may suddenly rupture, causing local pain, tenderness, swelling, and ecchymoses. A firm mass resulting from formation of a hematoma may appear in the popliteal fossa. Arteriography, CT, or ultrasonography may demonstrate the extent of the aneurysm.

Muscle cramps in the upper calf or lower thigh may be felt in the popliteal region. The pain is usually unilateral, but it may alternate sides. The painful site may be felt to tighten up. Massage and stretching relieve the pain. Such attacks are transient, and relief occurs within a few minutes, but residual movement-related pain provoked by walking may continue for several hours.

A *PCL and/or posterior joint capsule tear* may cause popliteal pain and tenderness. MRI of the knee or arthroscopic examination will demonstrate a partial or complete PCL rupture. Arthroscopy may demonstrate disruption of the posterior joint capsule.

Causes of bilateral knee pain are listed in Table 45-4.

Table 45-4
BILATERAL KNEE PAIN

Acute polyarthritis
  Septic arthritis
  Reactive arthritis
  Crystal-induced arthritis
  Hepatitis B-associated arthritis
  Lyme arthritis
  Rheumatoid arthritis
  Dermatitis-arthritis syndrome due to *N. gonorrhoeae*
  Serum sickness reaction to penicillin
  Viral arthritis
  Still's disease
Reflex sympathetic dystrophy
Medial meniscus tears
Hoffa's disease
Pes anserine bursitis
Iliotibial band syndrome
Lateral meniscus tears
Biceps femoris tendinitis
Patellar tendinitis
Prepatellar bursitis
Muscle cramps
Gastrocnemius muscle strain

☐ DESCRIPTION OF LISTED DISEASES

Generalized Knee Pain

1. Trauma

A. Fractures about the Knee

1. Supracondylar Fractures of the Femur A supracondylar fracture of the femur usually results from a high-velocity motor vehicle accident or a fall from a height. A similar injury may occur from a fall on a flexed knee in elderly persons. Some patients may have metaphyseal osteoporosis or a bone tumor. Severe pain,

swelling, tenderness, deformity, ecchymoses, and bony crepitus occur in the posterior and anterior aspects of the distal thigh. The condylar fragment may be rotated posteriorly by the pull of the gastrocnemius and hamstring muscles. Compression or laceration of the popliteal artery may occur and cause distal limb pallor, coldness, pain, paresis, paresthesias, and loss of the pedal pulses. Contusion or laceration of the sciatic nerve or its branches (the tibial nerve and the common peroneal nerve) may cause distal paresthesias, lower-extremity numbness, and weakness. Routine knee radiographs will usually demonstrate a supracondylar fracture, while an intercondylar fracture involving the articular surface (T or Y fractures) may require oblique views. Extension of the fracture into the knee results in acute joint swelling due to bleeding. Knee movements are limited, painful, and associated with palpable bony crepitus.

2. Patellar Fractures A patellar fracture may occur by direct impact or by traction forces exerted on the patella by a contracting quadriceps muscle. The latter occurs when the patient stumbles and tries to check his or her fall. As the patella fractures (usually transversely) under quadriceps traction, the lateral and medial quadriceps expansions may tear. The extent of this disruption determines the extent of fragment separation. Direct impact on the patella in a motor vehicle accident (knee striking the dashboard) or resulting from a fall from a height or from an erect posture to the ground while running may cause a stellate, comminuted, or vertical fracture. Diffuse swelling of the front of the knee is accompanied by severe pain, tenderness, crepitus, and a palpable patellar defect. A defect may be felt by the patient shortly after a transverse fracture. Undisplaced fractures may be associated with only slight swelling and local fracture line tenderness. Hemarthrosis frequently occurs, resulting in distension of the joint capsule. Dissection of blood into the subcutaneous tissues may produce extensive ecchymoses over the front and sides of the knee. Plain radiographs (anteroposterior and lateral) are usually diagnostic of transverse and stellate fractures. A skyline or axial view may be required to exclude a vertical fracture. A bipartite patella is not associated with point tenderness. This developmental variation appears on a radiograph as an apparent bone fragment in the superior lateral patella that is usually present on both sides. Round edges visible on a CT scan also help differentiate this radiographic finding from a patellar fracture. MRI will usually confirm preservation of intraarticular ligaments and menisci.

3. Fractures of the Proximal Tibia These injuries result when a pedestrian is struck by an automobile bumper or fender ("bumper" or "fender" fractures) (54 percent of cases). They may also occur with a fall from a height (17 percent of cases) or in a high-velocity motor vehicle accident. There may be diffuse pain and swelling of the knee secondary to soft tissue edema and a hemarthrosis. Pain and tenderness involve one or both sides of the injured knee (bicondylar fracture or a lateral condylar fracture and a medial collateral ligament injury). Plain radiographs may demonstrate a plateau fracture (compression, split-compression, total condylar depression, or bicondylar types). A stress film taken under anesthesia (valgus stress applied with knee extended) may reveal widening of the medial joint space indicating medial ligament disruption. It is important to monitor pedal pulses, skin color and temperature, sensory and motor nerve function, as well as lower leg and foot pain and tenderness after a condylar or bicondylar fracture because vascular injury or an anterior compartment syndrome may complicate proximal tibial fractures.

4. Fractures of the Tibial Spines or Intercondylar Eminence These fractures occur from forceful twisting or abduction-adduction knee injuries. Knee hyperextension may avulse the posterior cruciate ligament (PCL) with a fragment of bone. Injury is usually followed by pain and swelling due to a bloody intraarticular effusion. Associated cruciate or collateral ligament injuries should be excluded by physical examination and MRI. Routine radiographs usually reveal these fractures, but an intercondylar or tunnel view may be required to demonstrate minimally displaced fractures.

B. Acute Dislocation of the Knee Most cases of knee dislocation occur in high-velocity motor vehicle accidents or in athletic competition. Popliteal artery injury has been reported in up to 38 percent of cases, and peroneal nerve injury in 16 to 18 percent.

1. Anterior Dislocation A large force may cause severe knee hyperextension, resulting in a tear of the posterior capsule, the posterior and in some cases the anterior cruxiate ligament. There are severe pain, swelling, and tenderness, and the tibia and patella are displaced and palpable anterior to the distal femur. The lower leg is shortened, and there is marked deformity of the knee. Compression or laceration of the popliteal artery may result in distal pallor, paresthesias, coldness, loss of pedal pulses, and paresis of foot muscles. Reduction of the dislocation should be achieved at the scene or within a brief period of time to prevent popliteal artery occlusion or tibial and peroneal nerve injury.

2. Posterior Dislocation This injury occurs from a violent force. Knee pain, swelling, ecchymoses, diffuse tenderness, and deformity occur, and the tibia is displaced posteriorly. The femoral condyles are prominent and easily palpable subcutaneously. In both anterior and posterior dislocations, a knee effusion may not be present, since tears in the joint capsule allow synovial fluid and blood extravasation into the surrounding tissues. Plain radiographs will usually demonstrate a knee dislocation. Arteriographic evaluation of the popliteal artery should be completed prior to surgical intervention in a patient with knee dislocation.

3. Medial or Lateral Dislocation Such dislocations may also occur with violent lateral and rotational forces.

C. Acute Dislocation of the Patella This injury is sometimes confused with acute dislocation of the knee. It may result from a forceful quadriceps contraction or a direct blow to the patella with the knee flexed. Cutting during running may produce a valgus knee force and a rotational vector that results in lateral displacement of the patella. The patient may feel or hear a pop in the knee region with or without pain. Patellar dislocation produces a lateral knee deformity. The patella projects outward beyond the lateral femoral condyle. When first seen, the patient may have manually reduced the dislocation, or spontaneous reduction may have occurred. Patellar tenderness, a bloody knee effusion, and knee pain usually accompany an acute dislocation. Tenderness over the torn medial retinaculum may be present. Compression of the reduced patella against the femoral condyles elicits pain, and pushing the patella laterally as if to reproduce the dislocation makes the patient grab at the knee and at the examiner's hand (apprehension sign). If the patient is seen several hours or days after spontaneous reduction, pain and tenderness may be minimal.

Plain radiographs will demonstrate an unreduced dislocation and sometimes an associated osteochondral fracture of the lateral condyle of the femur. A patellar series consisting of a standing anteroposterior view, lateral views with the knee flexed 30 and 90°, a tangential view taken by the Hughston method, and a Merchant's view should be obtained. Oblique views taken with the leg in 45° of internal and external rotation are helpful in detecting osteochondral fractures of the condyles.

An intraarticular dislocation causes an anterior knee deformity and pain. Extension of the knee is blocked. Hemarthrosis may be present. A lateral radiograph will demonstrate the dislocation and the orientation of the patella in relation to the joint.

D. Ligament Injuries

1. Anterior Cruciate Ligament Tear Isolated complete or partial disruption of the ACL usually occurs in competitive sports. Up to 78 percent of such injuries may not involve contact with another player. ACL tears occur with rapid deceleration while running and are frequently associated with a simultaneous change in direction (e.g., the athlete lands on the leg and rapidly pivots in the opposite direction, producing forceful external rotation of the lower leg on the femur with a lateral-to-medial valgus stress on the knee). Noncontact injuries to the ACL may also occur when the athlete makes a rapid cutting movement on the extended knee. The tibia internally rotates as a varus force is applied to the joint. Hyperextension of the knee may sequentially tear the ACL, one or both menisci (30 percent of cases), and, if extreme, the PCL and posterior joint capsule. Hyperflexion of the knee and landing from a jump may also rupture the ACL. Contact injuries producing anterior cruciate disruption are characterized by a valgus force applied to the knee combined with simultaneous external rotation of the lower leg (e.g., a "clip" injury in football), or by hyperextension or external rotation of the fixed lower leg during tackling in football. Skiing has become a frequent cause of ACL tears.

Moderate-to-severe pain in the knee (70 percent of cases) and a popping sensation (36 percent) are felt at the time of injury. Pain may be mild or absent in 30 percent of cases with complete rupture. The knee becomes swollen within 1 to 4 h due to intraarticular bleeding. Aspiration of a tense hemarthrosis may be necessary to allow performance of the physical examination. The presence of fat globules in the aspirated bloody fluid is indicative of an associated osteochondral fracture of the joint surface. The knee is swollen, and there may be medial and/or lateral joint line tenderness. In the presence of a possible rupture of the ACL and a hemarthrosis, the following tests are most useful:

1. The *Lachman test* is performed with the patient supine and the knee flexed to 20 to 30°. The thigh is held fixed by one of the examiner's hands, and the tibia is subjected to an anteriorly directed force by the examiner's other hand. A positive test result is defined as an increase in the anterior displacement of the tibia on the injured side relative to the displacement on the normal side. This increase can be measured and reported quantitatively as the maximal displacement of the tibia at the joint line on the abnormal side minus the displacement on the normal side. A difference of 2.5 mm is considered diagnostic of ACL disruption.

2. The *flexion-rotation-drawer test* evaluates anterolateral instability and can be used in the acutely injured knee. The lower leg is held gently in the examiner's hands, and the knee is flexed to 15°. At 15°, the tibia is subluxed anteriorly, and the femur rotates externally. As flexion is increased to 30°, the tibia reduces posteriorly, and the femur rotates internally. These findings constitute a positive test result.

3. The *Losee test* is a modification of the pivot shift and jerk tests, and measures anterolateral instability. The lower leg is flexed to 45° or more, and the foot is externally rotated. The lower leg is gradually extended, and the foot is slowly internally rotated. As the lower leg is extended, a valgus force (lateral to medial) is exerted on the knee, and anterior pressure is applied behind the head of the fibula. The anterolateral surface of the tibia is subluxed forward. As the knee reaches full extension, a palpable clunk is produced by reduction of the tibia.

Physical examination of the knee with a painful acute hemarthrosis is unreliable. In this setting, only 9 to 24 percent of complete ACL tears found on arthroscopy were diagnosed by clinical examination. Use of clinical tests is more reliable when the patient is under general anesthesia. In one reported series of complete ACL tears, the anterior drawer test at 90° of flexion and the Lachman test had a sensitivity of 100 percent, and the pivot shift test, 90 percent in anesthetized patients. In alert patients examined at variable time intervals after an acute injury, the anterior drawer test was positive in 78 percent of cases and the Lachman test in 89 percent. The mean time interval after injury until examination was not available in this report. The anterior drawer test is performed in the same manner as the Lachman test, but at 90° of knee flexion. The pivot shift test of Gallway and MacIntosh is performed with the foot and tibia internally rotated, while a valgus stress (lateral to medial) is applied to the extended knee. The examiner's thumb puts anterior pressure on the posterior aspect of the fibula head, subluxing the anterolateral tibia forward. As knee flexion is gradually increased to 20 to 30°, the tibia is reduced, producing a palpable clunk. In patients with a partial ACL tear examined under anesthesia, the sensitivity of the Lachman test was only 23 percent; the anterior drawer test, 15 percent; and the pivot shift test, 0 percent. In two series of patients with acute painful hemarthrosis due to trauma who underwent arthroscopy, the frequency of ACL injuries was 42 and 54 percent, respectively. In one series, nearly 50 percent of the acute lesions were partial tears. Other associated injuries included medial and/or lateral meniscal tears, capsular tears, PCL tears, and chondral or osteochondral fractures.

The sensitivity of MRI for the diagnosis of a tear of the ACL is 61 to 100 percent, and the specificity is 82 to 98 percent when compared with arthroscopy as the "gold standard." Most series report sensitivities and specificities for MRI above 90 percent. No series were reported with studies restricted to acute injuries with hemarthrosis of the knee.

2. Posterior Cruciate Ligament Tear The most frequent cause of PCL injury is a posteriorly directed force applied to the proximal tibia with the knee flexed. This may occur as the proximal tibia strikes the dashboard in a motor vehicle collision or as a result of a motorcycle accident. A fall on the proximal tibia with the knee flexed will also disrupt the PCL. A severe hyperextension injury of the knee will tear the ACL, the PCL, and the posterior joint capsule. A torsional force that disrupts the arcuate complex laterally or the oblique popliteal ligament medially may also tear the PCL.

Patients have severe knee pain and swelling due to intraarticular bleeding. Range of motion may be limited to between 10 and 60° of flexion. Since the posterior drawer test requires flexion to 90°, a posterior Lachman test may be substituted when pain and swelling are severe. A posteriorly directed force is applied to the proximal tibia with the knee flexed to 30°. The posterior movement of the tibial articular surface is compared with that of the normal knee and the difference in millimeters recorded. The classic posterior drawer test may be performed when the patient is under anesthesia. More posterior tibial translation at 30° than at 90° of knee flexion may be secondary to damage to the posterolateral capsule and medial collateral ligament. The posterior "sag" sign of the tibia with the knee flexed to 90° is unlikely to be present in an acutely injured immobile knee.

An abduction stress test (Hughston) may be positive in 88 percent of patients with acute PCL injury and a negative or equivocal posterior drawer test. Compared with arthroscopy, MRI has been reported to be 100 percent sensitive and specific for the diagnosis of a PCL tear.

3. Multiple Ligament and Meniscus Injuries Simultaneous injury to both the medial and lateral menisci may follow an ACL tear. The tibia subluxes anteriorly beneath the femoral condyles, and longitudinal tears in the menisci may result. The joint is usually tensely swollen due to intraarticular bleeding. Joint line tenderness may be present medially and/or laterally, and joint mobility may be limited because of pain and bleeding. In one series, medial meniscus tears were reported in 13 percent of ACL ruptures and lateral meniscus tears in 5 percent. Five percent of patients with an ACL tear had tears of both menisci. Single-meniscus "bucket handle" tears were much more common than involvement of both menisci. Other causes of intraarticular pain included chondral and osteochondral fractures, many of which are demonstrable only by arthroscopy. Other injuries associated with acute hemarthrosis included PCL tears (3 percent), patellar dislocation (19 percent), and medial collateral ligament tears (14 percent).

Accurate assessment of all injuries in a patient with an acute hemarthrosis requires physical examination, knee examination under anesthesia, MRI, and arthroscopy. In some centers, examination under anesthesia and arthroscopy are considered the only reliable methods of assessing an acute knee injury.

E. "Dashboard Knee" When the rider on the passenger side of the front seat strikes his or her knee against the dashboard during a motor vehicle collision, one or more injuries may occur. These include a sprain and/or contusion of the patellar ligament; contusion of the fat pad and the anterior horns of the medial and lateral menisci; and contusion or fracture of the articular surface of the femoral condyles. Patellar injuries include dislocation, fracture, and/or contusion. "Dashboard knee" may progress and persist, causing chronic recurrent or persistent knee pain. Examination may reveal tenderness over the patellar ligament and patella; swelling and tenderness over the fat pad adjacent to the patella ligament; and tenderness and range-of-motion pain over the femoral condyles. Plain radiographs will exclude a fracture, and MRI will detect injuries of the ligaments and semilunar cartilages.

2. ACUTE MONARTHRITIS OF THE KNEE

A. Septic Arthritis

1. Neisseria gonorrhoeae Arthritis-Dermatitis Syndrome *N. gonorrhoeae* may cause an arthritis-dermatitis syndrome. Fever and chills may occur, but many patients have no systemic complaints. A migratory, and sometimes additive, polyarthralgia or polyarthritis occurs involving the knees, elbows, ankles, wrists, and fingers. Tenosynovitis or joint swelling may occur in two or more areas. The involvement is usually asymmetrical, with actual arthritis restricted to fewer than four joints. An eruption of discrete pustules and hemorrhagic purple vesicles on a 1- to 1.5-cm erythematous base appears on the distal portion of the arms and legs. The pain and tenderness may resolve spontaneously in most of the involved joints, but an acute arthritis with effusion may progress in the knee and one or two other joints. The involved knee may ache severely, and an excruciating throbbing pain may develop. The pain is intensified by any movement of the joint and by weight bearing. During the polyarthralgia or polyarthritis-dermatitis stage, *N. gonorrhoeae* may be isolated from the blood, but the joint fluid is usually sterile. When the knee joint becomes red, warm, and swollen, the synovial fluid leukocyte count usually exceeds 50,000 cells/mm^3 and the synovial fluid culture results are usually positive for *N. gonorrhoeae*. At this stage, the blood culture results are usually negative. Mucous membrane culture (i.e., throat, anorectum, cervix, and urethra) results are positive in 80 percent of patients. Results of mucosal site cultures from sexual contacts may also be positive, lending support to the clinical diagnosis. The arthritis responds to antibiotic therapy.

2. Neisseria gonorrhoeae Monarthritis Patients with an *N. gonorrhoeae* monarthritis of the knee present with severe knee pain and tenderness, redness, swelling, and warmth of the overlying skin. Fever, chills, and other systemic symptoms occur, but there is usually no rash or polyarthralgia. The diagnosis can be confirmed by joint fluid analysis, Gram's stain, and culture. Joint symptoms resolve within 2 to 4 days of initiating ceftriaxone therapy.

3. Nongonococcal Septic Arthritis Pain occurs at rest (87–100 percent of cases) and during the night in the affected knee. It may be a mild, dull ache or a severe, throbbing pain. Movement of the knee or weight bearing intensifies the pain. The knee is usually swollen, warm, and tender, and skin erythema may be present. Fever (68–90 percent of cases), chills, malaise, anorexia, and nausea are common accompanying symptoms. Most cases of septic arthritis of the knee are caused by *S. aureus*, streptococcal species, or gram-negative enteric bacteria.

The majority of patients developing nongonococcal septic arthritis of the knee have one or more of the following predisposing factors: immunosuppression due to corticosteroid administration, alcohol abuse, renal failure, malignancy, diabetes mellitus, intravenous drug abuse, collagen vascular disease, organ transplantation, or the acquired immunodeficiency syndrome; preexisting joint disease due to rheumatoid arthritis, osteoarthritis, or psoriatic arthritis; recent or past trauma or iatrogenic injury due to an intraarticular injection or joint surgery; and a local or distant site of recent or current infection (e.g., cellulitis, pyoderma, endocarditis, septic joint, visceral abscess, pneumonia, or meningitis).

Synovial fluid polymorphonuclear leukocytosis is usually present in patients with septic arthritis. The American Rheumatism Association has classified synovial fluid white blood cell counts as noninflammatory (total cell count, 200–2000 cells/mm³), inflammatory (total cell count, >2000 – 50,000 cells/mm³), and infectious (total cell count, >50,000 cells/mm³). Synovial fluid leukocyte counts in patients with culture-proven joint infection usually fall in the range 5200 to 156,000 or greater. In one reported series of 41 patients, the mean synovial fluid cell count was 46,500, and more than half the patients had counts in the inflammatory range (>2000–50,000 cells/mm³). Relatively low counts may be secondary to neoplastic disease, intravenous drug abuse, and corticosteroid administration. Polymorphonuclear leukocytes constituted a mean of 92 percent of the synovial fluid leukocytes in septic joints caused by *S. aureus, Streptococcus pyogenes*, other streptococcal species, or gram-negative rods. The etiologic agents of nongonococcal septic arthritis in adults are listed in Tables 45-1 and 45-2. A high polymorphonuclear leukocyte percentage is of minimal differential value, since inflammatory joint fluids may also have polymorphonuclear leukocyte counts exceeding 90 percent of the total cells. The sedimentation rate is elevated in 90 percent of patients with septic arthritis, and peripheral leukocytosis occurs in 57 percent. Synovial fluid glucose concentrations may be less than 40 percent of the simultaneously drawn blood glucose in patients with septic arthritis. Culture results may be falsely negative in up to 30 percent of cases. Infectious arthritis responds within 2 to 5 days to parenteral antibiotic therapy. Repeated aspiration or open surgical drainage of the knee facilitates recovery.

B. Mimics of Septic Arthritis of the Knee

1. Acute Pseudogout Severe pain, swelling, tenderness, erythema, and warmth of the overlying skin involve one knee. Weight bearing and walking may be intolerable or result in a limp. Synovial fluid aspirates are yellow-white and turbid. Leukocyte counts vary from 9000 to 58,000 cells/mm³, with a mean of 24,000 cells/mm³. The erythrocyte sedimentation rate may vary from 6 to 140 mm/h. Polarized light microscopy reveals large numbers of intracellular and extracellular rhomboid or rodlike crystals with positive birefringence. Patients without synovial fluid crystals may be diagnosed by making a wet preparation of articular cartilage obtained by arthroscopic biopsy. The presence of calcium pyrophosphate dihydrate crystals may be demonstrated by this procedure. Radiographs of the affected knee may demonstrate chondrocalcinosis.

Fever; mental confusion; and a red, tender, swollen knee may be misdiagnosed as an infectious arthritis. Such a misdiagnosis is more likely if neither calcium pyrophosphate dihydrate nor monosodium urate crystals are identified in the synovial fluid. Unless infection is superimposed on crystal-induced arthritis, culture results are negative, and calcium pyrophosphate dihydrate crystals are present in the joint fluid. Cases of pseudogout may be associated with bacterial infection and may be difficult to diagnose if synovial fluid culture results are negative. Acute arthritis involving more than one joint is frequent in pseudogout (42 percent of cases). Misdiagnosis of pseudogout as septic arthritis may lead to loss of knee range of motion, antibiotic complications, and iatrogenic joint sepsis from joint irrigation or synovectomy. Pseudogout of the knee responds to parenteral colchicine or an intraarticular injection of a microcrystalline glucocorticoid.

2. Acute Gout Pain, redness, heat, swelling, and tenderness of one knee occur. Fever and leukocytosis may accompany the knee pain. Chondrocalcinosis is not usually present on plain radiographs of the knee. The joint fluid contains increased concentrations of polymorphonuclear leukocytes. Compensated polarized light microscopy of synovial fluid demonstrates intracellular and extracellular monosodium urate crystals. The serum uric acid level is usually elevated but may be in the normal range in a small percentage of cases. There is usually a dramatic response to intravenous or oral colchicine or oral administration of indomethacin. Some patients have a history of prior attacks of acute podagra or arthritis involving the ankles. This disorder may be indistinguishable from pseudogout without synovial fluid examination.

3. Acute Leukemic Arthritis   Pain, swelling, and tenderness of the knee may be initial or late symptoms of acute leukemia. The diagnosis can be established by demonstrating blast cells in the synovial fluid or in a synovial tissue biopsy. Cell abnormalities in the peripheral blood and bone marrow are usually present. Bilateral arthritis involving the knees and ankles in an additive or migratory pattern is the most common form of leukemic joint involvement. Local irradiation or infiltration with corticosteroids is an effective method of controlling joint disease. Chemotherapy will also benefit this disorder. Less commonly, leukemic arthritis is caused by secondary gout, sepsis, or reactive synovitis produced by a leukemic cell infiltrate in the adjacent femur or tibia.

4. Traumatic Synovitis   This disorder follows an acute injury of the knee. Pain is the initial symptom, followed by local periarticular edema, warmth, and tenderness. A knee joint effusion may or may not occur. Intraarticular lesions associated with traumatic synovitis include meniscus injury, osteochondral fracture, and disruption of one or both cruciate ligaments. Arthroscopy may reveal a synovial inflammatory reaction. Biopsies reveal evidence of synovial tissue edema and infiltration by lymphocytes.

5. Foreign Body Synovitis ("Cactus Thorn or Plant Thorn Synovitis")   This disorder may present with fever, knee pain, swelling, warmth, tenderness, and sometimes redness. Wood splinters; sea urchin spines; silicone; starch; fiberglass; fragments of plastic, glass, brick, stone, or metal; or plant thorns may penetrate a knee joint and give rise to an acute synovitis. Plant thorns capable of causing acute synovitis may arise from date and sentinel palms, blackthorns, roses, yuccas, hawthorns, mesquite, bougainvillea, and cactus. In some cases, there is no recollection of knee penetration by a thorn or other foreign body.

In "cactus thorn synovitis," an entrance wound may be apparent. Arthroscopy may detect a thorn or other foreign body imbedded in the synovial membrane. Centrifugation of joint fluid and careful examination of the sediment under polarized light may reveal evidence of birefringent vegetable material. A CT study of the joint may reveal a thorn, since it has a greater radiodensity than synovial tissue.

The synovial fluid leukocyte count is usually in the inflammatory range, and cultures are negative. Synovial biopsies should be examined microscopically for foreign body giant cells and vegetable material when this disorder is suspected. Arthrotomy may be required to establish the diagnosis and for definitive therapy (e.g., extensive synovectomy in cases where the thorn or other foreign body cannot be located).

6. Acute Hemarthrosis   Acute hemorrhage into a knee may be caused by trauma or may be secondary to a hereditary bleeding disorder or anticoagulant therapy. The knee usually swells within 2 to 3 h and is painful, tender, and warm. Joint aspiration reveals blood. Some patients with hemophilia and recurrent hemarthrosis may develop an acute infectious arthritis. Fever, chills, prostration, and intense knee pain are clinical cues to aspirate the swollen knee and culture the synovial fluid.

7. Juvenile Rheumatoid Arthritis   This disorder may present with acute pain, swelling, and tenderness of one knee. In some cases, involvement of two or three more joints may follow. Systemic symptoms such as malaise, anorexia, and spiking fever may precede or accompany the arthritis. The characteristic evanescent maculopapular truncal and proximal extremity rash seen in polyarticular JRA rarely occurs with single joint involvement. This disorder usually occurs in small children, but cases may appear up to age 16. A similar disorder in adults (adult-onset Still's disease) has been described and occurs predominantly in women.

8. Acute Rheumatic Fever   Some cases of acute rheumatic fever in adults may cause monarthritis of the knee. The knee is usually painful at rest, swollen, red, warm, and tender. The levels of antistreptococcal antibodies (i.e., antihyaluronidase, antistreptolysin O, and anti-DNase B) are elevated in the serum. Other manifestations of rheumatic fever, such as chorea, erythema marginatum, and carditis, are uncommon in adults. A migratory polyarthritis may or may not follow monarthritis of the knee. There is a dramatic response to salicylate therapy.

9. Monarthritis of Unknown Etiology   Up to 30 percent of cases of acute or subacute monarthritis of the knee may go undiagnosed despite careful diagnostic evaluation and follow-up. Many of these attacks resolve spontaneously.

10. Acute Lyme Arthritis   This disorder usually begins with a painless, erythematous, annular skin lesion at the site of an ixodid tick bite. The lesion may gradually enlarge and may have a final diameter of 10 to 20 cm. This narrow pink or red annular lesion may be elevated or flat, and a central papule may remain at the site of the bite. Fever, chills, myalgias, arthralgias, malaise, headache, and meningismus may follow the onset of the rash. In children, intermittent attacks of pain and swelling of one or both knees and ankles may follow the onset of systemic symptoms. Acute arthritis is less common in adults. Older patients may develop a chronic destructive arthropathy in one or both knees. Acute Lyme arthritis usually allows ambulation without severe pain in the affected knee, a finding that distinguishes this disorder from suppurative arthritis caused by other bacteria. Skin erythema is also common in suppurative arthritis and is rarely seen in acute Lyme arthritis. The diagnosis of Lyme disease can be confirmed by serologic tests (i.e., enzyme-linked immunosorbent assay [ELISA]). IgM and IgG antibody titers to *B. burgdorferi* may also be measured by indirect immunofluorescence.

11. Acute Rheumatoid Arthritis of the Knee Aching knee pain, intensified by movement, is associated with swelling, warmth, and tenderness. Rheumatoid factor may be positive in only 33 percent of patients during the first 3 months of the illness. Within 1 year, 88 percent of patients are seropositive. In time, many of these patients develop symmetrical arthritis, hand and wrist arthritis, subcutaneous nodules, prolonged morning stiffness of the affected joints, involvement of three or more joint areas, and/or hand and wrist radiographic changes consistent with rheumatoid arthritis. Evolution from a monarthritis of the knee to a clinical picture characterized by four or more of the above-listed findings may take months or years.

3. ACUTE POLYARTICULAR DISORDERS INVOLVING THE KNEE

A. Septic Polyarthritis

1. Gonococcal Septic Polyarthritis Fever and other systemic symptoms may be mild or absent. A migratory polyarthralgia or polyarthritis occurs. Tenosynovitis may occur and involve the extensor tendons of one or both hands, feet, or wrists or the Achilles tendons of the ankles. Arthritis of the knees and wrists is most frequent. Ankle and hand involvement occurs but is less common. Papules, pustules, and hemorrhagic vesicles on a narrow, erythematous base appear on the distal portions of the arms and legs. Most joint effusions are sterile. This disorder may clear spontaneously or result in residual septic arthritis in one or more joints (e.g., knee or wrist). Culture of the blood during the polyarticular phase, urethra, cervix, throat, and anus may reveal *N. gonorrhoeae*. Culture of synovial fluid from persistently painful and swollen joints may reveal *N. gonorrhoeae*. Gonococcal arthritis and tenosynovitis clear rapidly after parenteral administration of ceftriaxone.

2. Nongonococcal Septic Polyarthritis

A. NEISSERIA MENINGITIDIS POLYARTHRITIS This disorder may cause a generalized polyarthritis, fever, chills, and a maculopapular and/or pustular rash. Synovial fluid (80–90 percent of cases) or blood cultures may yield *N. meningitidis*. In up to 50 percent of cases, arthritis is preceded by an upper respiratory infection. This disorder may mimic disseminated gonococcal infection

B. SEPTIC POLYARTHRITIS DUE TO SPECIES OTHER THAN NEISSERIA *S. aureus* is the com-

monest cause of polyarticular septic arthritis. In two reported series, it accounted for 70 and 82 percent of cases of septic polyarthritis, respectively. Other bacteria with a tendency to cause septic polyarthritis include *Streptococcus pneumoniae* (36 percent of cases of arthritis caused by this agent were polyarticular) and group G streptococcus (39 percent of cases of arthritis caused by this organism were polyarticular). Rare causes of septic polyarthritis include *Hemophilus influenzae* (36–48 percent of joint infections caused by this agent were polyarticular), anaerobic bacteria, gram-negative bacilli, *Pasteurella multocida*, *Streptococcus milleri*, and *Streptobacillus moniliformis*. Rare causes of septic arthritis and the disorders associated with these infectious agents are listed in Table 45-3.

Polyarticular septic arthritis occurs in 20 percent of patients with nongonococcal joint infection. Risk factors such as an underlying chronic inflammatory arthritis or prior joint trauma, immune suppression (e.g., from malignancy, alcoholism, or corticosteroids), and concurrent infection are associated with an increased likelihood of developing polyarticular septic arthritis. Isolation of the causative bacteria from one or more joints and/or the blood will confirm the diagnosis.

Rarely, intraarticular sepsis may produce gas visible on a plain radiograph. Infection with *S. milleri*, *Klebsiella* species, clostridial species, other anaerobes, and *Escherichia coli* have been associated with intraarticular gas production (i.e., emphysematous arthritis). Intraarticular gas may also result from an invasive joint procedure. The presence of joint space gas in the absence of such a procedure is indicative of joint infection.

B. Reactive Arthritis An asymmetrical oligoarthritis may follow a diarrheal illness (e.g., caused by species of *Salmonella*, *Shigella*, *Campylobacter*, and *Yersinia* or *Clostridium difficile*) or a urogenital infection (e.g., caused by *Chlamydia trachomatis*, *Ureaplasma urealyticum*, and possibly by *N. gonorrhoeae*). The male/female ratio is 10:1 in sexually acquired reactive arthritis and in *Shigella*-associated arthritis. The ratio is 1:1.6 in other forms of enterocolitic arthritis.

Arthritis usually begins within 1 to 4 weeks of the onset of gastrointestinal or urethral symptoms. There is a predilection for the larger joints of the lower extremity (knees, ankles, and hips) and the wrists and elbows. An asymmetrical distribution is frequent, and joints become inflamed in rapid succession. The knees become warm, painful, swollen, and sometimes red. The legs and feet are involved in 80 to 90 percent and the arms in 50 percent of cases. Enthesopathy (insertional tendinitis) occurs in 30 to 50 percent and may cause heel and buttock pain on one or both sides. Low back pain due to sacroiliitis and/

or spondylitis occurs in 20 to 30 percent. The metatarsophalangeal joints of the feet may become involved, resulting in forefoot and midfoot pain, swelling, warmth, and tenderness. Fever and malaise occur in up to 60 percent of cases.

Species of bacteria most commonly associated with postdysenteric reactive arthritis include *Shigella flexneri* types 1 and 2 (but not *Shigella sonnei*); *Salmonella typhimurium, Salmonella enteritidis, Salmonella heidelberg*, and *Salmonella blockley*; Yersinia enterocolitica serotypes 3, 6, 8, and 9 and *Yersinia pseudotuberculosis*; *Campylobacter* species; and, rarely *C. difficile*.

Sexually acquired reactive arthritis (SARA) follows or coincides with urethral and other infections with some *C. trachomatis* serovars, *U. urealyticum*, and in some cases *N. gonorrhoeae*. The role of *N. gonorrhoeae* in reactive arthritis is not accepted by all authors. Findings supporting a role for *N. gonorrhoeae* in some patients with reactive arthritis include culture-negative synovial fluid, positive synovial lymphocyte transformation test results in the presence of gonococcal antigens, and a positive gonococcal complement fixation test. Treatment for *N. gonorrhoeae* infection does not usually lead to resolution of the reactive arthritis attributed to this agent.

Up to 20 percent of patients with reactive arthritis who are infected with an enteric pathogen may be asymptomatic. Confirmation of the diagnosis of reactive arthritis in these cases requires a positive stool culture or a rise in antibody titer. Similarly, some patients with urogenital infection have few or no symptoms. Cultures for urogenital pathogens from mucosal sites (urethra, cervix, anus, and throat), serologic studies, and synovial lymphocyte blast transformation after exposure in vitro to a specific antigen provide evidence of etiology in patients with SARA.

The sterile synovial fluid in *Salmonella*-reactive arthritis may contain 300 to 61,000 cells/mm^3. The percentage of polymorphonuclear leukocytes varies from 20 to 93 percent (mean, 67 percent).

Extraarticular involvement may occur in reactive arthritis. Musculoskeletal lesions include enthesopathies (e.g., inflammation of tendinous insertions on the calcaneus and pelvic bones) causing heel and buttock pain and tenosynovitis of digits resulting in dactylitis ("sausage digits"). Genital inflammation may occur in postdysenteric reactive arthritis and cause diagnostic confusion. Urogenital involvement associated with reactive arthritis occurs with *Shigella* (70 percent), *Salmonella* (15 percent), *Campylobacter* (24 percent), and *Yersinia* species (13 percent). Conjunctivitis may occur in SARA (35 percent of cases) and in postdysenteric reactive arthritis (9–88 percent of cases). Circinate balanitis is seen in SARA (23 percent of cases) and in *Shigella*-related arthritis (24 percent). Keratoderma blennorrhagicum occurs in 12 percent of patients with SARA and is not usually seen after enteric infections.

On the other hand, diarrhea is uncommon in patients with SARA (12 percent). Less frequent manifestations include iritis (2–6 percent), myocarditis by electrocardiographic criteria (6–14 percent), and erythema nodosum (seen in 5 percent of patients with *Yersinia*-reactive arthritis).

Reiter's syndrome may occur after enterocolitic or urogenital infection. Many cases of the syndrome are incomplete, consisting of urethritis and arthritis, conjunctivitis and arthritis, and conjunctivitis and urethritis. The incidence of a complete Reiter's syndrome (urethritis, conjunctivitis, and arthritis) is probably less than 20 percent of patients with reactive arthritis.

HLA-B27 and sometimes -B7 antigen is present in a large percentage of patients with reactive arthritis. A subgroup of cases with similar clinical characteristics, HLA-B27 antigen positivity, and absence of a known infectious agent has been described.

Therapy consists of antimicrobial drugs to eradicate the associated microorganism and physiotherapy and nonsteroidal anti-inflammatory drugs for the arthritic symptoms.

C. Acute Rheumatic Fever   Acute rheumatic fever may cause a migratory asymmetrical polyarthritis involving the knees, ankles, wrists, elbows, shoulders, hands, and feet. The joints are often swollen, red, tender, and painful at rest and with movement. In adults, subcutaneous nodules may occur over extensor surfaces, but erythema marginatum, carditis, and chorea are rare. There is an increased level of serum antibody to streptolysin O, hyaluronidase, desoxyribonuclease B, and other streptococcal antigens (Streptozyme test); an elevated sedimentation rate; and in many cases leukocytosis. Clinical and serologic evidence of a recent streptococcal infection may be lacking in 5 to 10 percent of patients. There is a dramatic response to aspirin therapy with reduction of fever and joint complaints.

D. Crystal-Induced Polyarthritis   An oligoarticular or polyarticular pattern may occur. The knee on one or both sides may become swollen, red, tender, and painful. Weight bearing and passive movement increase pain. Ankles, metatarsophalangeal joints, wrists, elbows, and other joints may be involved in an asymmetrical or symmetrical distribution. Chondrocalcinosis may be present in the knees, wrists, shoulders, and other joints in pseudogout. Joint fluid contains an increased concentration of polymorphonuclear leukocytes, an elevated protein level, and intra- and extracellular monosodium urate (gout) or calcium pyrophosphate dihydrate (pseudogout) crystals. Fever, weakness, sweats, and anorexia may accompany severe episodes. Intravenous or oral colchicine, indomethacin, or prednisone will usually lead to symptom resolution in 1 to 3 days.

E. Hepatitis B-Associated Arthritis An acute migratory or additive polyarthritis occurs. The small joints of the fingers are inolved in up to 70 percent and the knees in 35 percent of cases. Up to 50 percent of patients develop urticaria or a pruritic maculopapular or petechial rash. Vasculitic (immune-complex) urticarial lesions often persist for more than 24 h, develop a central petechial area, and may cause burning discomfort as well as pruritus. Systemic complains such as fever, chills, myalgias, arthralgias, anorexia, and nausea may precede or accompany the arthritis. Hepatitis B surface antigen is usually present in the serum, and complement levels are depressed. Evidence of abnormal liver function may accompany the arthritis or develop within 1 to 4 weeks. Synovial fluid is sterile and contains an increased concentration of polymorphonuclear leukocytes and protein.

F. Lyme Arthritis This disorder most commonly affects the knees, but polyarthritis or polyarthralgias involving the shoulders, elbows, ankles, hips, hands, and feet may also occur. There is often a history of erythema chronicum migrans followed by a systemic illness (fever, chills, aseptic meningitis, and/or encephalitis). Serum antibody to *B. burgdorferi* is usually elevated. The joint symptoms usually respond to parenteral therapy with ceftriaxone.

G. Acute Rheumatoid Arthritis Up to 15 percent of patients with rheumatoid arthritis may present with an acute arthritis involving the metacarpophalangeal and proximal interphalangeal joints of the hands, the wrists, the elbows, the knees, and the ankles. Swelling, tenderness, warmth, and pain are common, but skin erythema over affected joints is not. Subcutaneous nodules may be palpable over extensor surfaces, and the serum test for rheumatoid factor may be positive. Joint involvement is usually symmetrical, but it may be asymmetrical early in the course of the disease. Some joints may be painful only on movement, with exertion of a force across the joint, or on weight bearing. Criteria for diagnosis, such as 1 h or more of morning stiffness, involvement of three or more joints, hand and wrist arthritis, symmetrical arthritis, subcutaneous nodules, a positive serum test result for rheumatoid factor, and radiographic evidence of juxtaarticular erosion and osteopenia of the hands and wrists, have been established by the American Rheumatism Association. The first four listed criteria must be present for at least 6 weeks. Early in the course of the disease, patients may lack one or more of the four criteria required for diagnosis. Fever in the 38 to 39°C (101 to 102°F) range, weight loss, anorexia, weakness, malaise, and other systemic complaints may occur in some cases.

H. Gonococcal Arthritis Disseminated gonococcal arthritis may be aseptic. It most commonly involves the knees and wrists. Ankles, finger joints, shoulders, and hips are less frequently affected. Skin lesions consisting of small yellow-green pustules or purple hemorrhagic vesicles on a 1- to 1.5-cm erythematous base occur predominantly on the distal arms and legs. Fever, weakness, and anorexia may occur but are usually mild or absent. Joint swelling and pain are commonly migratory. Tenosynovitis involving the dorsum of the hands and feet or the Achilles tendons occurs in up to 68 percent of cases. Synovial fluid cultures are negative for *N. gonorrhoeae*. There is usually an inflammatory-type synovial fluid with a predominance of polymorphonuclear leukocytes. Mucous membrane cultures have a sensitivity of 80 percent for *N. gonorrhoeae*. The joints are probably inflamed because of immune complex deposition. Ceftriaxone therapy leads to resolution of joint, tendon, and skin lesions.

Reactive arthritis due to *N. gonorrhoeae* is not associated with skin lesions and resembles the asymmetrical oligoarthritis associated with *C. trachomatis* and *U. urealyticum* infections.

I. Serum Sickness Response to Penicillin Treatment of an acute pharyngitis with penicillin may cause fever, myalgias, and a polyarthritis. Gross or microscopic hematuria may also occur. Angioedema or vasculitic urticaria, if present, suggest hypersensitivity as a basis for the clinical findings. Discontinuance of penicillin therapy results in resolution of symptoms, signs, and laboratory abnormalities within 5 to 14 days.

J. Viral Arthritis

1. Rubella Arthritis Symmetrical pain and stiffness involve the knees, wrists, metacarpophalangeal joints, and proximal interphalangeal joints. Swelling, redness, and warmth of the knees and other joints do not usually occur. Carpal tunnel syndrome, brachial neuritis, and tenosynovitis of the wrist and hands or feet may be associated. Posterior cervical painful and tender lymphadenopathy, fever, and a light pink maculopapular truncal rash may precede or follow the joint complaints. Rheumatoid factor is usually absent but may be present in a small percentage of cases. This disorder occurs in 15 to 60 percent of adult women with rubella. It is rare in men and children.

2. Rubella Vaccine-Induced Arthritis Live, attenuated rubella vaccine may cause joint complaints similar to those associated with rubella. In the vaccine-associated disorder, the knees are frequently the only joints affected. Joint symptoms follow vaccination within 2 to 4 weeks (range, 8–55 days). Arthritis lasts 1 to 46 days. Recurrent attacks of knee pain may occur for up to 3 years. This disorder is more common in adolescent girls and women than in children.

3. Varicella Arthritis This disorder usually occurs when the characteristic pox rash is present. It most commonly presents as a monarthritis of the knee or ankle. In some patients, both knees or multiple joints are involved. The synovial fluid cell counts range from 3500 to 51,700, and there is usually a mononuclear cell predominance. The glucose concentration in the synovial fluid may be low or normal. In two reported cases, varicella zoster virus was isolated from the joint fluid. All reported cases have been in children in the 2- to 11-year-old age group.

K. Still's disease

1. Acute Juvenile-Onset Rheumatoid Arthritis JRA may present as a polyarthritis (five or more joints) or as an oligoarthritis (four or fewer joints). The arthritis may be remittent and indolent. The knees, wrists, elbows, ankles, and small joints of the hands and feet are frequently involved. Asymmetrical joint involvement is uncommon but may occur. Pain at rest may be minimal, but palpation of the affected joint, weight bearing, and range-of-motion testing provoke discomfort.

In patients with polyarticular involvement, posterior neck pain and stiffness is caused by involvement of cervical facet joints. Temporomandibular joint inflammation may result in chewing difficulties and micrognathia.

High spiking fever, chills, and prostration may occur as unexplained symptoms or may be associated with arthritis and a rheumatoid rash. This exanthem consists of small, erythematous (salmon-colored) macules that appear on the trunk, upper arms, thighs, face, palms, and soles. The skin lesions appear for only a few hours and are often migratory. Some macules have a perilesional pallor but are nonpruritic. They may show central clearing and sometimes resemble urticaria. The rash occurs in patients with fever and chills or in those with polyarthritis. It seldom occurs in those with oligoarthritis. Skin lesions may be made to appear by rubbing or scratching the skin, or by a hot bath. Hepatosplenomegaly, lymphadenopathy, pericarditis, and pleuritis may accompany systemic complaints.

2. Adult-Onset Still's Disease This disorder begins in the 20- to 40-year-old age group and is more common in women than in men. It presents with daily spiking fever, systemic complaints, and polyarthritis. Enlargement of the liver and spleen; cervical, epitrochlear and axillary lymphadenopathy; a transient macular truncal rash; anemia; and leukocytosis are commonly present. Cervical spine involvement is frequent, causing pain, stiffness, and loss of neck mobility. Some adults also develop chest pain (pericarditis), pleural effusions (pleuritis), and unexplained abdominal pain. Results of the serum test for rheumatoid factor in juve-

nile-onset Still's disease may be positive in up to 20 percent of cases. Children under age 7 and adults are usually seronegative.

4. REFLEX SYMPATHETIC DYSTROPHY OF THE KNEE

Surgery (e.g., arthroscopic patellar debridement, patellectomy, and total knee arthroplasty), direct anterior knee trauma, knee manipulation, or a minor or major twisting or crush injury of the knee may cause severe, persistent, and disabling knee pain. This pain appears disproportionately intense and prolonged relative to the severity of the initiating trauma or the extent of the surgical procedure. The pain has been described as aching or burning. It may be felt in the entire knee (56 percent of cases), the anterior knee (36 percent), or the medial knee (8 percent). Rest pain is common; pain may be excruciating during weight bearing, rendering the patient incapable of walking unaided.

Initially, the skin over the affected knee may be warm and erythematous. After 2 to 3 weeks, it may become cool and mottled, and exhibit bluish discoloration. Hyperhidrosis, skin atrophy, and severe skin tenderness occur over the affected knee. Muscles involved in knee movement (quadriceps and hamstrings) become weak and atrophic. Passive and active range of knee motion is decreased because of joint stiffness and pain. Cold exposure intensifies knee pain. The skin in the periarticular region may be hypersensitive to touch (allodynia). Thermograms may reveal a reduced skin temperature in the knee region. Plain radiographs taken 3 or more weeks after pain onset may demonstrate osteopenia of the patella (49 percent of cases); the tibia, femur, and patella (39 percent); and the distal femur (12 percent). A three-phase radionuclide bone scan in reflex sympathetic dystrophy using technetium 99m methylene diphosphonate may demonstrate one of three reported patterns of blood velocity, blood pool, and early and delayed hyperfixation. The radionuclide findings are a function of the duration of pain and other symptoms. During weeks 0 to 20 of this disorder, there is an increase in blood velocity, blood pool, and early and delayed hyperfixation.

A sympathetic nerve block may be useful as a diagnostic test if it relieves pain. Lumbar sympathetic blocks (three or four blocks over a period of 4–5 days) have given a good or fair therapeutic response rate in 90 percent of cases. Persistent or frequently recurrent symptoms are an indication for lumbar sympathectomy. Definitive therapy for this disorder should be initiated as soon as possible, since results of treatment are poor if more than 6 months have elapsed without the use of sympathetic blockade or vasodilator drugs.

5. REFERRED PAIN TO THE KNEE

An acute synovitis of the hip may be referred to the knee. Examination may reveal hip joint tenderness, a decreased range of pain-free motion at the hip, and a normal range of pain-free motion at the knee.

An obturator hernia or another cause of compression of the obturator nerve may cause medial thigh and knee pain. A CT scan of the pelvis may be required to determine the site and cause of obturator nerve compression.

A lumbosacral plexopathy or intraspinal disease may involve the L2–L4 nerve roots, resulting in inguinal, anterior thigh, and/or knee pain on the ipsilateral side. A CT scan of the pelvis will detect tumor-related plexopathy. MRI of the lumbar region or a CT-enhanced myelogram may detect a space-occupying lesion of the spine or retroperitoneum. Retroperitoneal lesions that may cause lumbar plexopathy include tumor, aneurysm, abscess, or hematoma.

Medial Knee Pain

6. MEDIAL MENISCUS TEARS

A. Traumatic Tears   The partially flexed knee suffers a twisting injury, resulting in severe pain and sometimes a sensation of tearing or an audible pop within the joint. The foot is often fixed to the ground and externally rotated, while the thigh is violently twisted. This may happen when a football player is struck from the side; a soccer player kicking a ball catches his or her toe in the soft ground, trips, and falls while the foot and leg are externally rotated; or a squatting worker's knee is forcefully rotated without extension.

Some patients with an acute bucket-handle (bowstring) longitudinal tear of the medial meniscus may hear two pops at the time of injury. These pops correspond to dislocation and then reduction of the torn portion of cartilage.

Such injuries are usually vertical longitudinal, transverse, or oblique tears. At the instant of injury, the most severe pain occurs at the medial joint line, and weight bearing becomes intolerable. If walking becomes possible, a limp is usually present, and walking speed is severely reduced. The knee may swell within minutes (intraarticular hemorrhage) or an effusion may first appear after 12 to 24 h (traumatic synovitis), and this is usually an exudate. Warmth, swelling, and tenderness occur along the medial joint line at the site of maximal pain. Locking may occur at the time of the tear, limiting full knee extension because of interposition of the torn cartilage segment between the tibial and femoral articular surfaces. An episode of locking may be relieved by pulling, twisting, or shaking the leg.

More gradual development of limitation of knee exten-

sion or flexion may be associated with the accumulation of joint fluid, synovial hypertrophy, an intraarticular fracture, a loose body, or a tense popliteal cyst.

If the bowstring tear extends far enough posteriorly, knee flexion and medial rotation of the tibia may be restricted. A meniscal tear may be diagnosed by MRI. This procedure may demonstrate a linear, globular, or complex high-intensity meniscal signal. Such tears may be seen to extend partially or completely to the tibial surface. The sensitivity of MRI for medial meniscus tears has been reported as 77, 96, and 100 percent and specificity as 72, 100, and 88 percent in three published series, respectively. Confirmation of MRI findings and definitive therapy of the torn meniscus may be accomplished by arthroscopy.

B. Degenerative Tears   There is frequently no history of trauma other than a minor twist or sudden flexion of the knee when stumbling, jumping down from a height, or during a game of tennis or racquetball. Pain is felt in the medial joint line posterior to the medial collateral ligament. Initially it may be mild, but it becomes more severe within 12 to 24 h. Some tears cause pain in a limited range of knee motion (e.g., at 15–50° of flexion). The pain usually becomes more severe during weight bearing, walking, and jogging. Walking distance and speed are reduced. Early in the course, a constant pain may occur and persist into the night, interfering with sleep. Driving a car with the knee partially flexed may intensify the pain and may limit driving distance. This ache may be accomplished by medial joint line warmth, tenderness, and swelling. It may respond to aspirin or nonsteroidal antiinflammatory drugs and limitation of weight bearing. Locking (limitation of knee extension) or giving way (buckling) of the knee when walking on uneven terrain or during a sudden turn may occur. Degenerative tears usually occur in patients older than age 45 and involve the posterior horn of the medial meniscus. A joint effusion may occur but is uncommon.

Examination reveals medial joint line tenderness and sometimes localized warmth and swelling. Results of the McMurray test may be positive, but negative results do not exclude a degenerative posterior horn tear. In this test, the recumbent patient's painful knee is flexed until the heel contacts the gluteal region. The foot and leg are externally rotated, and valgus pressure is applied across the joint by the examiner's right hand as the knee is slowly extended. The point of the extension arc at which a painful click or snap is palpated defines the site of meniscus injury (i.e., posterior or middle segment). In many cases, weight-bearing and range-of-motion medial joint line pain are the only symptoms, and locking and giving way do not occur.

Meniscal clicks can be elicited by varus or valgus stress on the knee in the presence of a tear. The Apley grind test may be used to confirm meniscal injury. (This test is performed with the patient prone and the knee flexed to 90°. Downward compression of the knee is combined with internal or external rotation of the lower leg and foot. Induction of pain medially signals a medial meniscus injury.) MRI can be used to identify a posterior horn tear with a sensitivity of 95 percent.

7. TIBIAL COLLATERAL LIGAMENT BURSITIS (VOSHELL'S BURSITIS)

Medial joint line pain occurs at the site of the tibial collateral ligament. The diagnosis of bursitis is unlikely in the presence of knee locking. Examination reveals tenderness of the tibial collateral ligament at the joint line, with pain intensification by valgus stress on the knee. Local injection of lidocaine and a corticosteroid into Voshell's bursa provides rapid and usually complete pain relief. This approach is permanently effective in up to 62 percent of cases. Second injections may be required for patients with persistent or recurrent pain. MRI usually reveals a normal medial meniscus in most patients, but a tear of the medial meniscus unrelated to the pain may be detected in up to 23 percent of cases by MRI or arthroscopy. Voshell's bursitis has been mistaken for a medial meniscus tear and treated by unnecessary arthroscopic resection of the medial meniscus.

8. TIBIAL COLLATERAL LIGAMENT INJURY

A. Sprain (Partial Rupture)   This injury follows a twisting strain when the knee is flexed. Pain and tenderness occur over the medial aspect of the knee. Swelling is present over the medial condyle of the femur, and tenderness may be localized to the point of attachment of the tibial collateral ligament to the femoral condyle. Pain is intensified by lower leg abduction with the knee extended or by external rotation of the lower leg. There is no widening of the joint interval. Local injection of a corticosteroid and lidocaine provides immediate relief. Support and rest allows healing with 2 to 5 weeks.

B. Complete Rupture   This injury follows marked abduction and external rotation of the lower leg with the knee partially flexed (e.g., football clipping injury) or abduction of the leg with the knee extended. The joint fills with blood, and pain, tenderness, and edema develop over the medial portion of the knee. Testing for acute medial ligament rupture requires anesthesia. Test findings include increased external tibial rotation and valgus instability of the joint space with the knee flexed at 25° (i.e., a gap in the medial joint space of ≥10 mm is present). Severe tibial collateral ligament tears are often associated with one or more of the following injuries: a tear of the posteromedial joint capsule, rupture of the ACL, a medial meniscus tear, and fracture of the lateral tibial plateau.

9. EXTRAARTICULAR DISPLACEMENT OF THE MEDIAL MENISCUS

An abrupt or insidious onset may occur. Pain occurs during weight bearing and in a limited arc of knee motion. The discomfort can be provoked by weight bearing or external rotation of the lower leg. The area over the tibial collateral ligament is tender and may be swollen. The diagnosis may be confirmed by MRI or arthroscopy.

10. OSTEONECROSIS OF THE MEDIAL FEMORAL CONDYLE

There is an abrupt onset of persistent medial knee pain severe enough to disturb sleep. Weight bearing and walking intensify the pain. Diffuse swelling of the knee, intraarticular effusion, and stiffness may occur. Tenderness occurs over the medial condyle of the femur. Plain radiographs are usually negative at the onset of the pain. MRI or a radionuclide scan will demonstrate the area of osteonecrosis in the medial condyle within 2 to 3 weeks of the onset of symptoms. This disorder occurs most frequently in elderly persons. After 1 month or more, plain radiographs reveal a subchondral radiolucency beneath the weight-bearing surface of the medial femoral condyle. This osteolytic area is surrounded by a sclerotic halo.

11. HOFFA'S DISEASE

Pain and point tenderness occur over the anteromedial joint line. The patellar fat pad is swollen and tender and bulges forward on one or both sides of the patellar tendon. This disorder may respond to an extraarticular injection of lidocaine and corticosteroid.

12. PES ANSERINE BURSITIS

The pes anserinus ("goose's foot") is formed by the combined insertions of the sartorius, gracilis, and semitendinosus tendons on the proximal anteromedial surface of the tibia. The tibial collateral ligament is separated from these tendons by the pes bursa. Bursitis can cause pain, local tenderness, and sometimes diffuse swelling over the anteromedial portion of the upper tibia below the joint line. The pain is intensified by climbing stairs and walking. Pes anserine bursitis is often mistaken for osteoarthritis of the knee. Symptoms may respond to a local injection of corticosteroid and lidocaine.

13. PES ANSERINE–GASTROCNEMIUS-RELATED TENDINITIS

This disorder causes medial knee pain that mimics pes anserine bursitis. The tenderness is maximal between the pes anserine tendons and the gastrocnemius. This area is posterior to the bursa. This painful disorder is usually associated with prolonged ankle pronation.

14. SEMIMEMBRANOSUS TENDINITIS

Aching pain occurs over the posteromedial aspect of the knee and is provoked or intensified by walking, bending, lifting, climbing, or running. Posteromedial tenderness occurs just inferior to the joint line. Palpation of the semi-membranosus tendon reproduces the pain. This disorder may occur in endurance athletes (runners or triathletes), in patients with a medial meniscus tear, in association with chondromalacia patellae, or as an isolated entity.

If the tendinitis involves the fan-shaped insertion of the semimembranosus tendon into the proximal medial tibia, pes anserine bursitis may be mimicked. This tendon inserts proximal to the pes anserinus.

A bone scan may demonstrate increased uptake at the site of insertion of the tendon on the tibia in patients with persistent symptoms.

15. OSTEONECROSIS OF THE PROXIMAL TIBIA

This disorder causes proximal medial tibial pain and tenderness. The pain is persistent and is exacerbated by weight bearing and walking. It is associated with a positive radionuclide scan. MRI is a sensitive method for the demonstration of early osteonecrosis of the proximal tibia.

Lateral Knee Pain

16. ILIOTIBIAL BAND FRICTION SYNDROME

This disorder occurs in long-distance runners and is frequently associated with running on hills or banked terrain or with a crossover gait pattern.

Pain occurs over the lateral side of the knee and may be more severe during downhill running. Once the pain begins, it may be so severe that the runner may have to stop. Cessation of running results in rapid pain relief. Return to running results in abrupt recurrence of the same pain.

This disorder is caused by friction between the iliotibial band and the lateral epicondyle during running. The intervening bursa becomes inflamed. There is tenderness over the lateral femoral epicondyle. In severe and persistent cases, creaking occurs on flexion and extension of the knee. When thumb pressure is placed over the lateral epicondyle and the flexed knee is moved into extension (Noble's test), the posterior fibers of the iliotibial band move across the epicondyle beneath the thumb, and typical severe pain is provoked at 30° of knee flexion.

Ober's test (e.g., for abduction contracture) may reveal excessive tightness of the iliotibial band. This test is performed with the patient in the lateral decubitus position, lying on the asymptomatic side with the table-supported hip and knee flexed. The painful extremity is held by the lower leg; the hip is flexed to 90°, fully abducted and externally rotated, and the limb is passively moved into the neutral midline position of the body with the knee flexed to 90°. If the limb does not adduct toward the examining table after support is withdrawn (i.e., a positive test result), a tight iliotibial band should be suspected.

Predisposing disorders include calcaneal varus, tibia vara, cavus foot, and an abnormal valgus heel-forefoot alignment. In patients with these abnormalities, the lower leg does not absorb the forces generated during the stance phase of gait, and these forces are transmitted to the iliotibial band region.

17. POPLITEUS TENOSYNOVITIS

Pain is localized to the lateral side of the knee during weight bearing with the knee flexed 15 to 30°. A minority of patients feel pain during the early portion of the swing phase of the gait. Downhill running or walking often provokes symptoms. Symptoms usually improve on stopping the provoking activity. Some patients complain of pain when attempting to stand up from a cross-legged sitting position.

There is localized tenderness over the tendinous portion of the popliteus muscle-tendon unit just anterior to the insertion of the fibular collateral ligament on the lateral femoral condyle. To test for this disorder, the seated patient is instructed to flex the painful knee to 90° and to flex, abduct, and externally rotate the hip, placing the lateral side of the foot on the opposite knee. This position facilitates palpation of the popliteus tendon anterior to the fibular collateral ligament or provokes pain by placing stress on the tendon. Pain may also be provoked by external rotation of the tibia or by rotation of the femur internally on the fixed tibia with the knee flexed to 30°. Pain may be perceived as arising within the knee during running, since a portion of the tendon is intraarticular. Symptoms are relieved by running on flat terrain, local application of ice, and administration of a nonsteroidal anti-inflammatory drug.

18. POPLITEUS TENDON RUPTURE

Rupture rarely occurs as an isolated injury. It usually accompanies other lateral and posterolateral knee injuries. A sudden external rotation of the tibia with the knee flexed may rupture the tendon. A sudden crack or pop may be heard at the time of injury, accompanied by lateral knee pain, swelling, and inability to bear weight or walk because of the pain. A knee effusion may be present. Lateral joint line and diffuse posterolateral knee tenderness may be present. The diagnosis may be confirmed by arthroscopy. Probing of the popliteus tendon for laxity during this procedure may allow detection of tendon rupture.

19.   LATERAL MENISCUS TEAR

Lateral knee pain follows a twisting injury when the knee joint is flexed. There is local tenderness over the lateral joint line. Locking, preventing full knee extension, may occur but is less common than in medial meniscus tears. Other complaints include giving way and a small joint effusion. The Apley grind test may be positive. The diagnosis can be confirmed by MRI or arthroscopy. Pain may be referred medially, but joint line tenderness, clicking, and pain provoked by the Apley grind test are limited to the lateral side of the knee.

20.   LATERAL COLLATERAL LIGAMENT INJURY

Injury to the lateral ligamentous complex may result from a fall in a forward direction with the lower leg internally rotated and varus stress applied to the knee. Pain is felt over the lateral side of the knee and is usually associated with local tenderness over the ligament. Joint effusion is minimal. Walking causes little pain, but running and cutting or rapid deceleration may provoke a sensation of giving way of the knee. An adduction stress test at 30° of flexion may demonstrate lateral joint space widening. Flexion and internal rotation of the knee may allow detection of a tender defect in the lateral collateral ligament complex.

21.   TIBIOFIBULAR JOINT DISORDER

Instability or posttraumatic arthritis may follow direct or indirect trauma (ankle injury). Pain occurs over the lateral side of the knee. Walking, running, weight bearing on the flexed knee, and dorsiflexion of the ankle usually provoke pain.

The superior tibiofibular joint and the insertion of the biceps femoris tendon are usually tender.

Rocking the fibula head with the knee flexed and the ankle dorsiflexed, and walking with the toes turned in are painful. Forceful contraction of the biceps femoris against resistance reproduces typical pain. There is no knee pain through a full range of knee motion. Plain radiographs are not usually helpful. If the joint pain is due to arthritis, immediate relief results from an intraarticular injection of lidocaine.

22.   BICEPS FEMORIS TENDINITIS

Posterolateral knee pain and tenderness may result from inflammation of the biceps femoris tendon and/or the bursa situated beneath this tendon. A local injection of lidocaine and a corticosteroid may be both diagnostic and therapeutic.

23.   OSTEOCHONDRAL FRACTURE OF THE LATERAL FEMORAL CONDYLE

This injury follows a forceful twist of the flexed knee. There are lateral and anterior knee pain, tenderness, and swelling. Plain radiographs, MRI and arthroscopic examination will confirm the diagnosis.

Anterior Knee Pain

24.   PATELLAR TENDON INJURY

Trauma to the tendon as the knee strikes the dashboard during a motor vehicle accident causes pain on active knee extension and passive knee flexion. There are tenderness and swelling over the patellar tendon.

25.   PATELLAR TENDINITIS ("JUMPER'S KNEE")

Anterior knee pain occurs in an athlete after jumping, climbing, running, or kicking. The pain and tenderness are localized to the patellar tendon or the inferior pole of the patella. Initially, pain may occur only after activity, and it does not cause disability. As the disorder progresses, pain occurs during activity and persists for a prolonged period after rest is initiated. Pain occurs on extension against resistance, and there may be point tenderness and edema over the tendon near the patella. Tenderness may also occur under the inferior pole of the patella. Plain radiographs usually appear normal, but in some cases they may reveal a radiolucency in the inferior patella or prolongation of this region of the patella. In severe cases, an avulsion fracture of the inferior pole of the patella may occur. There may be tendon degeneration with fraying of fibers near the patellar attachment of the tendon. Surgical removal of painful granulation tissue in the tendon may be required for symptomatic relief. Patellar tendon rupture from the inferior pole of the patella may occur, preventing active knee extension. Local pain and tenderness and a palpable gap may be present with an acute rupture of the patellar tendon.

26. PREPATELLAR BURSITIS

Swelling, pain, and tenderness occur over the patella. These symptoms may follow direct trauma, recurrent frictional trauma, or pressure from long periods of kneeling (e.g., miners, housemaids, or people at prayer). The prepatellar location may be confirmed by straight leg raising. The dimensions of the swelling do not change with this maneuver, indicating that the bursal collection is not secondary to an intraarticular effusion.

Skin fissures over a swollen prepatellar bursa may result in introduction of infection, causing an acute septic bursitis. Antibiotic therapy and drainage of infected bursal fluid will usually lead to resolution.

27. CELLULITIS OF THE SKIN OVER THE KNEE

Cellulitis may cause local redness, pain, warmth, and swelling, and infection may spread to the underlying prepatellar bursa, resulting in a septic bursitis. Aspiration of fluid from the bursa for analysis of cell number and type and for culture should be performed, and antibiotic therapy should be initiated.

28. RETROPATELLAR BURSITIS

This disorder may follow direct trauma to the patellar tendon. There is a local, painful, tender, fluctuant swelling behind the patellar tendon.

29. INFRAPATELLAR FAT PAD INJURY

This injury may result from a dashboard injury or a fall on a hard surface with the knee flexed. There are local pain, tenderness, and swelling of the fat pad on one or both sides of the patellar tendon. The knee pain may become worse after activity, and a recurrent or persistent joint effusion may be present. Extension against resistance increases the pain.

30. HOFFA'S DISEASE (HYPERTROPHY AND INFLAMMATION OF THE INFRAPATELLAR FAT PAD)

Aching pain in the anterior knee is provoked by exercise and relieved by rest. The pain is most intense in extension and is partly relieved in flexion. High-heeled shoes may provide relief for some women, while flat shoes intensify the pain. Edema occurs on both sides of the patellar tendon, and the overlying skin may become warm. A joint effusion may occur, but it is generally small. There is tenderness over the swollen fat pad and patellar tendon.

Pain results from compression of the synovium between the articulating surfaces when the knee is extended. Causes include premenstrual water retention, a space-occupying lesion in the joint (e.g., displaced bucket-handle meniscus tear, synovioma, lipoma, or hemangioma), and a recurvatum deformity of the knee.

31. OSTEOCHONDRITIS DISSECANS OF THE PATELLA

Osteochondritis dissecans of the patella may follow a minor injury or may be idiopathic. The diagnosis can be confirmed by a plain radiograph showing a bony defect on the posterior surface of the patella. There is anterior knee pain and localized tenderness over the affected area of the patella. The fragment may detach and appear in the joint space as a loose body. This disorder can also be demonstrated by MRI or arthroscopy.

32. QUADRICEPS TENDON RUPTURE

Aching pain and soreness occur in the region of the proximal patella for several days prior to rupture. These symptoms may represent a low-grade tendinitis or a partial tear. Rupture occurs during forced flexion of the knee as the athlete attempts to extend the knee. It may occur in tennis players as they lose their balance and in weight lifters. A gap is palpable above the knee, and the patient is unable to extend the joint. A plain radiograph may sometimes demonstrate a fragment of bone avulsed from the superior pole of the patella.

33. OSTEOCHONDRAL FRACTURE OF THE PATELLA

These fractures occur during active extension of the knee with or without application of a twisting force to the joint. There is an abrupt onset of tearing anterior knee pain, and in some cases a breaking sound arising in the joint, followed by immediate swelling of the knee due to hemarthrosis. Tenderness at the site of patellar injury is usually present. Osteochondral fractures may also follow a direct impact. The diagnosis can be confirmed by plain radiography, MRI, or arthroscopy.

Posterior Knee Pain

34. GASTROCNEMIUS MUSCLE STRAIN

Tearing or ripping pain may occur in the posterior knee or upper calf after a sudden start or turn. The pain may be continuous or only present when walking or running. There are local tenderness and swelling over the painful area of muscle. Rest results in gradual improvement.

35. PLANTARIS MUSCLE TEAR

Sharp pain and/or a popping sensation occur behind the knee and in the upper calf. Walking becomes painful and results in a limp. Some authors believe that these symptoms are due to a gastrocnemius strain and not to disruption of the plantaris.

36. HAMSTRING MUSCLE AND TENDON DISORDERS

A. Hamstring Muscle Strain   Pain occurs in the region of the hamstring muscles in the popliteal fossa. It may be caused by forced extension of the partially flexed knee. Tenderness is localized to the muscle belly of the semimembranosus muscle medially or the biceps femoris muscle laterally. A local injection of lidocaine in the region of the inflamed muscle will provide immediate pain relief.

B. Hamstring Muscle Tendinitis   Inflammation of the semimembranosus tendon posteromedially or the biceps femoris tendon posterolaterally may cause local pain and tenderness that are responsive to an injection of lidocaine and a corticosteroid into the painful area.

37. POPLITEAL LYMPHADENITIS

There may be pain and an enlarged, tender lymph node in the popliteal fossa associated with a distal pyoderma, cellulitis, and/or lymphangitis.

38. RUPTURE OF A POPLITEAL ARTERY ANEURYSM

Sudden rupture of a popliteal aneurysm causes posterior knee pain and a tender popliteal hematoma. Pain and bleeding may extend into the calf and thigh. The diagnosis can be confirmed by arteriographic studies or a CT scan or MRI of the region. Compression of the popliteal artery by the hematoma may cause distal pallor, pain, weakness, paresthesias, and diminution or loss of the pedal pulses. Popliteal aneurysms almost always occur in men.

39. CRAMPS

Muscle cramps in the posterior calf and knee region may occur spontaneously, after plantar flexion of the foot while stretching, or during sexual intercourse. Symptoms are usually unilateral but may alternate sides and are relieved by massage, walking about, and stretching of the involved posterior leg muscle.

40. POSTERIOR CRUCIATE LIGAMENT AND POSTERIOR CAPSULE TEARS

A disruption of the PCL, and in some cases the posterior capsule of the knee, may cause popliteal fossa pain and tenderness. The causes of this injury, the physical findings, and the use of MRI and arthroscopy for diagnosis are described above.

Bilateral Knee Pain

Disorders that may occur bilaterally are listed in Table 45-4.

KNEE AND POPLITEAL FOSSA PAIN REFERENCES

Arthritis — Fungal

Bernreuter WK: Coccidioidomycosis of bone: A sequela of desert rheumatism. *Arthritis Rheum* 32:1608–1610, 1989.

Downs NJ, Hinthorn DR, Mhatre VR, et al: Intra-articular amphotericin B treatment of *Sporothrix schenckii* arthritis. *Arch Intern Med* 149:954–955, 1989.

Lantz B, Selakovich WG, Collins DN, et al: Coccidioidomycosis of the knee with a 26-year follow-up evaluation: A case report. *Clin Orthop Rel Res* 234:183–187, 1988.

Robert ME, Kauffman CA: Blastomycosis presenting as polyarticular septic arthritis. *J Rheumatol* 15:1438–1442, 1988.

Sinnott JT IV, Holt DA: Cryptococcal pyarthrosis complicating gouty arthritis. *South Med J* 82:1555–1556, 1989.

Smith SM, Lee EY, Cobbs CJ, et al: Unusual features of arthritis caused by *Candida parapsilosis*. *Arch Pathol Lab Med* 111:71–73, 1987.

Stead KJ, Klugman KP, Painter ML, et al: Septic arthritis due to *Cryptococcus neoformans*. *J Infect* 17:139–145, 1988.

Arthritis — Gout, Pseudogout

Bergström G, Bjelle A, Sorensen LB, et al: Prevalence of rheumatoid arthritis, osteoarthritis, chondrocalcinosis and gouty arthritis at age 79. *J Rheumatol* 13:527–534, 1986.

Geelhoed GW, Kelly TR: Pseudogout as a clue and complication in primary hyperparathyroidism. *Surgery* 106:1036–1042, 1989.

Horowitz MD, Abbey L, Sirota DK, et al: Intraarticular noninflammatory free urate suspension (urate milk) in 3 patients with painful joints. *J Rheumatol* 17:712–714, 1990.

Masuda I, Ishikawa K: Clinical features of pseudogout attack: A survey of 50 cases. *Clin Orthop Rel Res* 229:173–181, 1988.

Arthritis — Lyme Disease

Davidson RS: Orthopaedic complications of Lyme disease in children. *Biomed Pharmacother* 43:405–408, 1989.

Kahan A, Amor B, Menkes CJ: Lyme arthritis. *Biomed Pharmacother* 43:401–403, 1989.

Schoen RT, Aversa JM, Rahn DW, et al: Treatment of refractory chronic Lyme arthritis with arthroscopic synovectomy. *Arthritis Rheum* 34:1056–1060, 1991.

Snydman DR, Schenkein DP, Berardi VP, et al: *Borrelia burgdorferi* in joint fluid in chronic Lyme arthritis. *Ann Intern Med* 104:798–800, 1986.

Arthritis — Osteoarthritis

Burks RT: Arthroscopy and degenerative arthritis of the knee: A review of the literature. *Arthroscopy* 6:43–47, 1990.

Claessens AAMC, Schouten JSAG, van den Ouweland FA, et al: Do clinical findings associate with radiographic osteoarthritis of the knee? *Ann Rheum Dis* 49:771–774, 1990.

Kindynis P, Haller J, Kang HS, et al: Osteophytosis of the knee: Anatomic, radiologic, and pathologic investigation. *Radiology* 174:841–846, 1990.

Kozinn SC, Scott RD: Surgical treatment of unicompartmental degenerative arthritis of the knee. *Rheum Dis Clin North Am* 14:545–564, 1988.

Laskin RS: Rheumatologic and degenerative disorders of the knee, in Dee R, Mango E, Hurst LC (eds): *Principles of Orthopaedic Practice.* New York, McGraw-Hill, 1989, vol 2, pp 1371–1384.

Ostlere SJ, Seeger LL, Eckardt JJ: Subchondral cysts of the tibia secondary to osteoarthritis of the knee. *Skeletal Radiol* 19:287–289, 1990.

Smillie IS: Angular deformity: Aged, in Smillie IS (ed): *Diseases of the Knee Joint,* 2d ed. Edinburgh, Churchill Livingstone, 1980, pp 330–386.

Solomon L, Helfet AJ: Osteoarthritis, in Helfet AJ (ed): *Disorders of the Knee,* 2d ed. Philadelphia, Lippincott, 1980, pp 183–198.

Arthritis — Palindromic

Eliakim A, Neumann L, Horowitz J, et al: Palindromic rheumatism in Israel: A disease entity? A survey of 34 patients. *Clin Rheumatol* 8:507–511, 1989.

Arthritis — Protozoan

Lee MG, Rawlins SC, Didier M, et al: Infective arthritis due to *Blastocystis hominis. Ann Rheum Dis* 49:192–193, 1990.

Arthritis — Review

Brower AC: Appendicular arthropathy. *Orthop Clin North Am* 21:405–422, 1990.

Brown DG, Edwards NL, Greer JM, et al: Magnetic resonance imaging in patients with inflammatory arthritis of the knee. *Clin Rheumatol* 9:73–83, 1990.

Jenkinson ML, Bliss MR, Brain AT, et al: Peripheral arthritis in the elderly: A hospital study. *Ann Rheum Dis* 48:227–231, 1989.

Older J, Rollinson P, Pike C: Cytological assessment of knee effusions. *Arthroscopy* 4:174–178, 1988.

Arthritis — Rheumatoid

Björkengren AG, Geborek P, Rydholm U, et al: MR imaging of the knee in acute rheumatoid arthritis: Synovial uptake of gadolinium-DOTA. *AJR* 155:329–332, 1990.

Butler D, Tiliakos NA: Penicillamine-induced exacerbation of rheumatoid arthritis. *South Med J* 79:778–779, 1986.

Isacson J, Broström L-A, Allander E, et al: Radiological findings in the rheumatoid knee joint in a seventeen-year follow-up. *Scand J Rheumatol* 16:153–159, 1987.

Lambertus M, Thordarson D, Goetz MB: Fungal prosthetic arthritis: Presentation of two cases and review of the literature. *Rev Infect Dis* 10:1038–1042, 1988.

Ryczak M, Sands M, Brown RB, et al: Pneumococcal arthritis in a prosthetic knee: A case report and review of the literature. *Clin Orthop Rel Res* 224:224–227, 1987.

Schmerling RH, Parker JA, Johns WD, et al: Measurement of joint inflammation in rheumatoid arthritis with indium-111 chloride. *Ann Rheum Dis* 49:88–92, 1990.

Solomon L: The rheumatoid knee, in Helfet AJ (ed): *Disorders of the Knee,* 2d ed. Philadelphia, Lippincott, 1980, pp 283–292.

Taillan B, Leyge JF, Fuzibet JG, et al: Knee arthritis revealing acute leukemia in a patient with rheumatoid arthritis. *Clin Rheumatol* 10:76–77, 1991.

Walters MT, Stevenson FK, Goswami R, et al: Comparison of serum and synovial fluid concentrations of β_2-microglobulin and C reactive protein in relation to clinical disease activity and synovial inflammation in rheumatoid arthritis. *Ann Rheum Dis* 48:905–911, 1989.

Arthritis — Septic — Iatrogenic

Bernhang AM: *Clostridium* pyoarthrosis following arthroscopy. *Arthroscopy* 3:56–58, 1987.

D'Angelo GL, Ogilvie-Harris DJ: Septic arthritis following arthroscopy, with cost/benefit analysis of antibiotic prophylaxis. *Arthroscopy* 4:10–14, 1988.

Montgomery SC, Campbell J: Septic arthritis following arthroscopy and intraarticular steroids. *J Bone Joint Surg* 71-B:540, 1989.

Arthritis — Septic

Albornoz MA, Myers AR: Recurrent septic arthritis and Milroy's disease. *J Rheumatol* 15:1726–1728, 1988.

Andersson S, Krook A: Primary meningococcal arthritis. *Scand J Infect Dis* 19:51–54, 1987.

Balentine LT, Papasian CJ, Burdick C: Septic arthritis of the knee due to *Streptococcus anginosus. Diagn Microbiol Infect Dis* 12:189–191, 1989.

Borenstein DG, Simon GL: *Hemophilus influenzae* septic arthritis in adults: A report of four cases and a review of the literature. *Medicine* 65:191–201, 1986.

Broom MJ, Beebe RD: Emphysematous septic arthritis due to *Klebsiella pneumoniae. Clin Orthop Rel Res* 226:219–221, 1988.

Burdge DR, Reid GD, Reeve CE, et al: Septic arthritis due to dual infection with *Mycoplasma hominis* and *Ureaplasma urealyticum. J Rheumatol* 15:366–368, 1988.

Burkert T, Watanakunakorn C: Group G streptococcus septic arthritis and osteomyelitis: Report and literature review. *J Rheumatol* 18:904–907, 1991.

Carr DE, Frymoyer J: Septic arthritis: A case report. *Am J Sports Med* 15:517–518, 1987.

Chandrasekar PH, Narula AP: Bone and joint infections in intravenous drug abusers. *Rev Infect Dis* 8:904–911, 1986.

Christensen TH, Bliddal H, Westh H: Non-suppurative bacterial arthritis diagnosed by fine-needle aspiration biopsy. *Scand J Rheumatol* 18: 235–237, 1989.

Clarke HJ, Allum R: Anaerobic septic arthritis due to bacteroides: Brief report. *J Bone Joint Surg* 70-B:847–848, 1988.

Elliott TG, Burdge D, Reid GD: Factitious septic arthritis. *Arthritis Rheum* 32:352–354, 1989.

Fauser DJ, Zuckerman JD: Clostridial septic arthritis: Case report and review of the literature. *Arthritis Rheum* 31:295–298, 1988.

Finkelstein R, Raz R, Stein H, et al: Bone and joint infections due to *Pseudomonas aeruginosa:* Clinical aspects and treatment. *Isr J Med Sci* 25:123–126, 1989.

Flesher SA, Bottone EJ: *Eikenella corrodens* cellulitis and arthritis of the knee. *J Clin Microbiol* 27:2606–2608, 1989.

Graham MP, Barzaga RA, Cunha BA: Pneumococcal septic arthritis of the knee in a patient with multiple myeloma. *Heart Lung* 20:416–418, 1991.

Henderson RC, Rosenstein BD: Salmonella septic and aseptic arthritis in sickle-cell disease: A case report. *Clin Orthop Rel Res* 248:261–264, 1989.

Izraeli S, Flasterstein B, Shamir R, et al: *Branhamella catarrhalis* as a cause of suppurative arthritis. *Pediatr Infect Dis* J 8:256–257, 1989.

Lane JG, Falahee MH, Wojtys EM, et al: Pyarthrosis of the knee: Treatment considerations. *Clin Orthop Rel Res* 252:198–204, 1990.

Livneh A, Sewell KL, Barland P: Chronic gonococcal arthritis. *J Rheumatol* 16:245–246, 1989.

Massarotti EM, Dinerman H: Septic arthritis due to *Listeria monocytogenes:* Report and review of the literature. *J Rheumatol* 17:111–113, 1990.

Miller MI, Hoppmann RA, Pisko EJ: Multiple myeloma presenting with primary meningococcal arthritis. *Am J Med* 82:1257–1258, 1987.

Mitchell D, Duncan I, Brook A, et al: *Streptococcus faecalis* arthritis. *J Rheumatol* 16:138–139, 1989.

Morgan MG, Forbes KJ, Gillespie SG: Salmonella septic arthritis: A case report and review. *J Infect* 21:195–203, 1990.

Morley PK, Hull RG, Hall MA: Pneumococcal septic arthritis in rheumatoid arthritis. *Ann Rheum Dis* 46:482–484, 1987.

Newman ED, Davis DE, Harrington TM: Septic arthritis due to gram negative bacilli: Older patients with good outcome. *J Rheumatol* 15:659–662, 1988.

Rady M, Turner PG, Ross ERS: Group G streptococcal septic arthritis. *Br J Clin Pract* 44:287–289, 1990.

Samanta A, Turner A, Roy S, et al: Primary meningococcal arthritis associated with adult respiratory distress syndrome. *Ann Rheum Dis* 49:634–635, 1990.

Schonholtz GJ, Scott WO: *Moraxella* septic arthritis of the knee joint: A case report. *Arthroscopy* 2:96–97, 1986.

Smith MJ: Arthroscopic treatment of the septic knee. *Arthroscopy* 2:30–34, 1986.

Swischuk LE: Swelling of the knee. *Pediatr Emerg Care* 2:102–103, 1986.

Thiery JA: Arthroscopic drainage in septic arthritides of the knee: A multicenter study. *Arthroscopy* 5:65–69, 1989.

von Essen R, Kostiala AAI, Anttolainen I, et al: Arthritis caused by *Haemophilus paraphrophilus* and isolation of the organism by using an improved culture protocol. *J Clin Microbiol* 25:2447–2448, 1987.

Wilson J, Zaman AG, Simmons AV: Gonococcal arthritis complicated by acute pericarditis and pericardial effusion. *Br Heart J* 63:134–135, 1990.

Arthritis — Septic — Mimics

Deesomchok U, Tumrasvin T: Clinical pattern of females with crystal-induced arthritis: Gout and pseudogout. *J Med Assoc Thailand* 72:212–217, 1989.

Esposito PW, O'Malley D, Litaker D: Acute pseudogout mimicking septic arthritis following urologic manipulation. *Orthop Rev* 17:295–299, 1988.

Goupille P, Fouquet B, Favard L, et al: Two cases of plant thorn synovitis: Difficulties in diagnosis and treatment. *J Rheumatol* 17:252–254, 1990.

Heuijerjans W, Dandy DJ, Harris D: Arthroscopic excision of an intra-articular osteoid osteoma at the knee. *Arthroscopy* 2:215–216, 1986.

Kurosaka M, Ohno O, Hirohata K: Arthroscopic evaluation of synovitis in the knee joints. *Arthroscopy* 7:162–170, 1991.

Lindblad S, Wredmark T: Traumatic synovitis analysed by arthroscopy and immunohistopathology. *Br J Rheumatol* 29:422–425, 1990.

O'Connor CR, Reginato AJ, Delong WG Jr: Foreign body reactions simulating acute septic arthritis. *J Rheumatol* 15:1568–1571, 1988.

Scheib JS, Quinet RJ: Pellegrini-Stieda syndrome mimicking acute septic arthritis. *South Med J* 82:90–91, 1989.

Zoltan JS: Cactus thorn synovitis. *Arthroscopy* 7:244–245, 1991.

Arthritis — Septic — Review

Deesomchok U, Tumrasvin T: Clinical study of culture-proven cases of nongonococcal arthritis. *J Med Assoc Thailand* 73:615–623, 1990.

Joseph ME, Sublett KL, Katz AL: Septic arthritis in the geriatric population. *J Okla State Med Assoc* 82:622–625, 1989.

McCutchan HJ, Fisher RC: Synovial leukocytosis in infectious arthritis. *Clin Orthop Rel Res* 257:226–230, 1990.

Vincent GM, Amirault JD: Septic arthritis in the elderly. *Clin Orthop Rel Res* 251:241–245, 1990.

Arthritis — Still's Disease — Adult

Cabane J, Michon A, Ziza J-M, et al: Comparison of long-term evolution of adult onset and juvenile onset Still's disease, both followed up for more than 10 years. *Ann Rheum Dis* 49:283–285, 1990.

Arthritis — Tuberculous

Gimenez MH, Beltran JVT, Segui MIF, et al: Tuberculosis of the patella. *Pediatr Radiol* 17:328–329, 1987.

Linares LF, Valcarcel A, Del Castillo JM, et al: Tuberculous arthritis with multiple joint involvement (letter to editor). *J Rheumatol* 18:635–636, 1991.

Southwood TR, Hancock EJ, Petty RE, et al: Tuberculous rheumatism (Poncet's disease) in a child. *Arthritis Rheum* 31:1311–1313, 1988.

Valdazo J-P, Perez-Ruiz F, Albarracin A, et al: Tuberculous arthritis: Report of a case with multiple joint involvement and periarticular tuberculous abscesses. *J Rheumatol* 17:399–401, 1990.

Arthritis — Varicella

Gibson NF IV, Ogden WS: Varicella arthritis. *South Med J* 79:1028–1030, 1986.

Stabile A, Ranno O, Sopo SM, et al: Varicella arthritis: Report of a case. *Helv Paediatr Acta* 41:49–53, 1986.

Arthroscopy — Review

Christie WR, Sprague NF III, Kim L: Arthroscopic evaluation and treatment of the symptomatic previously operated knee. *Arthroscopy* 4:194–198, 1988.

Miller GK: Diagnostic and surgical arthroscopy. *Compr Ther* 16:25–28, 1990.

Minkoff J: The philosophy and application of arthroscopy in nonmeniscal problems of the knee. *Orthrop Clin North Am* 10:37–50, 1979.

Riddell RR: CO_2 arthroscopy of the knee. *Clin Orthop* 252:92–94, 1990.

Sherman OH, Fox JM, Snyder SJ, et al: Arthroscopy — "No-problem surgery": An analysis of complications in two thousand six hundred and forty cases. *J Bone Joint Surg* 68-A(2):256–265, 1986.

Injuries — Knee

Cohn SL, Sotta RP, Bergfeld JA: Fractures about the knee in sports. *Clin Sports Med* 9:121–139, 1990.

Dainer RD, Barrack RL, Buckley SL, et al: Arthroscopic treatment of acute patellar dislocations. *Arthroscopy* 4:267–271, 1988.

Harilainen A, Myllynen P, Antila H, et al: The significance of arthroscopy and examination under anaesthesia in the diagnosis of fresh injury haemarthrosis of the knee joint. *Injury* 19:21–24, 1988.

Hohl M, Larson RL, Jones DC: Fractures and dislocations of the knee, in Rockwood CA Jr, Green DP (eds): *Fractures in Adults,* 2d ed. Philadelphia, Lippincott, 1984, vol 2, pp 1429–1591.

Jensen DB, Johansen TP, Bjerg-Nielsen A, et al: Magnetic resonance imaging in the evaluation of sequelae after tibial plateau fractures. *Skeletal Radiol* 19:127–129, 1990.

Jones JR, Allum RL: Acute traumatic haemarthrosis of the knee: Expectant treatment or arthroscopy? *Ann R Col Surg Engl* 71:40–43, 1989.

Roberts JM: Operative treatment of fractures about the knee. *Orthop Clin North Am* 21:365–379, 1990.

Steiner ME, Grana WA: The young athlete's knee: Recent advances. *Clin Sports Med* 7:527–546, 1988.

Zairns B, Adams M: Knee injuries in sports. *N Engl J Med* 318:950–961, 1988.

Ligamentous Injuries—Cruciate, Anterior

Anderson AF, Lipscomb AB: Analysis of rehabilitation techniques after anterior cruciate reconstruction. *Am J Sports Med* 17:154–160, 1989.

Andersson C, Odensten M, Good L, et al: Surgical or non-surgical treatment of acute rupture of the anterior cruciate ligament: A randomized study with long-term follow-up. *J Bone Joint Surg* 71-A:965–974, 1989.

Buckley SL, Barrack RL, Alexander AH: The natural history of conservatively treated partial anterior cruciate ligament tears. *Am J Sports Med* 17:221–225, 1989.

Clancy WG Jr, Ray M, Zoltan DJ: Acute tears of the anterior cruciate ligament: Surgical versus conservative treatment. *J Bone Joint Surg* 70-A:1483–1488, 1988.

Fruensgaard S, Johannsen HV: Incomplete ruptures of the anterior cruciate ligament. *J Bone Joint Surg* 71-B:526–530, 1989.

Glashow JL, Friedman MJ: Diagnosis of knee ligament injuries: Magnetic resonance imaging, in Scott WN (ed): *Ligament and Extensor Mechanism Injuries of the Knee*. St. Louis, Mosby Yearbook, 1991, pp 121–134.

Glashow JL, Katz R, Schneider M, et al: Double-blind assessment of the value of magnetic resonance imaging in the diagnosis of anterior cruciate and meniscal lesions. *J Bone Joint Surg* 71-A:113–119, 1989.

Helfet AJ: Injuries of the capsular and cruciate ligaments, in Helfet AJ (ed): *Disorders of the Knee*, 2d ed. Philadelphia, Lippincott, 1980, pp 329–346.

Karzel RP Jr, Friedman MJ: Arthroscopic diagnosis and treatment of cruciate and collateral ligament injuries, in Scott WN (ed): *Arthroscopy of the Knee*. Philadelphia, Saunders, 1990, pp 131–154.

Lee JK, Yao L, Phelps CT, et al: Anterior cruciate ligament tears: MR imaging compared with arthroscopy and clinical tests. *Radiology* 166:861–864, 1988.

Pattee GA, Fox JM, Del Pizzo W, et al: Four- to ten-year follow-up of unreconstructed anterior cruciate ligament tears. *Am J Sports Med* 17:430–435, 1989.

Tria AJ Jr, Hosea TM: Diagnosis of knee ligament injuries: Clinical, in Scott WN (ed): *Ligament and Extensor Mechanism Injuries of the Knee*. St. Louis, Mosby-Year Book, 1991, pp 87–99.

Zarins B, Boyle J: Knee ligament injuries, in Nicholas JA, Hershman EB (eds): *The Lower Extremity and Spine in Sports Medicine*. St. Louis, Mosby, 1986, vol 2, pp 929–982.

Ligamentous Injuries, Cruciate, Posterior

Grover JS, Bassett LW, Gross ML, et al: Posterior cruciate ligament: MR imaging. *Radiology* 174:527–530, 1990.

Whipple TL, Ellis FD: Posterior cruciate ligament injuries. *Clin Sports Med* 10:515–527, 1991.

MRI—Knee

Adam G, Bohndorf K, Drobnitzky M, et al: MR imaging of the knee: Three-dimensional volume imaging combined with fast processing. *J Comput Assist Tomogr* 13:984–988, 1989.

Brunner MC, Flower SP, Evancho AM, et al: MRI of the athletic knee: Findings in asymptomatic professional basketball and collegiate football players. *Invest Radiol* 24:72–75, 1989.

Burk DL Jr, Mitchell DG, Rifkin MD, et al: Recent advances in magnetic resonance imaging of the knee. *Radiol Clin North Am* 28:379–393, 1990.

Herman LJ, Beltran J: Pitfalls in MR imaging of the knee. *Radiology* 167:775–781, 1988.

Jackson DW, Jennings LD, Maywood RM, et al: Magnetic resonance imaging of the knee. *Am J Sports Med* 16:29–38, 1988.

Mink JH, Deutsch AL: Magnetic resonance imaging of the knee. *Clin Orthop* 244:29–47, 1989.

Ng J, Baron M, Ng AC, et al: Traumatic knee injuries: The accuracy of MRI compared with arthroscopy. *Ind Med* 82:886–890, 1989.

Polly DW, Callaghan JJ, Sikes RA, et al: The accuracy of selective magnetic resonance imaging compared with the findings of arthroscopy of the knee. *J Bone Joint Surg* 70-A:192–198, 1988.

Stoller DW, Genant HK: Magnetic resonance imaging of the knee and hip. *Arthritis Rheum* 33:441–449, 1990.

Stull MA, Nelson MC: The role of MRI in diagnostic imaging of the injured knee. *Am Fam Physician* 41:489–500, 1990.

Tyrrell RL, Gluckert K, Pathria M, et al: Fast three-dimensional MR imaging of the knee: Comparison with arthroscopy. *Radiology* 166:865–872, 1988.

Vahey TN, Bennett HT, Arrington LE, et al: MR imaging of the knee: Pseudotear of the lateral meniscus caused by the meniscofemoral ligament. *AJR* 154:1237–1239, 1990.

Neoplastic Disorders

Malawer MM: Neoplasms affecting the lower extremity, in Dee R, Mango E, Hurst LC (eds): *Principles of Orthopaedic Practice*. New York, McGraw-Hill, 1989, vol 2, pp 1395–1419.

Smillie IS: Tumours and tumour-like conditions: Bone, in Smillie IS (ed): *Diseases of the Knee Joint,* 2d ed. Edinburgh, Churchill Livingstone, 1980, pp 463–502.

Osgood-Schlatter Disease

Krause BL, Williams JPR, Catterall A: Natural history of Osgood-Schlatter disease. *J Pediatr Orthop* 10:65–68, 1990.

Osteochondritis Dissecans

Vince KG: Osteochondritis dissecans of the knee, in Scott WN (ed): *Arthroscopy of the Knee*. Philadelphia, Saunders, 1990, pp 175–191.

Pain—Knee—Anterior

Bentley G: Anterior knee pain: Diagnosis and management. *J R Coll Surg Edinburgh* 34(suppl):52–53, 1989.

Bodne D, Quinn SF, Murray WT, et al: Magnetic resonance images of chronic patellar tendinitis. *Skeletal Radiol* 17:24–28, 1988.

Bourne MH, Hazel WA Jr, Scott SG, et al: Anterior knee pain. *Mayo Clin Proc* 63:482–491, 1988.

Busch MT, DeHaven KE: Pitfalls of the lateral retinacular release. *Clin Sports Med* 8:279–290, 1989.

Finsterbush A, Frankl U, Mann G: Fat pad adhesion to partially torn anterior cruciate ligament: A cause of knee locking. *Am J Sports Med* 17:92–95, 1989.

Fulkerson JP: Evaluation of the peripatellar soft tissues and retinaculum in patients with patellofemoral pain. *Clin Sports Med* 8:197–202, 1989.

Garrett JC: Osteochondritis dissecans. *Clin Sports Med* 10:569–593, 1991.

Helfet AJ: The "dashboard knee," in Helfet AJ (ed): *Disorders of the Knee,* ed. Philadelphia, Lippincott, 1980, pp 403–407.

Helfet AJ, Brookes Heywood AW: Dislocations of the patella, in Helfet AJ (ed): *Disorders of the Knee,* 2d ed. Philadelphia, Lippincott, 1980, pp 347–362.

Hughston JC: Patellar subluxation. *Clin Sports Med* 8:153–162, 1989.

Jackson RW: The patellofemoral joint, in Parisien JS (ed): *Arthroscopic Surgery*. New York, McGraw-Hill, 1988, pp 79–84.

Jacobson KE, Flandry FC: Diagnosis of anterior knee pain. *Clin Sports Med* 8:179–195, 1989.

Jørgensen U, Sonne-Holm S, Lauridsen F, et al: Long-term follow-up of meniscectomy in athletes: A prospective longitudinal study. *J Bone Joint Surg* 69-B:80–83, 1987.

Lombardo SJ, Bradley JP: Arthroscopic diagnosis and treatment of patellofemoral disorders, in Scott WN (ed): *Arthroscopy of the Knee*. Philadelphia, Saunders, 1990, pp 155–173.

Malek MM, Fanelli GC: Patellofemoral pain: An arthroscopic perspective. *Clin Sports Med* 10:549–567, 1991.

Merchant AC: Extensor mechanism injuries: Classification and diagnosis, in Scott WN (ed): *Ligament and Extensor Mechanism Injuries of the Knee*. St. Louis, Mosby-Year Book, 1991, pp 173–182.

Minkoff J, Fein L: The role of radiography in the evaluation and treatment of common anarthrotic disorders of the patellofemoral joint. *Clin Sports Med* 8:203–260, 1989.

Osgood JC, Kneisel JS, Barrack RL, et al: Arthroscopy in patients with recalcitrant retropatellar pain syndrome. *Orthop Rev* 18:1177–1183, 1989.

Schmidt DR, Henry JH: Stress injuries of the adolescent extensor mechanism. *Clin Sports Med* 8:343–355, 1989.

Pain—Knee—Lateral

Mayfield GW: Popliteus tendon tenosynovitis. *Am J Sports Med* 5:31–36, 1977.

Naver L, Aalberg JR: Avulsion of the popliteus tendon: A rare cause of chrondral fracture and hemarthrosis. *Am J Sports Med* 13:423–424, 1985.

Rettig A: Medial and lateral ligament injuries, in Scott WN (ed): *Ligament and Extensor Mechanism Injuries of the Knee.* St. Louis, Mosby-Year Book, 1991, pp 211–225.

Rose DJ, Parisien JS: Popliteus tendon rupture: Case report and review of the literature. *Clin Orthop* 226:113–117, 1988.

Pain—Knee—Medial

Busch MT: Meniscal injuries in children and adolescents. *Clin Sports Med* 9:661–680, 1990.

Clevers GJ, De Vries LS, Haarman HJTM: Diagnostic arthroscopy of the knee joint: Comparison of the accuracy of physical examination, contrast arthrography and arthroscopy. *Neth J Surg* 40:104–107, 1988.

Cooper DE, Arnoczky SP, Warren RF: Meniscal repair. *Clin Sports Med* 10:529–548, 1991.

Crues JV III, Ryu R, Morgan FW: Meniscal pathology: The expanding role of magnetic resonance imaging. *Clin Orthop* 252:80–87, 1990.

Dzioba RB: The classification and treatment of acute articular cartilage lesions. *Arthroscopy* 4:72–80, 1988.

Helfet AJ: Clinical features of injuries to the semilunar cartilages, in Helfet AJ (ed): *Disorders of the Knee,* 2d ed. Philadelphia, Lippincott, 1982, pp 109–122.

———: Differential diagnosis of tears of the semilunar cartilages, in Helfet AJ (ed): *Disorders of the Knee,* 2d ed. Philadelphia, Lippincott, 1982, pp 123–135.

Kerlan RK, Glousman RE: Tibial collateral ligament bursitis. *Am J Sports Med* 16:344–346, 1988.

Lantz B, Singer KM: Meniscal cysts. *Clin Sports Med* 9:707–723, 1990.

McGlade CT: Magnetic resonance imaging of the meniscus. *Clin Sports Med* 9:551–559, 1990.

Metcalf RW: The torn medial meniscus, in Parisien JS (ed): *Arthroscopic Surgery.* New York, McGraw-Hill, 1988, pp 93–110.

Parisien JS: Medial shelf syndrome, osteonecrosis of the knee, and tibial plateau fractures, in Parisien JS (ed): *Arthroscopic Surgery.* New York, McGraw-Hill, 1988, pp 85–92.

Pianka G, Combs J: Arthroscopic diagnosis and treatment of symptomatic plicae, in Scott WN (ed): *Arthroscopy of the Knee.* Philadelphia, Saunders, 1990, pp 83–95.

Poehling GG, Roch DS, Chabon SJ: The landscape of meniscal injuries. *Clin Sports Med* 9:539–549, 1990.

Ray JM, Clancy WG Jr, Lemon RA: Semimembranosus tendinitis: An overlooked cause of medial knee pain. *Am J Sports Med* 16:347–351, 1988.

Reikerås O: Arthroscopic resection of meniscal flaps of the knee. *Acta Orthop Scand* 60:28–29, 1989.

Van Heuzen EP, Golding RP, Van Zanten TEG, et al: Magnetic resonance imaging of meniscal lesions of the knee. *Clin Radiol* 39:658–660, 1988.

Woods GW, Whelan JM: Discoid meniscus. *Clin Sports Med* 9:695–706, 1990.

Pain—Knee—Posterior

Kimori K, Suzu F, Yamashita F, et al: Evaluation of arthrography and arthroscopy for lesions of the posteromedial corner of the knee. *Am J Sports Med* 17:638–643, 1989.

Mannino M, Marino C, Chawla K: Ruptured pyogenic Baker's cyst. *J Natl Med Assoc* 80:1018–1019, 1022, 1988.

Pain—Knee—Review

Boland AL Jr: Soft tissue injuries of the knee, in Nicholas JA, Hershman EB, (eds): *The Lower Extremity and Spine in Sports Medicine.* St. Louis, Mosby, 1986, vol 2, pp 983–1012.

Cherney S: Disorders of the knee, in Dee R, Mango E, Hurst LC

(eds): *Principles of Orthopaedic Practice.* New York, McGraw-Hill, 1989, vol 2, pp 1283–1330.

Cicuttini F, Littlejohn GO: Female adolescent rheumatological presentations: The importance of chronic pain syndromes. *Aust Paediatr J* 25:21–24, 1989.

Helfet AJ: Common derangements of the knee joint and their manner of production, in Helfet AJ (ed): *Disorders of the Knee,* 2d ed. Philadelphia, Lippincott, 1982, pp 85–108.

Henning CE, Lynch MA, Glick KR Jr: Physical examination of the knee, in Nicholas JA, Hershman EB (eds): *The Lower Extremity and Spine in Sports Medicine.* St. Louis, Mosby, 1986, vol 2, pp 765–800.

Kalund DN: Knee injuries in noncontact sports, in Helfet AJ (ed): *Disorders of the Knee,* 2d ed. Philadelphia, Lippincott, 1980, pp 363–390.

Nicholas JA, Scott WN: Major knee injuries in contact sports, in Helfet AJ (ed): *Disorders of the Knee,* 2d ed. Philadelphia, Lippincott, 1980, pp 391–402.

Rand JA: Arthroscopic diagnosis and management of articular cartilage pathology, in Scott WN (ed): *Arthroscopy of the Knee.* Philadelphia, Saunders, 1990, pp 113–130.

Smillie IS: Affectations of the synovial membrane: General, in Smillie IS (ed): *Diseases of the Knee Joint,* 2d ed. Edinburgh, Churchill Livingstone, 1980, pp 108–145.

———: Affectations of the synovial membrane: Local, in Smillie IS (ed): *Diseases of the Knee Joint,* 2d ed. Edinburgh, Churchill Livingstone, 1980, pp 146–171.

———: Problems of diagnosis in women, in Smillie IS (ed): *Diseases of the Knee Joint,* 2d ed. Edinburgh, Churchill Livingstone, 1980, pp 430–448.

Vigorita VJ: Synovial disorders, in Scott WN (ed): *Arthroscopy of the Knee.* Philadelphia, Saunders, 1990, pp 97–112.

Reflex Sympathetic Dystrophy

Cooper DE, DeLee JC, Ramamurthy S: Reflex sympathetic dystrophy of the knee: Treatment using continuous epidural anesthesia. *J Bone Joint Surg* 71-A:365–369, 1989.

Demangeat J-L, Constantinesco A, Brunot B, et al: Three phase bone scanning in reflex sympathetic dystrophy of the hand. *J Nucl Med* 29:26–32, 1988.

Katz MM, Hungerford DS: Reflex sympathetic dystrophy affecting the knee. *J Bone Joint Surg* 69-B:797–803, 1987.

Ogilvie-Harris DJ, Roscoe M: Reflex sympathetic dystrophy of the knee. *J Bone Joint Surg* 69-B:804–806, 1987.

Poehling GG, Pollock FE Jr, Koman LA: Reflex sympathetic dystrophy of the knee after sensory nerve injury. *Arthroscopy* 4:31–35, 1988.

Tietjen R: Reflex sympathetic dystrophy of the knee. *Clin Orthop Rel Res* 209:234–243, 1986.

Synovitis—Villonodular

Combe B, Krause E, Sany J: Treatment of chronic knee synovitis with arthroscopic synovectomy after failure of intraarticular injection of radionuclide. *Arthritis Rheum* 32:10–14, 1989.

Franssen MJAM, Boerbooms AMT, Karthaus RP, et al: Treatment of pigmented villonodular synovitis of the knee with yttrium-90 silicate: Prospective evaluations by arthroscopy, histology, and ^{99m}Tc pertechnetate uptake measurements. *Ann Rheum Dis* 48:1007–1013, 1989.

Goldman AB, DiCarlo EF: Pigmented villonodular synovitis: Diagnosis and differential diagnosis. *Radiol Clin North Am* 26:1327–1347, 1988.

Mandelbaum BR, Grant TT, Hartzman S, et al: The use of MRI to assist in diagnosis of pigmented villonodular synovitis of the knee joint. *Clin Orthop* 231:135–139, 1988.

Robinson DL, Blair DW, Lee SS, et al: Pigmented villonodular synovitis presenting as a large lateral knee mass: Case report and review of the literature. *Orthop Rev* 17:59–63, 1988.

Steinbach LS, Neumann CH, Stoller DW, et al: MRI of the knee in diffuse pigmented villonodular synovitis. *Clin Imag* 13:305–316, 1989.

CHAPTER 46

Acute Lower Leg and Ankle Pain

☐ DIAGNOSTIC LIST

GENERALIZED LOWER LEG PAIN

1. Fractures of the tibial shaft and/or fibula
   A. Traumatic
   B. Pathologic
2. Acute occlusion of the superficial femoral or popliteal artery
3. Acute infections of the lower leg
   A. Erysipelas
   B. Bacterial cellulitis
   C. Necrotizing fasciitis
   D. Gas gangrene (clostridial myonecrosis)
   E. Nonclostridial myositis
      1. Anaerobic streptococcal myonecrosis
      2. Synergistic necrotizing cellulitis
      3. Infected vascular gangrene
      4. *Aeromonas hydrophila* myonecrosis
   F. Clostridial anaerobic cellulitis
   G. Nonclostridial anaerobic cellulitis
   H. *Vibrio vulnificus* cellulitis
4. Sickle cell pain crisis
5. Delayed muscle soreness due to exercise

CALF PAIN

6. Deep vein thrombosis
   A. Effort-induced thrombosis
   B. Spontaneous thrombosis
7. Mimics of calf vein thrombosis
   A. Complications of a Baker's cyst
   B. Pyomyositis
   C. Hematoma of the calf
   D. Acute rhabdomyolysis
   E. Pseudo-pseudothrombophlebitis
   F. Rupture of the Achilles tendon
   G. Gastrocnemius muscle strain
   H. Soleus muscle strain
   I. Acute posterior compartment syndrome
8. Calf muscle cramps
   A. Benign
   B. Symptomatic of an underlying disorder

ANTEROLATERAL LOWER LEG PAIN

9. Anterior tibial vein thrombosis
10. Anterior compartment syndrome
11. Lateral compartment syndrome
12. Compression of the superficial peroneal nerve
13. Pyomyositis
14. Muscle strain and/or hematoma in the anterior compartment
15. Fracture of the shaft of the fibula
16. Maisonneuve fracture of the fibula

633

ANTEROMEDIAL LOWER LEG
PAIN

17. Stress fracture of the tibia
18. Stress microfractures of the tibia
19. Medial tibial stress syndrome
    (periostalgia)
20. Soleus syndrome
21. Anterolateral tibial margin pain
22. Distal, deep posterior
    compartment syndrome
23. Shin splints related to systemic
    disease
    A. Syphilis
    B. Paget's disease
24. Greater saphenous vein
    thrombophlebitis
25. Saphenous neuritis
26. Osteomyelitis of the tibia

DERMATOLOGIC DISORDERS OF
THE LOWER LEG

27. Nodular panniculitis
28. Erythema nodosum
29. Arterial and hypertensive ulcers
30. Systemic vasculitis with
    ulceration
31. Erythema induratum

GENERALIZED ANKLE PAIN

32. Acute injuries of the ankle
    A. Supination-adduction
    B. Supination-external rotation
       (eversion)
    C. Pronation-abduction
    D. Pronation-external rotation
       (eversion)
    E. Pronation-dorsiflexion
    F. Anterior dislocation
    G. Posterior dislocation
    H. Fracture of the neck of the
       talus
    I. Fracture of the body of the
       talus
33. Acute monarthritis of the ankle
    A. Septic arthritis
    B. Acute gout
    C. Acute pseudogout
    D. Acute rheumatoid arthritis
    E. Reflex sympathetic dystrophy
    F. Hemophilic arthropathy
    G. Acute hemarthrosis
34. Transient migratory osteoporosis
35. Osteochondritis dissecans of the
    talus
36. Ankle arthritis associated with
    acute polyarthritis
    A. Polyarticular septic arthritis
    B. Acute rheumatic fever

C. Lyme arthritis
D. Hepatitis B virus-associated
   arthritis
E. Rubella and rubella vaccine-
   associated arthritis
F. Arthritis associated with
   inflammatory bowel disease
G. Acute polyarticular gout
H. Calcium pyrophosphate
   deposition disease
I. Reiter's syndrome
J. Acute rheumatoid arthritis

37. Acute osteomyelitis

LATERAL ANKLE PAIN

38. Lateral collateral ligament injuries
    (anterior talofibular,
    calcaneofibular, and posterior
    talofibular ligaments)
39. Mimics of anterior talofibular
    ligament sprain
    A. Anterior tibiofibular ligament
       sprain
    B. Fracture of the lateral
       malleolus
    C. Fracture of the lateral process
       of the talus
    D. Fracture of the lateral tubercle
       of the posterior process of the
       talus
    E. Peroneal tendinitis
    F. Traumatic dislocation of the
       peroneal tendons
    G. Ganglion
    H. Stress fracture of the fibula
    I. Calcaneofibular ligament
       sprain (isolated)

ANTERIOR ANKLE PAIN

40. Peritendinitis of the extensor
    tendons of the foot and toes
41. Cruciate crural ligament
    (retinaculum) sprain
42. Sprain or rupture of the anterior
    tibiofibular ligament
43. Fracture of the anterior lip of the
    distal tibial articular surface

MEDIAL ANKLE PAIN

44. Deltoid ligament sprain
45. Fracture of the medial malleolus
46. Tibialis posterior tendinitis
47. Shin splints (stress fracture,
    periostitis, and musculotendinous
    pain)
48. Fracture of the sustentaculum tali
49. Tendinitis of the flexor hallucis
    longus and flexor digitorum
    communis

☐ SUMMARY

Generalized Lower Leg Pain

Tibial shaft fractures occur in motor vehicle accidents, falls from a height, and athletic competition. Pain, swelling, tenderness, bony crepitus, and deformity follow the injury. Open fractures may occur, resulting in bone protrusion or a contaminated open wound without visible bone. The diagnosis of fracture can be confirmed by a plain radiograph. The *fibula may be fractured* alone by a direct blow, but more often it is fractured by the same force that injures the tibia.

A *pathologic fracture* occurs on weight bearing or with a torsional force on the lower extremity. No trauma is involved. The patient feels a snap, sharp pain, and giving way of the limb, but a fall may not occur. Causes include lytic, cystic, or metabolic disorders of the tibia.

Acute occlusion of the superficial femoral or popliteal artery causes severe lower leg pain, muscle paresis, paresthesias, pallor or blanching of the skin, and loss of distal pulses. Causes include arterial compression or interruption due to trauma, an embolus, or thrombosis. Symptoms are reversed by removal of the obstructing arterial lesion or a bypass procedure leading to restoration of flow within 6 to 8 h.

Infections of the lower extremity may involve the upper dermis (erysipelas); the entire dermis and subcutaneous region (cellulitis); the skin and the deep fascia (necrotizing fasciitis); or the skin, subcutaneous fat, fascia, and muscle (myonecrosis).

Erysipelas causes an elevated, painful, fiery red, spreading plaque with a clearly demarcated border. The lesion is tender and may have a *peau d'orange* surface appearance. It is caused by a group A streptococcus and resolves with penicillin therapy. *Bacterial cellulitis* (streptococcal and staphylococcal species) causes burning and aching lower leg pain, redness, and tenderness. The erythematous region is tender and warm and has an irregular, advancing margin. The margin is not usually elevated, as it is in erysipelas. Centrally located small bullae, abscesses, or necrotic ulcers may appear. There is a prompt response to parenteral antibiotic therapy. *Necrotizing fasciitis* of the lower leg begins with shiny skin edema, erythema, warmth, severe local pain, and tenderness. The involved area has a poorly defined, irregular border. Systemic symptoms are severe and may lead to an alteration of mental status. Areas of skin become blue-gray or purplish, and hemorrhagic bullae soon appear. Skin hypesthesia or anesthesia in the affected area occurs and may antedate the development of gangrene. Skin gangrene soon develops, and necrotic skin may slough or require debridement. The underlying subcutaneous fat and fascia are necrotic and have a foul odor. This disorder may be caused by a synergistic infection involving obligate anaerobes and facultative anaerobes; or a group A streptococcal infection alone or in association with *Staphylococcus aureus*.

Gas gangrene (clostridial myonecrosis) follows a deep contaminated wound. Symptoms begin 1 to 3 days after the injury. Severe local wound pain is the initial complaint. Marked systemic symptoms and signs occur. The wound becomes markedly swollen and tender, and a malodorous, serosanguineous, dirty-appearing discharge appears. Skin crepitus due to subcutaneous gas may be present. The skin surrounding the wound soon becomes yellow or bronze in color; hemorrhagic bullae appear, as do patches of green-black skin gangrene. The leg may become diffusely edematous, and areas of skin black and anesthetic. The limb is extremely painful, but the pain may be overshadowed by the acute toxic delirium produced by the infection. *Clostridium perfringens* or other clostridial species are usually etiologic. These organisms can be isolated from bullae, wound drainage, or debrided tissue. Gram's stains of wound exudate may identify many large gram-positive rods. Wound exploration reveals evidence of myonecrosis.

Nonclostridial myonecrosis caused by anaerobic streptococci begins 3 to 4 days after a penetrating wound. This disorder begins with skin redness and swelling around the wound and a sour-smelling, copious, seropurulent discharge. Pain is initially absent, develops after 3 to 4 days, and gradually becomes more intense and generalized. This infection is caused by an anaerobic streptococcus and a group A streptococcus or a strain of *S. aureus*.

Synergistic necrotizing cellulitis begins with small, painful ulcers that drain foul-smelling, "dishwater" pus. Skin necrosis occurs adjacent to the ulcers. Severe leg pain and tenderness and severe toxemia occur. This disease is a synergistic infection that eventually causes necrosis of skin, fat, fascia, and muscle. The components of this mixed infection are usually anaerobic bacteria and facultative bacteria (Enterobacteriaceae). *Vascular gangrene may become secondarily infected* by a combination of anaerobic and aerobic bacteria. Tissue crepitus and foul-smelling drainage are prominent findings. Muscle necrosis is restricted to the region of ischemic gangrene. *Aeromonas hydrophila myonecrosis* follows wounding in a freshwater environment or in association with freshwater animals. This disorder mimics gas gangrene. It can be differentiated by the history of wounding in a freshwater environment and culture of the wound exudate. Extensive surgical debridement and antibiotic therapy are required.

Clostridial anaerobic cellulitis causes a wound infection with minimal systemic symptoms and signs; extensive gas production in the skin; and a thin, dark, sometimes malodorous wound drainage. Pain is mild, skin erythema minimal, and skin edema moderate. Surgical exploration excludes myonecrosis. Gram's stain and cultures identify a clostridial species. *Nonclostridial anaerobic cellulitis* causes a similar illness but can be differentiated by Gram's stain and culture of wound exudate and tissue. It is caused by anaerobic bacteria alone. *Vibrio vulnificus infection* follows wounding or wound contamination sustained in a saltwater environment. An extensive cellulitis involves the lower leg. Hemorrhagic skin bullae, necrotic ulcers, and skin gangrene may occur. Systemic toxicity may be severe. Debridement and doxycycline therapy lead to resolution.

Sickle cell anemia may cause unilateral or bilateral pain from the knee to the ankle or foot. This pain is deep, throbbing, or sharp and is associated with skin allodynia and hyperesthesia. Fever, knee effusions, and skin edema may accompany the pain and allodynia. Symptoms remit spontaneously in 3 to 14 days. A single episode or recurrent attacks involving the lower legs may occur. It is believed that the pain is due to a reversible sensory polyneuropathy and to ischemic bone marrow infarction. *Unaccustomed exercise* can cause generalized leg pain and tenderness that begins 24 to 48 h later. The pain is present at rest or only with muscle use. It resolves spontaneously over a period of 1 to 5 days.

Calf Pain

Effort-related calf vein thrombosis presents with the sudden onset of sharp calf pain during running. Swelling and tenderness of the painful area develop within hours. The pain is intensified by dependency and relieved by elevation. Contrast venography will establish the diagnosis.

Spontaneous venous thrombosis usually occurs in a patient with one or more risk factors for venous occlusion. These factors include recent surgery, pregnancy, leg injury, malignancy, leg immobilization, a hypercoagulable state, venous inflammation, obesity, and prior venous thromboses. Calf pain, edema, tenderness, and warmth are common symptoms but may be absent in a large percentage of patients with calf vein thrombosis proven by contrast venography. Calf pain associated with venous thrombosis is usually intensified by standing or walking and relieved by rest and elevation. Pain onset may be abrupt or gradual. Calf and popliteal fossa pain may be constant or may occur only with standing, walking, or other leg movements. Fever, myalgias, malaise, and leukocytosis may occur in some cases. Calf vein thrombosis may be imaged by color duplex flow imaging (CDFI; sensitivity, 48 percent)

or by contrast venography. Serial repetition of impedance plethysmography or CDFI studies will identify infrapopliteal thrombi that propagate to the femoropopliteal veins.

Calf pain, tenderness, swelling, redness, and warmth may result from *disorders that mimic deep venous thrombosis* of the calf and popliteal veins (pseudothrombophlebitis). An *enlarging, dissecting, or ruptured Baker's cyst* or a cyst that compresses the popliteal vein may cause calf symptoms that cannot be differentiated from thrombophlebitis without additional studies. Color duplex flow imaging can exclude thigh and some calf vein thrombi and identify a Baker's cyst. Arthrography or MRI can image an existing cyst and demonstrate leakage. Since sonographic studies may miss up to 30 percent of Baker's cysts, arthrography or MRI should be utilized to exclude this diagnosis in patients without risk factors for venous occlusive disease who have negative ultrasonographic study results for a Baker's cyst and negative venographic study results for calf and thigh vein thrombi.

Pyomyositis causes calf pain, swelling, and doughy calf induration or a fluctuant mass accompanied by fever, chills, sweats, and prostration. The diagnosis can be confirmed by ultrasonography or a CT scan. Aspiration reveals pus and gram-positive cocci (*S. aureus*).

A *hematoma of the calf* may result from direct trauma, a tear in the gastrocnemius or soleus muscles, or a fracture of the tibia. A CT scan or MRI will image the hematoma as a crescent-shaped mass lesion. A secondary posterior compartment syndrome may result from the presence of the hematoma. *Acute rhabdomyolysis* may rarely mimic an acute calf vein thrombophlebitis. Pain, tenderness, and swelling of the calf are associated with an elevated serum creatine kinase level and myoglobinuria. A markedly enlarged Baker's cyst may compress the popliteal vein, producing thrombosis, or bed rest required because of painful rupture of a Baker's cyst may result in calf vein thrombosis (*pseudo-pseudothrombophlebitis*).

Rupture of the Achilles tendon causes the sudden onset of sharp posterior calf pain and an audible pop, followed by paresis of plantar flexion. Walking on tiptoes reveals a heel drop, and results of the Thompson test are positive. A tender defect in the tendon is often palpable. "Tennis leg" refers to a *strain (tear) of the gastrocnemius or soleus muscle*. Passive dorsiflexion (stretching) of the foot or resisted plantar flexion intensifies the calf pain of "tennis leg." Pain, tenderness, swelling, warmth, and ecchymoses may be present over the medial calf, and a defect in the gastrocnemius muscle may sometimes be palpable. Pseudothrombophlebitis may also be caused by a soleus muscle tear. A hematoma in this muscle secondary to disruption of vessels may be imaged by MRI or a CT scan.

An *acute posterior compartment syndrome* may arise from a tibial shaft fracture, a muscle tear with posterior compartment bleeding, or excessive leg exercise by a usually sedentary person. Within minutes to hours after the injury, pain becomes constant and severe. Any leg movement increases the intensity of the pain. Paresthesias and hypesthesia of the feet may occur. The calf muscles are exquisitely tender and hard, and passive stretching of the muscles of the superficial posterior compartment (foot dorsiflexion) intensifies the pain. Similarly, stretching of the deep posterior compartment muscles by passive extension of the toes will provoke pain or intensify it if the pressure in the deep compartment is elevated. Paresis of plantar flexion (superficial compartment) or toe flexion (deep compartment) may be observed. Pulses may remain palpable even after myonecrosis has occurred. Decompression of the involved compartment after early confirmation of the diagnosis by intracompartmental pressure measurement relieves the pain and neurologic symptoms.

Calf muscle cramps occurring after effort, during pregnancy, or at night in elderly persons are usually benign and do not require further investigation. Cramps may also be secondary to a peripheral neuropathy, root or plexus lesion, hypocalcemia, hypomagnesemia, hyponatremia, or myositis. An increased frequency of cramps may also occur with lower motor neuron disease, cirrhosis, severe diarrheal disorders, renal salt wasting, alcohol abuse, tetanus, and sarcoidosis. Cramps have also been associated with hemodialysis and diuretic and phenothiazine therapy.

Anterolateral Lower Leg Pain

Anterolateral lower leg pain, swelling, and tenderness associated in some cases with skin redness and warmth may be secondary to *anterior tibial vein thrombosis*. This diagnosis can be confirmed in some cases by CDFI or contrast venography. Most patients with anterior tibial vein thrombosis also have femoropopliteal thrombi, easily detectable by CDFI.

An *acute anterior compartment syndrome* may complicate a tibial fracture or an anterior compartment muscle tear with bleeding. Excruciating, constant pain develops within minutes or hours after the injury. Swelling, exquisite tenderness, and increased tension (hardness) are present on palpation of the anterolateral compartment. Passive toe flexion and plantar flexion of the foot intensify the pain. Hypesthesia of the dorsum of the foot near the first web space may be present. Paresis of toe extension and foot dorsiflexion may be present. The diagnosis can be confirmed by measuring the intracompartmental pressure, and symptoms can be relieved by compartmental decompression.

An *acute lateral compartment syndrome* is rare. It may follow a contusion or tear of the peroneal muscles. Foot eversion may be paretic, and passive foot inversion intensifies the lateral calf pain. The lateral compartment may be swollen, tense, and tender. *Superficial peroneal nerve compression* may cause anterolateral lower leg pain with exercise or with certain rest positions of the lower leg and foot. Hypesthesia and paresthesia occur intermittently or persistently on the dorsum of the foot. Tinel's sign may be present over the nerve proximally, and lateral leg pain may be provoked when the ankle is passively flexed and supinated. Up to 50 percent of patients with this disorder have abnormal nerve conduction velocity of the superficial peroneal nerve. *Pyomyositis* may cause anterolateral

leg pain, swelling, tenderness, warmth, skin erythema, and fever. Sonographic studies or a CT scan will confirm the presence of an abscess. An *anterior compartment muscle strain and/or hematoma* causes local pain, swelling, and tenderness. Passive plantar flexion of the foot and dorsiflexion against resistance intensify the pain. If a hematoma is present, a CT scan or MRI will demonstrate its presence as a crescent-shaped mass. A *fibular shaft fracture* results from direct impact. It is associated with lateral leg pain, local tenderness, swelling, ecchymosis, and sometimes bony crepitus. A *Maisonneuve fracture of the proximal third of the fibula* causes anterolateral calf pain, tenderness, and crepitus associated with a distal tibiofibular diastasis and a severe ankle injury.

Anteromedial Lower Leg Pain

Anteromedial lower leg pain may begin after running or other exercise. It is intensified or provoked by exercise and relieved partially or completely by rest. The causes of such pain include stress fractures, periosteal inflammation, a reversible compartment syndrome or musculotendinous dysfunction of the muscles attached to the tibia. *Stress fracture of the tibia* occurs as a localized area of posteromedial tibial margin tenderness in the distal or middle third of the bone. A radionuclide scan shows increased uptake in a localized fusiform or round configuration. Results of plain radiographs may be negative or demonstrate an oblique or transverse fracture line. Similar pain and tenderness extending in a band along the margin of the tibia for 8 cm or more is usually caused by *stress microfractures of the tibia*. Bone tenderness corresponds to the linear band of increased radionuclide uptake seen on the scintigram. Results of plain radiographs are usually negative. The *medial tibial stress syndrome (periostalgia)* is associated with tenderness over the adjacent muscle at the tibial margin. Results of the radionuclide scan and plain radiographs are negative. Some patients may have *musculotendinous dysfunction* or a reversible *compartment syndrome*.

The *soleus syndrome* is associated with posteromedial tibial margin pain and tenderness that are provoked by running or jogging and relieved by rest. The radionuclide scan demonstrates evidence of periostitis. Plain radiographs seldom appear abnormal. Similar pain and tenderness may occur along the anterolateral tibial margin, due to a similar periosteal reaction. Longitudinal band tenderness along the tibial margin is associated with increased radionuclide uptake over the tender region.

A *distal, deep posterior compartment syndrome* may cause recurrent episodes of deep, distal calf pain and tenderness (without bone tenderness) that is provoked by running or jogging and relieved by rest. The pain may be acute and may persist if the cause is a tibial fracture, a muscle tear with a posterior compartment hematoma, or a large amount of unaccustomed leg exercise by an untrained person. Rarely, anteromedial pain may be secondary to *syphilis* (periostitis) or *Paget's disease of the tibia*.

A *greater saphenous thrombophlebitis* causes local medial lower leg ache and a tender "cord." *Saphenous neuritis* causes burning or aching anteromedial lower leg pain associated with hypesthesia and paresthesias. *Osteomyelitis of the tibia* causes fever, local bone pain, tenderness, and sometimes a draining sinus. A bone scan and plain radiographs or MRI will demonstrate the osteomyelitis with different degrees of sensitivity. A bone biopsy is required for a reliable culture. Most cases in children are hematogenous in origin, while those in adults result from an open fracture or open reduction of a closed fracture. Criteria for a positive diagnosis of osteomyelitis include characteristic radiographic changes, positive bone culture results, and histopathologic findings that support the diagnosis.

Dermatologic Disorders of the Lower Leg

Nodular panniculitis causes painful, tender, red patches, plaques, and nodules that simulate a cellulitis or a pyoderma. Multiple lesions occur and coalesce. Central necrosis leaves draining ulcers that exude a yellow-white, oily fluid that is often mistaken for pus. This fluid stains strongly for free fat with a Sudan stain. Fever, weight loss, weakness, malaise, and anorexia are associated. Systemic disorders associated with nodular panniculitis include connective tissue diseases, lymphoproliferative disorders, and pancreatic disease.

Erythema nodosum causes pretibial and anterior tibial tender, red, subcutaneous nodules that may occur alone or in association with ankle and knee pain, fever, and/or hilar adenopathy. Many systemic infections and diseases of unknown etiology are associated with this disorder.

Painful, punched-out, anterior tibial ulcers are caused by *hypertension and arterial ischemia*. *Systemic vasculitis* causes irregular, deep, purulent ulcers over the lower legs. These ulcers are associated with a collagen vascular disease or Wegener's granulomatosis. Sickle cell anemia may also cause lower-extremity ulceration.

Erythema induratum causes red or bluish, tender nodules over the calves. These nodules may ulcerate and become secondarily infected, causing pain. Biopsy of these lesions reveals granulomatous inflammation, vasculitis, and panniculitis.

Generalized Ankle Pain

Fractures and ligament ruptures at the ankle result *from abduction, adduction, internal or external rotation, or dorsiflexion forces*. Single injuries over the lateral or medial side of the ankle cause localized pain, swelling, tenderness, ecchymoses, sometimes bony crepitus, and radiographic evidence of fracture or diastasis between the talus and the articular surface of the tibia (i.e., indicating ligament rupture). Greater forces result in injuries to both the lateral and medial side of the ankle and, in some cases, to the anterior or posterior tibial articular mar-

ginal lips and the tibiofibular ligaments. Pain, swelling, and tenderness involve the lateral and medial aspects of the joint, and deformity of the foot-ankle articulation may be valgus or varus.

Dislocation of the ankle (*talotibial articulation*) requires disruption of the ankle capsule and most of the ligaments. *Anterior dislocation* causes diffuse ankle pain, dorsiflexion and elongation of the foot, and anterior prominence of the superior surface of the talus. *Posterior dislocation* results in plantar flexion and/or shortening of the foot. Plain radiographs will define the type and degree of dislocation and associated fractures.

Fracture of the neck or body of the talus may also cause diffuse ankle pain, tenderness, swelling, and ankle deformity due to talar dislocation. These fractures can be imaged by plain radiography (i.e., anteroposterior, lateral, and mortise views).

Acute septic monarthritis may cause ankle swelling, pain, tenderness, and erythema and warmth of the overlying skin. The synovial fluid contains an increased number of polymorphonuclear leukocytes, and culture results are positive for *S. aureus*, a streptococcal species, or a gram-negative bacterium. Sexually active adults may develop joint infection caused by *N. gonorrhoeae*. Diagnosis of this infection may require mucous membrane, blood, and/or synovial fluid cultures.

Acute gout or pseudogout may mimic joint sepsis, producing a red, painful, tender, swollen ankle. Synovial fluid will contain monosodium urate or calcium pyrophosphate dihydrate crystals and increased numbers of polymorphonuclear leukocytes.

Acute rheumatoid arthritis may begin as a monarthritis of the ankle with pain, swelling, and tenderness. In time, serum rheumatoid factor test results become positive, and other criteria for a diagnosis of rheumatoid arthritis appear.

Reflex sympathetic dystrophy may follow a relatively minor ankle or foot injury. Burning or aching pain involves the ankle and/or foot. The pain is out of proportion to the injury or existing local disease. Skin warmth, erythema, tenderness, and allodynia occur. Within weeks, joint pain and stiffness limit extremity use. The skin then becomes edematous, cold, and shiny, and use of the ankle or foot is avoided. Allodynia and skin hyperesthesia become worse, and hyperhidrosis may be present. A bone scan will show increased periarticular uptake, and radiographs will reveal patchy or diffuse osteoporosis of the ankle joint.

An *acute intraarticular hemorrhage* presents with the sudden onset of joint pain, swelling, tenderness, and inability to walk without severe pain. Joint aspiration reveals blood, and there is no evidence of a coagulopathy. Some cases of *ankle hemarthrosis* are *associated* with *hemophilia*.

Transient migratory osteoporosis causes local ankle pain and diffuse swelling without pitting edema, warmth, and redness. Joint mobility is preserved. Bone scan results are strongly positive, and radiographs reveal diffuse osteoporosis of all bones comprising the ankle joint. Corticosteroid therapy may be effective. Migration to the joints of the foot or knee may follow.

Osteochondritis dissecans of the talus occurs in older children, adolescents, and young adults. Anteromedial ankle pain and tenderness impair running or jogging. The diagnosis can be confirmed by MRI or arthroscopy.

Diffuse ankle pain, swelling, tenderness, skin warmth, and erythema may occur as part of an *acute inflammatory polyarthritis*. Causes include *polyarticular septic arthritis*, *acute rheumatic fever*, *Lyme disease*, *hepatitis B-associated arthritis*, *rubella and rubella vaccine–associated arthritis*, *arthritis associated with inflammatory bowel disease*, *polyarticular gout*, *calcium pyrophosphate deposition disease*, *Reiter's syndrome*, *and acute rheumatoid arthritis*.

Acute osteomyelitis causes severe ankle pain, tenderness, swelling, fever and chills. MRI or a radionuclide bone scan will be abnormal before plain radiographic changes appear. This disorder is more common in children and is seldom seen in adults.

Lateral Ankle Pain

An adduction force on the plantar-flexed ankle joint may *sprain the anterior taliofibular ligament* (ATFL) and in some cases the *calcaneofibular ligament* (CFL), major components of the lateral collateral ligament of the ankle. ATFL injury causes pain, tenderness, and swelling anterior and inferior to the lateral malleolus, and CFL injury causes the same symptoms inferior to the tip of the lateral malleolus. The anterior drawer and inversion tests are used to detect ligament rupture and require local or general anesthesia if they are performed on an acutely injured ankle. Radiographic measurements of talar tilt (i.e., stress inversion test) and anterior movement of the talus (i.e., anterior drawer test) are abnormal with ATFL rupture, with or without associated CFL disruption. Arthrography is more accurate than the inversion and anterior drawer tests for the diagnosis of ATFL and/or CFL rupture.

Mimics of ATFL and CFL injury include *anterior tibiofibular ligament sprain* and *lateral malleolus fracture*. The tenderness in an anterior tibiofibular ligament sprain is more medial and superior to the lateral malleolus. Complete rupture of the anterior tibiofibular ligament may sometimes be detected on an external rotation stress film of the ankle. Fracture of the lateral malleolus produces tenderness over the distal fibula and radiographic evidence of fracture. Fractures of the talus produce point tenderness and swelling inferior to the tip of the lateral malleolus and radiographic evidence of a *fracture of the lateral process of the talus or the lateral tubercle of the posterior process of the talus*.

Peroneal tendinitis causes local tendon-associated pain, tenderness, and swelling below and posterior to the lateral malleolus. Passive plantar inversion and flexion intensify the pain. Ankle eversion against resistance also increases the pain. Lidocaine injection into the painful region of the tendon immediately relieves rest- and movement-related pain and is of diagnostic value. *Traumatic dislocation of the peroneal tendons* presents with an acute pain and a snap over the lateral aspect of the ankle. If the tendons remain dislocated, the diagnosis is straightforward. If not, attempted dorsiflexion against resistance with the foot plantar-flexed and everted should be attempted in order to cause the tendons to redislocate to a position anterior to the lateral malleolus. Local edema may occur over the posterolateral aspect of the ankle. A *ganglion* may present as a cystic, tender mass below the lateral malleolus. A *fibular stress fracture* causes pain and localized tenderness over the posterolateral aspect of the lower fibula. A radionuclide scan or plain radiograph will confirm the diagnosis of fibular stress fracture. A *CFL sprain* is an uncommon isolated injury. There are localized lateral ankle pain, swelling, and tenderness over the anatomic site of the ligament.

Anterior Ankle Pain

Peritendinitis involves the extensor tendons of the foot and toes. The tendons are locally tender, and passive stretch (plantar flexion and toe flexion) intensifies local pain, as does local tendon palpation. An *injury to the cruciate crural ligament* may cause similar symptoms and examination findings, but local tenderness is maximal over the region of the ligament. *Injury to the anterior tibiofibular ligament* causes pain and tenderness medial and superior to the lateral malleolus. *Fracture of the anterior lip of the tibial articular surface* follows a pronation-dorsiflexion injury. Anterior ankle tenderness and swelling occur, and the fracture can be visualized by routine radiographic studies of the ankle.

Medial Ankle Pain

Medial ankle pain immediately following an abduction or external rotation injury of the ankle may be due to a *deltoid ligament sprain*. Medial ankle joint tenderness, swelling, and sometimes ecchymoses may occur. Rupture of the deltoid ligament may be detected on a mortise view of the ankle showing a diastasis of more than 4 mm between the inner surface of the medial malleolus and the talus. *Fracture of the medial malleolus* by a similar type of injury results in local pain, tenderness, and swelling over the fracture site, and the diagnosis can be confirmed by a plain radiograph. *Tibialis posterior tendinitis* causes pain over the medial foot, the medial malleolus, and the region posterior to the medial malleolus. The tendon may be tender and swollen, filling in the concave space normally present posterior to the medial malleolus. Resisted supination of the foot or passive pronation intensifies the medial ankle pain.

Posteromedial distal tibial pain, or *shin splints*, arise from a *stress fracture*, *periostitis*, or a *disorder in the musculotendinous tissue just posterior to the posteromedial tibial margin*. These causes of pain can be differentiated by clinical examination, a radionuclide bone scan, and plain radiographs.

Fracture of the sustentaculum tali may mimic a medial ankle sprain. Passive inversion of the foot causes pain below the medial malleolus. Passive hyperextension of the great toe may also provoke or intensify the pain. An axial radiograph of the calcaneus is useful in detecting the fracture. *Tendinitis of the flexor hallucis longus muscle and/or flexor digitorum communis muscle* may cause pain and tenderness posterior to the medial malleolus. Passive extension or resisted flexion of the toes intensifies the pain. Local crepitus and tenderness may be present over the involved tendons.

Posterior Ankle Pain

Achilles tendinitis is associated with tendon enlargement, tenderness, crepitus, and, in a small percentage of cases, rheumatoid arthritis and gout. *Bursitis* may occur *between the Achilles tendon and the skin* or between the Achilles tendon and the calcaneous (*retrocalcaneal bursitis*). The retrocalcaneal bursa may be swollen and tender anterior and adjacent to both sides of the Achilles tendon. Pressure applied to the bursal tissue anterior and parallel to the Achilles tendon elicits tenderness. A *partial tear in the Achilles tendon* may cause tenderness and pain with resisted plantar flexion or passive dorsiflexion of the ankle. *Complete rupture of the Achilles tendon* causes the sudden onset of posterior ankle and calf pain and tenderness associated with a snapping sensation. A tender gap in the tendon may be palpable. Plantar flexion is impaired. An *avulsion fracture of the calcaneal tuberosity* may follow a fall from a step by an elderly person. Posterior heel and ankle pain and tenderness occur. Plantar flexion of the foot is impaired. A plain lateral radiograph will confirm the diagnosis of fracture of the calcaneal tuberosity.

Bilateral Lower Leg and Ankle Pain

The disorders listed in Table 46-1 may cause *bilateral*, as well as unilateral, *lower leg and ankle pain*.

☐ DESCRIPTION OF LISTED DISEASES

Generalized Lower Leg Pain

1. FRACTURES OF THE TIBIAL SHAFT AND/OR FIBULA

A. Traumatic Tibial shaft fractures may result from indirect or direct impact during a motor vehicle accident (dashboard injury) or a motor vehicle-pedestrian accident, or from a low- or high-velocity gunshot wound. Such fractures are usually transverse or comminuted, and up to 30 percent may be open. Severe fractures are accompanied by a fracture of the fibula. A fall with the foot

Table 46-1
CAUSES OF BILATERAL LOWER LEG AND ANKLE PAIN

Generalized leg pain
  Sickle cell pain crisis
  Delayed muscle soreness due to exercise
  Bilateral tibial shaft and/or fibula fractures due to trauma
Calf pain
  Acute rhabdomyolysis
  Gastrocnemius muscle strain
  Soleus muscle strain
  Muscle cramps (benign or symptomatic)
  Deep calf vein thrombosis
Anterolateral lower leg pain due to anterior compartment muscle
  strain
Anteromedial lower leg pain
  Stress fracture of the tibia
  Stress microfracture of the tibia
  Medial tibial stress syndrome
  Soleus syndrome
  Anterolateral tibial margin pain
  Shin splints related to early acquired syphilis or Paget's disease
  Saphenous neuritis
Dermatologic disorders
  Nodular panniculitis
  Erythema nodosum
  Arterial and ischemic ulcers
  Systemic vasculitis with ulceration
  Erythema induratum
Generalized ankle pain
  Bilateral ankle fractures and ligament disruption due to trauma
  Reflex sympathetic dystrophy
  Osteochondritis dissecans
  Polyarthritis due to septic arthritis, acute rheumatic fever, Lyme
    arthritis, hepatitis B virus, rubella virus, inflammatory bowel
    disease, gout, pseudogout, Reiter's syndrome, or acute
    rheumatoid arthritis
Lateral ankle pain
  Bilateral lateral fractures or ligament sprains due to trauma
  Stress fracture of the fibula
Anterior ankle pain due to peritendinitis of the extensor tendons of
  the foot and toes
Medial ankle pain
  Bilateral medial fractures or ligament sprains due to trauma
  Stress fractures of the tibia
  Periostitis of the tibia
  Musculotendinous pain arising in the posterior compartment
    muscles
Posterior ankle pain
  Achilles tendinitis
  Retrocalcaneal bursitis
  Subcutaneous Achilles bursitis

anchored or during skiing may result in a torque-related spiral or oblique fracture of the tibia and fibula.

Pain occurs at the site of the fracture in the upper, mid, or lower portion of the lower leg and is severe when the tibia is fractured. Lateral pain and tenderness may be secondary to an associated fracture of the fibula. Weight bearing is poorly tolerated and avoided in patients with undisplaced fractures, and is not possible in those with angulation and displacement.

TABLE OF DISEASE INCIDENCE

INCIDENCE PER 100,000 (APPROXIMATE)

Common (>100)	Uncommon (>5–100)	Rare (>0–5)
	GENERALIZED LOWER LEG PAIN	
Traumatic fracture of the tibial shaft and/or fibula	Acute femoropopliteal arterial occlusion	Pathologic fracture of the tibial shaft and/or fibula
Bacterial cellulitis	Erysipelas	Necrotizing fasciitis
Delayed muscle soreness due to exercise	Infected vascular gangrene	Gas gangrene
	Sickle cell pain crisis	Nonclostridial myositis: anaerobic streptococcal myonecrosis, synergistic necrotizing cellulitis, and *Aeromonas hydrophila* myonecrosis
		Clostridial anaerobic cellulitis
		Nonclostridial anaerobic cellulitis
		Vibrio vulnificus cellulitis
	CALF PAIN	
Spontaneous deep vein thrombosis	Effort-induced deep vein thrombosis	Pyomyositis
Baker's cyst complications	Hematoma of the calf	Acute rhabdomyolysis
Gastrocnemius muscle strain	Pseudo-pseudothrombophlebitis	
Benign muscle cramps	Rupture of the Achilles tendon	
	Soleus muscle strain	
	Acute posterior compartment syndrome	
	Symptomatic muscle cramps	
	ANTEROLATERAL LOWER LEG PAIN	
Muscle strain and/or hematoma in the anterior compartment	Anterior tibial vein thrombosis	Lateral compartment syndrome
	Anterior compartment syndrome	Pyomyositis
	Compression of the superficial peroneal nerve	
	Fracture of the fibula shaft	
	Maisonneuve fracture of the fibula	
	ANTEROMEDIAL LOWER LEG PAIN	
Stress fracture of the tibia	Distal deep posterior compartment syndrome	Shin splints due to syphilis or Paget's disease
Stress microfractures of the tibia	Osteomyelitis of the tibia	
Medial tibial stress syndrome (periostalgia)	Greater saphenous vein thrombophlebitis	
Soleus syndrome	Saphenous neuritis	
Anterolateral tibial margin pain		
DERMATOLOGIC DISORDERS OF THE LOWER LEG		
Erythema nodosum	Nodular panniculitis	Erythema induratum
	Arterial or hypertensive ulcers	
	Systemic vasculitis with ulceration	
	GENERALIZED ANKLE PAIN	
Fractures of the medial and/or lateral malleolus	Fracture of the neck of the talus	Anterior dislocation of the ankle
Disruption of the medial and/or lateral ligaments of the ankle	Fracture of the body of the talus	Posterior dislocation of the ankle
Acute gout	Fracture of the anterior or posterior lips of the tibial articular surface	Acute hemarthrosis
Acute pseudogout	Septic arthritis	Transient migratory osteoporosis
Rubella and rubella vaccine-associated arthritis	Acute rheumatoid arthritis	Acute osteomyelitis
	Reflex sympathetic dystrophy	
	Hemophilic arthropathy	
	Osteochondritis dissecans of the talus	
	Polyarticular septic arthritis	
	Acute rheumatic fever	
	Lyme arthritis	
	Hepatitis B virus-associated arthritis	
	Arthritis associated with inflammatory bowel disease	
	Acute polyarticular gout	
	Calcium pyrophosphate deposition disease	
	Reiter's syndrome	
	Acute rheumatoid arthritis	

TABLE OF DISEASE INCIDENCE

INCIDENCE PER 100,000 (APPROXIMATE)

Common (>100)	Uncommon (>5–100)	Rare (>0–5)
	LATERAL ANKLE PAIN	
ATFL sprain with or without a CFL sprain	Anterior tibiofibular ligament sprain	
Fracture of the lateral malleolus	Fracture of the lateral process of the talus	
	Fracture of the lateral tubercle of the posterior process of the talus	
	Peroneal tendinitis	
	Traumatic dislocation of the peroneal tendons	
	Ganglion	
	Stress fracture of the fibula	
	CFL sprain (isolated)	
	ANTERIOR ANKLE PAIN	
Peritendinitis of the extensor tendons of the foot and toes	Cruciate crural ligament sprain	
	Anterior tibiofibular ligament sprain	
	Fracture of the anterior lip of the distal tibial articular surface	
	MEDIAL ANKLE PAIN	
Fracture of the medial malleolus	Deltoid ligament sprain	
Shin splints due to stress fracture of the tibia, periostitis, or musculotendinous pain	Tibialis posterior tendinitis	
	Fracture of the sustentaculum tali	
	Tendinitis of the flexor hallucis longus muscle and/or flexor digitorum communis muscle	
	POSTERIOR ANKLE PAIN	
Achilles tendinitis	Subcutaneous Achilles bursitis	Fracture of the calcaneal tuberosity
	Retrocalcaneal bursitis	
	Achilles tendon partial or complete rupture	

Limb shortening and deformity occur secondary to angulation and fragment rotation and displacement. Swelling, crepitus, tenderness, and ecchymoses may be present over the area of deformity in the fracture region.

Open fractures may present as a skin puncture wound from a tibial fracture fragment penetrating the skin surface, or a large fragment of tibia may protrude through the skin of the medial portion of the lower leg. Plain anteroposterior or lateral radiographs will demonstrate fractures of the tibia and/or fibula, their location (proximal, middle, or lower third), the type of fracture (transverse, oblique, spiral, segmental, or comminuted), the degree and type of angulation (valgus or varus), the degree of lateral and/or anteroposterior displacement of the distal to the proximal fragments, and the amount of fragment overlap or distraction.

B. Pathologic Localized aching pain, often intensified when the limb is dependent, may sometimes precede a pathologic fracture. Most patients are asymptomatic until they report an abrupt snapping or giving way in the lower leg during weight bearing or walking. This feeling is accompanied by the onset of localized pain and tenderness and an inability to bear weight without increasing the severity of the pain.

Plain radiographs may reveal an osteolytic or cystic lesion of the tibia and an associated fracture. Some patients have a history and/or physical, laboratory, or radiologic findings of metastatic malignancy, leukemia, a cystic bone lesion, or localized osteoporosis. The diagnosis may be established by the associated clinical findings or by bone biopsy.

2. ACUTE OCCLUSION OF THE SUPERFICIAL FEMORAL OR POPLITEAL ARTERY

Sudden distal occlusion of the superficial femoral or popliteal artery may cause diffuse lower leg pain, paresthesias, muscle paresis, skin pallor and coldness (a line of demarcation between normal, warm skin and cold, pale, white skin may be observed), and absence of pedal and/or popliteal pulses. A fracture of the proximal tibia or distal femur, an embolus (arising in the heart, aorta, or proximal vessels), or arterial thrombosis may be responsible for the arterial obstruction. Symptoms may be completely reversed if arterial occlusion is relieved within 6 to 8 h.

3. ACUTE INFECTIONS IN THE LOWER LEG

A. Erysipelas This disorder is a superficial streptococcal cellulitis of the skin involving the upper dermis and cutaneous lymphatic channels. The skin of the foot, ankle, and lower leg becomes acutely painful, fiery red, tender, and indurated. The lesion has a clearly demarcated, elevated, spreading border. A *peau d'orange* appearance in the erythematous region may be present. Fever, chills, diaphoresis, malaise, and leukocytosis may occur. Up to 80 percent of cases involve the legs, and only 15 to 20 percent are confined to the face. Local trauma, skin ulcers, preexisting dermatologic lesions, or cutaneous fungal infections may serve as portals of entry for the responsible group A streptococcus (rarely, group C or G streptococci may be etiologic). Parenteral penicillin therapy will result in resolution of pain and regression of skin abnormalities within 48 to 72 h.

B. Bacterial Cellulitis Involvement of the deep dermis and subcutaneous tissue causes foot and leg pain, diffuse erythema, and local tenderness. The advancing irregular lesional margin is flat and poorly demarcated. Fever, chills, and malaise may be associated. Most cases arise in a chronic ulcer, abrasion, or fissure. Superficial cutaneous edema adjacent to the advancing margin occurs. Superficial abscesses or bullous hemorrhagic lesions, 1 to 4 cm in diameter, may develop within the erythematous region. These lesions may drain, leaving a necrotic ulcer.

C. Necrotizing Fasciitis This disorder begins with erythema, pain, tenderness, and edema of the skin of the foot and lower leg. Spiking fever, chills, tachycardia, alteration of mental status (e.g., drowsiness), and severe toxicity occur. Examination reveals a warm, red lower leg and foot. The edema is firm and nonpitting, and may extend beyond the erythematous margins. Because of the swelling, the skin may appear smooth, shiny, and tense. Within 48 to 96 h, the skin color becomes blue-gray or purplish in some areas. Vesicles and bullae containing reddish-brown fluid may appear in the involved region. Skin hypesthesia or anesthesia may develop in the affected region secondary to involvement of cutaneous sensory nerves by the deep inflammatory process. Within 5 to 8 days, the involved skin becomes leathery and black and may begin to slough, exposing malodorous necrotic fascia and fat. Lymphangitis or lymphadenitis may occur but is uncommon. Subcutaneous gas may be palpable (skin crepitus) or detectable on a plain radiograph. If the developing lesion is explored through an adjacent skin incision, a long hemostat can be easily passed along a space superficial to the deep fascia. This finding does not occur in an uncomplicated cellulitis. Criteria for the diagnosis of necrotizing fasciitis include necrosis of the superficial fascia and undermining of surrounding tissue, systemic symptoms and altered mental status, absence of myonecrosis, absence of vascular occlusion, absence of clostridial species on culture, histopathologic findings on debrided tissue of polymorphonuclear leukocyte infiltration, thrombosis of microvasculature, and focal necrosis of subcutaneous fat and the superficial fascia. Type I necrotizing fasciitis is caused by a synergistic infection involving one or more anaerobes (e.g., a *Bacteroides* or peptostreptococcal species) and one or more facultative anaerobes, such as non-group A streptococci and members of the Enterobacteriaceae. Type II necrotizing fasciitis is caused by group A streptococci alone or in association with *S. aureus*. Early differentiation from a case of uncomplicated cellulitis requires a deep skin biopsy, allowing identification of fat and fascial necrosis. Extensive, frequent debridement and the use of antibiotics offer the best hope of patient survival. Up to 75 percent of patients with necrotizing fasciitis may have diabetes mellitus. There is also a high prevalence of obesity, and peripheral arterial disease. There is usually a history of minor trauma prior to onset, although some patients do not report a prior injury.

D. Gas Gangrene (Clostridial Myonecrosis) This infection is usually secondary to deep trauma involving muscle injury and contamination with soil or foreign bodies. Open fractures, severe gunshot wounds, and arterial insufficiency of the leg provide settings for the initiation of clostridial myonecrosis. Rare cases may occur in the absence of wounding. These cases arise in an ulceration in the bowel and reach a peripheral site by hematogenous dissemination.

Symptoms begin within 1 to 3 days of injury. Some patients have had an onset after only 6 h. Severe local wound pain is the initial complaint. The patient is usually extremely ill, with pallor, diaphoresis, faintness, and hypotension. Apathy, drowsiness, prostration, and agitation may occur and may progress to stupor or coma. Fever may appear, but the temperature tends to remain less than 38°C (101°F). Early changes in the wound include intense edema, tenderness, and pallor, accompanied by a serosanguineous, dirty-appearing, malodorous discharge. Skin crepitus is usually present but may be difficult to detect because of extensive skin edema. The skin surrounding the wound becomes yellow or bronze in color; and tense vesicles and bullae containing dark fluid, and greenish-black, necrotic skin patches appear. Within hours, the lower leg may become diffusely and massively swollen, and large areas of the skin black and anesthetic. The entire limb may be severely painful, but this discomfort may be overshadowed by the severity of the systemic symptoms (i.e., fever and delirium). Leukocytosis and hemolytic anemia frequently occur, but results of blood cultures for *Clostridium perfringens* are positive in only

15 percent of cases. Wound exploration reveals evidence of myonecrosis. A Gram stain of the wound exudate or bulla fluid reveals many large gram-positive rods. Radiographs reveal gas in muscle and in fascial planes. *C. perfringens* is isolated from wound exudate or debrided tissue in 80 to 96 percent of cases. *Clostridium novyi* and *Clostridium septicum* account for the remaining cases. Isolation of other bacteria, such as *Escherichia coli*, other Enterobacteriaceae, or enterococci, from the same wound indicates a mixed infection resulting from the initiating injury.

E. Nonclostridial Myositis

1. Anaerobic Streptococcal Myonecrosis This disorder begins 3 to 4 days after a penetrating leg wound. Early symptoms are skin erythema and edema around the wound and a copious, sour-smelling, seropurulent wound discharge. Pain is initially absent, but it develops late and gradually becomes more intense and diffuse. Without treatment, skin and muscle gangrene, toxemia, and shock develop. Involved muscles are discolored but react to stimulation. This disorder is a mixed infection caused by anaerobic streptococci and group A streptococci or *S. aureus*. Surgical exploration and debridement of necrotic tissue and antibiotic therapy will lead to resolution.

2. Synergistic Necrotizing Cellulitis This disorder is most likely to occur in a setting of diabetes mellitus, cardiovascular or renal disease, obesity, or advanced age. The initial lesions are small, painful skin ulcers that drain reddish-brown, foul-smelling (''dishwater'') pus. Pain is accompanied by skin areas of gray-green gangrene that surround the initial draining lesions. Severe toxemia and diffuse pain and tenderness of the leg are characteristic findings. Tissue gas is noted in up to 25 percent of cases. Blood cultures may be positive in up to 50 percent of cases. This disease results from a mixed infection of anaerobes (*Bacteroides* species and anaerobic streptococci) and facultative bacteria (Enterobacteriaceae). Radical debridement or extremity amputation and antibiotic therapy offer the best chance for survival.

3. Infected Vascular Gangrene Infection occurs in an ischemic leg. *Proteus* species, *Bacteroides* species, and anaerobic streptococci may be isolated from the necrotic tissue. Crepitus due to gas production and malodorous pus are prominent findings. Infection is restricted to the region of necrotic ischemic muscle. *Bacillus cereus* may be associated with infection of necrotic muscle after acute closure of an arterial graft.

4. Aeromonas hydrophila *Myonecrosis This disorder occurs after wounding in fresh water or during handling of fish, shellfish, or other aquatic animals. It mimics gas gangrene because of a rapid onset (1–2

days) of severe, generalized lower leg pain and edema, with serosanguineous bullae and toxicity. Plain radiographs demonstrate gas in fascial spaces and muscle. The diagnosis can be suspected from the setting in which the wound occurred and confirmed by a Gram stain and culture of drainage or bulla fluid.

F. Clostridial Anaerobic Cellulitis This disorder begins in a skin wound 3 to 5 days after the injury. Moderate local swelling, mild leg pain, and minimal toxicity occur. A thin, dark, malodorous wound drainage, sometimes containing free fat globules, and extensive gas formation in the skin are characteristic findings. Gram-stained smears show gram-positive bacilli. Soft tissue radiographs reveal tissue gas. Surgical exploration is required to exclude myonecrosis. Debridement of necrotic tissue and antibiotic therapy lead to recovery.

G. Nonclostridial Anaerobic Cellulitis This disorder presents 3 or more days after wounding, with local edema and mild lower leg pain. A dark, foul-smelling wound discharge occurs, but there is minimal skin discoloration. Systemic symptoms are mild to moderate in severity. Surgical exploration is required to exclude acute myonecrosis. This disorder is caused by anaerobic bacteria alone or as part of mixed infection with facultative bacteria (streptococcal species, staphylococcal species, or coliform bacilli). It resembles the anaerobic cellulitis caused by clostridial species. Debridement of necrotic tissue and antibiotic therapy result in recovery. This infection is more commonly seen in diabetics.

H. *Vibrio vulnificus* Cellulitis Wounding or wound contamination in warm ocean water may cause an extensive cellulitis of the leg with hemorrhagic skin bullae, necrotic ulcers, and skin necrosis. This infection may progress rapidly and may be accompanied by fever, chills, diaphoresis, and severe signs of toxicity. There is a good response to doxycycline and debridement of necrotic tissue.

4. SICKLE CELL PAIN CRISIS

Severe, diffuse lower leg pain; skin allodynia; hyperesthesia; and deep muscle, bone, and joint tenderness may occur in patients with sickle cell anemia. This pain has an abrupt onset, with or without paresthesias. Fever and associated pain in the low back, arms, chest, or abdomen may be present or soon appear. The leg pain and skin allodynia are frequently circumferential, and the pain is described as an ache or as throbbing and sharp. The pain is partially relieved by meperidine. There is gradual spontaneous resolution of the painful crisis over a period of 3 to 15 days. Pain may extend from the knees or below the knees to the ankles, or it may include the ankles and feet.

We believe that this pain represents a reversible sensory neuropathy. Some patients have recurrent attacks of lower leg pain every 2 to 4 weeks, while others may only experience a single episode in this region.

5. DELAYED MUSCLE SORENESS DUE TO EXERCISE

Aching pain and tenderness of the leg muscles in the thigh and/or below the knees may result from unaccustomed exercise. The pain begins 24 to 48 h after the exercise and may be present at rest or may be only provoked by walking, running, or stair climbing. Rhabdomyolysis and myoglobinuria may occur in severe cases. The outcome is usually benign, and most cases resolve spontaneously in 1 to 5 days.

Calf Pain

6. DEEP VEIN THROMBOSIS

A. Effort-Induced Thrombosis This disorder occurs most frequently in middle-aged joggers. There is an abrupt onset during running of sharp calf pain. The pain continues and worsens if the jogger continues to run in an attempt to work out or run through the pain. Calf swelling and tenderness develop within hours. The pain is intensified by dependency and relieved by leg elevation. Examination reveals calf enlargement and tenderness. Skin warmth, erythema, and ecchymoses may be present in some cases. Contrast venography will establish the diagnosis, and symptoms resolve with heparin therapy.

B. Spontaneous Thrombosis Spontaneous thrombosis has a more gradual onset than does effort-induced thrombosis and usually occurs in a patient with one or more risk factors for venous thrombosis. Risk factors for deep vein thrombosis in the calf and thigh include recent surgery; malignancy (e.g., pancreas, lung, ovary, testes, urinary tract, breast, or stomach); trauma (e.g., fracture of the pelvis, femur, or tibia); prolonged immobilization (e.g., a long airplane or automobile ride, or bed rest for a nonsurgical illness such as acute myocardial infarction, cerebrovascular accident, or spinal cord injury); pregnancy; estrogen use; a hypercoagulable state (e.g., deficiency of antithrombin III, protein C, or protein S; circulating lupus anticoagulant; myeloproliferative disorders; dysfibrinogenemia; and disseminated intravascular coagulation); venous inflammation (e.g., thromboangiitis obliterans or Behçet's disease); obesity; congestive heart failure; and prior venous thromboses.

Calf pain occurred in 57 percent, edema in 28 percent, and localized calf tenderness in 21 percent of patients with venographic evidence of acute popliteal or calf vein thrombosis in one reported series. Local calf swelling, with only moderate induration, tenderness, and skin warmth, is a common presentation. Calf pain is usually intensified by standing or walking and relieved by rest and elevation. The pain of an acute deep venous thrombosis may begin gradually over a period of hours or suddenly (e.g., during jogging or running). Constant, unremitting aching pain in the calf and popliteal fossa may be present, or pain may occur only with activity. Fever, malaise, diaphoresis, and leukocytosis may occur in some cases.

Confirmation of isolated calf vein thrombosis usually requires contrast venography. Impedance plethysmography has only a 17- to 33-percent sensitivity for the detection of an isolated deep calf vein thrombosis. This method detects venous obstruction due to proximal segment thrombosis by measuring the venous capacitance of the limb and the rate of venous outflow after deflation of a compressing thigh cuff. In contrast with its low sensitivity for the diagnosis of calf vein thrombosis, impedance plethysmography is reported to have a sensitivity of 87 to 100 percent and a specificity of 92 to 100 percent for the diagnosis of proximal deep vein thrombosis.

Gray-scale ultrasonography has a sensitivity of 88 to 100 percent for the detection of iliofemoral venous occlusion and less than 25 percent for the diagnosis of calf vein thrombosis.

Color duplex flow imaging (CDFI) has been used for the diagnosis of calf and above-the-knee deep vein thrombosis. CDFI provides a real-time image of the vein and the direction and flow rate of the contained blood. CDFI uses color and hue to represent blood velocity and direction relative to the transducer. In one study, when CDFI was used to display calf veins, a technically adequate study was performed in 60 percent of extremities. The remaining group of lower extremities had severe calf swelling; were large, fat legs; or had adjacent veins that obscured the signal from the vein being studied. In the 60 percent of extremities where the calf veins were adequately imaged, sensitivity was 95 percent. Up to 20 percent of infrapopliteal deep vein thromboses may extend proximally. CDFI has a poor sensitivity (<25 percent) for the diagnosis of small, nonocclusive thrombi. The overall sensitivity of CDFI for the diagnosis of calf vein thrombosis varies from 25 to 48 percent. CDFI allows direct observation of a venous thrombus as a flow void within the imaged vein (e.g., black color) and permits testing of venous compressibility using gentle pressure with the ultrasound probe held transverse to the artery and veins. Thrombosis is diagnosed when a dilated, noncompressable vein is imaged.

One recent proposal to limit the use of venography for the diagnosis of calf vein occlusion is to reserve its use for patients without sonographic evidence of above-the-knee deep vein thrombosis and a technically inadequate CDFI study of the calf.

Another strategy designed to avoid venography is to repeat impedance plethysmographic, B-mode sonographic, or CDFI studies every 2 to 3 days to detect propagation of an infrapopliteal thrombosis into the popliteal and/or femoral vein. CDFI has a sensitivity of 92 percent, a specificity of 100 percent, and an accuracy of 97 percent for the diagnosis of thrombi located between the knee and inguinal ligament.

Contrast venography may be of help in identifying new thrombi in patients with a history of deep vein thrombosis and CDFI evidence of deep vein thrombosis of indeterminate age. The symptoms and signs of deep vein thrombosis usually resolve on anticoagulant therapy.

7. MIMICS OF CALF VEIN THROMBOSIS (PSEUDOTHROMBOPHLEBITIS)

A. Complications of a Baker's Cyst These cysts appear in the popliteal fossa and may be asymptomatic or cause mild discomfort or a pressure sensation. They arise secondary to intraarticular disorders such as osteoarthritis, meniscal tears, and rheumatoid arthritis or without apparent knee joint disease. Less common causes of Baker's cyst include crystal-induced arthritis, reactive arthritis, the spondyloarthropathies, septic arthritis, posttraumatic arthritis, and Still's disease.

A Baker's cyst may cause calf pain, swelling, warmth, tenderness, and skin erythema if it ruptures, spilling cyst fluid into the soft tissues of the calf and thigh; if it enlarges and dissects without rupturing into the muscle planes of the calf, producing a rise in compartmental pressure; or by compressing the popliteal vein. The latter effect may result in deep vein thrombosis. An enlarged cyst may compress or entrap the tibial nerve, causing dysesthesias and hypesthesia of the sole and/or weakness of the ankle plantar flexors.

Larger cysts may be palpable. Ultrasonography has a sensitivity of 60 to 70 percent and a specificity of 80 to 90 percent. This procedure is usually performed initially to exclude a deep vein thrombosis in the femoropopliteal veins. A contrast venogram in patients with a Baker's cyst may be entirely normal or may demonstrate lateral deviation and/or compression of the popliteal vein. Arthrography has been used to detect Baker's cysts and to confirm rupture when the clinical evidence is supportive and results of sonographic and venographic studies are negative. Ultrasonography may miss a ruptured cyst when it is small or filled with debris or when calf swelling is extensive. MRI may be used instead of arthrography. MRI can image the cyst and detect evidence of rupture. Patients with a clinical picture of deep vein thrombosis of the calf who do not have risk factors for venous thrombosis are as likely to have pseudothrombophlebitis due to a Baker's cyst as they are to have deep vein thrombosis. Rest, an-

algesics, and intraarticular corticosteroid drugs may be used to treat Baker's cyst enlargement or rupture.

B. Pyomyositis Severe calf pain, swelling, tenderness, and doughy calf induration or a fluctuant mass are accompanied by high fever, chills, diaphoresis, and prostration. Risk factors for this disorder are trauma and poorly controlled diabetes mellitus. Leukocytosis is frequently present. Sonographic studies of the calf reveal an anechoic mass or a hypoechoic, irregular, sometimes septated mass lesion. CT studies of the calf will also reveal the abscess. Pus may be aspirated, Gram stained, and cultured. This disorder responds to incision and drainage of the abscess and antibiotic therapy. It occurs most commonly in tropical countries. *S. aureus* is the responsible organism in 90 percent of cases.

C. Hematoma of the Calf Pain, swelling, and tenderness occur in the calf and mimic thrombophlebitis. A sudden, abrupt onset while running or jumping suggests an acute muscle strain as the cause, but other cases related to muscle tears have a more gradual onset. Some cases follow direct calf trauma (e.g., a blow or kick) or a fracture of the tibia. A CT scan of the calf will demonstrate a crescent-shaped band of variable attenuation. High attenuation suggests a recent hemorrhage, while low attenuation indicates a subacute or chronic hematoma.

Transaxial MRI will demonstrate a crescent-shaped area of high signal, sometimes containing one or more small irregular areas of low signal intensity. The adjacent muscle may appear as an area of increased signal on a T_1-weighted image due to necrosis, edema, and interstitial bleeding. Such lesions can be clearly defined prior to surgical intervention by the use of coronal, as well as transaxial, MRI images. Symptoms associated with a large calf hematoma include pain on passive dorsiflexion of the foot, weakness of the toe and foot flexors, and hyperesthesia of the sole of the foot. A large hematoma may result in elevation of intracompartmental pressure above 35 torr, leading to an acute posterior compartment syndrome.

D. Acute Rhabdomyolysis In rare cases, calf pain, swelling, and tenderness, with loss of the ability to bear weight on the affected limb, may be the initial symptoms of rhabdomyolysis. The urine may be dark and contain myoglobin, and a marked elevation of the serum creatine kinase enzyme activity is usually present. A case of rhabdomyolysis-associated calf pain and swelling has been reported secondary to alcohol abuse and leg compression during sleep and another secondary to severe hypokalemia associated with Conn's syndrome (primary aldosteronism due to an aldosterone-producing tumor).

E. Pseudo-pseudothrombophlebitis A ruptured or markedly enlarged Baker's cyst and deep vein thrombosis of the calf may occur simultaneously. Bed rest or pressure from the enlarged cyst may be responsible for thrombosis of one or more calf veins.

F. Rupture of the Achilles Tendon   Spontaneous rupture occurs in racquet sports, football, and basketball. Sudden dorsiflexion of the foot with the gastrocnemius contracted may result in the abrupt onset of sharp lower calf pain, an audible pop, and in some cases loss of plantar flexion strength. A tender defect in the Achilles tendon may be palpable. Plantar flexion may be possible if the posterior tibial, flexor digitorum longus, and peroneal muscles compensate. Walking on tiptoes may reveal a heel drop in patients with Achilles tendon rupture. The Thompson squeeze test may also be positive. (This test is carried out with the patient prone and the knee flexed to 90°. When the calf is squeezed on the normal side, the foot plantar flexes toward the ceiling. If the Achilles tendon is ruptured, plantar flexion does not occur with calf muscle compression on the painful side.)

G. Gastrocnemius Muscle Strain   A sudden pain occurs in the posterior calf on rapid acceleration from a stance position. There are medial calf tenderness, warmth, diffuse swelling, and sometimes ecchymoses in the overlying skin. Walking intensifies the calf pain with each step. Passive dorsiflexion of the foot or resisted plantar flexion has a similar effect. "Tennis leg" is caused by a partial tear in the gastrocnemius muscle, usually occurring during a sudden start or cutting movement. At the time of injury, the knee is usually extended and the ankle dorsiflexed. A defect in the gastrocnemius muscle may be palpable. Conservative therapy results in recovery in 1 to 12 weeks.

H. Soleus Muscle Strain   Pain, swelling, warmth, and tenderness in the calf, mimicking a thrombophlebitis, may result from a tear or rupture of the soleus muscle. Pain and tenderness are deep in the calf anterior to the gastrocnemius muscle. A hematoma in the muscle can be detected by MRI or CT scan. Rest usually results in healing.

I. Acute Posterior Compartment Syndrome   This syndrome may arise from a fracture of the shaft of the tibia with hemorrhage into the posterior compartment or from a tear in the gastrocnemius or soleus muscles, resulting in the formation of an intracompartmental hematoma. A posterior compartment syndrome may result from a calf muscle tear because of intracompartmental bleeding caused by the use of heparin after an incorrect diagnosis of acute deep vein thrombosis.

"Tennis leg," or a gastrocnemius muscle tear, usually begins with an acute pain occurring on jumping or after sudden dorsiflexion of the ankle with the knee extended. Other injury mechanisms include falls, stretching exercises, or simply getting out of bed. The tenderness is usually localized to the medial aspect of the calf. Local ecchymoses may occur. MRI will demonstrate a hematoma produced by a severe tear as a mass lesion of high signal intensity. A venogram will show extrinsic pressure on the medial calf veins but no evidence of thrombosis.

Formation of a large hematoma in the posterior compartment may produce a rise in intracompartmental pressure above 50 to 70 torr. A kick in the calf region (e.g., in a soccer game) or excessive leg exercise by an untrained person may also provoke an acute compartment syndrome.

Constant pain begins gradually after an injury or during unaccustomed exercise but may develop as long as 12 h later. Within a brief period of time, the initial ache becomes an excruciating pain. Any movement of the leg or foot intensifies the pain. Paresthesias and hypesthesia of the plantar region frequently occur. Palpation of the calf muscles reveals evidence of increased compartment tension (muscle hardness) and tenderness. The overlying skin may be warm, red, and edematous. Marked intensification of pain occurs on passive stretching of the affected muscles (e.g., foot dorsiflexion for the gastrocnemius and soleus muscles in the superficial posterior compartment and passive toe extension for the toe flexors in the deep posterior compartment).

Weakness of plantar flexion (superficial posterior compartment syndrome) or toe flexion (deep posterior compartment syndrome) may be observed. Pulses may remain palpable until irreversible muscle necrosis has occurred. The diagnosis can be established clinically and confirmed by measurement of intracompartmental pressure with a wick catheter. A rest pressure above 35 torr supports the diagnosis.

Evacuation of a hematoma or abscess and fasciotomy will decompress the involved posterior compartment and lead to resolution of pain, muscle pareses, and sensory changes.

8. CALF MUSCLE CRAMPS

A. Benign   Severe pain occurs in the calf either spontaneously or during active use of the involved muscles (e.g., plantar flexion of the feet during coitus). The pain is associated with sustained muscle contraction and palpable induration and tightness of the affected muscle group (e.g., gastrocnemius and soleus muscles). Massage and passive or active stretching of the affected muscles (e.g., forced dorsiflexion of the foot for a calf cramp) result in pain relief. Such pain may last only 1 to 2 min or as long as 15 to 20 min. Residual soreness during walking may remain for several hours and may be associated with local tenderness. Calf cramps may occur on one side only or affect both sides, but simultaneous attacks in both calves are uncommon.

Most patients with muscle cramps have no underlying disorder. Their cramps may occur with increased frequency at rest, after or during exercise, and at night during sleep. Use of the legs for unaccustomed exercise may result in an increased frequency of cramps for 1 to 2 days afterward. Pregnancy-associated cramps and cramps following excessive use of the calf muscles in athletics (effort cramps), as well as the nocturnal leg cramps of elderly persons, are considered benign and do not require intensive investigation.

B. Symptomatic Cramps Calf muscle cramps may also be symptomatic of significant pathologic states. Studies of cancer patients have demonstrated a specific association of recurrent cramps and tumor or chemotherapy-related peripheral neuropathy (45 percent), root and plexus lesions (21 percent), myositis (4 percent), and hypomagnesemia (2 percent).

Muscle cramps were the initial symptom of an underlying pathologic disorder in 64 percent of cancer patients with this complaint.

Cramps have also been reported with motor neuron disease, hypocalcemia, cirrhosis of the liver, renal salt wasting, severe diarrhea, alcoholism, and tetanus. Diuretic therapy and hemodialysis may be responsible for muscle cramps, and an increased incidence has been reported in patients taking phenothiazines. An unusual case of muscle involvement in sarcoid, resulting in a painful 2-cm calf nodule, presented with calf muscle cramps. Biopsy of the nodule confirmed the diagnosis.

Anterolateral Lower Leg Pain

9. ANTERIOR TIBIAL VEIN THROMBOSIS

Pain, swelling, and tenderness may occur in the anterolateral lower leg. Skin warmth and erythema may be present in some cases. The anterior tibial veins may be imaged in up to 65 percent of cases by CDFI. Almost all patients with anterior tibial vein occlusion also have venographic evidence of femoropopliteal venous thrombosis. Impedance plethysmography and CDFI will detect thigh vessel occlusion with an accuracy of 99 percent. Symptoms resolve with anticoagulant therapy.

10. ANTERIOR COMPARTMENT SYNDROME

This disorder may complicate a relatively minor tibial fracture or a muscle strain and intracompartmental hemorrhage. It may follow a minimal undisplaced closed tibial fracture or, less commonly, a severe open fracture. Excruciating pain occurs in the anterior tibial region. Swelling, increased muscle tension, and exquisite tenderness

are present over the anterior compartment of the lower leg. Passive flexion of the toes or plantar flexion of the foot intensifies the pain. Hypesthesia may be present on the dorsum of the foot between the first and second toes. Weakness or paralysis of the tibialis anterior muscle and the extensors of the toes may follow. The diagnosis can be confirmed by measuring the intracompartmental pressure. Symptoms respond to fasciotomy.

11. LATERAL COMPARTMENT SYNDROME

Severe pain, tenderness, and increased tension over the peroneal muscles are present. These muscles may be weak or paralysed. Stretch of these muscles by passive inversion of the foot intensifies the pain. The intracompartmental pressure is elevated, and symptoms respond to fasciotomy.

12. COMPRESSION OF THE SUPERFICIAL PERONEAL NERVE

Pain may occur in the anterolateral lower leg during exercise or when the foot and ankle are held in a particular position at rest. Hypesthesia and paresthesias over the dorsum of the foot and the second to fourth toes occur during exercise or are persistent. Tenderness over the anterior intramuscular septum 8 to 15 cm proximal to the lateral malleolus while the patient is dorsiflexing and everting the foot is a sign of nerve compression.

Tinel's sign may be present over the nerve, and pain may be provoked or intensified by passive flexion and supination of the ankle. Up to 50 percent of patients have a normal nerve conduction velocity. Nerve compression has been associated with a fascial defect and muscle herniation; a lipoma; a long peroneus tunnel; an ankle sprain; fasciotomy of the anterior compartment; and an anomalous course of the superficial peroneal nerve.

13. PYOMYOSITIS

Pain, swelling, tenderness, and skin erythema may occur over the anterior compartment. Fever and toxicity may be present. A CT scan or MRI will usually image the intramuscular abscess. Drainage and antibiotic therapy lead to symptom resolution.

14. MUSCLE STRAIN AND/OR HEMATOMA

Pain and tenderness over the anterior compartment muscles occur. Passive plantar flexion of the foot and dorsiflexion against resistance intensify the pain. If a hematoma results from the muscle tear, the anterolateral lower leg may be swollen and warm. A CT scan or MRI will demonstrate a crescent-shaped hematoma. With a severe strain, a defect in the belly of the tibialis anterior muscle may be palpable.

15. FRACTURE OF THE SHAFT OF THE FIBULA

These fractures are uncommon unless associated with a tibial or ankle injury. There is usually a history of direct impact to the bone when the fracture is an isolated injury. Local pain, tenderness, and swelling occur, and ecchymoses may appear within 48 h or less. A plain radiograph will confirm the diagnosis.

16. MAISONNEUVE FRACTURE OF THE FIBULA

This proximal fibula fracture follows an external rotation force applied to the foot and ankle joint. The syndesmotic ligaments (anterior and posterior tibiofibular) and the interosseous membrane are disrupted. The deltoid ligament is usually severely damaged, or the medial malleolus is avulsed. The fracture is located at the proximal third of the fibula. It is a marker for syndesmotic disruption. An external rotation stress radiograph will demonstrate the resulting diastasis between tibia and fibula.

Proximal lateral calf pain, tenderness, and swelling due to the fibular fracture is associated with medial ankle pain and edema caused by disruption of the deltoid ligament or an avulsion fracture of the medial malleolus.

Anteromedial Lower Leg Pain

17. STRESS FRACTURE OF THE TIBIA

Pain occurs along the posteromedial border of the tibia. It is provoked or intensified by running or jogging, and relieved completely or partially by rest. Finger pressure and/or percussion tenderness is localized over a 2- to 3-cm area of the medial tibia. This disorder occurs during training in military recruits and in athletes involved in running or jogging. The onset of pain in conditioned runners usually follows an increase in the distance run, speed, or hours of training.

A radionuclide technetium bone scan reveals localized uptake in a fusiform or round configuration in the tender area. Plain anteroposterior or oblique radiographs may be normal or demonstrate a nondisplaced or, less commonly, a displaced linear fracture. Discontinuance of running or other exacerbating activities for 6 to 10 weeks leads to resolution of symptoms.

18. STRESS MICROFRACTURES OF THE TIBIA

Pain occurs along the posteromedial border of the tibia. It is provoked or exacerbated by running or jumping. The tenderness is confined to the bone and may extend longitudinally for 6 to 10 cm. A radionuclide scan will show increased uptake in a linear band along the posteromedial tibial margin extending for 6 to 10 cm. Results of plain radiographs are usually negative. This type of shin splint also responds to rest for 6 to 10 weeks.

19. MEDIAL TIBIAL STRESS SYNDROME (PERIOSTALGIA)

Pain occurs along the posteromedial or anteromedial tibial margin. The tenderness is localized, not to the bone, but to the soft tissue junction with the periosteum. It may extend for 10 to 12 cm along the tibial edge or the entire length of the bone. Results of radionuclide scans and radiographs are usually normal. Rest, taping, use of an orthosis and anti-inflammatory medication lead to symptom resolution. Some patients have musculotendinous dysfunction or a reversible compartment syndrome.

20. SOLEUS SYNDROME

This disorder arises in the attachments of the soleus muscle and its enveloping fascia to the periosteum of the posteromedial tibial margin. Pain and tenderness are provoked by running or jogging and relieved completely or partially by rest. Tenderness occurs over an extended length of the posteromedial tibia (middle and lower third of the bone) and the adjacent soleus muscle. The radionuclide angiogram and blood pool images are normal (phases 1 and 2), but the delayed phase demonstrates a long, narrow band of uptake along the posteromedial margin of the tibia that extends for one-third or more of the length of the bone. The uptake is of variable intensity. Plain radiographs usually appear normal, but in rare cases they may show cortical thickening and scalloping of the periosteal surface of the tibia. Bone biopsies (i.e., performed during experimental studies) have demonstrated periostitis and new bone formation. Intracompartmental pressures are usually normal.

21. ANTEROLATERAL TIBIAL MARGIN PAIN

Pain may follow a sudden burst of running activity in an unconditioned person. Patients have diffuse pain and tenderness of the musculotendinous attachment of the anterior compartment muscles to the tibia. Rest for 2 to 14 days usually results in resolution of pain and tenderness.

There are no bone tenderness and no increase in radio-nuclide uptake. Pain associated with bone tenderness may also occur along the anterolateral margin of the tibia. Localized tenderness indicates a stress fracture, and more diffuse linear tenderness extending 8 cm or more along the bone edge suggests periostitis. These impressions can be confirmed by radionuclide studies and radiographs.

22. DISTAL DEEP POSTERIOR COMPARTMENT SYNDROME

Aching or sharp pain occurs in the distal lower leg during running and is relieved or persists after rest. A sensation of tightness may occur during exercise, and up to 39 percent of patients with this disorder may experience paresthesias over the instep of the foot. Tenderness is localized to the deep distal calf muscles and is absent over the tibia and its adjacent musculotendinous posteromedial attachment to the deep calf muscles. The pain is referred to the posteromedial calf, deep behind the tibia. Resting pressures in the deep posterior compartment are elevated even hours after exercise and increase to higher levels during exercise. Discomfort may last for up to 24 h after exercise or may persist indefinitely. Some patients experience symptoms only during running, and this discomfort is promptly relieved by stopping. Other patients may continue to run, despite the pain, only to experience severe pain and tightness over the next 24 h. This syndrome tends to recur with each attempt at exercise and is relieved by avoidance of the provoking activity. An acute compartment syndrome may accompany a fracture, a muscle tear and hematoma, or a marked amount of leg exercise performed by a usually sedentary individual.

23. SHIN SPLINTS RELATED TO SYSTEMIC DISEASE

A. Syphilis In a single case report, the following findings were described. Pain appeared over the tibia with associated tenderness. Bilateral symptoms were present and were intensified or precipitated by vigorous exercise. There was diffuse tenderness over the tibia, and nocturnal pain occurred. Walking or leg movement partially relieved the pain. The serologic tests for syphilis were positive. A radionuclide bone scan revealed increased uptake over the length of both tibias. Symptoms resolved in 7 to 10 days after the initiation of penicillin therapy. Acute periostitis is a rare presentation of early acquired syphilis.

B. Paget's Disease of the Tibia In a single case report, the following findings were presented. Pain and swelling

over the tibial region on one side occurred with exercise. A radionuclide scan revealed diffuse uptake over the painful tibia. A plain radiograph demonstrated tibial cortical thickening; a coarsened, irregular trabecular pattern; and enlargement and anterior bowing.

24. GREATER SAPHENOUS THROMBOPHLEBITIS

This disorder causes local pain, redness, swelling, warmth, and tenderness over the medial lower leg. A palpable, tender cord is usually present. Fever and malaise may occur. A history of trauma or use of the vein for intravenous access may be obtained.

25. SAPHENOUS NEURITIS

Pain, hypesthesia, hyperesthesia, and/or paresthesias occur over the medial aspect of the lower leg. This disorder may occur as part of a femoral neuropathy associated with anterior thigh pain. It also occurs after surgical removal of the saphenous vein for use as a graft in coronary artery bypass surgery.

26. OSTEOMYELITIS OF THE TIBIA

This infection is most common in infants and children and usually occurs in the distal or proximal aspect of the tibia in the metaphyseal and epiphyseal regions. Local pain, skin warmth, swelling, and bone tenderness are usually accompanied by fever and leukocytosis. There is a good response to parenteral antibiotic therapy. Infections localizing to these regions of the tibia are usually hematogenous in origin. *S. aureus,* streptococcal species, or gram-negative bacteria are the usual isolates from bone biopsies.

Nonhematogenous osteomyelitis of the tibia results from an open fracture or as a complication of an open reduction. Symptoms may begin weeks or months after the initial injury or surgical procedure. They may include fever, chills, local pain, skin redness, and edema. Signs may include, purulent drainage, localized bone tenderness, skin erythema, and a limp. Plain radiographs may show only the fracture site or may demonstrate bone erosion, osteopenia, bone lucencies, and a periosteal reaction. Reliable cultures require bone biopsy. Criteria for diagnosis include positive bone culture results, histopathologic findings supportive of the diagnosis, and radiographic signs of osteomyelitis. The usual isolates are *S. aureus* and/or gram-negative bacteria.

Symptoms and signs resolve with antibiotic therapy. Surgical debridement of necrotic, infected bone may be required in up to 83 percent of cases.

Dermatologic Disorders of the Leg

27. NODULAR PANNICULITIS

Red, painful, and tender plaques and nodules (0.5–10 cm in diameter) appear over the lower legs and ankle region on one or both sides. These lesions may coalesce. The nodules are firm to fluctuant and may necrose centrally, draining a yellow-white, oily fluid that is often mistaken for pus. This drainage stains strongly for free fat with a Sudan stain. Some patients have only skin lesions, while others develop fever, ecchymoses, marked leukocytosis, nodular pulmonary lesions, and elevated serum amylase and lipase levels. This disorder is most commonly mistaken for a cellulitis or a superficial thrombophlebitis. Systemic causes include connective tissue diseases (e.g., scleroderma or lupus erythematosus), lymphoproliferative disorders (e.g., lymphoma or histiocytoma), alpha$_1$-antitrypsin deficiency, pancreatic disease (e.g., pancreatitis or carcinoma of the pancreas), generalized lipodystrophy, and paraproteinemia with a C1 inhibitor deficiency.

Histiocytic cytophagic panniculitis is associated with fever, pleuritis, liver and spleen enlargement, pancytopenia, coagulation defects, and nodular panniculitis. Nodular panniculitis may appear at any skin site, but it has a predilection for the lower extremities.

28. ERYTHEMA NODOSUM

Bilateral, tender, red, subcutaneous nodules occur over the anterior tibial and pretibial regions. Similar lesions, in less abundance, may occur on the forearms. Pain may occur but is less common than lesion tenderness. Fever, malaise, and ankle and knee pain and swelling may occur. Unilateral or bilateral hilar adenopathy may occur. These lesions do not usually ulcerate. Cases associated with group A streptococcal respiratory infection, sarcoidosis, inflammatory bowel disease, nonspecific respiratory infections, and an idiopathic group are most common.

Rare etiologies include tuberculosis; histoplasmosis; coccidioidomycosis; blastomycosis; deep *Trichophyton* infections; drugs (e.g., oral contraceptives or sulfa drugs); psittacosis; cat-scratch fever; Behçet's syndrome; infections with *Chlamydia*, *Yersinia*, or *Salmonella* species; and leprosy (erythema nodosum leprosum).

29. ARTERIAL AND HYPERTENSIVE ULCERS

Unilateral or bilateral, punched-out, painful, tender ulcers, several millimeters to 1 to 2 cm in size, occur over the anterior tibial or pretibial region. Hypertension and peripheral vascular disease are associated.

30. SYSTEMIC VASCULITIS WITH ULCERATION

Painful ulceration of the lower legs may occur due to a vasculitis associated with systemic lupus erythematosus, polyarteritis nodosa, rheumatoid arthritis, or Wegener's granulomatosis. These lesions may begin as subcutaneous, erythematous, painful nodules and evolve into irregular, deep, purulent ulcerations over the lower legs. Ischemic lower leg ulcers may also occur in sickle cell anemia.

31. ERYTHEMA INDURATUM

Subcutaneous, brownish-red or bluish nodules occur over the calves and anterior lower legs. Bilateral lesions are usually present. Flat, subcutaneous plaques may also appear. Necrosis of the nodules and secondary infection may cause painful ulcerations that may persist for a long time. Biopsy reveals granulomatous inflammation, vasculitis, and panniculitis. This disease has a predilection for the calves, while erythema nodosum primarily occurs on the anterior aspect of the lower legs.

Generalized Ankle Pain

32. ACUTE INJURIES OF THE ANKLE

Pain on the medial and lateral aspect of the ankle may follow trauma. It may be caused by bone fracture or by a combination of ligament disruption and fracture. Four types of ankle injuries are designated in the Lauge-Hansen classification system (see sections A through D below). The first word describes the position of the foot at the time of injury and the second the direction of the force causing the injury. Five additional types of ankle injuries are also discussed.

A. Supination-Adduction Initially there is a transverse fracture of the lateral malleolus or a tear of the lateral collateral ligament. With more severe force, this injury is combined with an oblique fracture of the medial malleolus. There are pain, swelling, and tenderness over the medial and lateral aspects of the ankle. Disruption of the ring of the ankle mortise at two sites results in a varus deformity of the foot as the talus is displaced medially. Plain radiographs will reveal a transverse fracture of the fibula, a vertical oblique fracture of the medial malleolus, and, in severe cases, medial displacement of the malleoli and the talus.

B. Supination-External Rotation (Eversion) Pain, swelling, diffuse tenderness, and ecchymoses may occur about the entire circumference of the ankle. External rotation of the foot or internal rotation of the leg on the fixed foot may initially rupture the anterior tibiofibular ligament. More severe force may cause a spiral or oblique fracture of the lateral malleolus, fracture of the posterior tibial margin, and rupture of the deltoid ligament or fracture of the medial malleolus. The talus may shift laterally, producing a valgus deformity of the ankle. A radiograph demonstrating a fracture of the lateral malleolus may show a fracture of the medial malleolus or widening of the medial clear space between the medial malleolus and the talus due to a tear of the deltoid ligament.

C. Pronation-Abduction This type of injury may cause only rupture of the deltoid ligament or fracture of the medial malleolus. More severe force results in rupture of both anterior inferior and posterior inferior tibiofibular ligaments, fracture of the posterior lip of the articular surface of the tibia, and a fibular fracture just proximal to the ankle joint or 8 to 10 cm proximal to the joint (Dupuytren type). The talus is shifted laterally, resulting in a valgus deformity of the foot. The medial malleolus may penetrate the skin, resulting in an open fracture.

D. Pronation-External Rotation (Eversion) An avulsion fracture of the medial malleolus or a tear of the deltoid ligament is the initial injury. More severe force may cause disruption of the anterior inferior tibiofibular ligament and interosseous ligaments, an interosseous membrane tear and a spiral fracture of the fibula 7 to 8 cm proximal to the lateral malleolus, and an avulsion fracture of the posterior lip of the tibia associated with ligamentous avulsion of the posterior inferior and inferior transverse tibiofibular ligaments. A valgus deformity of the foot occurs as the talus tilts and shifts laterally.

E. Pronation-Dorsiflexion This type of injury was added to the Lauge-Hansen classification by Pettrone. Increasingly severe force may fracture the medial malleolus or rupture the deltoid ligament, fracture the anterior lip of the tibial articular surface, cause a supramalleolar fracture of the fibula, and cause a transverse fracture of the posterior lip of the tibial articular surface.

Fractures should be suspected when localized point or linear tenderness occur over bone, bony crepitus is palpable, swelling and ecchymoses are extensive, and a valgus or varus deformity of the foot is present. Anteroposterior, lateral, and mortise views of the ankle will usually demonstrate most fractures and dislocations. Disruption of the ring of the ankle mortise at one site may allow weight bearing with a limp, but disruption at two or more sites makes walking impossible because of pain and the instability of the ankle mortise.

F. Anterior Dislocation of the Ankle This injury results from a posteriorly directed force that displaces the tibia on the foot. All ligaments and capsular attachments of the tibia and fibula to the talus are torn, except in some cases the posterior talofibular ligament. The foot appears slightly dorsiflexed and elongated anteriorly relative to the other foot. The grooves that parallel the Achilles tendon are absent. The talus may be palpable anteriorly. Ankle motion is limited and painful, and diffuse swelling and pain may occur.

G. Posterior Dislocation of the Ankle This injury follows an anteriorly directed blow to the posterior tibia, resulting in plantar flexion and shortening of the foot. Plain radiographs will demonstrate both types of dislocation. Ankle dislocations may be reduced by manual traction.

H. Fracture of the Neck of the Talus This deceleration injury occurs with the foot hyperdorsiflexed. It occurs in motor vehicle accidents or during a fall from a height. There are severe ankle and foot pain and diffuse ankle swelling and tenderness. Deformity of the ankle and foot region results from subluxation or dislocation of the talus. Medial or lateral malleolar fractures may be associated in up to 28 percent of cases. Plain radiographs (anteroposterior, oblique, and lateral) will demonstrate talar body displacement from the ankle mortise and the fracture line through the neck of the talus. Dislocation of both the subtalar and tibiotalar joints may occur.

I. Fracture of the Body of the Talus This is an uncommon type of fracture. It usually follows a fall from a height that results in axial compression of the talus between the tibial plafond and the calcaneus. Pain and swelling occur at the ankle, and local tenderness may be present over the talus. Inversion and eversion of the foot are extremely painful, as is flexion of the ankle.

33. ACUTE MONARTHRITIS OF THE ANKLE

A. Septic Arthritis Pain, swelling, skin erythema and warmth, and diffuse ankle tenderness occur. Fever, chills, and diaphoresis may be prominent symptoms in some cases. Other patients are afebrile and have minimal systemic signs. Synovial fluid cell counts may be as low as 5000 cells/mm^3 or may exceed 250,000 cells/mm^3. Some patients have a low synovial glucose level. Culture results are positive in 60 to 90 percent of cases. Patients in the sexually active age group may have *N. gonorrhoeae* arthritis. This organism may be isolated from the joint fluid or from mucous membrane sites. Other patients with septic arthritis usually have another local or remote site of active infection, a history of prior ankle joint trauma or disease, and/or evidence of immunosuppression. *S. aureus,* streptococcal species, and gram-negative bacteria are the organisms usually isolated from synovial fluid in patients with a nongonococcal etiology. There is a good response to antibiotic therapy and to some type of joint drainage procedure.

B. Acute Gout   Severe ankle pain, swelling, redness, warmth, tenderness, and fever may be caused by a crystal-induced arthritis. In gout, there may be a history of po-dagra or knee joint arthritis. The synovial fluid contains increased numbers of polymorphonuclear leukocytes and intra- and extracellular monosodium urate crystals. The serum uric acid level may be elevated or, less commonly, in the normal range.

C. Acute Pseudogout   This disorder may cause ankle arthritis clinically indistinguishable from gout. Synovial fluid contains intra- and extracellular calcium pyrophos-phate dihydrate crystals and increased numbers of poly-morphonuclear leukocytes. Chondrocalcinosis of the an-kles, knees, wrists, or shoulders may be present on plain radiographs of these joints.

D. Acute Rheumatoid Arthritis   Ankle pain, swelling, and tenderness without skin erythema or warmth develop over a period of several weeks. Serum rheumatoid factor may be present, and synovial fluid cell counts are in the inflammatory range (2000–50,000 cells/mm^3). Synovial fluid analysis may reveal a polymorphonuclear predomi-nance and a poor mucin clot. Synovial fluid C3 and C4 levels are decreased, and the glucose level may be slightly diminished or normal. Culture results are negative. In time, morning stiffness, symmetrical joint involvement, finger and wrist arthritis, involvement of three or more joint areas, subcutaneous nodules, and radiographic evi-dence of juxtaarticular erosions and osteopenia may occur in the fingers, hands, and wrists.

E. Reflex Sympathetic Dystrophy   Severe and per-sistent burning, throbbing, or aching ankle and/or foot pain occur 1 day or more after a relatively minor distal extremity injury. Early in the course, the skin of the distal leg and foot is warm and swollen; erythema is present diffusely or only over joints. Increased hair growth and sweating occur. The skin is tender, and allodynia is present. After 2 to 5 weeks, the distal portion of the limb becomes cool, pale, mottled, and cyanotic. Joint move-ments in the ankle and foot are impaired by stiffness and pain, and the swollen skin becomes shiny and smooth. Radiographs show diffuse osteopenia and cortical bone resorption. With progression, the joints become immobile and nonfunctional. Some cases are not associated with trauma. Triphasic radionuclide bone scans show increased periarticular uptake. The sensitivity of this test is 86 to 96 percent, and the specificity is 68 to 98 percent. Sym-pathetic blocks are the most reliable method of treating lower extremity reflex sympathetic dystrophy.

F. Hemophilic Arthropathy   An acute, painful hemar-throsis may occur. The ankle is third, behind the knee and elbow, as a site of intraarticular hemorrhage. Symp-toms respond to splinting, joint aspiration, and factor VIII replacement.

G. Acute Hemarthrosis   There is an abrupt onset of spontaneous swelling and ankle pain and tenderness, im-pairing ambulation. Aspiration reveals blood. The cause is rupture of a subsynovial vein or a synovial heman-gioma. There is no historical or other evidence of a coag-ulopathy.

34. TRANSIENT MIGRATORY OSTEOPOROSIS

Pain, swelling, and tenderness occur over the ankle joint. There is no pitting edema, warmth, or erythema, and joint mobility is preserved, in contrast to reflex sympathetic dystrophy. Ankle symptoms gradually resolve sponta-neously in 6 to 9 months. Within 1 to 2 years, pain and swelling may develop at another site (e.g., foot or knee). A radionuclide bone scan shows increased uptake in the ankle region, and there is radiographic evidence of diffuse osteoporosis of all bones adjacent to the ankle. The os-teoporosis in reflex sympathetic dystrophy is more spotty and subchondral. Symptoms may be relieved by salicy-lates or corticosteroids.

35. OSTEOCHONDRITIS DISSECANS OF THE TALUS

This disorder usually occurs in older children, adoles-cents, and young adults. Unilateral ankle pain and swell-ing are intensified by walking or jogging. There may be limitation of ankle mobility. Local tenderness may affect the anterior portion of the ankle joint, and there may be local tenderness over the anteromedial aspect of the talus. Plain radiographs show a small area of partially detached bone surrounded by a radiolucent margin. Such lesions may be more easily imaged by a CT scan or MRI. Healing may occur spontaneously with avoidance of weight bear-ing, or surgical intervention may be required. Some cases require arthroscopy for diagnosis and treatment.

36. ANKLE ARTHRITIS ASSOCIATED WITH ACUTE POLYARTHRITIS

A. Polyarticular Septic Arthritis   Up to 15 percent of cases of joint sepsis may involve two or more joints. *N. gonorrhoeae* may present as a monarthritis or as a migratory polyarthritis associated with vesiculopustular skin lesions on the arms and legs. *S. aureus,* streptococcal species, and gram-negative bacteria may also cause polyarthritis involving the ankle. There is a therapeutic response to antibiotic therapy.

B. Acute Rheumatic Fever   Fever, sweats, migratory arthritis, and subcutaneous nodules may occur. The joints may be swollen, red, warm, tender, and painful. There is a dramatic response to aspirin therapy. Serum levels of antistreptolysin O, antihyaluronidase, and antideoxyribonuclease B are elevated. The Streptozyme hemagglutination titer may show a rise during the course of the illness.

C. Lyme Disease   This disorder follows exposure to ticks in an endemic area. Up to 80 percent of patients develop an annular, erythematous skin lesion at the site of the tick bite. This lesion may be pruritic and may enlarge. Satellite ring lesions appear in some cases. The patient may develop an acute febrile illness during the 4 weeks following exposure, with myalgias, arthralgias, headache, and neck pain and stiffness (aseptic meningitis). Impaired ability to concentrate, memory deficits, and mild confusion indicate an encephalitic component of the acute illness. Swelling and pain may involve one or both knees (76 percent) and/or the ankles (12 percent), elbows (20 percent), and shoulders (28 percent). Demonstration of antibody to *Borrelia burgdorferi* and a therapeutic response to ceftriaxone therapy support the diagnosis.

D. Hepatitis B Virus-Associated Arthritis   This viral disease may cause an urticarial or maculopapular rash and a migratory or additive polyarthritis that involves the ankles in up to 25 percent of cases. Hepatitis B surface antigen is present in the serum, and liver function test results are often abnormal.

E. Rubella Arthritis   Natural infection or the rubella vaccine may both cause polyarticular joint pain and stiffness. A painful occipital lymphadenitis and a faint, pink macular rash usually precede joint symptoms but may follow them. The ankles are involved in up to 40 percent of the disease-associated disorder.

F. Arthritis Associated with Inflammatory Bowel Disease   Arthritis is more likely to occur in patients with colonic disease and other complications. The usual presentation is an acute polyarthritis with red, warm, swollen, painful joints. The knees, ankles, wrists, and elbows are more commonly involved than are the small hand and finger joints. Migratory arthritis occurs in up to 50 percent of cases. Synovial fluid cell counts are in the inflammatory range, and there is a polymorphonuclear predominance. The joint disease responds to successful therapy for the bowel disease.

G. Acute Polyarticular Gout   Fever and symmetrical

or asymmetrical acute arthritis occur. The lower extremities are involved most frequently. Redness, warmth, pain, swelling, and tenderness occur over the joints of the feet, ankles, knees, elbows, and wrists. Subdeltoid or olecranon bursitis may occur. Retrocalcaneal bursitis and Achilles tendinitis are also common and may be confused with arthritic involvement of the ankle.

The joint fluid contains monosodium urate crystals, and the serum uric acid level is elevated in most, but not all, cases. There is usually a dramatic response to colchicine or indomethacin therapy.

H. Calcium Pyrophosphate Deposition Disease   This disorder may present as an acute inflammatory polyarthritis with joint pain, swelling, and tenderness involving the wrists, hands, hips, shoulders, elbows, and ankles. Synovial fluid contains polymorphonuclear leukocytes in concentrations in the inflammatory range and calcium pyrophosphate dihydrate crystals. There may be radiographically demonstrable chondrocalcinosis in the knees, ankles, wrists, and shoulders. Acute attacks respond to colchicine or indomethacin therapy.

I. Reiter's Syndrome   This disorder causes an asymmetrical acute arthritis involving the hips, knees, ankles, shoulders, and wrists. Articular involvement may be accompanied by conjunctivitis or iridocyclitis and urethritis. Diarrhea may occur in some cases. Reiter's syndrome is a form of reactive arthritis and may follow an episode of urethritis or a bowel infection caused by a species of *Shigella*, *Salmonella*, *Yersinia*, *Campylobacter*, or *Clostridium difficile*. Mucocutaneous manifestations include oral ulcers, balanitis circinata, and psoriasis-like lesions of the soles (keratoderma blennorrhagicum). Heel pain may reflect an Achilles tendinitis at the site of tendon insertion into the calcaneus.

J. Acute Rheumatoid Arthritis   Up to 15 percent of cases may present as an acute polyarthritis with ankle involvement as described above.

37. ACUTE OSTEOMYELITIS

Fever, chills, ankle swelling, pain, and tenderness may suggest an acute arthritis or osteomyelitis of the tibia. An MRI or radionuclide bone scan is more sensitive than plain radiographs for confirmation of bone infection. This disorder usually occurs in infants and children and is rare in adults in the absence of significant local trauma (i.e., open fracture). Bone biopsy may be required to identify the responsible organism prior to initiating antibiotic therapy. Early cases usually respond well to parenteral antibiotic therapy.

Lateral Ankle Pain

38. LATERAL COLLATERAL LIGAMENT INJURIES (ANTERIOR TALOFIBULAR LIGAMENT, CALCANEOFIBULAR LIGAMENT, AND POSTERIOR TALOFIBULAR LIGAMENT)

The majority of ankle ligament sprains affect the lateral side of the ankle. Up to 97 percent of ligament ruptures leading to instability involve the anterior talofibular ligament (ATFL). Up to 25 percent of ATFL injuries are associated with sprains of the calcaneofibular ligament (CFL, middle ligament) and 10 percent involve the anterior tibiofibular ligament.

In an ATFL sprain, an adduction force is exerted on the plantar-flexed ankle joint. There is a sudden, sharp pain over the anterolateral aspect of the joint and well-localized tenderness over the ATFL (anterior and slightly inferior to the lateral malleolus). Within minutes, localized swelling appears, and in some cases ecchymosis is evident within 12 to 24 h along the lateral side of the heel and foot. Weight bearing intensifies the pain.

Some patients with prior injuries may adduct the ankle yet feel no pain for 1 to 2 days. The resultant inflammatory reaction during this latent period leads to the apparent spontaneous appearance of lateral ankle pain and localized tenderness and local or diffuse ankle swelling (40 percent of cases). These patients and their physicians may consider the pain to be due to arthritis in the absence of a history of injury. Most talofibular ligament tears are partial and do not result in ankle instability.

Testing for ligament rupture with associated instability requires local anesthesia (e.g., injection of lidocaine or bupivacaine into the painful site) or general anesthesia. The extent of anterior instability can be evaluated by the anterior drawer test. In this test, the patient lies supine with the hip and knee flexed (knee at 45° of flexion). One hand pulls the heel forward, and the opposite hand exerts stabilizing pressure on the lower tibia. A positive test result demonstrates forward movement of the talus in the ankle mortise of more than 8 mm on a lateral radiograph and is diagnostic of an ATFL tear. Anterior displacement may also be compared with the normal side.

Increased inversion of the heel on the affected side may also be demonstrable. The patient lies prone with the ankles extending beyond the edge of the examining table. Passive supination of the heels is performed on both sides, and the extent of movement on the injured and normal sides may be compared. Results of this test are most frequently positive when the CFL is also disrupted.

There is usually no tenderness over the lateral malleolus. In up to 5 percent of cases, a talar dome osteochondral fracture may occur, resulting in persistent ankle pain. Plain anteroposterior and lateral radiographs are taken to exclude a talar dome or a fibula avulsion or transverse fracture.

Stress radiographs are performed to determine the extent of ligament disruption and potential ankle instability. Anteroposterior stress films are taken with the ankle in 15° of internal rotation. Heel inversion is passively produced on both sides and the extent of talar tilt (i.e., the angle subtended by lines drawn along the tibial plafond and the dome of the talus on an anteroposterior radiograph) measured and compared. Talar tilt may be as great as 25° in normal ankles without a history of prior injury. It is less than 5° in 98 percent of normal ankles. There may be ankle-to-ankle variation in the same individual. Some authors cite a talar tilt value of twice the normal side, or over 9°, as evidence of lateral ligament rupture. Disruption of the anterior talofibular ligament may increase talar tilt in plantar flexion but not in a neutral position of the ankle. If both the talofibular ligament and CFL are torn, talar tilt is increased in both ankle positions and to a greater degree in plantar flexion.

Inversion stress testing is 68-percent accurate using local anesthesia and 92-percent accurate using general anesthesia.

The lateral stress film demonstrates the anterior drawer test radiographically. The distance from the talar dome to the posterior part of the tibial articular surface is measured. A distance exceeding 5 mm is considered abnormal. The lateral stress film is taken with the patient supine and the knee flexed to 30°. A static load of 4 kg is applied to the anterior tibia for 2 min before the film is obtained. (This test is a version of the anterior drawer test described above.) Neither the inversion nor the anterior drawer test can distinguish single or double ligament tears accurately. Isolated CFL tears are uncommon. Arthrography will demonstrate extraarticular dye anterior to the lateral malleolus with an ATFL tear, and dye in the peroneal tendon sheath with rupture of the CFL. Arthrography is superior to the inversion and drawer tests for diagnosis of ligament ruptures (96 percent accuracy).

39. MIMICS OF ANTERIOR TALOFIBULAR LIGAMENT SPRAIN

A. Anterior Tibiofibular Ligament Sprain Local pain, tenderness, and swelling occur over the area of this ligament. The extent of injury to the syndesmotic ligaments may be assessed using external rotation stress films of both ankles.

Abduction or abduction-external rotation injuries, in which all the syndesmotic ligaments are disrupted, are usually associated with tibiofibular separation apparent on routine radiographs. Diastasis occurs when the clear space between the medial cortex of the fibula and the posterior edge of the peroneal groove exceeds 5.5 mm in an anteroposterior view of the ankle.

B. Fracture of the Lateral Malleolus (Fibula) Pain, tenderness, and swelling occur over the surface of the fibula, and the ATFL is not tender. Plain radiographs will establish the diagnosis.

C. Fracture of the Lateral Process of the Talus Pain, swelling, and tenderness occur over the lateral ankle. Point tenderness occurs over the lateral process of the talus, slightly anterior and inferior to the tip of the lateral malleolus.

A lateral process fracture can be visualized clearly on a mortise view of the ankle. Careful and clear definition of the extent of the fracture can be determined by a CT scan. Delay in diagnosis and treatment can result in persistent ankle pain due to nonunion and posttraumatic arthritis of the subtalar joint. This fracture usually occurs when the foot is dorsiflexed and inverted.

D. Fracture of the Lateral Tubercle of the Posterior Process of the Talus These fractures may occur after inversion of the ankle as the posterior talofibular ligament avulses the lateral tubercle of the posterior process of the talus or after compression of the lateral tubercle with the ankle in an exaggerated equinus position. The patient presents as an ankle sprain with posterolateral ankle tenderness and pain. Movement of the ankle and subtalar joints causes pain. Active flexion of the big toe may also be painful as the flexor hallucis longus contracts in the vicinity of the fracture. The fracture can be demonstrated on a plain lateral radiograph. In some cases, confirmation by plain radiography may not be possible, and a CT scan may be useful. A missed diagnosis can result in persistently painful nonunion and posttraumatic arthritis.

E. Peroneal Peritendinitis The major cause of peroneal peritendinitis is trauma, including lateral malleolar fractures, inversion ankle injuries, direct trauma to the peroneal tubercle, and calcaneal fractures alone or associated with calcaneofibular impingement of the peroneal tendon sheaths.

There is a gradual onset of pain and edema below the lateral malleolus, with point tenderness over the peroneal tendons at the inferior peroneal retinaculum. Passive plantar flexion and inversion, and active eversion against resistance intensify the pain. Walking barefoot or on irregular ground may also increase symptoms. Point tenderness is present over one or both peroneal tendons, and subtalar motion is decreased. The pain may be eliminated for a short period by an injection of lidocaine into the tendon sheath. Peroneal contrast tenography usually demonstrates a block or constriction of the tendon sheath at the level of the inferior peroneal retinaculum.

F. Traumatic Dislocation of the Peroneal Tendons Anterior dislocation of the peroneal tendons from their retromalleolar groove occurs most commonly as an athletic injury. Sports associated with this disorder include skiing, ice-skating, soccer, basketball, and football.

This injury usually results from forceful passive dorsiflexion of the inverted foot with strong reflex contraction of the peroneal tendons. There is an abrupt onset of posterolateral ankle pain, accompanied by a snapping sensation. Swelling and tenderness soon occur posterior and superior to the tip of the lateral malleolus.

Injury to the posterior talofibular ligament may result in similar findings on inspection and palpation.

Attempted dorsiflexion against resistance with the foot plantar flexed and everted causes retromalleolar pain and may reproduce tendon dislocation. A severe injury with a rim avulsion fracture of the lateral malleolus confirms dislocation. Unless the dislocation is seen at the time of injury or can be reproduced on examination, the diagnosis is difficult to confirm. A CT scan may be of use in evaluating peroneal tendon dislocation.

G. Ganglion A mildly painful, cystic lesion (0.5–1.5 cm) may form over the lateral ankle below the lateral malleolus. This cyst may decrease in size after a night in bed. The pain is mild, or the lesion may be painless. It may follow an inversion injury of the ankle.

H. Stress Fracture of the Fibula Pain and tenderness occur over a localized portion of the posterolateral distal fibula. A radionuclide scan demonstrates localized round or fusiform uptake. Plain radiographs are frequently negative in the presence of a positive bone scan but may show a nondisplaced fracture line.

I. Calcaneofibular Ligament Sprain (Isolated) Pain, tenderness, and swelling occur over the lateral ankle inferior to the midportion of the lateral malleolus. There is point tenderness over the ligament on the fibula, on the calcaneus, or in the intervening space. Isolated tears are uncommon, and sprain of this ligament usually accompanies an ATFL injury.

Anterior Ankle Pain

40. PERITENDINITIS OF THE EXTENSOR TENDONS OF THE FOOT AND TOES

Pain occurs over the anterior aspect of the ankle. Swelling, tenderness, and skin erythema or crepitus may be present. The anterior ankle pain may be intensified by passive plantar flexion of the ankle (i.e., stretching the inflamed tendons), or by resisting extension of toes 2 to 5 (extensor digitorum longus) or the great toe (extensor hallucis longus), or ankle dorsiflexion (tibialis anterior and peroneus tertius). One or more of the extensor tendons of the toes and the foot may be involved. Direct palpation of individual tendons during resisted active movement for tenderness may be helpful in diagnosis.

41. CRUCIATE CRURAL LIGAMENT SPRAIN

This crural ligament is the major extensor retinaculum of the ankle joint. It prevents bow-stringing of the foot and toe extensor tendons that cross the anterior aspect of the ankle during ankle dorsiflexion. An injury to this ligament may occur in association with trauma to the extensor tendon. It may be torn during a fall or directly contused by an impact force delivered during a soccer or football game. The instep may become swollen, and tenderness is present over the ligament (retinaculum). Resisted toe extension will intensify the pain, as will local palpation of the ligament. Rest and use of a nonsteroidal anti-inflammatory drug may provide relief within 1 to 4 weeks.

42. ANTERIOR TIBIOFIBULAR LIGAMENT SPRAIN

Pain, tenderness, and swelling occur medial and superior to the lateral malleolus. Isolated injury of this ligament may cause a partial diastasis visible only on an external rotation stress radiograph.

43. FRACTURE OF THE ANTERIOR LIP OF THE DISTAL TIBIAL ARTICULAR SURFACE

This fracture follows a pronation-dorsiflexion injury. The anterior tibial injury may be associated with a fracture of the medial malleolus or rupture of the deltoid ligament. There are anterior ankle pain, tenderness, swelling, and sometimes ecchymoses. Plain radiographs will identify a fracture of the anterior lip of the tibial articular surface.

Medial Ankle Pain

44. DELTOID LIGAMENT SPRAIN

A deltoid ligament injury occurs with an abduction or external rotation force. Partial tears involving the anterior fibers of the ligament are more frequent than complete rupture. A fall in a hole with abduction or external rotation of the foot may injure this ligament. Medial ankle pain,

tenderness, ecchymoses, and edema follow the injury. Rupture of the ligament may be associated with a lateral malleolar fracture and/or disruption of the syndesmotic ligaments. A diagnosis of deltoid ligament rupture can be supported by a plain radiograph showing widening of the clear space between the inner surface of the medial malleolus and the talus to more than 4 mm (e.g., mortise view). Occasionally, abduction-external rotation stress films or arthrography are required to confirm the diagnosis.

45. FRACTURE OF THE MEDIAL MALLEOLUS

An isolated injury of the medial malleolus may follow an abduction or external rotation force applied to the pronated foot and ankle. There are local pain, swelling, and direct tenderness over the fracture line within the first hour after the injury. Within the first day, extensive swelling and diffuse tenderness may occur. The diagnosis can be confirmed by a plain radiograph.

46. TIBIALIS POSTERIOR TENDINITIS

Pain occurs over the medial aspect of the midfoot with radiation to the medial malleolus and posteromedial border of the distal tibia. Ankle movement intensifies the pain during activity. The posterior tibial tendon is tender, and swelling may be great enough to obliterate the normal concavity posterior to the medial malleolus. Crepitus may be palpable as the tendon moves during supination of the foot.

Resisted supination of the foot or passive pronation intensifies the pain. Tenderness over the tendon itself suggests an overuse-related disorder. If tenderness and pain are more prominent in the midfoot, an accessory navicular bone or a tendon-bone avulsion should be considered.

47. SHIN SPLINTS

Pain and tenderness over the distal posteromedial border of the tibia may be confused with a tibialis posterior tendinitis. There is local tenderness over the tibial margin (stress fracture) or more diffuse tenderness over one-third or more of the distal posteromedial tibial margin (periostitis) or over the muscle and fascia adjacent to the posteromedial tibial border (musculotendinous stress injury). These disorders can be differentiated by clinical findings and a radionuclide bone scan. A stress fracture produces a localized, round or fusiform, 2- to 3-cm area of increased radionuclide uptake; a periostitis causes a longitudinal band of irregular uptake, extending 8 cm or more along the medial tibial margin; and musculotendinous stress injuries do not show an increase in radionuclide uptake over the tibia.

48. FRACTURE OF THE SUSTENTACULUM TALI

This fracture may result from a fall on the heel with marked inversion of the foot. It is an uncommon isolated injury. Pain and tenderness occur over the medial ankle, heel, and hindfoot. Passive inversion of the foot causes pain below the medial malleolus. This injury is often mistaken for an ankle sprain. The diagnosis depends on the history of injury and localization of pain and tenderness just below the medial malleolus. Passive hyperextension of the great toe may also intensify the pain. An axial radiograph of the calcaneus should be obtained if this injury is suspected.

49. TENDINITIS OF THE FLEXOR HALLUCIS LONGUS AND FLEXOR DIGITORUM COMMUNIS

Medial ankle pain and tenderness occur posterior to the medial malleolus. Sprinting or attempts to jump provoke pain. Passive extension or resisted flexion of the small toes and/or great toe intensifies the pain. Local edema and tenderness over the tendons may be present. These tendons are more lateral (i.e., closer to the Achilles tendon) than the tendon of the tibialis posterior muscle.

Posterior Ankle Pain

50. ACHILLES TENDINITIS

Pain occurs over the Achilles tendon from its insertion on the calcaneus to a point 3 to 6 cm proximal to the insertion. The pain is intensified by activity, the tendon is tender, and palpable crepitus with movement may be present. Increased thickness of the tendon may be noted when the symptomatic tendon is compared to that on the asymptomatic side. Dorsiflexion may be limited to less than 25 to 45°. Radiographs may reveal calcification of the tendon or increased size of the superior tuberosity of the calcaneus. Systemic disorders that may be associated with Achilles tendinitis include rheumatoid arthritis and gout.

51. SUBCUTANEOUS ACHILLES BURSITIS

Local pain, swelling, and tenderness occur posterior to the Achilles tendon. A fluctuant, tender bursa may be palpable.

52. RETROCALCANEAL BURSITIS

This bursa occurs between the calcaneus and Achilles tendon. Pain, tenderness, and swelling occur anterior and to either side of the Achilles tendon just proximal to its insertion on the calcaneus. Light pinch pressure applied to the tissue anterior to the tendon elicits pain. This disorder may be associated with gout.

53. PARTIAL RUPTURE OF THE ACHILLES TENDON

Severe pain and tenderness over the Achilles tendon may begin abruptly. A nodule may be palpated in the tendon.

54. COMPLETE RUPTURE OF THE ACHILLES TENDON

This tendon usually ruptures 2 to 6 cm proximal to its insertion in the calcaneus. Severe pain in the posterior heel, ankle, and calf and a snap signal the rupture. A gap is palpable in the tendon, and local swelling, ecchymoses, and tenderness occur. Plantar flexion of the foot is impaired because of weakness, and this impairment can be confirmed by the Thompson test (failure of the ankle to plantar flex when the calf is squeezed). The standing patient has difficulty raising the affected heel.

55. FRACTURE OF THE CALCANEAL TUBEROSITY

This rare fracture produces functional loss similar to that produced by an Achilles tendon rupture. Avulsion is the usual cause. Elderly patients are susceptible to this injury. The usual event is a fall from a curb or down a step. The fragment is avulsed by a sudden pull of the Achilles tendon. Posterior heel and ankle pain, tenderness, swelling, and ecchymoses occur. Standing on tiptoe may be impaired. A plain lateral radiograph will confirm the diagnosis. The single-heel rise test (i.e., rising to tiptoe on one leg with the knee extended) may also be impaired with rupture of the tibialis posterior tendon.

Bilateral Lower Leg and Ankle Pain

The causes of bilateral ankle pain are listed in Table 46-1. These disorders may cause unilateral or bilateral pain.

LOWER LEG AND ANKLE PAIN REFERENCES

Ankle Pain—Anterior

Jones BH: Overuse injuries of the lower extremities associated with marching, jogging, and running: A review. *Mil Med* 148:783–787, 1983.

Nair UR, Griffiths G, Lawson RAM: Postoperative neuralgia in the leg after saphenous vein coronary artery bypass graft: A prospective study. *Thorax* 43:41–43, 1988.

Panni AS, Maiotti M, Burke J: Osteoid osteoma of the neck of the talus. *Am J Sports Med* 17:584–588, 1989.

Ankle Pain—General

Barber FA, Britt BT, Ratliff HW, et al: Arthroscopic surgery of the ankle. *Orthop Rev* 17:446–451, 1988.

Clanton TO: Instability of the subtalar joint. *Orthop Clin North Am* 20:583–592, 1989.

Ferkel RD, Fischer SP: Progress in ankle arthroscopy. *Clin Orthop* 240:210–220, 1989.

Goldie I: Talar and peritalar injuries, in Helal B, Wilson D (eds): *The Foot*. Edinburgh, Churchill Livingstone, 1988, vol 2, pp 916–931.

Hardaker WT Jr: Foot and ankle injuries in classical ballet dancers. *Orthop Clin North Am* 20:621–627, 1989.

Jackson P: Ankle injuries, in Helal B, Wilson D (eds): *The Foot*. Edinburgh, Churchill Livingstone, 1988, vol 2, pp 868–893.

Jahss MH: The subtalar complex in Jahss MH (ed): *Disorders of the Foot and Ankle,* 2d ed. Philadelphia, Saunders, 1991, vol 2, pp 1333–1371.

Mann RA, Baumgarten M: Subtalar fusion for isolated subtalar disorders: Preliminary report. *Clin Orthop* 226:260–265, 1988.

Mendel F, Gordin A, Herness D, et al: Transient bilateral peroneal palsy in a painter's model. *J Occupat Med* 29:109–111, 1987.

Schon LC, Ouzounian TJ: The ankle, in Jahss MH (ed): *Disorders of the Foot and Ankle,* 2d ed. Philadelphia, Saunders, 1991, vol 2, pp 1417–1460.

Waugh W: Ankle disorders, in Helal B, Wilson D (eds): *The Foot*. Edinburgh, Churchill Livingstone, 1988, vol 1, pp 550–566.

Wilson FC: Fractures and dislocations of the ankle, in Rockwood CA Jr, Green DP (eds): *Fractures in Adults*. Philadelphia, Lippincott, 1984, vol 2, pp 1665–1701.

Ankle Pain—Lateral

Airaksinen O, Kolari PJ, Miettinen H: Elastic bandages and intermittent pneumatic compression for treatment of acute ankle sprains. *Arch Phys Med Rehabil* 71:380–383, 1990.

Bassett FH III, Gates HS III, Billys JB, et al: Talar impingement by the anteroinferior tibiofibular ligament: A cause of chronic pain in the ankle after inversion sprain. *J Bone Joint Surg (Am)* 72A:55–59, 1990.

Dee R: Rheumatological and degenerative disorders of the foot and ankle, in Dee R, Mango E, Hurst LC (eds): *Principles of Orthopaedic Practice*. New York, McGraw-Hill, 1989, vol 2, pp 1385–1394.

Hocutt JE Jr, Jaffe R, Rylander CR, et al: Cryotherapy in ankle sprains. *Am J Sports Med* 10:316–319, 1982.

Larsen E, Aru A: Synovitis in chronically unstable ankles. *Acta Orthop Scand* 60:340–344, 1989.

Lassiter TE, Malone TR, Garrett WE Jr: Injury to the lateral ligaments of the ankle. *Orthop Clin North Am* 20:629–640, 1989.

Ryan JB, Hopkinson WJ, Wheeler JH, et al: Office management of acute ankle sprain. *Clin Sports Med* 8:477–493, 1989.

Sammarco GJ, DiRaimondo CV: Surgical treatment of lateral ankle instability syndrome. *Am J Sports Med* 16:501–511, 1988.

Ankle Pain—Medial

Dubey L, Krasinski K, Hernanz-Schulman M: Osteomyelitis secondary to trauma or infected contiguous soft tissue. *Pediatr Infect Dis J* 7:26–34, 1988.

Johnson DP, Hill J: Fracture-dislocation of the ankle with rupture of the deltoid ligament. *Injury* 19:59–61, 1988.

Kerr HD: Posterior tibial tendon rupture. *Ann Emerg Med* 17:649–650, 1988.

Shelbourne KD, Fisher DA, Rettig AC, et al: Stress fractures of the medial malleolus. *Am J Sports Med* 16:60–63, 1988.

Short LA, Mattana GW, Benton VG: Osteoid osteoma in the medial malleolus. *J Foot Surg* 27:264–267, 1988.

Wu KK: Unicameral bone cyst of the medial malleolus of the ankle. *J Foot Surg* 29:183–187, 1990.

Ankle Pain—Posterior

Krackow KA: Acute, traumatic rupture of a flexor hallucis longus tendon: A case report. *Clin Orthop Rel Res* 150:261–262, 1980.

Nelimarkka O, Lehto M, Järvinen M: Soleus muscle anomaly in a patient with exertion pain in the ankle: A case report. *Arch Orthop Trauma Surg* 107:120–121, 1988.

Calf—Muscle Cramps

Janssen M, Dijkmans BAC, Eulderink F: Muscle cramps in the calf as presenting symptom of sarcoidosis. *Ann Rheum Dis* 50:51–52, 1991.

Konikoff F, Theodor E: Painful muscle cramps: A symptom of liver cirrhosis? *J Clin Gastroenterol* 8:669–672, 1986.

Steiner I, Siegal T: Muscle cramps in cancer patients. *Cancer* 63:574–577, 1989.

Claudication—Neurogenic

Conley FK, Cady CT, Lieberson RE: Decompression of lumbar spinal stenosis and stabilization with Knodt rods in the elderly patient. *Neurosurgery* 26:758–763, 1990.

Dodge LD, Bohlman HH, Rhodes RS: Concurrent lumbar spinal stenosis and peripheral vascular disease: A report of nine patients. *Clin Orthop* 230:141–148, 1988.

Dong GX, Porter RW: Walking and cycling tests in neurogenic and intermittent claudication. *Spine* 14:965–969, 1989.

Downs SE: Unilateral intermittent claudication of the lower left extremity. *J Manipulative Physiol Ther* 11:322–324, 1988.

Eskola A, Alaranta H, Pohjolainen T, et al: Calcitonin treatment in lumbar spinal stenosis: Clinical observations. *Calcif Tissue Int* 45:372–374, 1989.

Health JM: The clinical presentation of lumbar spinal stenosis. *Ohio Med* 85:484–487, 1989.

Jensen OH, Schmidt-Olsen S: A new functional test in the diagnostic evaluation of neurogenic intermittent claudication. *Clin Rheumatol* 8:363–367, 1989.

Lipson SJ: Spinal stenosis. *Rheum Dis Clin North Am* 14:613–618, 1988.

Morgenlander JC, Massey EW: Neurogenic claudication with positionally dependent weakness from a thoracic disk herniation. *Neurology* 39:1133–1134, 1989.

Porter RW, Miller CG: Neurogenic claudication and root claudication treated with calcitonin: A double-blind trial. *Spine* 13:1061–1064, 1988.

Young S, Veerapen R, O'Laoire SA: Relief of lumbar canal stenosis using multilevel subarticular fenestrations as an alternative to wide laminectomy: Preliminary report. *Neurosurgery* 23:628–633, 1988.

Claudication — Vascular

Coffman JD: New drug therapy in peripheral vascular disease. *Med Clin North Am* 72:259–265, 1988.

Collins PS, McDonald PT, Lim RC: Popliteal artery entrapment: An evolving syndrome. *J Vasc Surg* 10:484–490, 1989.

Dorigo B, Bartoli V, Grisillo D, et al: Fibrositic myofascial pain in intermittent claudication: Effect of anesthetic block of trigger points on exercise tolerance. *Pain* 6:183–190, 1979.

Jelnes R, Bülow J, Tønnesen KH: A pitfall in the evaluation of medical therapy for occlusive arterial disease using the xenon wash-out technique. *Scand J Clin Lab Invest* 47:229–231, 1987.

Jørgensen B, Henriksen LO, Karle A, et al: Percutaneous transluminal angioplasty of iliac and femoral arteries in severe lower-limb ischaemia. *Acta Chir Scand* 154:647–652, 1988.

Lundgren F, Dahllöf A-G, Lundholm K, et al: Intermittent claudication: Surgical reconstruction or physical training? A prospective randomized trial of treatment efficiency. *Ann Surg* 209:346–355, 1989.

Mukherjee D, Inahara T: Endarterectomy as the procedure of choice for atherosclerotic occlusive lesions of the common femoral artery. *Am J Surg* 157:498–500, 1989.

Prevention of Atherosclerotic Complications with Ketanserin claudication substudy investigators: Randomized placebo-controlled, double-blind trial of ketanserin in claudicants: Changes in claudication distance and ankle systolic pressure. *Circulation* 80:1544–1548.

Shestak KC, Fitz DG, Newton ED, et al: Expanding the horizons in treatment of severe peripheral vascular disease using microsurgical techniques. *Plast Reconstr Surg* 8:406–411, 1990.

Compartment Syndrome — Lower Leg

Anouchi YS, Parker RD, Seitz WH Jr: Posterior compartment syndrome of the calf resulting from misdiagnosis of a rupture of the medial head of the gastrocnemius. *J Trauma* 27:678–680, 1987.

Turnipseed W, Detmer DE, Girdley F: Chronic compartment syndrome: An unusual cause for claudication. *Ann Surg* 210:557–563, 1989.

Fractures — Tibial Shaft

Holbrook JL, Swiontkowski MF, Sanders R: Treatment of open fractures of the tibial shaft: Ender nailing versus external fixation, a randomized, prospective comparison. *J Bone Joint Surg (Am)* 71A:1231–1238, 1989.

Peter RE, Bachelin P, Fritschy D: Skiers' lower leg shaft fracture: Outcome in 91 cases treated conservatively with Sarmiento's brace. *Am J Sports Med* 16:486–491, 1988.

Leg Pain — Review

Crisci C, Baker MK, Wood MB, et al: Trochanteric sciatic neuropathy. *Neurology* 39:1539–1541, 1989.

Provan JL, Moreau P, MacNab I: Pitfalls in the diagnosis of leg pain. *Can Med Assoc J* 121:167–171, 1979.

Lower Leg Pain — Anterior

Bates P: Shin splints: A literature review. *Br J Sports Med* 19:132–137, 1985.

DeCamp JR: Radiology Clinic: Female runner with shin pain. *Indiana Med* 81:1021–1022, 1988.

Detmer DE: Chronic leg pain. *Am J Sports Med* 8:141–144, 1980.

———: Chronic shin splints: Classification and management of medial tibial stress syndrome. *Sports Med* 3:436–446, 1986.

Golding DN: Pain and periostitis. *R Soc Med* 78:706–707, 1985.

Mason BA, Kressel BR, Cashdollar MR, et al: Periostitis associated with myelofibrosis. *Cancer* 43:1568–1571, 1979.

Meier JL, Mollet E: Acute periostitis in early acquired syphilis simulating shin splints in a jogger. *Am J Sports Med* 14:327–328, 1986.

Michael RH, Holder LE: The soleus syndrome: A cause of medial tibial stress (shin splints). *Am J Sports Med* 13:87–94, 1985.

Milgrom C, Giladi M, Stein M, et al: Medial tibial pain: A prospective study of its cause among military recruits. *Clin Orthop* 213:167–171, 1986.

Styf J: Chronic exercise-induced pain in the anterior aspect of the lower leg: An overview of diagnosis. *Sports Med* 7:331–339, 1989.

———: Diagnosis of exercise-induced pain in the anterior aspect of the lower leg. *Am J Sports Med* 16:165–169, 1988.

Lower Leg Pain — General

Carpenter CCJ: Other pathogenic vibrios, in Mandell GL, Douglas RG Jr, Bennett JE (eds): *Principles and Practice of Infectious Diseases,* 3d ed. New York, Churchill Livingstone, 1990, pp 1646–1649.

Goldstein EJC: Bites, in Mandell GL, Douglas RG Jr, Bennett JE (eds): *Principles and Practice of Infectious Diseases,* 3d ed. New York, Churchill Livingstone, 1990, pp 834–837.

Leach RE: Fractures of the tibia and fibula, in Rockwood CA Jr, Green DP (eds): *Fractures in Adults.* Philadelphia, Lippincott, 1984, vol 2, pp 1593–1663.

Swartz MN: Cellulitis and superficial infections, in Mandell GL, Douglas RG Jr, Bennett JE (eds): *Principles and Practice of Infectious Diseases,* 3d ed. New York, Churchill Livingstone, 1990, pp 796–807.

Swartz MN: Lymphadenitis and lymphangiitis, in Mandell GL, Douglas RG Jr, Bennett JE (eds): *Principles and Practice of Infectious Diseases,* 3d ed. New York, Churchill Livingstone, 1990, pp 818–825.

Swartz MN: Myositis, in Mandell GL, Douglas RG Jr, Bennett JE (eds): *Principles and Practice of Infectious Diseases,* 3d ed. New York, Churchill Livingstone, 1990, 812–818.

Swartz MN: Subcutaneous tissue infections and abscesses, in Mandell GL, Douglas RG Jr, Bennett JE (eds): *Principles and Practice of Infectious Diseases,* 3d ed. New York, Churchill Livingstone, 1990, pp 808–812.

Lower or Posterior Lower Leg Pain

Greenfield LJ: Venous and lymphatic disease, in Schwartz SI (ed): *Principles of Surgery,* 5th ed. New York, McGraw-Hill, 1989, pp 1011–1040.

Imparato AM, Riles TS: Peripheral arterial disease, in Schwartz SI (ed): *Principles of Surgery,* 5th ed. New York, McGraw-Hill, 1989, pp 933–1010.

Pseudothrombophlebitis

Chaudhuri R, Salari R: Baker's cyst simulating deep vein thrombosis. *Clin Radiol* 41:400–404, 1990.

Churgin P: Acute calf pain: Is MRI overkill? *Hosp Prac* 27:12, 1992.

Hall S, Littlejohn GO, Brand C, et al: The painful swollen calf: A comparative evaluation of four investigative techniques. *Med J Aust* 144:356–358, 1986.

Kashani SR, Moon AH, Gaunt WD: Tibial nerve entrapment by a Baker cyst: Case report. *Arch Phys Med Rehabil* 66:49–51, 1985.

Mahdyoon H, Mermiges DN, Wisgerhof M: Conn's syndrome with rhabdomyolysis mimicking deep vein thrombophlebitis. *South Med J* 83:346–347, 1990.

Pakter RL, Fishman EK, Zerhouni EA: Calf hematoma: Computed tomographic and magnetic resonance findings. *Skeletal Radiol* 16:393–396, 1987.

Prosser AJ, Brenkel IJ, Pearse M, et al: Popliteal vein obstruction by an osteochondroma of the proximal tibia. *Postgrad Med J* 63:657–659, 1987.

Reilly PA, Maddison PJ: Painful, swollen calf in a patient with SLE. *Br J Rheumatol* 26:319–320, 1987.

Small M, Alzaid A, Gray HW: Rhabdomyolysis mimicking deep vein thrombosis. *Postgrad Med J* 63:653–655, 1987.

Unger EC, Glazer HS, Lee JKT, et al: MRI of extracranial hematomas: Preliminary observations. *AJR* 146:403–407, 1986.

Yagupsky P, Shahak E, Barki Y: Non-invasive diagnosis of pyomyositis *Clin Pediatr* 27:299–301, 1988.

Venous Occlusive Disease

Appelman PT, DeJong TE, Lampmann LE: Deep venous thrombosis of the leg: US findings. *Radiology* 163:743–746, 1987.

Baxter GM, McKechnie S, Duffy P: Colour Doppler ultrasound in deep venous thrombosis: A comparison with venography. *Clin Radiol* 42:32–36, 1990.

Cohen JR, Tymon R, Pillari G, et al: Regional anatomical differences in the venographic occurrence of deep venous thrombosis and long-term follow-up. *J Cardiovasc Surg* 29:547–551, 1988.

Foley WD, Middleton WD, Lawson TL, et al: Color Doppler ultrasound imaging of lower-extremity venous disease. *AJR* 152:371–376, 1989.

Jennings AM, Walker M, Ward JD: Diabetic neuropathic bladder associated with clinical features of iliofemoral venous thrombosis. *Diabetic Med* 5:391–392, 1988.

Killewich LA, Bedford GR, Beach KW, et al: Diagnosis of deep venous thrombosis: A prospective study comparing duplex scanning to contrast venography. *Circulation* 79:810–814, 1989.

Krupski WC, Bass A, Dilley RB, et al: Propagation of deep venous thrombosis identified by duplex ultrasonography. *J Vasc Surg* 12:467–475, 1990.

Polak JF, Culter SS, O'Leary DH: Deep veins of the calf: Assessment with color Doppler flow imaging. *Radiology* 171:481–485, 1989.

Rose SC, Zwiebel WJ, Nelson BD, et al: Symptomatic lower extremity deep venous thrombosis: Accuracy, limitations, and role of color duplex flow imaging in diagnosis. *Radiology* 175:639–644, 1990.

Stringer MD, Steadman CA, Hedges AR, et al: Deep vein thrombosis after elective knee surgery: An incidence study in 312 patients. *J Bone Joint Surg (Br)* 71B:492–497, 1989.

Totterman S, Francis CW, Foster TH, et al: Diagnosis of femoropopliteal venous thrombosis with MR imaging: A comparison of four MR pulse sequences. *AJR* 154:175–178, 1990.

Vaughan BF: CT of swollen legs. *Clin Radiol* 41:24–30, 1990.

Vogel P, Laing FC, Jeffrey RB Jr, et al: Deep venous thrombosis of the lower extremity: US evaluation. *Radiology* 163:747–751, 1987.

Ward PE, Bradley FB, Brown JG, et al: Impedance plethysmography: A noninvasive screening method to detect deep-vein thrombosis. *Clin Orthop Rel Res* 248:195–199, 1989.

Acute Foot Pain

☐ DIAGNOSTIC LIST

GENERALIZED FOOT PAIN

1. Trauma
   A. Crush injury
   B. Compartment syndrome of the foot
   C. Traumatic amputation of the foot
2. Infection
   A. Cellulitis
      1. Cellulitis due to *Staphylococcus aureus* and streptococcal species
      2. Cellulitis due to *Aeromonas hydrophila*
      3. Cellulitis due to *Vibrio vulnificus*
      4. Cellulitis at a saphenous vein donor site
   B. Necrotizing fasciitis
   C. Abscess of the foot
   D. Osteomyelitis of the foot
3. Arthritis of the foot
   A. Septic arthritis
   B. Seropositive rheumatoid arthritis
      1. Forefoot pain
      2. Midfoot pain
      3. Hindfoot pain
   C. Seronegative spondyloarthropathies
      1. Ankylosing spondylitis
      2. Reiter's syndrome

3. Psoriatic arthritis
   4. Arthritis associated with inflammatory bowel disease
   D. Acute gout
   E. Acute pseudogout
   F. Acute rheumatic fever
   G. Systemic lupus erythematosus
   H. Sickle cell pain crisis
   I. Hepatitis B-associated arthritis
   J. Rubella-associated arthritis
4. Vascular pain
   A. Acute arterial occlusion
   B. Nocturnal rest pain
   C. Ulceration and gangrene
      1. Cholesterol embolism
      2. Arteriosclerosis obliterans and progressive ischemia
      3. Systemic vasculitis
         a. Polyarteritis nodosa
         b. Allergic angiitis and granulomatosis (Churg-Strauss disease)
         c. Systemic lupus erythematosus
         d. Rheumatoid arthritis
         e. Hypersensitivity vasculitis
         f. Thromboangiitis obliterans (Buerger's disease)
      4. Erythromelalgia

5. Phlegmasia cerulea dolens (venous gangrene of the foot)
5. Reflex sympathetic dystrophy
6. Foot cramps
7. Peripheral polyneuropathy
   A. Endocrine
      1. Diabetic polyneuropathy
         a. Acute sensory polyneuropathy
         b. Subacute or chronic sensorimotor polyneuropathy
         c. Mononeuritis multiplex
      2. Hypothyroid polyneuropathy
   B. Toxic
      1. Alcoholic polyneuropathy
      2. Heavy metal poisoning
         a. Arsenic polyneuropathy
         b. Mercury polyneuropathy
         c. Thallium polyneuropathy
      3. Drugs
         a. Disulfiram
         b. Isoniazid
         c. Hydralazine
         d. Other drugs (Table 47-3)
      4. Chemicals (Table 47-4)
   C. Systemic disorders
      1. Carcinoma
         a. Subacute sensory polyneuropathy
         b. Sensorimotor polyneuropathy
      2. Acute leukemia
      3. Chronic leukemia
      4. Lymphoma
      5. Myeloma
         a. Lytic
         b. Osteosclerotic
         c. POEMS syndrome
      6. Waldenstrom's macroglobulinemia
      7. Cryoglobulinemia
      8. Primary amyloidosis
      9. Connective tissue diseases
         a. Polyarteritis nodosa
         b. Other collagen vascular diseases (rheumatoid arthritis, systemic lupus erythematosus, and Churg-Strauss disease)

      10. Renal failure (uremic neuropathy)
      11. AIDS (distal symmetrical polyneuropathy)
      12. Sarcoidosis
   D. Hereditary
      1. Fabry's disease
      2. Intermittent acute porphyria
8. Nerve and root compression syndromes
   A. Tarsal tunnel syndrome
   B. Superficial peroneal nerve entrapment
   C. Deep peroneal nerve entrapment
   D. Sural nerve entrapment
   E. L5 and S1 root compression
9. Cold injury
   A. Frostbite
      1. First degree
      2. Second degree
      3. Third degree
   B. Trench foot
   C. Immersion foot
   D. Pernio (chilblains)
10. Bites
   A. Human bites
   B. Dog bites
   C. Cat bites
   D. Venomous snake bites
   E. Recluse spider bites
   F. Sea urchin stings
   G. Venomous fish stings
11. Cutaneous disorders
   A. Palmoplantar pustulosis with or without psoriasis
   B. Dyshidrotic eczema (pompholyx)
   C. Pustular bacterid of hands and feet
   D. Acrodermatitis continua
   E. Infectious eczematoid dermatitis
   F. Hand-foot-and-mouth disease
   G. Herpes zoster
   H. Vesicular type of tinea pedis
   I. Atopic dermatitis
   J. Contact dermatitis (shoe dermatitis)
   K. Vitamin B deficiencies
   L. Fixed drug eruption
   M. Erosive lichen planus

FOREFOOT PAIN
12. Metatarsalgia of rays 2 to 4 (metatarsal head overload)

A. High-heeled shoes
B. Equinus foot
C. Cavus foot
D. First-ray insufficiency syndrome (Morton's syndrome)
   1. Deutschlander's disease (march fractures)
   2. Chronic first-ray insufficiency
E. Central-ray overload syndrome
13. Freiberg's disease
14. Second metatarsal space syndrome
15. Morton's neuroma (plantar interdigital neuroma)
16. Idiopathic synovitis of the second metatarsophalangeal joint
17. Inflammatory arthritis of the metatarsophalangeal joints
18. Arterial insufficiency
19. Traumatic metatarsal fractures
20. Forefoot sprain
21. Bursitis (submetatarsal and interdigital)
22. Submetatarsal cysts
23. Self-inflicted trauma

GREAT TOE AND MEDIAL FOREFOOT PAIN

24. Trauma
A. First metatarsophalangeal joint injury
   1. Sprain
   2. Dislocation
   3. Sesamoid fracture
B. Fracture of the great toe
C. Dislocation of the interphalangeal joint
D. Subungual hematoma
E. Crush injury of the distal toe (soft tissue injury)
25. Plantar cutaneous lesions
A. Calluses
B. Plantar warts
C. Corns
26. Nail lesions of the hallux
A. Ingrown toenail
B. Infected ingrown toenail
C. Subungual melanocarcinoma
D. Subungual glomus tumor
E. Other subungual tumors
F. Paronychia
G. Pulp space infection
H. Infected blister
27. Hallux valgus
28. Bunion of the great toe

29. Hallux limitus or rigidus
30. Hallucal sesamoid disorders
31. First metatarsophalangeal joint arthritis
A. Septic arthritis and osteomyelitis
B. Podagra
32. Joplin's neuroma
33. Gangrene or ulceration of the great toe
34. Radicular pain (L5 root)
35. Shoe vamp ulcer and bursitis
36. First-ray overload syndrome
37. Calcific tendinitis of the flexor hallucis tendons

SMALL TOE PAIN

38. Hard corns
39. Soft corns
40. Heloma verruca (mosaic warts)
41. End corns
42. Mallet toe deformity
43. Hammer toe deformity
44. Periungual corn of the fifth toe
45. Ulcerations of the toes
A. Ischemic
B. Neuropathic
46. Tophus
47. Arthritis of the small toes
48. Tinea pedis
49. Candidiasis
50. Dorsal interphalangeal joint area pain and inflammation
51. Trauma (contusions and fractures)
52. "Tailor's bunion" (bunionette of the fifth toe)
53. Raynaud's disease and phenomenon
54. Osler's nodes
55. Subungual tumors
A. Glomus tumor
B. Osteoid osteoma
C. Subungual wart

MIDFOOT PAIN

56. Longitudinal arch strain
57. Trauma
A. Tarsometatarsal joints
   1. Sprain
   2. Dislocation or fracture-dislocation
B. Midtarsal region (Chopart's or the transverse tarsal joint)
   1. Medial injuries
   2. Longitudinal injuries
   3. Lateral injuries
   4. Plantar injuries
   5. Crush injuries
C. Navicular fractures

1. Traumatic fractures
2. Stress fractures
D. Fracture of the fifth metatarsal
    1. Avulsion fractures
    2. Diaphysial fractures (true Jones fractures)
58. Aseptic necrosis of the navicular bone
59. Tendinitis
    A. Flexor hallucis longus tendinitis
    B. Peroneal tendinitis
60. Subtalar osteochondral fracture
61. Interosseous myositis or strain
62. Stress fracture of one or more metatarsal or tarsal bones
63. *Pseudomonas* osteomyelitis
64. Acquired flatfoot
    A. Rupture of the tibialis posterior tendon
    B. Ligamentous or bone failure
65. Osteoarthritis
    A. First metatarsocuneiform joint
    B. Cuboideometatarsal joint
66. Plantar fascial pain
    A. Plantar fasciitis
    B. Heel pain syndrome
67. Plantar abscess

DORSAL FOOT PAIN

68. Tendinitis
    A. Extensor hallucis longus muscle
    B. Extensor digitorum longus muscle
    C. Tibialis anterior muscle
69. Cruxiate crural ligament injury
70. Other causes (Table 47-6)

HINDFOOT PAIN

71. Generalized hindfoot pain
    A. Calcaneal fractures
        1. Intraarticular
        2. Extraarticular
            a. Fracture of the medial calcaneal process
            b. Fracture of the superior portion of the calcaneal tuberosity
            c. Fracture of the sustentaculum tali
    B. Ischemic necrosis of the heel
72. Plantar hindfoot pain
    A. Fat pad disorders
        1. Atrophy
        2. Inflammation
        3. Fat pad separation from the calcaneus

4. Piezogenic papules
B. Glomus tumor
C. Stress fracture of the calcaneus
D. Heel pain syndrome due to overuse ("plantar fasciitis")
E. Rupture of the plantar fascia
F. Heel pain syndrome associated with systemic disorders
G. Entrapment neuropathy of the first branch of the lateral plantar nerve
H. True plantar fasciitis
I. Flexor tendinitis
    1. Flexor hallucis longus tendinitis
    2. Flexor digitorum longus tendinitis
73. Posterior hindfoot pain
    A. Superficial Achilles bursitis ("pump bump")
    B. Retrocalcaneal bursitis
    C. Haglund's syndrome
    D. Achilles tendinitis
    E. Achilles tendon rupture
    F. Calcaneal periostitis and osteitis
    G. Calcaneal osteomyelitis
    H. Fracture of the posterosuperior calcaneal tuberosity
74. Medial hindfoot pain
    A. Tibialis posterior tendinitis
    B. Flexor hallucis longus tendinitis
    C. Tarsal tunnel syndrome
    D. Calcaneal fractures (medial calcaneal process or sustentaculum tali)
    E. Calcaneal branch neurodynia
75. Lateral hindfoot pain
    A. Peroneal muscle strain
    B. Peroneal tendinitis
    C. Lateral ankle sprain
    D. Fracture of the lateral process of the talus
    E. Osteochondral fracture of the talar dome
    F. Sural nerve entrapment
    G. Stress fracture of the lateral malleolus

BILATERAL FOOT PAIN
(Table 47-7)

☐ SUMMARY

Generalized Foot Pain

Crush injuries of the foot may avulse soft tissue because of shear forces (e.g., a tire passing over a foot); may impact and damage soft tissue and fracture bone (e.g., a falling object causing a brief impact); or may compress soft tissue, crush bone, and produce a bursting effect in the distal forefoot (e.g., injury from a static load pinning the foot against a surface). Blood vessel and nerve injuries associated with crushing forces may be significant, and they are important determinants of prognosis.

A *compartment syndrome of the foot* may result from a crush injury or from less severe trauma (e.g., a calcaneal fracture with a subfascial plantar hematoma). Progressively severe and persistent foot pain, appearing at times too severe for the causative trauma, is an important clue to the possibility of a compartment syndrome of the foot. The foot is swollen, and affected compartments (medial, lateral, central, or interosseous) are tense and tender. Any active or passive movement (toe extension) exacerbates pain. Distal paresthesia, hypesthesia, and/or anesthesia of the foot and toes is an important clue to the diagnosis. Intracompartmental pressure will exceed 30 mmHg, and relief is obtained by a decompressive fasciotomy and evacuation of any large subfascial hematomas.

Traumatic amputation of the foot may result from lawn mower injuries, land mines or other explosions, a shotgun blast at close range, or severe mangling of the foot in an industrial or motor vehicle accident.

Cellulitis of the foot causes pain, erythema, edema, tenderness, and sometimes ascending lymphangitis. Fever, chills, and sweating may be associated. The advancing erythematous margin has an irregular outline and is flat. Centrally located bullae or superficial abscesses may occur. Most cases are caused by *streptococci* or *staphylococci*. *Aeromonas hydrophila* infection is encountered after wounding in fresh water. Sever cellulitis, fasciitis, and myonecrosis may occur. A bullous and necrotizing cellulitis of the foot may follow saltwater wounding or wound contamination by *Vibrio vulnificus*. Septicemia may accompany a severe cellulitis. *Saphenous vein donor sites* are sometimes associated with a severe form of recurrent *cellulitis*.

Necrotizing fasciitis may complicate acute trauma. It begins as a cellulitis, and then skin necrosis, crepitus, bullae formation, and cutaneous anesthesia develop, indicating deep involvement. Radiographs may demonstrate subcutaneous gas. Systemic symptoms may be severe. The diagnosis can be confirmed by exploration of the infected area to debride necrotic subcutaneous and fascial tissue and exclude myonecrosis. This disorder may be caused by obligate and facultative anaerobes (type I) or group A streptococcus with or without *Staphylococcus aureus* (type II).

An *abscess of the foot* usually involves one or more of the plantar spaces of the central compartment of the foot. Local swelling of the sole, pain, erythema, warmth, and tenderness may occur. The abscess can be imaged by MRI or a radionuclide scan. It responds to drainage and antibiotic therapy.

Osteomyelitis of the foot may cause localized pain, tenderness, swelling, erythema, and warmth of the overlying skin. The calcaneus and metatarsals are the bones most frequently involved. The diagnosis can be confirmed by MRI or supported by a radionuclide scan. MRI is more specific than a radionuclide scan. Bone biopsy will provide a specific diagnosis and define the type of antibiotic therapy to be administered.

Septic arthritis of the foot is usually monarticular. Aching and/or throbbing pain, edema, and redness occur over the affected joint. Intraarticular foot infection may arise as part of a disseminated gonococcal infection in a sexually active young adult. Staphylococci and gram-negative bacteria are the usual isolates in older patients with preexisting joint disease, immunosuppression, and/or an infection at an adjacent (e.g., osteomyelitis of the foot) or a distant site (e.g., skin or urinary tract infection). Synovial fluid analysis and culture will establish the diagnosis. Symptoms and signs resolve with joint drainage and/or irrigation and parenteral antibiotic therapy.

Rheumatoid arthritis may cause painful metatarsalgia and swelling due to synovitis of the metatarsophalangeal (MTP) joints and secondary toe deformities such as claw or hammer toes, hallux valgus, and hallux rigidus. Interphalangeal (IP) toe arthritis may also occur. Subtalar rheumatoid arthritis and tenosynovitis of the peroneal and tibialis posterior tendons may cause hindfoot pain. Retrocalcaneal bursitis may be responsible for posterior hindfoot pain. Midfoot pain may arise medially in the talonavicular joint. Foot involvement may be a major cause of limited ambulation in a patient with rheumatoid arthritis. Other criteria required for the diagnosis of rheumatoid arthritis are usually present or develop within 2 years.

Seronegative spondyloarthropathies may affect the foot. *Ankylosing spondylitis* may cause an erosive arthritis of the MTP, IP, midtarsal, and/or subtalar joints. Achilles tendinitis and a heel pain syndrome due to an enthesitis at the site of insertion of the plantar fascia on the medial calcaneal tuberosity may occur. Ankylosing spondylitis can be diagnosed if radiographic evidence of sacroiliitis is present and either inflammatory back pain, restriction of back motion, or restriction of chest expansion is present. HLA-B27 antigen positivity is associated with ankylosing spondylitis and Reiter's syndrome.

Reiter's syndrome (urethritis, conjunctivitis, and arthritis) may occur in a complete or incomplete form (i.e., only two components present). Asymmetrical involvement of MTP and IP joints occurs. Dactylitis (''sausage digits'') of one or two toes may be present. Mucous membrane and cutaneous lesions may develop in some patients. Late radiographic changes include osteopenia, joint space narrowing, and erosions. Soft tissue involvement includes plantar fasciitis and Achilles tendinitis.

Psoriatic arthritis may cause metatarsalgia and dactylitis of one or more toes due to tenosynovitis, periostitis, and arthritis. Distal interphalangeal (DIP) joint involvement is frequent and sometimes severe. Plantar fasciitis and Achilles tendinitis may occur. The diagnosis is suggested by the presence of psoriatic skin and nail lesions and an asymmetrical oligoarthritis with prominent involvement of the DIP joints.

A *migratory and/or additive polyarthritis* that may affect the MTP and IP joints of the feet, ankles, and knees may be associated with *inflammatory bowel disease*. No destructive radiographic changes occur, and symptoms resolve after successful treatment of the bowel disease.

Acute gout may cause severe pain, swelling, redness, and tenderness over the first MTP joint, dorsum of the foot, and ankle region. The serum uric acid level is usually elevated, and the synovial fluid contains monosodium urate crystals and an increased concentration of polymorphonuclear leukocytes. A similar first MTP arthritis may be caused by *pseudogout, psoriasis, Reiter's syndrome, and sarcoidosis.* Synovial fluid obtained from a pseudogout synovial effusion contains intra- and extracellular calcium pyrophosphate dihydrate crystals and an increased concentration of polymorphonuclear leukocytes.

Other disorders that may involve the small joints of the feet include *acute rheumatic fever, systemic lupus erythematosus, hepatitis B-associated arthritis,* and *rubella-associated arthritis. Sickle cell pain crisis* may be associated with severely painful lower legs and feet. Swelling of the knees and diffuse edema of the feet may occur and resolve spontaneously. Extensive allodynia and skin hyperesthesia suggest that sickle cell pain crisis has a neuropathic component.

Acute arterial occlusion causes pallor, pain, paresthesias, paresis, and loss of pulses in the foot and lower leg. Removal of a clot in the popliteal or tibial artery within 4 to 8 h results in resolution of all symptoms and signs. *Nocturnal pain* in the toes and feet that is relieved by dependency or walking may be *caused by arterial insufficiency.* The pedal pulses are diminished or absent, and the foot is cool and pale.

Ulceration and gangrene of the toes may be caused by *cholesterol embolization,* progressive ischemia due to *severe arteriosclerosis,* or a *systemic vasculitis.* The diagnosis of *cholesterol embolism* is dependent on a history of a recent diagnostic or therapeutic intraarterial intervention and positive results of tissue biopsy. *Arteriosclerosis obliterans* occurs in diabetic and elderly patients. Popliteal and pedal pulses are absent. A femoral arteriogram will help establish the diagnosis. *Polyarteritis nodosa* is a systemic disease that may cause toe and finger ulcers or gangrene. A renal or mesenteric angiogram showing aneurysms of small or medium-sized vessels and/or a tissue biopsy is required for the diagnosis of this disorder. Elevated serum levels of C-ANCA (antineutrophil cytoplasmic antibody) or P-ANCA may be associated with microscopic polyarteritis nodosa.

Allergic angiitis and *granulomatosis* is another cause of finger and toe gangrene and ulceration. Severe asthma, pulmonary infiltrates, and eosinophilia are associated with the systemic symptoms and multisystem involvement (e.g., nervous, rheumatologic, or cardiac).

Other diseases that may be associated with vasculitis resulting in painful finger and toe ulceration and gangrene include *systemic lupus erythematosus, rheumatoid arthritis, Sjögren's syndrome, Schönlein-Henoch purpura, essential mixed cryoglobulinemia,* and *lymphoid and reticuloendothelial malignancies.*

Thromboangiitis obliterans (Buerger's disease) may cause toe gangrene and ulceration of the digits, arm and leg claudication, rest pain in the fingers and feet, and migratory thrombophlebitis in young adult males of Asian or eastern European descent who abuse tobacco. Distal pulses are weak or absent, and proximal pulses are usually present. An arteriogram of the legs will demonstrate smooth, tapering, distal, segmental arterial lesions, and a biopsy of an involved artery will confirm the diagnosis.

Erythromelalgia is a disorder that causes attacks of foot and toe burning or throbbing pain, redness, warmth, and sometimes swelling. The attack may occur spontaneously or may be provoked by warming the extremity, exercise, or dependency. Cooling, elevation of the foot, and in some cases use of aspirin will abort the episode or prevent it. Primary erythromelalgia consists of hereditary cases and secondary cases that have not yet revealed an underlying disorder. Thrombocythemia and polycythemia vera and other diseases may be responsible for secondary erythromelalgia. A dose of aspirin may prevent attacks for 3 to 4 days in patients with a platelet-associated disorder. Some toe lesions may progress to coldness, pallor, and gangrene. Not all cases of idiopathic and secondary erythromelalgia respond to aspirin prophylaxis.

Phlegmasia cerulea dolens is characterized by massive lower extremity swelling and pain, distal coldness and cyanosis, and gangrene of some toes and portions of the foot. Hemorrhagic bullae may form in the involved area of venous gangrene.

Reflex sympathetic dystrophy may follow minor or major trauma or surgery or may begin without a precipitating event. The burning, aching, or throbbing pain that occurs is more severe and persistent than expected for the amount of trauma or the extent of surgery. Edema, warmth, erythema of the overlying skin, hyperhidrosis, joint pain and stiffness, and skin hyperesthesia affect all or a part of the foot. Within weeks, the foot becomes cool and the edema more persistent. The skin becomes shiny and taut, and allodynia more severe. Plain radiographs reveal patchy osteoporosis, and a triphasic radionuclide bone scan reveals increased bone uptake over juxtaarticular areas of the foot. Sympathetic blockade relieves pain and permits joint mobility. *Foot cramps* cause acute pain in the arch of the foot that is relieved by massage or walking. Benign and secondary types of cramps related to muscle disease, neurological disease, or electrolyte disturbances occur.

Symmetrical acute sensory polyneuropathy, with burning pain of the toes and the plantar surfaces of the feet, paresthesias, and allodynia, may occur with *diabetes mellitus.* Electric shock-like, sharp, shooting lower leg and foot pains may be superimposed. Symptoms are worse at night and after walking or weight bearing, and may be improved by bed rest. This disorder may be associated with weight loss, fatigue, and poor diabetic control. It improves with time and treatment of the glucose intolerance. A *subacute sensorimotor neuropathy* in the legs with distal weakness and wasting may also occur in diabetics. Sensory symptoms and findings (e.g., decreased superficial and deep sensation) are similar to those of the acute sensory polyneuropathy. *Mononeuritis multiplex* causes lower leg and foot pain, dysesthesias, sensory and motor deficits in the distribution of two or more distal lower extremity nerves (e.g., posterior tibial nerve, or superficial peroneal nerve), and sometimes upper extremity nerves. It may be caused by diabetes mellitus. *Hypothyroidism* may also present with distal pain and sensory and motor changes. *Alcohol abuse* is second to diabetes mellitus as a cause of neuropathic foot pain, paresthesias, weakness, and sensory loss. *Heavy metal poisoning by arsenic, mercury, or thallium* may cause neuropathic foot and hand pain, paresthesias, painful dysesthesias, and distal motor weakness. Measurement of serum levels or urine excretion of these metals will establish the diagnosis.

Therapeutic drugs (e.g., disulfiram, isoniazid, cis-platinum, gold, metronidazole, and vincristine) may cause painful sensory or sensorimotor polyneuropathies. Similarly, *industrial chemicals* such as acrylamide, carbon disulfide, and *n*-hexane may cause a sensory or sensorimotor polyneuropathy. *Systemic diseases* such as *carcinoma, leukemia, lymphoma, myeloma, macroglobulinemia, cryoglobulinemia,* and *amyloidosis* may cause painful sensory or sensorimotor polyneuropathy. *Vasculitis, renal failure, AIDS,* and *sarcoidosis* are other systemic disorders that may cause polyneuropathy. Renal failure related foot pain and paresthesias respond to hemodialysis or renal transplantation. Sarcoidosis-associated neuropathy may respond to prednisone, and vasculitis to prednisone and cyclophosphamide.

Hereditary causes of painful neuropathy include *Fabry's disease* and *intermittent acute porphyria*. These disorders can be diagnosed from the clinical findings and by measurement of leukocyte enzyme levels. *Mononeuropathy multiplex*, with multiple episodes of painful sensory or sensorimotor peripheral nerve involvement, may also be caused by vasculitis, sarcoidosis, AIDS, amyloidosis, coagulopathies, or hypothyroidism.

The *tarsal tunnel syndrome* causes burning pain on the plantar surface of the foot. The entire sole, the medial or lateral side, or the anterior two-thirds may be painful. Paresthesias and dysesthesias may be associated. Pressure over the medial foot (i.e., posterior tibial nerve) may provoke pain and paresthesias (Tinel's sign). Motor symptoms are uncommon. Sensation may be impaired over part of the sole or may be intact. Electrophysiologic studies are useful in confirming the diagnosis. Some cases are associated with electric shock-like or stabbing pains that radiate into the foot. Causes include space-occupying lesions, tight ligaments and fascial bands, pes planus and hindfoot valgus, poorly fitting shoes, and acute eversion injuries of the ankle. Conservative therapy often leads to resolution, but surgery may be required.

Superficial peroneal nerve entrapment may occur at the ankle and cause pain and paresthesias over the dorsum of the foot. *Deep peroneal nerve compression* over the anterior ankle causes pain and paresthesias over the first dorsal web space.

Plantar flexion with toe extension may provoke symptoms, and Tinel's sign may be present. *Sural nerve entrapment* may cause pain and paresthesias on the lateral border of the foot. Tenderness over the region of compression and Tinel's sign may be present. *S1 or L5 root compression* causes back pain and sciatica. S1 root compression may cause lateral plantar pain, paresthesias, hypesthesia, and a depressed ankle jerk. L5 compression may result in dorsal foot and great toe pain and paresthesias. Dejerine's sign (i.e., sciatic pain provoked by coughing or straining) may be present and/or there may be positive results on the straight leg-raising test, and a contrast-enhanced CT or MRI may demonstrate a root-compressing lesion (e.g., disc, tumor, narrow foramen, or abscess).

Frostbite follows exposure of the feet to subzero temperatures for a prolonged period. First-degree injury results in erythema and edema of the foot, pain, and paresthesias followed by spontaneous recovery and gradual resolution of symptoms. Pain on future cold exposure may recur, and this problem may persist. Second-degree frostbite results in bullae formation and superficial skin necrosis. Third-degree frostbite causes distal numbness and gangrene and proximal erythema, pain, and bullae formation. Pain begins 3 to 14 days after cold injury and may be burning, throbbing, and, later, shooting or electric-like. Spontaneous relief of pain occurs after weeks or months.

Trench foot occurs at above-freezing temperatures when the feet are kept in wet socks and shoes. On rewarming and drying, paresthesias and foot pain occur in association with skin hyperemia, edema, and bullae formation. Skin necrosis may develop in severe cases. The pain is usually aching or burning and may have a lightning-like or sharp, shooting component that begins 1 to 2 weeks after rewarming.

Immersion foot occurs after prolonged immersion of the feet in warm or chilly water. On rewarming and drying, throbbing, burning, or aching pain occurs. Within 1 week, sharp, shooting pains may occur. The feet become swollen, red, and tender; bullae may develop, and areas of skin necrosis may occur. Pain is relieved spontaneously in 6 to 10 weeks.

Pernio (chilblains) refers to a raised, erythematous rash over the feet, associated with burning pain and/or pruritus. This disorder is caused in some individuals by outdoor activities in cold weather. It resolves spontaneously during warm weather, resulting from a change in the season or a vacation trip.

Human and some animal bites lacerate and crush tissue and inoculate the bite wound with aerobic and anaerobic bacteria. Sequelae may include local infection with redness and swelling around the wound and purulent drainage; spreading cellulitis, lymphangitis, and femoral and inguinal lymphadenitis; and septicemia. Major local complications of the bite include septic tenosynovitis, septic arthritis, or osteomyelitis. Human bite isolates include many aerobic and anaerobic bacteria and *Eikenella corrodens*.

Dog bites can also cause cellulitis, lymphangitis, and local tendon, bone, or joint sepsis. *Pasteurella multocida* is a common cause of dog bite infection. *Cat bites* are usually small puncture wounds, and *P. multocida* is a common isolate. *Venomous snakebites* cause severe pain and edema that occur within minutes of envenomation. Skin gangrene at the site of venom injection occurs and is associated with sloughing of tissue. Secondary bacterial infection from organisms in the snake's mouth may occur. A *recluse spider bite* causes extensive skin redness and edema and a central bulla that evolves into a painful, necrotic ulcer. A *sea urchin sting* occurs while wading in the ocean. The foot swells and is painful, red, and tender, and ulceration may occur. The sea urchin spine may be retained under the skin. *Venomous fish stings* may occur when a swimmer is wading or swimming. Pain and paresthesias occur at the time of the underwater sting. The site swells and becomes red and tender. Ecchymoses, skin necrosis, and sloughing may occur. Stone fish envenomation may cause cardiac toxicity, hypotension, dyspnea, and death.

Skin disorders of the foot include *palmoplantar pustulosis and pustular psoriasis*. Painful pustules occur on the hands and feet and, in the case of psoriasis, at other cutaneous sites as well. *Dyshidrotic eczema* causes plantar and palmar epidermal vesicles that may rupture and sting. Pustular lesions of the hands and feet (i.e., *pustular bacterid*) may be caused by a distant focal infection (e.g., tonsillitis, sinusitis, or dental abscess). *Acrodermatitis continua* begins on a single digit and causes subungual pus, erosions, and additional pustules on the hands and sometimes on the feet. *Infectious eczematoid dermatitis* may cause foot redness, pustules, fissures, and erosions that respond to antibiotic therapy. *Hand-foot-and-mouth disease* is a mild viral illness (coxsackie A and B or enterovirus 71) that causes mildly tender, ovoid, football-shaped vesicles on the hands and feet, and ulcers and vesicles in the mouth. *Herpes zoster* causes burning and aching leg and foot pain associated with the eruption of clusters of vesicles and crusted ulcers. *Tinea pedis* may cause mildly painful and tender plantar vesicles. *Atopic dermatitis* of the feet causes weeping and crusted erosions, redness, swelling, and painful fissures. Culture results are negative. *Contact dermatitis* causes stinging pain and itching, with erythema, vesicles, and bullae. Examples are poison ivy and shoe dermatitis. *Vitamin B deficiency* may cause burning foot pain. A *fixed drug eruption* causes an ovoid, red, well-circumscribed, painful, tender plaque that disappears when the responsible drug is discontinued. *Erosive lichen planus* causes large, confluent, ulcerations on the feet. Typical violaceous polygonal papules usually occur adjacent to the erosions or at another skin site.

Forefoot Pain

Metatarsalgia of the heads of rays 2 to 4 is associated with plantar tenderness over the involved metatarsal heads. The dorsal aspect of the joint is usually not tender unless a synovitis is present.

High-heeled shoes increase metatarsal load, prevent weight bearing by the lesser toes, and may cause acute and recurrent metatarsalgia. An *equinus foot* or a *cavus foot* also causes mechanical overload of the metatarsal heads. The *first-ray in-*

sufficiency syndrome (Morton's syndrome) results from a short first ray, varus deviation of the first ray, or functional shortening of the first ray due to posterior placement of the sesamoid bones. Pes planus and valgus deformity of the heel may also cause first-ray insufficiency and metatarsalgia of the heads of metatarsals 2, 3, and/or 4.

Stress (march) fracture of metatarsals 2, 3, and/or 4 may result from repetitive overload and cause acute forefoot pain and tenderness. Such fractures can be demonstrated by a radionuclide scan and/or plain radiograph.

Persistent first-ray insufficiency may cause aching metatarsalgia over the heads of metatarsals 2 to 4, the formation of painful callus in this area, and bursal enlargement and/or bursitis of the associated intermetatarsal bursae.

Central-ray overload may result when the affected metatarsal is unusually long, there is an increased downward angle of one or more metatarsals with the horizontal, or when metatarsal dorsiflexion at the tarsometatarsal joint is impaired by trauma or arthritis. Mechanical pain and/or pain due to formation of a callus, corn, or bursa over the overloaded metatarsal head occurs. *Freiberg's disease* causes pain, swelling, and tenderness over the head of metatarsal 2 or 3. A radionuclide scan or MRI will detect early cases of this disorder, caused by osteonecrosis of the metatarsal head. The *second metatarsal interspace syndrome* is associated with pain, tenderness, swelling, and sometimes redness of the skin in that area. There may be dorsal tenderness and pain on range-of-motion testing of the second or third MTP joint. The pain is aching and does not radiate into the toes. It is intensified by weight bearing and walking. A local injection of lidocaine and a corticosteroid provides dramatic pain relief. The cause is an inflammatory reaction in and around the second or third MTP joint and the adjacent intermetatarsal bursa.

Morton's neuroma causes burning or shooting, electric-like pain in the second or third metatarsal interspace with radiation into the third, fourth, or sometimes the second toe. Severe, spontaneous, nocturnal episodes and attacks provoked by walking or foot movements occur. Patients find some relief by manipulating and massaging the foot or cooling it with cold water. Medial-lateral compression of the forefoot or anteroposterior or dorsoplantar compression of the painful interspace may reproduce the pain and allow palpation of a tender nodule or a click (Mulder's click) in the web space. Conservative measures or surgical excision will lead to symptom relief.

Synovitis of the second MTP joint causes local pain, tenderness, and swelling, and range-of-motion testing may intensify or provoke pain. The synovitis may be caused by weight bearing, overload, or recurrent subluxation of the proximal phalanx.

Inflammatory arthritis (e.g., rheumatoid arthritis, the seronegative spondyloarthropathies, and the peripheral arthritis associated with inflammatory bowel disease) may cause aching MTP joint pain, swelling, and plantar and dorsal joint tenderness. Psoriasis and Reiter's syndrome may cause dactylitis ("sausage digit") of one or two toes. Rheumatoid arthritis-related changes at the MTP joints may cause claw or hammer toes and plantar displacement of the metatarsal heads, resulting in a mechanical, as well as an inflammatory, type of metatarsalgia.

Atherosclerotic obstruction or vasculitis may cause calf or foot claudication, rest pain, and toe gangrene and ulceration. A direct blow to the forefoot may *fracture* one or more metatarsals, and these fractures can be observed on a plain radiograph. Athletes are subject to painful *forefoot sprain*. Symptoms may be subtle and often neglected. Stress of the foot (e.g., placing weight on the toes and leaning forward) causes pain, as do running, cutting, or jumping. Walking may be deceptively pain free. Intermetatarsal *bursitis* causes fluctuant localized swelling, pain, and tenderness under the MTP joint of one or more toes. *Cysts* in the skin of the same region may sometimes be confused with bursal swelling and inflammation. They may discharge sebaceous material intermittently through a small central pore. *Local scratching* of a pruritic sole may cause excoriation and painful local infection that responds to avoidance of scratching and to antibiotics.

Great Toe and Medial Forefoot Pain

A *sprain of the first MTP joint* causes local pain, tenderness, and swelling. It may be caused by axial loading of the heel with the foot in equinus. This results in hyperextension of the joint and stretching of the plantar capsule and volar plate. Hyperflexion, abduction, or adduction sprains may also occur but are less common.

Dislocation of the first MTP joint follows motor vehicle trauma or a fall from a height. There are local pain, swelling, tenderness, and dorsal deformity. *Sesamoid bone fractures* can cause plantar pain and localized tenderness and can be identified on ''sesamoid'' views. Differentiation from sesamoid partition is required and may be facilitated by a radionuclide bone scan. *Traumatic fracture of the phalanges of the great toe* results from a direct blow or stubbing the toe. *Phalangeal dislocation* is less common but may follow kicking a hard object or surface.

A *subungual hematoma* follows a direct blow to the nail. Excruciating pain and exquisite tenderness occur. The nail is blue but usually intact. Drainage of the hematoma relieves the pain. *Contusion of the soft tissue on the dorsum of the toe* may cause pain, ecchymoses, and swelling without an associated fracture. *Calluses* (opalescent center after paring), *plantar warts* (central punctate reddish-black capillary thrombi visible after paring), and *corns* (conical hyperkeratosis) are painful and tender cutaneous lesions that may appear over the plantar aspect of the MTP joint of the great toe or other toes.

An *ingrown toenail* causes local nail margin pain, tenderness, and redness. *Infection of the margin of the ingrown nail* causes increased pain, redness, swelling, tenderness, and subungual pus. Drainage relieves pain. Granulation tissue forms at the nail margin and may require excision to allow drainage of pus. A *melanocarcinoma of the nail bed or edge* can mimic

local infection and requires biopsy for diagnosis. A *glomus tumor* is a painful, 2- to 3-mm, blue-red nail bed lesion. Pain is provoked by cold or direct pressure. Other painful subungual lesions include *osteoid osteoma* and *warts*.

Paronychia causes nail margin redness, pain, swelling, tenderness, and purulent or watery drainage. Causes include an ingrown nail, a local abrasion or laceration, or a retained foreign body. *Pulp space infection* due to a puncture wound and *an infected blister* are other painful lesions of the great toe.

Hallux valgus causes forefoot pain by producing a medial bunion and by dislocating the proximal phalanx of the second and sometimes the third toe by underlapping them. This dislocation may cause synovitis of the second and third MTP joints, callus formation beneath these joints, and bursal swelling in the same area. These disorders may become symptomatic with weight bearing. *Bunion* formation at the medial aspect of the first MTP joint results from uncovering of the medial portion of the first metatarsal head, thickening of the overlying skin, and formation of an adventitial bursa. This bursa may become painful, tender, swollen, and red. *Hallux limitus or rigidus* causes pain on extension of the hallux and limitation of movement. It may be caused by an injury to the dorsal surface of the articular cartilage of the first metatarsal head or may be secondary to osteoarthritis, osteochondritis dissecans, or an inflammatory form of arthritis. *Sesamoid pain*, tenderness, and swelling are sharply localized to the affected bone. Causes include fracture, osteonecrosis, sesamoiditis, and arthritis. Radiographs and radionuclide bone scans are helpful in establishing the diagnosis. *MTP septic arthritis* may cause local pain, swelling, tenderness, redness, and systemic symptoms. Synovial fluid culture results are positive. *Podagra* refers to an intensely painful, red, and swollen first MTP joint. The most common cause is gout, but pseudogout and inflammatory forms of arthritis may also cause first MTP joint inflammation. *Joplin's neuroma* causes pain and paresthesias along the medial plantar surface of the first MTP joint. Local pressure on the involved nerve reproduces pain and paresthesias.

Pain, *ulceration, and gangrene of the great toe* may result from ischemia due to vasculitis, microemboli, or larger emboli or thromboses involving two or more infrapopliteal arteries. A *root lesion involving L5* may cause back pain, sciatic or calf pain, and pain and paresthesias over the dorsum of the foot and great toe. Dejerine's sign and results of the straight leg-raising test are positive. MRI of the spine will usually reveal the cause of the root lesion. A *shoe vamp ulcer* may form a local area of inflammation over the dorsum of the base of the first toe. The *first-ray overload syndrome* may cause metatarsalgia due to a large hallux and first metatarsal. Plantar callus, bursitis, and sesamoid pain may occur. Relief of first-ray weight bearing leads to symptom relief.

Calcific tendinitis of the flexor hallucis tendons may cause plantar pain, redness, swelling, and tenderness beneath the first MTP joint. Great toe passive extension or active flexion result in pain. Tendon calcification is visible on a plain radiograph of the foot.

Small Toe Pain

Hard corns are round, elevated, and sometimes conical, localized, hyperkeratotic lesions that cause pain and tenderness of the toes and foot. They appear on the dorsal surface of the toes or the end of a toe (*end corn*), between the toes (*soft corn*), or on the plantar, weight-bearing areas (over metatarsal heads). *Soft corns* may be associated with skin maceration and may be mimicked by tinea pedis and *mosaic warts*. *Mallet toe, hammer toe, and claw toe* deformities result in frictional contact of the dorsum and/or end of the toes with the shoe and result in the formation of painful, red areas of friction-induced inflammation, blisters, or corns. *Periungual corns* may form at the tip of the fifth toe and cause pain in this area. Painful toe *ulceration* may be caused by *ischemia or neuropathy*. A *tophus* may appear as a furuncle-like lesion on a toe, causing pain, redness, and a white, chalky discharge that resembles pus. Microscopic examination of the discharge reveals monosodium urate crystals. *Arthritis of the lesser toes* may take the form of IP joint inflammation with pain, redness, and swelling (e.g., rheumatoid arthritis) or a "sausage toe" (e.g., Reiter's syndrome or psoriatic arthritis). *Tinea pedis* causes pruritus, odor, and macerated and fissured skin in the third and fourth web spaces. Local pain and tenderness may result from fissures, erosions, and skin ulceration. Results of cultures for *Trichophyton* species and bacteria are usually positive. A *Candida* species may also affect the web spaces and cause a disorder similar to that produced by *Trichophyton* species. Hallux valgus may cause *dorsal displacement of the second and sometimes the third toe*, resulting in friction with the toe box of the shoe, resulting in blister or corn formation. Similarly, *overlapping of the fourth toe by the fifth* can cause frictional irritation on the dorsal surface of the fifth toe. *Direct trauma* or stubbing can cause toe pain, swelling, and ecchymoses due to a fracture. An inflamed *bunionette* may occur over the fifth MTP joint due to bursitis at this site. *Raynaud's phenomenon* may affect both the fingers and toes. Well-demarcated digit pallor, followed by cyanosis and painful hyperemia, occurs in 20- to 30-min episodes. Attacks are produced by cold or emotional upset. Some cases are idiopathic, while others are caused by collagen vascular disorders, occlusive vascular disease, blood dyscrasias, neurologic disorders, and drugs. *Osler's nodes* are slightly painful, tender, red macules occurring on the tips of fingers and toes in patients with bacterial endocarditis.

Subungual pain may be caused by tumors, including the 1- to 3-mm, round, red-blue, cold-sensitive *glomus tumor*; the continuously painful *osteoid osteoma*; and the mildly painful *subungual wart*.

Midfoot Pain

Longitudinal arch strain results in medial midfoot pain that is intensified by weight bearing and foot dorsiflexion and relieved by rest and plantar flexion. The cause is muscle or tendon fatigue or ligament injury of the foot.

Tarsometatarsal joint (Lisfranc's joint) injury results from axial loading of the heel of the foot fixed in equinus, a crush injury, or a forefoot twist. *Sprain* is associated with local pain, tenderness, and swelling over Lisfranc's joint. Passive supination or pronation of the midfoot with the heel fixed provokes or intensifies the pain.

Tarsometatarsal fracture-dislocation causes diffuse midfoot pain, swelling, ecchymoses, tenderness, and sometimes deformity. Weight bearing is not possible or is intensely painful. Radiographs will define the type and extent of fracture-dislocation.

Midtarsal joint (Chopart's joint) injuries are classified by the direction of the injuring force and resultant forcefoot displacement. Pain, swelling, ecchymoses, tenderness, and deformity occur in the proximal midfoot. Medial, longitudinal, lateral, plantar, or crushing forces can cause fracture-sprains, fracture-dislocations, and swivel dislocations. These injuries are identified by clinical findings and plain radiographs.

Traumatic fractures of the navicular bone follow an eversion force on the foot and result in dorsomedial midfoot pain and swelling. Fracture of the body of the navicular bone is usually associated with other midtarsal joint injuries. *Stress fracture of the navicular bone* results from overuse caused by running, jogging, or prolonged walking. Local dorsomedial pain and tenderness are increased by activity. The diagnosis can be confirmed by a radionuclide scan, a CT scan, or, less frequently, plain radiographs (e.g., only 24-percent sensitive in one study).

Fracture of the base of the fifth metatarsal can cause pain, swelling, and tenderness over the cuboid metatarsal articulation. It results from sudden inversion of the foot and is usually an *avulsion fracture* of the tuberosity of the fifth metatarsal.

Tenderness and swelling localized 1.5 to 2 cm distal to the fifth metatarsal-cuboid articulation are associated with *true Jones fractures of the metatarsal diaphysis*. This fracture has a high delayed union, nonunion, and refracture rate.

Aseptic necrosis of the navicular bone in adults causes mediodorsal foot pain associated with swelling, redness, and warmth. Early cases may be demonstrable only by MRI or a radionuclide scan. Advanced cases are easily seen on a plain radiograph.

Flexor hallucis longus tendinitis causes medial plantar midfoot pain and tenderness that are intensified by weight bearing and walking. The plantar portion of the tendon is locally tender. *Peroneal tendinitis* causes lateral midfoot pain and tenderness. Active eversion of the foot against resistance or passive inversion of the foot intensifies the pain.

Subtalar articular injury can cause lateral midfoot pain and tenderness that are intensified by weight bearing. This injury can be confused with peroneal tendinitis. It can be diagnosed by MRI, and pain can be relieved by arthrodesis. *Interosseous muscle strain or myositis* causes midfoot pain and tenderness on weight bearing in bare feet. Shoes alleviate weight-bearing pain to some extent. Tenderness is maximal on palpation of the involved muscles in the spaces between metatarsals. In some cases, MRI may show an edematous interosseous muscle on a T_2-weighted image of the foot, confirming the clinical diagnosis.

Stress fracture of a metatarsal or tarsal bone causes activity-related, localized bone pain and tenderness. The diagnosis can be confirmed during the first 2 to 3 weeks by a radionuclide bone scan. Evidence of fracture on a plain radiograph may not appear for 4 to 12 weeks.

A nail puncture wound of the foot may cause a streptococcal or staphylococcal cellulitis or a *Pseudomonas osteomyelitis*. Bone infection can be established by a radionuclide scan or plain radiography and needle biopsy of the involved bone.

Acquired flatfoot may result from *rupture of the tibialis posterior tendon*. Rupture is often preceded by tendinitis with associated medial ankle and midfoot pain and tenderness. Once flatfoot is acquired, lateral foot pain may result from impingement of the calcaneus on the talus and on the lateral malleolus. Acquired flatfoot may also result from *trauma with ligamentous injury or from arthritic changes in the midtarsal and tarsometatarsal joints*. Medial and sometimes lateral midfoot and ankle pain result.

Medial pain and tenderness may be caused by *osteoarthritis of the first metatarsocuneiform joint*. Pressure from an exostosis at this site may cause redness and tenderness of the overlying dorsal skin and tenderness of the extensor hallucis longus tendon.

Osteoarthritis or a sprain of the cuboideometatarsal joint may cause dorsolateral pain and joint line tenderness that is provoked or exacerbated by weight bearing, walking, and jogging.

True *plantar fasciitis* results from overuse of the foot and is associated with diffuse plantar midfoot pain and tenderness that is intensified by passive or active toe dorsiflexion. Pain is intensified by weight bearing or walking and relieved by rest.

The *heel pain syndrome* is sometimes called "plantar fasciitis." Maximal pain and well-localized tenderness occur at the point of insertion of the plantar fascia on the medial calcaneal tuberosity. Toe dorsiflexion does not provoke or intensify the pain. The cause is an enthesitis of the insertion of the plantar fascia. It may result from overuse or be caused by a seronegative spondyloarthropathy.

A *plantar abscess* causes midfoot, dorsal, and plantar edema, pain, and tenderness associated with fever, chills, sweats, and toxicity. The abscess and its extent can be imaged by MRI. Symptoms resolve with incision and drainage of the abscess and antibiotic therapy.

Dorsal Foot Pain

Tendinitis of one or more of the dorsal tendons (i.e., *tibialis anterior, extensor hallucis longus, or extensor digitorum longus*) may cause dorsal foot pain that is intensified by walking. Palpation of the involved tendon during active use of the corresponding muscle reveals tenderness. Passive flexion of the

toes or plantar flexion of the foot may provoke or intensify dorsal foot pain. *Crural ligament (i.e., retinaculum) injury* is associated with local tenderness over the ligament.

Other causes of dorsal foot pain include *compression neuropathy of the superficial or deep peroneal nerve, inflammatory disorders* (e.g., gout, pseudogout, cellulitis, abscess, osteomyelitis, or septic arthritis), *peripheral neuropathy, trauma* (e.g., bites or fracture-dislocations of the metatarsal and tarsal bones), *stress fractures, degenerative disorders* (e.g., osteoarthritis, acquired flatfoot, or osteonecrosis of the navicular bone), and *skin disorders* (e.g., herpes zoster or shoe dermatitis).

Hindfoot Pain

Calcaneal fractures usually result from a fall from a height. *Intraarticular fractures* account for 85 percent of cases, as the talus is driven into the calcaneous on impact. Diffuse, severe pain in the heel is associated with plantar swelling, ecchymoses, tenderness, and widening of the heel. Rarely, excruciating heel pain and tenderness may be caused by an acute compartment syndrome of the foot caused by the fracture and an associated hematoma. Plain radiographs will define the type and extent of calcaneal fractures.

Extraarticular calcaneal fractures may cause medial foot pain and swelling (e.g., *fracture of the medial calcaneal process or fracture of the sustentaculum tali*). Pain may be intensified by forced dorsiflexion of the ankle or toes (medial calcaneal process fracture) or inversion of the foot (sustentaculum tali fracture). Axial radiographs will demonstrate both types of fractures.

A *fracture of the superior portion of the calcaneal tuberosity* may cause posterior heel pain and swelling and weakness of plantar flexion similar to the findings of Achilles tendon rupture. A plain lateral radiograph will demonstrate the fracture fragment. Plantar flexion weakness occurs when the Achilles tendon is detached from the calcaneus by the fracture.

Pressure necrosis of the heel occurs in elderly comatose or stroke patients. The heel is black, indurated, and tender. Sloughing occurs after several weeks or months, leaving a painful and/or tender infected, ulcerated heel region requiring debridement and grafting.

Plantar Hindfoot Pain

Fat pad atrophy occurs in elderly persons and in long-distance runners who train on hard surfaces. Examination reveals thinning of the fat pad and tenderness of the heel. Symptoms respond to cushioning of the plantar surface of the heel.

Heel *fat pad inflammation* results from repetitive impact on a normal calcaneal fat pad. Rest and use of a semirigid, plastic heel pad without cushioning results in gradual resolution of pain and tenderness. *Separation of the fat pad from the cal-*

caneus by a fluid-filled cyst may also cause heel pain, tenderness, and swelling. This cyst can be detected by MRI. Aspiration of the cyst allows the fat pad to readhere to the calcaneus and relieves the pain.

Piezogenic papules are nodules of fat in the heel fat pad that become tender and cause heel pain. The pain is relieved by use of a heel arthrosis.

A rare cause of localized heel pain, often made worse by cold or pressure, is a *glomus tumor. Stress fracture of the calcaneus* occurs in military recruits. Local or diffuse heel pain is intensified by weight bearing. A radionuclide scan will usually detect an early stress fracture.

The *heel pain syndrome* causes medial distal hindfoot pain and localized tenderness over the medial calcaneal tuberosity and the proximal 5 mm of the plantar fascia. Dorsiflexion of the toes does not intensify the pain. A triphasic radionuclide bone scan may show early soft tissue blood pool uptake (fasciitis), delayed uptake (periostitis), or no significant uptake.

Rupture of the plantar fascia usually occurs in a patient with heel pain syndrome who has received one or more local corticosteroid injections. There is an abrupt onset of a severe, tearing, medial heel pain that makes further activity unbearable. Within 1 to 2 days, ecchymoses may appear in the painful, tender region of the heel. The preexistent heel pain syndrome is "cured" as a result of the rupture. *The heel pain syndrome* is an enthesitis and can occur *as part of the clinical course of certain systemic disorders*, including rheumatoid arthritis, a seronegative spondyloarthropathy, gonococcal arthritis, osteoarthritis, DISH, sarcoidosis, osteomalacia, and the arthritis associated with inflammatory bowel disease.

Entrapment of the first branch of the lateral plantar nerve can cause pain and tenderness medial and anterior to the medial tuberosity of the calcaneus. Tinel's sign may be present on pressing on the nerve where it crosses from the medial side of the foot to the sole.

True plantar fasciitis causes diffuse pain and tenderness over the plantar extent of the fascia. The pain is intensified by toe dorsiflexion. This overuse syndrome responds to rest.

Flexor hallucis longus tendinitis causes pain and medial hindfoot or midfoot localized tenderness over the tendon on the plantar aspect of the foot. Passive great toe dorsiflexion and active plantar flexion against resistance intensify or provoke pain. The latter test has no effect on true plantar fasciitis.

Flexor digitorum longus tendinitis may cause medial hindfoot pain, which is intensified by lesser toe flexion against resistance, and local tenderness of the tendon.

Posterior Hindfoot Pain

Pain, erythema, swelling, and tenderness can occur superficial to the Achilles tendon in a localized area. It is caused by friction between the heel and the shoe counter (*"pump bump"*). A superficial bursa may develop at this site and become inflamed. *Retrocalcaneal bursitis* causes pain and tenderness anterior and adjacent to the Achilles tendon. Dorsiflexion

of the foot compresses the bursa and intensifies the pain, while plantar flexion has minimal effect on the pain. Tenderness medial, lateral, and anterior to the Achilles tendon supports the diagnosis. Retrocalcaneal bursitis may result from heel counter friction, overuse, or inflammatory joint disease (e.g., gout, rheumatoid arthritis, or a seronegative spondyloarthropathy). *Haglund's syndrome* is a disorder defined by radiographic criteria. It consists of superficial Achilles bursitis, retrocalcaneal bursitis, Achilles tendinitis, and a prominent posterosuperior tuberosity of the calcaneus defined by the parallel pitch lines of Pavlov. *Achilles tendinitis* causes swelling, tendon enlargement, pain, and tenderness that are intensified by passive dorsiflexion or active plantar flexion of the foot against resistance. An insertional tendinitis or a severe inflammatory calcific tendinitis may occur in some cases. Achilles tendinitis may result from overuse, an irritating heel counter, gout, acute injury, or a seronegative spondyloarthropathy. *Rupture of the Achilles tendon* causes the abrupt onset of posterior heel and lower calf pain and tenderness. Plantar flexion is impaired, and standing on tiptoe is not usually possible. A tender gap in the tendon may be palpable, and results of Thompson's test are positive. Local pain, swelling, and tenderness over the calcaneus may be due to *periostitis*. This disorder is usually caused by injury or inflammatory arthritis. *Calcaneal osteomyelitis* causes heel pain, swelling, tenderness, and redness associated with fever, chills, and sweats. The diagnosis can be confirmed by a radionuclide bone scan or MRI early in the course and by plain radiographs when the disease has been present for 3 to 4 weeks.

Fracture of the posterosuperior calcaneal tuberosity causes posterior heel pain, swelling, and tenderness associated with paresis of plantar flexion. It may mimic rupture of the Achilles tendon. The tibialis posterior and toe flexors can produce some plantar flexion, making the diagnosis of tendon rupture or an avulsion fracture including the tendon less reliable when based on paresis of plantar flexion. Results of Thompson's test will be positive if the tendon is ruptured or avulsed from the calcaneus.

Medial Hindfoot Pain

Tendinitis of the tibialis posterior tendon causes medial hindfoot pain and tenderness along the course of the tendon or at its insertion on the navicular bone. Resisted inversion with the foot plantar flexed will provoke or intensify the pain. Swelling may occur in the retromalleolar area or inferior to the medial malleolus.

Flexor hallucis longus tendinitis may cause pain, swelling, and tenderness in the same area of the foot affected by tibialis posterior tendinitis. Passive dorsiflexion of the great toe or resisted flexion intensify the pain. Retromalleolar swelling and tenderness may be present.

The *tarsal tunnel syndrome* may cause medial foot pain and tenderness, as well as medial and/or lateral burning pain, paresthesias, and sometimes hypesthesia of part of the sole.

Tinel's sign may be elicited over the medial ankle. Medial ankle pain, swelling, and tenderness may occur from a *fracture of the medial calcaneal process or sustentaculum tali.*

Calcaneal branch neurodynia causes medial heel pain that is intensified by weight bearing. There is tenderness below and posterior to the tarsal tunnel. This disorder is caused by irritation or entrapment of the medial calcaneal branch of the posterior tibial nerve.

Lateral Hindfoot Pain

Peroneal muscle strain or tendinitis causes lateral foot pain and tenderness over the peroneal tendons. Passive inversion or eversion of the foot against resistance provokes or intensifies the pain.

Lateral ankle sprains can cause upper lateral foot pain and tenderness. The pain may be intensified by passive inversion of the foot. Tenderness is localized over the anterior talofibular and/or calcaneofibular ligaments.

Fracture of the lateral process of the talus or the talar dome can cause lateral ankle and foot pain. Talar dome fractures may require MRI or arthroscopy for diagnosis.

Sural nerve entrapment may cause lateral foot pain and paresthesias that are relieved by neurolysis.

Stress fracture of the lateral malleolus may cause lateral foot ache and localized tenderness over the lateral malleolus. A bone scan or plain radiographs will confirm the diagnosis. This disorder may be confused with peroneal tendinitis.

Bilateral Foot Pain

The causes of *bilateral foot pain* are listed in Table 47-7.

☐ DESCRIPTION OF LISTED DISEASES

Generalized Foot Pain

1. TRAUMA

A. Crush Injury   Extensive soft tissue and/or bone injury may result from a crush injury. The type of injury produced is dependent on the amount of force and time of tissue contact with that force.

A motor vehicle tire passing over a foot usually crushes the soft tissues and shears and avulses the dorsal skin and subcutaneous tissue from the deep fascial compartments. The usual result is a large, open wound on the dorsum of the foot containing varying amounts of crushed and devitalized tissue.

A heavy object striking the foot for a brief period (e.g.,

less than a millisecond) may cause severe soft tissue injury and fracture of the underlying bone. The soft tissue may initially appear relatively uninvolved except for superficial abrasion, pain, tenderness, and swelling. Within days, the overlying soft tissues may necrose and slough.

Crushing of the foot secondary to a static load applied to the dorsal aspect (e.g., the foot is trapped under a beam or a forklift) may result in crushing injury to soft tissue and bone directly under the applied weight. In addition, the subcutaneous tissue may be separated from the underlying deep fascia by shear forces, and a bursting effect may occur in the distal portion of the foot (e.g., forefoot region), with disruption of the skin, swelling, and extrusion of soft tissue from the burst wound.

Blood vessel and nerve injury, as well as wound contamination, may be significant determinants of the outcome of surgical management.

B. Compartment Syndrome of the Foot   This complication of blunt trauma is associated with crush injury of the foot. It may also occur with less severe forms of localized foot trauma (e.g., calcaneal fracture and a subfascial plantar hematoma).

Severe persistent and progressive pain in the foot is the major complaint. The foot is usually swollen, and the soft tissues are tender and tense. The pain is not relieved by rest, immobilization, or elevation. Any active or passive movement of the foot (e.g., extension of the toes) intensifies the pain. Hypesthesia to light touch, two-point discrimination, and pinprick sensation testing of the foot and toes are early sensory findings. Pulses and capillary refill time may remain normal, despite severe intracompartmental muscle ischemia. Intracompartmental pressure in one or all four compartments of the foot (e.g., medial, lateral, central, and interosseous) are elevated above 30 mmHg and are often in excess of 70 mmHg.

Intermediate surgical decompression with evacuation of hematomas and fasciotomy of one or more compartments results in relief of pain and resolution of sensory deficits.

C. Traumatic Amputation of the Foot   Lawn mower injuries may result in laceration and avulsion of soft tissue from the dorsal aspect of the forefoot and/or midfoot and multiple comminuted fractures of the metatarsals. There are massive edema, severe pain and tenderness, and necrotic tissue and clot in the surface wounds. Survival of the distal foot is dependent upon the degree of soft tissue damage, the number and severity of fractures, and neurovascular deficits present. Replantation of a completely or partially amputated foot may be successful, but experienced surgical teams available only at major surgical centers are required to ensure a reasonable possibility of success. Penetrating and blast trauma, such as a land mine or other explosion, a shotgun wound at close range, or severe mangling of the foot in a machine or motor vehicle accident, may also result in traumatic amputation.

2. INFECTION

A. Cellulitis   Pain, skin erythema, swelling, warmth, and tenderness occur on the dorsum and sides of the foot and extend above the ankle. The advancing margin is flat and has an irregular, ill-defined margin. Linear pink or reddish streaks may occur over the skin of the lower leg above the advancing erythematous margin, and a tender femoral and/or inguinal lymphadenitis may be present. Fever, chills, malaise, and weakness may accompany the local signs of infection. The usual entry site is a skin fissure (e.g., dermatophytosis of the toes), an ulceration, or a traumatic abrasion. Edema of the foot due to venous insufficiency, heart failure, cirrhosis, nephrotic syndrome, or lymphatic obstruction is a significant risk factor for bacterial cellulitis.

1. Cellulitis Due to **Staphylococcus aureus** *or a* **Streptococcal Species**   *Staphylococcus aureus, Streptococcus pyogenes*, and nongroup A beta-hemolytic streptococci (groups B, C, and G) are the most common pathogens. Less commonly, *Streptococcus pneumoniae, Pasteurella multocida*, or *Pseudomonas aeruginosa* are responsible. There is prompt response to antibiotic therapy.

2. Cellulitis Due to **Aeromonas hydrophila**   *Aeromonas hydrophila* may cause a severe cellulitis of the foot following an injury sustained in a freshwater environment or after foot injury associated with freshwater animals. Severe pain, redness, and swelling of the foot are associated with skin necrosis, ulcers, and hemorrhagic bullae formation. Severe systemic symptoms and bacteremia may be associated.

TABLE OF DISEASE INCIDENCE

INCIDENCE PER 100,000 (APPROXIMATE)

Common (>100)	Uncommon (>5–100)	Rare (>0–5)
	GENERALIZED FOOT PAIN	
Cellulitis due to streptococcal or staphylococcal species	Crush injury of the foot	Compartment syndrome of the foot
Cellulitis at a saphenous vein donor site	Traumatic amputation of the foot	Cellulitis due to *Aeromonas hydrophila*
Seropositive rheumatoid arthritis	Abscess of the foot	Cellulitis due to *Vibrio vulnificus*
Ankylosing spondylitis	Osteomyelitis of the foot	Necrotizing fasciitis
Reiter's syndrome	Septic arthritis of the foot	Ulceration and gangrene due to polyarteritis
Acute gout	Psoriatic arthritis	nodosa, allergic angiitis and
Sickle cell pain crisis	Arthritis associated with inflammatory bowel	granulomatosis, thromboangiitis
Nocturnal rest pain	disease	obliterans, erythromelalgia, or venous
Ulceration and gangrene due to	Acute pseudogout	gangrene
arteriosclerosis obliterans and progressive	Acute rheumatic fever	Heavy metal poisoning-related
ischemia	Systemic lupus erythematosus	polyneuropathy due to arsenic, mercury,
Foot cramps	Hepatitis B-associated arthritis	or thallium
Diabetic polyneuropathy	Rubella-associated arthritis	Drug-related polyneuropathy due to
Alcoholic polyneuropathy	Acute arterial occlusion	disulfiram, hydralazine, amiodarone,
Drug-related polyneuropathy caused by	Ulceration and gangrene due to cholesterol	metronidazole, misonidazole, phenytoin,
vincristine or *cis*-platinum	embolism, systemic lupus erythematosus	perhexilene, pyridoxine (high doses), or
Polyneuropathy due to systemic disorders:	vasculitis, rheumatoid arthritis vasculitis,	8-hydroxyquinolines
carcinoma, rheumatoid arthritis, and renal	or hypersensitivity vasculitis	Chemical-related polyneuropathy
failure	Reflex sympathetic dystrophy	Polyneuropathy due to systemic disorders:
Tarsal tunnel syndrome	Hypothyroid polyneuropathy	leukemias (acute and chronic),
Root compression of L5 and S1	Drug-related polyneuropathy caused by	lymphomas, POEMS syndrome,
Cold injury: frostbite and pernio	isoniazid, nitrofurantoin, or gold	osteosclerotic myeloma,
Human bites	Polyneuropathy due to systemic disorders:	cryoglobulinemia, Waldenström's
Dog bite	osteolytic myeloma, systemic lupus	macroglobulinemia, primary amyloidosis,
Cat bites	erythematosus, and AIDS	polyarteritis nodosa, Churg-Strauss
Dyshidrotic eczema	Intermittent acute porphyria neuropathy	disease, or sarcoidosis
Infectious eczematoid dermatitis	Superficial peroneal nerve entrapment	Fabry's disease and neuropathy
	Trench foot	Deep peroneal nerve entrapment
	Immersion foot	Sural nerve entrapment
	Snake bites	Palmoplantar pustulosis
	Recluse spider bites	Pustular bacterid of the hands and feet
	Sea urchin stings	Herpes zoster
	Venomous fish stings	Atopic dermatitis
	Pustular psoriasis	Vitamin B deficiencies
	Acrodermatitis continua	Fixed drug eruption
	Hand-foot-and-mouth disease	Erosive lichen planus
	Vesicular tinea pedis	
	Contact dermatitis	

(continued)

TABLE OF DISEASE INCIDENCE

INCIDENCE PER 100,000 (APPROXIMATE)

Common (>100)	Uncommon (>5–100)	Rare (>0–5)
	FOREFOOT PAIN	
Metatarsalgia due to high-heeled shoes	Metatarsalgia due to equinus foot, cavus	
Morton's neuroma	foot, first-ray insufficiency (acute march	
Inflammatory arthritis of the MTP joints	fracture and chronic first-ray	
Arterial insufficiency of the forefoot	insufficiency) or central-ray overload	
Traumatic fractures	syndrome	
Forefoot sprain	Freiberg's disease	
Self-inflicted trauma	Second metatarsal space syndrome	
	Idiopathic synovitis of second MTP joint	
	Bursitis (submetatarsal and interdigital)	
	Submetatarsal cyst	
	GREAT TOE AND MEDIAL FOREFOOT PAIN	
First MTP joint injury due to sprain	First MTP joint injuries due to dislocation or	Subungual melanocarcinoma
Fracture of the great toe	fracture of the sesamoids	Subungual glomus tumor
Subungual hematoma	Dislocation of the IP joint of the great toe	Subungual tumor
Crush injury of the distal toe resulting in	L5 radicular pain	Pulp space infection
soft tissue injury	First-ray overload syndrome	First MTP joint arthritis (septic) with or
Calluses		without associated osteomyelitis
Plantar warts		Joplin's neuroma
Corns		Calcific tendinitis of flexor hallucis tendons
Ingrown toenail		
Infected ingrown toenail		
Paronychia		
Infected blister		
Hallux valgus		
Bunion of the great toe		
Hallux limitus or rigidus		
Hallucal sesamoid disorder		
MTP joint arthritis (podagra)		
Gangrene or ulceration of the great toe		
Shoe vamp ulcer and bursitis		
	SMALL TOE PAIN	
Hard corns	Mallet toe	Tophus
Soft corns	Periungual corn (fifth toe)	Osler's nodes
Mosaic warts	Ulceration of the toes due to neuropathy	Subungual tumors: glomus tumor and
End corns	Candidiasis of the small toes	osteoid osteoma
Hammer toe	"Tailor's bunion"	
Ulceration of the toes due to vasculitis	Raynaud's disease and phenomenon	
Arthritis of the small toes	Subungual wart	
Tinea pedis		
Dorsal IP joint area pain and inflammation		
Contusions and fractures of the small toes		
	MIDFOOT PAIN	
Longitudinal arch strain	Tarsometatarsal joint sprain	Tarsometatarsal joint dislocation and/or
Subtalar osteochondral fracture	Navicular fractures: traumatic fractures and	fracture
Stress fracture of one or more metatarsals	stress fractures	Injury to the midtarsal joints
Osteoarthritis: first metatarsocuneiform joint	Fracture of the fifth metatarsal: avulsion and	Aseptic necrosis of the navicular bone
and cuboideometatarsal joint	diaphyseal	
Plantar fasciitis	Tendinitis of the flexor hallucis longus and	
Heel pain syndrome	peroneus longus and brevis	
	Interosseous myositis	
	Stress fracture of one or more tarsal bones	
	Pseudomonas osteomyelitis	
	Acquired flatfoot due to rupture of the	
	tibialis posterior tendon or ligamentous or	
	bone failure	
	Plantar abscess of the foot	

Common (>100)	Uncommon (>5–100)	Rare (>0–5)
	DORSAL FOOT PAIN	
Cellulitis	Acute pseudogout	Abscess of the foot
Acute gout	Reflex sympathetic dystrophy	Osteomyelitis
Peripheral polyneuropathy	Superficial peroneal nerve entrapment	Septic arthritis
Metatarsal trauma	Deep peroneal nerve entrapment	Herpes zoster
Stress fracture of the metatarsal	Bites	Aseptic necrosis of the navicular bone
Osteoarthritis of the tarsometatarsal joints	Shoe dermatitis	
Tendinitis of the tibialis anterior and toe extensor tendons	Tarsal bone trauma	
	Subtalar arthritis or osteochondral fracture	
	Interosseous muscle strain	
	Acquired pes planus	
	Cruxiate crural ligament sprain	
	GENERALIZED HINDFOOT PAIN	
Calcaneal fracture (intraarticular)	Calcaneal fracture (extraarticular)	
Ischemic necrosis of the heel		
	PLANTAR HINDFOOT PAIN	
Heel pain syndrome due to overuse	Fat pad disorders: atrophy, inflammation, fat pad separation due to a cyst, and piezogenic papules	Glomus tumor
Heel pain syndrome due to systemic disorders	Stress fracture of the calcaneus	
	Rupture of the plantar fascia	
	Entrapment neuropathy of the first branch of the lateral plantar nerve	
	True plantar fasciitis	
	Flexor tendinitis	
	POSTERIOR HINDFOOT PAIN	
Superficial Achilles bursitis	Haglund's syndrome	Calcaneal osteomyelitis
Retrocalcaneal bursitis	Achilles tendon rupture	
Achilles tendinitis	Calcaneal periostitis and osteitis	
	Fracture of the posterosuperior calcaneal tuberosity	
	MEDIAL HINDFOOT PAIN	
Tarsal tunnel syndrome	Tibialis posterior tendinitis	Calcaneal branch neurodynia
	Flexor hallucis longus tendinitis	
	Calcaneal fractures of the medial calcaneal process or sustentaculum tali	
	LATERAL HINDFOOT PAIN	
Lateral ankle sprain	Peroneal muscle strain	Sural nerve entrapment
	Peroneal tendinitis	
	Fracture of the lateral process of the talus	
	Osteochondral fracture of the talar dome	
	Stress fracture of the lateral malleolus	

A deeper injury may be associated with myonecrosis (e.g., gas in fascial planes and cutaneous crepitus). Surgical exploration to confirm or exclude myonecrosis and debride necrotic tissue, and parenteral antibiotic therapy lead to resolution. *A. hydrophila* may be isolated from the blood, wound drainage, debrided tissue, or bullae fluid.

3. Cellulitis Due to Vibrio vulnificus This infection causes a severely painful, red, warm, swollen foot with areas of skin necrosis, hemorrhagic bullae, and superficial ulceration. The infection follows wounding or wound contamination in warm ocean water. Systemic symptoms caused by bacteremia may be associated. There is a response to antibiotic therapy, incision and drainage, and debridement.

4. Cellulitis at a Saphenous Vein Donor Site One or more attacks of cellulitis caused by streptococcal species occur in up to 6 percent of patients who have had saphenous veins removed for use as coronary artery bypass grafts. Acute erythema, pain, swelling, and tenderness affect the proximal foot and lower leg. High fever, rigors, and toxicity are associated.

B. Necrotizing Fasciitis This disorder follows acute trauma or may complicate a cutaneous foot ulcer. Diabetes mellitus and alcohol and/or intravenous drug abuse are important risk factors. The foot becomes diffusely edematous, red, and hot, and the skin shiny and tense. The pain and tenderness are severe. Skin color changes appear during the first 2 to 4 days, resulting in irregular patches of blue-gray skin discoloration. Bullae containing hemorrhagic fluid may form. These bullae may rupture and collapse, leaving granular, deep-red, weeping superficial ulcerations. The involved area may become anesthetic in up to 16 percent of cases secondary to ischemia and destruction of the cutaneous nerves in the necrotic skin and subcutaneous tissue. Discolored areas of skin may progress to become black, leathery patches of skin gangrene (50 percent of cases). Subcutaneous gas may be demonstrable by palpation or on a plain radiograph. High fever, chills, rigors, diaphoresis, prostration, malaise, delirium, and a toxic appearance accompany the local changes in the foot. The wound and wound drainage may be very malodorous. Debridement reveals necrosis of the subcutaneous fat and the deep fascia and absence of myonecrosis. Type I necrotizing fasciitis is caused by a mixed infection consisting of an obligate anaerobic (e.g., *Bacteroides* or *Peptostreptococcus* species) and one or more facultative anaerobic bacteria (e.g., non-group A streptococci and members of the Enterobacteriaceae). Type II necrotizing fasciitis is caused by a group A streptococcus acting alone or in association with *S. aureus*. Extensive and frequent debridement and, in some cases, amputation are required. Antibiotic therapy is helpful in early cases and when used in patients receiving careful and frequent excision of necrotic tissue.

C. Abscess of the Foot　There is usually a toe or web space infection, a plantar ulcer, toe gangrene, or a contaminated deep, penetrating wound. Most abscesses occur in the central plantar compartment. Medial or lateral compartment infections result from ulceration of a bunion or bunionette, respectively. Diabetes and arteriosclerosis obliterans are important risk factors.

The dorsum of the foot becomes swollen and tender and the sole of the foot painful, tender, and flattened (e.g., loss of longitudinal arch due to edema). Local redness and warmth of the overlying skin may be present. The pain may be severe, deep, and throbbing, but in patients with severe diabetic polyneuropathy, the pain may be mild because of loss of sensory innervation. Fever, chills, malaise, anorexia, and delirium are sometimes associated. The abscess may be delineated most clearly by a T_2-weighted MRI. It may also be detected on a CT or an indium 111 labeled leukocyte scan. Drainage and antibiotic therapy may lead to resolution. The central plantar compartment contains four potential spaces layered one above the other (M1–M4) and partitioned by the bellies of the flexor and adductor muscles of the toes. One or all of these fascial spaces of the central compartment may contain pus.

D. Osteomyelitis of the Foot　Hematogenous osteomyelitis of the foot is uncommon in both children and adults. There are localized pain and tenderness and localized or diffuse swelling, erythema, and warmth. The calcaneus is most commonly involved (51 percent of cases), followed by the metatarsal bones (23 percent), tarsal bones (10 percent), and phalanges (7 percent). In adults, fever and leukocytosis may not occur. The sedimentation rate, however, is usually elevated.

Confirmation of the diagnosis requires evidence of the disease by imaging studies and bone biopsy. Plain radiographs with or without tomography may not demonstrate any abnormality for 7 to 15 days. Radionuclide studies such as triple-phase technetium 99m methylene diphosphonate (^{99m}Tc-MDP), indium 111 labeled leukocyte, and gallium 67-citrate scans are sensitive and accurate methods of detecting bone infection. Radionuclide scans often fail to differentiate soft tissue infection from osteomyelitis.

False-positive results may occur in the feet of patients with osteoarthritis or diabetic neuroarthropathy. MRI is as sensitive as ^{99m}Tc-MDP and gallium 67-citrate scans and is more specific (false-positive rate, 11 percent vs. 82 percent). In one report, osteomyelitis in the foot was best demonstrated on T_1-weighted or short-tau inversion recovery (STIR) images. There is a therapeutic response to parenteral antibiotic therapy. Surgical intervention is required when fever and local tenderness persist and there is evidence of a subperiosteal abscess, sequestra, and necrotic soft tissue.

3. ARTHRITIS OF THE FOOT

A. Septic Arthritis　This disorder is usually monarticular. Oligoarticular involvement may occur, but it is rare. Aching and/or throbbing pain, swelling, and tenderness occur over the affected joint. Skin erythema and warmth may be present. Hematogenous spread, an adjacent osteomyelitis, or a penetrating wound (nail puncture) may be the cause. Risk factors for septic arthritis in patients without gonococcal infection include local trauma, immunosuppression, preexisting joint disease (e.g., osteoarthritis and rheumatoid arthritis), and infection at another site.

In sexually active adults, *Neisseria gonorrhoeae* is a frequent cause of septic arthritis. Involvement of the foot is uncommon in disseminated gonococcal disease. Migratory polyarthralgias; tenosynovitis of the wrists, hands, feet, and ankles; pustular, necrotic, or hemorrhagic vesicular, 1- to 1.5-cm, red-based skin lesions on the distal portion of the arms and legs; localized arthritis in one to three joints; positive results of blood, synovial fluid, or mucous membrane cultures for *N. gonorrhoeae*; and a dramatic response to parenteral ceftriaxone therapy are characteristic findings in disseminated gonococcal infection.

Older adults are infected by *S. aureus*, streptococcal species, and gram-negative bacteria.

Synovial fluid contains 5000 to over 250,000 cells/mm³ with a polymorphonuclear leukocyte predominance. Cultures are positive in 70 to 90 percent of cases. Results of a Gram stain of synovial fluid may be falsely negative in up to 50 percent of cases. Parenteral antibiotic therapy and needle aspiration, open surgical drainage, or continuous irrigation of the joint lead to resolution of joint symptoms.

B. Seropositive Rheumatoid Arthritis

1. Forefoot Pain   Metatarsalgia is an early complaint. The lateral metatarsophalangeal (MTP) joints are usually the first to be affected, and eventually all MTP joints are involved. The forefoot is usually tender and swollen. Local palpation over the MTP joints, movement of the joints, and lateral compression of the foot provoke or intensify the pain.

Ligamentous laxity in the forefoot leads to spreading of the metatarsals and splaying of the forefoot (33 percent of cases) on weight bearing. Subluxation of the metatarsals downward and laterally occurs. The metatarsal heads may protrude on the plantar surface of the forefoot and may cause the development of painful calluses, inflamed bursae, or plantar ulcers.

Claw toes (hyperextension of the MTP joint and flexion of both interphalangeal [IP] joints) and hammer toes (hyperextension of the MTP joint, flexion of the proximal interphalangeal [PIP] joint, and extension of the distal interphalangeal [DIP] joint) frequently develop (53 percent of cases) secondary to MTP joint involvement due to downward subluxation of the metatarsal heads and intrinsic muscle imbalance. Hyperextension of the phalanges occurs at the arthritic MTP joints. Painful calluses and ulcers may develop over the dorsum of the PIP joints due to friction with a closely fitting shoe toe box. The skin over the joint becomes red, swollen, and tender and may form a fissure or ulcer.

Hallux valgus (59 percent of cases) occurs, and the great toe passes below or above the second and third toes. Hallux rigidus may also develop and cause great toe pain.

2. Midfoot Pain   Midfoot pain is usually minimal. The talonavicular joint is the most common site. There may be local swelling and tenderness over the joint. Asymptomatic midfoot involvement is frequent, occurring in 58 to 72 percent of cases. Valgus deformity of the hindfoot and flattening of the longitudinal arch may occur.

3. Hindfoot Pain   Subtalar joint pain, swelling, stiffness, and tenderness occur. Foot inversion or eversion movements are painful and may be limited. Palpation of the sinus tarsi reveals tenderness. Acquired flatfoot may occur, causing medial and/or lateral hindfoot and midfoot pain. Other causes of hindfoot pain include tenosynovitis of the peroneal and/or tibialis posterior tendons. In most cases, however, rheumatoid tenosynovitis is painless. Retrocalcaneal bursitis and plantar calcaneal rheumatoid nodules may occur.

The feet may be the initial site of symptomatic joint involvement. In such cases, other criteria for the diagnosis of rheumatoid arthritis (e.g., serum rheumatoid factor) develop within 2 years.

Achilles tendinitis and plantar fasciitis seldom occur with seropositive rheumatoid arthritis. Diagnostic criteria for rheumatoid arthritis include (1) morning stiffness for 1 h or more and present for 6 weeks; (2) arthritis involving three or more joints for at least 6 weeks; (3) swelling and pain of wrist, metacarpophalangeal, or PIP joints for 6 or more weeks; (4) symmetrical joint swelling and pain; (5) rheumatoid nodules; (6) positive serum test results for rheumatoid factor; and (7) hand radiographic changes showing juxtaarticular erosion and osteopenia. Radiographic changes in the feet may precede those in the hands, allowing for earlier definitive diagnosis. The presence of four of the seven American Rheumatism Association criteria listed above allows classification of a case as rheumatoid arthritis.

C. Seronegative Spondyloarthropathies

1. Ankylosing Spondylitis   This disorder usually presents with a history of inflammatory back pain (e.g., pain with onset before age 40; duration of more than 3 months before help is sought; morning back pain and stiffness; insidious mode of onset; and improvement with exercise and activity). Other diagnostic criteria for ankylosing spondylitis include limitation of motion of the lumbar spine in the sagittal and frontal planes, limited chest expansion, and definite radiographic evidence of sacroiliitis. The presence of radiographic evidence of sacroiliitis and one other criterion is sufficient for a diagnosis of ankylosing spondylitis. The HLA-B27 gene is present in 90 percent of white and 50 percent of black patients with ankylosing spondylitis. Forefoot involvement includes the MTP joints (resulting in metatarsalgia) and toe deformities (hammer toes). Erosive arthritis may involve the MTP and IP joints. Involvement is asymmetrical, in contrast to seropositive rheumatoid arthritis. Midfoot involvement includes painless fusion of the intertarsal joints. Subtalar arthritis, resulting in marked limitation of foot inversion or eversion, plantar fasciitis, and Achilles tenosynovitis may cause midfoot and hindfoot pain. Bone erosions may occur at the Achilles tendon insertion site, and a calcaneal spur may be present on a plain radiograph of the heel. Radiographic characteristics that help separate the seronegative spondyloarthropathies from rheumatoid arthritis include asymmetry of joint involvement, less juxtaarticular osteopenia, more osteosclerosis, new periosteal bone formation, and atypical punched-out, and sometimes large, peripheral erosions.

Acute anterior uveitis, with eye pain, redness, photophobia, and tearing is the most common extraarticular manifestation of ankylosing spondylitis (20 percent of cases). Attacks of uveitis are usually unilateral and tend to be recurrent.

2. Reiter's Syndrome This form of reactive arthritis may follow an episode of diarrheal disease (e.g., caused by *Salmonella, Shigella, Yersinia,* or *Campylobacter* species or *Clostridium difficile*) or urethritis (e.g., caused by *Chlamydia trachomatis, Ureaplasma urealyticum,* or *N. gonorrhoeae*). A complete syndrome with arthritis, urethritis, and conjunctivitis, may occur (20 percent of cases), or more commonly only two of the syndrome components may be present (80 percent of cases).

Forefoot findings include asymmetrical MTP and IP arthritis, dactylitis (sausage digits) due to periostitis, and flexor tenosynovitis. Dactylitis may at times be painless. Sesamoiditis may cause first metatarsal region pain and tenderness. Painful or painless tarsal joint disease may occur, leading to bony rigidity of the midfoot region. Hindfoot pain may result from subtalar arthritis, periostitis, plantar fasciitis, Achilles tendinitis, calcaneal erosions, and spurs. Radiographic evidence of new bone formation at the insertion of the Achilles tendon or the plantar fascia on the calcaneus may be present. A "fluffy" periostitis results at the heel and other sites. The heel abnormalities associated with postvenereal Reiter's syndrome have been called "lover's heels." Early in the course of this disorder, radiographs may show periarticular soft tissue swelling and joint effusions, or they may appear normal. With progression, juxtaarticular osteoporosis, joint space narrowing, and erosions develop. Periostitis may appear in the feet, pelvis, and at other sites, and calcaneal spurs may occur. Reiter's syndrome may also be associated with iridocyclitis, balanitis circinata, keratoderma blennorrhagicum, and oral ulcers. Reiter's syndrome is considered a subset of reactive arthritis. The HLA-B27 gene is associated with reactive arthritis (75 percent of patients in most ethnic groups with reactive arthritis). Patients with reactive arthritis may also have spondylitis, which begins at any point along the lumbar spine. The syndesmophytes are coarse and nonmarginal, arising at times from the middle of a vertebral body, a pattern seldom seen in ankylosing spondylitis.

3. Psoriatic Arthritis Psoriasis may be associated with painful swelling of one or more toes. Dactylitis, or "sausage toe," may involve the fifth toe alone or several toes. This lesion is caused by PIP and DIP joint involvement, flexor tenosynovitis, and periostitis. Heel pain due to insertional tendinitis or plantar fasciitis may also occur. Midfoot pain may be due to intertarsal arthritis or to plantar fasciitis. DIP arthritis is more prominent than MTP involvement. Osteolysis may occur at the ends of metatarsals and phalanges, resulting in "pencil-in-cup" radiographic deformities. Digit shortening may result from osteolysis, and severe osteolysis may cause an "opera glass" deformity of all the digits of the foot. Hammer or claw toes and downward dis-

placement of the metatarsal heads is uncommon. New bone formation of the base of the great toe can cause a painful hallux rigidus. Arthritis involving the great toe may simulate acute gout.

Nail changes (i.e., pitting, ridging, onychodystrophy, subungual hyperkeratosis, onycholysis, and yellow pigmentation of the nails) may occur in psoriasis or in Reiter's syndrome. Radiologic findings that differentiate psoriatic arthritis from rheumatoid arthritis include DIP joint lesions with erosions and expansion of the bases of the terminal phalanges, distal phalangeal osteolysis, oligoarthritis, sacroiliitis, spondylitis, and arthritis mutilans ("pencil-in-cup" appearance at one or more DIP joints).

4. Arthritis Associated with Inflammatory Bowel Disease Arthritis may occur with inflammatory bowel disease (9–20 percent of cases). It is more often associated with large-bowel disease and occurs in patients with such complications of their intestinal disease as abscesses, pseudomembranous polyposis, anal fistulae, bleeding, uveitis, stomatitis, erythema nodosum, and pyoderma gangrenosum. Fifty percent of patients have a migratory polyarthritis. MTP joint pain, swelling, and tenderness may occur. The knee, ankle, elbow, wrist, and hand joints may be affected. Synovial fluid cell counts are in the 5000 to 12,000 range, with a polymorphonuclear cell predominance. Radiographs show soft tissue edema and joint effusions without erosions. Joint symptoms respond to treatment of the bowel disease by colectomy or drugs.

D. Acute Gout An attack of acute arthritis may be precipitated by alcohol abuse, dehydration, trauma, surgery, septic arthritis, protein fasting, diuretic therapy, excessive purine ingestion, and introduction of allopurinol or uricosuric agents.

Severe pain, swelling, heat, redness, and exquisite local tenderness may involve the first MTP joint area (podagra), the instep region, the ankle joint, and the heel (retrocalcaneal bursitis and Achilles tendinitis). Fever, chills, sweating, and malaise may be associated findings. One or more of these sites may be involved in an acute attack. Any jarring or movement of the limb may provoke pain. Involvement is usually limited to one foot and ankle region but may be bilateral. Synovial fluid cell counts may exceed 100,000 cells/mm^3, with a polymorphonuclear cell predominance. Intra- and extracellular monosodium urate crystals may be seen in the synovial fluid and identified by their characteristic shape and negative birefringence. The serum uric acid level is usually elevated. Some cases mimic a cellulitis or phlebitis.

Podagra is not specific for acute gout. First MTP joint inflammation may occur in calcium pyrophosphate deposition disease, psoriatic arthritis, Reiter's syndrome, sarcoidosis, and with septic arthritis. Acute gout will usually respond dramatically to colchicine or indomethacin.

E. Acute Pseudogout   A similar acute arthritis may occur and mimic gout. The ankle, the dorsum of the foot, and the first MTP joint may be involved serially or simultaneously. Attacks may be less severe than in gout. Surgery or trauma may provoke an attack. Synovial fluid contains extra- and intracellular calcium pyrophosphate dihydrate crystals (positive birefringence) and an increased concentration of polymorphonuclear leukocytes. Chondrocalcinosis may be demonstrable in plain radiographs of the knees, wrists, shoulders, and ankles.

F. Acute Rheumatic Fever   An acute migratory polyarthritis occurs, primarily involving the ankles and knees. The wrists, elbows, fingers, MTP, and toe joints may be affected. The joints are usually swollen, warm, red, and tender. Walking may be extremely painful because of ankle and foot pain. Fever, generalized aching, diaphoresis, and weight loss may be associated. The acute arthritic syndrome usually begins within 2 to 5 weeks of an acute streptococcal tonsillitis or pharyngitis. Subcutaneous nodules may be palpable over extensor surfaces. Joint involvement is frequently asymmetrical. Symptoms and signs of carditis and neurologic dysfunction (i.e., chorea) are rare in adults. There is a dramatic response of fever and joint symptoms to aspirin therapy. Mild anemia and leukocytosis may be present. Antistreptolysin O, antihyaluronidase, and anti-DNase B titers are elevated, as is the Streptozyme agglutination titer.

G. Systemic Lupus Erythematosus   Arthralgias or arthritis in the MTP joints, midfoot, and ankles may occur. The Achilles tendon may rupture, causing posterior hindfoot pain and tenderness and weakness of plantar flexion. Pain in the toes and fingers may result from Raynaud's phenomenon or from digital ischemia with or without gangrene due to vasculitis. Paresthesias, pain, and dysesthesias in the digits may also result from a peripheral polyneuropathy. The serum antinuclear antibody level is usually elevated, and anti-ds-DNA and anti-Smith antibody levels may be elevated. Arthritic symptoms respond dramatically to prednisone therapy.

H. Sickle Cell Pain Crisis   Severe pain may occur in the lower legs, feet, and ankles, associated with skin allodynia and hyperesthesia. Subcutaneous edema may be present over the small joints and bones of the feet. Any movement or light touch to the skin intensifies the pain. MRI may reveal normal bones or a small area of bone marrow infarction, as well as edema of the skin and subcutaneous tissue. The pain appears to be due to a reversible sensory neuropathy and, in some areas of the feet, to bone marrow infarction. Spontaneous remission of pain and edema occur in 1 to 3 weeks.

I. Hepatitis B-Associated Arthritis   Fever, malaise, sore throat, myalgias, nausea, and vomiting precede the onset of joint pain by 1 to 12 weeks. A symmetrical migratory or additive polyarthritis occurs. The toes are involved in 15 percent and the fingers in 65 percent of cases.

Joint complaints may persist for a few days or several months. Up to 50 percent of patients develop an urticarial or maculopapular rash that may be pruritic. Angioedema of the soles of the feet may occur. Hepatitis B surface antigen (HB_sAg) is usually present in the serum, and liver function test results may be abnormal.

J. Rubella-Associated Arthritis   A faint maculopapular rash; a painful, tender occipital lymphadenitis; and low-grade fever precede or follow complaints of symmetrical polyarthralgia and joint stiffness. Pain is mild at rest but is intensified by joint movement and use. The toes are involved in up to 25 percent of cases.

4.   VASCULAR PAIN

A. Acute Arterial Occlusion   There is an abrupt onset of aching, deep, and/or burning superficial pain in the foot and lower leg. Skin pallor and coldness, weakness of the distal limb muscles, acroparesthesias, decrease or loss of light touch and two-point discrimination, and absence of pulses are other associated findings. A skin line of demarcation separating ischemic pallor from normal skin color may be present. Cyanotic mottling of the toes and plantar aspect of the foot may develop. Sudden occlusion may follow trauma (e.g., due to arterial disruption, compression, or thrombosis), an embolus (e.g., arising in the aorta or heart), or a thrombosis. Surgical restoration of blood flow to the distal extremity within 6 h leads to resolution of all symptoms without residual weakness, sensory loss, or gangrene.

B. Nocturnal Rest Pain   Severe, aching pain in the foot and/or lower leg occurs during sleep and wakes the patient. Dangling the foot over the edge of the bed or standing and walking about provides partial or complete relief. The ankle/brachial index is usually less than 0.5. Nocturnal pain is associated with a sleep-related fall in mean arterial blood pressure and decreased perfusion in the subcutaneous tissue of the foot.

C. Ulceration and Gangrene

1. Cholesterol Embolism   Risk factors include hypercholesterolemia, diabetes mellitus, tobacco use, hypertension, a history of vascular disease at other sites (e.g., cerebrovascular disease, angina or myocardial infarction, intermittent claudication), and an aortic or popliteal aneurysm. Precipitating events include angiography (i.e., aortic arch, aorta, and coronary), trauma, aortitis, angioplasty, use of an intraaortic balloon, vascular surgery (e.g., femoropopliteal or aortofemoral bypass and aortic aneurysm resection), and use of heparin, streptokinase, or warfarin. Most embolic events occur within the first 2 weeks after a diagnostic or therapeutic intervention. In some cases, no precipitating event can be identified. Foot pain may be associated with the ''blue toe'' syndrome, areas of blue-black plantar infarction, foot and toe gangrene, foot ulcers, and foot and toe ischemia. Renal emboli may be associated. Flank and back pain, gross hematuria, accelerated hypertension, and rapidly progressive renal insufficiency may occur with renal embolization. Penile gangrene, bowel infarction, and spinal cord infarction may occur in a small percentage of cases. Laboratory abnormalities include eosinophilia, leukocytosis, microhematuria, albuminuria, thrombocytopenia, and hypocomplementemia. Histologic confirmation of the diagnosis is required using resected tissue (i.e., for gangrene) or biopsy of foot or lower leg skin, subcutaneous tissue, or muscle. Unilateral or bilateral foot involvement may occur.

2. Arteriosclerosis Obliterans and Progressive Ischemia
The extremities are cool, pale, and hairless, and evidence of calf and sometimes thigh muscle atrophy is present. Trophic nail changes may occur. A history of intermittent claudication and/or nocturnal or persistent rest pain may be obtained. One or more toes become painful and then black and mummified. In some cases, necrotic toe ulcers develop. Pulses are usually absent in the feet and popliteal space and may be present or barely palpable in the femoral region. Unilateral or bilateral pain and necrosis may occur.

3. Systemic Vasculitis

A. POLYARTERITIS NODOSA   Bilateral or unilateral toe gangrene, skin infarcts, ischemic ulcers (e.g., over the lateral malleolus or plantar surface), arthralgias, and Raynaud's phenomenon are the more frequent causes of foot pain associated with this disorder. Symptoms and signs of a systemic disorder are usually present. They may include fever, weakness, weight loss, anorexia, malaise, myalgias, headache, arthralgias, and abdominal pain.

Renal involvement may result in microscopic hematuria, albuminuria, cylindruria, an elevated creatinine level, and hypertension. Renal ischemia and infarction and glomerulitis occur. Cardiac involvement may cause acute myocardial infarction, pericarditis, and congestive heart failure. Cerebral infarction, delirium, and seizures result from ischemic damage to the central nervous system. Peripheral polyneuropathy and mononeuropathy multiplex result from ischemic injury to peripheral nerves. Intraabdominal vasculitis may cause abdominal pain, nausea, vomiting, bleeding, bowel infarction, perforation, peritonitis, cholecystitis, and pancreatic and hepatic infarction.

Leukocytosis, an elevated sedimentation rate, anemia, and hypergammaglobulinemia are common findings. Total serum complement and C3 and C4 levels may be depressed. Hepatitis B surface antigen may be detected in 10 to 54 percent of cases. The diagnosis is supported by detection of aneurysms of small and medium-sized arteries in the renal, hepatic, or gastrointestinal vascular beds. Biopsy of a skin nodule, a tender testicle, or a painful and tender muscle will frequently confirm the diagnosis. Symptoms and signs respond to combined treatment with cyclophosphamide and prednisone.

B. ALLERGIC ANGIITIS AND GRANULOMATOSIS (CHURG-STRAUSS DISEASE)   This disorder is similar to polyarteritis nodosa. Differences include severe pulmonary symptoms with asthma and pulmonary infiltrates and only mild renal involvement. Purpura and skin nodules occur in 70 percent of cases. Peripheral eosinophilia (10 percent or greater) is a frequent finding and is helpful in supporting the diagnosis and in distinguishing this disorder from polyarteritis nodosa. Confirmation of the diagnosis requires a tissue biopsy demonstrating granulomatous vasculitis and tissue infiltration by eosinophils. Mononeuropathy or polyneuropathy and paranasal sinus abnormalities are also associated. Toe and foot gangrene may occur from small vessel occlusion in the feet. Symptoms and signs respond to therapy with cyclophosphamide and prednisone.

Antineutrophil cytoplasmic antibodies (ANCA) have been used to differentiate types of vasculitis. C-ANCA is a cytoplasmic immunofluorescence staining pattern associated with antiproteinase 3 antibodies. This pattern occurs with microscopic polyarteritis nodosa, Wegener's granulomatosis, and primary necrotizing and crescentic glomerulonephritis. The P-ANCA pattern associated with antimyeloperoxidase antibodies occurs with the same three diseases and Churg-Strauss disease.

C. SYSTEMIC LUPUS ERYTHEMATOSUS   Gangrene of the toes or fingers, plantar region, and foot and painful ischemic foot and lower leg ulcers are associated with vasculitis. The sedimentation rate is elevated, and total serum complement, C3, and C4 levels are decreased. Clinical and laboratory features of systemic lupus erythematosus include the following: (1) nonerosive polyarthritis; (2) malar rash; (3) discoid rash; (4) photosensitivity; (5) oral ulcers; (6) hematologic abnormalities (e.g., anemia of chronic disease, hemolytic anemia, lymphopenia, leukopenia, and thrombocytopenia); (7) neurologic disease (e.g., psychoses and seizures); (8) cardiopulmonary disease (e.g., pleurisy, pericarditis, and myocarditis); (9) renal disease (e.g., proteinuria, cylindruria, nephrotic syndrome, and renal failure);

(10) positive anti-nuclear antibody (ANA) test results; and (11) confirming test results (positive LE cell slide test, anti-ds-DNA titer, or anti-Sm titer results or a false-positive VDRL test). A combination of a positive ANA test result and a confirming test or a total of four or more of the above-listed clinical and laboratory disease criteria makes a diagnosis of systemic lupus erythematosus highly probable.

D. RHEUMATOID ARTHRITIS Vasculitis may cause digital pain and gangrene in the feet and/or hands, nail fold infarcts, and painful ischemic ulcers on the feet and toes. Visceral involvement in the form of intestinal ischemia and infarction, pericarditis, and coronary occlusion may be associated. Serum total hemolytic complement and C3 and C4 levels are depressed. Peripheral neuritis and mononeuritis multiplex may be associated findings. Vasculitis occurs in patients with severe arthritis, rheumatoid nodules, and a high titer of circulating rheumatoid factor. Therapy with prednisone and cyclophosphamide may control the vasculitis.

E. HYPERSENSITIVITY VASCULITIS This disorder may result in areas of cutaneous necrosis and painful ulceration on the feet and toes. It may occur as Schönlein-Henoch purpura (palpable purpuric skin lesions on the legs and buttocks, joint and abdominal pain, and glomerulonephritis) or as a small-vessel vasculitis associated with Sjögren's syndrome or with essential mixed cryoglobulinemia (glomerulonephritis, joint pain, hepatosplenomegaly, lymphadenopathy, and palpable purpura).

Hypersensitivity vasculitis may also be associated with an underlying lymphoid or reticuloendothelial neoplasm. The diagnosis can be confirmed by biopsy of cutaneous lesions. Schönlein-Henoch purpura may respond to glucocorticoid therapy or resolve spontaneously.

F. THROMBOANGIITIS OBLITERANS (BUERGER'S DISEASE) This disorder occurs predominantly in young men (male/female ratio, 9:1) in the 20- to 40-year-old age group. Most cases occur in Asians and eastern Europeans. Raynaud's phenomenon and ischemic finger and/or toe pain associated with pallor, skin mottling, and coldness are common complaints. Digital ulceration and/or gangrene may also occur. Ischemic neuropathy may cause shooting pains in the lower legs and feet. Intermittent claudication involving the lower calf or arch of the foot may occur. Claudication of the forearms and hands may also be present. Migratory thrombophlebitis involving the superficial veins of the feet, legs, and arms may occur. Examination reveals absent or diminished pedal, radial, and ulnar pulses and normal proximal pulses. The digits may be pale and cold, or mottled and painful toe and plantar surface ulcers and gangrene

may occur. Visceral infarction may be associated. There is strong association with smoking tobacco. Clinical findings supporting the diagnosis include evidence of upper and lower extremity ischemia and migratory superficial thrombophlebitis. Arteriograms showing smooth, tapering, segmental distal arterial lesions and prominent collateral vessels at sites of vascular occlusion are characteristic. Excisional biopsy and histopathologic examination of an involved vessel will confirm the diagnosis. Cessation of smoking may or may not retard disease progression. There is no effective therapy.

4. Erythromelalgia This disorder causes episodes of intense burning and throbbing pain in the toes and soles, accompanied by redness, warmth, and in some cases swelling of the affected foot. Less commonly, the fingers and palms may be involved. In the primary or idiopathic type, symmetrical involvement of the sole of the forefoot and the toes is the rule. Exposure to warmth (e.g., a warm room, a heating blanket, or sunlight), dependency, or exercise may precipitate an attack, while cold water, an ice bath, use of aspirin, or elevation of the foot relieves it. Some attacks are spontaneous. Episodes may last a few minutes, hours, or several days. Symptoms can be provoked in the laboratory by increasing the skin temperature of the foot or hand to 32 to 36°C.

Secondary forms of erythromelalgia caused asymmetrical symptoms in 48 percent of cases, while the idiopathic type is asymmetrical in only 5 to 10 percent. Foot involvement alone occurs in 65 to 75 percent of cases, while palm and finger involvement as the only complaint occurs in only 5 to 9 percent.

Secondary erythromelalgia is associated with essential thrombocythemia, polycythemia vera, agnogenic myeloid metaplasia, and, rarely, with chronic myelogenous leukemia. Symptoms of erythromelalgia precede the clinical onset of the myeloproliferative disease by a median interval of $2\frac{1}{2}$ years, but this period may be as long as 16 years. Less commonly, erythromelalgia may follow the onset of the myeloproliferative disease. Secondary erythromelalgia may also occur in hypertension, venous insufficiency, diabetes mellitus, systemic lupus erythematosus, rheumatoid arthritis, gout, multiple sclerosis, and spinal cord disease. Drug-related erythromelalgia has also been reported (e.g., bromcriptine, ergot, and nifedipine).

Toe pain and erythema may progress to cyanosis, coldness, and gangrene. Necrosis of toes, portions of the forefoot, or the entire foot may develop. Ischemic foot ulcers and secondary septicemia may occur.

Peripheral pulses are usually normal, and thermography has been used to map erythromelalgic areas, but this technique does not provide specific diagnostic information.

Aspirin relieves thrombocythemia-related erythromelalgia for 3 to 4 days, while indomethacin is effective for less than 24 h. Aspirin may also provide relief in some cases of primary or idiopathic erythromelalgia and to some patients with secondary erythromelalgia not related to thrombocythemia. Platelet-mediated arteriolar inflammation and thrombosis may be responsible for many cases. These histopathologic changes may be observed on skin biopsies.

Cases of erythromelalgia beginning during the first two decades of life may have a hereditary basis. This type may be refractory to aspirin and other forms of therapy.

5. *Phlegmasia Cerulea Dolens*   Nearly all of the deep veins draining the leg are occluded. The leg is cool, cyanotic, and markedly swollen. Foot and calf pain are severe. Necrosis of the skin of the foot and ankle may occur, and hemorrhagic bullae may form over the dorsum of the foot and sides of the ankle. Salvage of the foot is possible with anticoagulant and systemic thrombolytic therapy.

5. REFLEX SYMPATHETIC DYSTROPHY

This disorder may begin spontaneously or follow mild or severe trauma or surgery. The predominant symptom is severe burning, aching, or throbbing pain in the entire foot or in a localized portion of the foot (e.g., medial forefoot, plantar surface, or dorsum of the foot). Swelling and skin warmth with diffuse or periarticular erythema are common accompanying signs during the first few days or weeks. The pain appears to be too severe to be explained by previous trauma, surgery, or physical examination findings. The joints are painful and stiff. Initially, the edema is pitting and resolves with foot elevation. Hyperhidrosis of the painful foot may be present. Hypertrichosis may first become apparent after 2 to 4 weeks. Skin hyperesthesia and allodynia are severe. Emotional stress, noise, jarring, air currents, or the pressure of bed sheets may intensify the foot pain. The first stage, described above, may continue for 1 to 3 months. During the latter part of the first month, the skin may become cold, pale, and shiny. During stage 2, cyanotic mottling of the foot and lower leg develop. Hyperhidrosis persists, but the rate of hair and nail growth decreases. Joint range of motion continues to be limited by pain and stiffness. Hyperesthesia remains severe, and walking or even standing without crutches is not tolerated. Plain radiographs at 4 to 6 weeks reveal patchy, mottled osteoporosis in the painful area, and a radionuclide bone scan reveals increased periarticular uptake. Sympathetic blockade relieves pain and allodynia and allows increased range of joint motion. Physiotherapy made possible by sympathetic blockade leads to improved function and resolution of pain, edema, and abnormalities of skin color and temperature. Patients with reflex sympathetic dystrophy may appear anxious,

unstable, and withdrawn. These symptoms may persist after the pain and other abnormalities have been successfully treated.

6. FOOT CRAMPS

Severe, sharp pain may occur in the arch of the foot following unaccustomed exercise involving the lower extremity, in association with pregnancy, or secondary to a number of disorders. These include peripheral polyneuropathy, polymyositis, radiculitis or radicular compression, lower motor neuron disease, hyponatremia, hypocalcemia, hypomagnesemia, and hypocapnia (carpopedal spasm) secondary to hyperventilation and cirrhosis of the liver. A painful foot cramp may be relieved by manual stretching of the involved muscle, by massage, or by walking on the painful foot, which stretches the contracted muscle.

7. PERIPHERAL NEUROPATHY

The causes of mononeuritis multiplex and symmetrical polyneuropathy are summarized in Tables 47-1 and 47-2, respectively.

A. Endocrine

1. *Diabetic Polyneuropathy*

A. ACUTE SENSORY POLYNEUROPATHY   This disorder has an acute onset with constant burning pain in the feet and, in some cases, the lower leg and ankle region. Painful paresthesias, allodynia, and skin hyperesthesia are associated. Both feet and

Table 47-1
MONONEURITIS MULTIPLEX ASSOCIATED WITH ASYMMETRICAL DISTAL LEG AND FOOT PAIN

Vasculitis
  Polyarteritis nodosa
  Rheumatoid arthritis
  Wegener's granulomatosis
  Sjögren's syndrome
  Churg-Strauss disease
  Systemic lupus erythematosus
  Giant cell arteritis
  Systemic sclerosis
  Hypersensitivity vasculitis
Sarcoidosis
AIDS
Amyloidosis
Coagulopathies
Diabetes mellitus
Hypothyroidism

Table 47-2
SYMMETRICAL POLYNEUROPATHY ASSOCIATED WITH FOOT PAIN SENSORY OR SENSORIMOTOR

Endocrine
  Diabetes mellitus
  Hypothyroidism
Toxic
  Alcohol abuse and nutritional deficiencies
  Heavy metal poisoning
    Arsenic
    Mercury
    Thallium
  Drugs
    Disulfiram
    Isoniazid
    Hydralazine
    Other drugs (Table 47-3)
  Chemicals (Table 47-4)
Systemic disorders
  Carcinoma
  Acute leukemia
  Chronic leukemia
  Lymphoma
  Myeloma (osteolytic, osteosclerotic, and POEMS syndrome)
  Waldenström's macroglobulinemia
  Cryoglobulinemia
  Connective tissue diseases
    Polyarteritis nodosa
    Rheumatoid arthritis
    Systemic lupus erythematosus
    Churg-Strauss disease
  Renal failure
  AIDS
  Sarcoidosis
Hereditary
  Fabry's disease
  Intermittent acute porphyria

lower legs are involved, symmetrically. Sharp, stabbing, or electric-like shooting pains occur in the lower legs and feet at irregular intervals. Symptoms are more severe at night and after standing or walking for a prolonged period. Patchy sensory loss for light touch, pinprick sensation, and vibration may affect the toes and distal feet, but the motor system remains intact. Weight loss, fatigue, and depression are associated. Good diabetic control leads to symptom improvement and resolution within weeks or months.

B. SUBACUTE OR CHRONIC SENSORIMOTOR POLYNEUROPATHY   This disorder has a more insidious onset than acute sensory polyneuropathy, with sensations of numbness, prickling or tingling paresthesias, and/or burning pain on the soles. Symptoms are usually confined to the feet, although episodic numbness and paresthesias of the fingers may be reported. Burning discomfort may involve the dorsum and plantar surface of the feet or only the latter. The pain may be precipitated by prolonged standing and walk-

ing. Sharp, electric-like pains may radiate down or up the legs and involve the feet. Symptoms are usually more severe at night. Skin hyperesthesia and allodynia may be intermittent. Sensory loss is more severe over the forefoot and may be partial or complete. All sensory modalities may be lost. A "painful-painless" foot may occur. A patient with this problem feels pain but demonstrates loss of pain sensation, placing the foot at risk of injury. Atrophy of small foot muscles and depressed reflexes also occur. Burning and stabbing foot pain may be present every day or may occur in episodes. Truncal polyneuropathy with abdominal or flank pain and hyperesthesia may be associated. Tricyclic drugs (e.g., imipramine and amitriptyline) may provide complete or partial relief.

C. MONONEURITIS MULTIPLEX   This disorder involves multiple peripheral nerves. It causes painful dysesthesias, pain, paresthesias, and sensory and motor deficits in the distribution of the involved nerves (e.g., posterior tibial nerve, superficial peroneal nerve, or sural nerve). The feet and lower legs are involved on one or both sides. Similar symptoms may occur in the arms and hands.

2. Hypothyroid Polyneuropathy   Pain and paresthesias in the feet and hands occur. Distal sensory loss and depressed reflexes occur in the arms and legs. Muscle dysfunction may also develop, resulting in a slowing of muscle contraction and relaxation. Decreased nerve conduction velocity may be detected in the motor and sensory nerves of the arms and legs. In severe cases, distal muscle weakness may be present, and painful muscle cramps may occur. Pain and other symptoms resolve with thyroid replacement therapy.

B. Toxic

1. Alcoholic Polyneuropathy   Alcohol abuse and dietary deficiency are both involved in the pathogenesis of this disorder. In severe cases, patients complain of burning feet, paresthesias, and skin hypesthesia of the stocking areas of the legs. The legs are affected before the arms, and in most cases the upper extremities are spared. The pain in the feet may be described as a burning discomfort over the soles or as a deep, dull, constant ache. Sharp, stabbing, brief pains may shoot down or up the leg and into the feet.

Allodynia and tactile hyperesthesia may be severe. Contact of the feet with the bed sheets may provoke severe discomfort and prevent sleep. Physical examination may reveal distal and/or proximal muscle weakness, and muscle tenderness (i.e., in the feet and calves). Ankle and knee reflexes are diminished. Hyperhidrosis of the feet and hands is common and reflects sympathetic overactivity. Sensory loss includes touch;

pain; temperature (superficial sensation); and deep pressure, vibration, and position senses (deep sensation). Most patients show a combination of both superficial and deep sensory loss, but superficial loss alone may occur in up to 25 percent and deep loss alone in up to 10 percent.

Alcoholic polyneuropathy may be associated with cerebellar degeneration (tremors and limb-gait ataxia), Wernicke's disease (nystagmus, lateral rectus muscle weakness or paralysis, paralysis of conjugate gaze, gait ataxia, and a global confusional state), or Wernicke-Korsakoff syndrome (Wernicke's disease combined with an amnestic confabulatory psychosis).

Abstinence from alcohol, thiamine and other B vitamin replacement, and a good diet may lead to gradual resolution of the neuropathic and central nervous system manifestations of alcohol abuse.

2. Heavy Metals

A. ARSENIC POLYNEUROPATHY   Acute poisoning may be preceded by an acute gastrointestinal illness, with anorexia, nausea, vomiting, abdominal pain, and diarrhea within 1 to 3 weeks of the onset of limb pain, paresthesias, and weakness.

Burning pain and paresthesias or paresthesias alone involve the feet and hands. Motor weakness may interfere with walking and use of the arms and hands. Both distal and proximal muscles may be affected. Superficial and deep sensation in the feet and lower legs and hands may be impaired. Anemia and leukopenia may be associated. The diagnosis of arsenic poisoning can be confirmed by measurement of arsenic concentrations in blood, urine, hair, or nails; by atomic absorption spectrophotometry; or by neutron activation methods. Urine arsenic levels are less than 5 μg/24 h in the absence of poisoning. Dimercaprol therapy is ineffective in the treatment of an established neuropathy. Gradual resolution of the neuropathy may occur without specific therapy. Unexplained arsenic poisoning may be the result of an attempted homicide or accidental contamination of food, drink, or dishes.

B. MERCURY POLYNEUROPATHY   The metal may be absorbed during industrial or agricultural exposures. It may be responsible for a sensory or sensorimotor neuropathy similar to that produced by arsenic. Urine mercury levels above or greater than 150 μg/liter are associated with toxicity. Normal urinary excretion is less than 20 μg/liter.

C. THALLIUM POLYNEUROPATHY   A sensory neuropathy occurs, with bilateral aching leg and foot pain and paresthesias. Arthralgias may also develop and may be migratory. Deep and superficial sensation may be impaired. Gait ataxia and a motor neuropathy with limb and respiratory weakness may oc-

cur. Fever and such gastrointestinal symptoms as nausea, vomiting, abdominal pain, and watery or bloody diarrhea may be associated with the acute ingestion of thallium.

Loss of hair occurs within 2 to 4 weeks of poisoning and suggests the diagnosis. Thallium levels in the urine range from 10 to 20 μg/liter with severe poisoning.

3. Drugs

A. DISULFIRAM (ANTABUSE)   This drug is used to treat alcohol abuse. It may cause a sensorimotor neuropathy that initially involves the feet. Paresthesias, burning pain, and weakness may occur. Muscle pain and tenderness do not develop. Superficial and deep sensation may be impaired. Discontinuance of the drug may result in slow or no improvement. This disorder may be confused with alcoholic polyneuropathy, but patients under institutional care while receiving the drug have developed neuropathy at a time when they were not drinking alcohol and were receiving a good diet and vitamin supplements.

B. ISONIAZID   The initial complaints are numbness and paresthesias of the fingers and toes. These complaints may extend proximally to involve the feet and lower legs and the hands. Burning pain and dysesthesias may occur in the feet and hands, and distal weakness in the legs may develop. Pyridoxine given with isoniazid prevents the development of neuropathy.

C. HYDRALAZINE   Peripheral sensory or sensorimotor neuropathy is a rare effect of hydralazine therapy and can be prevented by pyridoxine supplementation.

D. OTHER DRUGS   Table 47-3 lists other drugs associated with sensory or sensorimotor polyneuropathy.

4. Chemicals   Table 47-4 lists chemicals used in and around the home and in industry that may cause painful sensory or sensorimotor neuropathy.

C. Systemic Disorders

1. Carcinoma

A. SUBACUTE SENSORY NEUROPATHY   This disorder results from degeneration of neuronal cell bodies in the dorsal root ganglia. Symptoms include paresthesias, numbness, and burning or aching pain in the feet and sometimes the hands. A sensory ataxia may occur. Neuropathic symptoms usually precede clinical manifestations of the primary malignancy by a few months to as long as $3\frac{1}{2}$ years. Oat cell carcinoma of the lung is the usual cause, but carcinomas of the esophagus, stomach, cecum, and other organs have also been associated with this disorder.

Table 47-3
DRUGS ASSOCIATED WITH SENSORY (S) AND SENSORIMOTOR (SM) PERIPHERAL NEUROPATHY

Amiodarone	SM
Cis-platinum	S
Ethionamide	SM
Disulfiram	SM
Gold	SM
Hydralazine	SM
8-Hydroxyquinolines (clioquinol and iodoquinol)*	SM
Isoniazid	SM
Metronidazole	S
Misonidazole	S
Nitrofurantoin	SM
Pyridoxine in high doses (>500 mg/day)	S
Phenytoin	S > M
Perhexilene	SM
Vincristine	S > M

*Cause subacute myeloptic neuropathy.

B. SENSORIMOTOR POLYNEUROPATHY Symptoms include numbness, paresthesias, and pain in the feet, lower legs, and hands, and distal limb weakness and wasting. The onset may precede or follow the clinical manifestations of the malignancy. Primary sites include the lung (oat cell), breast, stomach, pancreas, bladder, kidney, and uterus.

A relapsing or remitting polyneuropathy may occur in some cases and antedate detection of the tumor by 2 to as long as 8 years. Remitting types of neuropathy may resolve after successful therapy of the underlying tumor (e.g., renal carcinoma or seminoma of testis).

2. Acute Leukemia Rarely, leukemic infiltration of peripheral nerves may cause a symmetrical polyneuropathy with numbness, paresthesias, distal extremity pain, and proximal and distal weakness and wasting.

Table 47-4
CHEMICALS ASSOCIATED WITH SENSORY AND SENSORIMOTOR PERIPHERAL NEUROPATHY

Acrylamide (monomer used in production of polyacrylamide)
Carbon disulfide (solvent)
Dichlorophenoxyacetic acid (herbicide)
Ethylene oxide (disinfectant gas)
n-Hexane (solvent)
Methyl bromide (fumigating agent)
Sodium cyanide (insecticides, rodenticides, metallurgy, and electroplating)

3. Chronic Leukemia An acute sensory or sensorimotor polyneuropathy may develop in patients with chronic lymphatic leukemia. Neuropathy may occur with chronic myelogenous leukemia, but it is rare.

4. Lymphoma Hodgkin's disease may be associated with an acute sensory polyneuropathy with limb weakness, tingling paresthesias, and foot and/or hand pain. A subacute sensorimotor polyneuropathy has been reported with Hodgkin's and non-Hodgkin's lymphoma. Relapsing and remitting polyneuropathy may also occur with these disorders.

5. Myeloma

A. LYTIC MULTIPLE MYELOMA A subacute or chronic sensorimotor polyneuropathy occurs in 5 percent of cases of lytic or diffuse osteoporotic myeloma. Pain in the feet, lower legs, arms, and hands is characteristic of myelomatous neuropathy, although bone pain may also be responsible for some of the discomfort. Paresthesias, numbness, weakness, and wasting of the distal extremities are other symptoms. Osteosclerotic myeloma has a strong association with neuropathy (50 percent of cases of this disorder). Only 3 percent of myeloma cases are osteosclerotic.

B. OSTEOSCLEROTIC MYELOMA Polyneuropathy associated with osteosclerotic myeloma or a solitary plasmacytoma often improves with therapy for the primary disorder, is likely to be demyelinating, is associated with various monoclonal proteins and light chains (mostly lambda); and may occur as part of the POEMS syndrome.

C. POEMS SYNDROME The POEMS syndrome consists of *p*olyneuropathy, *o*rganomegaly (hepatosplenomegaly), *e*ndocrinopathy, *M* protein, and *s*kin changes (skin thickening, hyperpigmentation, hypertrichosis, and clubbing of the fingers).

6. Waldenström's Macroglobulinemia This disorder presents with weakness, fatigue, visual disturbances, recurrent infections, and a bleeding diathesis (e.g., epistaxis or gastrointestinal bleeding). Adenopathy, hepatosplenomegaly, and abnormal retinal veins may be observed on examination. Peripheral neuropathy causes paresthesias, pain, and cramps in the lower legs and feet, and partial or complete loss of superficial and deep sensation. Muscle weakness, wasting, and fasciculations occur in both the upper and lower extremities. Footdrop with a steppage gait may occur. The usual onset of the neuropathy is insidious or subacute. Early in its course, the polyneuropathy may be asymmetrical. A serum M component is present in excess of 3 g/dl. The light-chain isotype is kappa in 80 percent of cases. Remission of the polyneuropathy with therapy may occur but is unusual.

7. Cryoglobulinemia   Essential mixed cryoglobulinemia may cause peripheral neuropathy, Raynaud's phenomenon, toe gangrene, gastrointestinal bleeding, arthralgias, purpura, glomerulonephritis, and ulceration of the toes and feet. Pain, paresthesias, weakness, and wasting may involve the feet and, less frequently, the fingers and hands. Sensory symptoms may be precipitated by exposure to cold. Cryoglobulinemia associated with lymphoma, myeloma, chronic infection, or polyarteritis nodosa may also cause a progressive sensorimotor neuropathy.

8. Primary Amyloidosis   Pain, paresthesias, unpleasant dysesthesias, and loss of light touch and temperature sense occur in the toes and feet. Neuropathy may occur a median of 4 years before a diagnosis of AL (amyloid of light-chain origin) amyloidosis is established.

Neuropathy occurs in 35 percent of patients with AL amyloidosis. Cardiac involvement resulting in refractory heart failure; gastrointestinal infiltration with weight loss, obstruction, malabsorption, and bleeding; and renal involvement with the nephrotic syndrome and renal failure are other manifestations of this disorder. Sural nerve biopsy may confirm the diagnosis by demonstrating amyloid deposition in a peripheral nerve. Clinical trials with melphalan, prednisone, and colchicine suggest that life may be prolonged by such therapy.

9. Connective Tissue Diseases

A. POLYARTERITIS NODOSA   This disorder may cause mononeuropathy multiplex, with pain and paresthesias involving the foot and lower leg on one or both sides. A motor deficit in the foot and lower leg may follow within hours or days. Sensory loss, skin hyperesthesia, and weakness may be demonstrable in the foot and lower leg. A symmetrical polyneuropathy may also occur in polyarteritis nodosa. The upper extremities are involved as frequently as the lower extremities.

B. OTHER COLLAGEN VASCULAR DISEASES (RHEUMATOID ARTHRITIS, SYSTEMIC LUPUS ERYTHEMATOSUS, AND CHURG-STRAUSS DISEASE)   A symmetrical sensorimotor polyneuropathy with bilateral burning foot pain and cramps may also occur in rheumatoid arthritis, systemic lupus erythematosus, and some cases of Churg-Strauss disease. Vasculitis may be demonstrated on a sural nerve biopsy.

Mononeuropathy multiplex, with sharp, shooting pain over the distribution of one or more peripheral nerves of the lower extremity, may also occur in rheumatoid arthritis, Churg-Strauss disease, and systemic lupus erythematosus when vasculitis is present. Other disorders associated with mononeuropathy multiplex include diabetes mellitus, AIDS, amyloidosis, and sarcoidosis.

10. Renal Failure (Uremic Neuropathy)   Early symptoms include burning feet in 6 percent of cases and pedal dysesthesias and paresthesias, which may be described as tingling, a raw sensation, constrictive pressure about the ankles, or a sensation of puffiness or swelling of the fingers or toes. Loss of the ankle jerk, followed by loss of the knee reflex, is characteristic. Rapid progression may occur without treatment of the renal failure. The result may be complete limb anesthesia and paralysis. Such cases are unusual and do not occur with hemodialysis. Hemodialysis or renal transplantation will usually lead to recovery, with complete clearing of neuropathic symptoms.

11. AIDS (Distal Symmetrical Polyneuropathy)   This disorder may present with toe and foot pain, paresthesias, and dysesthesias that spread proximally. Superficial and deep sensory deficits are present in the toes and feet. Ankle jerks are depressed, while other reflexes are preserved. Nerve biopsy reveals axonal degeneration and some areas of segmental demyelination. Distal muscles may be weak. Electromyographic studies reveal partial denervation of clinically weak distal muscles. Mononeuropathy multiplex may also occur in some cases.

12. Sarcoidosis   This disorder may be associated with a symmetrical pattern of paresthesias, pain, and hyperesthesia in the feet and lower legs. Distal limb weakness may develop. A mononeuropathy multiplex pattern of leg and foot pain, paresthesias, weakness, and sensory loss may also occur. A sural nerve biopsy may demonstrate noncaseating sarcoid granulomas. Acute polyneuropathy may respond dramatically to corticosteroid therapy.

D. Hereditary

1. Fabry's Disease   Intense pain in the feet and lower legs is the most severe complaint. These pain crises may last minutes to days. Excruciating burning pain occurs in the soles, the lower legs, and sometimes the hands and more proximal regions of the extremities. Fever may accompany the attacks of pain. Paresthesias of the feet and hands may be associated. Pain crises usually begin in childhood or early adulthood.

Angiokeratomas (telangiectasis) occur as small, dark-red to blue-black, flat to slightly elevated, discrete lesions over the "bathing trunk" region in a symmetrical pattern. Lesions on the lips and oral mucosa may also occur. Corneal opacities are observed, and retinal veins may show tortuosity, aneurysmal dilatation, and segmental areas of dilation. Cardiac involvement results in angina pectoris, myocardial infarction, and congestive heart failure. The urine contains albumin, erythrocyte casts, and renal cells, and the associated renal disease leads to azotemia before age 40. The diagnosis may be confirmed by demonstrating a decreased level of alpha-galactosidase A in serum, leukocytes, biopsied tissue, or cultured fibroblasts.

2. Intermittent Acute Porphyria An attack of abdominal pain with minimal tenderness is a common symptom. The pain may be localized or generalized, but the abdomen is usually soft, with normal bowel sounds. Associated fever, vomiting, and leukocytosis lead to consideration of an intraabdominal inflammatory disorder and, in some cases, exploratory surgery.

Neuropathy may occur, with burning or aching foot and/or hand pain, paresthesias, numbness, and unpleasant dysesthesias. Distal extremity light touch and pain sensation may be decreased or absent. Sensory impairment may be "glove or stocking" or proximal ("bathing trunk") in distribution. Thigh or upper arm sensory impairment may also occur.

Proximal limb weakness is more severe than distal weakness, and the arms are more severely involved than the legs. Weakness of the extensors of the toes and foot (footdrop) and the fingers and wrists (wristdrop) may occur on one or both sides. Myalgias and cramps may occur in the distal portion of the lower extremities. The painful muscles may be tender. Reflexes may be depressed, absent, or normal.

Behavioral changes may also occur, including anxiety states, emotional instability, or an organic brain syndrome with confusion, restlessness, delusions, and visual hallucinations. Some patients may become combative.

There may be a tachycardia up to 160 beats per minute, a low-grade fever, and labile hypertension. Cardiac or respiratory failure–related sudden death may occur during an acute attack.

The urine color varies from pink to dark, reddish-brown (port-wine color) in patients with acute hepatic porphyria. Acute attacks may last from a few days to 1 month or more. Recovery of the neuropathy during remission proceeds from proximal to distal regions. There is increased excretion of delta-aminolevulinic acid (ALA) and porphobilinogen (PBG) during attacks. In some cases, urinary PBG becomes normal after an attack. In asymptomatic cases, the diagnosis may sometimes be confirmed by measuring the activity of PBG deaminase in erythrocytes or lymphocytes. Intravenous infusion of glucose (500 g/day) or hematin may lead to remission of symptoms within 48 h. Prevention of future attacks is essential and can be accomplished by avoidance of attack-precipitating drugs, steroids, alcohol, and fasting.

8. NERVE AND ROOT COMPRESSION SYNDROMES

A. Tarsal Tunnel Syndrome Burning pain, numbness, and paresthesias may occur over the entire sole, the me-

dial and lateral sole with sparing of the heel, and either the medial or lateral anterior two-thirds of the sole. Retrograde spread of pain into the calf may occur. The pain may be spontaneous and continuous or present only at night. It may be intensified or provoked by weight bearing and walking, being exacerbated by each step. Pressure over the posterior tibial nerve at the medial aspect of the ankle reproduces pain and paresthesias. These symptoms may also be provoked by application of a tourniquet about the ankle. The pain may have a burning quality at rest and an electric shock-like quality with each step. Nocturnal pain may be partially relieved by placing the affected leg in a dependent position. Motor symptoms are rarely present. Sensation on the sole may be decreased but is often intact. Electrophysiologic studies may detect increased distal latencies (normal, 4.4–4.6 ± 0.5 ms) on the affected side, and electromyography may demonstrate sharp positive wave spikes and fibrillation potentials in the abductor hallucis or abductor digiti quinti pedis muscles. Latencies may be compared to the pain-free side or to standard normal values. Pressure on the posterior tibial nerve at the medial ankle may be caused by a synovial sarcoma, a neurilemoma, a ganglion, an exostosis or osteophyte, an adjacent fracture fragment, callus, arthritis, tenosynovitis, bursitis, an edema-producing disorder, plantar fasciitis, an anomalous abductor hallucis, an os trigonum or an os intermetatarsum (accessory bones), prolonged indirect pressure, or poorly fitting, tight shoes. The posterior tibial nerve may be compressed by a tight flexor retinaculum as it passes beneath the medial malleolus. Compression may also occur after branching into medial and lateral plantar branches along the inferomedial midfoot. Distal points of compression include the calcaneonavicular ligament or the abductor hallucis muscle region. Some patients with this disorder have flexible or fixed pes planus and hindfoot valgus. In patients with pes planus and hindfoot valgus, a minor eversion twist of the ankle may precipitate the tarsal tunnel syndrome. Pes planus and hindfoot valgus may also place the posterior tibial nerve on stretch with each step, and this may result in nerve injury. Generalized benign joint hypermobility may be present. The tarsal tunnel syndrome may be associated with a carpal tunnel syndrome and sciatica. Reflex sympathetic dystrophy may occur as a secondary event in some patients with this disorder and may lead to diagnostic confusion. Relief has followed use of an orthosis to correct pes planus or surgical resection of constricting elements associated with the flexor retinaculum and the abductor hallucis muscle. Common misdiagnoses have included ankle sprains, arthritis, and sciatica. In up to 50 percent of cases, no etiology may be apparent.

B. Superficial Peroneal Nerve Entrapment Compression over the lateral ankle by a tight-fitting boot may cause pain and tingling paresthesias on the dorsum of the foot and lateral toes. It may also occur after an ankle sprain. More proximal compression may result from a chronic lateral compartment syndrome or from an adjacent fibula fracture. Tinel's sign may be present in the area of compression.

C. Deep Peroneal Nerve Entrapment (Anterior Tarsal Tunnel Syndrome) Compression may occur at the anterior tibiotalar joint or underneath the inferior extensor retinaculum. It also may occur in patients wearing high-heeled shoes or tight-fitting boots. Other associations include ankle fractures and dislocations or sprains. Paresthesias, pain, and numbness occur at the first dorsal web space. Nocturnal pain may occur when the foot is held in plantar flexion with the toes extended. This pain may be decreased or eliminated by everting and dorsiflexing the foot, which relieves retinaculum compression. Tinel's sign may be present. Hypesthesia or anesthesia is present over the first web space, and there is minimal motor loss. The diagnosis can be confirmed by electrophysiologic studies. Failure of conservative therapy requires surgical decompression.

D. Sural Nerve Entrapment Pain, paresthesias, and hypesthesia occur over the lateral border of the foot. Tenderness over the region of nerve compression and Tinel's sign may be present. Fractures of the calcaneus or fifth metatarsal or compression by a ganglion or, rarely, an aponeurotic band are possible causes of sural nerve entrapment. Conservative therapy may be successful, but some patients require surgical decompression.

E. L5 and S1 Root Compression S1 root compression may cause posterolateral thigh and calf pain and low back pain. In some cases with calf and foot pain, confusion with a tarsal tunnel syndrome may occur. S1 radiculopathy may cause pain, paresthesias, and hypesthesia over the sole and the lateral side of the foot. The ankle jerk is depressed or absent. Posterior tibial nerve latencies across the ankle are normal. A contrast-enhanced CT scan or MRI of the lumbosacral spine will demonstrate a lesion compressing the ipsilateral S1 root.

L5 root compression may cause pain and paresthesias over the dorsum of the foot and the great toe. Great toe extension may be weak. Pain may also occur in the posterior thigh and lower leg and may be intensified or provoked by straining, coughing, or straight leg raising. Imaging studies of the lumbosacral spine will identify the root-compressing lesion.

9. COLD INJURY

A. Frostbite During the first minutes of cold exposure, the feet and toes may develop pain and paresthesias. With prolonged exposure, the pain ceases and the feet and toes feel numb and insensitive (i.e., "frostnip"). Rapid re-

warming at this stage (e.g., going indoors) will cause a feeling of burning discomfort, warmth, and redness of the feet and other affected parts. After cold injury, the foot may become pale, cool, and waxy white. During rewarming at 40 to 42°C, severe pain may occur. Frostbite is classified in a manner similar to burns, and this classification is presented below.

1. First Degree Erythema and edema of the feet occur. Pain and paresthesias begin after 3 to 13 days but may not occur in all cases. Excessive sweating may begin after 2 or 3 weeks and continue for months. No tissue loss occurs, but the skin desquamates after 5 days. Pain on future cold exposure may occur for months or years.

2. Second Degree During the first 24 h after rewarming, hyperemia, edema, and bullae formation occur on the toes and dorsum of the feet. These tense bullae rupture and collapse into dry, black eschars. Aching pain in the feet may develop after the third day, as may hyperhidrosis. Cold sensitivity, pain, paresthesias, hypesthesia, and coldness of the feet may follow due to increased sympathetic activity and cold-related nerve injury.

3. Third Degree Changes over the toes include cyanosis, pallor, and hypesthesia or anesthesia. Proximal edema, hyperemia, and bullae are present. The skin over the fingers, toes, or more proximal parts of the hands and feet becomes dry, shriveled, and black. Necrotic skin may slough. Severe aching or shooting, knifelike pain may occur after the first 5 days. Joint pain and stiffness may develop due to cold injury. Radiographs may demonstrate juxtaarticular, punched-out, cystic vascular infarcts involving the painful joints. First- and second-degree frostbite develop within 2 h in average winter subfreezing temperatures. Third- and fourth-degree injuries usually require more time. Severe full-thickness injuries involving muscle and bone (fourth degree) usually require amputation.

B. Trench Foot This disorder develops with temperatures in the 0.5 to 10°C (33 to 50°F) range when the feet are exposed to constant moisture (e.g., wet socks and boots).

The feet are pale and swollen and feel leaden and numb. Paresthesias and a sensation of coldness are felt. Pulses are decreased and reflexes depressed. Walking causes pain, and the toes and ankles are stiff. After rewarming, the skin becomes red, warm, and swollen, and bullae and ecchymotic areas appear. Distal areas (forefoot) that remain pale or cyanotic may blacken. Gangrene is usually superficial. Continuous aching or burning pain occurs in the feet, and within 1 to 2 weeks severe shooting, lightning-like, or stabbing pains that radiate into the toes may occur. These pains and numbness may persist for weeks. Hyperemia may last for up to 10 weeks.

Other symptoms include cold sensitivity, hyperhidrosis, coldness, and paresthesias. Hypesthesia may be demonstrable.

C. Immersion Foot This disorder is a nautical version of trench foot and results from prolonged immersion of the feet in chilly seawater.

During immersion, the feet feel numb, cool, and weak. Muscle cramps in the feet or calves may occur. In cool sea water, the feet are red, while in warmer water they appear yellow-white or cyanotic.

On rewarming, the feet become red, and pulses become bounding. Throbbing, burning, constant pain develops, and brief, shooting pains occur after 1 week. The feet become edematous and beefy red, and bullae and ecchymoses appear over the dorsum of the foot and calf. Skin hyperesthesia may occur. Weakness and wasting of the intrinsic foot muscles may appear. Superficial areas of gangrene may develop in pale or cyanotic areas. Hyperemia of the feet, accompanied by aching, burning, and/or shooting pains, may last for 6 to 10 weeks.

D. Pernio (Chilblains) Raised red lesions occur over the dorsum of the toes, the heads of the first and fifth metatarsals, the heels, and other areas of the feet. The rash is accompanied by burning discomfort and pruritus. Superficial ulceration may occur. This disorder is associated with outdoor activities in cold weather. Remission occurs in a warm climate. An angiitis of small skin vessels is present on skin biopsy.

10. BITES

A. Human Bites Crush and shear injury and inoculation of anaerobic and aerobic bacteria occur. The wound becomes surrounded by erythema and edema. A diffuse cellulitis of the foot may develop with fever, pain, and tenderness. Lymphangitis and femoral or linguinal lymphadenitis may accompany the pedal infection. Septic arthritis or osteomyelitis may result from a human bite. Aerobic isolates from human bite wounds include viridans streptococci, group A streptococci, alpha-hemolytic streptococci, *Staphylococcus aureus*, *Hemophilus parainfluenzae*, *Klebsiella pneumoniae*, and *Eikenella corrodens*. The most frequent anaerobic isolates are *Bacteroides* species, *Fusobacterium* species, and anaerobic gram-positive cocci. *E. corrodens* may occur as part of a mixed infection with streptococcal species, staphylococci, *Bacteroides* species, and/or gram-negative bacteria. *E. corrodens* may be associated with more severe forms of wound sepsis and complications. It may be eradicated by intravenous administration of penicillin. Debridement and parenteral antibiotic therapy are required to treat infected human bite wounds. Infected wounds should be left open for at least 3 to 5 days after therapy is initiated.

B. Dog Bites Crush injury and shear damage are combined with inoculation of canine oral flora. Cellulitis, lymphangitis, lymphadenitis, and septicemia may occur. Pain and tenderness occur in the area of edema and erythema surrounding the bite site. A purulent discharge may flow from the wound. Septic arthritis, osteomyelitis, tenosynovitis, or a subcutaneous abscess may develop as a complication. Severe septicemia may occur following a dog bite contaminated with a *Bacteroides* species or dysgonic fermenter (DF-2 bacillus) (e.g., in patients with severe liver disease or splenectomy). The most frequent isolates in dog bites are streptococcal species. Other frequent infecting organisms include *Pasteurella multocida* (30 percent of cases), *Bacteroides* species (19 percent of cases), *S. aureus* (30 percent of cases), and *Fusobacterium* species (19 percent of cases). Anaerobic organisms are usually always isolated in mixed culture.

C. Cat Bites These are usually small puncture wounds or scratches. *P. multocida* is a common isolate from infected cat bites. Infected bites usually respond to irrigation, debridement when appropriate, and antibiotic therapy.

D. Venomous Snake Bites Pit viper and cobra bites cause burning, local pain within a short time after the bite. Severe local edema, ecchymoses, and bullae may develop, and gangrene of the skin may occur near the site of envenomation. Sloughing of necrotic skin and subcutaneous tissue follows necrosis. Secondary infection may result from microorganisms in the mouth of the snake.

Common isolates from the mouths of rattlesnakes include *Pseudomonas aeruginosa*, *Proteus* species, coagulase-negative staphylococci, and *Clostridium* species. Supportive care and administration of antivenin may limit the development of pain, edema, and necrosis. Antibiotics may be used to prevent progression of wound contamination to clinical infection.

E. Recluse Spider Bites Severe local pain begins at the site of the bite after 2 to 8 h. Diffuse redness surrounds the bite, and one or more bullae may form at the bite site. Bulla rupture results in the formation of a deep, necrotic ulcer (within 3 to 7 days). Lesions larger than 1 cm at 12 h usually progress to central necrosis. Dapsone may prevent progression to severe necrosis and lessens pain and tenderness.

F. Sea Urchin Stings After stepping on a sea urchin spine, the affected foot may become painful, red, and tender. Ulceration may occur. Systemic neurotoxic symptoms such as paresis of the oral musculature may develop.

G. Venomous Fish Stings These injuries occur in a watery environment when a bather steps on a venomous fish or is stung on the foot while swimming. The foot rapidly becomes painful and blanched and then red and edematous. Local necrosis, ecchymoses, and tissue sloughing may occur. Pain results from the venom, the spine, or retained foreign material.

In severe envenomations (e.g., from a stonefish), shock, dyspnea, cardiac toxicity, and death may occur. Venomous fish include stingrays, weever fish, toadfish, lionfish, stonefish, zebra fish, catfish, and sturgeon.

Pain and local edema are maximal in 60 to 90 min and then resolve during the next 12 h. Local necrosis and sloughing are particularly common after lionfish and catfish stings.

11. CUTANEOUS DISORDERS

A. Palmoplantar Pustulosis   Small (1–2 mm) pustules on red plaques occur on the soles and palms. These pustules may rupture or simply dry, producing a crust. Recurrent crops of pustules occur. Open lesions may be mildly painful.

Similar lesions may occur on the palms and soles in patients with typical psoriatic skin and nail lesions at other sites. This disorder has been called pustular psoriasis of Barber.

B. Dyshidrotic Eczema (Pompholyx)   Small, painful intraepidermal vesicles occur with or without surrounding redness and may cause stinging hand and foot pain and tenderness. The vesicles may be associated with hyperhidrosis of the palms and soles.

C. Pustular Bacterid of the Hands and Feet   The initial lesion is a pustule that occurs in the sole of the midfoot or midportion of the palm. More pustules follow. Local pain and itching may occur. The pustules dry, and scaling and exfoliation follow. Criteria for diagnosis include a pustular eruption of the palms and soles; an intraepidermal location; a peripheral leukocytosis; and a relationship to a focal infection (e.g., tonsillitis, dental abscess, or sinusitis). This disorder resolves after treatment of the associated infection.

D. Acrodermatitis Continua   This disease begins on the foot or hands, usually on a digit. There is an eruption of pustules that coalesce and form lakes of pus. A common site is the skin about a nail. Necrosis of skin and sloughing may occur, leaving denuded and crusted areas. Erosions, pustules, and crusted ulcers are present. The affected nails are loosened, lifted off by a lake of pus, and pustules may form on denuded nail beds. Eroded areas and pustules may cause pain and tenderness.

This disorder may remain confined to one hand or may spread to the other and to the feet. It tends to start at the tips of digits and involve the perionychial tissue and nail beds.

E. Infectious Eczematoid Dermatitis   This disorder may cause skin erythema, vesicles, erosions, pustules, and fissures. There is good response to antimicrobial therapy. Eroded areas and fissures are usually painful and tender.

F. Hand-Foot-and-Mouth Disease   There is an eruption of vesicles and ulcers on the buccal mucosa and tongue. Some vesicles may coalesce and form bullae. Oval-shaped subepithelial vesicles on an erythematous base occur on the palms and soles or the extensor surfaces of the hands and feet. The lesions are not usually painful unless subjected to light pressure (e.g., palpation or weight bearing). A sore throat and/or mouth is a common complaint. This disorder occurs as an acute illness in the first decade of life but may occur in older children and adults. Coxsackie A16 and other A strains, Coxsackie B5, and enterovirus 71 are known etiologic agents of this self-limited disorder.

G. Herpes Zoster   Pain, grouped vesicles, and crusted ulcers occur in one lower leg and foot. Herpes zoster rarely occurs on the foot alone. The pain is aching or burning and may be mistaken for sciatica until the characteristic skin eruption occurs.

H. Vesicular Type of Tinea Pedis   *Trichophyton rubrum* infection may occur on the soles as a vesicular eruption with surrounding erythema. Rupture of vesicles to form ulcers and fissuring or excoriation from scratching may cause local pain. Examination and culture of skin scrapings for fungi will confirm the diagnosis. A dermatophytic reaction may affect the palms secondarily. Erythema, pustules, and vesicles occur, presumably by dissemination of fungi from the feet to the hands by a hematogenous route. Results of cultures of hand vesicles and pustules are negative for fungi. Treatment of the pedal infection results in resolution of the palmar lesions.

I. Atopic Dermatitis   Erythema, edema, vesicles, weeping erosions and fissures, crusting, scaling, and lichenification occur on the soles. Other sites of involvement in adults include the neck, hands, antecubital and popliteal fossae, and periorbital and oral areas. Results of cultures for fungi are negative, and there is a good response to corticosteroid ointment. Secondary bacterial infection may occur in some cases.

J. Contact Dermatitis   Early lesions are characterized by erythema, edema, papulovesicles, and bullae. Secondary changes include erosions, fissures, crusting and excoriation, lichenification, and thickening of the skin. This disorder may result from a primary skin irritant (e.g., a chemical such as salicylic, benzoic, or monochloracetic acid) or an allergen (e.g., poison ivy or shoe dermatitis from rubber).

Shoe dermatitis is an example of contact dermatitis that affects the feet exclusively. Erythema, edema, vesicles, bullae, and pustules occur on the dorsum of the foot. Chemical allergens leaking out of rubber in the shoe may initiate this contact type of dermatitis. Chemicals used to ''tan'' shoes are rarely the cause.

Some cases of shoe dermatitis may affect only the soles. Shoe dermatitis is most frequently caused by catalysts, such as mercaptobenzothiazole and tetramethylthiaram, used in synthesizing rubber; adhesives; and dichromates in rubber. Shoe dermatitis may sometimes resemble psoriasis. Patch testing of the chemicals involved in the production of the shoe or by use of a piece of the suspected portion of the shoe will establish the diagnosis.

If the patient discontinues wearing the offending shoes and/or applies a corticosteroid ointment, the rash resolves.

K. Vitamin B Deficiencies   Burning pain on the soles and erythematous skin mottling may occur.

L. Fixed Drug Eruption   A red, edematous, painful, tender, circumscribed area may form on the foot secondary to oral ingestion of a drug. Recognition of the cause and discontinuance of the drug lead to resolution.

M. Erosive Lichen Planus   This disorder begins as multiple, small, polygonal, violaceous, flat-topped papules. A thin, white scale may cover the papules. Lesions may be pruritic. Extensive painful ulceration of the soles and sides of the feet may occur. Papules on the sole appear yellowish and resemble pustules. Koebner's phenomenon may be demonstrable (i.e., appearance of lesions at sites of trauma, e.g., where the skin has been scratched).

Forefoot Pain

12. METATARSALGIA OF RAYS 2 TO 4 (METATARSAL HEAD OVERLOAD)

A. High-Heeled Shoes   Aching pain occurs over the metatarsal area. Tenderness may be present on the plantar aspect of the MTP joints and metatarsal heads, but there is no edema or redness. Dorsal tenderness is not usually noted unless a synovitis is present. The incidence of metatarsalgia in women is 89 percent and in men 12 percent. The difference in frequency is probably related to the use of high-heeled shoes by women. High heels increase the weight-bearing load on the forefoot threefold or more, depending on the height of the heels. The narrow toe of stylish female footwear also contributes to this painful disorder, since the dorsiflexed and compressed toes fail to provide additional weight-bearing support to the metatarsal heads. It is estimated that most women wear a shoe that is one size too small for their feet.

B. Equinus Foot   Metatarsalgia occurs with shortening (contracture) of the Achilles tendon, which may occur with spasticity or after poliomyelitis.

C. Cavus Foot   The high plantar arch and higher heel place excessive weight bearing on the ball of the foot, leading to metatarsalgia. The toes and external arch of the foot do not support the foot during walking. Initial contact of the foot with the ground surface during walking is accomplished, not by the heel, but by the ball of the foot.

D. First-Ray Insufficiency Syndrome (Morton's Syndrome)   The first metatarsal head does not carry out its normal support function. The second and third metatarsals are overloaded, resulting in pain and tenderness over the heads of these rays on the plantar surface.

The causes of first-ray insufficiency include congenital shortening of the first metatarsal relative to the second (≥ 2 cm), varus deviation of the first metatarsal more than 15° in relation to the direction of the second ray, and posterior placement of the sesamoid bones, which causes functional shortening of the first metatarsal.

Laxity of the Lisfranc ligament and the forefoot muscles allows the first metatarsal to tilt upward (e.g., hypermobility syndrome of the first ray). Weight bearing shifts to the second and third metatarsal heads. Radiographs may demonstrate a diastasis between the first and second cuneiforms.

Other causes of first-ray insufficiency include lateral dislocation of the sesamoid bones and pes planus. The latter deformity may be associated with a valgus deformity of the heel. Heel valgus may result in forefoot supination, elevating the first ray and interfering with its weight-bearing function. Some hallux valgus operations have also resulted in first-ray insufficiency.

The consequences of first-ray insufficiency may be acute or chronic, recurrent pain (e.g., metatarsalgia).

1. Deutschlander's Disease (March Fracture)   Severe pain in the forefoot occurs abruptly following a long march. The patient is forced to stop walking. Swelling may appear on the dorsum of the foot. The fracture usually occurs in the second metacarpal at the juncture of the middle and distal thirds of the bone. It may also occur in the third or fourth metatarsal and may affect more than one ray. Bilateral fractures are less common. During the first 2 to 4 weeks, a radionuclide bone scan may be required to demonstrate the fracture. After this time, radiographs may demonstrate the fracture line and the bulblike callus formed in the reparative process. Shortening of the metatarsal may occur. This disorder may occur in athletes, dancers, soldiers, or middle-aged and elderly patients without the clear-cut history of a long march or repetitive overload that is found in younger patients.

2. Chronic First-Ray Insufficiency This disorder causes persistent metatarsalgia over the heads of the second and third metatarsals; formation of hyperkeratosis of the plantar skin beneath the heads of the second, third, and fourth rays; formation of a swollen bursa beneath the hyperkeratotic area and in some cases episodes of bursitis; dorsal subluxation of the proximal phalanx of the second or third toe; and periostitis of the second or third metatarsal, visible on a plain radiograph as periosteal new bone synthesis.

E. Central-Ray Overload Syndrome Isolated overload of the head of one of the central metatarsals may result from a long metatarsal that exceeds the length of adjacent rays; when the angle formed by the metatarsals with the horizontal is excessive in a downward direction; and when the capacity for ray dorsiflexion is lost at the tarsometatarsal articulation. Mechanical pain occurs over the head of the third or fourth metatarsal. A corn may form in the skin over it. Bursitis in a sac formed between the skin and the metatarsal head may cause local pain, heat, redness, and tenderness. Surgical correction of the abnormal metatarsal may be required.

13. FREIBERG'S DISEASE

This disorder has a male/female ratio of 1:3 and does not usually occur before age 11 without local trauma. It causes pain, swelling, and tenderness over the second or third metatarsal heads. It usually occurs in the second decade of life and is more common in girls than in boys, but it may first appear in middle age. In stage 1, a fissure fracture of the epiphysis of the metatarsal head appears. This fracture may result in alteration of the radiographic surface contour by bone absorption (stage 2). In stage 3, the central portion of the involved metatarsal head becomes more depressed, sinking into the proximal portion of the head. In stage 4, a loose body separates from the head. In stage 5, flattening of the head and secondary arthritis of the MTP joint occur. Pain is relieved by rest and intensified by weight bearing. The pain can be reproduced by palpation of the metatarsal head. Early diagnosis can be achieved by a radionuclide bone scan or MRI. Most cases are advanced when first seen and require surgical treatment. The most likely etiology is avascular necrosis of the metatarsal head.

14. SECOND METATARSAL INTERSPACE SYNDROME

Pain occurs in the anterior portion of the second metatarsal interspace, associated with tenderness and sometimes swelling and redness in the front portion of the interspace. Pinching the space with the thumb and index finger will confirm the tenderness. There may be dorsal tenderness and pain on range-of-motion testing of the second or third MTP joint. The pain is relieved by rest, does not radiate into the toes, and is exacerbated by walking. Shortness of the first ray may be demonstrable on x-ray. Local injection of lidocaine and a corticosteroid into the painful area produces dramatic relief of the pain and tenderness. The cause is an inflammatory reaction in the vicinity of the MTP joint and adjacent intermetatarsal bursa.

15. MORTON'S NEUROMA (PLANTAR INTERDIGITAL NEUROMA)

Sharp, electric shock-like, or burning pain that is provoked by certain foot movements, prolonged walking, or wearing shoes occurs in the second or third interspace and radiates into the second, third, or fourth toe. Nocturnal crises, with severe spontaneous pain, occur. The fourth toe is most severely affected. Pain in the second toe, as well, may be due to two lesions in separate metatarsal interspaces. Referred pain may extend upward into the calf. Pain during walking requires the patient to stop, rest, remove the shoe, and manipulate and massage the foot. Several attacks during walking may occur in a single day. Certain foot movements (e.g., by dancers or pressing on a motorcycle acceleration pedal) may provoke pain. Rest pain and nocturnal pain may improve more rapidly by cooling the foot with cold water. Unless seen during an attack of pain, the patient appears normal. Night pain or provoked pains may be so severe that emergency aid is sought.

When the examiner compresses the forefoot with one hand and presses upward and backward in the second or third interspace, local soft tissue tenderness is elicited in one or, less commonly, two of the interspaces. Pain may also be reproduced by medial-lateral compression of the forefoot and/or bidigital dorsoplantar palpation of the involved intermetatarsal soft tissue space. Using this method, the examiner may palpate a tender nodule. The pain is reproduced by pressing the lesion against the distal margin of the deep transverse ligament. A click (Mulder's click) may sometimes be detected during interspace compression when the nodule escapes from the intermetatarsal space into the sole. Such clicks may be absent in thin lesions or when advanced larger lesions are adherent to the transverse ligament. Conservative treatment with a metallic insole and local injections of 2% procaine hydrochloride and a corticosteroid may be successful in up to 50 percent of cases. Resection of the enlarged nerve between the third and fourth metatarsal heads provides complete or partial relief in cases refractory to nonsurgical treatment. This disorder is probably caused by microtrauma to the affected nerve associated with compression of the forefoot by a tight shoe. This may explain a male/female disease ratio of 1:5. The usual age of onset is age

40 to 60 years. An increased incidence may also occur with hallux valgus and as an early manifestation of rheumatoid arthritis.

Most lesions are found in the third intermetatarsal space, but some authors have reported a significant number of lesions in the second space.

The histopathologic findings and clinical course of this lesion suggest that it results from microtrauma and represents a traumatic neuritis with proliferative elements due to nerve entrapment. Less likely are the hypotheses stating that these are true neoplasms (neuromas and neurofibromas) or the result of vascular injury.

16. IDIOPATHIC SYNOVITIS OF THE SECOND MTP JOINT

The second MTP joint is most frequently involved. This disorder may be differentiated from metatarsalgia by the presence of swelling and tenderness over the dorsal aspect of the affected MTP joint. With metatarsalgia, there is usually only plantar tenderness. Passive movement of a joint affected by synovitis is usually painful. In some cases, a short first ray may cause chronic overload of the second MTP joint and hyperextension, which causes MTP synovial trauma.

Instability of the second MTP joint due to subluxation of the phalanx may result in mechanically induced synovitis. This type of instability may follow forefoot trauma. Subluxation can be tested for by a "Lachman test." The metatarsal is stabilized, and the examiner attempts to dorsally subluxate the phalanx.

17. INFLAMMATORY ARTHRITIS OF MTP JOINTS

Metatarsalgia may be caused by synovitis associated with rheumatoid arthritis, the seronegative spondyloarthropathies (ankylosing spondylitis, Reiter's syndrome, reactive arthritis, and psoriatic arthritis), or arthritis associated with inflammatory bowel disease.

Involvement of the entire digit in the inflammatory process is seen most frequently in Reiter's syndrome and psoriatic arthritis. The dactylitis (i.e., "sausage digit") usually involves only one or two toes and is due to periostitis, flexor tenosynovitis, and DIP and PIP synovitis. The MTP joints are tender on the dorsal and plantar sides, and passive movement through a range of motion produces pain. The joints may or may not be swollen. Decreased mobility may also be demonstrable. In rheumatoid arthritis, the MTP joints may be the only joints affected by synovitis. MTP subluxation may produce claw toes, with hyperextension of the proximal phalanx and flexion at both IP joints, or hammer toes, with MTP hyperextension and PIP flexion, plantar displacement of the metatarsal heads, migration of the protective plantar forefoot

fat pad, and hallux valgus. These changes result in mechanical, as well as inflammatory, metatarsalgia.

18. ARTERIAL INSUFFICIENCY

Ischemia causing forefoot and toe pain, ulceration, and gangrene may result from arteriosclerosis obliterans, thromboangiitis obliterans, or some form of vasculitis. Ischemic pain is characterized by nocturnal occurrence and relief by dependency; and is associated with a pale, atrophic, cold, hairless foot, and absent pulses below the knee or femoral region. Pulses in the feet may be retained when the ischemia is due to small vessel vasculitis.

19. TRAUMATIC METATARSAL FRACTURES

The usual mechanism is a direct blow to the forefoot. Soft tissue injury, with pain, swelling, and ecchymoses, occurs over the dorsum of this region. The pain is increased by dependency or weight bearing. There is localized tenderness over the fracture site if the injury is seen early. Plantar palpation of the involved metatarsal shaft will produce pain and sometimes bony crepitus. Axial loading pressure on the corresponding toe will also provoke metatarsal pain. Anteroposterior, oblique, and lateral radiographs will identify one or more metatarsal fractures and/or tarsometatarsal dislocations.

20. FOREFOOT SPRAIN

Forefoot sprains cause pain that is most severe when the patient places weight on the toes and leans forward (e.g., football running back or lineman's stance). Pain may occur during running or cutting but may be absent when walking. Swelling and tenderness over the involved intermetatarsal muscles may occur. Difficulty in "pushing off" is a common complaint. This injury is common in sports among running backs, basketball players, and high jumpers. Application of ice, immobilization, and prevention of activity for a prolonged period to allow healing are usually required.

21. BURSITIS (SUBMETATARSAL AND INTERDIGITAL)

Swelling, pain, and tenderness may occur under the first (associated with sesamoid bones), second, or third metatarsal head. Such lesions are fluctuant and only mildly painful and tender. A large intermetatarsal bursa may be evidenced by splaying of the toes and swelling of the web space, visible clinically and radiographically. Medial-to-lateral compression of the foot may compress the inflamed bursa and cause pain. Rarely, compression of the plantar digital nerves by a distended bursa may cause neuritic pain that radiates into a toe, simulating Morton's neuroma. Intermetatarsophalangeal bursitis may be an early symptom of rheumatoid arthritis. Infection may follow needle aspiration or spread from a web space abscess. Bursae may result from excessive walking and weight bearing or inflammatory arthritis. Avoidance of exercise and weight bearing and use of metatarsal or sesamoid pads and/or rubber wedgie shoes lead to a decrease in swelling and tenderness. Intrabursal injection of a corticosteroid may also provide dramatic relief of symptoms.

22. SUBMETATARSAL CYSTS

A slightly painful and tender plantar dermal cyst may mimic a submetatarsal bursa. Sebaceous material may be periodically discharged through a small pore, and the cyst is usually adherent to the dermis.

23. SELF-INFLICTED TRAUMA

Pruritus of the sole due to fungal infection or foot dryness may lead to scratching and excoriation of an area of the plantar surface. This area may become locally infected, causing disabling pain, swelling, and tenderness or a local cellulitis. The infection responds to prevention of further scratching and use of antibiotics.

Great Toe and Medial Foot Pain

24. TRAUMA

A. First MTP Joint Injury

1. Sprain (Capsule Injury)   This injury occurs in football ("turf toe") and in ballet. Use of flexible-soled shoes on artificial turf has increased the frequency of "turf toe." The injury mechanism is forced hyperextension of the joint when the player's foot is in equinus with the toe against the ground. Loading over the posterior aspect of the foot causes the injury. Brief subluxation of the proximal phalanx occurs, with stretching of the plantar capsule and volar plate during the applied force. The joint is swollen, painful, and tender. Range-of-motion testing or passive extension during the push-off phase of walking or running increases the pain.

Hyperflexion injuries of the first MTP joint may occur as a ballet dancer falls forward. The dorsal capsule is torn as the body weight falls over the extended great toe. Abduction forces injure the lateral capsular liga-

ments and often avulse a small fragment of bone from the base of the proximal phalanx. These soft tissue injuries respond to rest, application of ice, and use of nonsteroidal anti-inflammatory drugs.

2. Dislocation   This rare injury usually occurs in a high-energy motor vehicle accident or as a result of a fall from a height. It is frequently associated with other foot injuries. Local pain, swelling, tenderness, and deformity of the MTP joint occur. The proximal phalanx is displaced dorsal to the first metatarsal, producing toe shortening, an elevation of the dorsum of the great toe, and plantar prominence of the metatarsal head. Associated sesamoid bone fractures may occur. The diagnosis may be confirmed by plain radiographs.

The dislocation can usually be reduced without surgery using traction and manipulation.

3. Sesamoid Fractures   Fractures of the sesamoid bones result from direct trauma, an avulsion force, or repetitive loading (repetitive forces applied through the flexor tendons of the great toe during ballet dancing or running may cause avulsion or stress fractures). Pain and tenderness occur over the involved sesamoid (usually the medial). Passive hyperextension of the great toe intensifies the pain. Most fractures are transverse. Tangential views may show a small avulsion fracture. Many patients have bipartite sesamoids (8–33 percent of cases), and partition occurs 10 times more often in the medial sesamoid bone than in the lateral sesamoid bone. In up to 15 percent of cases, partition is unilateral, making comparison with the asymptomatic side unreliable. Irregular fragment edges, evidence of callus formation within 2 to 3 weeks, and a transverse fracture line suggest fracture rather than a partite sesamoid bone. A bone scan may be confirmatory before radiographic changes are definitive.

B. Fracture of the Great Toe   A direct blow to the dorsum of the great toe from a falling object or stubbing of the toe are the usual causes of fracture. Pain, swelling, local tenderness, ecchymoses, and a subungual hematoma are usually present. Fracture of the proximal or distal phalanx will be demonstrated on a plain radiograph.

C. Dislocation of the IP Joint   Pain, swelling, and tenderness occur over the IP joint. Dorsal deformity occurs due to subluxation of the distal phalanx. The usual injury mechanism is an axial load applied to the toe (e.g., kicking against a hard surface with the toe extended).

D. Subungual Hematoma   Severe throbbing pain and tenderness confined to the subungual area can occur within seconds of injury by a falling object or a crushing force applied to the nail bed. The nail is blue and exquisitely tender. The pain can be rapidly relieved by using a small drill hole to drain a subungual collection of blood.

E. Crush Injury of the Distal Toe (Soft Tissue Injury) This injury may cause pain, tenderness, swelling, and blue-black nail discoloration that resolves within 1 to 2 days. Soft tissue injury is prominent, but no fractures occur.

25. PLANTAR CUTANEOUS LESIONS

A. Calluses A hard, dense, flat callus beneath the first metatarsal may cause disabling pain on weight bearing and local tenderness. Pain can be relieved by paring the callus. This leaves an avascular, homogeneous, opalescent center without central bleeding points. A conical, hard corn may occur in the center of a painful callus.

B. Plantar Warts These callus-like lesions cause local pain and tenderness of the plantar surface beneath the head of the first or fifth metatarsal. Paring the wart leaves a central core with multiple, reddish-black, punctate, thrombosed bleeding points. Normal papillary lines may be seen up to the edge of the wart. These lesions may be associated with warts at other sites.

C. Corns These are small, hard, conical, hyperkeratotic lesions caused by friction and pressure. They may occur on the dorsum of the toes or on the sole of the foot beneath the metatarsal heads, or on the underside of the proximal phalanx of the great toe. They cause local pressure and weight bearing-induced pain, and they are tender when compressed.

26. NAIL LESIONS OF THE HALLUX

A. Ingrown Toenail of the Hallux This disorder may result from short or tight shoes with a narrow toe box, overcurvature of the nail plate, incorrect cutting of the nail, or a combination of these factors. The lateral nail fold of the great toe is most frequently involved. Growth of the curved nail into the soft tissue at the nail margin causes local pain, tenderness, redness, and swelling. Medial nail edge ingrowth may also occur but is less frequent.

B. Infected Ingrown Toenail The ingrown nail incises the soft tissue and provides access for local skin bacteria and fungi. Infection results in local redness, swelling, tenderness, and purulent discharge associated with collected pus under the distal corner of the nail on the affected side. Pressure on the nail plate intensifies the pain.

Granulation tissue over the dorsal edge of the nail may restrict drainage from a deep, subungual abscess. With further production of nail edge granulation tissue, drainage may become completely blocked. The subungual abscess enlarges and spreads proximally. Pain becomes intense and throbbing.

Packing cotton under the nail edge or resecting the nail margin facilitates drainage. This allows the lesion to heal and symptoms to resolve. Local or systemic use of antimicrobial drugs is helpful but will be ineffective without adequate subungual drainage.

C. Subungual Melanocarcinoma This lesion may mimic the granulation tissue of an infected nail bed. It appears at the nail edge and may be amelanotic or pigmented. If the nail is partially destroyed, a malignancy should be suspected. Differentiation from a pyogenic granuloma can be made by biopsy.

D. Subungual Glomus Tumor A small (3 mm) painful and tender, blue-red lesion occurs in the nail bed. Exposure to cold or pressure causes severe pain. Local excision relieves symptoms.

E. Other Subungual Tumors Other subungual lesions may cause local pain and tenderness. Osteoid osteoma can cause nocturnal pain that is relieved by aspirin. It can be identified by a plain radiograph or radionuclide bone scan. Other subungual lesions include warts and fibromas.

F. Paronychia Pain, redness, and tenderness occur at the nail margin on the medial or lateral side of the nail. Purulent drainage may occur. The cause may be an ingrown toenail, an embedded foreign body, or a skin infection occurring by inoculation through a minor scratch or abrasion (e.g., caused by eponychial injury with a scissors). Pus may dissect beneath the nail or spread around the edge. Drainage and antibiotic administration lead to resolution.

Paronychia in a diabetic patient may be caused by *Candida albicans,* staphylococci, gram-negative bacteria, enterococci, or anaerobes. Mixed infections are common.

G. Pulp Space Infection This rare lesion usually follows a puncture wound. The plantar aspect of the great toe becomes red, swollen, painful, and tender. Drainage and antibiotic therapy lead to resolution.

H. Infected Blister A blister may form on the great toe due to friction with the shoe during walking or running. The blister causes local burning pain and tenderness. Purulence or cloudiness of the blister fluid suggests infection. Unroofing the blister provides drainage and leads to resolution. Antibiotics may be required if local infection is severe.

27. HALLUX VALGUS

Lateral deviation of the great toe occurs. The proximal phalanx is displaced laterally on the medially displaced first metatarsal head. The medial joint surface of the first metatarsal head becomes uncovered and becomes the site of bunion formation. Progressive increase in the valgus angle of the proximal phalanx results in medial rotation of the hallux and lateral subluxation of the sesamoid complex into the intermetatarsal space. This deformity has a male/female ratio of 1:9, and footwear has been cited as an important cause.

Mild forms of hallux valgus may be asymptomatic. As the great toe deviates laterally, it presses against or underlaps the second toe and may cause pain in the second MTP joint. When the great toe underlaps the second toe, subluxation of the second proximal phalanx may occur due to stretching of its plantar joint capsule. This subluxation can be demonstrated by physical examination. Pain occurs when the second toe is moved through its range of motion at the MTP joint. This discomfort is caused by a traumatic synovitis produced at this site by forces generated during walking and weight bearing. The second toe and its MTP joint may become swollen. The second toe may dislocate from the MTP joint and become a hammer toe. The third toe may similarly dislocate dorsally, giving rise to displacement of the third metatarsal head in a plantar direction. Weight bearing gives rise to metatarsalgia at the base of the second and third toes, and the wearing of tight and narrow shoes can cause painful, traumatic irritation of the skin and soft tissue over the dorsum of the PIP joints of the second and third toes and/or an inflammatory swelling of the medial bunion at the first MTP joint. Hallux valgus is associated with hypermobile pes planus, pes planovalgus (in patients with cerebral palsy), wearing of high-heeled shoes with a narrow toe box, wide forefeet or splay feet and hypermobile pes planus, metatarsus primus varus, joint hyperlaxity (Down's syndrome and Ehlers-Danlos syndrome), and rheumatoid arthritis.

28. BUNION OF THE GREAT TOE

Formation of a hallux valgus deformity stretches the medial MTP joint capsule. The medial portion of the first metatarsal head becomes exposed as a bunion. Medially, some reactive bone formation occurs. Local pressure from shoes results in thickening of the medial joint capsule and the production of a superficial adventitial bursa. Bursal inflammation may occur, resulting in local pain, swelling, redness, and tenderness. Infection of a bursa may result from needle aspiration to remove fluid, and this procedure should be avoided. An inflamed bursa will become asymptomatic if an open shoe or a shoe with a cutout in the area of the bursa is worn.

29. HALLUX LIMITUS OR RIGIDUS

Acute pain can follow a stubbed toe. The dorsum of the first MTP joint may be swollen and tender, and dorsiflexion of the toe causes pain. Push-off during walking causes great toe passive dorsiflexion and intensifies the pain, while plantar flexion is pain free. The cause is a contusion or a chondral or osteochondral fracture of the dorsal portion of the articular surface of the metatarsal head.

Persistent symptoms over the first MTP joint may result from osteoarthritis. This condition may cause pain and limited dorsiflexion, although normal plantar flexion is painless. An osteochondral fracture may be identified by MRI or plain radiographs and osteoarthritis by plain radiographs. Osteophytes may be palpable on the dorsum of the joint in patients with severe osteoarthritis.

Juvenile hallux rigidus may result from osteochondritis dissecans or from severe pes planovalgus and a hypermobile first metatarsal and metatarsus primus elevatus.

While most cases of adult hallux rigidus are the result of trauma or osteoarthritis, some are caused by gout, one of the seronegative spondyloarthropathies, or rheumatoid arthritis. In most cases due to systemic arthritis, there is bilateral disease with asymmetry in the severity of involvement. Males are more commonly affected than females. Hallux rigidus may also develop secondary to a hallux valgus deformity.

Radiographs in long-standing cases may reveal a prominent dorsal or lateral exostosis. Dorsal or lateral bursal enlargements over the first MTP joint may develop.

30. HALLUCAL SESAMOID DISORDERS

Pain, tenderness, and swelling occur on the plantar side of the first MTP joint. Weight bearing and walking intensify the pain and may be voluntarily limited by the patient. The sesamoid bones (medial and lateral) may be palpated near the head-neck junction of the first metatarsal. Tenderness may be localized to the area of a single sesamoid bone.

Causes of local pain and sesamoid tenderness include sesamoiditis; sesamoid contusion; sesamoid fractures, usually associated with significant falls from a height and sometimes confused radiographically with partite sesamoids; aseptic necrosis, detectable by a bone scan with pin-hole collimation; bursitis under the first metatarsal head, which may occur from prolonged walking or standing; and an enlarged arthritic medial sesamoid bone.

Tangential ''sesamoid'' radiographic views are useful for the identification of fractures, avascular necrosis, osteomyelitis, and degenerative arthritis. Radiographically negative, painful sesamoid area disorders include chondromalacia, sesamoid bursitis, first MTP joint synovitis, a symptomatic bipartite sesamoid bone, or tendinitis of the flexor hallucis longus. Sesamoid fractures may require surgery for nonunion or intraarticular displacement. Infected or necrotic sesamoid bones may also require excision.

31. FIRST MTP JOINT ARTHRITIS

A. Septic Arthritis and Osteomyelitis
Septic arthritis may have a hematogenous origin, may follow penetrating trauma (e.g., needle aspiration) or an open fracture or fracture-dislocation, or may result from joint penetration by a plantar ulcer. Plantar ulcers are usually trophic and secondary to severe peripheral neuropathy. Sesamoid infection and lysis may be associated, or the metatarsal head may become infected. The region over the first MTP joint may be diffusely tender, swollen, warm, and red. Pain may be mild to severe, depending on the degree of prior neuropathic involvement. Fever, sweats, and an elevated leukocyte count and sedimentation rate may be associated findings. Plain radiographs or MRI will demonstrate the extent of soft tissue and bone involvement. Synovial fluid has a high concentration of polymorphonuclear leukocytes, and synovial fluid cultures are usually positive. Surgical debridement or amputation, as well as a prolonged course of intravenous antibiotic therapy, may be required.

B. Podagra
Severe-to-excruciating pain, redness, warmth, swelling, and exquisite tenderness occur over the medial forefoot and first MTP joint. Aspiration of joint fluid may reveal monosodium urate (gout) or calcium pyrophosphate dihydrate (pseudogout) crystals. Rarely, hydroxyapatite or calcium oxalate crystal deposition in the joint may cause a similar clinical picture. Other disorders that may occasionally cause an acute synovitis of the first MTP joint include rheumatoid arthritis, Reiter's syndrome, ankylosing spondylitis, and the arthritis associated with inflammatory bowel disease. These systemic disorders may be identified by clinical history and associated physical and laboratory findings.

32. JOPLIN'S NEUROMA

Pain and paresthesias occur along the medial plantar surface of the first MTP joint and radiate into the great toe. The cause is perineural fibrosis of the plantar proper digital nerve of the great toe. Local palpation over the digital nerve at the MTP joint may reproduce the pain and paresthesias. Symptoms are increased by wearing shoes or weight bearing. Local trauma to the first MTP joint, bunion surgery, and hallux valgus-related nerve entrapment are possible causes of this disorder. Surgical excision of the involved nerve may be required.

33. GANGRENE OR ULCERATION OF THE GREAT TOE

Pain, blackening, and tenderness of the great toe may occur. Ulceration results when the necrotic area sloughs. Erythema may surround the blackened area. The foot is cool, pale, and usually pulseless, unless the cause is small vessel vasculitis or cholesterol emboli. The pain may begin abruptly and persist. The cause may be arterial embolism by clot or cholesterol, a local thrombosis in a distal vessel, or vasculitis and small artery occlusion. In patients with vasculitis, systemic symptoms and multiple organ involvement are usually present. The diagnosis of arteriosclerosis obliterans can be confirmed by arteriography. Transesophageal echocardiography may be utilized to determine whether there is a cardiac source of embolic material. Cholesterol embolization usually results from arteriography, angioplasty, or use of an intraaortic balloon.

34. RADICULAR PAIN (L5 ROOT)

An L5 radiculopathy due to an L4–L5 disc herniation may cause sciatic and back pain, calf pain, or dorsomedial foot and great toe pain. Weakness of great toe extension may be present. The diagnosis can be confirmed by finding pain provocation or exacerbation with cough or straining and/or with the straight leg-raising test. A lumbar lesion can be identified by MRI or contrast-enhanced CT.

35. SHOE VAMP ULCER AND BURSITIS

Pressure from a tight shoe vamp over the dorsum of the proximal hallux may cause redness, tenderness, and superficial ulceration. An adventitial bursa may form, become red and tender, and, in some cases, drain fluid through a sinus tract.

36. FIRST-RAY OVERLOAD SYNDROME

First metatarsal pain and tenderness occur secondary to an enlarged first ray and a long great toe that abuts the toe box of the shoe and transmits forces back to the MTP joint, resulting in articular injury and osteoarthritis. Sudden loading of the MTP region may be caused by a fall on the tiptoes, plantar pressure on a brake during a motor vehicle accident, or overuse resulting from repetitive jumps on the tiptoes (e.g., as in dancers). An angle of more than 25° between the first metatarsal and the floor can also cause overload. This can occur when the shoes being worn have excessively high heels or there is downward displacement of the first metatarsal in an anterior cavus foot.

Examination findings include first MTP joint tenderness, metatarsal head prominence on the plantar side, and great toe hyperextension during walking. The consequences of this overload are plantar calluses and/or corns, adventitial bursitis, sesamoiditis, fracture or aseptic necrosis of the sesamoid bones, and synovitis of the first MTP joint. Lateral radiographs may demonstrate vertical orientation of the first metatarsal (i.e., on non-weight-bearing views).

37. CALCIFIC TENDINITIS OF FLEXOR HALLUCIS TENDONS

Pain, swelling, redness, and tenderness occur near the first MTP joint on the plantar aspect. The pain is provoked or exacerbated by walking, flexion of the great toe against resistance, or passive extension of the hallux and direct pressure over the painful site. Plain radiographs will reveal a soft tissue calcification in the region of the flexor hallucis tendons. Rest and nonsteroidal anti-inflammatory drugs usually result in resolution.

Small Toe Pain

38. HARD CORNS

These round (3–10 mm), conical, hyperkeratotic lesions form secondary to external pressure (i.e., from a shoe) over sites of bony prominence, such as a prominent condyle on a phalanx or an exostosis. The common locations are on the lateral side of toe 5, the dorsal aspect of the other toes over the IP joints (e.g., hammer or claw toes), or at the tip of the toes (end corns). After paring, the conical portion of the corn has a lighter center than the surrounding skin. Corns often result from a poorly fitting shoe (too large or too small) or a preexisting foot deformity (e.g., pes planus with elevation of the lateral border of the foot). Paring and enucleation of the corn will relieve pain and pressure-related tenderness. Recurrent corns may require removal of the underlying bony prominence for cure.

39. SOFT CORNS

These painful and tender lesions usually occur between the fourth and fifth or the third and fourth toes. Pressure of one condyle against an adjacent condyle results in corn formation. Associated skin maceration in the web space may mimic a fungal infection. A soft corn may also occur in the web space, caused by pressure of the base of a proximal phalanx on the metatarsal head of the adjacent toe. A kissing lesion on the adjacent toe favors a diagnosis

of soft corn. A bony prominence palpable in the bed of a macerated lesion also supports a diagnosis of soft corn. An unreduced joint dislocation (MTP or PIP) may also result in soft corn formation.

40. HELOMA VERRUCA

A mosaic wart, consisting of a group of tiny warts, may mimic the appearance of a soft corn. This lesion may be tender and painful.

41. END CORNS

These painful, hyperkeratotic lesions occur at the end of the toe near the nail margin. Claw or mallet toe deformities may be responsible for the location of the corn at the end of the toe. The skin may be impinged upon by the nail, the underlying bony tuft of the distal phalanx, and the inner surface of the shoe.

42. MALLET TOE DEFORMITY

There is a dynamic flexion deformity of the DIP joint of a toe. An associated flexion deformity of the PIP joint may be associated in some cases. This deformity is known as claw toe.

Painful disorders resulting from a mallet toe deformity include an end corn; a dorsal corn; nail-toe-pulp irritation and pain; friction-induced redness, pain, and tenderness over the dorsal aspect of one or both IP joints; and an ingrown toenail with associated infection.

43. HAMMER TOE DEFORMITY

There is a flexion deformity at the PIP joint, with extension or hyperextension of the DIP joint. The joint deformities may be flexible or fixed.

Redness, local pain and tenderness, and blister formation may occur over the dorsal prominence of the PIP joint due to frictional contact with a tight shoe. A painful corn may form at this site and/or at the end of the toe.

Hammer toes can result from wearing shoes that are too short for the foot, intrinsic muscle imbalance, a cavus foot, and neurologic disorders affecting the anterior muscle power of the foot.

44. PERIUNGUAL CORN OF THE FIFTH TOE

This corn causes pain and tenderness over the distal portion of the lateral or medial side of the small toe adjacent to the nail. It is often caused by dorsolateral shoe pressure.

In some cases, this lesion results from downward rotation of the fifth toe, so that the nail edge rubs against the inner sole of the shoe. In such cases, corrective surgery is required.

45. ULCERATION OF THE TOES

A. Ischemic These ulcerations may be caused by ischemia secondary to an embolus, thrombosis, vasculitis, or obstructive arteriosclerotic disease. Toe blackening on the same and/or other toes may be associated.

B. Neuropathic Neuropathy, causing pain, paresthesias, and anesthesia of the toes, may lead to the formation of a relatively painless neuropathic ulcer.

46. TOPHUS

A firm, red, tender lesion may form on the dorsum of a small toe and mimic a corn or a skin abscess because of its white center. The lesion may rupture and drain a whitish, chalky material. Microscopic examination of the discharge reveals masses of monosodium urate crystals. The lesion resembles a furuncle, but the discharge is chalky white and not yellow. A radiograph of the foot may reveal erosive, gouty lesions of the phalanges and metatarsals.

47. ARTHRITIS OF THE SMALL TOES

Isolated DIP or PIP joint pain, tenderness, and swelling may be a sign of early rheumatoid arthritis or may occur as a dactylitis ("sausage digit") with psoriatic arthritis or Reiter's syndrome. "Sausage toe" is associated with radiographic evidence of periostitis, IP joint synovitis, and sometimes flexor tenosynovitis.

48. TINEA PEDIS

This disorder may be asymptomatic or may cause itching of the third and fourth web spaces or sharp, stinging pain due to erosion and fissuring of the skin. Neglected cases may progress to involve all the web spaces, and erosion or ulceration of the proximal plantar surface of the toes may occur. The web spaces are wet and macerated, and a cheesy discharge may be wiped from the surface. Common fungal organisms isolated include *Trichophyton rubrum* or *mentagrophytes*. Superinfection with diphtheroids and gram-negative bacteria (*Pseudomonas* and *Proteus* species) may occur.

Aeration of the feet (by wearing sandals or open shoes) and use of antifungal solutions and powders lead to reso-

lution. Wet or vesicular lesions may be treated with wet dressings of Burow's solution (1:20) or potassium permanganate (1:10,000).

49. CANDIDIASIS

This infection may occur between the toes and cause maceration, weeping, burning pain, and itching. The skin of the toes may become erythematous, and vesicular lesions may appear. Obesity, diabetes mellitus, and alcoholism are associated. Other skin areas, such as nail edges (paronychia), the axillae, inframammary areas, and groins may also be affected. Topical therapy is usually effective.

50. DORSAL IP JOINT AREA PAIN AND INFLAMMATION

This friction-related symptom may result from hammer toes; claw toes; subluxation of the MTP joints, resulting in hammer toes; crossover of the second and sometimes the third toe on the hallux due to subluxation at the MTP joint; dislocation of the second MTP joint; or a rotational deformity of the fifth toe such that it overlaps the fourth toe. Metatarsalgia (e.g., related to MTP joint subluxation) may be associated with dorsal PIP joint region inflammation, blister formation, callus and/or corn formation, or ulceration.

51. TRAUMA (CONTUSIONS AND FRACTURES)

Direct injury by a falling object or stubbing the toes against a hard surface can cause soft tissue injury, subungual hematoma, fracture, or dislocation of the phalanges. Plain radiographs will determine the presence of a fracture or dislocation.

52. "TAILOR'S BUNION" (BUNIONETTE)

Pain, swelling, and tenderness occur over the lateral side of the fifth MTP joint. There is varus deviation at the MTP joint of the proximal phalanx, producing uncovering of the lateral articular surface of the fifth metatarsal head and formation of a lateral prominence. Friction with the shoe may result in formation of a callus and a subcutaneous bursa over this bony prominence. Traumatic bursitis, with swelling, redness, and tenderness, can cause pain at this site. Relief of friction with the shoe usually leads to resolution of the inflammatory reaction. Metatarsal osteotomy may be required for refractory cases.

53. RAYNAUD'S DISEASE AND PHENOMENON

This disorder affects the fingers and may affect the toes in up to 40 percent of patients (i.e., with Raynaud's disease). Exposure to cold or emotional upset may provoke an attack. One or more fingers and one or more toes may be affected. Initially, the digits become mildly painful and white. This pallor may be sharply demarcated at one of the palmar or plantar creases of the digits. After 10 or 15 min of pallor, the fingers and toes become congested and cyanotic and finally red, hyperemic, and painful. Although this color sequence (white, blue, and red) is characteristic, some patients experience only pallor and cyanosis or cyanosis alone. Tingling paresthesias may occur during the white phase and the hyperemic recovery period. Episodes last 20 to 30 min and recovery can sometimes be accelerated by warming the digits in warm water. Patients with frequent attacks may develop digital ulcers, sclerodactyly, and skin infarction. Raynaud's disease is the name applied to this disorder when no associated disease is apparent. Cases associated with an underlying disease are considered to have Raynaud's phenomenon. The causes of Raynaud's phenomenon are listed in Table 47-5.

54. OSLER'S NODES

Small red macules with a punctate central elevation appear on the tips of one or more fingers or toes. These lesions are tender and feel like "paper cuts." They are associated with bacterial endocarditis. Fever, musculoskeletal pain, pallor, petechiae, splinter hemorrhages, a heart murmur, anorexia, and encephalopathy are associated findings. The diagnosis is confirmed by one or more positive blood culture results and transesophageal echocardiography of the heart valves (e.g., by imaging valve vegetations).

55. SUBUNGUAL TUMORS

A. Glomus Tumor   This 1- to 3-mm, reddish-blue lesion may cause subungual pain and tenderness. The pain is provoked by cold exposure or pressure. Pain is relieved after excision.

B. Osteoid Osteoma   Subungual aching pain occurs and is more severe at night. Aspirin rapidly and dramatically relieves the pain. Soft tissue swelling of the distal portion of the toe may be present. The lesion can sometimes be identified on a plain radiograph or tomogram as an osteosclerotic phalangeal tumor with a central radiolucent nidus. If plain radiographs are negative or equivocal, a radionuclide bone scan will usually demonstrate the lesion.

C. Subungual Wart   This lesion may appear at the nail

Table 47-5
CAUSES OF RAYNAUD'S PHENOMENON AND PREVALENCE IN PATIENTS WITH THE LISTED DISEASE (%)

Fibromyalgia	30
Collagen vascular diseases	
Systemic sclerosis	80–90
Systemic lupus erythematosus	30
Dermatomyositis and polymyositis	30
Mixed connective tissue disease	81
Rheumatoid arthritis	4–17
Sjögren's syndrome	16–42
Polyarteritis nodosa	5–10
Occlusive arterial disease	
Arteriosclerosis obliterans	
Thrombonagiitis obliterans	
Acute arterial embolus	
Pulmonary hypertension	50
Blood dyscrasias	
Cryoglobulinemia	
Cold agglutinins	
Cryofibrinogenemia	
Waldenström's macroglobulinemia	33
Myeloproliferative disorders	
Cold injury	
Neurologic disorders	
Intervertebral disc disease	
Spinal cord tumors	
Drugs	
Beta-blocking drugs	
Ergot derivatives	
Bleomycin	
Vinblastine } combined therapy for germ cell cancer	44
Cis-platinum	
Migraine headache	22–33
Raynaud's disease*	
Women	4
Men	1–2

*Raynaud's phenomenon in the general population without any underlying disease.

edge and grow beneath the nail, causing local discomfort. An invasive wart may erode the underlying bony tuft.

Midfoot Pain

56. LONGITUDINAL ARCH STRAIN

Aching pain occurs over the medial aspect of the plantar midfoot. This pain is intensified by weight bearing and dorsiflexion of the foot and relieved by rest and plantar flexion. This disorder results from muscle and tendon fatigue and/or ligament injury. Foot disorders associated with longitudinal arch strain precipitated by prolonged weight bearing include pes planus, pes cavus, rigid feet with limited tarsal mobility, and lax ligaments. Treatment with rest and a flexible arch support frequently relieve the pain.

57. TRAUMA

A. Tarsometatarsal Joints (Lisfranc's Joint) Injury occurs by axial loading of the fixed foot, crushing, or a forefoot twist. An axial load can be applied to the heel of a football player with the foot in equinus, or the patient's own body weight can overload the midfoot with the foot in extreme equinus. This type of force can also occur with a missed step off a curb. A vertical load on the tarsometatarsal articulation may cause a sprain, a dislocation, or a fracture-dislocation.

1. Sprain Midfoot swelling, pain, and tenderness occur along Lisfranc's joint. Passive supination or pronation of the forefoot with the heel held in the examiner's hand will elicit pain.

2. Dislocation or Fracture-Dislocation In addition to local pain, ecchymoses, tenderness, and swelling, there will be a deformity in the midfoot region. Weight bearing is impossible or intensely painful. Three patterns of tarsometatarsal dislocation include (1) dislocation of all metatarsals laterally; (2) dislocation of one or two metatarsals from the others; and (3) dislocation of the metatarsals in different directions and planes. Rarely, disruption of the anterior and posterior tibial arteries may result in forefoot gangrene. Plain radiographs will allow detection of significant fractures and dislocations at the tarsometatarsal joint level.

B. Injury of the Midtarsal Region (Chopart's or the Transverse Tarsal Joint) This joint is composed of the talonavicular and calcaneocuboid articulations. Midtarsal joint injuries have been classified into five types. The names describe the direction of the applied injuring force and the direction of displacement.

1. Medial Injuries Medial forces may produce fracture-sprains, fracture-subluxation, or swivel dislocations.

A fracture-sprain may cause an avulsion fracture of the dorsal surface of the talar head, the navicular and lateral margin of the cuboid, or the anterior process of the calcaneus. Dorsal midfoot pain, swelling, and tenderness extend from the medial to the lateral side.

Fracture-subluxation or -dislocation causes similar findings, with the addition of medial displacement of the forefoot. Swivel dislocations result from falls from a height. The talonavicular joint is medially displaced. Medial rotation of the forefoot results in dislocation of the talonavicular articulation. The talocalcaneal interosseous ligament and calcaneocuboid joint remain intact. Maximum tenderness and swelling occur medially over the talonavicular joint.

2. Longitudinal Injuries These injuries occur when the foot is plantar-flexed and axial loading of the meta-

tarsal heads occurs. The navicular bone is compressed by the cuneiforms and the talus. This produces a compression fracture of the navicular bone and/or crushing of the talus. Medial forefoot displacement may occur with calcaneocuboid joint disruption if similar forces are applied to the lateral cuneiforms. Fracture of the lateral portion of the navicular bone and the talus may be associated. Dorsal midfoot pain, edema, and tenderness are extensive and involve the entire instep.

3. Lateral Injuries These injuries result from a motor vehicle accident or a fall from a height. Severe pronation of the front of the foot occurs. Fracture-sprain may result in an avulsion fracture of the navicular bone and talus medially and impaction fractures of the articular margins of the cuboid bone or calcaneus laterally.

Fracture subluxation of the talonavicular joint laterally and comminuted fractures of the anterior portion of the calcaneus or cuboid bone occur. The longitudinal arch is lost, and the cuboid bone may be extruded. Lateral swivel dislocations cause lateral dislocation of the talonavicular joint, while other midfoot joints are not disrupted.

4. Plantar Injuries Fracture-sprains cause avulsion injuries of the navicular bone, talus, or calcaneus. Plantar displacement of the navicular bone, the cuboid bone, and the forefoot may occur. This displacement is best seen on a lateral radiograph. Motorcycle accidents and falls are usually responsible for these injuries.

5. Crush Injuries Crush injuries may cause multiple compression fractures, open fractures, and a compartment syndrome of the foot. Isolated fractures of the navicular bone, cuboid bone, calcaneus, or talus cause localized tenderness and swelling and can be detected by plain radiographs.

C. Navicular Fractures

1. Traumatic Fractures Local pain and tenderness occur over the dorsomedial region of the midfoot secondary to a dorsal avulsion fracture. The usual injury mechanism is forceful eversion of the ankle. Less commonly, a direct blow may fracture the navicular bone. A dorsal avulsion fracture is often mistaken for a deltoid ligament sprain before radiographs are taken. Medial midfoot pain, dorsal tenderness, and swelling occur. Avulsion fracture of the navicular tuberosity follows excessive ankle eversion and has a similar clinical presentation to a dorsal navicular fracture. Plain radiographs will demonstrate the fracture. Body fractures of the navicular bone are usually associated with other midtarsal joint injuries, as described above. Isolated body fractures are rare.

2. Stress Fractures This is a disorder of young athletes (e.g., basketball players). Stress fracture of the navicular bone causes medial midfoot pain and tenderness without edema. There is no history of injury. Pain is provoked by weight bearing or running. There may be no evidence of fracture on a plain radiograph (76 percent of cases). The diagnosis can usually be established by a bone scan. A CT scan may detect the fracture line before a plain radiograph can. A missed diagnosis and continued activity may result in nonunion or delayed union and significant disability.

D. Fracture of the Base of the Fifth Metatarsal (Jones Fracture)   Two types of fractures occur at the base of the fifth metatarsal: avulsion fractures and diaphyseal fractures.

1. Avulsion Fractures   A sudden inversion of the foot, combined with reflex contraction of the peroneus brevis, results in avulsion of the tuberosity of the fifth metatarsal. Tenderness occurs over the base of the fifth metatarsal laterally at the joint line with the cuboid. Active eversion of the foot is painful. This fracture is sometimes confused with an ankle sprain. Immobilization in a walking cast for 2 to 3 weeks leads to union.

2. Diaphyseal Fractures (True Jones Fractures) Diaphyseal fractures also follow inversion of the plantar-flexed foot. Loading of the lateral aspect of the foot occurs. The Jones diaphyseal fracture usually occurs in a male athlete (e.g., basketball player). There is localized tenderness 1 to 2 cm distal to the metatarsal base. Radiographs reveal a transverse linear fracture across the metatarsal. This fracture has a high delayed union, nonunion, and refracture rate. Some of these injuries may be stress fractures of the base of the fifth metatarsal and not acute fractures.

58. ASEPTIC NECROSIS OF THE NAVICULAR BONE (MULLER-WEISS DISEASE)

This disorder occurs in adults with severe pes planus and a prominent navicular bone. Severe dorsomedial midfoot pain is associated with edema and sometimes erythema and warmth of the overlying skin. Radiographs reveal accordion-like narrowing of the navicular bone, with a dense sclerotic lateral portion of the bone. A fracture line may be observed. Degenerative changes may be present in the talonavicular joint. MRI or a radionuclide scan will detect early lesions. Arthrodesis may be required in adults with refractory symptoms.

59. TENDINITIS

A. Flexor Hallucis Longus Tendinitis   During walking, pain occurs in the medial plantar aspect of the midfoot distal to the tender area associated with the heel spur

syndrome. Passive or active dorsiflexion of the hallux allows palpation of the tendon. A focal area of tendon tenderness may be present in the midfoot region. This disorder most frequently results from overuse (e.g., prolonged walking or jogging). It responds to limitation of walking and use of rubber-soled wedgies.

B. Peroneal Tendinitis   Pain occurs over the lateral aspect of the midfoot near the insertion of the peroneus brevis on the base of the fifth metatarsal bone. Active eversion against resistance or passive inversion intensifies the pain. Pain due to peroneus longus tendinitis may radiate from the area of the cuboid bone under the arch of the foot to the medial side, where it is inserted on the base of the first metatarsal. Local tenderness is present over one or both tendons near their points of insertion. Rarely, acute peroneal tendinitis can be due to *N. gonorrhoeae* infection, a seronegative spondyloarthropathy, or seropositive rheumatoid arthritis. Fractures of the calcaneus may cause peroneal tendon irritation and tendon sheath constriction.

60. SUBTALAR OSTEOCHONDRAL FRACTURE

Pain and tenderness occur over the region of the sinus tarsi or just distal to the tip of the lateral malleolus or at both sites. A fixed valgus deformity of the hindfoot may be present, and there may be spastic, painful, subtalar motion. In many cases, the cause of the pain is, not compression and irritation of the peroneal tendons that result in peroneal muscle spasm, but an unsuspected subtalar articular surface injury. Subtalar arthrodesis, not peroneal tendon release, relieves the symptoms. MRI can image the peroneal tendons and the degree of subtalar joint damage.

The presence of a calcaneal spur adjacent to the peroneal tendons on a CT or MRI does not mean that the spur is the cause of lateral midfoot symptoms. Spur removal may have no effect if subtalar damage is the cause of the pain. Subtalar articular pain may require arthrodesis for relief.

61. INTEROSSEOUS MYOSITIS OR STRAIN

Pain occurs on weight bearing in the midfoot region. It may be most intense on arising in the morning and is improved by wearing shoes. Lateral-to-medial side compression of the midfoot and forefoot by the examiner provokes or intensifies the pain. Rest, without weight bearing, relieves the discomfort. Tenderness occurs over the soft tissue between the second and third or the third and fourth metatarsals and not over a metatarsal bone.

MRI may show increased signal intensity of the affected inflamed interosseous muscle on a T_2-weighted image. This disorder responds to avoidance of weight bearing for 2 to 4 weeks.

62. STRESS FRACTURE OF ONE OR MORE METATARSAL OR TARSAL BONES

Stress fracture of a metatarsal shaft, the navicular bone, or another midfoot bone may cause aching pain that is provoked or intensified by weight bearing and running and relieved by rest. Plain radiographs may appear negative or reveal a fracture on ray 2, 3, or 4. A radionuclide bone scan is usually positive within 2 to 4 weeks of pain onset. The increased radionuclide uptake on the scan is focal, as is the tenderness associated with this lesion. One or more stress fractures may be present. Symptoms usually improve and resolve with restriction of weight bearing and activity for 3 to 5 weeks.

63. PSEUDOMONAS OSTEOMYELITIS OF THE MIDFOOT

A nail puncture wound may result in midfoot pain, swelling, and tenderness at the site of the wound. The nail may inoculate *Pseudomonas aeruginosa* into one of the metatarsals, resulting in an osteomyelitis. Early evidence of bone infection may be obtained by MRI or a radionuclide bone scan. Local pain, swelling, and tenderness respond to antibiotic therapy. Most nail puncture wounds do not cause osteomyelitis. Cellulitis or an abscess due to a staphylococcal species is more common. Rarely, *Mycobacterium fortuitum* may be the cause of puncture wound-associated infection.

64. ACQUIRED FLATFOOT

A. Rupture of the Tibialis Posterior Tendon This disorder often occurs in a patient with a history of mild-to-moderate congenital pes planus. Pain, swelling, and tenderness occur over the tendon in the medial forefoot near the medial malleolus, and there is flattening of the longitudinal arch in the affected foot. Standing on tiptoes on the painful foot is not possible. When the foot is viewed from behind, a hindfoot valgus deformity is present, as is a ''too-many-toes'' sign. The ability of the examiner to see four or five toes from the rear on the affected foot reflects severe pronation. Inversion strength of the foot is weak.

With time, pain also occurs over the lateral mid- and forefoot, possibly due to impingement of the anterior portion of the posterior subtalar facet upon the sinus tarsi area of the calcaneus. In severe cases, the calcaneus may impinge upon the lateral malleolus. This disorder occurs predominantly in women (male/female ratio, 1:2) in the 40- to 75-year-old age group. Two-thirds of ruptures of the tibialis posterior occur on the left, and 5 percent are bilateral. MRI may visualize the tibialis posterior tendon and may demonstrate attenuation or a split in the tendon or a heterogeneous signal due to degeneration, but MRI may be equivocal or falsely negative. Up to 20 percent of cases are associated with a seronegative spondyloarthropathy or rheumatoid arthritis.

In advanced cases with complete tendon rupture, the talus subluxates medially on weight bearing and forms a prominent bony mass below the medial malleolus.

B. Ligamentous or Bone Failure Acquired flatfoot may result from trauma with ligamentous injury or from arthritic changes in the talonavicular, navicular cuneiform, or metatarsocuneiform joints. Midtarsal fracture-dislocation may also result in acquired flatfoot, causing medial midfoot pain and, when severe, lateral midfoot and ankle pain.

65. OSTEOARTHRITIS

A. First Metatarsocuneiform Joint Osteoarthritis of the first metatarsocuneiform joint can produce a dorsal exostosis that can cause pressure irritation of the overlying dorsal skin or tenosynovitis of the extensor hallucis longus tendon.

Adventitial bursitis may occur over the exostosis. Medial midfoot pain and tenderness occur. Tendinitis is confirmed by detecting focal tenderness of the involved tendon and pain intensification by passive stretching or active use of the tendon.

B. Cuboideometatarsal Joint Pain related to jogging or running occurs in the lateral midfoot. Tenderness occurs along the joint line of the cuboideometatarsal articulation. Results of plain radiographs may be negative. The cause of this pain is mild osteoarthritis of the articulation between the cuboid and the fourth and fifth metatarsals. Sprain of the associated ligaments near this articulation is difficult to differentiate in the absence of radiographic evidence of osteoarthritis. This disorder responds to abstinence from running or jogging for 2 to 4 weeks.

66. PLANTAR FASCIAL PAIN

A. Plantar Fasciitis Pain occurs over the plantar aspect of the midfoot on getting out of bed in the morning. After a few steps, the pain improves or disappears, only to return later in the day. The plantar fascia is diffusely tender, and pain is intensified by passive or active dorsiflexion of the toes. Local tenderness over the calcaneal insertion of the plantar fascia may be minimal or absent. There is no localized tenderness over the tendon of the flexor hallucis longus, a structure that can be made easily palpable by extension of the great toe. Plantar fasciitis is usually an overuse syndrome, but it may be associated with systemic disorders. Pain is intensified by weight bearing or jogging. Improvement occurs with rest, non-steroidal anti-inflammatory drugs, and circumferential taping of the foot. Refractory cases may respond to a rigid orthosis designed at the University of California Bio-mechanics Laboratory (e.g., UCBL insert).

B. Heel Pain Syndrome In the heel pain syndrome, often confused with true plantar fasciitis, described above, there are localized pain and tenderness over the medial plantar aspect of the heel and no intensification of pain on toe dorsiflexion. The plantar fascia is seldom diffusely tender in the midfoot. The onset of heel pain syndrome is usually gradual and is due to overuse. It is caused by microtrauma to the origin of the plantar fascia with a reparative inflammatory reaction. Similar injury occurs to the more superior flexor digitorum brevis muscle at its insertion on the calcaneus. Microscopic stress fractures of the medial calcaneal tuberosity may also occur in asso-ciation with the microtears in the fascia and muscle. These bone changes may be identified, in some cases, by a radionuclide bone scan (e.g., the delayed phase shows increased uptake over the calcaneus). Acute midfoot pain may arise from rupture of the plantar fascia or fracture of a large heel spur. The heel pain syndrome is an enthesitis, and similar symptoms and signs may be associated with one of the seronegative spondyloarthropathies.

67. PLANTAR ABSCESS

This severe infection may involve the forefoot and mid-foot or the midfoot alone. Diabetes or peripheral vascular disease are commonly associated. Fever, chills, sweats, and malaise are associated with midfoot pain, swelling, and tenderness. The dorsum of the foot may also be swol-len and tender. Leukocytosis is usually present. Common isolates include *S. aureus* or a mixed flora. Weight bear-ing is difficult or impossible. Any movement of the foot intensifies the pain. The central compartment of the foot is usually involved. MRI can localize pus in the plantar spaces deep to the plantar fascia. Symptoms resolve with incision, drainage, and antibiotic therapy.

Dorsal Foot Pain

68. TENDINITIS

A. Extensor Hallucis Longus Muscle Pain occurs on the dorsomedial aspect of the foot during walking. Local

tenderness is present over the tendon. Extension of the hallux against resistance or passive flexion may provoke the pain.

B. Extensor Digitorum Longus Muscle Pain occurs over this tendon during walking and the tendon is tender. Small toe extension against resistance or passive flexion causes pain.

C. Tibialis Anterior Muscle There is local pain during walking. Palpation of the tendon during resisted dorsi-flexion of the foot elicits tenderness and supports the diag-nosis. Passive plantar flexion of the ankle may be painful.

69. CRUXIATE CRURAL LIGAMENT INJURY

Cruciate crural ligament sprain is usually caused by direct or indirect trauma. Palpation of the ligament during toe dorsiflexion will result in pain and tenderness. Severe tenderness over the ligament with minimal intensification of pain by toe dorsiflexion suggests ligament injury.

70. OTHER CAUSES

The other causes of dorsal foot pain are listed in Table 47-6 and are discussed in previous sections of this chapter.

Table 47-6
CAUSES OF DORSAL FOOT PAIN

Cellulitis
Abscess of the foot
Osteomyelitis
Septic arthritis
Acute gout or pseudogout
Reflex sympathetic dystrophy
Peripheral polyneuropathy
Superficial peroneal nerve entrapment
Deep peroneal nerve entrapment
Bites
Herpes zoster
Shoe dermatitis
Trauma to the metatarsal and tarsal bones (fracture and dislocation)
Aseptic necrosis of the navicular bone
Subtalar osteochondral fracture
Interosseous myositis or strain
Stress fracture of a metatarsal or tarsal bone
Acquired flatfoot
Osteoarthritis of the tarsal metatarsal joints (first metatarsocuneiform joint and cuboideometatarsal joint)
Tendinitis of the tibialis anterior, the extensor hallucis longus, and/or the extensor digitorum longus
Cruxiate crural ligament sprain

Hindfoot Pain

71. GENERALIZED HINDFOOT PAIN

A. Calcaneal Fractures

1. Intraarticular   A fall from a height is the usual cause. The talus is driven downward into the calcaneus on impact (85 percent of cases). In 5 to 9 percent of cases, fractures of the calcaneus are bilateral, and 10 percent are associated with fractures of the lumbar spine.

Severe, diffuse pain in the heel is associated with extensive plantar ecchymoses, swelling, and tenderness. In many cases, the heel is widened, and a valgus deformity occurs. Excruciating pain that is unrelieved by analgesics may on rare occasions result from hematoma formation and a compartment syndrome of the foot. In this situation, any toe movement may intensify the pain, and the central compartment may become tense and exquisitely tender. Distal foot paresthesias and sensory loss occur. The diagnosis can be confirmed by finding elevated intracompartmental pressures. The intense pain can be relieved by surgical decompression of the central and other involved fascial compartments.

Anteroposterior, lateral, axial, calcaneal, and oblique radiographic views will identify and define most calcaneal fractures. Lateral radiographs usually demonstrate tongue and joint depression-type fractures. An anteroposterior view allows detection of associated fractures of the navicular and cuboid bone and assessment of the calcaneocuboid and talonavicular joints. The axial view will demonstrate heel widening, impingement on the peroneal space by a lateral fragment, and the amount of displacement and comminution of fragments. Complex fractures are best examined by a CT scan of the heel.

2. Extraarticular

    A. FRACTURE OF THE MEDIAL CALCANEAL PROCESS   There are medial inframalleolar pain, swelling, tenderness, and ecchymoses. Joint range of motion is preserved, but forced dorsiflexion of the ankle or toes may provoke pain. An axial view demonstrates the fracture and the degree of displacement.

    B. FRACTURE OF THE SUPERIOR PORTION OF THE CALCANEAL TUBEROSITY   Pain, swelling, tenderness, and ecchymoses occur over the posterior portion of the heel near the insertion of the Achilles tendon. This fracture may be produced by avulsion of a bone fragment at the insertion of the Achilles tendon during a fall from a step as the calf muscles suddenly contract. This type of fracture occurs primarily in older women with osteoporosis. Active plantar flexion is impaired or absent. Standing on tiptoe is difficult (e.g., loss of plantar flexion) but may be possible if the tibialis posterior muscle and the toe flexors produce some plantar flexion. Results of Thompson's test, however, are positive if the Achilles tendon and attached bone fragment are disconnected from the calcaneus. A lateral radiograph will reveal the fracture.

    C. FRACTURE OF THE SUSTENTACULUM TALI   A fall on the heel, combined with forceful inversion of the foot, is the usual mechanism of fracture. Swelling, pain, and tenderness occur on the inframalleolar region of the medial hindfoot. Pain is intensified by inversion of the foot. Tenderness of the heel is usually absent or minimal. Passive hyperextension of the great toe may also intensify the pain. An axial view will demonstrate the fracture.

B. Ischemic Necrosis of the Heel
Elderly patients may develop pain, redness, and blackening of one or both heels secondary to pressure necrosis of the unprotected skin. Such ischemia occurs in comatose, stroke, or other bedridden patients. Similar findings may occur, less commonly, in younger patients in deep coma. Examination reveals a small-to-large area of skin induration and blackening over the heel, surrounded by a narrow margin of skin erythema. Systemic symptoms do not usually occur. Pain may be mild or provoked only by movement-induced pressure on the heel or palpation of the infarcted region. Within weeks, partial sloughing of the blackened area occurs, leaving a residual infected ulceration. Debridement and grafting may be required for reconstruction of the heel. In milder cases, spontaneous healing may occur.

72. PLANTAR HINDFOOT PAIN

A. Fat Pad Disorders

1. Atrophy   Heel pain occurs on the plantar surface and is intensified by hard-soled shoes and walking on hard surfaces. The adipose tissue of the heel pads is softened, thinned, and flattened. The calcaneal tubercles are easily palpable through the skin. Compression of this area by the examiner reproduces the pain. Use of soft-soled shoes, a shock-absorbent heel cup, and elevation of the heel provide partial or complete relief. Elderly people and runners who train on hard surfaces are susceptible to this disorder.

2. Inflammation   Heel pain and tenderness occur on the plantar surface, but the heel pad is not atrophic. Symptoms result from repetitive impact loading, prolonged weight bearing, or direct trauma to the heel. Treatment consists of the use of a semirigid plastic heel cup without the cushion used for patients with atrophy. Resolution will usually occur within 6 months.

3. Fat Pad Separation from the Calcaneus   Fat pad separation from the calcaneus by a fluid-filled bursa may cause heel pain, tenderness, and swelling. This diagnosis can be confirmed by MRI. Aspiration of the bursal sac or cyst or excision allows the fat pad to readhere to the calcaneus, thus relieving the pain.

4. Piezogenic Papules   These painful pressure papules are larger than nonpainful papules. They may represent herniations of subcutaneous fat into the dermis with associated ischemia of the papule, causing tenderness of the papule and pain. A heel orthosis to relieve pressure is usually required.

B. Glomus Tumor   Well-localized plantar heel pain and tenderness that are made worse by cold may be caused by a glomus tumor. The tumor may not be palpable. This rare lesion requires excision for pain relief.

C. Stress Fracture of the Calcaneus   Diffuse pain occurs about the heel in a military recruit or an athlete undergoing extensive training (e.g., a recruit training over 16 h/day). Heel pain begins after several weeks of training and persists. It is relieved by rest and exacerbated by activity. Swelling and redness of the overlying skin may occur, and the calcaneus is tender. Results of a plain radiograph are negative or demonstrate a vertical, dense line that begins at the posterosuperior plateau of the calcaneus and runs downward toward the plantar surface. A radionuclide bone scan or a CT scan provides greater sensitivity for the early diagnosis of a calcaneal stress fracture.

D. Heel Pain Syndrome due to Overuse   Pain occurs over the medial plantar aspect of the heel. There is local tenderness over the medial calcaneal tuberosity and the plantar fascia for up to 5 mm distal to this point. Most of the distal plantar fascia is nontender, and there is no increase in pain with passive dorsiflexion of the toes. Onset is gradual. Pain is initially noticed on walking barefoot in the morning, and it resolves with activity as the day progresses. Prolonged standing, jogging, or running exacerbates the pain. A relationship to pes planus and pes cavus has been reported. The usual cause of this disorder is overuse, which results in microscopic tears in the attachment of the plantar fascia to the calcaneus and tears in the fibers of the adjacent flexor digitorum brevis muscle.

Granulation tissue forms at the site of these tears. Periostitis or microfracture of the calcaneus also occurs. A radionuclide bone scan may show increased uptake in the soft tissue blood pool phase (fasciitis) or in the late phase (periostitis and microfractures). Some patients have normal bone scan results. Plain radiographs may demonstrate a calcaneal spur in up to 50 percent of patients with heel pain. Similar spurs occur in 16 percent of patients without pain. The heel spur is not considered the cause of heel pain in most patients with this finding. Failure of conservative therapy (rest, nonsteroidal anti-inflammatory drugs, orthotic devices, and soft-soled shoes) requires surgical release of the plantar fascia.

E. Rupture of the Plantar Fascia   There is usually a history of plantar fasciitis-related pain of several weeks or months. One or more local injections of corticosteroid into the painful area may have been given in the preceding weeks. Rupture has an abrupt onset during walking, running, or climbing stairs. A tearing or ripping pain in the midfoot and hindfoot occurs that makes further activity or weight bearing intolerable. Within 1 to 2 days, a plantar ecchymoses may appear on the sole and medial plantar area of the heel. Symptoms resolve spontaneously within 3 to 4 weeks, and the previous symptoms of "plantar fasciitis" or the heel pain syndrome do not recur.

F. Heel Pain Syndrome Associated with Systemic Disorders   Pain and tenderness occur over the medial tuberosity of the calcaneus and the attachment of the plantar fascia at that site. Disorders responsible include rheumatoid arthritis, the seronegative, spondyloarthropathies (e.g., Reiter's syndrome, ankylosing spondylitis, and psoriatic arthritis), arthritis associated with inflammatory bowel disease, gonococcal arthritis, osteoarthritis, osteomalacia, osteomyelitis, sarcoidosis (e.g., associated with acute polyarthritis, fever, erythema nodosum, and hilar adenopathy), and diffuse idiopathic skeletal hyperostosis (DISH).

G. Entrapment Neuropathy of the First Branch of the Lateral Plantar Nerve (the Abductor Digiti Quinti Muscle)   Pain occurs over the plantar surface of the heel. Tenderness occurs over the nerve as it passes around the medial surface of the foot to the plantar side. This area is slightly anterior and medial to the point of insertion of the plantar fascia on the calcaneus. In 20 percent of cases, paresthesias and pain will be reproduced by palpation of the nerve. This disorder can be treated conservatively or by surgical decompression. Flexor digitorum tendinitis may cause medial plantar hindfoot pain and tenderness that are intensified by toe dorsiflexion and active flexion against resistance.

H. True Plantar Fasciitis   Pain occurs in the anterior plantar aspect of the heel and the midfoot. Passive extension of the toes tenses the plantar fascia and intensifies the pain. Tenderness of the plantar fascia is widespread, extending from the heel into the midfoot. This is an overuse syndrome and responds to rest. It is differentiated from the heel pain syndrome, which is an enthesopathy involving the insertion of the plantar fascia.

I. Flexor Tendinitis

1. Flexor Hallucis Longus Tendinitis   Plantar hindfoot and midfoot pain may occur in the medial side.

Passive dorsiflexion of the great toe may intensify the pain of tendinitis and plantar fasciitis. Resisted flexion only intensifies the pain of tendinitis. The tendon is the site of local tenderness in flexor tendinitis.

2. *Flexor Digitorum Longus Tendinitis*   Flexor tendinitis may also cause medial heel pain with local tenderness of the tendon and exacerbation of pain by lesser toe flexion against resistance. Toe flexion against resistance does not increase the pain of plantar fasciitis.

72. POSTERIOR HINDFOOT PAIN

A. Superficial Achilles Bursitis   Mild posterior heel pain results from irritation by the upper edge of a shoe counter of the skin over the Achilles tendon, resulting in the formation of an adventitious bursa. Tenderness occurs posterior (i.e., superficial) to the Achilles tendon. The skin and underlying bursa produce a bumplike erythematous thickening over the region of maximum heel counter friction with the foot. This area is firm and tender and may show evidence of fissuring of the overlying skin. Removal of the offending shoes provides some relief. The posterior prominence is referred to as a ''pump bump.'' Removal or softening of the heel counter leads to resolution.

B. Retrocalcaneal Bursitis   Pain and swelling occur anterior and parallel to the Achilles tendon. Overuse, gout, rheumatoid arthritis, and a seronegative spondyloarthropathy may be responsible for this disorder. The tender, fluid-filled bursa can be squeezed between the thumb and middle finger to elicit tenderness and fluctuance. An associated superficial bursitis may be present, or a posterior prominence may occur as the retrocalcaneal bursa displaces the Achilles tendon posteriorly. Medial and lateral tenderness adjacent and anterior to the Achilles tendon, as described above, supports the diagnosis. Redness, warmth, and swelling of the posterior heel may occur. Active or passive dorsiflexion of the foot causes the Achilles tendon to compress the bursa, and this may produce more pain than plantar flexion. Runners complain of increased pain when running up hills, compared to running on a level surface. MRI can visualize the enlarged retrocalcaneal bursa. Erosive changes in the calcaneus suggest the possibility of an inflammatory form of arthritis as the cause.

C. Haglund's Syndrome   Prominence of the posterior superior calcaneal tuberosity is a risk factor for the development of retrocalcaneal bursitis. The bursitis results from compression of the prominent tuberosity by a rigid heel counter. This syndrome has been defined radiographically by four criteria: (1) retrocalcaneal bursitis, (2) Achilles tendinitis (>9-mm diameter of the tendon 2

cm above the posterosuperior tuberosity), (3) superficial Achilles bursitis, and (4) a prominent posterosuperior tuberosity of the calcaneus that extends above the upper parallel pitch line of Pavlov and Heneghan. Failure of conservative therapy requires excision of the retrocalcaneal bursa and an osteotomy of the posterior superior tuberosity.

D. Achilles Tendinitis   Pain, enlargement of the tendon, and tenderness occur over a segment of tendon 2 to 3 cm proximal to the posterosuperior tuberosity of the calcaneus. Similar findings may occur at the site of tendon insertion into the calcaneus (insertional tendinitis). Crepitus over the tendon may be felt with movements of the foot. Calcium deposition in the tendon may be detected on a lateral radiograph. Calcification can cause severe, acute inflammation with overlying skin redness, edema, warmth, tenderness, and severe, constant pain.

Achilles tendinitis-related pain is intensified by plantar flexion against resistance and passive dorsiflexion of the foot. Achilles tendinitis may result from overuse, irritating shoes, a seronegative spondyloarthropathy, gout, or an acute injury.

Superficial bursitis, retrocalcaneal bursitis, and Achilles tendinitis may occur simultaneously, resulting in severe posterior heel pain, swelling, and tenderness.

E. Achilles Tendon Rupture   Pain of abrupt onset, followed by swelling and tenderness, occurs over the posterior heel. A gap in the tendon may be palpable. Plantar flexion is impaired such that standing on tiptoe is impossible or difficult. Results of Thompson's test are positive. A partial rupture may sometimes be diagnosed by sonographic studies or MRI.

F. Calcaneal Periostitis and Osteitis   Posterior heel pain, tenderness, and swelling occur. Calcaneal periostitis may follow injury, rheumatoid arthritis, or a seronegative spondyloarthropathy. The diagnosis can be supported by a radionuclide bone scan showing increased uptake over the calcaneus.

G. Calcaneal Osteomyelitis   Severe pain, swelling of the hindfoot, and tenderness occur. Fever, chills, and sweats may be associated, or systemic symptoms may be absent. Diabetes mellitus, renal failure, or some other disorder causing immunosuppression may be associated. The sedimentation rate is usually elevated, and leukocytosis may occur. Radiographs may show osteolytic bone areas and periosteal elevation. Falsely negative radiographs may be associated with increased late uptake in the infected portion of the calcaneus on a triphasic radionuclide bone scan. A CT scan may more clearly define the extent of bone lysis and necrosis. A needle or open bone biopsy and culture will confirm the diagnosis. Antibiotic therapy alone or combined with surgical debridement will result in resolution.

H. Fracture of the Posterosuperior Calcaneal Tuberosity This disorder causes symptoms similar to those of Achilles tendon rupture. Results of Thompson's test are positive if the tendon is detached from the calcaneus by an avulsion fracture. This injury is discussed above.

74. MEDIAL HINDFOOT PAIN

A. Tibialis Posterior Tendinitis Medial hindfoot and proximal arch pain may be caused by posterior tibial tendinitis. Pain and tenderness occur posterior to the medial malleolus and follow the course of the tendon distally into its insertion on the navicular bone in the medial aspect of the midfoot. Pain is intensified by resisted inversion with the foot plantar-flexed. Swelling posterior to the medial malleolus may fill in the normal concavity in the retromalleolar area. Distal tenderness over the navicular bone may be caused by an accessory navicular bone. Acute tendinitis may result from sudden, forceful pronation of the foot.

B. Flexor Hallucis Longus Tendinitis Pain occurs behind and below the medial malleolus. Passive extension of the great toe or resisted flexion intensifies the pain. Local swelling and tenderness may occur over the tendon posterior and inferior to the medial malleolus. Stenosing tenosynovitis can result in loss of great toe extension.

Pain and tenderness that are localized to the retromalleolar area may result from impingement on the tendon by an enlarged os trigonum. A CT scan and/or a tenogram may define the relationship between the os trigonum and the flexor tendon. Osteoarthritic changes between the os trigonum and the talus may also be defined by a CT scan.

C. Tarsal Tunnel Syndrome Medial plantar pain may be caused by posterior tibial nerve entrapment. The heel and the medial side of the forefoot and midfoot may be the site of pain and paresthesias. Nocturnal pain and pain that is intensified by walking or standing are common. Tapping or direct pressure over the medial side of the foot may reproduce pain and paresthesias. This disorder is discussed in more detail in an earlier section of this chapter.

D. Fracture of the Medial Calcaneal Process or Sustentaculum Tali These fractures may cause medial ankle and foot pain, swelling, and tenderness. They are discussed above.

E. Calcaneal Branch Neurodynia Aching pain that is intensified by weight bearing occurs along the medial border of the heel. A mild degree of planovalgus deformity occurs, and tenderness is present posteroinferior to the tarsal tunnel. No anterior pain radiation occurs. Medial elevation of the heel with a pad relieves pain. Refractory cases require surgery.

75. LATERAL HINDFOOT PAIN

A. Peroneal Muscle Strain Pain occurs over the lateral foot, and the peroneal tendons are tender. Eversion against resistance or passive inversion intensifies the pain.

B. Peroneal Tendinitis The tendons may be swollen and tender, and inversion-eversion movements provoke pain. Pain may radiate into the arch of the foot.

C. Lateral Ankle Sprain Anterior talofibular and calcaneofibular ligament sprains may cause lateral ankle and foot pain, tenderness, and swelling. Passive inversion provokes pain. Stress radiographs will confirm complete disruption of one or more of the lateral ankle ligaments.

D. Fracture of the Lateral Process of the Talus This fracture may cause local lateral ankle and foot pain, swelling, and tenderness that may mimic a lateral ankle sprain. This fracture can be demonstrated on a plain radiograph.

E. Osteochondral Fracture of the Talar Dome This lesion may cause lateral and central ankle and lateral foot pain. The diagnosis can be confirmed by plain radiographs, MRI, or ankle arthroscopy.

F. Sural Nerve Entrapment Posttraumatic scarring occurs posterior to the lateral malleolus and entraps the sural nerve. Less commonly, compression occurs proximally in the deep fascia of the lower leg. There are localized pain and paresthesias over the lateral aspect of the heel. Symptoms can be relieved by neurolysis. This disorder is discussed in an earlier section of this chapter.

G. Stress Fracture of the Lateral Malleolus Local pain may occur over the lateral malleolus and adjacent foot. Localized tenderness occurs over the lateral malleolus. Inversion-eversion has no pain-intensifying effect. The diagnosis can be confirmed in early cases by a radionuclide bone scan and in chronic cases by plain radiography. This disorder has been confused with peroneal tendinitis.

Bilateral Foot Pain

Disorders that may occur bilaterally are listed in Table 47-7. Many of these disorders usually occur on one side only.

Table 47-7
CAUSES OF BILATERAL FOOT PAIN

GENERALIZED FOOT PAIN
Trauma
Arthritis
  Seronegative spondyloarthropathies
  Rheumatoid arthritis
  Acute gout
  Acute pseudogout
  Acute rheumatic fever
  Systemic lupus erythematosus
  Sickle cell pain crisis
  Hepatitis B-associated arthritis
  Rubella-associated arthritis
Vascular
  Nocturnal rest pain
  Cholesterol embolism
  Arteriosclerosis obliterans and
    ischemic pain
  Systemic vasculitis
  Thromboangiitis obliterans
  Erythromelalgia
Reflex sympathetic dystrophy
Peripheral polyneuropathies
Tarsal tunnel syndrome
Frostbite
Trench foot
Immersion foot
Pernio
Cutaneous disorders
  Palmoplantar pustulosis with or
    without psoriasis
  Dyshidrotic eczema
  Pustular bacterid of hands and feet
  Acrodermatitis continua
  Infectious eczematoid dermatitis
  Hand-foot-and-mouth disease
  Vesicular tinea pedis
  Atopic dermatitis
  Contact dermatitis
  Vitamin B deficiencies
  Erosive lichen planus

FOREFOOT PAIN
Metatarsalgia due to
  High-heeled shoes
  Equinus foot
  Cavus foot
  First-ray insufficiency syndrome
  Central-ray overload
Freiberg's disease
Morton's neuroma
Idiopathic synovitis of second MTP joint
Inflammatory arthritis of the
  metatarsophalangeal joints
Arterial insufficiency
Forefoot sprain

GREAT TOE AND MEDIAL FOREFOOT PAIN
Calluses
Plantar warts
Corns
Hallux valgus
Bunion of the great toe
Hallux limitus and rigidus
Hallucal sesamoid disorders
MTP joint arthritis (podagra)
Gangrene or ischemic ulceration
Shoe vamp ulcer
First-ray overload syndrome

SMALL TOE PAIN
Corns
Mosaic warts
Hammer toes
Periungual corn of the fifth toe
Ischemic and neuropathic ulcers
Tophi
Arthritis of MTP and IP joints
Tinea pedis
Candidiasis
Dorsal IP area pain and inflammation
Trauma (contusions and fractures)
"Tailor's bunion"
Raynaud's phenomenon or disease
Osler's nodes

MIDFOOT PAIN
Longitudinal arch strain
Trauma of the tarsometatarsal and midtarsal joints
Subtalar osteochondral fractures
Interosseous myositis or strain
Stress fractures of the metatarsal bones
Acquired flatfoot due to tibialis posterior rupture
Osteoarthritis of the tarsal joints
True plantar fasciitis
Heel pain syndrome

DORSAL FOOT PAIN
Acute gout
Acute pseudogout
Reflex sympathetic dystrophy
Peripheral polyneuropathy
Deep peroneal nerve entrapment
Shoe dermatitis
Trauma to metatarsals
Subtalar arthritis
Interosseous myositis or strain
Metatarsal stress fracture
Acquired flatfoot
Osteoarthritis of tarsometatarsal joints
Tendinitis of the tibialis anterior and the toe
  extensors

HINDFOOT PAIN
Calcaneal fractures
Ischemic heel necrosis

PLANTAR HINDFOOT PAIN
Fat pad disorders
  Atrophy
  Inflammation
  Piezogenic papules
Heel pain syndrome due to overuse
Heel pain syndrome due to systemic
  disorders
True plantar fasciitis
Flexor tendinitis
  Flexor hallucis longus
  Flexor digitorum longus
Entrapment of first branch of lateral plantar
  nerve

POSTERIOR HINDFOOT PAIN
Superficial Achilles bursitis
Retrocalcaneal bursitis
Haglund's syndrome
Achilles tendinitis
Calcaneal periostitis and osteitis

MEDIAL HINDFOOT PAIN
Tibialis posterior tendinitis
Flexor hallucis longus tendinitis
Tarsal tunnel syndrome

LATERAL HINDFOOT PAIN
Lateral ankle sprain
Peroneal tendinitis
Osteochondral fracture of the talar dome
Stress fracture of the lateral malleolus

FOOT PAIN REFERENCES

Compartment Syndrome

Starosta D, Sacchetti AD, Sharkey P: Calcaneal fracture with compartment syndrome of the foot. *Ann Emerg Med* 17:856–858, 1988.

Dermatologic Disorders

Conklin RJ: Common cutaneous disorders in athletes. *Sports Med* 9:100–119, 1990.

Gibbs RC: The skin, in Jahss MH (ed): *Disorders of the Foot and Ankle,* 2d ed. Philadelphia, Saunders, 1991, vol 2, pp 1540–1572.

———: Skin diseases of the feet, in Gibbs RC (ed): *Skin Diseases of the Feet.* St. Louis, W.H. Green, 1974, pp 3–219.

Omura EF: Dermatologic disorders, in Gould JS (ed): *The Foot Book.* Baltimore, Williams & Wilkins, 1988, pp 70–88.

Shuster S, Daly M: Skin disorders, in Helal B, Wilson D (eds): *The Foot.* Edinburgh, Churchill Livingstone, 1988, vol 2, pp 802–836.

Smith RW: Calluses: Nonsurgical treatment, in Gould JS (ed): *The Foot Book.* Baltimore, Williams & Wilkins, 1988, pp 89–97.

Erythromelalgia

Drenth JPH: Erythromelalgia induced by nicardipine. *BMJ* 298:1582, 1989.

Kraus A: Erythromelalgia in a patient with systemic lupus erythematosus treated with clonazepam (letter to the editor). *J Rheum* 17:120, 1990.

Kurzrock R, Cohen PR: Erythromelalgia and myeloproliferative disorders. *Arch Intern Med* 149:105–109, 1989.

Levesque H, Moore N, Wolfe LM, et al: Erythromelalgia induced by nicardipine (inverse Raynaud's phenomenon). *BMJ* 298:1252–1253, 1989.

Michiels JJ, van Joost T: Erythromelalgia and thrombocythemia: A causal relation. *J Am Acad Dermatol* 22:107–111, 1990.

Michiels JJ, van Joost T, Vuzevski VD: Idiopathic erythermalgia: A congenital disorder. *J Am Acad Dermatol* 21:1128–1130, 1989.

Millard FE, Hunter CS, Anderson M, et al: Clinical manifestations of essential thrombocythemia in young adults. *Am J Hematol* 33:27–31, 1990.

Foot Deformity

Mutoh K, Okuno T, Ito M, et al: MR imaging of a group I case of Hallervorden-Spatz disease. *J Comput Assist Tomogr* 12:851–853, 1988.

Fractures/Dislocations

Davis AW, Alexander IJ: Problematic fractures and dislocations in the foot and ankle of athletes. *Clin Sports Med* 9:163–181, 1990.

Neoplasms

Goldman FD, Dayton PD, Hanson CJ: Renal cell carcinoma and osseous metastases: Case report and literature review. *J Am Podiatr Med Assoc* 79:618–625, 1989.

Harrelson JM: Tumors of the foot, in Jahss MH (ed): *Disorders of the Foot and Ankle,* 2d ed. Philadelphia, Saunders, 1991, vol 2, pp 1654–1677.

Kirby EJ, Shereff MJ, Lewis MM: Soft-tissue tumors and tumor-like lesions of the foot: An analysis of eighty-three cases. *J Bone Joint Surg (Am)* 71A:621–628, 1989.

Revell PA, Sommerlad BC: Tumours, In Helal B, Wilson D (eds): *The Foot.* Edinburgh, Churchill Livingstone, 1988, vol 2, pp 739–769.

Osteomyelitis

Speer KP, Fitch RD: *Neisseria gonorrhoeae* foot abscess: A case report. *Clin Orthop* 234:209–210, 1989.

Yuh WTC, Corson JD, Baraniewski HM, et al: Osteomyelitis of the foot in diabetic patients: Evaluation with plain film, ^{99m}Tc-MDP bone scintigraphy, and MR imaging. *AJR* 152:795–800, 1989.

Zahari DT, Bakst S: Disseminated gonococcal infection involving the foot. *J Foot Surg* 28:405–409, 1989.

Pain—Dorsum

Giorgini RJ, Bernard RL: Sinus tarsi syndrome in a patient with talipes equinovarus. *J Am Podiatr Med Assoc* 80:218–222, 1990.

Levin KH, Stevens JC, Daube JR: Superficial peroneal nerve conduction studies for electromyographic diagnosis. *Muscle Nerve* 9:322–326, 1986.

Warren RF: Ganglion of the sinus tarsi: A case report. *Am J Sports Med* 8:133–134, 1980.

Pain—Forefoot

Barnes C: Systemic disease, in Helal B, Wilson D (eds): *The Foot.* Edinburgh, Churchill Livingstone, 1988, vol 2, pp 777–801.

Black JR: Stress fractures of the foot in female soldiers: A two-year survey. *Mil Med* 147:861–862, 1982.

Brahms MA: The small toes: Corns and deformities of the small toes, in Jahss MH (ed): *Disorders of the Foot and Ankle,* 2d ed. Philadelphia, Saunders, 1991, vol 2, pp 1175–1198.

Chioros PG, Frankel SL, Sidlow CJ: Sesamoid pain secondary to a plantar neuroma. *J Foot Surg* 26:296–300, 1987.

Fu FH, Gomez W: Bilateral avascular necrosis of the first metatarsal head in adolescence: A case report. *Clin Orthop* 246:282–284, 1989.

Gainor BJ, Epstein RG, Henstorf JE, et al: Metatarsal head resection for rheumatoid deformities of the forefoot. *Clin Orthop* 230:207–213, 1988.

Gould JS: Metatarsalgia. *Orthop Clin North Am* 20:553–562, 1989.

Jahss MH: The small toes: Other disorders of the small toes, in Jahss MH (ed): *Disorders of the Foot and Ankle,* 2d ed. Philadelphia, Saunders, 1991, vol 2, pp 1198–1204.

Kaufman JL, Leather RP: Vascular diseases of the foot, in Jahss MH (ed): *Disorders of the Foot and Ankle,* 2d ed. Philadelphia, Saunders, 1991, vol 2, pp 1787–1827.

Kitaoka HB, Leventen EO: Medial displacement metatarsal osteotomy for treatment of painful bunionette. *Clin Orthop* 243:172–179, 1989.

Mann RA, Coughlin MJ: Lesser-toe deformities, in Jahss MH (ed): *Disorders of the Foot and Ankle,* 2d ed. Philadelphia, Saunders, 1991, vol 2, pp 1205–1228.

Merkel KD, Johnson KA: Developmental disorders: Adult foot—interdigital neuroma, in Gould JS (ed): *The Foot Book.* Baltimore, Williams & Wilkins, 1988, pp 268–279.

Myerson MS: Injuries to the forefoot and toes, in Jahss MH (ed): *Disorders of the Foot and Ankle,* 2d ed. Philadelphia, Saunders, 1991, vol 2, pp 2233–2273.

Rana NA: Rheumatoid arthritis, other collagen diseases, and psoriasis of the forefoot, in Jahss MH (ed): *Disorders of the Foot and Ankle,* 2d ed. Philadelphia, Saunders, 1991, vol 2, pp 1719–1751.

Reese RC Jr, Burruss TP: Athletic training techniques and protective equipment, in Nicholas JA, Hershman EB (eds): *The Lower Extremity and Spine in Sports Medicine.* St. Louis, Mosby, 1986, pp 289–293.

Reynolds JC: Developmental disorders: Adult foot—metatarsalgia, in Gould JS (ed): *The Foot Book.* Baltimore, Williams & Wilkins, 1988, pp 219–227.

Rhodes RA, Stelling CB: Calcific tendinitis of the flexors of the forefoot. *Ann Emerg Med* 15:751–753, 1986.

Shereff MJ: Disorders of the toes: Acquired disorders of the toes, in Gould JS (ed): *The Foot Book.* Baltimore, Williams & Wilkins, 1988, pp 98–104.

Stockley I, Betts RP, Eng C, et al: A prospective study of forefoot arthroplasty. *Clin Orthop* 248:213–218, 1989.

Thomas N, Nissen KI, Helal B: Disorders of the lesser rays, in Helal B, Wilson D (eds): *The Foot.* Edinburgh, Churchill Livingstone, 1988, vol 1, pp 485–510.

Viladot A Sr: The metatarsals, in Jahss MH (ed): *Disorders of the Foot and Ankle*, 2d ed. Philadelphia, Saunders, 1991, vol 2, pp 1229–1268.

Pain — Generalized

Angier N: The shoe problem: What looks good doesn't feel good. *New York Times*, March 7, 1991, pp B1, B8.

Black JR: The survey of foot and ankle morbidity during a National Guard Reserve annual training period. *Mil Med* 146:694–695, 1981.

Mann RA: Pain in the foot: 1. Evaluation of foot pain and identification of associated problems. *Postgrad Med* 82:154, 156–157, 160, 162, 1987.

Milburn PB, Brandsma JL, Goldsman CI, et al: Disseminated warts and evolving squamous cell carcinoma in a patient with acquired immunodeficiency syndrome. *J Am Acad Dermatol* 19:401–405, 1988.

Rudicel S: Arthritis of the foot: Pinpointing the disease process involved. *Postgrad Med* 86:122–125, 128–129, 132, 1989.

Santoro JP, Sartoris DJ, Cachia VV, et al: Nonspecific inflammation in the foot demonstrated by magnetic resonance imaging. *J Foot Surg* 27:478–483, 1988.

Stevens DL, Tanner MH, Winship J, et al: Severe group A streptococcal infections associated with a toxic shock-like syndrome and scarlet fever toxin A. *N Engl J Med* 321:1–7, 1989.

Pain — Generalized/Localized — Review

Adelaar RS: Developmental disorders: Adult foot — running injuries of the foot and ankle, in Gould JS (ed): *The Foot Book*. Baltimore, Williams & Wilkins, 1988, pp 313–324.

Aguayo AJ: Neuropathy due to compression and entrapment, in Dyck PJ, Thomas PK, Lambert GH (eds): *Peripheral Neuropathy*. Philadelphia, Saunders, 1975, vol 2, pp 688–713.

Alexander IJ: The foot: Examination and diagnosis, in Alexander IJ (ed): *The Foot*. New York, Churchill Livingstone, 1990, pp 1–160.

Asbury AK: Uremic neuropathy, in Dyck PJ, Thomas PK, Lambert GH (eds): *Peripheral Neuropathy*. Philadelphia, Saunders, 1975, vol 2, pp 982–992.

Bastron JA: Neuropathy in diseases of the thyroid, in Dyck PJ, Thomas PK, Lambert GH (eds): *Peripheral Neuropathy*. Philadelphia, Saunders, 1975, vol 2, pp 999–1011.

Baxter DE: Running injuries, in Jahss MH (ed): *Disorders of the Foot and Ankle*, 2d ed. Philadelphia, Saunders, 1991, vol 2, pp 2446–2465.

Brady RO, King FM: Fabry's disease, in Dyck PJ, Thomas PK, Lambert GH (eds): *Peripheral Neuropathy*. Philadelphia, Saunders, 1975, vol 2, pp 914–927.

Cohen AS, Benson MD: Amyloid neuropathy, in Dyck PJ, Thomas PK, Lambert GH (eds): *Peripheral Neuropathy*. Philadelphia, Saunders, 1975, vol 2, pp 1067–1091.

Coker P: Sports injuries to the foot and ankle, in Jahss MH (ed): *Disorders of the Foot and Ankle*, 2d ed. Philadelphia, Saunders, 1991, vol 2, pp 2415–2445.

Creager MA, Dzav VJ: Vascular diseases of the extremities, in Wilson JD, Braunwald E, Isselbacher RJ, et al (eds): *Harrison's Principles of Internal Medicine*, 12th ed. New York, McGraw-Hill, 1991, vol 1, pp 1018–1026.

Evanski PM: The geriatric foot, in Jahss MH (ed): *Disorders of the Foot and Ankle*, 2d ed. Philadelphia, Saunders, 1991, vol 2, pp 1643–1653.

Fauci AS: The vasculitis syndrome, in Wilson JD, Braunwald E, Isselbacher RJ, et al (eds): *Harrison's Principles of Internal Medicine*, 12th ed. New York, McGraw-Hill, 1991. vol 2, pp 1457–1463.

Fleming LL: Developmental disorders: Adult foot — tendinitis and bursitis, in Gould JS (ed): *The Foot Book*. Baltimore, Williams & Wilkins, 1988, pp 303–312.

Frey CC, Shereff MJ: Chemical, environmental and foreign-body injuries to the foot and ankle, in Jahss MH (ed): *Disorders of the Foot and Ankle*, 2d ed. Philadelphia, Saunders, 1991, vol 2, pp 2564–2583.

Gilliland BC: Relapsing polychondritis and miscellaneous arthritides, in Wilson JD, Braunwald E, Isselbacher RJ, et al (eds): *Harrison's Principles of Internal Medicine*, 12th ed. New York, McGraw-Hill, 1991, vol 2, pp 1484–1490.

Goldstein NP, McCall JT, Dyck PJ: Metal neuropathy, in Dyck PJ, Thomas PK, Lambert GH (eds): *Peripheral Neuropathy*. Philadelphia, Saunders, 1975, vol 2, pp 1227–1262.

Hahn BH: Systemic lupus erythematosus, in Wilson JD, Braunwald E, Isselbacher RJ, et al (eds): *Harrison's Principles of Internal Medicine*, 12th ed. New York, McGraw-Hill, 1991, vol 2, pp 1432–1437.

Hoffman GS: Arthritis due to deposition of calcium crystals, in Wilson JD, Braunwald E, Isselbacher RJ, et al (eds): *Harrison's Principles of Internal Medicine*, 12th ed. New York, McGraw-Hill, 1991, vol 2, pp 1479–1482.

Hopkins A: Toxic neuropathy due to industrial agents, in Dyck PJ, Thomas PK, Lambert GH (eds): *Peripheral Neuropathy*. Philadelphia, Saunders, 1975, vol 2, pp 1207–1226.

Jacobs RL: The diabetic foot: The avascular diabetic foot, in Jahss MH (ed): *Disorders of the Foot and Ankle*, 2d ed. Philadelphia, Saunders, 1991, vol 2, pp 1926–1936.

————: The diabetic foot: Diabetic neuropathy, in Jahss MH (ed): *Disorders of the Foot and Ankle*, 2d ed. Philadelphia, Saunders, 1991, vol 2, pp 1908–1925.

Jahss MH, Luskin R: Miscellaneous peripheral neuropathies and neuropathy-like syndromes, in Jahss MH (ed): *Disorders of the Foot and Ankle*, 2d ed. Philadelphia, Saunders, 1991, vol 2, pp 2125–2155.

Johnson KA, Alexander IJ: Reflex sympathetic dystrophy, in Jahss MH (ed): *Disorders of the Foot and Ankle*, 2d ed. Philadelphia, Saunders, 1991, vol 2, pp 2187–2191.

LeQuesne PM: Neuropathy due to drugs, in Dyck PJ, Thomas PK, Lambert GH (eds): *Peripheral Neuropathy*. Philadelphia, Saunders, 1975, vol 2, pp 1263–1280.

Lipsky PE: Rheumatoid arthritis, in Wilson JD, Braunwald E, Isselbacher RJ, et al (eds): *Harrison's Principles of Internal Medicine*, 12th ed. New York, McGraw-Hill, 1991, vol 2, pp 1437–1443.

Lusskin R, Battista A: Peripheral neuropathies affecting the foot: Traumatic ischemic and compressive disorders, in Jahss MH (ed): *Disorders of the Foot and Ankle*, 2d ed. Philadelphia, Saunders, 1991, vol 2, pp 2089–2124.

Maggiore P, Echols RM: Infections in the diabetic feet, in Jahss MH (ed): *Disorders of the Foot and Ankle*, 2d ed. Philadelphia, Saunders, 1991, vol 2, pp 1937–1957.

————: Nonsurgical and surgical infections of the foot and ankle: Nonsurgical infections, in Jahss MH (ed): *Disorders of the Foot and Ankle*, 2d ed. Philadelphia, Saunders, 1991, vol 2, pp 1828–1851.

————: Nonsurgical and surgical infections of the foot and ankle: Surgical infections, in Jahss MH (ed): *Disorders of the Foot and Ankle*, 2d ed. Philadelphia, Saunders, 1991, vol 2, pp 1851–1863.

Mann RA: Pain in the foot: 2. Causes of pain in the hindfoot, midfoot, and forefoot. *Postgrad Med* 82:167–171, 174, 1987.

Matheson GO, MacIntyre JG, Taunton JE, et al: Musculoskeletal injuries associated with physical activity in older adults. *Med Sci Sports Exerc* 21:379–385, 1989.

McLeod JG: Carcinomatous neuropathy, in Dyck PJ, Thomas PK, Lambert GH (eds): *Peripheral Neuropathy*. Philadelphia, Saunders, 1975, vol 2, pp 1301–1313.

McLeod JG, Walsh JC: Neuropathies associated with paraproteinemias and dysproteinemias, in Dyck PJ, Thomas PK, Lambert GH (eds): *Peripheral Neuropathy*. Philadelphia, Saunders, 1975, vol 2, pp 1012–1029.

————: Peripheral neuropathy associated with lymphomas and other reticuloses, in Dyck PJ, Thomas PK, Lambert GH (eds): *Peripheral Neuropathy*. Philadelphia, Saunders, 1975, vol 2, pp 1314–1325.

Moutsopoulos HM: Behçet's syndrome, in Wilson JD, Braunwald E, Isselbacher RJ, et al (eds): *Harrison's Principles of Internal Medicine*, 12th ed. New York, McGraw-Hill, 1991, vol 2, pp 1455–1456.

Myerson MS, Burgess AR: The initial evaluation and treatment of the acutely traumatized foot and ankle, in Jahss MH (ed): *Disorders of the Foot and Ankle*, 2d ed. Philadelphia, Saunders, 1991, vol 2, pp 2209–2232.

Orava S: Overexertion injuries in keep-fit athletes: A study on over-exertion injuries among non-competitive keep-fit atheletes. *Scand J Rehabil Med* 10:187–191, 1978.

Ridley A: Porphyric neuropathy, in Dyck PJ, Thomas PK, Lambert GH (eds): *Peripheral Neuropathy*. Philadelphia, Saunders, 1975, vol 2, pp 942–955.

Sammarco GJ: The foot and ankle in dance, in Jahss MH (ed): *Disorders of the Foot and Ankle*, 2d ed. Philadelphia, Saunders, 1991, vol 2, pp 2483–2513.

Schur PH: Psoriatic arthritis and arthritis associated with gastrointestinal diseases, in Wilson JD, Braunwald E, Isselbacher RJ, et al (eds): *Harrison's Principles of Internal Medicine*, 12th ed. New York, McGraw-Hill, 1991, vol 2, pp 1482–1484.

Singer KM, Jones DC: Ligament injuries of ankle and foot, in Nicholas JA, Hershman EB (eds): *The Lower Extremity and Spine in Sports Medicine*. St. Louis, Mosby, 1986, pp 475–497.

———: Soft tissue conditions of the ankle and foot, in Nicholas JA, Hershman EB (eds): *The Lower Extremity and Spine in Sports Medicine*. St. Louis, Mosby, 1986, pp 498–525.

Stern SH: Ankle and foot pain. *Prim Care* 15:809–826, 1988.

Taurog JD, Lipsky PE: Ankylosing spondylitis and reactive arthritis, in Wilson JD, Braunwald E, Isselbacher RJ, et al (eds): *Harrison's Principles of Internal Medicine*, 12th ed. New York, McGraw-Hill, 1991, vol 2, pp 1451–1456.

Turco VJ, Spinella AJ: Occult trauma and unusual injuries in the foot and ankle, in Nicholas JA, Hershman EB (eds): *The Lower Extremity and Spine in Sports Medicine*. St. Louis, Mosby, 1986, pp 541–559.

Victor M: Polyneuropathy due to nutritional deficiency and alcoholism, in Dyck PJ, Thomas PK, Lambert GH (eds): *Peripheral Neuropathy*. Philadelphia, Saunders, 1975, vol 2, pp 1030–1066.

Wood B: The painful foot, in Kelley WN, Harris ED Jr, Ruddy S (eds): *Textbook of Rheumatology*. Philadelphia, Saunders, 1981, vol 1, pp 472–484.

Pain — Hallux

Foulston J: Ingrowing toe nail, in Helal B, Wilson D (eds): *The Foot*. Edinburgh, Churchill Livingstone, 1988, vol 1, pp 858–867.

Jahss MH: Disorders of the hallux and first ray, in Jahss MH (ed): *Disorders of the Foot and Ankle*, 2d ed. Philadelphia, Saunders, 1991, pp 943–1174.

Lapidus PW: The toe nails, in Jahss MH (ed): *Disorders of the Foot and Ankle*, 2nd ed. Philadelphia, Saunders, 1991, vol 2, pp 1573–1594.

Mirra JM, Kameda N, Rosen G, et al: Primary osteosarcoma of toe phalanx — first documented case: Review of osteosarcoma of short tubular bones. *Am J Surg Pathol* 12:300–307, 1988.

Rana NA: Gout, in Jahss MH (ed): *Disorders of the Foot and Ankle*, 2d ed. Philadelphia, Saunders, 1991, vol 2, pp 1712–1718.

Wilson DW: Hallux valgus and rigidus, in Helal B, Wilson D (eds): *The Foot*. Edinburgh, Churchill Livingstone, 1988, vol 1, pp 411–483.

Pain — Hindfoot

Ahstrom JP Jr: Spontaneous rupture of the plantar fascia. *Am J Sports Med* 16:306–307, 1988.

Bateman JE: The adult heel, in Jahss MH (ed): *Disorders of the Foot and Ankle*, 2d ed. Philadelphia, Saunders, 1991, vol 2, pp 1372–1381.

Baxter DE, Pfeffer GB, Thigpen M: Chronic heel pain: Treatment rationale. *Orthop Clin North Am* 20:563–569, 1989.

Beito SB, Krych SM, Harkless LB: Recalcitrant heel pain: Traumatic fibrosis versus heel neuroma. *J Am Podiatr Med Assoc* 79:336–339, 1989.

Connolly JF: Persistent heel pain twenty years after calcaneal fracture and triple arthrodesis relieved by lateral decompression. *J Trauma* 27:809–810, 1987.

Dee R: Miscellaneous disorders of the foot, in Dee R, Mango E, Hurst LC (eds): *Principles of Orthopaedic Practice*. New York, McGraw-Hill, 1989, vol 2, pp 1431–1460.

Devas M: Stress fractures, in Helal B, Wilson D (eds): *The Foot*. Edinburgh, Churchill Livingstone, 1988, vol 2, pp 967–993.

Didia BC, Horsefall AU: Medial calcaneal nerve: An anatomical study. *J Am Podiatr Med Assoc* 80:115–119, 1990.

Downey DJ, Simkin PA, Mack LA, et al: Tibialis posterior tendon rupture: A cause of rheumatoid flat foot. *Arthritis Rheum* 31:441–446, 1988.

Fisk GR: Calcaneal fractures, in Helal B, Wilson D (eds): *The Foot*. Edinburgh, Churchill Livingstone, 1988, vol 2, pp 894–915.

Freeman C Jr: Heel pain, in Gould JS (ed): *The Foot Book*. Baltimore, Williams & Wilkins, 1988, pp 228–238.

Gurtowski J, Ries M, Levin PE: Fractures and dislocation of the foot, in Dee R, Mango E, Hurst LC (eds): *Principles of Orthopaedic Practice*. New York, McGraw-Hill, 1989, vol 2, pp 1242–1260.

Hansen ST Jr: Trauma to the calcaneus and its tendon: Trauma to the heel cord, in Jahss MH (ed): *Disorders of the Foot and Ankle*, 2d ed. Philadelphia, Saunders, 1991, vol 3, pp 2355–2360.

Heckman JD: Fractures and dislocations of the foot, in Rockwood CA Jr, Green DP (eds): *Fractures in Adults*, 2d ed. Philadelphia, Lippincott, 1984, vol 2, pp 1703–1832.

King JB, Levack B: Hindfoot disorders, in Helal B, Wilson D (eds): *The Foot*. Edinburgh, Churchill Livingstone, 1988, vol 1, pp 542–549

Kitaoka HB: Rheumatoid hindfoot. *Orthop Clin North Am* 20:593–604, 1989.

Kulund DN: Pain under the heel in runners. *Va Med* 115:340–342, 1988.

Lutter LD: Sports injuries, in Helal B, Wilson D (eds): *The Foot*. Edinburgh, Churchill Livingstone, 1988, vol 2, pp 994–1006.

———: Surgical decisions in athletes' subcalcaneal pain. *Am J Sports Med* 14:481–485, 1986.

Meltzer EF: A rational approach to the management of heel pain: A protocol proposal. *J Am Podiatr Med Assoc* 79:89–92, 1989.

Misoul C: Nerve injuries and entrapment syndromes of the lower extremity, in Dee R, Mango E, Hurst LC (eds): *Principles of Orthopaedic Practice*. New York, McGraw-Hill, 1989, vol 2, pp 1420–1430.

Ott H, Van Linthoudt D: Heel pain in sarcoidosis: Is sarcoid a cause of spondarthropathy? (letter to the editor). *Br J Rheum* 26:468, 1987.

Pfeffer GB, Baxter DE: Surgery of the adult heel, in Jahss MH (ed): *Disorders of the Foot and Ankle*, 2d ed. Philadelphia, Saunders, 1991, vol 2, pp 1396–1416.

Plattner P, Johnson K, Tendons and bursae, in Helal B, Wilson D (eds): *The Foot*. Edinburgh, Churchill Livingstone, 1988, vol 2, pp 581–613.

Sanders R, Hansen ST Jr, McReynolds IS: Trauma to the calcaneus, in Jahss MH (ed): *Disorders of the Foot and Ankle*, 2d ed. Philadelphia, Saunders, 1991, vol 3, pp 2326–2354.

Schepsis AA, Leach RE: Surgical management of Achilles tendinitis. *Am J Sports Med* 15:308–315, 1987.

Shikoff MD, Figura MA, Postar SE: A retrospective study of 195 patients with heel pain. *J Am Podiatr Med Assoc* 76:71–75, 1986.

Solomon G: Inflammatory arthritis, in Jahss MH (ed): *Disorders of the Foot and Ankle*, Philadelphia, Saunders, 1991, vol 2, pp 1681–1702.

Spiera H: Diffuse connective-tissue diseases, in Jahss MH (ed): *Disorders of the Foot and Ankle*, 2d ed. Philadelphia, Saunders, 1991, vol 2, pp 1703–1711.

Sundberg SB, Johnson KA: Painful conditions of the heel, in Jahss MH (ed): *Disorders of the Foot and Ankle*, 2d ed. Philadelphia, Saunders, 1991, vol 2, pp 1382–1395.

Pain — Midfoot

Cachia VV, Santoro JP, Grumbine NA, et al: Spontaneous rupture of the peroneus longus tendon with fracture of the os peroneum. *J Foot Surg* 27:328–333, 1988.

Cass JR: Disorders of the anterior tarsus, midtarsus, and Lisfranc's joint: Overview of injuries to the anterior tarsus and navicular, in Jahss MH (ed): *Disorders of the Foot and Ankle,* 2d ed. Philadelphia, Saunders, 1991, vol 2, pp 1321–1332.

Hooper, G, Hughes S: Midfoot and navicular injuries, in Helal B, Wilson D (eds): *The Foot.* Edinburgh, Churchill Linvingstone, 1988, vol 2, pp 933–943.

Jahss MH: Disorders of the anterior tarsus, midtarsus, and Lisfranc's joint: The anterior tarsus, midtarsus, and Lisfranc's joint, in Jahss MH (ed): *Disorders of the Foot and Ankle,* 2d ed. Philadelphia, Saunders, 1991, vol 2, pp 1284–1320.

————: Tendon disorders of the foot and ankle, in Jahss MH (ed): *Disorders of the Foot and Ankle,* 2d ed. Philadelphia, Saunders, 1991, vol 3, pp 1461–1513.

Johnson KA: Developmental disorders: Adult foot—acquired flatfoot, in Gould JS (ed): *The Foot Book.* Baltimore, Williams & Wilkins, 1988, pp 291–302.

King RE, Powell DF: Injury to the talus, in Jahss MH (ed): *Disorders of the Foot and Ankle,* 2d ed. Philadelphia, Saunders, 1991, vol 3, pp 2293–2325.

Scranton PE: Osteochondritides, in Helal B, Wilson D (eds): *The Foot.* Edinburgh, Churchill Linvingstone, 1988, vol 2, pp 524–534.

Shelton MH, Pedowitz WJ: Injuries to the talar dome, subtalar joint, and midfoot, in Jahss MH (ed): *Disorders of the Foot and Ankle,* 2d ed. Philadelphia, Saunders, 1991, vol 3, pp 2274–2292.

Villadot A Sr, Villadot A Jr: Osteochondroses: Aseptic necrosis of the foot, in Jahss MH (ed): *Disorders of the Foot and Ankle,* 2d ed. Philadelphia, Saunders, 1991, vol 1, pp 617–638.

Zahari DT, Bakst S: Disseminated gonococcal infection involving the foot. *J Foot Surg* 28:405–409, 1989.

Polyneuropathy

Albers JW, Kelly JJ Jr: Acquired inflammatory demyelinating polyneuropathies: Clinical and electrodiagnostic features. *Muscle Nerve* 12:435–451, 1988.

Argov Z, Steiner I, Soffer D: The yield of sural nerve biopsy in the evaluation of peripheral neuropathies. *Acta Neurol Scand* 79:243–245, 1989.

Boulton AJM, Ward JD: Diagnostic neuropathies in pain. *Clin Endocrinol Metabol* 15:917–931, 1986.

Charnock E, Newton N: Case report: AIDS peripheral neuropathy. *Am J Med Sci* 298:256–260, 1989.

Cohen JA, Gross KF: Peripheral neuropathy: Causes and management in the elderly. *Geriatrics* 45:21–34, 1990.

Denning DW: The neurological features of acute HIV infection. *Biomed Pharmacother* 42:11–14, 1988.

Duston MA, Skinner M, Anderson J, et al: Peripheral neuropathy as an early marker of AL amyloidosis. *Arch Intern Med* 149:358–360, 1989.

Golbus J, McCune WJ: Giant cell arteritis and peripheral neuropathy: A report of 2 cases and review of the literature. *J Rheumatol* 14:129–134, 1987.

Greene DA, Sima AAF, Pfeifer MA, et al: Diabetic neuropathy. *Annu Rev Med* 41:303–317, 1990.

Harati Y: Diabetic peripheral neuropathies. *Ann Intern Med* 107:546–559, 1987.

Jarratt JA: The electrophysiological diagnosis of peripheral neuropathy: A brief review. *Bull Eur Physiopathol Respir* 23(suppl 1): 195S–198S, 1987.

Leedman PJ, Davis S, Harrison LC: Diabetic amyotrophy: Reassessment of the clinical spectrum. *Aust N Z J Med* 18:768–773, 1988.

Masson EA, Hunt L, Gem JM, et al: A novel approach to the diagnosis and assessment of symptomatic diabetic neuropathy. *Pain* 38:25–28, 1989.

McArthur JC, Griffin JW, Cornnblath DR, et al: Steroid-responsive myeloneuropathy in a man dually infected with HIV-1 and HTLV-I. *Neurology* 40:938–944, 1990.

Naidu S, Chatterjee S, Murphy M, et al: Rett syndrome: New observations. *Brain Dev* 9:525–528, 1987.

Poser CM: The peripheral nervous system in multiple sclerosis: A review and pathogenetic hypothesis. *J Neurol Sci* 79:83–90, 1987.

Schenone A, DeMartini I, Tabaton M, et al: Direct immunofluorescence in sural nerve biopsies. *Eur Neurol* 28:262–269, 1988.

Smith T, Trojaborg W: Somatosensory evoked potentials in the evaluation of patients with stocking/glove paresthesias. *Acta Neurol Scand* 79:63–67, 1989.

Tan WD, Macfarlane JD, Eulderink F: Leg claudication and peripheral neuropathy as main features of systemic necrotizing vasculitis (letter to editor). *Arthritis Rheum* 32:510–511, 1989.

Woo C-C: Neurological features of acromegaly: A review and report of two cases. *J Manipulative Physiol Ther* 11:314–321, 1988.

Reflex Sympathetic Dystrophy

Ameratunga R, Daly M, Caughey DE: Metastatic malignancy associated with reflex sympathetic dystrophy. *J Rheumatol* 16:406–407, 1989.

Klenerman L: Reflex sympathetic dystrophy: A neglected cause of foot pain. *Bull Hosp Joint Dis Orthop Inst* 47:211–215, 1987.

Ladd AL, DeHaven KE, Thanik J, et al: Reflex sympathetic imbalance: Response to epidural blockade. *Am J Sports Med* 17:660–668, 1989.

Lemahieu R-A, VanLaere C, Verbruggen LA: Reflex sympathetic dystrophy: An underreported syndrome in children? *Eur J Pediatr* 147: 47–50, 1988.

Paulson RR: Reflex sympathetic dystrophy in a teenaged girl. *Postgrad Med* 81:66–67, 1987.

Schiller JE: Reflex sympathetic dystrophy of the foot and ankle in children and adolescents. *J Am Podiatr Med Assoc* 79:545–551, 1989.

Schwartzman RJ, McLellan TL: Reflex sympathetic dystrophy: A review. *Arch Neurol* 44:555–561, 1987.

Tarsal Coalition

Wheeler R, Guevera A, Bleck EE: Tarsa coalitions: Review of the literature and case report of bilateral dual calcaneonavicular and talocalcaneal coalitions. *Clin Orthop* 156:175–177, 1981.

Tarsal Tunnel Syndrome

Francis H, March L, Terenty T, et al: Benign joint hypermobility with neuropathy: Documentation and mechanism of tarsal tunnel syndrome. *J Rheumatol* 14:577–581, 1987.

Stern DS, Joyce MT: Tarsal tunnel syndrome: A review of 15 surgical procedures. *J Foot Surg* 28:290–294, 1989.

Stuart JD, Morgan RF, Persing JA: Nerve compression syndromes of the lower extremity. *AFP* 40:101–112, 1989.

Vascular Disease—Ischemic

Andros G, Harris RW, Salles-Cunha SX, et al: Bypass grafts to the ankle and foot. *J Vasc Surg* 7:785–794, 1988.

Clifford EJ, Fry RE, Clagett GP, et al: Results of in-situ saphenous vein bypass to the foot. *Am J Surg* 158:502–504, 1989.

Dahlberg PJ, Frecentese DF, Cogbill TH: Cholesterol embolism: Experience with 22 histologically proven cases. *Surgery* 105:737–746, 1989.

Jelnes R, Bulow J, Tønnesen KH, et al: Why do patients with severe arterial insufficiency get pain during sleep? *Scand J Clin Lab Invest* 47:649–654, 1987.

Matos MH, Amstutz HC, Machleder HI: Ischemia of the lower extremity after total hip replacement: Report of four cases. *J Bone Joint Surg (Am)* 61A:24–27, 1979.

Myers KA: Management of the severely ischaemic leg. *Aust Fam Physician* 8:733–745, 1979.

Parkhouse N, LeQuesne PM: Impaired neurogenic vascular response in patients with diabetes and neuropathic foot lesions. *N Engl J Med* 318:1306–1309, 1988.

Piecuch T, Jaworski R: Resting ankle-arm pressure index in vascular diseases of the lower extremities. *Angiology* 40:181–185, 1989.

Walsh JJ Jr, Cofelice M, Lumpkin D, et al: Is screening for vascular disease a valuable proposition? *J Cardiovasc Surg* 29:306–309, 1988.

P|A|R|T T|E|N
Acute Generalized Pain

Acute Generalized Pain

☐ DIAGNOSTIC LIST

1. Muscle-related (myopathic) pain
   - A. Acute polymyositis
     1. Idiopathic
     2. Toxoplasmosis
   - B. Acute myalgia and rhabdomyolysis associated with viral infection
     1. Influenza A virus
     2. Epstein-Barr virus
     3. Coxsackievirus
     4. Herpes simplex virus
   - C. Exertional myalgias and rhabdomyolysis in normal individuals
   - D. Myalgias due to inherited metabolic disorders of muscle
     1. Carbohydrate metabolism
        a. Myophosphorylase deficiency (McArdle's disease)
        b. Other enzyme deficiencies affecting carbohydrate metabolism
     2. Lipid metabolism: carnitine palmityl transferase deficiency
     3. Nucleotide metabolism: myoadenylate deaminase deficiency
     4. Mitochondrial disorders: NADH-coenzyme-Q reductase deficiency
   - E. Endocrine disorders
     1. Hypothyroidism
     2. Hyperthyroidism
     3. Hypoadrenalism (Addison's disease)
     4. Panhypopituitarism
     5. Hypoparathyroidism and hypocalcemia
   - F. Myalgias and rhabdomyolysis associated with alcohol and drug abuse (heroin, amphetamines, cocaine, and phencyclidine)
   - G. Myalgias and rhabdomyolysis associated with therapeutic drugs
     1. Clofibrate
     2. Lovastatin
     3. Emetine
     4. Epsilon-aminocaproic acid
   - H. Myalgias without rhabdomyolysis associated with therapeutic drugs and immunizations
   - I. Nonspecific myalgias due to systemic infection or overexertion
   - J. Myalgias and/or cramps due to electrolyte and mineral deficiencies
     1. Acute hypokalemia
     2. Acute hypocalcemia
     3. Acute hypomagnesemia
     4. Acute hyponatremia
     5. Acute hypophosphatemia
   - K. Trichinosis
   - L. Tetanus
   - M. Strychnine poisoning
   - N. Black widow spider bite
   - O. Eosinophilia-myalgia syndrome
   - P. Mimics of the eosinophilia-myalgia syndrome

1. Eosinophilic polymyositis
2. Relapsing eosinophilic perimyositis
3. Toxic oil syndrome
4. Cysticercosis
5. Sarcoidosis
6. Eosinophilic fasciitis
7. Idiopathic polymyositis
8. Idiopathic dermatomyositis
9. Polymyositis and dermatomyositis associated with malignancy
10. Churg-Strauss disease
11. Trichinosis
   Q. Fibromyalgia
2. Nerve-related (neuropathic) pain: Acute polyneuropathy
   A. Arsenic poisoning
   B. Thallium poisoning
   C. Diabetes mellitus
   D. AIDS
   E. Intermittent acute porphyria
   F. Alcohol abuse and/or nutritional deficiencies
   G. Hypothyroidism
   H. Renal failure
   I. Malignancy
   J. Myeloma and POEMS syndrome
   K. Cryoglobulinemia
   L. Guillain-Barré syndrome

   M. Therapeutic drugs
3. Joint-related pain
   A. Polyarthralgias
   B. Psychogenic rheumatism
4. Muscle-, joint-, and/or nerve-related pain
   A. Polyarteritis nodosa
   B. Allergic angiitis and granulomatosis (Churg-Strauss disease)
   C. Rheumatoid arthritis and vasculitis
   D. Systemic lupus erythematosus and vasculitis
   E. Behçet's disease
   F. Lyme disease
   G. Polymyalgia rheumatica
   H. Mimics of polymyalgia rheumatica
      1. Secondary polymyalgia rheumatica due to neoplasm or infection
      2. Seronegative rheumatoid arthritis
      3. Collagen vascular disorders with polymyalgia rheumatica-like symptoms
   I. Pseudolupus due to human immunodeficiency virus (HIV-1) infection

☐ SUMMARY

Idiopathic polymyositis may sometimes begin as an acute illness. Proximal muscle pain, tenderness, and weakness may occur bilaterally in both upper and lower extremities. Arthralgias involving the knees, elbows, wrists, and hands may occur, but actual arthritis is uncommon. Creatine phosphokinase and/or aldolase levels are elevated in 95 to 99 percent of cases of recent onset. The electromyogram may reveal findings of myopathy and denervation (70–90 percent), and a muscle biopsy will show evidence of fiber destruction, regeneration, and/or interstitial and perivascular inflammation (65 percent of cases). Rarely, *toxoplasmosis* may present a similar clinical picture. Serum antibody studies may demonstrate an acute rise in IgM antibody for *Toxoplasma gondii*. In some cases, fever, chills, sweats, and cervical or generalized lymphadenopathy may accompany the myalgias and muscle tenderness. Muscle biopsy may rarely demonstrate toxoplasma organisms.

Acute viral infections, with fever, arthralgias, weakness, malaise, and respiratory and/or gastrointestinal symptoms, may present with or soon cause shoulder and upper arm and/or hip and thigh myalgias. In some cases, mild hyperesthesia of the skin is present. In rare instances, the myalgic pain is severe, and the involved muscles are tender and weak; the serum creatine phosphokinase and aldolase levels are markedly elevated; and severe myoglobinuria is present. The viral agents that have been associated with severe myalgias and muscle damage include *influenza A virus*, *Epstein-Barr virus*, *coxsackievirus*, *and herpes simplex virus*. The diagnosis can be confirmed by serial antibody studies or viral isolation from throat washings, stool, or cutaneous lesions (e.g., herpes simplex).

Severe myalgias, muscle tenderness, and weakness have been described in military recruits undergoing *intensive physical training* as well as in "out-of-shape" civilians participating in a physical conditioning program. The pain is intensified by muscle use and is probably related to fiber injury. A small percentage of these individuals develop myoglobinuria and renal insufficiency. The amount of exercise involved is usually excessive and prolonged. The incidence of this disorder can be reduced by more gradual training.

Exercise-related myalgia and muscle tenderness may be due to a muscle enzyme deficiency. *Myophosphorylase deficiency (McArdle's disease)* causes myalgias and cramp-related pain in exercised muscles. Fatigue, stiffness, and muscle weakness also occur, and all symptoms subside with rest. Some patients experience a "second wind" phenomenon after the initial episode of weakness, pain, and fatigue if they are able to continue exercising after pain begins. Creatine phosphokinase levels are usually elevated at rest. Severe cramping during exercise may result in rhabdomyolysis with myoglobinuria, but renal failure is uncommon.

Other disorders of muscle carbohydrate metabolism due to enzyme deficiency present a similar clinical picture (e.g., phosphofructokinase and phosphoglycerate mutase).

Carnitine palmityl transferase (CPT) deficiency produces exertional myalgia and stiffness without cramps, precipitated by fasting or prolonged exercise. The creatine phosphokinase level at rest is normal. Results of the ischemic forearm exercise test and electromyographic studies are normal. Muscle pain and tenderness may be associated with myoglobinuria and, in severe cases, a rise in creatinine level. Muscle biopsy reveals lipid storage and CPT deficiency on biochemical assay.

Myoadenylate deaminase (MADA) deficiency is associated with postexercise myalgias, muscle tenderness, cramps, and weakness of exercised muscles. No rise in venous ammonia levels occurs after ischemic forearm exercise.

NADH-coenzyme-Q reductase deficiency may cause exertional myalgia, tenderness, and weakness associated with severe neurologic problems (e.g., dementia and ataxia).

Myalgias and/or muscle stiffness and/or weakness may occur in *hypothyroidism, hyperthyroidism, Addison's disease, and panhypopituitarism.*

Hypoparathyroidism results in hypocalcemia and severe muscle pain due to muscle spasm. Chvostek's and/or Trousseau's signs may be present, and carpopedal spasm may occur.

Myalgias, muscle tenderness, and swelling may occur with *alcohol and/or drug abuse* (heroin, amphetamines, cocaine, or phencyclidine), and result in marked elevations of creatine kinase levels, myoglobinuria, and renal failure. Direct toxic effects on muscle and/or crushing of muscle by body weight during prolonged periods of stupor or unconsciousness are believed to be responsible for the rhabdomyolysis.

Drugs associated with myalgias, muscle tenderness, stiffness, weakness, and *rhabdomyolysis* include *clofibrate, lovastatin* (e.g., when taken with gemfibrozil), *emetine, and epsilon-aminocaproic acid.*

Myalgias may also result from *diuretic-induced hypokalemia* and the *administration of isoetharine, danazol, vincristine, trazodone, cimetidine, lithium, and some cytotoxic drugs.* Some *immunizations* may cause low-grade fever and/or myalgias.

Nonspecific myalgias, with or without local tenderness, may occur in febrile illnesses caused by viruses, bacteria, fungi, or parasites or in normal individuals 12 to 48 h after unaccustomed exercise.

Electrolyte and mineral deficiencies may cause myalgias and, in severe cases, rhabdomyolysis (e.g., hypokalemia or hypophosphatemia) or painful muscle cramps (e.g., hyponatremia, hypocalcemia, or hypomagnesemia).

Trichinosis is acquired by eating infected and inadequately cooked pork, bear meat, or walrus. Symptoms include fever, chills, severe myalgias, muscle tenderness, weakness, and periorbital edema. Eosinophilia is frequently present. Splinter hemorrhages and small hemorrhages at the insertions of the extraocular muscles may be detected. The diagnosis can be confirmed by examination of involved muscle as a fresh specimen or after fixation and staining. Serologic tests (e.g., enzyme-linked immunosorbent assay [ELISA], indirect fluorescent antibody, and bentonite flocculation) may also provide diagnostic confirmation.

Tetanus is caused by wound contamination with *Clostridium tetani.* Puncture wounds, foreign bodies, soil contamination, and lack of immunization are risk factors for development of tetanus after penetrating trauma. The initial symptoms may begin at the wound site. Pain and local stiffness progress to generalized myalgias and stiffness. Trismus and risus sardonicus soon occur. Severe aching pain is associated with generalized muscle rigidity. Attacks of excruciating pain occur due to localized or generalized muscle spasms. Prevention of spasms by physical isolation, diazepam, and use of neuromuscular blockade and mechanical ventilation may be required.

Strychnine poisoning may be accidental, suicidal, or homicidal. Severe generalized pain occurs due to tetanic muscle contractions. Stiffness first affects head and neck muscles. Because of heightened reflex excitability, minimal sensory stimulation results in a forceful extensor thrust of the entire body or tetanic convulsions resulting in opisthotonos and respiratory arrest. Recurrent seizures occur and are often provoked by noise, touching, or movement of the patient. Before severe hypoxia develops, the patient is usually alert and may complain of severe pain during and following the muscle contractions. Diazepam will prevent seizures.

Within ½ to 3 h after a *black widow spider bite*, severe pain and muscle cramping occur at the bite site. These painful muscle spasms spread to the abdomen, chest, and extremities. Muscle fasciculations, sweating, nausea, and vomiting may occur. Patients may writhe from the pain. Severe hypertension and tachycardia may occur due to catecholamine release; or, in lethal envenomations, hypotension, delirium, and coma ensue. Calcium gluconate or diazepam may prevent painful spasms, while beta-blocking drugs will control hypertension and tachycardia.

The *eosinophilia-myalgia syndrome* appeared in 1989 in persons ingesting over-the-counter L-tryptophan as a hypnotic. These patients developed severe generalized myalgias and muscle stiffness, exercise-related cramps, a skin rash, localized or generalized edema, fever, arthralgias, and respiratory symptoms. Eosinophilia was associated with these symptoms.

A number of disorders may be confused with eosinophilia-myalgia syndrome. *Eosinophilic polymyositis* may be mistaken for eosinophilia-myalgia syndrome, but in this disorder there is no history of L-tryptophan ingestion. Myalgias, eosinophilia, and evidence of myositis are present. *Relapsing eosinophilic perimyositis* is a rare disorder. Myalgia and muscle tenderness are associated with eosinophilia and evidence of perimysial infiltration by eosinophils or other inflammatory cells on biopsy, but there is no relationship to L-tryptophan ingestion. The *toxic oil syndrome* occurred in Spain in 1982, and no cases have followed that epidemic. Myalgias occurred 4 months after a respiratory illness, and eosinophilia was present.

Cysticercosis may cause myalgia and eosinophilia during dissemination to skeletal muscle. Most cases occur in Mexico and South America and are rarely symptomatic. Evidence of infection may be obtained by muscle biopsy, stool examination for eggs, and serologic tests.

Rarely, *sarcoidosis* may present with acute myalgia and tenderness and mild eosinophilia. Bilateral hilar adenopathy, with or without diffuse parenchymal changes, may be present, and serum angiotensin-converting enzyme levels may be elevated. Muscle biopsy reveals noncaseating granulomas. *Eosinophilic fasciitis* causes skin swelling, induration, pain, and tenderness on the extremities and trunk but few, if any, myalgias. Pain and stiffness are localized to areas of skin involvement.

Idiopathic polymyositis causes proximal and, less commonly, distal limb weakness, myalgias, muscle tenderness, and stiffness. Muscle enzyme levels are elevated, electromyographic studies reveal evidence of myopathy and denervation, and muscle biopsy reveals degenerating fibers and an inflammatory infiltrate. Patients with dermatomyositis have similar muscle pain and tenderness associated with erythematosus, knuckle plaques, periungual erythema and telangiectasia, finger ulcers, heliotrope discoloration of the upper lids, and in some cases diffuse edema and redness of large areas of skin.

Polymyositis or dermatomyositis may begin before, simultaneously with, or after the symptoms of a *malignant tumor*. Polymyositis and dermatomyositis are not associated with eosinophilia or L-tryptophan ingestion.

Churg-Strauss disease is a variant of polyarteritis nodosa. Myalgias and muscle tenderness, arthralgias, and neuropathic pain may occur in association with systemic symptoms, severe asthma, pulmonary infiltrates, and eosinophilia. Biopsies reveal evidence of granulomatous vasculitis and tissue infiltration by eosinophils.

Trichinosis may also cause myalgias, muscle tenderness, swelling, and eosinophilia and requires exclusion in patients with myalgia and eosinophilia. Fibromyalgia may initially cause localized and then widespread, constant, severe, myalgic pain, with normal laboratory values and demonstrable, palpable, tender points. The pain is exacerbated by activity, cold, and stress; sleep is poor, and fatigue is prevalent. The diagnosis is clinical and requires exclusion of many rheumatic disorders.

Neuropathic pain may be burning and superficial or deep and aching. Lancinating jabs of pain may occur alone or superimposed on constant aching or burning pain. Cramping muscles caused by the neuropathy are another cause of pain. Neuropathic pain is associated with paresthesias, unpleasant dysesthesias, allodynia, hyperpathia, and loss or impairment of one or more modalities of peripheral sensation. Pain, paresthesias, and sensory loss may occur in a stocking-glove, stocking only, boot, or entire leg distribution. Symptoms and signs may be symmetrical or asymmetrical and may involve both the upper and the lower extremities equally or unequally or, more commonly, the lower extremities exclusively. Motor weakness and wasting may be associated with pain, paresthesias, and sensory loss.

Arsenic poisoning may cause a painful sensorimotor neuropathy that begins 1 to 2 weeks after a gastrointestinal illness. Accidental poisoning or attempted homicide may be responsible. The diagnosis can be established by analysis of the serum or urine for arsenic content. *Thallium poisoning* may also be accidental or homocidal. Alopecia beginning 2 to 3 weeks after the onset of painful arthralgias, myalgias, and neuralgias requires measurement of the urinary excretion of thallium.

Diabetes mellitus may cause a painful sensory or sensorimotor neuropathy affecting the stocking or stocking-glove regions of the extremities. Symptoms improve with better control of hyperglycemia and/or the use of tricyclic antidepressant drugs for their analgesic effects.

Patients with AIDS may develop a symmetrical sensorimotor polyneuropathy in a stocking-glove distribution or an asymmetrical neuropathy (i.e., mononeuropathy multiplex).

Intermittent acute porphyria may cause a painful sensorimotor polyneuropathy; abdominal pain mimicking a surgical abdomen; and/or delirium, a behavior disorder, neurosis, or psychosis. The diagnosis can be confirmed by detection of a high concentration of porphobilinogen in the urine and/or by measuring the red blood cell or lymphocyte activity of porphobilinogen deaminase.

Other causes of painful polyneuropathy include *alcohol abuse and nutritional deficiency*, *hypothyroidism*, *renal failure*, *malignancy*, *myeloma and POEMS syndrome*, *amyloidosis*, *drugs*, *Lyme disease*, *mercury poisoning*, *industrial chemicals*, *the Guillain Barré syndrome*, *Fabry's disease*, *sickle cell anemia*, *Waldenström's macroglobulinemia*, *cryoglobulinemias*, and *systemic vasculitis*.

Joint-related pain may take the form of *nonspecific polyarthralgia*s. Pain occurs in multiple joints and may be intensified or provoked by joint movement or weight bearing. Results of radiographic studies are normal, as are those of laboratory tests. The sedimentation rate may be elevated. Results of a joint scintiscan may be positive in up to 63 percent of cases. Many cases resolve spontaneously, while others with positive scintiscan results may go on to develop an arthritic disorder. Patients with joint pain that is not aggravated by palpation or movement and with negative laboratory and imaging study results are often considered to have *psychogenic rheumatism*.

Some disorders may cause myalgias, arthralgias, and/or neuropathic pain. *Polyarteritis nodosa* may cause ischemic myopathy, arthralgias, or arthritis, and neuropathy in the form of a symmetrical polyneuropathy or mononeuropathy multiplex. This multisystem disorder causes systemic complaints such as fever, anorexia, weakness, weight loss, and malaise. Criteria for the diagnosis (i.e., requiring three or more of the ten listed) of polyarteritis nodosa include: weight loss; livedo reticularis; testicular pain; myalgias or muscle tenderness; neuropathy; diastolic hypertension; renal insufficiency; hepatitis B surface antigen in the serum; aneurysms of renal or visceral arteries; and a positive biopsy showing a granulocytic arteritis. Arthralgias or arthritis may also occur. This disorder improves and/or resolves after therapy with prednisone and cyclophosphamide.

Churg-Strauss disease causes a systemic illness similar to polyarteritis nodosa with only mild or no renal involvement. Severe asthma, pulmonary infiltrates, eosinophilia, and a biopsy showing granulomatous arteritis and tissue infiltration by eosinophils distinguishes this disorder from polyarteritis nodosa.

Patients with *rheumatoid arthritis* or *systemic lupus erythematosus* may have arthralgias or arthritis, diffuse myalgias, and a painful symmetrical polyneuropathy or asymmetrical pain due to mononeuropathy multiplex.

Behçet's disease causes painful oral and genital ulcers and eye pain and redness. Abdominal pain may result from colitis, limb pain from erythema nodosum or thrombophlebitis, muscle pain from myositis, headache and neck pain from meningoencephalitis, and joint pain from arthritis. Criteria for the diagnosis of Behçet's disease include involvement of the oral mucosa, genitalia, eyes, and skin. Involvement of all four sites confirms the presence of Behçet's disease. Disease at fewer than four sites is classified as incomplete Behçet's disease.

Lyme disease is acquired from an *Ixodes* tick bite in an endemic region. The initial symptom is usually a painless skin rash with an annular appearance that spreads (erythema migrans). The rash is accompanied by fever, myalgias, arthralgias, and headaches in up to 50 percent of cases. Treatment with amoxicillin or doxycycline leads to rapid disappearance of all symptoms and cure. Up to 15 percent of untreated patients develop neurologic disease with a unilateral or bilateral Bell's palsy, meningitis or meningoencephalitis, truncal or limb radiculoneuropathy, plexopathy, or neuropathy.

Recurrent arthritis or arthralgias (50–60 percent of cases) occur in the early months of the untreated illness. Late in the course, up to 10 percent of patients with joint complaints develop a persistent arthritis, usually of one or both knees. Ceftriaxone therapy will lead to improvement and/or resolution of neurologic and arthritic manifestations. The diagnosis of Lyme disease is based on clinical criteria. An ELISA test showing rising levels of antibody or, in chronic cases, a high titer of IgG antibody is supportive of the clinical diagnosis. Low titer test results may still represent *Borrelia burgdorferi* infection, and ELISA test specificity may be improved by performance of a Western blot.

Polymyalgia rheumatica is a disease of elderly people. Fever, malaise, and anorexia occur prior to or at the time of myalgic symptoms. Pain and tenderness occur over the shoulders, posterior neck and upper arms, low back, buttocks, and proximal legs and knees. Sometimes more distal joints may be painful, and the knees may develop effusions. The sedimentation rate is elevated and may exceed 100 mm/h. There is a

dramatic and rapid improvement after 10 to 15 mg/day of oral prednisone. Up to 15 percent of patients with this disorder have a temporal artery biopsy that reveals granulomatous arteritis.

A disorder that is clinically similar to polymyalgia rheumatica may occasionally be *associated with an underlying neoplasm* (e.g., breast or gastrointestinal carcinoma) *or an infection* (e.g., subacute bacterial endocarditis). *Seronegative rheumatoid arthritis* in an elderly person may be indistinguishable from polymyalgia rheumatica. The early symptoms of *polymyositis*, *systemic lupus erythematosus*, *Sjögren's syndrome*, *and the necrotizing vasculitides* may be difficult to differentiate clinically from polymyalgia rheumatica.

Human immunodeficiency virus (HIV-1) infection may mimic systemic lupus erythematosus. Multisystem involvement in AIDS may include arthritis or arthralgias, nephritis, hematologic abnormalities (i.e., leukopenia, thrombocytopenia, and anemia), neurologic abnormalities (i.e., seizures, dementia, and neuropathies), malar rash, and immunologic abnormalities (e.g., antinuclear antibody, lupus anticoagulant, and anticardiolipin antibodies). Patients with clinical findings that may occur in both disorders should have HIV infection excluded by ELISA and/or antigen detection techniques.

☐ DESCRIPTION OF LISTED DISEASES

1. MUSCLE-RELATED PAIN

A. Acute Polymyositis

1. Idiopathic   Most cases of idiopathic polymyositis develop slowly progressive symptoms over a period of 3 months or more. Some patients with this disorder develop acute generalized muscle pain. The involved muscles are usually tender and weak. Proximal muscle involvement is the most frequent finding, and it is usually symmetrical, but it can be asymmetrical in up to 17 percent of cases. Ten to 14 percent of patients may have both proximal and distal muscle weakness. Serum levels of aldolase and creatinine phosphokinase are usually elevated, but either or both may be normal. A muscle biopsy will usually confirm the diagnosis. Prednisone in doses of 60 to 80 mg/day will usually lead to improvement or resolution of symptoms.

Rarely, severe myalgia and muscle tenderness may be associated with myoglobinuria.

2. Toxoplasmosis   Patients may have generalized or bilateral cervical adenopathy, fever, and a painful, tender polymyositis. An elevated or rising titer of IgM antibody to toxoplasmosis will confirm the diagnosis. The clinical picture is otherwise indistinguishable from acute idiopathic polymyositis. Muscle biopsies may sometimes demonstrate *Toxoplasma* organisms. It is unclear whether

TABLE OF DISEASE INCIDENCE

INCIDENCE PER 100,000 (APPROXIMATE)

Common (>100)

Myalgias associated with viral and other infections

Myalgias in normal individuals after exertion

Myalgias associated with therapeutic drugs and immunizations

Myalgias and/or cramps due to hyponatremia or hypokalemia

Fibromyalgia

Polyneuropathy due to diabetes mellitus

Polymyalgia rheumatica

Seronegative rheumatoid arthritis

Polyneuropathy due to alcohol abuse and/or nutritional deficiencies

Uncommon (>5–100)

Idiopathic polymyositis

Rhabdomyolysis in normal individuals after extreme exertion

Myoadenylate deaminase deficiency

Myalgias due to hypothyroidism or hypoparathyroidism

Rhabdomyolysis with alcohol or drug abuse

Myalgias and/or cramps due to hypocalcemia with or without hypoparathyroidism

Idiopathic polymyositis and dermatomyositis

Polymyositis and dermatomyositis associated with malignancy

Polyarthralgias

Rheumatoid arthritis and vasculitis

Systemic lupus erythematosus and vasculitis

Lyme disease

Polymyalgia rheumatica secondary to neoplasia or infection

Polymyalgia rheumatica-like disease with collagen vascular disorders

Pseudolupus due to HIV infection

Polyneuropathy due to hypothyroidism, malignancy, therapeutic drugs, Lyme disease, AIDS, renal failure, Guillain-Barré syndrome, sickle cell anemia, or vasculitis

Polyarthralgias

Rare (>0–5)

Toxoplasma polymyositis

Rhabdomyolysis due to influenza A virus, Epstein-Barr virus, coxsackievirus, or herpes simplex virus

Myophosphorylase deficiency and other carbohydrate enzyme deficiencies

Carnitine palmityl transferase deficiency

NADH-coenzyme-Q reductase deficiency

Myalgias due to hyperthyroidism, hypoadrenalism, or panhypopituitarism

Rhabdomyolysis associated with therapeutic drugs

Myalgias and/or cramps due to hypomagnesemia or hypophosphatemia

Trichinosis

Tetanus

Strychnine poisoning

Black widow spider bite

Eosinophilia-myalgia syndrome

Eosinophilic polymyositis

Relapsing eosinophilic perimyositis

Toxic oil syndrome

Cysticercosis

Sarcoidosis

Eosinophilic fasciitis

Churg-Strauss disease

Polyneuropathy due to arsenic, thallium, or intermittent acute porphyria

Psychogenic rheumatism

Polyarteritis nodosa

Behçet's disease

Polyneuropathy due to insulinoma, amyloidosis, myeloma and POEMS syndrome, mercury, industrial chemicals, Fabry's disease, or cryoglobulinemia

---

toxoplasmosis causes the polymyositis or occurs because of reactivation of infection in an immunocompromised host with idiopathic polymyositis. Specific therapy may cause a fall in IgM antibody, but it seldom cures the polymyositis, which usually persists and requires prednisone therapy for control.

B. Acute Myositis and Rhabdomyolysis Associated with Viral Infections

1. Influenza A Virus Diffuse myalgias occur frequently in patients with influenza virus infection. These myalgias involve the neck, shoulders, upper arms, lower back, and thighs. Muscles are usually not tender. There may be mild hyperesthesia of the skin. In rare cases, severe myalgias, muscle tenderness, and weakness occur, and the serum creatinine phosphokinase level becomes markedly elevated and the urine dark brown due to myoglobin excretion. Unless adequate hydration is provided, such patients may develop oliguric renal failure.

2. Epstein-Barr Virus Infection with the Epstein-Barr virus has also been associated with muscle injury, myoglobinuria, and renal failure. Most cases of infection-related muscle injury and myoglobinuria have been reported with influenza A virus.

3. Coxsackievirus It has also been reported that coxsackievirus causes a similar syndrome with muscle pain and injury.

4. Herpes Simplex Virus Oral mucosal and lip ulceration, fever, and polymyositis with painful, tender muscles may be caused by herpes simplex virus.

C. Exertional Rhabdomyolysis in Normal Individuals

Military recruits and others in physical conditioning programs have been the source of reports on this disorder. Only a small percentage of individuals undergoing the same training develop myoglobinuria (23 of 586 military recruits in one series).

In those affected, muscles become painful, swollen,

tender, and weak. Use momentarily increases the pain. The overlying skin may become edematous and sometimes ecchymotic. Fever and malaise may occur. The urine may become a dark reddish-brown because of myoglobin excretion.

Myoglobinuria can result in acute oliguric renal failure. This can be prevented by giving large volumes of fluid to increase urine flow rates and alkali to raise urine pH, increasing the solubility of myoglobulin. Other problems that can arise from rhabdomyolysis include elevation of the serum concentration of potassium and phosphorus (due to release from muscle) and lowering of the serum calcium level (due to calcium deposition in injured muscle). Serum uric acid levels become very elevated (as high as 50 mg/dl). Disseminated intravascular coagulation can occur, giving rise to bleeding in the skin, urine, or gastrointestinal or respiratory tract.

A syndrome similar to exertional rhabdomyolysis may occur after generalized involuntary muscular activity related to uncontrolled seizures, tetanus, or strychnine poisoning.

D. Myalgias Due to Inherited Metabolic Disorders of Muscle

1. Carbohydrate Metabolism

A. MYOPHOSPHORYLASE DEFICIENCY (MCARDLE'S DISEASE) Many cases (42 percent) develop symptoms before age 20. Inheritance is autosomal recessive. Pain occurs during exercise in the active muscles. Cramps typically occur after exercise or during exercise if the patient continues without resting. Pain and associated muscle stiffness, fatigue, and weakness subside with rest. Some patients experience a "second wind" phenomenon after pain, weakness, and fatigue begin, if they can continue to exercise. Muscle necrosis with persistent pain and tenderness and myoglobinuria may occur after exertion in up to 50 percent of patients, but renal failure has been reported in only 7 percent of cases. Myoglobinuria is associated with severe cramping of the exercising muscles. Following ischemic forearm testing, there is no rise in venous lactate and a normal or exaggerated rise in blood ammonia. Creatine phosphokinase levels may be elevated at rest (94 percent). McArdle's disease is the most common disorder of muscle carbohydrate metabolism.

B. OTHER ENZYME DEFICIENCIES Deficiencies of phosphofructokinase, phosphoglycerate kinase, phosphoglycerate mutase, and lactate dehydrogenase may be clinically similar to McArdle's disease. Muscle biopsy and enzyme assays are required for specific diagnosis of these deficiencies. A normal ischemic forearm exercise test excludes McArdle's disease but not some of the glycolytic cycle enzyme deficiencies.

2. Lipid Metabolism: Carnitine Palmityl Transferase Deficiency
Exertional myalgia and stiffness, without cramps, occurs after prolonged exercise or fasting. Myoglobinuria is frequent and provoked by exertion, fasting, infection, cold exposure, or emotional upset. It may be associated with severe persistent myalgias, tenderness, and muscle weakness. The creatine phosphokinase level at rest is usually normal, and there is no pain or muscle tenderness between attacks. Results of the ischemic exercise test and electromyographic studies are normal. The muscle biopsy reveals normal histology or demonstrates lipid storage, but there is an absence of carnitine palmityl transferase (CPT) activity. This enzyme is involved in the transport of lipid substrate into mitochondria for energy production by oxidation. A muscle deficient in CPT is solely dependent on carbohydrate for energy. This disorder may begin in childhood or in early adulthood. Inheritance is autosomal recessive.

3. Nucleotide Metabolism: Myoadenylate Deaminase Deficiency
This enzyme deficiency is highly prevalent (1–2 percent of biopsies). It is associated with recurrent myalgias, muscle tenderness, cramps, weakness, and fatigue after exertion (88 percent of cases). The creatine phosphokinase level may be elevated, but rhabdomyolysis does not occur. There is no rise in venous ammonia after an ischemic forearm exercise test. Some patients with myoadenylate deaminase (MADA) deficiency are asymptomatic and the clinical significance of this deficiency has been questioned.

4. Mitochondrial Disorders: NADH-Coenzyme-Q Reductase Deficiency
Patients may have muscle discomfort and fatigue with exercise. Muscle contracture and myoglobinuria do not occur. Onset is in childhood, and other neurologic problems are associated (e.g., dementia, ataxia, ophthalmoparesis, positive Babinski signs, and areflexia). Persistent low-intensity work may be restricted by fatigue.

Metabolic disorders of muscle may present initially in adolescence or adult life as an acute exercise-provoked painful disorder (i.e., myalgias and/or cramps). Most of these deficiencies then cause recurrent symptoms of variable severity.

E. Endocrine Disorders Myalgias, muscle stiffness, and cramps may occur in several endocrine disorders.

1. Hypothyroidism
Myalgic pain, tenderness, and stiffness may occur. The creatinine phosphokinase level is usually elevated. Myopathic abnormalities may be found on electromyographic study. The diagnosis can be confirmed by detecting low levels of T_3 and T_4 and an elevated level of thyroid-stimulating hormone (TSH).

2. Hyperthyroidism
This disorder may cause proximal muscle weakness. "Myalgias" may be secondary to associated bone disease.

3. Hypoadrenalism (Addison's Disease)
This disorder may present with generalized myalgias, muscle weak-

ness, and arthralgias. Weakness and pain may be so severe that walking is not possible. Flexion contractures affecting the knees or hips may occur. Myalgias may be constant or intermittent and can be generalized or involve only the back or legs. Corticosteroid administration relieves myalgic pain and muscle tenderness. Rarely, an acute myopathy with elevated serum muscle enzymes may occur. Myalgia and muscle tenderness are uncommon symptoms of Addison's disease.

4. Panhypopituitarism This disorder may be associated with diffuse myalgias and muscle weakness secondary to deficiency of thyroid and/or adrenal hormones.

5. Hypoparathyroidism and Hypocalcemia This disorder may cause severe muscle pain due to muscle spasm. Carpopedal spasm, facial distortion, seizures, and laryngospasm may occur. Chvostek's or Trousseau's signs may be present. Parathyroid hormone deficiency may be hereditary, secondary to thyroid surgery with parathyroid gland removal, or related to hypomagnesemia.

F. Rhabdomyolysis Associated with Alcohol and Drug Abuse Rhabdomyolysis and myoglobinuria have been associated with alcohol and narcotic and/or other types of drug abuse. A large amount of alcohol or the use of heroin, cocaine, amphetamines, or phencyclidine can cause generalized myalgias, muscle swelling and tenderness, myoglobinuria, and renal failure. Creatine phosphokinase levels are markedly elevated, reflecting severe muscle cell damage. Biopsies of involved muscles have shown fiber necrosis and early fiber regeneration. Some alcoholic or narcotic abuse patients may remain unconscious for a prolonged period, causing limb ischemia from the weight of the body compressing one or more limbs. Such ischemia can result in a compartment syndrome with local swelling and tender, tense muscles with or without diminished distal pulses and distal sensory loss and paresthesias. Measured intracompartmental pressures exceed 33 mmHg and may be greater than 70 mmHg. Failure to decompress such a compartment by immediate fasciotomy can result in muscle necrosis and rhabdomyolysis. In many cases related to prolonged unconsciousness, necrosis has already occurred, and fasciotomy is of no benefit. In other cases, direct toxic effects of alcohol or drugs on muscle are likely. Other risk factors for the development of rhabdomyolysis are often present in drug-intoxicated patients. These risk factors include excessive muscular activity, seizures, coma, hyperthermia, and hypovolemia.

G. Myalgias and Rhabdomyolysis Associated with Therapeutic Drugs

1. Clofibrate Some patients may have an acute syndrome consisting of bilateral thigh and shoulder muscle pain, tenderness, stiffness, and weakness. The serum creatine phosphokinase (CPK) and aspartate aminotransferase (AST), levels are usually elevated, and myoglobinuria may occur. Discontinuance of the drug relieves symptoms, while challenge precipitates muscle complaints, usually with the initial dose.

2. Lovastatin A small percentage of patients (0.2 percent) may develop acute generalized muscle pain, tenderness, and weakness. Severe rhabdomyolysis and renal failure may occur in patients taking gemfibrozil or cyclosporine in addition to lovastatin. These drugs may impair the catabolism of lovastatin.

3. Emetine Used in the past to treat amebiasis, emetine can cause diffuse muscle pain, tenderness, stiffness, and weakness secondary to myonecrosis. Rhabdomyolysis, myoglobinuria, and renal failure occur in severe cases.

4. Epsilon-aminocaproic Acid Some patients may develop myositis with myalgias, muscle tenderness, and rhabdomyolysis.

H. Myalgias without Rhabdomyolysis Associated with Therapeutic Drugs and Immunizations Diuretics (e.g., thiazides, furosemide, bumetanide, and metolazone) may cause severe hypokalemia, resulting in muscle aching, tenderness, and weakness, but myoglobinuria does not usually occur. Myalgias can also result from the use of isoetharine, phenytoin, danazol, procainamide, vincristine, trazodone, cimetidine, penicillin, lithium, nalidixic acid, nicotinic acid, chloroquine, and other cytotoxic drugs. The administration of vaccines such as typhoid, cholera, hepatitis B, yellow fever, and plague can cause generalized myalgias and malaise. In the case of most vaccines, the myalgias last 1 to 2 days. The myalgias associated with yellow fever vaccine may last 2 to 3 weeks.

I. Nonspecific Myalgias Diffuse myalgias, with or without local muscle tenderness, may occur in acute infectious diseases due to viral agents (e.g., influenza virus, coxsackievirus, and echoviruses), bacteria (e.g., streptococcal tonsillitis and bacterial endocarditis), fungal diseases (e.g., acute histoplasmosis), and parasitic diseases (e.g., malaria and trichinosis). These myalgias usually are transient and resolve with the underlying infection.

Myalgias may also occur in normal individuals within 12 to 48 h after unaccustomed physical activity. Pain may occur only during muscle use. Such myalgias are usually mild and transient, clearing in 24 to 48 h.

J. Myalgias and/or Cramps Due to Electrolyte and Mineral Deficiencies

1. Acute Hypokalemia Myalgias, weakness, muscle tenderness, and, in severe cases, myoglobinuria and an elevated serum CPK level may accompany this disturbance.

2. *Acute Hypocalcemia* Severe, painful muscle spasms and tetany occur. Metabolic or respiratory alkalosis may decrease the ionized calcium level and cause similar painful muscle spasms in the trunk and extremities.

3. *Acute Hypomagnesemia* Hypocalcemia is usually associated. Painful muscle cramps and tetany occur. Weakness, tremor, myoclonus, hyperreflexia, and an exaggerated startle response may also be present.

4. *Acute Hyponatremia* Painful muscle cramps may occur when sweat is replaced with water without salt.

5. *Chronic Hypophosphatemia* Patients may have myalgias, muscle tenderness, and muscle necrosis with myoglobinuria.

K. Trichinosis This disorder may follow the ingestion of uncooked or inadequately cooked pork products or walrus, bear, or horse meat. Within 48 h of ingestion of contaminated meat, abdominal pain, nausea, vomiting, diarrhea, and sometimes fever begin. Some patients do not experience these initial symptoms. Within 5 to 14 days after the onset of gastrointestinal complaints, generalized muscle pain, tenderness, stiffness, and weakness occur. Fever, periorbital edema, conjunctival redness, and subconjunctival bleeding may accompany the diffuse myalgias. A maculopapular, petechial, or urticarial rash appears in some cases. Small hemorrhages may be noted at the sites of insertion of extraocular muscles onto the globe and under the nails as "splinter" hemorrhages.

Eosinophilia (absolute count, >500 cells/mm^3, or >5 percent of the total leukocytes) is usual, as is leukocytosis. Serum enzyme levels of CPK, aldolase, and AST are usually elevated. Hypocalcemia, associated with hypoalbuminemia and a polyclonal hypergammaglobulinemia, may occur. The hypoalbuminemia occurs in severe cases due to diffuse capillary damage and leakage of albumin into the extracellular spaces of the inflamed muscles.

Antibodies to *Trichinella* may be detected by an indirect fluorescent antibody test, an enzyme-linked immunosorbent assay (ELISA), or the bentonite flocculation test. Symptomatic infections generally are associated with muscle larvae counts of 50 to 100/g. If taken from painful, tender muscles, gastrocnemius or biceps muscle biopsies result in positive confirmation of the diagnosis in 60 to 80 percent of patients tested. Muscle should be examined as a crush preparation, after pepsin digestion, and as a fixed and stained section. Peptic digestion is the most sensitive method of larval detection. The ELISA test for IgE and IgM antibodies to *Trichinella spiralis* is 100-percent sensitive and specific and can be used to confirm less specific tests, such as the indirect fluorescent antibody and bentonite flocculation tests. Antibodies can usually be detected by the third week of illness, but ELISA tests may be positive after 1 week of symptoms.

Most infections acquired in the United States are asymptomatic or mild and are misdiagnosed as some other illness (e.g., influenza). Symptomatic infections, however, may be severe, causing considerable morbidity and even death. Pulmonary, cardiac, and central nervous system involvement may develop in severe cases, but such involvement is relatively uncommon. Pulmonary involvement is signaled by cough, hemoptysis, and pulmonary infiltrates. Myocardial injury can be detected by the presence of electrocardiographic abnormalities, a gallop rhythm, and signs of heart failure or cardiovascular collapse. Nervous system involvement occurs in less than 1 percent of cases and may include meningitis and/or encephalitis. Central nervous system involvement may result in mono-, hemi-, or quadriparesis; aphasia; cortical blindness; delirium; seizures; cranial nerve deficits; and myelopathy. Retinal and choroidal hemorrhages may occur. A diffuse central nervous system disorder associated with myalgias, elevated serum AST and/or CPK levels, and eosinophilia should prompt a search for *Trichinella* infection by serological techniques and muscle biopsy.

Patients with a confirmed diagnosis should be treated with mebendazole to eradicate intestinal and tissue larvae. Corticosteroids have been used to treat myocardial and nervous system disease. The overall mortality is now less than 1 percent. Trichinosis is an entirely preventable disease if meat is prepared by cooking all portions of the meat to 77°C (170°F), which may require a prolonged time on a barbecue grill and thin-slicing of the meat. Freezing pork at $-15°C$ for 20 days or at $-18°C$ for 1 day kills infectious larvae. This approach does not work for walrus or bear meat from Alaska or other arctic regions, since cold-region strains of *Trichinella spiralis* have been shown to be resistant to freezing. Polar bear meat frozen at $-18°C$ for 24 months has remained infectious.

L. Tetanus This disease may be produced by introduction of toxin-generating strains of *Clostridium tetani* into a wound. Foreign bodies, such as wood or soil, in the wound and a low level of O_2 (e.g., in closed puncture wounds or necrotic tissue) increase the likelihood of clinical tetanus. Incomplete or no immunization or lack of a booster within the previous 5 to 10 years increases the risk of clinical tetanus. The severity of the disease is usually less if initial symptoms begin more than 9 days after injury and if muscle spasms are absent or occur more than 48 h after onset of muscle stiffness.

Local pain and muscle stiffness near the wound (i.e., localized tetanus) is followed by generalized myalgias and stiffness. The jaw muscles may become stiff or rigid, resulting in trismus (i.e., lockjaw). Rigidity of other facial muscles may alter the patient's appearance. The mouth can barely be opened. Spasm of the facial muscles may cause a sneering grimace (i.e., risus sardonicus). The patient may appear to be lying at attention in bed, or the spine may be so extended that the patient is balanced on the vertex of his or her skull and heels (opisthotonos). Spasm of pharyngeal muscles may cause painful dysphagia and may lead to aspiration.

Severe tetanus causes generalized muscle rigidity accompanied by diffuse aching pain. Intense, sudden paroxysmal muscle spasms occur, producing excruciating pain. Opisthotonos may be extreme. Vertebrae may fracture from the intense muscle contractions, causing persistent back pain. Prolonged severe spasms, with apnea and cyanosis, can lead to death. These attacks of sustained muscle contraction can be provoked by noise, cold air, or touching the patient.

Labile hypertension and tachycardia may occur. The systolic pressure may rise to over 300 mmHg. Peripheral vasoconstriction occurs, and diaphoresis may be profuse. Cardiac arrhythmias, profound hypotension, and cardiac arrest may result from autonomic involvement.

Admission to an intensive care unit is required once the diagnosis has been made. Muscle spasms can be controlled with diazepam. Neuromuscular blockade (e.g., pancuronium bromide), intubation, and mechanical ventilation are required for severe spasms that impair ventilation. Sympathetic overactivity can be controlled by the use of beta blockers with alpha-blocking activity or morphine sulfate. Wound excision, passive immunization with human tetanus antitoxin, and administration of large amounts of penicillin are measures directed at minimizing the amount of toxin remaining in the body by preventing further production in the wound and neutralizing free toxin that has not been taken up by nerve cells.

M. Strychnine Poisoning   Patients who abuse intravenous drugs are at risk, since street drugs may be cut with strychnine. This poison has also been used for homicidal and suicidal purposes.

Soon after ingestion or injection, facial and neck muscle stiffness develops. There is heightened reflex excitability. Any stimulus produces a forceful extensor thrust. Shortly thereafter, tetanic convulsions occur. The back arches in hyperextension (opisthotonos) such that only the top of the head and heels are in contact with the surface of the table or bed. All muscles contract, and the patient is unable to breathe. Death may result rapidly from impaired respiration. Recurrent seizures occur provoked by sensory stimuli. Early in this syndrome, the patient is alert and may complain of extreme generalized pain due to the convulsions. Death may occur after one to five seizures.

Seizures can be terminated by intravenous diazepam. Intubation and mechanical ventilation, and neuromuscular blockade may be required. Tetanus may be confused with strychnine poisoning. Dystonic reactions to phenothiazine drugs may resemble a mild form of these disorders because of a tendency to mild opisthotonos and complaints of neck and back stiffness. Patients with a dystonic reaction may complain that their tongue feels too big for their mouth. They may grimace frequently. Torticollis may occur, as may oculogyric crisis. These patients are not usually in pain, and they respond to anticholinergic antiparkinsonian drugs (i.e., benztropine mesylate) or meperidine.

N. Black Widow (*Latrodectus* Species) Spider Bite
Two punctate, red lesions usually mark the bite site on the legs, arms, or buttocks. The latter location is related to the use of outdoor toilets, often frequented by these spiders. Within a brief period after a bite, localized pallor or redness, edema, stinging or aching pain, and numbness may occur at the site of envenomation. Neurotoxins present in the venom release acetylcholine at motor end plates and synapses and catecholamines from adrenergic nerve endings. Within 30 min to 3 h, severe local pain and muscle cramping begin near the bite wound and may spread to the abdomen, flanks, back, chest, and all extremities.

Abdominal wall muscle spasm and pain may mimic an acute abdominal emergency. Chest pain may be described as a pressure or constricting, or it may be sharp and pleuritic. Pain in the legs, shoulders, and arms is associated with muscle spasms. Muscle fasciculations and tremors may be observed in areas of pain and spasm. Generalized sweating, nausea, and vomiting are often present, and a marked rise in blood pressure and pulse rate are frequent findings. Patients may writhe from severe pain rather than lie still, as a patient with an acutely inflamed abdomen usually does.

Death may occur from respiratory muscle weakness. In patients with cardiovascular disease, the hypertension and tachycardia may precipitate a stroke, acute cardiac failure, or myocardial ischemia. In severe cases, hypotension and delirium may progress to coma. Death occurs in less than 5 percent of cases and is more common in young children and elderly people. Recovery may be protracted with fatigue, headache, paresthesias, insomnia, and impotence, often continuing for months. Calcium gluconate, methocarbamol, or diazepam given intravenously usually provide relief of painful muscle spasms. Narcotics are also useful. Antivenin should be given to small children, pregnant women, and older patients with cardiovascular disease. Propranolol is effective for the treatment of hypertension and cardiac arrhythmias.

O. Eosinophilia-Myalgia Syndrome   This disorder has been related to the ingestion of specific lots of over-the-counter L-tryptophan used for the treatment of insomnia, migraine, or depression. It appeared in epidemic proportions in October 1989. During the ensuing 8 months, 1536 cases were reported to the Centers for Disease Control.

Symptoms occurring during the first 2 months of the illness include severe and sometimes incapacitating myalgias (100 percent of cases) and stiffness; localized erythema; a diffuse maculopapular or erythematous rash or a sclerodermiform rash (72 percent); localized edema of the hands, feet, or face or generalized edema (52 percent); arthralgias (35 percent); fever (41 percent); and respiratory symptoms (32 percent). Muscle tenderness usually accompanies myalgias. Muscle cramps are associated with activity. Eosinophilia exceeds 1×10^9/liter and may range from 1.2×10^9/liter to 12.1×10^9/liter. Acute manifestations, such as edema and myalgia, respond to prednisone. Localized tissue involvement may occur and progress. Eosinophilic fasciitis, pneumonitis and restrictive pulmonary disease, sensorimotor neuropathy, pleural effusion, myocarditis, intraabdominal fibrosis, and encephalopathy may occur in some patients. Biopsies reveal fascial and perimyseal inflammation by mononuclear cells and sometimes eosinophils but minimal or no muscle degeneration. An inflammatory and/or occlusive microangiopathy occurs. Some muscle fiber atrophy and endomyseal inflammation may be noted. The skin may show scleroderma-like changes. Muscle-associated inflammatory changes predominantly involve epimyseal and perimysial connective tissue and resemble changes seen in eosinophilic fasciitis. The serum CPK level is usually normal, but aldolase activity may be increased, and the sedimentation rate may be normal or elevated. A weakly reactive antinuclear antibody test (speckled pattern) may be present.

The cause is believed to be a contaminant present in L-tryptophan produced by a single manufacturer (Showa-Denko, Japan) in association with abnormalities in tryptophan metabolism present in some patients. The identity of the contaminant and the role of the metabolic abnormality remain unknown. This disorder may progress despite discontinuance of L-tryptophan and prednisone therapy. Death may occur in severe cases. The differential diagnosis of the eosinophilia-myalgia syndrome is given in Table 48-1.

P. Clinical Mimics of the Eosinophilia-Myalgia Syndrome

1. Eosinophilic Polymyositis Myalgias, proximal weakness, elevated creatine phosphokinase levels, and electromyographic evidence of myositis occur. Muscle biopsy reveals muscle necrosis and regeneration and tissue inflammation by eosinophils. Systemic manifestations respond to prednisone, methotrexate, or leukapheresis.

2. Relapsing Eosinophilic Perimyositis Myalgias, muscle tenderness, and swelling occur with normal or elevated serum levels of aldolase and creatine phospho-

Table 48-1
DIFFERENTIAL DIAGNOSIS OF THE EOSINOPHILIA-MYALGIA SYNDROME

Eosinophilic polymyositis
Relapsing eosinophilic perimyositis
Toxic oil syndrome (Spain)
Cysticercosis
Sarcoidosis
Eosinophilic fasciitis
Idiopathic polymyositis
Idiopathic dermatomyositis
Polymyositis and dermatomyositis associated with malignant disease
Collagen vascular disease (Churg-Strauss disease)
Trichinosis

kinase. Electromyographic studies may show evidence of myositis. Symptoms respond to prednisone.

3. Toxic Oil Syndrome This disorder occurred in Spain in 1981 and caused an epidemic affecting 20,000 people. It was caused by use of an illegally marketed cooking oil. Disabling myalgias followed 3 to 4 months after an initial illness characterized by cough, dyspnea, pulmonary infiltrates, and eosinophilia. Skin and gastrointestinal symptoms were common. This disorder occurred as a single epidemic and subsequent cases have not occurred.

4. Cysticercosis When ingested, eggs hatch in the upper intestinal tract or after retrograde transport of egg-filled proglottids to the same region by reverse peristalsis. Larvae may produce fever, myalgias, tender muscles, and eosinophilia as they invade muscle. This disorder occurs in Mexico and South America and is rare in the United States. Calcified cysts visible on a plain radiograph may be present in affected muscles months or years later as evidence of this disorder. An ELISA test is useful in confirming the diagnosis.

5. Sarcoidosis Patients may present with an acute, generalized myositis with myalgias, tenderness, and weakness, associated with elevation of CPK and aldolase and electromyographic evidence of myositis. Mild eosinophilia, an elevated sedimentation rate, hyperglobulinemia, and an elevated serum level of angiotensin-converting enzyme (ACE) may be associated. A pulmonary radiograph may reveal bilateral hilar adenopathy and/or diffuse parenchymal changes. Muscle biopsy reveals noncaseating granulomas.

6. Eosinophilic Fasciitis Pain, swelling, induration, thickening, and tenderness of the skin occur on the extremities. Similar lesions may occur on the trunk. Eosinophilia, an elevated sedimentation rate and CPK level, and electromyographic evidence of myositis may be present. Biopsies may show evidence of involvement of epimysium and perimysium.

Diffuse myalgic pain does not occur, and pain and stiffness are associated only with areas of skin involvement. Histopathologic changes may be difficult to differentiate from the findings in the eosinophilia-myalgia syndrome.

7. Idiopathic Polymyositis The major symptom is weakness of proximal limb muscles, trunk, and neck. Difficulty rising from a chair, crossing the legs, or climbing the stairs reflects thigh and pelvic muscle weakness; and difficulty lifting and placing objects on a shelf or combing the hair reflects proximal arm weakness. Myalgic pain in a symmetrical (57 percent of cases) or asymmetrical distribution (17 percent) is accompanied by muscle tenderness. Dysphagia (17 percent) and dysphonia may also occur. Eosinophilia does not usually occur. Arthralgia is frequent, but frank arthritis seldom occurs. The serum CPK level is elevated in 95 to 99 percent of cases. In more chronic cases, the false-negative rate for muscle enzyme elevation may be as high as 33 percent. Distal limb involvement may occur in 10 to 14 percent of cases. Electromyographic studies reveal evidence of myopathy (i.e., short duration, low amplitude, and polyphasic potentials) after voluntary contraction. Fibrillation potentials reflect involvement of neuronal processes in the muscle. Electromyography has a sensitivity of 70 to 90 percent. The sensitivity of muscle biopsy may be only 65 percent, and 17 percent of biopsies may be completely normal on histologic examination.

8. Idiopathic Dermatomyositis   Muscle involvement is similar to that occurring in polymyositis. An erythematous or violaceous rash occurs on the face, neck, chest, and limbs and may precede the onset of muscle symptoms. The rash on the extremities takes the form of erythematous plaques over the knuckles (Grotton's papules), wrists, elbows, knees, and medial ankle region. A whitish scale may adhere to these plaques. Hyperemia of the periungual skin of some or all of the fingers occurs. Edema of the lower legs or the skin beneath rash covered regions may occur. Cutaneous nodules, periungual infarction, and digital ulceration represent vasculitic changes. An erythematous, lilac or heliotrope rash occurs over the upper eyelids and may also occur on the neck, shoulders, and chest. Periorbital and facial edema may be associated.

9. Polymyositis and Dermatomyositis Associated with Malignancy   Two-thirds of cases related to neoplasms are associated with dermatomyositis and one-third with polymyositis. The incidence of an underlying malignancy with polymyositis is 2 to 3 percent and with dermatomyositis, 15 to 20 percent. It is highest in individuals older than age 60.

The tumor will be observed within 2 years after onset of skin and muscle symptoms (59 percent of cases) or at the time of onset (10 percent). In 31 percent, the skin and/or muscle disease begins after the tumor is discovered. Muscle and/or skin symptoms may improve with treatment of the tumor and may return or worsen with tumor recurrence.

Muscle weakness, myalgias, tenderness, and rash are not associated with eosinophilia. Primary tumors associated with these disorders include carcinomas of the lung, breast, colon, stomach, nasopharynx, ovary, and uterus; lymphomas; sarcomas; and myeloproliferative disorders.

10. Churg-Strauss Disease   This variant of polyarteritis nodosa may be associated with myalgias, arthralgias, and muscle tenderness. Severe asthma, pulmonary infiltrates, and eosinophilia occur. Biopsies show evidence of granulomatous vasculitis and tissue infiltration with eosinophils.

11. Trichinosis   This disorder may cause myalgias, muscle tenderness, fever, and eosinophilia. There may be a history of ingestion of inadequately cooked pork or bear meat. The diagnosis can be confirmed by muscle biopsy or serologic tests. This disease is discussed more thoroughly in Section 1K.

Q. Fibromyalgia   Obligatory criteria for the diagnosis of fibromyalgia include (1) generalized myalgias persistent for 3 months or more at three or more anatomic sites; (2) absence of traumatic injury or other underlying inflammatory, endocrine, or infectious disease; and (3) normal laboratory test results (e.g., normal sedimentation rate, absence of rheumatoid factor or antinuclear antibody, normal serum muscle enzyme levels, normal electromyographic study results, and normal muscle biopsy results).

In addition, five or more tender points should be present, with the patient usually unaware of their existence before palpation (this is a major criterion). Minor diagnostic criteria include (1) increase in pain or stiffness with activity, (2) increase of symptoms with cold weather and improvement with warm weather, (3) increase of symptoms with anxiety or stress, (4) nonrestorative sleep, (5) fatigue during the day, (6) anxiety, (7) chronic headaches, (8) irritable bowel syndrome, (9) subjective swelling or dysesthesias, (10) vague numbness unrelated to dermatomal patterns, and (11) electroencephalographic evidence of alpha intrusion in non-REM sleep.

The number and sites of tender points required for a diagnosis is controversial. The required number has varied from 3 to 5 of 40, 7 of 14, 12 of 14, 10 of 25, and 7 of 15. A list of testable tender points appears in Table 48-2. Use of pressure algometers or dolorimeters has been advocated for evaluation of tender points. Fibromyalgia patients may have a lower pain threshold at all sites relative to pain-free control patients. There is a marked female predominance in this disorder (male/female ratio, 1:9) and the age range of highest frequency is 40 to 60 years. Sleep disturbance occurs in 60 to 90 percent of cases, and this problem requires recognition and treatment. Back pain may cause confusion with lumbar disc disease, and joint pain and stiffness with rheumatoid arthritis. Limb paresthesias, coldness, and aching with weakness suggest a neuropathic or vascular disorder of the extremities. Local pain can mimic many other disorders, and the diagnosis may not become apparent until pain is widespread. Some cases of fibromyalgia may occur secondary to rheumatoid arthritis or to infectious diseases (e.g., Lyme disease or chronic Coxsackie B2 infection).

Symptom onset in primary fibromyalgia may be abrupt in 33 percent of cases, and it may be localized to one anatomic region in 87 percent of cases when the disorder begins. Up to 60 percent of patients do not associate an injury, strain, or other illness with the onset of fibromyalgia. The cause of fibromyalgia is unknown. Hypotheses include a psychologic disturbance, a sleep disorder, a

Table 48-2
TENDER POINTS USEFUL FOR DIAGNOSIS OF FIBROMYALGIA

Occiput: bilateral; at suboccipital muscle origins
Low cervical: bilateral; at anterior regions of interspinous spaces C4–C7
Trapezius muscles: bilateral; midpoint of upper border
Supraspinatus muscle: bilateral; origins above the scapular spine at the medial border of the scapula
Paraspinous: bilateral; 3 cm lateral to the midline at the level of the midscapula over the rhomboid muscles
Second rib: bilateral; at the upper margin of the costochondral junction
Lateral pectoral: bilateral; at the level of rib four at the anterior axillary line
Lateral epicondyle: bilateral; 2 cm distal to the epicondyle
Medial epicondyle: bilateral; at the epicondyle
Gluteal: bilateral; in the upper, outer quadrant of the buttock in the gluteus medius muscle
Greater trochanter: bilateral; posterior to the trochanteric prominence
Knees: bilateral; at the medial fat pad proximal to the joint line
Low lumbar: interspinous ligaments in the midline L4–S1

---

poorly defined connective tissue disease, and a chronic infection or metabolic disorder of muscle.

2. NERVE-RELATED PAIN: ACUTE PAINFUL NEUROPATHY

Neuropathic pain may be superficial, burning, and constant. The stocking-glove areas are usually involved bilaterally, but symptoms and signs may be restricted to portions of the distal extremities (e.g., the toes, fingers, and soles of the feet). Deep, aching, constant pain may also be a manifestation of neuropathy. Brief jabs of pain may radiate down a limb into the fingers or toes. These pains are described as sharp, knifelike, or electric-like, and they often travel over a path 1 to 2 inches wide. Pains beginning in the foot or hand and shooting up the extremity may occur less frequently. Shooting pain may occur as a single event or in a series of jabs separated by seconds, minutes, or hours.

Myopathies and neuropathies, as well as radiculopathies and lower motor neuron disorders (e.g., amyotrophic lateral sclerosis), may cause mildly to severely painful muscle cramps in the extremities or on the trunk. Neuropathic pain may be constant, with superimposed lancinating pain, as described, or may consist only of shooting or jabbing pains. Paresthesias (e.g., tingling, prickling, and crawling sensations), annoying dysesthesias (e.g., coldness, burning, and painful prickling), and numbness may be present in or near the painful regions. There may be a subjective feeling of swelling and tightness of the feet or of walking on crushed glass or cotton. Mild-to-severe allodynia (pain produced by stroking the skin lightly) and hyperpathia may be present.

Two-point discrimination; light-touch, pinprick, pain, temperature, and vibration sensation; and proprioceptive sense may be uniformly or selectively impaired in the affected region. Muscle weakness, fasciculation, and wasting may occur in association with sensory complaints. Neuropathic pain is often worse at night and after cold exposure or use of the affected extremities. Pain, paresthesias, and dysesthesias may occur symmetrically or asymmetrically and may involve the lower or upper extremities predominantly or both equally. Some disorders (e.g., porphyria) involve the bathing trunk area. Polyneuropathy caused by the disorders discussed below may or may not always be painful. The prevalence of pain in most of these polyneuropathies has not been systematically studied. Table 48-3 lists important causes of acute painful polyneuropathy.

A. Arsenic Poisoning Symptoms of arsenic ingestion may begin within minutes or hours. Initially, a patient may note a metallic taste and the examiner a garlicky breath. Dry mouth and burning throat discomfort may occur. Severe, generalized, crampy abdominal pain associated with nausea, vomiting, and diarrhea soon begin. A plain radiograph of the abdomen taken at this time may show the presence of radiopaque arsenic in the stomach or intestine. Its appearance may be similar to that of an upper gastrointestinal series with barium. Gastrointestinal symptoms may last 2 to 3 days and are often attributed to intestinal flu.

Generalized extremity pain, headache, vertigo, and oliguria may develop. Liver toxicity may become apparent within 48 h, beginning with dark urine and jaundice and possibly resulting in a misdiagnosis of viral hepatitis. Levels of liver enzymes, such as serum alanine aminotrans-

Table 48-3
CAUSES OF ACUTE PAINFUL POLYNEUROPATHY

Diabetes mellitus
Insulinoma
Alcohol abuse and/or nutritional deficiencies
Hypothyroidism
Amyloidosis
Myeloma
Carcinoma
Drug-related (isoniazid, cis-platinum, gold, misonidazole, disulfiram, vincristine, nitrofurantoin, metronidazole, and hydralazine)
Infection-related (AIDS and Lyme disease)
Toxin-related (arsenic, mercury, thallium, and industrial chemicals)
Intermittent acute porphyria
Guillain-Barré syndrome
Waldenström's macroglobulinemia
Cryoglobulinemia
Fabry's disease
Sickle cell anemia
Vasculitis associated with polyarteritis nodosa, Churg-Strauss disease, systemic lupus erythematosus, hypersensitivity angiitis, or rheumatoid arthritis

ferase (ALT), and alkaline phosphatase, may be elevated in patients without jaundice. The urine may contain increased numbers of red blood cells and protein. Sweating, lacrimation, and salivation may be increased.

Vasodilation and capillary leakage may lead to hypotension, irreversible circulatory failure, and death during the first 24 to 48 h. Arsenic is toxic to the myocardium and can cause such electrocardiographic abnormalities as a widened QT interval and ST segment prolongation. Cardiac arrhythmias, such as ventricular tachycardia and torsades de pointes, may occur.

Encephalopathy due to cerebral edema and arsenic effects on the central nervous system may ensue. Delirium, confusion, uncooperative and combative behavior, and psychoses have been reported.

Erythematous maculopapular or vesicular rashes may occur during the first week after ingestion. Diffuse skin pigmentation may follow within 3 to 8 weeks, with palm and sole hyperkeratosis and desquamation. Fissuring and cracking of hyperkeratotic areas may be painful and are a common occurrence. Aldrich-Mees lines (i.e., transverse white bands on the nails) may be found after 4 to 6 weeks.

Numbness and paresthesias of the toes and fingers begin 1 to 3 weeks after the initial gastrointestinal complaints. These sensations may be accompanied by burning pain of the soles of the feet and shooting, stabbing pains in the forearms, hands, lower legs, and feet. The numbness may progress up the limbs, resulting in a stocking-glove distribution of sensory complaints. Distal motor loss is manifested by weakness of foot and hand muscles and foot- and/or wristdrop. In severe cases, proximal muscles may become weak. Severe allodynia and hyperpathia of the limbs may occur, such that gentle stroking or the wearing of clothing may cause intense discomfort in the affected areas.

Sensory loss is usually present and severely involves vibration and position sense (deep sensation), while light-touch, pinprick, and temperature sensation (superficial sensation) are variably impaired. An ascending paralysis mimicking the Guillain-Barré syndrome may occur in severe cases.

During the first 2 weeks, normochromic anemia, leukopenia, and thrombocytopenic purpura may develop, reflecting bone marrow toxicity. Leukocytosis, monocytosis, and eosinophilia have been described in a small percentage of cases.

The diagnosis can be confirmed by measuring arsenic concentrations in the blood and urine (normal, < 5 μg/day). Arsenic can also be measured in the hair and nails and in the ingested food or water.

Arsenic poisoning usually represents a recognized accidental or suicidal ingestion or a covert homicidal act. Other sources of poisoning have included contaminated well water, beer (the Staffordshire, England, beer epidemic), and moonshine whiskey and the burning of arsenate-treated wood. Industrial accidents may cause severe poisoning due to the inhalation of arsine gas. Chronic ingestion of me-

dicinals (i.e., Fowler's solution) containing arsenic has also had toxic effects.

The use of dimercaprol (British antilewisite [BAL]) may correct the bone marrow toxicity, but it is ineffective in preventing neuropathy unless it is started within 18 to 24 h of arsenic ingestion. Despite this fact, many physicians still treat established neuropathy with BAL in the hope of preventing further neural damage. The effectiveness of such an approach has not been proven. D-Penicillamine can also be used if dimercaprol cannot be tolerated. Arsine poisoning may require exchange transfusion and hemodialysis if renal failure occurs.

If homicidal poisoning is suspected, the police should be notified and a thorough investigation carried out. Some victims have been fatally poisoned after an initial, sublethal dose has led to illness and hospitalization. Other unexplained cases of arsenic poisoning should have a thorough epidemiologic investigation, since others at the same factory or in the community may be at risk.

B. Thallium Poisoning Accidental (grain impregnated with thallium), suicidal, or homicidal ingestion of thallium may occur. Toe and foot pain, paresthesias, and dysesthesias are associated with severe, generalized myalgias and arthralgias. A bilateral sensorimotor polyneuropathy occurs and may progress. Visual loss can result from optic neuritis. Sensory ataxia may occur. Alopecia beginning 3 weeks after the onset of neurologic complaints usually suggests the diagnosis. It can be confirmed by measurement of urinary thallium excretion. Severe poisoning is associated with a urinary excretion of 10 to 20 μg/day.

C. Acute Diabetic Polyneuropathy Patients with undiagnosed diabetes mellitus and those who are noncompliant in relation to dietary control and insulin usage may develop severe, burning and/or aching pain; paresthesias; and superimposed sharp, shooting, or lancinating pains in all extremities. Examination reveals only patchy sensory loss in the feet and sometimes allodynia. Polyuria, polydipsia, weight loss, postural dizziness, visual blurring, and drowsiness may be associated. Such patients have elevated blood sugar levels and may or may not be ketotic and acidotic. The limb pains respond within 1 to 10 weeks to insulin administration and dietary control.

D. Polyneuropathy with AIDS Patients with human immunodeficiency virus infection may develop a symmetrical, stocking-glove sensorimotor polyneuropathy, with limb pains and distal paresthesias and painful dysesthesias.

Mononeuropathy multiplex may occur, causing asymmetrical pain, paresthesias, and dysesthesias, with sensory and motor loss in the distribution of two or more peripheral nerves. These neuropathic lesions improve and resolve spontaneously or persist. Intravenous drug abusers and homosexuals are the major risk groups presenting with HIV-related neuropathies.

E. Intermittent Acute Porphyria   This disorder may initially present with abdominal pain. Flank, back, and limb pain may also be present. Anorexia, nausea, vomiting, and intense constipation are usually associated with the abdominal distress. The pain is usually generalized and may be constant or colicky. It may localize to a portion of the upper or the lower abdomen and can mimic acute surgical disorders, such as cholecystitis or appendicitis. The abdomen is only mildly tender, and guarding does not usually occur. Fever may occur as part of this disorder. Its occurrence should initiate a search for infection. Leukocytosis can occur and may often influence a surgeon to operate. Plain abdominal radiographs may reveal an ileus with dilated segments of the small and large bowel.

A moderate-to-severe peripheral neuropathy may accompany the abdominal pain. Numbness, paresthesias, and dysesthesias occur in a stocking-glove distribution. Sensory loss may follow this distribution or may involve the bathing trunk area and/or both thighs. The limb pain may be aching or burning, and there may be superimposed lancinating jabs of pain. Pain and light-touch sensation are the most severely impaired sensory modalities, while position sense and vibration may be spared. Motor weakness may be distal or proximal, or both portions of the limbs may be involved. Paraplegia or quadriplegia may occur, and diaphragmatic weakness may lead to respiratory insufficiency and death. Cranial nerve involvement may cause loss of vision (nerve II), diplopia (nerves III, IV, and VI), and dysphagia (nerves IX and X).

In addition to abdominal pain and a sensorimotor polyneuropathy, these patients may develop involvement of the central nervous system. This involvement may take the form of a delirium, with confusion and disorientation, or a depression. Some patients may have delusions and hallucinations and may mimic schizophrenia. Others may have neurotic complaints, hypochondriasis, or conversion reactions. Seizures of a grand mal type occur in 20 percent of cases and pose a problem as to drug management, since phenytoin may worsen porphyria. Bromides, magnesium sulfate, and diazepam have been used to control seizures without worsening the neurologic and abdominal symptoms.

Hyponatremia may occur and is usually secondary to inappropriate secretion of antidiuretic hormone. The urinalysis and routine blood chemistries are usually normal. Urine left at room temperature in sunlight may darken to a dark red-burgundy color due to nonenzymatic conversion of porphobilinogen (PBG) to the dark-brown compound porphobilin. A similar conversion can occur in the bladder, leading to excretion of a dark-red urine in a small percentage of cases. During attacks, the urine concentrations of PBG and delta-aminolevulinic acid (ALA) are elevated. False-negative test results for PBG in asymptomatic patients or carriers occur with a frequency of 20 to 30 percent. Results of qualitative screening tests, such as the Watson-

Schwartz or the Hoesch test, for PBG are usually positive in symptomatic patients.

If the concentration of PBG in the urine is found to be normal between attacks, this disorder can still be diagnosed by measuring the level of the red blood cell enzyme PBG deaminase (uroporphyrinogen I synthase). The red blood cell and lymphocyte contents of this enzyme are depressed in patients with symptomatic disease and in carriers. Familial studies have indicated a role for restriction fragment length polymorphism studies of the PBG deaminase gene for a more accurate diagnosis of the carrier state for intermittent acute porphyria.

Less than 20 percent of carriers have symptoms in the absence of such precipitants as drugs, starvation (e.g., severe dieting), alcohol, or endocrine factors (e.g., menstrual cycle). Abdominal pain is the most common manifestation of intermittent acute porphyria, while sensory and/or motor neuropathy occurs in 40 to 50 percent of cases. Seizures affect 10 to 20 percent, and behavioral disorders, emotional instability, psychoses, and neuroses occur in 30 to 40 percent. Most patients do not exhibit the triad of abdominal pain, neuropathy, and mental disturbances. Drugs that may precipitate an acute attack or worsen an attack include barbiturates, chlordiazepoxide, chloroquine, ergotamine, estrogens, griseofulvin, phenytoin, imipramine, methyldopa, sulfonamides, and oral contraceptives.

Therapy involves the use of analgesics and intravenous glucose to provide a high carbohydrate intake (400 g/day). Propranolol can counter the hypertension and tachycardia and may reverse abdominal complaints if used in high dosages. Intravenous hematin can be used to alter the course of the abdominal pain, neuropathy, and encephalopathy. Improvement begins in 48 to 72 h. Hematin may arrest a progressing neuropathy but it cannot usually correct an already established neuropathy. Death can occur from nervous system involvement, but the use of intravenous hematin and respiratory support with intubation and mechanical ventilation have improved the likelihood of survival.

F. Alcohol Abuse and/or Nutritional Deficiencies   Patients with a long history of alcoholism, poor nutrition, and numbness and paresthesias of the feet and ankle region may gradually or abruptly develop burning and aching pain in the feet and legs. Burning feet is a frequent complaint in this group of patients. Symptoms gradually respond to abstinence from alcohol and administration of B vitamin supplements.

G. Hypothyroidism   These patients may have generalized myalgias due to myopathy. Pain and paresthesias in the legs may also occur due to neuropathy. Pain and paresthesias in the hands may be caused by a carpal tunnel syndrome. Symptoms vanish with thyroid hormone replacement.

H. Renal Failure   Pain and paresthesias in the feet and lower legs, burning pain on the soles, and muscle cramps may be due to the polyneuropathy of renal failure. Symptoms resolve with hemodialysis or renal transplantation.

I. Malignancy   Aching pain, paresthesias, and dysesthesias occur in the distal portions of the arms and legs. Symptoms of neuropathy often antedate those of the associated tumor by months or years (e.g., 1–5 years). Severe sensory impairment may occur. Small-cell carcinoma of the lung is the most frequent cause, but gastrointestinal carcinomas, other carcinomas, and lymphomas may also be responsible.

J. Myeloma and POEMS Syndrome   The osteosclerotic form of myeloma accounts for less than 3 percent of all cases of myeloma. However, it is commonly (50–67 percent of cases) associated with a painful polyneuropathy. The POEMS syndrome (i.e., *p*olyneuropathy, *o*rganomegaly [hepatosplenomegaly], *e*ndocrinopathy, *M* protein, and *s*kin abnormality) is a variant of this form of myeloma. A plasmacytoma may also cause a painful polyneuropathy.

The painful polyneuropathies occurring with osteosclerotic myeloma are usually demyelinating and are associated with different monoclonal proteins and light chains than are osteolytic forms of myeloma. Polyneuropathy associated with plasmacytoma may respond to treatment of the underlying disease.

K. Cryoglobulinemias   Essential and secondary types of cryoglobulinemia may cause a painful polyneuropathy.

L. Guillain-Barré Syndrome   Patients with this syndrome develop ascending weakness or paralysis and sometimes proximal aching and/or burning pain. The CPK level may be elevated, suggesting associated myopathic changes.

M. Therapeutic Drugs   Isoniazid, disulfiram, *cis*-platinum, nitrofurantoin, gold, hydralazine, vincristine, misonidazole, and metronidazole may give rise to a painful polyneuropathy in some patients.

3. JOINT-RELATED PAIN

Polyarthralgias and polyarthritis are discussed more extensively in Chap. 50.

A. Polyarthralgias   Joint pains occur and are sometimes intensified or provoked by movement of the involved joints. There is no swelling, redness, or warmth of the overlying skin and no joint effusions. Clinical examination may be normal or reveal mild joint tenderness. Rheumatoid factor and antinuclear antibody assays on serum are negative, and results of joint radiographs are normal. The sedimentation rate may be normal or increased. A joint scintiscan with technetium 99m polyphosphate may reveal increased synovial uptake in symptomatic joints in up to 65 percent of such patients. Symptoms may respond to nonsteroidal anti-inflammatory drugs.

Patients with negative scintiscan results will probably not go on to develop an erosive, deforming arthritis but may still have significant disorders (e.g., systemic lupus erythematosus or polymyalgia rheumatica). Scans are useful, since they prevent misdiagnosis of patients with mild synovitis as having a functional disorder.

B. Psychogenic Rheumatism   Patients have polyarthralgias and myalgias, but there is no clinical, laboratory, or imaging evidence of synovitis or myositis. Results of all joint radiography and scintiscans are normal. Patients complain of joint pain but have no increase of pain on weight bearing or joint use. A subset of these patients may go on to develop significant joint and/or muscle disease, but most do not, and symptoms subside spontaneously.

4. MUSCLE-, JOINT-, AND/OR NERVE-RELATED PAIN

The disorders discussed in this section cause pain by involving joints, muscles, and/or nerves. Two or more of these tissues are involved in pain production.

A. Polyarteritis Nodosa   Mononeuropathy multiplex causes distal extremity pain of a deep, aching, or burning nature, associated with weakness, paresthesias, and painful dysesthesias. Two or more limbs are involved, and the symptoms may be asymmetrical in distribution (e.g., with one leg and foot and the opposite arm and hand involved). A symmetrical peripheral polyneuropathy may develop acutely or result from multiple episodes of peripheral nerve ischemia and infarction. Generalized myalgias are frequent, and they are usually not associated with significant weakness unless the muscle pain and tenderness are the results of an ischemic neuropathy. Joint pain and soreness without significant swelling are common and involve the knees and ankles most frequently. Arthralgia or arthritis accompanying polyarteritis is usually mild and of short duration.

Hypertension results from renal ischemia and/or infarction. Renal infarction may also cause flank and costovertebral angle pain and gross or microscopic hematuria. Glomerulitis is suggested by the presence of hematuria, red blood cell casts, proteinuria, and progressive renal failure.

Abdominal pain localized to the umbilical area may be due to bowel infarction, resulting in ileus and peritonitis. Right hypochondriac pain can result from ischemic injury of the gallbladder, and arteritis of the appendix can cause right iliac pain that can mimic acute appendicitis. Chest pain in the substernal area can result from coronary vasculitis, resulting in an acute myocardial infarction or coronary insufficiency. Chest pain that is intensified by a deep breath or lying flat in bed may be due to pericarditis.

Headache can result from cerebral arteritis or from subarachnoid bleeding. Such an event may be signaled by the sudden onset of a severe headache or worsening of a mild headache. Associated symptoms include a painful, stiff neck and photophobia. Seizures, hemiparesis, and aphasia can accompany headache in victims of this disorder.

Testicular pain or tenderness may occur with vasculitis of the testis. Finger or toe tip gangrene, and ecchymoses involving the upper arms and thighs or the trunk, may occur. Urticaria and erythema multiforme-like lesions may occur on the skin. Painful, subcutaneous nodules may also appear, persist, or regress. These nodules are 0.5 to 3 cm in size and can cause inflammation (redness and tenderness) or ulceration of the overlying skin. They usually occur along the course of small, subcutaneous arteries.

Fever, anorexia, weight loss, weakness, and malaise accompany the other, more local complaints. Leukocyte and platelet counts, sedimentation rate, liver enzyme levels, and creatinine levels may be elevated. Anemia, sometimes severe, is commonly present. The urine may contain increased numbers of red blood cells, casts, and an increased concentration of protein. The diagnosis depends on demonstrating periarteritis in muscle, testis, or some other site by biopsy. Biopsy of a painful, tender area in a muscle or testis provides a higher diagnostic yield than does blind biopsy of an asymptomatic region. Demonstration of medium or small renal or hepatic artery aneurysms by angiography can be used to support the diagnosis without biopsy. Survival rates have improved with combination cyclophosphamide-prednisone therapy.

Hepatitis B surface antigen (HB_sAg) may form part of the immune complexes deposited in the arterial walls in up to 30 percent of patients with polyarteritis nodosa. HB_sAg can be detected in the serum in 10 to 30 percent of cases.

Criteria for the diagnosis of polyarteritis nodosa are presented in Table 48-4.

Table 48-4
1990 AMERICAN COLLEGE OF RHEUMATOLOGY CRITERIA FOR THE CLASSIFICATION OF POLYARTERITIS NODOSA

Weight loss ≥4 kg
Livedo reticularis
Testicular pain or tenderness
Myalgias, weakness, or tenderness of leg muscles
Mononeuropathy or polyneuropathy
Diastolic blood pressure >90 mmHg
Elevated blood urea nitrogen or creatinine
HB_sAg in serum
Arteriographic abnormality showing aneurysms or occlusions of medium- and small-sized arteries
Biopsy of small- or medium-sized artery showing granulocytes or granulocytes and mononuclear cells in the arterial wall

Note: The diagnosis of polyarteritis nodosa is established, with a sensitivity of 82 percent and a specificity of 87 percent, if three or more of these criteria are present.

B. Allergic Angiitis and Granulomatosis (Churg-Strauss Disease) Patients have severe and often intractable asthma associated with transient pulmonary infiltrates and peripheral eosinophilia. There may be segmental or lobar areas of consolidation, or there may be pulmonary cavitation. Upper and lower lung fields may be equally involved. These patients also have generalized multisystem disease due to an arteritis that is similar or equivalent to that found with polyarteritis nodosa. Systemic symptoms such as fever, anorexia, weakness, weight loss, and malaise occur, as in classic polyarteritis nodosa, but renal involvement is less frequent and severe. Biopsy of involved tissue reveals distinctive findings that differ from those in polyarteritis nodosa (e.g., granulomatous arteritis and tissue infiltration by eosinophils are present in Chung-Strauss disease).

The associated arteritis may cause generalized myalgias and arthralgias or arthritis. It can also cause ischemic neuropathic pain associated with unpleasant dysesthesias. In addition, regional pain syndromes can involve the abdomen (e.g., bowel ischemia and pain, diarrhea, bowel or stomach ulceration with gastrointestinal bleeding, and intestinal obstruction), chest (e.g., myocardial ischemia, infarction, or pericarditis), and limbs, producing ischemic infarction of the digits (e.g., pain, gangrene, and ulceration).

C. Rheumatoid Arthritis and Vasculitis Vasculitic neuropathic changes can occur in patients with classical rheumatoid arthritis. Patients may have severe myalgias, a symmetrical sensorimotor polyneuropathy, and/or mononeuropathy multiplex. They also have severe arthritis, typical rheumatoid nodules, and a high titer of rheumatoid factor in the serum. In contrast, patients with polyarteritis nodosa have a mild and transient arthritis or only arthralgias, do not have rheumatoid nodules, and usually do not have positive serum test results for rheumatoid factor. Patients with rheumatoid arthritis and arteritis may develop extensive granulating ulcerations on one or both lower legs.

D. Systemic Lupus Erythematosus and Vasculitis Arthralgias and arthritis are usually symmetrical and most often involve the small joints of the fingers, metacarpophalangeal joints, wrists, and knees. The majority of patients with this disorder have arthralgias or arthritis. Up to 30 percent have symmetrical myalgias. Pleuritis and pericarditis may cause sharp, sticking chest pain that is intensified by a deep breath or a change in position (e.g., lying down increases pericardial pain). A butterfly facial rash, a discoid lupus rash, photosensitivity of the skin, and painful oral ulcers are common findings.

Renal involvement may take the form of the nephrotic syndrome, a nephritic syndrome, or rapidly progressive renal failure. The urine contains an increased concentration of protein and may contain red blood cells and granular casts.

There may be depression of leukocyte, red blood cell, and platelet counts. Antinuclear antibody is present, and speckled, homogeneous, or peripheral immunofluorescent staining patterns may occur. Positive LE cell tests occur in 80 percent and anti-ds-DNA antibodies are present in the majority of patients with active disease.

Neurologic involvement occurs, with grand mal or temporal lobe seizures. Mild dementia, manifested by impaired memory, poor judgment, and difficulty learning new information, occurs. A symmetrical peripheral sensory polyneuropathy with stocking-glove paresthesias, numbness, and pain may be present. Mononeuropathy multiplex, leading to extremity pain, dysesthesias, weakness, and hypesthesia in the region of distribution of two or more peripheral nerves, may occur.

Vasculitis should be treated with prednisone, combined with cyclophosphamide or azathioprine. A sensory polyneuropathy occurs in up to 15 percent of cases, while vasculitis and mononeuropathy multiplex occur in less than 5 percent of patients with systemic lupus erythematosus. Other manifestations of vasculitis include bowel infarction with abdominal pain, myocardial infarction with chest pain, and cerebral infarction with hemiparesis, aphasia, and seizures.

E. Behçet's Disease   Oral ulcers involving the buccal and lingual mucosa occur in crops and are painful. Ulcerations of the penis and scrotum are also usually tender and cause aching or stinging discomfort. Vaginal and labial ulcers may be painful, but they are often painless. Joint pain may involve one or both knees, ankles, wrists, or elbows, and actual arthritis may occur.

Abdominal pain, vomiting, diarrhea, passage of gross or occult blood, and increased flatus reflect ileal and colonic inflammation and ulceration. Eye pain and blurred vision may be due to an iritis or iridocyclitis. Recurrent hypopyon may occur, as may chorioretinitis. Skin involvement may take the form of an acute thrombophlebitis of a leg or arm or painful erythema nodosum of both legs. Acneform lesions may involve the face and upper trunk.

Meningoencephalitis, with headache and a painful, stiff neck, may develop. Vasculitis of the central nervous system, leading to paraplegia, hemiplegia, aphasia, or cerebellar ataxia and incoordination, can occur. Dementia and personality changes may also result from central nervous system involvement. Generalized myalgias may result from myositis, but this is an unusual symptom in this disease.

Behçet's disease should be considered in patients with mouth and genital pain from ulcers; eye redness and pain, and blurred vision; and a generalized symmetrical pattern of joint pain and arthritis. In addition, regional pain syndromes related to colon (e.g., lower abdominal pain and diarrhea) or skin involvement (e.g., tender, superficial phlebitis of the limbs and erythema nodosum of the legs) occur in some, but not all, patients. Pathergy of the skin occurs after a needle stick. The skin responds to such an injury by forming a papule or pustule at the puncture site. This finding is typical but not pathognomonic.

Oral, skin, eye, and genital lesions are considered major criteria for the diagnosis. A diagnosis of Behçet's disease requires the presence of lesions at all four sites. Involvement at fewer than four sites is classified as incomplete Behçet's disease.

Corticosteroids may ameliorate some symptoms. Cyclophosphamide, azathioprine, or chlorambucil may be used with corticosteroids for severe complications (e.g., nervous system or eye involvement).

F. Lyme Disease   This multisystem disorder has been reported in 43 states of the United States, but 97 percent of cases occur in the northeast (New England states to Maryland), the upper midwest (Wisconsin and Minnesota), and Pacific coastal regions (California, Oregon, Nevada, and Utah). It has also been reported from Europe.

There is usually a history of exposure by being in a brushy, wooded, or grassy area in an endemic county (i.e., a county in which at least two cases of Lyme disease have been acquired or in which a tick vector has been demonstrated to be infected with the etiologic agent, *Borrelia burgdorferi*) less than 30 days before the onset of erythema migrans.

Erythema migrans begins 3 to 30 days after an *Ixodes* tick bite. It occurs in 60 to 83 percent of cases. The lesion begins as a small, red papule or indurated macule at the location of the bite. This erythematous lesion then expands to form an annular, flat rash that results from central clearing. A red punctum or slightly larger macule remains at the site of the bite. The flat or slightly raised border migrates outward, reaching an average size of 15 cm (minimum acceptable size for diagnosis, ≥5 cm). Lesions as large as 68 cm have been reported. Erythema migrans is usually asymptomatic, but itching and burning pain, tenderness, hyperesthesia, and dysesthesia have been reported.

In more than 50 percent of cases, erythema migrans is accompanied by a febrile illness, with generalized myalgias; bone pain; arthralgias; headache; a painful, stiff neck; photophobia; fatigue; and malaise. Without therapy, erythema migrans fades within 1 month or more, leaving scaling or pigmentation as a residual finding. Antibiotic therapy leads to disappearance of the lesion in a few days. Variations in the appearance of erythema migrans include a homogeneous, erythematous patch without central clearing; a target lesion; or a lesion with central purpura, vesiculation, necrosis, and ulceration. Oval, triangular, and linear lesions may occur. Secondary annular lesions occur in 6 to 48 percent of cases at the site of a faded primary lesion or at distant sites (satellite lesions). Secondary erythema migrans lesions are usually smaller, migrate less, and do not have a firm center.

Early disseminated infection begins weeks to months after the rash. Up to 15 percent of patients develop involvement of the nervous system. Headache; a painful, stiff neck; nausea; vomiting; and irritability represent an acute meningitis. Sleep disturbances, impaired memory and concentration, emotional lability, chorea, irritability, and fibromyalgia are caused by encephalitis. Up to 50 percent of patients with meningeal symptoms develop unilateral or, less commonly, bilateral seventh nerve paralysis (Bell's palsy). Diplopia may result from involvement of the oculomotor or abducens nerves.

Sensory or sensorimotor radiculopathies, plexopathies, or peripheral neuropathies may cause limb pain, paresthesias, painful dysesthesias, numbness, and weakness. Mononeuropathy multiplex, transverse myelitis, cerebellar ataxia, and a Guillain-Barré neuropathy have been described in a few patients.

Cerebrospinal fluid findings include a normal pressure, lymphocytic pleocytosis, an elevated protein level, a normal glucose level, and an increase in the IgM, and sometimes the IgG, index for *B. burgdorferi* antibodies. The antibody index is not always positive in the presence of central nervous system disease. Rarely, *B. burgdorferi* may be cultured from the cerebrospinal fluid.

Musculoskeletal symptoms consist of myalgias, arthralgias, and bone, tendon, and bursal pain. Up to 60 percent of untreated patients develop articular inflammation weeks or months after the onset of erythema migrans. Early symptoms are intermittent. Most common is a recurrent, monarticular or oligoarticular arthritis involving the larger joints. Pain, swelling, and warmth of the overlying skin occur, but ambulation remains relatively unimpaired despite lower extremity involvement. Less commonly, a seronegative rheumatoid arthritis-like polyarthritis occurs, affecting large and small joints. Arthritic episodes may last 1 to 12 weeks, with symptom-free periods of 1 to 4 weeks. The knee is most frequently affected, and pseudothrombophlebitis from a ruptured or dissecting Baker's cyst may occur. Rarely, fever, joint pain, swelling, and heat mimic septic arthritis. In up to 10 percent of cases with intermittent arthritis, a persistent erosive arthritis develops, which eventually makes ambulation painful and difficult.

Cardiac involvement is a late manifestation and occurs in 8 percent of untreated cases. It occurs weeks or months after onset. Dizziness, fainting, dyspnea, and central chest pain are the predominant complaints. A pericardial friction rub, rhythm disturbances, and an S3 gallop may be observed. The major electrocardiographic abnormality is a variable degree of atrioventricular block. Myocarditis is the cause of the clinical and electrocardiographic findings.

Laboratory confirmation of the disease involves measurement of serum antibody to whole-organism antigens. An ELISA is used in most clinical laboratories. IgM antibody develops within 2 to 4 weeks and declines by 4 to 6 months. IgG antibody appears within 6 to 8 weeks and persists in patients with continued infection.

Serologic tests for Lyme disease (e.g., ELISA) are not standardized, and various laboratories report varying sensitivities and specificities. The same sample sent to several laboratories may yield different qualitative and/or quantitative results. True seronegativity is rare in patients with clinical manifestations of disseminated or chronic Lyme disease. Antibody responses may be delayed for months in some cases. True-positive results may be differentiated from false-positive results by Western blotting. The latter may remain falsely negative for months, until antibodies to outer-surface proteins (OspA and OspB) appear.

The specificity of serologic tests varies with the pretest probability of Lyme disease. Routine use of the test without regard for clinical findings increases the false-positive rate. False-positive results have been reported in infectious mononucleosis, rheumatoid arthritis, systemic lupus erythematosus, periodontal disease, and syphilis.

Serologic testing is useful in patients living in or recently visiting an endemic area, who develop a systemic illness without erythema migrans, or who develop arthritic, neurologic, or cardiac disease compatible with *B. burgdorferi* infection. A true-positive test means only previous immunologic exposure and may have no relationship to current patient complaints.

The sedimentation rate may be normal in 50 percent of patients with symptoms. If serum IgM levels are elevated, serial measurements of the IgM level provide an indicator of disease activity. Mild anemia, slight leukocytosis, an elevated serum AST level, and microhematuria and proteinuria may occur. Serum C3 and C4 levels are normal. Antinuclear antibody and rheumatoid factor titers are usually normal in adults.

Early Lyme disease responds to amoxicillin or doxycycline, administered orally for 10 to 21 days. Disseminated or late disease (e.g., neurologic disorder; arthritis; or carditis) responds to ceftriaxone therapy.

G. Polymyalgia Rheumatica with or without Granulomatous Arteritis This disorder is rare before age 50 and has a mean age of onset of 70 years. The incidence is twice as great in women as in men. Systemic symptoms include low-grade fever, anorexia, weakness, weight loss, lassitude, apathy, and malaise. These complaints usually precede rheumatic manifestations.

Severe arthralgias and myalgias involve the shoulders and/or hips initially. Unilateral shoulder or hip girdle pain soon becomes bilateral. The involved muscles and joints ache and are tender, and movement or use intensifies the pain. Myalgias may involve the neck, upper back, shoulders, upper arms, low back, hips, and thighs. Rising from a chair, getting out of an automobile, or putting on a coat unassisted becomes difficult or impossible because of pain and paresis. Gelling is severe, and morning stiffness a persistent and prominent complaint. Muscle tenderness is present in the trapezius and other neck muscles, and in the hip girdle and thigh muscles. Synovitis may occur in one or both knees, with a joint effusion, and local tenderness. Knee pain may occur at rest or with weight bearing or may only be provoked by range-of-motion testing.

The erythrocyte sedimentation rate is elevated and often exceeds 100 mm/h. A normochromic normocytic anemia may occur, and the platelet count may be increased. The leukocyte and differential counts are usually normal. Liver function test abnormalities occur in up to 30 percent of cases (e.g., elevated alkaline phosphatase and AST levels). Granulomatous hepatitis may sometimes be seen on liver biopsy. Muscle enzyme levels and biopsies are usually normal. Synovial fluid analysis reveals an inflammatory-type fluid ($1-20 \times 10^9$ cells/liter). The synovial fluid mucin clot is poor, but complement levels are normal. Synovial biopsy reveals a mild lymphocytic synovitis. Polymyalgia rheumatica responds dramatically to low doses of prednisone (10–15 mg/day). Symptoms and signs rapidly vanish. Polymyalgia rheumatica may be associated with granulomatous arteritis (15 percent of cases are temporal artery biopsy-positive). Symptoms of this disorder include temporal or occipital headache and scalp tenderness, jaw claudication, and abrupt partial or complete loss of vision in one or both eyes. This disorder responds to high doses of prednisone (40–60 mg/day).

H. Mimics of Polymyalgia Rheumatica

1. Secondary Polymyalgia Rheumatica   A similar disorder may occur secondary to an underlying neoplasm (e.g., breast or gastrointestinal tract) or infection (e.g., subacute bacterial endocarditis). The response to corticosteroids may initially suppress symptoms, but relapse or breakthrough commonly occurs with passage of time. Endocarditis may reveal itself on examination by the presence of a heart murmur, petechiae, splinter hemorrhages, Roth's or cotton-wool spots in the retina, microhematuria, and positive blood culture results.

2. Seronegative Rheumatoid Arthritis   This disorder may appear to be similar to polymyalgia rheumatica and may not be separable by clinical and laboratory findings. Manifestations of seronegative rheumatoid arthritis in elderly people that result in difficulty in differentiating it from polymyalgia rheumatica include proximal myalgias, more involvement of proximal joints, acute onset, a lower prevalence of seropositivity, and less evidence of erosive disease. Four of the American College of Rheumatology criteria for the diagnosis of rheumatoid arthritis (morning stiffness, arthritis at three or more sites, sym-

metrical joint involvement, and involvement of one hand or wrist joint) would be satisfied by many patients now labeled as having polymyalgia rheumatica. Seropositive rheumatoid arthritis is associated with the HLA-DR4 gene (subtypes DW4 and DW14), while polymyalgia rheumatica and seronegative rheumatoid arthritis are not.

3. Collagen Vascular Disorders with Polymyalgia Rheumatica-like Symptoms   Polymyalgia-like symptoms may occur in early systemic lupus erythematosus, polymyositis, Sjögren's syndrome, and in various forms of necrotizing systemic vasculitis. In the latter disorders, demonstration of vasculitis by biopsy may be required. The presence of antineutrophil cytoplasmic antibodies (ANCA) may be of aid in the diagnosis of some forms of vasculitis.

I. Pseudolupus due to HIV Infection   A malar, erythematous rash can occur in HIV-infected patients due to seborrheic dermatitis. HIV-positive patients may also have arthralgias and arthritis; nephritis (i.e., with albuminuria, cylindruria, an elevated serum creatinine, and intraglomerular immune deposits); hematologic changes (thrombocytopenia, leukopenia, lymphopenia, neutropenia, and hemolytic anemic [Coombs-positive]); neurologic disease (headaches, seizures, dementia, symmetrical peripheral neuropathy, mononeuropathy multiplex, myelopathy, and progressive multifocal encephalopathy); Sjögren's syndrome involving the eyes; vasculitis; systemic symptoms (fever, lymphadenopathy, and weight loss); and immunologic abnormalities (antinuclear antibodies, lupus anticoagulant, anticardiolipin antibodies, circulating immune complexes, and rheumatoid factor). An HIV-infected patient may satisfy five or more of the American Rheumatism Association criteria for the diagnosis of systemic lupus erythematosus.

Rarely, patients with both HIV infection and systemic lupus erythematosus have been reported. Some patients with HIV-related rheumatologic and immunologic manifestations have been incorrectly diagnosed as having Sjögren's syndrome or systemic lupus erythematosus. HIV infection should be excluded in patients with one or more of the described clinical and/or laboratory findings that may occur in both systemic lupus erythematosus and AIDS.

GENERALIZED PAIN REFERENCES

Bone Disease

Coburn JW, Norris KC: Diagnosis of aluminum-related bone disease and treatment of aluminum toxicity with deferoxamine. *Semin Nephrol* 6(suppl 1):12–21, 1986.

Coburn JW, Norris KC, Nebeker HG: Osteomalacia and bone disease arising from aluminum. *Semin Nephrol* 6:66–89, 1986.

Cushner HM, Adams ND: Review: Renal osteodystrophy: Pathogenesis and treatment. *Am J Med Sci* 4:264–275, 1986.

Fukumoto Y, Tarui S, Tsukiyama K, et al: Tumor-induced vitamin D-resistant hypophosphatemic osteomalacia associated with proximal renal tubular dysfunction and 1,25-dihydroxyvitamin D deficiency. *J Clin Endocrinol Metab* 49:873–878, 1979.

Greditzer HG III, McLeod RA, Unni KK, et al: Bone sarcomas in Paget disease. *Radiology* 146:327–333, 1983.

Hadjipavlou A, Lander P, Srolovitz H: Pagetic arthritis: Pathophysiology and management. *Clin Orthop* 208:15–19, 1986.

Kaplan FS, Soriano S, Fallon MD, et al: Osteomalacia in a night nurse. *Clin Orthop* 205:216–221, 1986.

Malee MP: Multiple myeloma in pregnancy: A case report. *Obstet Gynecol* 75:513–515, 1990.

McGuire MH, Merenda JT, Etzkorn JR, et al: Oncogenic osteomalacia: A case report. *Clin Orthop* 244:305–308, 1989.

Merkow RL, Lane JM: Paget's disease of bone. *Orthop Clin North Am* 21:171–189, 1990.

Middleton S, Rowntree C, Rudge S: Bone pain as the presenting manifestation of secondary syphilis. *Ann Rheum Dis* 49:641–642, 1990.

Nebeker HG, Coburn JW: Aluminum and renal osteodystrophy. *Annu Rev Med* 37:79–95, 1986.

Nuovo MA, Dorfman HD, Sun C-CJ, et al: Tumor-induced osteomalacia and rickets. *Am J Surg Pathol* 13:588–599, 1989.

Parker MS, Klein I, Haussler MR, et al: Tumor-induced osteomalacia: Evidence of a surgically correctable alteration in vitamin D metabolism. *JAMA* 245:492–493, 1981.

Quarles LD, Gitelman HJ, Drezner MK: Aluminum: Culprit or accessory in the genesis of renal osteodystrophy. *Semin Nephrol* 6:90–101, 1986.

Renal osteodystrophy. Coburn, JW, principal discussant. *Kidney Int* 17:677–693, 1980.

Seret P. Basle MF, Rebel A, et al: Sarcomatous degeneration in Paget's bone disease. *J Cancer Res Clin Oncol* 113:392–399, 1987.

Sudhaker D, Parfitt AM, Villanueva AR, et al: Hypophosphatemic osteomalacia and adult Fanconi syndrome due to light-chain nephropathy: Another form of oncogenous osteomalacia. *Am J Med* 82:333–338, 1987.

Tzamaloukas AH: Diagnosis and management of bone disorders in chronic renal failure and dialyzed patients. *Med Clin North Am* 74:961–974, 1990.

Wallach S: Chronic joint pain: Arthritis or osteitis? *Hosp Pract* 20:29–39, 1985.

Eosinophilia-Myalgia Syndrome and Mimics

Dicker RM, James N, Cunha BA: The eosinophilia-myalgia syndrome with neuritis associated with L-tryptophan use. *Ann Intern Med* 112:957–958, 1990.

Fang MA, Verity A, Paulus HE: Subacute perimyositis. *J Rheumatol* 15:1291–1293, 1988.

Gibbons RB, Metzger JR: Eosinophilia-myalgia syndrome: Recognition of a distinct clinicopathologic entity. *Arch Intern Med* 150:2175–2177, 1990.

Kazura JW: Eosinophilia-myalgia syndrome: Unresolved questions *Cleveland Clin J Med* 57:415–416, 1990.

Lakhanpal S, Duffy J, Engel AG: Eosinophilia associated with perimyositis and pneumonitis. *Mayo Clin Proc* 63:37–41, 1988.

Martin RW, Duffy J, Engel AG, et al: The clinical spectrum of the eosinophilia-myalgia syndrome associated with L-tryptophan ingestion: Clinical features in 20 patients and aspects of pathophysiology. *Ann Intern Med* 113:124–134, 1990.

Strongwater SL, Woda BA, Yood RA, et al: Eosinophilia-myalgia syndrome associated with L-tryptophan ingestion: Analysis of four patients and implications for differential diagnosis and pathogenesis. *Arch Intern Med* 150:2178–2186, 1990.

Varga J, Vitto J, Jimenez: The cause and pathogenesis of the eosinophilia—myalgia syndrome. *Ann Intern Med* 116:140–147, 1992.

Verity MA, Bulpitt KJ, Paulus HE: Neuromuscular manifestations of L-tryptophan—associated eosinophilia-myalgia syndrome: A histomorphologic analysis of 14 patients. *Hum Pathol* 22:3–11, 1991.

Fibromyalgia

Alfici S, Sigal M, Landau M: Primary fibromyalgia syndrome: A variant of depressive disorder? *Psychother Psychosom* 51:156–161, 1989.

Bengtsson A, Henriksson KG: The muscle in fibromyalgia: A review of Swedish studies. *J Rheumatol* 16(suppl 19):144–149, 1989.

Bennett RM: Confounding features of the fibromyalgia syndrome: A current perspective of differential diagnosis. *J Rheumatol* 16(suppl 19):58–61, 1989.

———:Current issues concerning management of the fibrositis/fibromyalgia syndrome. *Am J Med* 81(suppl 3A):15–18, 1986.

Boulware DW, Schmid LD, Baron M: The fibromyalgia syndrome: Could you recognize and treat it? *Postgrad Med* 87:211–214, 1990.

Buckelew SP: Fibromyalgia: A rehabilitation approach–a review. *Am J Phys Med Rehabil* 68:37–42, 1989.

Calabrese LH, Mitsumoto H, Chou SM: Inclusion body myositis presenting as treatment-resistant polymyositis. *Arthritis Rheum* 30:397–403, 1987.

Campbell SM: Is the tender point concept valid? *Am J Med* 81(suppl 3A):33–37, 1986.

Campbell SM, Bennett RM: Fibrositis. *Dis Mon* 32:653–722, 1986.

Dinerman H, Goldenberg DL, Felson DT: A prospective evaluation of 118 patients with the fibromyalgia syndrome: Prevalence of Raynaud's phenomenon, sicca symptoms, ANA, low complement, and Ig deposition at the dermal-epidermal junction. *J Rheumatol* 13:368–373, 1986.

Fischer AA: Pressure tolerance over muscles and bones in normal subjects. *Arch Phys Med Rehabil* 67:406–409, 1986.

Gatter RA: Pharmacotherapeutics in fibrositis. *Am J Med* 81(suppl 3A):63–66, 1986.

Goldenberg DL: Fibromyalgia syndrome: An emerging but controversial condition. *JAMA* 257:2782–2787, 1987.

———:Psychological symptoms and psychiatric diagnosis in patients with fibromyalgia. *J Rheumatol* 16(suppl 19):127–130, 1989.

———:Psychologic studies in fibrositis. *Am J Med* 81(suppl 3A):67–70, 1986.

———:A review of the role of tricyclic medications in the treatment of fibromyalgia syndrome. *J Rheumatol* 16(suppl 19):137–139, 1989.

Gupta MA, Moldofsky H: Dysthymic disorder and rheumatic pain modulation disorder (fibrositis syndrome): A comparison of symptoms and sleep physiology. *Can J Psychiatry* 31:608–616, 1986.

Hadler NM: A critical reappraisal of the fibrositis concept. *Am J Med* 81(suppl 3A):26–30, 1986.

Hartz A, Kirchdoerfer E: Undetected fibrositis in primary care practice. *J Fam Pract* 25:365–369, 1987.

Hench PK: Evaluation and differential diagnosis of fibromyalgia: Approach to diagnosis and management. *Rheum Dis Clin North Am* 15:19–29, 1989.

———:Secondary fibrositis. *Am J Med* 81(suppl 3A):60–62, 1986.

Hench PK, Mitler MM: Fibromyalgia: 1. Review of a common rheumatologic syndrome. *Postgrad Med* 80:47–50, 52–53, 55–56, 1986.

———:Fibromyalgia: 2. Management guidelines and research findings. *Postgrad Med* 80:57–64, 1986.

McCain GA: Role of physical fitness training in the fibrositis/fibromyalgia syndrome. *Am J Med* 81(suppl 3A):73–77, 1986.

Moldofsky H: Sleep and musculoskeletal pain. *Am J Med* 81(suppl 3A):85–89, 1986.

Molony RR, MacPeek DM, Schiffman PL, et al: Sleep, sleep apnea and the fibromyalgia syndrome. *J Rheumatol* 13:797–800, 1986.

Müller W: The fibrositis syndrome: Diagnosis, differential diagnosis and pathogenesis. *Scand J Rheumatol* (suppl 65):40–53, 1987.

Reilly PA, Littlejohn GO: Current thinking on fibromyalgia syndrome. *Aust Fam Phys* 19:1505–1506, 1508, 1511–1512, 1516, 1990.

Rice JR: "Fibrositis" syndrome. *Med Clin North Am* 70:455–468, 1986.

Rogers, EJ, Rogers R: Fibromyalgia and myofascial pain: Either, neither, or both? *Orthop Rev* 18:1217–1224, 1989.

Rollman GB: Measurement of pain in fibromyalgia in the clinic and laboratory. *J Rheumatol* 16(suppl 19):113–119, 1989.

Simms RW, Goldenberg DL, Felson DT, et al: Tenderness in 75 anatomic sites: Distinguishing fibromyalgia patients from controls. *Arthritis Rheum* 31:182–187, 1988.

Smythe H: Fibrositis syndrome: A historical perspective. *J Rheumatol* 16(suppl 19):2–6, 1989.

————:Referred pain and tender points. *Am J Med* 81(suppl 3A):90–92, 1986.

————:Tender points: Evolution of concepts of the fibrositis/fibromyalgia syndrome. *Am J Med* 81(suppl 3A):2–6, 1986.

Truta MP, Santucci ET: Head and neck fibromyalgia and temporomandibular arthralgia. *Otolaryngol Clin North Am* 22:1159–1171, 1989.

Tunks, E, Crook J, Norman G, et al: Tender points in fibromyalgia. *Pain* 34:11–19, 1988.

Turk DC, Flor H: Primary fibromyalgia is greater than tender points: Toward a multiaxial taxonomy. *J Rheumatol* 16(suppl 19):80–86, 1989.

Wolfe F: The clinical syndrome of fibrositis. *Am J Med* 81(suppl 3A):7–14, 1986.

————:Development of criteria for the diagnosis of fibrositis. *Am J Med* 81(suppl 3A):99–104, 1986.

————:Fibromyalgia: The clinical syndrome. *Rheum Dis Clin North Am* 15:1–18, 1989.

Yunus MB, Kalyan-Raman UP, Kalyan-Ran K, et al: Pathologic changes in muscle in primary fibromyalgia syndrome. *Am J Med* 81(suppl 3A):38–42, 1986.

Lyme Disease

Duffy J: Lyme disease. *Infectious Dis Clin North Am* 1:511–527, 1987.

Kovanen J, Schauman K, Valpas J: Bannwarth's syndrome and Lyme disease in Finland. *Scand J Infect Dis* 18:421–424, 1986.

Malane MS, Grant-Kels JM, Feder HM Jr, et al: Diagnosis of Lyme disease based on dermatologic manifestations. *Ann Intern Med* 114:490–498, 1991.

Rahn DW, Malawista SE: Lyme disease: Recommendations for diagnosis and treatment. *Ann Intern Med* 114:472–481, 1991.

Sigal LH: Summary of the first 100 patients seen at a Lyme disease referral center. *Am J Med* 88:577–581, 1990.

Metabolic Myopathies

Byrne E: Chronic myalgia, a personal approach. *Aust N Z J Med* 16:745–748, 1986.

Elliot DL, Buist NRM, Goldberg L, et al: Metabolic myopathies: Evaluation by graded exercise testing. *Medicine* 68:163–172, 1989.

Gospe SM Jr, Lazaro RP, Lava NS, et al: Familial X-linked myalgia and cramps: A nonprogressive myopathy associated with a deletion in the dystrophin gene. *Neurology* 39:1277–1280, 1989.

Hers H-G, Van Hoff F, Barsy Tde: Glycogen storage diseases, in Scriver CR, Beavdet AL, Sly W, et al (eds): *The Metabolic Basis of Inherited Disease.* New York, McGraw-Hill, 1989, vol 1, pp 443–444.

Mendell JR, Griggs RC: Muscular dystrophy: Disorders of muscle energy metabolism, in Wilson JD, Braunwald E, Isselbacher KJ, et al (eds): *Harrison's Principles of Internal Medicine,* 12th ed. New York, McGraw-Hill, 1991, vol 2, pp 2112–2118.

Myalgias—Chronic Fatigue Syndrome

Bryan CS: Managing chronic fatigue syndrome: What's practical and what isn't. *Consultant* 32:33–40, 1992.

Buchwald D, Cheney PR, Peterson DL, et al: A chronic illness characterized by fatigue, neurologic and immunologic disorders, and active human herpesvirus type 6 infection. *Ann Intern Med* 116:103–113, 1992.

Myalgias—Drug-Associated

Carmichael AJ, Martin AM: Acute painful proximal myopathy associated with nalidixic acid. *BMJ* 297:742, 1988.

Esplin DW, Zablocka-Esplin B: Central nervous system stimulants: 1. Strychnine, in Goodman LS, Gilman A (eds): *The Pharmacologic Basis of Therapeutics,* 4th ed. London, Macmillan, 1970, pp 348–350.

Halla JT, Fallahi S, Koopman WJ: Penicillamine-induced myositis: Observations and unique features in two patients and review of the literature. *Am J Med* 77:719–722, 1984.

Knodel LC, Talbert RL: Adverse effects of hypolipidaemic drugs. *Med Toxicol* 2·10–32, 1987.

Litin SC, Anderson CF: Nicotinic acid-associated myopathy: A report of three cases. *Am J Med* 86:481–483, 1989.

Myalgias—Endocrine Disorders

Mor F, Green P, Wysenbeek AJ: Myopathy in Addison's disease. *Ann Rheum Dis* 46:81–83, 1987.

Roy EP III, Gutmann L: Myalgia. *Neurol Clin* 6:621–636, 1988.

Shapiro MS, Trebich C, Shilo L, et al: Myalgias and muscle contractures as the presenting signs of Addison's disease. *Postgrad Med J* 64:222–223, 1988.

Turken SA, Cafferty M, Silverberg SJ, et al: Neuromuscular involvement in mild, asymptomatic primary hyperparathyroidism. *Am J Med* 87:553–557, 1989.

Myalgias—Infection-Related

Byrne E: Idiopathic chronic fatigue and myalgia syndrome (myalgic encephalomyelitis): Some thoughts on nomenclature and aetiology. *Med J Aust* 148:80–82, 1988.

Gaines H, von Sydow M, Pehrson PO, et al: Clinical pictures of primary HIV infection presenting as a glandular-fever-like illness. *BMJ* 297:1363–1368, 1988.

Hierholzer JC, Stewart JA, Himmelwright JP, et al: Herpes type 2 infection with unusual generalised manifestations and delayed diagnosis in an adult male. *J Infect* 6:187–192, 1983.

Pun KK, Wong WT, Wong PHC: The first documented outbreak of trichinellosis in Hong Kong Chinese. *Am J Trop Med Hyg* 32:772–775, 1983.

Sawyer LA, Fishbein DB, McDade JE: Q fever: Current concepts. *Rev Infect Dis* 9:935–946, 1987.

Myalgic Pain—Envenomation

Theakston RDG, Phillips RE, Warrell DA, et al: Envenoming by the common trait *(Bungarus caeruleus)* and Sri Lankan cobra *(Naja naja naja):* Efficacy and complications of therapy with Haffkine antivenom. *Trans R Soc Trop Med Hyg* 84:301–308, 1990.

Myofascial Pain

Fischer AA: Documentation of myofascial trigger points. *Arch Phys Med Rehabil* 69:286–291, 1988.

Skootsky SA, Jaeger B, Oye RK: Prevalence of myofascial pain in general internal medicine practice. *West J Med* 151:157–160, 1989.

Myopathy—Sarcoidosis

Heck AW, Phillips LH II: Sarcoidosis and the nervous system. *Neurol Clin* 7:641–654, 1989.

Wolfe SM, Pinals RS, Aelion JA, et al: Myopathy in sarcoidosis: Clinical and pathologic study of four cases and review of the literature. *Semin Arthritis Rheum* 16:300–306, 1987.

Pain and Malignancy

Gildenberg PL: Myelotomy and percutaneous cervical cordotomy for the treatment of cancer pain. *Appl Neurophysiol* 47:208–215, 1984.

Patchell RA, Posner JB: Neurologic complications of systemic cancer. *Neurol Clin* 3:729–750, 1985.

Polymyalgia Rheumatica

Bennett RM: Confounding features of the fibromyalgia syndrome: A current perspective of differential diagnosis. *J Rheumatol* 16(suppl 19):58–61, 1989.

Cohen MD, Ginsburg WW: Polymyalgia rheumatica. *Rheum Dis Clin North Am* 16:325–329, 1990.

Davison S, Spiera H: Polymyalgia rheumatica. *Clin Orthop* 57:95–99, 1968.

Ehrlich GE: Diagnosis and management of rheumatic diseases in older patients. *J Am Geriatr Soc* 30(suppl 11):S45–S51, 1982.

Espinoza LR, Vidal L, Pastor C: Diagnosis and management of polymyalgia rheumatica. *Compr Ther* 12:19–23, 1986.

Manolios N, Schrieber L: Polymyalgia rheumatica. *Aust Fam Phys* 15:1298–1300, 1986.

Stander PE: Polymyalgia rheumatica: Clinical features and management. *Postgrad Med* 86:131–133,136,138, 1989.

Polymyalgia Rheumatica and Giant Cell Arteritis

Andersson R, Malmvall B-E, Bengtsson B-A: Long-term survival in giant cell arteritis including temporal arteritis and polymyalgia rheumatica: A follow-up study of 90 patients treated with corticosteroids. *Acta Med Scand* 220:361–364, 1986.

Boesen P, Sørensen SF: Giant cell arteritis, temporal arteritis, and polymyalgia rheumatica in a Danish county: A prospective investigation, 1982–1985. *Arthritis Rheum* 30:294–299, 1987.

Dasgupta B, Duke O, Kyle V, et al: Antibodies to intermediate filaments in polymyalgia rheumatica and giant cell arteritis: A sequential study. *Ann Rheum Dis* 46:746–749, 1987.

Ettlinger RE, Hunder GG, Ward LE: Polymyalgia rheumatica and giant cell arteritis. *Ann Rev Med* 29:15–22, 1978.

Golbus J, McCune WJ: Giant cell arteritis and peripheral neuropathy: A report of 2 cases and review of the literature. *J Rheumatol* 14:129–134, 1987.

Larson TS, Hall S, Hepper NGG, et al: Respiratory tract symptoms as a clue to giant cell arteritis. *Ann Intern Med* 101:594–597, 1984.

Nuessle WF, Miller HE, Norman FC: Polymyalgia rheumatica, giant-cell arteritis and blindness: A review and case report. *J Am Geriatr Soc* 14:566–577, 1966.

Smith AJ, Kyle V, Cawston TE, et al: Isolation and analysis of immune complexes from sera of patients with polymyalgia rheumatica and giant cell arteritis. *Ann Rheum Dis* 46:468–474, 1987.

Polymyositis/Dermatomyositis — Idiopathic

Bradley WG: Inflammatory diseases of muscle, in Kelley WN, Harris ED Jr, Ruddy S, et al (eds): *Textbook of Rheumatology*. Philadelphia, Saunders, 1981, vol 2, pp 1255–1276.

Bradley WG, Tandan R: Dermatomyositis and polymyositis, in Wilson JD, Braunwald E, Isselbacher KJ, et al (eds): *Harrison's Principles of Internal Medicine,* 12th ed. New York, McGraw-Hill, 1991, vol 2, pp 2108–2111.

Edwards RHT, Round JM, Jones DA: Needle biopsy of skeletal muscle: A review of 10 years experience. *Muscle Nerve* 6:676–683, 1983.

Hochberg MC, Feldman D, Stevens MB: Adult onset polymyositis/dermatomyositis: An analysis of clinical and laboratory features and survival in 76 patients with a review of the literature. *Semin Arthritis Rheum* 15:168–178, 1986.

Kagen LJ: Polymyositis/dermatomyositis, in McCarty DJ (ed): *Arthritis and Allied Conditions: A Textbook of Rheumatology,* 11th ed. Philadelphia, Lea & Febiger, 1989, pp 1092–1117.

Mastaglia FL, Ojeda VJ: Inflammatory myopathies: 1. *Ann Neurol* 17:215–227, 1985.

Rhoades DW, Pascucci RA: Cardiac involvement in polymyositis: Report of case and review of literature. *J Am Osteopath Assoc* 87:310–313, 1987.

Strongwater SL, Annesley T, Schnitzer TJ: Myocardial involvement in polymyositis. *J Rheumatol* 10:459–463, 1983.

Tymms KE, Webb J: Dermatopolymyositis and other connective tissue diseases: A review of 105 cases. *J Rheumatol* 12:1140–1148, 1985.

Polymyositis/Dermatomyositis and Neoplasia

Dowsett RJ, Wong RL, Robert NJ, et al: Dermatomyositis and Hodgkin's disease: Case report and review of the literature. *Am J Med* 80:719–723, 1986.

Peters WA III, Andersen WA, Thornton WN Jr: Dermatomyositis and coexistent ovarian cancer: A review of the compounding clinical problems. *Gynecol Oncol* 15:440–446, 1983.

Polymyositis and Toxoplasmosis

Adams EM, Hafez GR, Carnes M, et al: The development of polymyositis in a patient with toxoplasmosis: Clinical and pathologic findings and review of literature. *Clin Exp Rheumatol* 2:205–208, 1984.

Behan WMH, Behan PO, Draper IT, et al: Does toxoplasma cause polymyositis? Report of a case of polymyositis associated with toxoplasmosis and a critical review of the literature. *Acta Neuropathol* 61:246–252, 1983.

Polyneuropathy

Archer AG, Watkins PJ, Thomas PK, et al: The natural history of acute painful neuropathy in diabetes mellitus. *J Neurol Neurosurg Psychiatry* 46:491–499, 1983.

Asbury AK: Diseases of the peripheral nervous system, in Wilson JD, Braunwald E, Isselbacher KJ, et al (eds): *Harrison's Principles of Internal Medicine,* 12th ed. New York, McGraw-Hill, 1991, vol 2, pp 2096–2107.

Bishopric G, Bruner J, Butler J: Guillain-Barré syndrome with cytomegalovirus infection of peripheral nerves. *Arch Pathol Lab Med* 109:1106–1108, 1985.

Britland ST, Young RJ, Sharma AK, et al: Association of painful and painless diabetic polyneuropathy with different patterns of nerve fiber degeneration and regeneration. *Diabetes* 39:898–908, 1990.

Kang WH, Chun SI, Lee S: Generalized anhidrosis associated with Fabry's disease. *J Am Acad Dermatol* 17:883–887, 1987.

Lightfoot RW Jr, Michel BA, Bloch DA, et al: The American College of Rheumatology 1990 criteria for the classification of polyarteritis nodosa. *Arthritis Rheum* 33:1088–1093, 1990.

Portenoy RK: Painful polyneuropathy. *Neurol Clin* 7:265–288, 1989.

Schaumburg HH: Diseases of the peripheral nervous system, in Wyngaarden JB, Smith LH Jr (eds): *Cecil Textbook of Medicine,* 18th ed. Philadelphia, Saunders, 1988, vol 2, pp 2258–2268.

Young RJ, Ewing DJ, Clarke BF: Chronic and remitting painful diabetic polyneuropathy: Correlations with clinical features and subsequent changes in neurophysiology. *Diabetes Care* 11:34–40, 1988.

Repetitive Strain Disorders

Hagberg M: Occupational musculoskeletal stress and disorders of the neck and shoulder: A review of possible pathophysiology. *Int Arch Occup Environ Health* 53:269–278, 1984.

Matoba T, Sakurai T: Physiological methods used in Japan for the diagnosis of suspected hand-arm vibration syndrome. *Scand J Work Environ Health* 13:334–336, 1987.

Matsumoto T: Tests employed in Japan for the investigation of peripheral circulatory disturbances due to hand-arm vibration exposure. *Scand J Work Environ Health* 13:356–357, 1987.

McDermott FT: Repetition strain injury: A review of current understanding. *Med J Aust* 144:196–200, 1986.

Rhabdomyolysis

Younger DS, Hays AP, Uncini A, et al: Recurrent myoglobinuria and HIV seropositivity: Incidental or pathogenic association? *Muscle Nerve* 12:842–843, 1989.

Rhabdomyolysis — Alcohol-/Drug-Related

Averbukh Z, Modai D, Leonov Y, et al: Rhabdomyolysis and acute renal failure induced by paraphenylenediamine. *Hum Toxicol* 8:345–348, 1989.

Brody SL, Wrenn KD, Wilber MM, et al: Predicting the severity of cocaine-associated rhabdomyolysis. *Ann Emerg Med* 19:1137–1143, 1990.

Miller LG, Bowman RC, Mann D, et al: A case of fluoxetine-induced serum sickness. *Am J Psych* 146:1616–1617, 1989.

Rubin RB, Neugarten J: Cocaine-induced rhabdomyolysis masquerading as myocardial ischemia. *Am J Med* 86:551–553, 1989.

Rheumatologic Symptoms and Infection

Azevedo J, Ribeiro C, Loureira O, et al: Rheumatic symptoms and signs in subacute infective endocarditis. *Eur Heart J* 5(suppl C):71–75, 1984.

Kaye BR: Rheumatologic manifestations of infection with human immunodeficiency virus (HIV). *Ann Intern Med* 111:158–167, 1989.

Moldofsky H: Nonrestorative sleep and symptoms after a febrile illness in patients with fibrositis and chronic fatigue syndromes. *J Rheumatol* 16(suppl 19):150–153, 1989.

Nash P, Chard M, Hazleman B: Chronic Coxsackie B infection mimicking primary fibromyalgia. *J Rheumatol* 16:1506–1508, 1989.

Shirouzu K, Miyamoto Y, Yasaka T, et al: *Vibrio vulnificus* septicemia. *Acta Pathol Jpn* 35:731–739, 1985.

49   Acute Hemibody Pain

☐ DIAGNOSTIC LIST

1. Thalamic syndrome
2. Mimics of the thalamic syndrome
   A. Cortical or subcortical infarction
   B. Wallenberg's lateral medullary syndrome
   C. Spinal cord lesion
3. Acute asymmetrical arthritis

   A. Gonococcal arthritis
   B. Acute rheumatic fever
   C. Hepatitis B-associated arthritis
   D. Inflammatory bowel disease-associated arthritis
   E. Reiter's syndrome
   F. Yersiniosis
4. Acute trauma involving one side

☐ SUMMARY

The *thalamic syndrome* usually follows a mild stroke. One day to 6 months after the vascular accident, severe, persistent, and/or paroxysmal pain occurs on the side of the body contralateral to the thalamic lesion. The pain is described as burning, aching, boring, stabbing, crushing, gnawing, or shooting. A mild hemianesthesia is present on the affected side, but the initial hemiparesis may clear completely. Hyperalgesia, hyperpathia, and dysesthesias occur on the painful side. Mild sensory stimuli or an emotional upset may intensify or provoke the pain. The entire side of the body, the limbs only, or the face, hand, and foot may be painful and dysesthetic. A vascular lesion of the posterior ventral, lateral, and medial nuclei of the thalamus is the usual cause, but neoplasms, arteriovenous malformations, or trauma may cause a similar syndrome. MRI or a CT scan may image the causative lesion.

Lesions of the parietal cortex or subcortex, lateral medullary region, or spinal cord may masquerade as the thalamic syndrome. Cortical and subcortical lesions can be identified by MRI or a CT scan. Patients with a lateral medullary syndrome usually have dysarthria, dysphagia, hoarseness, contralateral hemianesthesia, ipsilateral facial hypesthesia, ataxia, diplopia, vertigo, nausea, and an ipsilateral Horner's syndrome.

TABLE OF DISEASE INCIDENCE

INCIDENCE PER 100,000 (APPROXIMATE)

Common (>100)	Uncommon (>5–100)	Rare (>0–5)
	Asymmetrical polyarthritis due to gonococcal arthritis, acute rheumatic fever, hepatitis B-associated arthritis, inflammatory bowel disease-associated arthritis, or Reiter's syndrome	Thalamic syndrome Mimics of the thalamic syndrome: cortical or subcortical infarction, Wallenberg's lateral medullary syndrome, or spinal cord lesion
	Acute trauma involving one side	Asymmetrical polyarthritis due to yersiniosis

An *asymmetrical polyarthritis* may cause unilateral arm and leg pain that is localized to the joints. The causes of an acute asymmetrical polyarthritis include acute gonococcal arthritis, acute rheumatic fever, hepatitis B-associated arthritis, inflammatory bowel disease-associated arthritis, Reiter's syndrome, and yersiniosis. *Trauma to one side of the body* may cause hemibody pain because of fractures, fracture-dislocations, sprains, and contusions.

☐ DESCRIPTION OF LISTED DISEASES

1. THALAMIC SYNDROME

This disorder follows an acute stroke by 1 day to as long as 6 months. The vascular accident is usually characterized by an abrupt onset of a mild hemiparesis and superficial hemianesthesia. Hemiataxia, unilateral choreoathetoid movements, and cortical sensory deficits (e.g., astereognosis) may occur in some cases.

Pain may involve the contralateral half of the body, the contralateral arm and leg only, or the face and contralateral hand and foot. The pain has been described as burning, aching, icy, boring, stabbing, crushing, gnawing, or shooting. It is of mild-to-excruciating severity. The pain is often spontaneous and persistent, but it may be intensified or provoked by stimuli such as a touch, hot or cold air or liquids, bright light, loud noise, music, fear, an argument, or odors. Some degree of residual sensory loss is usually detectable, while the initial hemiparesis may resolve partly or completely on the painful side. The sensory loss is most marked for touch and position sense. Hyperesthesia and hyperpathia of the painful side are usually present. Sensory abnormalities may cross the midline of the body and may alter sensation for 1 to 3 cm on the normal side. Painful stimuli may be felt over an area wider than that subjected to the painful stimulus.

Sharp jabs of pain may be superimposed upon the constant hemibody pain. There may be a lag time in the response to a sensory stimulus, and the pain may outlast the stimulus. Limb movement may provoke pain, so that some patients prefer to keep their arms at their sides and may avoid walking, since leg movement may induce twinges of pain. Spontaneous paresthesias and dysesthesias may occur on the painful side. Cortical sensation is frequently affected. Astereognosis, inability to distinguish weight differences, impaired two-point discrimination, and abnormal sensory localization may occur on the painful side. Tactile inattention to the affected side may be present.

Infarction or bleeding in the region of the posterior ventral, lateral, and medial nuclei of the thalamus is the usual cause. Rarely, trauma, tumors, an arteriovenous malfor-mation, or surgical lesions of the thalamus are the cause of this disorder. Infarction or hemorrhage can usually be demonstrated by MRI or a CT scan. The pain is resistent to narcotic therapy. Naloxone infusions or apomorphine may relieve pain in some cases. Neurosurgical procedures relieve pain in less than 25 percent of cases.

2. MIMICS OF THE THALAMIC SYNDROME

A. Cortical or Subcortical Infarction An ischemic lesion in this region may cause contralateral hemiparesis and hemianesthesia. Thalamic syndrome-like pain may begin after a variable time interval. MRI or a CT scan will demonstrate a large lesion interrupting radiating fibers from the thalamic nuclei to the cerebral cortex.

B. Wallenberg's Lateral Medullary Syndrome This ischemic brain stem syndrome begins abruptly, with some or all of the following symptoms: hoarseness, dysphagia, and dysarthria (due to a lesion of nerves IX and X); loss of pain and temperature sense on the contralateral half of the body (due to a lesion of the spinothalamic and quintothalamic tracts); an ipsilateral Horner's syndrome (due to a lesion of sympathetic fibers); ataxia (due to a lesion of the inferior cerebellar peduncle); impaired sensation of the ipsilateral side of the face (due to a lesion of the nucleus and tract of nerve V); vomiting (due to a lesion of the nucleus ambiguous); hiccups (due to a lesion of the reticular formation); and diplopia, vertigo, and nausea (due to a lesion of the inferior vestibular nucleus). Spontaneous pain in the ipsilateral ear, eye, or head has been reported in up to 23 percent of cases, and contralateral limb and trunk pain in 18 percent. The limb pain has been described as burning or stinging. Some patients may have pain only in the contralateral arm and leg or hand and foot. Skin hyperalgia and hyperpathia may be present on the painful side. An incorrect diagnosis of a thalamic lesion has been made in patients with lateral medullary infarction. MRI will usually show a normal thalamic region and may demonstrate the brain stem infarction.

C. Spinal Cord Lesions Such lesions may cause hemibody pain below the level of the neck. Dysesthesias, hyperpathia, and hyperalgesia may occur on the painful side. Acute spinal cord lesions that may masquerade as a thalamic syndrome include a trauma-related Brown-Sequard syndrome or a spinal cord concussion.

3. ACUTE ASYMMETRICAL ARTHRITIS

Joint pain, swelling, tenderness, and loss of mobility may be asymmetrical and migratory or additive. Asymmetrical arthritis may occur in the following disorders.

A. Acute Gonococcal Arthritis   Arthritis may involve the elbow, wrist, knee, and ankle on one side and few or no joints on the other. Skin pustules and hemorrhagic vesicles may occur on the forearms, hands, lower legs, and feet. Fever, chills, and malaise may occur, but many patients have few systemic symptoms. Mucous membrane cultures have a sensitivity of 80 percent and blood or synovial fluid cultures less than 50 percent for *Neiserria gonorrhoeae*. There is a prompt response to intravenous penicillin therapy.

B. Acute Rheumatic Fever   This disorder causes high fever; diaphoresis; chills; and warm, swollen, red, painful joints in the arms and legs on one or both sides. A migratory polyarthritis is characteristic. The joints usually ache, and movement intensifies the pain. There is often a history of a recent ''cold'' or ''sore throat.'' The serum Streptozyme titer or antistreptolysin O titer is usually elevated. There is dramatic response to salicylate therapy.

C. Hepatitis B-Associated Arthritis   Joint pain, swelling, redness, warmth, and tenderness may be preceded by an urticarial or maculopapular prurutic rash. The polyarthritis is migratory and may be asymmetrical. Results of serum assays for hepatitis B surface antigen (HB$_s$Ag) are usually positive, and/or abnormal levels of liver enzymes are frequently present. Clinical hepatitis may never occur, despite the prodromal illness, or severe jaundice may develop 1 to 3 weeks after the onset of joint symptoms.

D. Inflammatory Bowel Disease-Associated Arthritis   An asymmetrical migratory polyarthritis may occur in patients with Crohn's colitis or with idiopathic ulcerative colitis. Joints become swollen, tender, red, and painful. Marked asymmetry of involvement can cause pain on one side of the body. Salicylates may reduce pain, but remission is dependent on treatment of the bowel disease.

E. Reiter's Syndrome   Conjunctivitis, urethritis, and an asymmetrical arthritis are associated. Some patients also develop iridocyclitis, diarrhea, balanitis circinata, and keratoderma blennorrhagicum. The joint disease may be confused with gonococcal polyarthritis, but there is no responses to penicillin therapy.

F. Yersiniosis   This disorder may mimic acute rheumatic fever. The migratory polyarthritis may be asymmetrical. A history of diarrhea or acute right lower abdominal pain and tenderness may be present. *Yersinia enterocolitica* agglutinin levels are elevated. Stool cultures on special media may grow *Y. enterocolitica*. Antibiotic therapy has little effect on the course of the joint disease.

4. ACUTE TRAUMA INVOLVING ONE SIDE

Fractures, fracture-dislocations, sprains, and contusions may occur on one side of the body if the injuring force is directed at that side. Involvement of the arm, leg, and trunk on one side may result from a fall, an assault, or a motor vehicle accident.

HEMIBODY PAIN REFERENCES

Painful Ataxic Hemiparesis
Bogousslavsky J, Regli F, Ghika J, et al: Painful ataxic hemiparesis. *Arch Neurol* 41:892–893, 1984.

Spinal Cord/Brain Stem Central Pain
Pagni CA: Central pain due to spinal cord and brain stem damage, in Wall PD, Melzack R (eds): *Textbook of Pain*, 2d ed. Edinburgh, Churchill Livingstone, 1989, pp 634–655.

Thalamic Pain Syndrome
Adams RD, Victor M: Other somatic sensations, in Adams RD, Victor M (eds): *Principles of Neurology,* 4th ed. New York, McGraw-Hill, 1989, pp 118–133.
———: Pain, in Adams RD, Victor M (eds): *Principles of Neurology,* 4th ed. New York, McGraw-Hill, 1989, pp 103–117.
Agnew DC: Thalamic pain. *Bull Clin Neurosci* 49:93–98, 1984.
Ghose K: Pizotifen in deafferentation pain. *Postgrad Med J* 65:79–82, 1989.
Levin AB, Ramirez LF, Katz J: The use of stereotaxic chemical hypophysectomy in the treatment of thalamic pain syndrome. *J Neurosurg* 59:1002–1006, 1983.

Nuzzo JLJ, Warfield CA: Thalamic pain syndrome. *Hosp Pract* 20:32C-D, 32H-J, 1985.
Ray DAA, Tai YMA: Increasing doses of naloxone hydrochloride by infusion to treat pain due to the thalamic syndrome. *BMJ* 296:969–970, 1988.
Siegfried J: Sensory thalamic neurostimulation for chronic pain. *PACE* 10:209–212, 1987.

Wallenberg's Lateral Medullary Syndrome
Adams RD, Victor M: Cerebrovascular diseases (lateral medullary syndrome), in Adams RD, Victor M (eds): *Principles of Neurology,* 4th ed. New York, McGraw-Hill, 1989, pp 617–692.
Currier RD, Giles CL, DeJong RN: Some comments on Wallenberg's lateral medullary syndrome. *Neurology* 11:778–791, 1961.
Luker J, Scully C: The lateral medullary syndrome. *Oral Surg Oral Med Oral Pathol* 69:322–324, 1990.
Moffie D, Hamburger HL: Pain and neuroma formation in Wallenberg's lateral medullary syndrome. *Clin Neurol Neurosurg* 88:217–220, 1986.

CHAPTER 50

Acute Generalized Joint Pain

☐ DIAGNOSTIC LIST

1. Reactive arthritis and Reiter's syndrome
2. Gonococcal arthritis (arthritis-dermatitis syndrome)
3. Polyarticular nongonococcal septic arthritis
4. Acute rheumatic fever (poststreptococcal arthritis)
5. Viral arthritis: common causes in the United States
   A. Hepatitis B-associated polyarthritis
   B. Rubella-associated arthritis
   C. Parvovirus B19 polyarthralgia and polyarthritis
   D. Human immunodeficiency virus (HIV)-associated arthritis
6. Syndrome of remitting seronegative symmetric synovitis with pitting edema (RS₃PE)
7. Acute seropositive rheumatoid arthritis
8. Adult-onset Still's disease
9. Systemic lupus erythematosus
10. Polyarthritis and vasculitis
    A. Polyarteritis nodosa
    B. Allergic angiitis and granulomatosis (Churg-Strauss disease)
    C. Polyangiitis overlap syndrome
    D. Wegener's granulomatosis
11. Subacute bacterial endocarditis
12. Lyme disease
13. Crystal-induced polyarthritis
    A. Polyarticular gout

B. Calcium pyrophosphate dihydrate deposition disease
14. Polyarthritis and bowel disease
    A. Polyarthritis associated with inflammatory bowel disease
    B. Bowel-associated dermatosis-arthritis syndrome
    C. Whipple's disease
15. Sarcoid arthritis
16. Polychondritis
17. Behçet's syndrome
18. Polyarthritis associated with malignant disease
    A. Leukemia
    B. Carcinoma polyarthritis
    C. Lymphoma
19. Polyarthritis associated with familial hypercholesterolemia
20. Rare causes of infectious polyarthralgia and polyarthritis
    A. Secondary syphilis
    B. Brucellosis
    C. Rat-bite fever
    D. Viral arthritis: rare causes in the United States
    E. Poncet's disease (tuberculous rheumatism)
21. Allergic synovitis
    A. Food-induced polyarthralgia and polyarthritis
    B. Serum sickness
    C. Drug-associated polyarthralgia and polyarthritis
    D. Schönlein-Henoch purpura
22. Subcorneal pustular dermatosis with polyarthritis

☐ SUMMARY

An attack of *reactive arthritis* usually begins 1 to 3 weeks after an episode of urethritis (uroarthritis) or a diarrheal illness (enteroarthritis). Fever occurs most commonly in patients with reactive arthritis following enteric infection. Pain, swelling, and tenderness occur in 1 to 13 joints (mean, 5) in an asymmetrical distribution. The weight-bearing joints of the lower extremity (e.g., knees, ankles, metatarsophalangeal, and interphalangeal joints) are affected in 80 to 90 percent of patients, while upper extremity articulations (e.g., wrists, shoulders, hands, and fingers) are involved in 50 percent of cases. Low back and buttock pain may result from spondylitis and sacroiliitis, while heel discomfort is commonly caused by plantar fasciitis or Achilles tendinitis and knee pain by patellar tendinitis. Anterior chest pain, mimicking pleuritis or cardiac disease, may result from costochondritis or inflammation of the costosternal joints. Arthritis and enthesitis are the only findings in up to 50 percent of cases.

Reactive arthritis may be associated with conjunctivitis alone (9 percent of cases); with urethritis (22 percent); or with urethritis and conjunctivitis (complete Reiter's syndrome, 22 percent). The former syndromes are referred to as incomplete Reiter's syndromes. When Reiter's syndrome follows enteric infection, the urethritis is sterile and is considered reactive. Skin and mucosal involvement occur in a minority of patients with Reiter's syndrome. Oral ulceration (10–20 percent), balanitis circinata (23 percent), and keratoderma blennorrhagicum (12 percent of patients with sexually acquired reactive arthritis) are the most frequent manifestations. Antibiotic therapy has no effect on the immediate clinical course of the arthritis or mucous membrane lesions, which resolve spontaneously in 2 to 4 months. Antibiotic administration may have a role in preventing chronic reactive arthritis by eradicating the causative microorganism.

Gonococcal arthritis results from disseminated gonococcal infection. Migratory polyarthralgia (70 percent of cases) or polyarthritis (10 percent) is usually accompanied by tenosynovitis of the distal extremity regions (67 percent) and small cutaneous papules, pustules, and hemorrhagic vesicles on an erythematous base. Fever, chills, diaphoresis, and other systemic symptoms may be prominent in some cases and minimal in others. Symptoms of urogenital, pharyngeal, and anorectal disease are uncommon, despite cultural evidence of *Neisseria gonorrhoeae* at these sites in 80 percent of cases. The diagnosis can be confirmed by blood culture during the first 3 days of illness. Patients with negative blood cultures can be diagnosed by synovial fluid culture, and mucous membrane cultures. Skin, joint, and tendon symptoms and signs respond within 48 h to parenteral ceftriaxone therapy. *Neisseria meningitidis* septicemia may mimic gonococcal polyarthritis and dermatitis but can be differentiated by blood and synovial fluid cultures.

Polyarticular nongonococcal septic arthritis occurs most frequently in the very young and the elderly. Up to 19 percent of patients with septic arthritis have oligo- or polyarticular involvement. Large joints, such as the knees, ankles, wrists, shoulder, and hips, are most frequently involved. The joints are painful, swollen, red, and warm, and rest and movement- or use-provoked pain is prominent. An asymmetrical pattern of joint inflammation is most common. Elderly patients frequently have underlying joint disease (e.g., rheumatoid arthritis or severe osteoarthritis), an adjacent or distant focus of infection, and/or a medical disorder that impairs immune defenses. *Staphylococcus aureus* is the most frequent cause. *Streptococcus pneumoniae*, group G streptococci, and *Hemophilus influenzae* have a propensity to cause polyarticular septic arthritis. Polyarticular septic arthritis may be diagnosed by aspiration of two or more joints and analysis and culture of the synovial fluids. Blood culture results may also be positive. Therapy with parenteral antibiotics, joint aspiration, and/or open surgical drainage results in gradual improvement, but residual damage and functional loss in one or several joints is a common outcome.

Acute rheumatic fever follows within 2 to 5 weeks of a "cold" or sore throat due to group A streptococci. Fever, chills, sweats, malaise, and weakness are associated with a migratory polyarthritis. The involvement is usually asymmetrical, and joints often improve spontaneously in 2 to 7 days. Up to 16 joints may be affected. The involved joints are painful, tender, mildly swollen, warm, and sometimes red. Walking and range-of-motion testing are painful and restricted. Carditis occurs in only 15 percent of adults and may cause mitral and/or aortic valve insufficiency, pericardial chest pain, heart failure, and variable degrees of atrioventricular block on the electrocardiogram. Antibodies to streptococcal antigens (streptolysin O, hyaluronidase, or DNase B) are demonstrable in 86 to 100 percent (Streptozyme test) of cases, and/or results of a throat culture are positive for *Streptococcus pyogenes* (50 percent of cases). Joint symptoms improve dramatically with aspirin therapy.

Hepatitis B virus infection causes a migratory or additive symmetrical polyarthritis in 10 to 30 percent of patients infected by this virus. Joint symptoms are associated with a maculopapular or urticarial skin eruption in 50 percent of cases. The serum contains hepatitis B surface antigen (HB$_s$Ag), and during subsequent weeks the levels of hepatic enzymes in the serum rise. In most cases, arthritis resolves spontaneously within 2 to 3 weeks, but it may persist for up to 6 months. Anicteric or icteric hepatitis usually follows the disappearance of joint symptoms within 1 to 4 weeks.

Rubella-associated arthritis causes a symmetrical polyarthralgia or polyarthritis with joint stiffness and movement- or use-related pain that precedes or follows clinical rubella. Women are affected in 16 to 33 percent of cases of rubella, while arthritis seldom occurs in men and children. Some patients may develop an elevated titer of serum rheumatoid factor or persistent joint pain lasting for a year or more. In most cases, arthritic complaints resolve spontaneously in 2 to 4 weeks. Rubella arthritis may also be vaccine-induced.

Parvovirus B19 may cause facial erythema ("slapped cheeks rash"); a reticular, maculopapular, erythematous extremity rash; and a symmetrical seronegative polyarthralgia or polyarthritis. Women are affected twice as often as men, and polyarthralgia or polyarthritis has a high incidence in adults (77 percent) and a low rate of occurrence in children (8 percent). Joint symptoms usually resolve spontaneously in 2 weeks but may persist for up to 6 months. The diagnosis can be confirmed by a parvovirus B19 IgM antibody capture enzyme-linked immunosorbent assay (ELISA). IgG antibody levels may also be elevated at the time of onset of joint complaints.

Human immunodeficiency virus (HIV) infection may be associated with arthritis in 71 percent of cases. Reiter's syndrome is responsible in 54 percent, psoriatic arthritis in 17 percent, undifferentiated arthritis in 13 percent, and an acute symmetrical polyarthritis (ASP) resembling rheumatoid arthritis in 17 percent. ASP associated with HIV infection is usually, but not always, seronegative and is associated with radiographic evidence of periostitis, an uncommon finding in rheumatoid arthritis.

The *syndrome of remitting seronegative symmetric synovitis with pitting edema* (RS₃PE) occurs in middle-aged and elderly men (male/female ratio, 4:1). There is a sudden onset of symmetrical arthritis of the wrists and the carpal and small finger joints and tenosynovitis of the flexor tendon sheaths of the hands. Patients have severe pitting edema of the dorsa of the hands and wrists, or "boxing glove hands." Large joints in the arms and legs may also be affected, and pedal and pretibial edema may occur. Low-dose prednisone or hydroxychloroquine-salicylate therapy induces a remission that persists after drug withdrawal.

Seropositive rheumatoid arthritis may begin acutely in up to 15 percent of cases. This disorder causes a symmetrical polyarthritis (involving more than four joints) with prolonged morning stiffness, hand and wrist joint involvement, subcutaneous nodules, seropositivity for rheumatoid factor, and in some cases radiographic evidence of erosions and juxtaarticular osteopenia of hand, wrist, and foot joints. The presence of four or more of these manifestations is considered diagnostic of rheumatoid arthritis. Low-grade fever, fatigue, paresthesias, and malaise may occur in some cases.

Adult-onset Still's disease causes an evanescent, salmon-pink, macular rash on the trunk and the proximal extremities, spiking fevers, and polyarthralgia or polyarthritis. The involvement is symmetrical, and there is a predilection for the small joints of the hands and feet, the knees, the elbows, and the shoulders. Joint pain may be spontaneous and/or movement- or use-related. The joints are tender, swollen, and warm but seldom red. Morning stiffness, myalgias, sore throat, and abdominal pain are common associated complaints. Examination reveals an elevated temperature, a rash, lymphadenopathy, hepatomegaly (38–48 percent of cases), and splenomegaly (52–65 percent). These patients are usually seronegative for rheumatoid factor and antinuclear antibody.

Other manifestations of this disease include pleuritis, pericarditis, glomerulitis, meningoencephalitis, neuropathy, and myocarditis. Prednisone therapy leads to control of systemic and joint complaints. Rare case reports have associated coxsackievirus (B4) with a similar disorder.

Systemic lupus erythematosus may cause a symmetrical polyarthralgia or polyarthritis that is sometimes mistaken for rheumatoid arthritis. Persistent morning stiffness may occur in up to 50 percent of cases. Knee effusions contain less than 3000 cells/mm³, with a lymphocytic predominance and low synovial fluid complement levels. Eleven criteria are currently considered specific enough to be useful in diagnosing systemic lupus erythematosus: a malar rash, discoid lupus, photosensitivity, oral ulcers, nonerosive polyarthritis, cardiopulmonary disease (pleuritis, pericarditis, and/or myocarditis), renal disease, neurologic disease (seizures or a psychosis), hematologic abnormalities, immunologic abnormalities (anti-ds-DNA and anti-Sm antibodies, false-positive serologic test results for syphilis), and an elevated titer of antinuclear antibody. The presence of four or more of these criteria allows classification of a patient as having systemic lupus erythematosus.

Polyarteritis nodosa may cause such nonspecific systemic symptoms as fever, anorexia, weakness, weight loss, and malaise. Polyarthralgia occurs in up to 70 percent of cases. Less commonly, an asymmetrical, nondeforming polyarthritis involving larger joints may develop early in the disease and then subside spontaneously. Skin lesions include painful, tender, red subcutaneous nodules; painful ulcers and infarcts; livedo reticularis; and petechiae. Peripheral neuropathy, dementia or delirium, hemiparesis, and aphasia indicate involvement of peripheral and central nervous system vessels. Hypertension, nephritis, and renal infarction may occur. Intraabdominal ischemia or infarction may cause generalized or localized abdominal pain and tenderness (infarction of the appendix or gallbladder), gastrointestinal bleeding, or perforation. Criteria for the diagnosis of polyarteritis nodosa include involuntary weight loss (≥4 kg) livedo reticularis; testicular pain and tenderness; myalgias, weakness, or leg tenderness; mononeuropathy or polyneuropathy; diastolic pressure greater than 90 mmHg; elevated blood urea nitrogen and creatinine levels; detection of HBₛAg in the serum; an arteriogram showing multiple saccular or fusiform aneurysms of the renal, hepatic, or mesenteric arteries; and a biopsy of a medium or small artery showing granulocytic infiltration and necrosis of the vessel wall. The presence of three or more of these criteria supports a diagnosis of polyarteritis nodosa.

Churg-Strauss disease is a variant of polyarteritis nodosa. It begins with pulmonary infiltrates, severe asthma, and eosinophilia, and in time systemic symptoms and evidence of arteritis develop. Renal involvement is less frequent and milder than in classic polyarteritis nodosa. Arthritis or arthralgia occurs in 21 percent of cases.

The *polyangiitis overlap syndrome* includes patients with polyarteritis nodosa, Churg-Strauss disease, and hypersensitivity vasculitis components of their illness.

Wegener's granulomatosis may cause polyarthralgia or polyarthritis in up to 44 percent of cases. Purulent sinusitis and rhinitis, nasal ulceration, cough, hemoptysis, and pleuritic chest pain may occur. Systemic symptoms include fever, anorexia, and weight loss, but only a minority of patients have these complaints. Chest radiographs show bilateral pulmonary infiltrates, which may be diffuse, nodular, or tumorlike. Cavitation of pulmonary lesions is common, and pleural effusion may occur in up to 20 percent of cases. Renal involvement results in proteinuria, microhematuria, cylindruria, and a rising creatinine level. Antineutrophil cytoplasmic antibodies occur in high titer, and up to 50 percent of patients may be seropositive for rheumatoid factor. Biopsy of sinus or nasal mucosa or lung tissue will establish a specific diagnosis.

Subacute bacterial endocarditis may cause low back pain, polyarthralgias, or polyarthritis in up to 35 percent of cases. The larger proximal joints, including the knees, elbows, ankles, wrists, and shoulders, are most commonly affected. The diagnosis should be considered in the presence of fever, weakness, anorexia, encephalopathy, petechiae and splinter hemorrhages, a mitral or aortic regurgitant murmur, and positive blood cultures. Symptoms resolve with intravenous antibiotic therapy.

Lyme disease initially presents with an asymptomatic, annular, erythematous rash that expands to a diameter of 5 to 68 cm. Fever, myalgias, and polyarthralgias may accompany the onset of the rash in up to 50 percent of cases. This flulike illness is usually self-limited. Untreated patients may develop a recurrent oligoarthritis or, less commonly, a symmetrical polyarthritis 1 or more months after the appearance of the rash. Up to 15 percent of patients develop facial palsy, aseptic meningitis and/or encephalitis, and a painful plexopathy or radiculoneuropathy. These neuropathic lesions may cause trunk and extremity pain and dysesthesias. An ELISA test for *Borrelia burgdorferi* antibodies, with confirmation by Western blot, can be used to confirm the clinical diagnosis. Treatment with parenteral ceftriaxone usually leads to improvement or resolution of rheumatologic and neurologic symptoms.

Polyarticular gout causes a symmetrical or asymmetrical polyarthritis with predominant involvement of the lower extremities. The joints are painful and tender, and movement is restricted voluntarily. Swelling, heat, and redness may occur due to effusions and periarticular soft tissue inflammation. Fever, anorexia, and chilly sensations may occur as associated symptoms. The serum uric acid level is elevated above 7 mg/dl in 97 percent of cases, and the synovial fluid contains an increased concentration of polymorphonuclear leukocytes and intra- and extracellular sodium monourate crystals. Joint pain, swelling, heat, and redness respond within 48 to 72 h to colchicine or indomethacin therapy. Gout is predominantly a disease of middle-aged and elderly men (93–97 percent of cases). An attack of gouty arthritis may be provoked by surgery, a medical illness, trauma, exercise, alcohol, or drugs.

Calcium pyrophosphate dihydrate (CPPD) deposition disease is a disease of elderly men and women (male/female ratio, 1.5:1). Up to 40 percent of attacks are polyarticular. Two or more joints may become involved simultaneously, or a single joint may be affected, followed by a cluster attack of arthritis at two or more nearby joints. Painful joints are usually swollen, warm, erythematous, and tender. Fever, headache, weakness, mental confusion, and dizziness may be associated symptoms. Synovial fluid contains an increased concentration of polymorphonuclear leukocytes and calcium pyrophosphate dihydrate crystals. Plain radiographs of the knees, wrists, shoulders, and ankles may demonstrate chondrocalcinosis. CPPD arthritis may be precipitated by trauma, surgery, or a medical illness and may be relieved by colchicine or indomethacin therapy.

Polyarthritis may be associated with *inflammatory bowel disease*. The incidence is higher in patients with severe disease and complications. A migratory or additive polyarthritis accompanies the symptoms of intestinal disease or, less commonly, precedes them. The weight-bearing joints of the lower extremities are most frequently involved. The skin manifestations include erythema nodosum or pyoderma gangrenosum. Bowel resection may lead to improvement or complete resolution of the arthritis.

The *bowel-associated dermatosis-arthritis syndrome* occurs in 20 percent of patients who have had a jejunoileal bypass procedure for obesity. Fever, chills, myalgias, polyarthralgia, and malaise are accompanied by an eruption of 2- to 4-mm erythematous papules and pustules on the upper trunk and extremities. Symptoms resolve spontaneously in 2 to 6 days but recur every 1 to 6 weeks. Rarely, a case may follow gastric or colorectal surgery or occur in the absence of surgery. Reversal of the bypass procedure or intensive treatment of continuing inflammatory bowel disease, the disorder originally responsible for the colorectal surgery, leads to resolution of symptoms.

Whipple's disease may cause an acute polyarthritis or polyarthralgia. The joints may appear normal, or they may be acutely inflamed. Attacks last 3 to 14 days and recur once or twice a month. Fever, chills, sweating, and malaise accompany the joint symptoms. Diarrhea, malabsorption and fatty stools, weight loss, and abdominal pain may develop months or years after joint symptoms begin. The diagnosis can be confirmed by a peroral jejunal, synovial, or lymph node biopsy revealing periodic acid-Schiff (PAS)-positive macrophages containing bacilliform structures. Four weeks of tetracycline therapy leads to resolution of bowel and joint symptoms.

Sarcoidosis may cause polyarthralgia or polyarthritis, erythema nodosum, and bilateral hilar adenopathy (Lofgren's syndrome). The serum angiotensin-converting enzyme level may be elevated, and a gallium citrate (^{67}Ga) scan may show increased uptake over the salivary and lacrimal glands. A biopsy of a lymph node, muscle, or lung tissue may reveal noncaseating granulomas. Symptoms improve or resolve with prednisone therapy.

Polychondritis causes painful and tender, red, swollen auricles associated with nontender, white ear lobes; a symmetrical or asymmetrical polyarthritis; costochondritis; ocular inflammation; and laryngotracheobronchial inflammation. The arthritis is nonerosive and resolves spontaneously or with prednisone therapy. The diagnosis may be made on the basis of the distinctive clinical findings involving the auricles, nasal cartilages, and trachea and can be confirmed, if required, by an auricular cartilage biopsy.

Behçet's syndrome causes painful oral ulcers, skin lesions (e.g., erythema nodosum, superficial thrombophlebitis, folliculitis, and pathergy), eye lesions (e.g., iridocyclitis and hypopyon), and genital ulcers. Polyarthralgia or polyarthritis occur in up to 60 percent of cases. Colitis, epididymitis, arteritis with occlusion, and neurologic disease may also occur. Symptoms may improve with chlorambucil therapy.

Polyarthritis and polyarthralgia may be associated with *malignant disease*. *Acute leukemia* may cause a symmetrical and/or migratory polyarthritis or polyarthralgia. Joint disease is more common in children. Pain seems unusually severe given the appearance of symptomatic joints. Chemotherapy for the leukemia may result in remission of the joint pain.

Carcinoma of the breast in women and other carcinomas may cause a symmetrical or an asymmetrical seronegative polyarthritis. The lower extremity joints are most commonly involved. Joint symptoms may be acute. Treatment of the associated tumor may result in relief of the joint symptoms. Polyarthritis associated with *lymphoma* is rare. T-cell lymphoma with erythroderma may be associated with polyarthritis or polyarthralgia.

Familial hypercholesterolemia may cause a recurrent migratory polyarthritis and a heart murmur due to aortic stenosis. Tendinous xanthomas of the hands, tuberous xanthomas of the knees, and hypercholesterolemia are associated findings.

Secondary syphilis follows 2 to 8 weeks after the appearance of a primary lesion on the penis or vulva. Fever, malaise, a generalized maculopapular rash involving the palms and soles, polyarthralgias, and mucous membrane lesions (condylomata lata and mucous patches) occur. Polyarthritis is rare. Results of a VDRL or RPR test for syphilis are positive, and all symptoms vanish with penicillin therapy.

Brucellosis may cause a monoarticular or polyarticular migratory or additive polyarthritis, with the knees and hips most frequently involved. Spondylitis and sacroiliitis may occur. Ingestion of unpasteurized dairy products or work in an abattoir is associated with this disease. Serologic tests are the usual method of diagnostic confirmation. Results of cultures of blood, bone marrow, or synovial fluid may be positive, but the sensitivity of cultures is low in subacute cases. Symptoms respond to antibiotic therapy.

Rat-bite fever due to *Streptobacillus moniliformis* causes fever, chills, headache, vomiting, and severely painful migratory polyarthralgias and myalgias that begin 1 to 22 days after a rat bite. Laboratory workers, farmers, homeless people, and people from lower socioeconomic groups living in rat-infested dwellings are at risk. A generalized maculopapular rash occurs in 93 percent of cases and may involve the palms and soles. An asymmetrical migratory polyarthritis occurs. The diagnosis can be established by culture of blood or synovial fluid. A false-positive biological test for syphilis may occur in up to 25 percent of cases. Treatment with penicillin is rapidly effective.

Rarely, polyarthritis in the United States may result from infection with *adenovirus*, *mumps virus*, *echovirus*, *or coxsackievirus*. Fever, rash, and polyarthritis occur in Africa from chikungunya virus and in Australia from Ross River virus.

Poncet's disease is a rare manifestation of primary tuberculosis. Fever and a painful polyarthritis occur. The purified protein derivative (PPD) skin test is usually positive. The chest radiograph is most commonly negative, but it may demonstrate parenchymal infiltrates and hilar adenopathy. Symptoms respond to antituberculous drug therapy.

Food-induced polyarthralgia follows within hours of ingestion of certain foods by atopic individuals. Skin tests, a radioallergosorbent test (RAST), an elimination diet, and food challenge may identify the causative food.

Serum sickness may follow administration of equine serum (antivenin for snake bite) or a drug (e.g., penicillin or other antimicrobial drugs). Symptoms and signs include fever, chills, polyarthralgia or polyarthritis, myalgias, an erythematous maculopapular or urticarial rash, leg edema, and lymph node enlargement. Symptoms resolve spontaneously with discontinuance of the causative substance.

Polyarthralgia and polyarthritis may occur in a small number of patients given such *drugs* as amphotericin B, cimetidine, and beta blockers.

Schönlein-Henoch purpura causes palpable purpura on the legs and buttocks, abdominal pain, polyarthralgia or polyarthritis, and nephritis. It may be associated with a recent respiratory infection, a drug, or some other unknown antigen. Palpable purpura may occur with systemic lupus erythematosus, rheumatoid arthritis, and essential mixed cryoglobulinemia. Prednisone may improve joint and other symptoms in some cases of Schönlein-Henoch purpura.

Subcorneal pustular dermatosis may be associated with a low-grade fever and polyarthralgia or polyarthritis. The etiology of the dermatosis is unknown. Symptomatic treatment with nonsteroidal anti-inflammatory drugs relieves arthralgic and arthritic symptoms.

☐ DESCRIPTION OF LISTED DISEASES

1. REACTIVE ARTHRITIS AND REITER'S SYNDROME

Reactive arthritis occurs 1 to 3 weeks after an episode of urethritis (uroarthritis) in a male or following an acute diarrheal illness (enteroarthritis) in members of either sex. Fever occurs in up to 60 percent of patients with diarrhea-associated arthritis but is less common in uroarthritis. The lower extremity weight-bearing joints (e.g., toe, metatarsophalangeal, subtalar, ankle, and knee and hip joints) are affected most commonly (80–90 percent of cases), and involvement is usually asymmetrical. Joints become involved in rapid succession or simultaneously. A mean of 5 joints (range, 1–13) are affected, and inflammation persists at the involved joints for 2 to 16 weeks or more. Insertional tendinitis (enthesis) affects the heel (plantar fasciitis and Achilles tendinitis), knees (patellar tendini-

TABLE OF DISEASE INCIDENCE

INCIDENCE PER 100,000 (APPROXIMATE)

Common (>100)	**Uncommon (>5–100)**	**Rare (>0–5)**
Reactive arthritis and Reiter's syndrome	Gonococcal arthritis	Adult-onset Still's disease
Rubella-associated arthritis	Polyarticular nongonococcal septic arthritis	Polyarteritis nodosa
HIV-associated arthritis	Acute rheumatic fever	Churg-Strauss disease
Acute seropositive rheumatoid arthritis	Hepatitis B-associated polyarthritis	Polyangiitis overlap syndrome
Crystal-induced polyarthritis due to gout or calcium pyrophosphate dihydrate deposition disease	Parvovirus B19 polyarthritis	Wegener's granulomatosis
	RS$_3$PE	Bowel associated dermatosis-arthritis syndrome
	Systemic lupus erythematosus	Whipple's disease
	Subacute bacterial endocarditis	Polychondritis
	Lyme disease	Behçet's syndrome
	Polyarthritis associated with inflammatory bowel disease	Leukemic polyarthritis
	Sarcoid arthritis	Lymphoma polyarthritis
	Carcinoma polyarthritis	Polyarthritis associated with familial hypercholesterolemia
	Secondary syphilis	Brucellosis
	Serum sickness due to serum or drug administration	Rat-bite fever
	Schönlein-Henoch purpura	Viral arthritis (rare causes in United States)
		Poncet's disease
		Food-induced polyarthralgia or polyarthritis
		Drug-associated polyarthralgia or polyarthritis
		Subcorneal pustular dermatosis with polyarthritis

tis), and buttocks. Bilateral or unilateral buttock and low back pain may occur in up to 50 percent of cases due to sacroiliitis and spondylitis. Dactylitis (''sausage toe'') of one or more toes suggests reactive or psoriatic arthritis. Chest pain may result from costochondritis or from inflammatory changes at the manubriosternal or sternoclavicular joints.

The involved joints may be spontaneously painful at rest or painful only during weight bearing or joint movement. Joint swelling with effusion may occur (e.g., in the knees and shoulders), and local tenderness and range-of-motion testing pain are usually present. In some patients, the overlying skin is red, warm, and swollen. The upper extremities are affected in up to 50 percent of cases, and the shoulders, wrists, and fingers are most frequently involved. Arthritis without other organ or tissue involvement occurs in 45 to 50 percent of cases, and these patients are classified as having reactive arthritis.

Reiter's syndrome may be complete (urethritis, conjunctivitis, and arthritis) or incomplete (arthritis and conjunctivitis; arthritis and urethritis; or urethritis and conjunctivitis). In one series of *Salmonella* species-associated enteroarthritis, a complete Reiter's syndrome occurred in 22 percent of cases, arthritis and conjunctivitis in 9 percent, and arthritis and urethritis in 22 percent, while arthritis alone occurred in 48 percent.

The urethritis following bowel infection is considered reactive (i.e., urethral culture results are negative), but in rare cases a urethral pathogen may be isolated. Urethritis may occur in up to 50 percent of patients with enteroarthritis. It may be asymptomatic, cause mild dysuria, stain the underwear, produce morning discharge, or cause a ''watering can effect'' during the first morning urination due to dried urethral exudate.

Uroarthritis (sexually acquired reactive arthritis [SARA]) is caused by *Chlamydia trachomatis* (40 percent of cases) or *Ureaplasma urealyticum* (40 percent of cases). Some authors consider *Neisseria gonorrhoeae* to be a cause of reactive arthritis. *C. trachomatis*, *U. urealyticum*, or *N. gonorrhoeae* can be cultured from the urethra of some patients with SARA if antibiotics have not been given and the time interval from urethral symptoms to attempted isolation is less than 3 weeks.

Enteroarthritis may affect both sexes and is caused by an enteric infection that may cause fever and watery or bloody diarrhea. In up to 20 percent of cases, there are no enteric symptoms, and the diagnosis can be established only by stool culture or serologic methods (e.g., *Yersinia* species or *Salmonella* species). *Shigella flexneri* types 1 and 2; *Yersinia enterocolitica* types 3, 6, 8, and 9; *Yersinia pseudotuberculosis*; many serotypes of *Campylobacter jejuni*, *Campylobacter coli*, or *Campylobacter fetus* subspecies *fetus*; and *Salmonella typhimurium*, *Salmonella enteritidis*, *Salmonella blockly*, and *Salmonella heidelberg* (groups B, C, and D) have been associated with reactive arthritis and Reiter's syndrome. Rarely (10 reported cases), *Clostridium difficile* may cause reactive arthritis in a patient being treated with antibiotics for pharyngitis, urethritis, or diarrhea. The diagnosis of *C. difficile* colitis can be established by culture of the stool and a tissue culture assay for *C. difficile* toxin (the more specific test). Enteroarthritis begins a mean of 12 days after the onset of diarrhea, but 10 to 20 percent of patients may first become symptomatic after an interval exceeding 30 days.

Mucocutaneous lesions may occur in patients with Reiter's syndrome. Balanitis circinata may appear in 23 percent, keratoderma blennorrhagicum in 12 percent (usually only with SARA), and painless or painful oral ulcers and stomatitis in 10 to 20 percent of cases.

The male/female ratio of reactive arthritis varies with the associated microbial agent. The ratio for *Shigella* species is 9:1; for *Salmonella* species, 1.6:1; for *Campylobacter* species, 1.3:1; for *Yersinia* species 0.9:1; and for SARA, 28:1.

The sedimentation rate and leukocyte count may be normal or elevated, and the hemoglobin concentration low or normal. HLA-B27 antigen is present in 80 to 100 percent of patients with reactive arthritis or Reiter's syndrome, and a low-titer rheumatoid factor (1:32–1:64) may be present in 20 percent.

Synovial fluid cell counts vary between 5000 and 30,000 cells/mm^3, with an initial polymorphonuclear leukocyte predominance. Gram stain and cultures of synovial fluid are negative, and synovial fluid lymphocytes may increase (^{3}H) thymidine uptake when exposed to antigens derived from the causative organism. This lymphocyte stimulation index is currently being investigated for its diagnostic usefulness and is not an established diagnostic procedure.

Antibiotic therapy has no immediate effect on the course of the arthritis or the extraarticular manifestations. Some authors believe that it may prevent a chronic form of reactive arthritis or Reiter's syndrome by eradicating the associated microorganism. Joint pain and tenderness respond partially or completely to nonsteroidal anti-inflammatory drugs.

2. GONOCOCCAL ARTHRITIS (ARTHRITIS-DERMATITIS SYNDROME)

Disseminated gonococcal infection may cause a migratory or additive polyarthritis (10 percent of cases) and/or polyarthralgias (70 percent). Tenosynovitis involving the extensors of the wrists and fingers, the ankles and toes, and/or the Achilles tendon occurs in 67 percent of cases. Dermatitis, in the form of necrotic papules, pustules, or hemorrhagic purple vesicles surrounded by an erythematous rim, occurs in 67 percent of cases. These lesions occur most frequently on the extremities and less often on the trunk. Tenosynovitis and dermatitis may occur alone or in association with a poly- or oligoarthritis.

In patients with disseminated gonococcal infection culture proven mucous membrane infections are usually not symptomatic [e.g., urethral (87 percent), pharyngeal (80 percent), and anorectal area (100 percent) isolates are not associated with local symptoms.] The male/female ratio is 1:4.

The involved joints may be painful, tender, swollen, warm, and red. Fever, chills, and leukocytosis may occur in up to 50 percent of cases, but their absence has no diagnostic significance. Resolution of inflammation and pain occurs spontaneously at most sites, but one or more joints (most often the knees or wrists) may remain swol-

len, red, warm, and severely painful. Synovial fluid analysis reveals a leukocyte count in the range of 35,000 to 65,000 cells/mm^3, with a polymorphonuclear leukocyte predominance. Counts as high as 200,000 cells/mm^3 or as low as 1000 cells/mm^3 may occur. Gram stains reveal extracellular and intracellular gram-negative diplococci in 25 to 30 percent of cases, and results of cultures for *N. gonorrhoeae* are positive in 30 to 50 percent.

Despite the relative infrequency of symptoms related to the urethra, cervix and uterus, pharynx, and anorectal area, results of cultures of these mucosal sites are positive in 80 percent of cases. Results of cultures of skin vesicle fluid are positive in 5 percent of cases and those of blood cultures in 13 to 30 percent during the first 4 days of illness. A positive mucous membrane culture result from a sexual partner may provide supportive evidence for a clinical diagnosis. Parenteral administration of ceftriaxone results in clinical improvement within 48 h in 90 percent of cases. This therapeutic response supports the clinical diagnosis.

3. POLYARTICULAR NONGONOCOCCAL SEPTIC ARTHRITIS

Polyarticular septic arthritis occurs in 19 percent of reported cases of nongonococcal septic arthritis in adults. The commonest etiologic agent is *Staphylococcus aureus* (70–82 percent of cases). Polyarticular septic arthritis usually involves two to five joints. The knees, wrists, ankles, shoulders, elbows, and hips are most frequently involved. The arthritis is usually asymmetrical and begins at all sites simultaneously or in rapid succession. The affected joints are swollen, painful, and tender, and the overlying skin is usually warm, red, and swollen.

Patients with oligo- or polyarticular joint sepsis are usually elderly, have underlying rheumatoid arthritis and/or some other medical disorder that causes immunosuppression (e.g., diabetes mellitus, chronic renal failure, alcoholism, cirrhosis of the liver, malignancy, and/or immunosuppressive therapy), and/or have an adjacent or distant focus of infection. Bacteria may be cultured from the blood and the synovial fluid obtained from two or more joints. There is a gradual response to parenteral antibiotic therapy and joint drainage, but persistent pain and loss of joint mobility may occur despite intensive antimicrobial therapy. Relative to septic involvement of a single joint, polyarticular septic arthritis occurs more often with *Streptococcus pneumoniae* (39 percent), group G streptococci (36 percent), and *Hemophilus influenzae* (36 percent), and less often with gram-negative bacilli (3 percent).

Mortality is highest in patients with rheumatoid arthritis (56 percent of cases), while it is only 8 percent in the absence of this underlying disease.

Rare cases of primary meningococcal polyarthritis have been reported. They are associated with fever, chills, myalgia, headache, sore throat, a maculopapular rash, and skin pustules resembling the lesions of disseminated gon-ococcal infection. The knees, ankles, shoulders, elbows, and wrists may be involved. A synovial fluid Gram stain may demonstrate gram-negative diplococci, and synovial fluid cultures for *Neisseria meningitidis* are positive in 80 to 90 percent of cases. Therapy with parenteral penicillin or ceftriaxone will lead to improvement.

4. ACUTE RHEUMATIC FEVER (POSTSTREPTOCOCCAL ARTHRITIS)

A migratory polyarthritis may involve up to 16 joints. The involvement is usually asymmetrical, and symptoms consist of pain, tenderness, slight swelling of the affected joints, and loss of pain-free range of motion. Swelling, erythema, and heat of the overlying skin are less common but may occur.

The lower extremity joints (e.g., metatarsophalangeal, subtalar, ankle, knee, and hip) are most frequently affected, but upper extremity sites (e.g., carpal and finger joints, wrists, elbows, and shoulders) may also be affected. The joint pain and tenderness persist for 2 to 7 days and then resolve spontaneously. The entire episode of polyarthritis usually resolves without sequelae in 2 to 4 weeks without specific therapy. Adults and adolescents have a high rate of migratory polyarthritis (82–100 percent). The joint symptoms and associated fever, chills, and sweating respond dramatically to aspirin therapy.

Carditis occurs in 32 percent of teenagers (age, 13–17 years) and in only 15 percent of adults. It is usually less severe in older patients than in children. Mitral regurgitation (i.e., a long, loud apical systolic murmur that may vary in intensity from day to day), aortic insufficiency (aortic decrescendo, blowing, high-pitched diastolic murmur), and a Carey-Coombs apical mid-diastolic murmur are common clinical manifestations of carditis. Other findings suggestive of carditis include tachycardia, muffled heart sounds, a friction rub, loud S1 and S2 sounds, an S3 or S4 gallop, and cardiomegaly. Signs of congestive heart failure occur in 5 to 10 percent and pericarditis in 10 percent of those with carditis. Doppler echocardiography may be used to detect clinically silent mitral and aortic regurgitation and to exclude mitral valve prolapse and valve vegetations. The diagnosis of carditis is currently based on clinical findings and not Doppler echocardiography, but these criteria may be modified in the future. Chorea does not occur in adults, except rarely during pregnancy, and erythema marginatum and subcutaneous nodules are seldom observed in adults.

A history of a "cold" or "sore throat" within 5 weeks prior to the onset of fever, joint pain, and carditis is obtained in 33 to 38 percent of cases. Initial throat cultures may be positive in up to 50 percent of cases for *Streptococcus pyogenes*. Antistreptolysin O titers are elevated in 91 percent of cases and antideoxyribonuclease (anti-DNase) B and antihyaluronidase in 86 percent of cases when fever and migratory polyarthritis are present.

The Streptozyme agglutination test is a rapid, highly sensitive test (100 percent) for antibody to a mixture of streptococcal antigens. In some cases, reproducibility of test results has caused problems and confirmatory tests (i.e., antistreptolysin O and anti-DNase B) are required. The modified Jones criteria for the diagnosis of acute rheumatic fever are presented in Table 50-1.

Some cases of adult-onset rheumatic fever may be recurrent attacks and not primary episodes. Such patients have clinical evidence of established rheumatic heart disease or a history of one or more prior attacks of fever, migratory polyarthritis, carditis, and/or chorea.

Migratory polyarthritis may occur with disorders other than disseminated gonococcal arthritis and rheumatic fever. The differential diagnosis of acute migratory polyarthritis is presented in Table 50-2.

5. VIRAL ARTHRITIS: COMMON CAUSES IN THE UNITED STATES

A. Hepatitis B-Associated Polyarthritis   A symmetrical or, less commonly, an asymmetrical polyarthritis occurs involving the proximal interphalangeal, distal interphalangeal, and metacarpophalangeal joints of the hands as well as the knees, shoulders, ankles, elbows, and wrists. There are mild-to-severe rest- and movement-related pain, tenderness, and joint swelling. In some cases,

Table 50-1
REVISED JONES CRITERIA FOR THE DIAGNOSIS OF ACUTE RHEUMATIC FEVER

Major Manifestations	Minor Manifestations	Supporting Evidence of Streptococcal Infection
Carditis (15% in adults)	Clinical history of prior episode(s) of rheumatic fever or rheumatic carditis	Increased titer of antistreptococcal antibodies
Polyarthritis (100% in adults)		Positive results of throat culture for *S. pyogenes*
Chorea (0% in adults and rare in pregnant adults)	Arthralgia	Recent scarlet fever
Erythema marginatum (<1% in adults)	Fever	
Subcutaneous nodules (<1% in adults)	Elevated sedimentation rate, leukocyte count, or C-reactive protein level	
	Prolonged PR interval on electrocardiogram	

Note: The presence of two major or one major and two minor manifestations, plus confirmatory evidence of preexisting streptococcal infection, indicates a high likelihood of rheumatic fever.

Table 50-2
DIFFERENTIAL DIAGNOSIS OF ACUTE MIGRATORY POLYARTHRITIS

Cause	Possible Historical Findings	Possible Examination Findings	Possible Laboratory Findings	Therapeutic Response of Polyarthitis to
Gonococcal	Sexual activity, urethritis, pelvic inflammatory disease, polyarthralgia	Fever, skin pustules, and/or hemorrhagic vesicles on an erythematous base, oligo- or polyarthritis	Mucous membrane, blood, and/or synovial fluid cultures positive for *N. gonorrhoeae*	Ceftriaxone
Acute rheumatic fever	Cold or sore throat 2–5 weeks before onset, prior rheumatic fever, polyarthralgia	Fever, subcutaneous nodules (<1%), carditis with mitral or aortic insufficiency murmurs and/or S3 or S4 gallop and cardiomegaly (<15% in adults), polyarthritis	Throat culture positive for group A streptococci (50%), antistreptococcal antibodies elevated (90–100%)	Aspirin
Hepatitis B	Intravenous drug abuse, sexual exposure, use of blood products for therapy, polyarthralgia	Fever; maculopapular or urticarial rash (50%), sometimes pruritic; polyarthritis	HB$_s$Ag positive in serum, abnormal liver function test results	No specific therapy available, aspirin may ameliorate symptoms
Parvovirus B19	Exposure to child with rash or fifth disease, polyarthralgia	Fever; rash on trunk, extremities, and face ("slapped cheeks rash"); polyarthritis	Positive IgM antibody capture ELISA for parvovirus B19 or IgG antibody to parvovirus B19	No specific therapy available
Inflammatory bowel disease-associated	Diarrhea, abdominal pain, fever before or after onset of joint symptoms, polyarthralgia	Fever, erythema nodosum, pyoderma gangrenosum, endoscopic or radiographic evidence of inflammatory bowel disease, polyarthritis	Occult blood in stool, leukocytes in stool, bacterial pathogens and pathogenic *Entamoeba histolytica* absent from stool (negative cultures and microscopic stool examination), negative serologic test results for amebiasis (indirect hemagglutination antiamoeba antibody test)	Colectomy, medical therapy for inflammatory bowel disease
Familial hypercholesterolemia	Family history, xanthomas, recurrent attacks of polyarthritis beginning during first two decades, polyarthralgia	Fever, xanthomas, xanthelasma, polyarthritis	Hypercholesterolemia	Cholesterol reduction
Rat-bite fever	Rat bite; patient is a farmer or laboratory worker, or dwelling is rat-infested, polyarthralgia	Fever, maculopapular rash, polyarthritis	Synovial fluid and/or blood cultures positive for *Streptobacillus moniliformis*	Penicillin
Brucella-associated arthritis	Patient is a veterinarian, farmer, or abattoir worker; has ingested unpasteurized milk or other dairy products, back and buttock pain, polyarthralgia	Fever, spondylitis, sacroiliitis, polyarthritis	Brucella agglutinins positive, culture of blood and/or synovial fluid positive, but culture sensitivity low in subacute cases	Streptomycin and tetracycline, or doxycycline and rifampin
Acute leukemia	Most frequent in first decade, polyarthralgia	Fever, pallor, petechiae, and ecchymoses, splenomegaly, polyarthritis	Peripheral smear and bone marrow positive for leukemia	Antileukemic chemotherapy

the overlying skin is warm and erythematous. A migratory or additive arthritis is the usual clinical pattern. Tendinitis of the hands and feet may be associated. The arthritis may be preceded or accompanied in up to 50 percent of cases by an urticarial or sometimes a macular, papular, or pe- techial rash. The rash may be pruritic and usually involves the legs, but other regions may also be affected. Nonspecific symptoms, such as fever, chills, myalgias, malaise, anorexia, weakness, nausea, and vomiting, may begin 1 day to as much as 3 months before the onset of joint symptoms. The diagnosis depends on detection of HB_sAg in the serum, but several blood samples may be required because of a high false-negative rate. As the arthritis and rash resolve, HB_sAg is replaced in the serum by anti-HB antibody; the serum aspartate aminotransferase (AST) and alanine aminotransferase (ALT) levels may rise; and an-icteric or icteric hepatitis, with fever and right upper abdominal pain and/or tenderness, may follow within 1 to 4 weeks. In some cases, liver enzyme levels may remain normal. Serum complement levels (e.g., C_3, C_4, and CH_{50}) may be depressed when the arthritis first appears (28–45 percent of cases). Synovial fluid leukocyte counts vary from 465 to 90,000 cells/mm^3, with a polymorphonuclear leukocyte predominance. HB_sAg may be detected in synovial fluid. Articular symptoms may respond to salicylate therapy. The rash and arthritis usually resolve spontaneously in 2 to 3 weeks, but in a small percentage of cases joint symptoms may persist for up to 6 months.

B. Rubella-Associated Arthritis   Arthritis may precede symptoms of rubella (i.e., low-grade fever; painful, tender occipital adenopathy; and a faint pink macular truncal rash) or follow them by as much as 6 days. The arthritis associated with rubella begins abruptly with symmetrical stiffness and joint use- and/or movement-related pain in the fingers, knees, wrists, elbows, ankles, and toes. Tenosynovitis in the hands and wrists or a carpal tunnel syndrome may occur. The incidence in women with rubella is 16 to 33 percent. Arthritis rarely occurs in adult men with rubella. Joint symptoms are resolved spontaneously in 1 month but may persist for more than a year in a small percentage of patients.

Rheumatoid factor may be detected in the serum in some patients. Synovial fluid cell counts range from 14,600 to 60,000 cells/mm^3, and there may be a polymorphonuclear leukocyte or mononuclear cell predominance. Rubella virus has sometimes been cultured from synovial fluid in patients with joint pain and stiffness.

Rubella-associated arthritis may be vaccine-induced. The joint symptoms begin 2 to 4 weeks after vaccination and are similar to those associated with natural infection. Arthritis restricted to the knees and carpal tunnel syndrome are more frequent with vaccine-induced arthritis. The usual duration of joint symptoms is 1 to 3 weeks (range, 1 day to 7 weeks). Recurrent attacks of arthritis have been reported in 10 to 33 percent of patients with knee involvement and may continue for as long as 3 years.

C. Parvovirus B19 Polyarthralgia or Polyarthritis Children and some adults develop a bright-red rash on the face that has been described as having a "slapped cheeks" appearance. Erythematous macules may also occur on the chin, frontal area, and neck. The rash may be pruritic. A lacelike rash may develop on the extensor surfaces of the arms and legs and on the buttocks. Rashes may recur intermittently for up to 10 months after initial resolution.

Adults do not usually have a typical "slapped cheeks

rash." There may be diffuse erythema of the entire face or a faint malar flush and a truncal and/or extremity rash that may be reticular, morbilliform, macular, maculopapular, or, rarely, vesiculopustular. Polyarthralgia and fever begin suddenly and may be incapacitating, leaving the patient bedridden. The polyarthralgia may be migratory or additive. Morning stiffness, joint swelling, tenderness, and rest- and movement- or use-related pain occur. Symmetrical involvement of the small joints of the hands, wrists, shoulders, hips, knees, and ankles and/or the metatarsophalangeal joints is common. Most patients are seronegative for rheumatoid factor. Women are affected twice as frequently as men. Adults becoming ill with this disorder often give a history of exposure to a child with a rash or a confirmed case of fifth disease. Joint symptoms resolve spontaneously in 70 percent of cases within 2 weeks but may persist for up to 6 months. Parvovirus B19 causes fifth disease (erythema infectiosum) in children and adults, but the incidence of polyarthralgia is 77 percent in adults and only 8 percent in children.

Parvovirus B19 is an important cause of epidemic arthritis and may be misdiagnosed as acute seronegative rheumatoid arthritis. The diagnosis of acute parvovirus B19 infection can be confirmed by an IgM antibody capture enzyme-linked immunosorbent assay (ELISA). IgG antibody may also be detectable at the time joint symptoms begin. A rising or falling antibody titer on serial assays may also support the diagnosis. There is no specific therapy, and the arthritis spontaneously resolves.

D. HIV-Associated Polyarthritis   Joint symptoms occurred in 71 percent of 101 patients with HIV infection in one report. In another study of HIV infection and arthritis, 54 percent of the patients had Reiter's syndrome, 17 percent psoriatic arthritis, 13 percent undifferentiated arthritis, and 17 percent an acute symmetrical polyarthritis. The latter disorder resembles rheumatoid arthritis and affects the arms and hands predominantly. Synovial involvement and proliferative periostitis occur. Radiographic findings include osteoporosis, soft tissue edema, joint effusions, joint space narrowing, marginal erosions, periosteal reaction, and, in advanced cases, deformities (ulnar deviation of the fingers and swan neck deformities). In patients with acute symmetrical polyarthritis, serum rheumatoid factor titers may occasionally be elevated. Proliferative periostitis is uncommon in rheumatoid arthritis. Its presence should suggest the possibility of HIV-associated symmetrical polyarthritis.

6. SYNDROME OF REMITTING SERONEGATIVE SYMMETRIC SYNOVITIS WITH PITTING EDEMA

RS$_3$PE affects patients in the 48- to 86-year-old age range (mean age, 71 years) who live in rural or semirural environments. The male/female ratio is 4:1. There is an abrupt onset, with symmetrical arthritis of the wrist and carpal joints and tenosynovitis of the flexor tendon sheaths. Pitting edema of the hands occurs, producing "boxing glove hands." Joint pain and swelling may affect the elbows, shoulders, hips, knees, and ankles, as well as the joints of the feet. Pretibial and pedal edema may occur. The sedimentation rate is usually elevated, and a mild anemia occurs, but the serum tests negative for rheumatoid factor. Treatment with small doses of prednisone (10 mg/day) or hydroxychloroquine and salicylate may result in a remission that is maintained when the drugs are withdrawn, in contrast to what occurs in seropositive rheumatoid arthritis. Up to 70 percent of patients test positive for HLA-B27 antigen, compared with 24 percent of the general population. Restriction of motion may occur in the wrists, elbows, and hands after remission, and this diminished range of movement may persist.

7. ACUTE SEROPOSITIVE RHEUMATOID ARTHRITIS

Eight to 15 percent of patients may have an acute onset of arthritis. There is symmetrical or asymmetrical involvement of the metacarpophalangeal joints (63 percent of cases), proximal interphalangeal joints (58 percent), wrists (58 percent), metatarsophalangeal joints (48 percent), shoulders (40 percent), knees (33 percent), ankles (24 percent), and elbows (18 percent). Morning stiffness, movement- or use-related pain, and joint tenderness may precede spontaneous rest pain. Symptoms persist, and joint enlargement may occur due to effusions (e.g., in the knees) or edema of the periarticular tissues (spindle-shaped or fusiform enlargement of the proximal interphalangeal joints). The overlying skin may be warm, but it is seldom erythematous. Fever, anorexia, malaise, depression, fatigue, myalgia, lymphadenopathy, and splenomegaly may occur in patients with an acute onset of this disorder. Seropositivity may be present in only 33 percent of cases during the first 3 months, but after a year, 88 percent of patients are seropositive. Seropositivity may antedate the onset of joint symptoms.

The erythrocyte sedimentation rate is elevated, and the leukocyte and platelet counts may also be increased. A normocytic or microcytic anemia may be present. Serum complement levels are normal or elevated, and α_2 globulins and gamma globulins may be increased. Synovial fluid contains 5000 to 25,000 leukocytes/mm^3, and there is a polymorphonuclear leukocyte predominance. Elderly patients have a lower rate of seropositivity (48 percent) and appear to have a better prognosis. Revised criteria for the diagnosis of rheumatoid arthritis were published in 1987 by the American Rheumatism Association. These criteria include the following:

1. *Morning stiffness:* Stiffness in and around joints, lasting 1 h before maximal improvement, occurs in 98

percent of patients. It worsens with inactivity and lessens with activity.
2. *Arthritis of three or more joint areas:* At least three joint areas observed by a physician at one examination have soft tissue swelling or joint effusions, not just bone overgrowth. The 14 possible joint areas involved are the right or left proximal interphalangeal, metacarpophalangeal, elbow, wrist, knee, ankle, and MTP joints.
3. *Arthritis of hand joints:* There is arthritis of the wrist, metacarpophalangeal, or proximal interphalangeal joints.
4. *Symmetrical arthritis:* The same joint areas on both sides of the body are simultaneously involved.
5. *Rheumatoid nodules:* Subcutaneous nodules over bony prominences, extensor surfaces, or juxtaarticular areas are observed by a physician (prevalence, 20–30 percent). They are located over the olecranon bursa, the proximal ulna, the Achilles tendon, the occipital region, and other sites.
6. *Serum rheumatoid factor:* An abnormal amount of serum rheumatoid factor is demonstrated by any method for which the result has been positive in less than 5 percent of normal control subjects. In patients over age 65, the seropositivity rate in the general population without rheumatoid arthritis is 10 to 20 percent.
7. *Radiographic changes:* Typical changes of rheumatoid arthritis on a posteroanterior hand and wrist radiograph. These changes must include erosions or bony decalcification localized in or most severe adjacent to the involved joints.

Four of these criteria are required for classification of a patient as having rheumatoid arthritis. The sensitivity of these criteria is 91 to 94 percent, and the specificity 89 percent. Those with more than one diagnosis are not excluded. Some patients with early rheumatoid arthritis may fail to meet these criteria (e.g., low seropositivity rate in first 3 months, asymmetrical joint involvement, absence of erosive changes in early cases, and absence of subcutaneous nodules). Further abnormalities may develop with time and can be detected through continued observation.

8. ADULT-ONSET STILL'S DISEASE

Fever exceeds 39°C (102.2°F) in 81 percent of cases. It follows a quotidian or double quotidian pattern (i.e., a single or double daily temperature spike). A typical rash occurs in 85 to 90 percent of cases. It consists of 2- to 5-mm salmon-colored macules that are most frequently distributed over the trunk and proximal extremities but may appear on the palms, soles, and face. Individual macules may be encircled by a narrow zone of pallor, and the larger lesions may show central clearing. The skin rash may mimic urticaria, but it is not pruritic. The rash is typically evanescent in any one location, migratory, and associated with fever. It may be present only late in the evening and be gone by morning.

Polyarthralgia may occur in up to 100 percent of cases. Definite evidence of joint enlargement occurs in 76 percent of patients at the onset of the illness. The joints are enlarged due to periarticular edema and/or intraarticular effusion. Polyarthritis (more than four joints) and polyarthralgia are bilaterally symmetrical. The small joints of the hands and feet, the knees, the ankles, the elbows, and the shoulders are most commonly affected. Rest pain may occur, but joint discomfort may only appear on weight bearing, movement, or other use. Swelling, heat, and tenderness occur, but erythema of the overlying skin is uncommon. Morning stiffness occurs in 95 percent, myalgia in 76 percent, abdominal pain in 48 percent, sore throat in 90 percent, and weight loss (>10 percent of body weight) in 67 percent of cases. Tenosynovitis may affect the extensor tendons of the fingers, wrists, ankles, and toes.

Examination reveals fever; an evanescent rash; lymphadenopathy (69–90 percent) involving nodes in the cervical, axillary, inguinal, submandibular, and supraclavicular areas; hepatomegaly (38–48 percent); and splenomegaly (52–65 percent). Laboratory findings at presentation include negative test results for rheumatoid factor (94 percent of cases) and antinuclear antibody (93 percent), an elevated erythrocyte sedimentation rate (>40 mm/h; 96 percent), anemia (hemoglobin <10 g; 59 percent), leukocytosis (89 percent), granulocytosis (83 percent), liver dysfunction (elevated AST, ALT, and alkaline phosphatase levels), and hyperferritinemia (82 percent). Serum complement levels may be increased in 67 percent.

During the course of the disease, pleuritis may occur in 12 to 43 percent, pericarditis in 10 to 33 percent, and pneumonitis in 6 to 10 percent of cases. Glomerulitis, with albuminuria, cylindruria, and microhematuria, may develop in 15 percent, peripheral neuropathy in 6 percent, and meningoencephalitis in 8 percent. Myocarditis leading to cardiac failure is a rare complication. Symptoms respond to oral corticosteroids and less well to nonsteroidal anti-inflammatory drugs.

Coxsackie B4 infection has been reported to cause an illness that is clinically indistinguishable from adult-onset Still's disease, with rash, spiking fever, and polyarthritis. Other viruses reported to cause a similar polyarticular disorder include adenovirus, mumps virus, and rubella virus.

9. SYSTEMIC LUPUS ERYTHEMATOSUS

Polyarthralgia or symmetrical polyarthritis is present at onset in the majority of patients. Arthralgia or arthritis occurs in the proximal interphalangeal joints (82 percent), knees (76 percent), wrists and metacarpophalangeal joints (50–70 percent), ankles (55 percent), elbows (54 percent), and shoulders (45 percent). Morning stiffness may

occur in 50 percent of cases. Knee effusions contain less than 3000 cells/mm^3, with a lymphocyte predominance. Antinuclear antibodies and LE cells may be present in synovial fluid, and synovial fluid complement levels are depressed. The American Rheumatism Association criteria for the classification of systemic lupus erythematosus are listed below. Four of the 11 are required for diagnosis. Prevalence is given in percent in parentheses after each criterion.

The 11 criteria are (1) malar rash (40–64 percent); (2) discoid lupus (17–32 percent); (3) photosensitivity (17–41 percent); (4) oral ulcers (15–36 percent); (5) arthritis (86–90 percent) in two or more peripheral joints, with tenderness, swelling, or effusion and absence of erosion on plain joint radiographs; (6) cardiopulmonary disease with serositis in the form of pleuritis (50 percent) or pericarditis (30 percent), and/or myocarditis (10 percent); (7) renal disease, with proteinuria (>500 mg/24 h; 50 percent), cellular casts (50 percent), nephrotic syndrome (25 percent), and renal failure (5–10 percent); (8) neurologic disorder with seizures (20 percent) or psychosis (10 percent); (9) hematologic disorder, with hemolytic anemia (10 percent), anemia of chronic disease (50–70 percent), leukopenia (17–65 percent), lymphopenia (50 percent), or thrombocytopenia (5 percent); (10) an immunologic disorder with LE cells in the peripheral blood and/or anti-ds-DNA (40 percent), and anti-Sm (Smith; 30 percent) antibodies in the serum, or a false-positive serologic test result for syphilis (25 percent); and (11) an elevated titer of antinuclear antibody (85–95 percent). The presence of one component of a criterion (e.g., leukopenia for the hematologic disorder criterion) satisfies the requirements of that criterion. The presence of four or more criteria allows classification of a patient as having systemic lupus erythematosus.

Joint and other symptoms frequently improve dramatically with corticosteroid therapy.

10. POLYARTHRITIS AND VASCULITIS

A. Polyarteritis Nodosa Nonspecific symptoms, such as fever (71 percent), weight loss (54 percent), malaise, anorexia, weakness, and fatigue, occur. Polyarthralgia (53–70 percent) and myalgia (31 percent) are common, but polyarthritis with joint swelling and tenderness is infrequent. An asymmetrical nondeforming polyarthritis, primarily involving the larger joints (knees and ankles) of the lower extremities, may occur early in the disease. This polyarthritis often subsides spontaneously as the disease progresses. It may sometimes be mistaken for rheumatoid arthritis. Skin involvement includes livedo reticularis; tender, 0.5- to 1-cm skin infarcts; painful, tender, erythematous, 0.5- to 3-cm subcutaneous nodules (due to inflammation of small subcutaneous arteries; 30 percent of cases); skin ulceration; and petechiae. The peripheral nervous system may be involved, producing mononeuropathy multiplex or a symmetrical sensory polyneuropathy (51 percent of cases). Central nervous system disease (32 percent of cases) may occur in the form of hemiplegia (11 percent), aphasia, dementia or delirium (10 percent), and/or seizures (4 percent). Hypertension occurs in 54 percent, congestive heart failure in 12 percent, and usually silent myocardial infarction in 6 percent. Renal involvement develops in 70 percent of cases in the form of proteinuria, microhematuria, red blood cell casts, and progressive renal failure. Gastrointestinal symptoms are caused by organ ischemia or infarction. Localized pain may be caused by gallbladder, appendix, or bowel infarction. Gastrointestinal bleeding occurs in 6 percent, bowel perforation in 5 percent, and bowel infarction in 1.4 percent. The mean age of onset is 45, and the male/female ratio is 2.5:1. Laboratory abnormalities include an elevated erythrocyte sedimentation rate (94 percent), leukocytosis (74 percent), anemia (66 percent), thrombocytosis (53 percent), depression of C3 (70 percent) and C4 (30 percent), a rheumatoid factor titer of $\geq$ 1:160 (40 percent), circulating immune complexes (63 percent), and cryoglobulins (25 percent). HB_sAg is present in the serum in 10 to 30 percent of cases.

The diagnosis can be supported by angiography demonstrating multiple aneurysms of small and medium-sized renal and visceral arteries and confirmed by a biopsy of a painful muscle, testis, or skin nodule that demonstrates granulocytic infiltration of the wall of a small or medium-sized artery and vessel necrosis.

The American College of Rheumatology criteria published in 1990 for the classification of polyarteritis nodosa include the following: (1) involuntary weight loss of at least 4 kg; (2) livedo reticularis; (3) testicular pain and/or tenderness not due to infection, injury, or other causes; (4) myalgias, weakness, or leg tenderness; (5) mononeuropathy or polyneuropathy; (6) diastolic pressure greater than 90 mmHg of recent onset; (7) elevated blood urea nitrogen (BUN) or creatinine levels not caused by dehydration or obstruction; (8) detection of hepatitis B virus (i.e., HB_sAg) or recent appearance of anti-HB in serum; (9) an arteriogram showing saccular or fusiform aneurysms of renal, hepatic, and visceral arteries not due to fibromuscular dysplasia, arteriosclerosis, other nonvasculitic causes, an overlap syndrome, or systemic lupus erythematosus; and (10) biopsy of a small or medium-sized artery demonstrating a necrotizing vasculitis with granulocytes or granulocytes and monocytes in the artery wall.

The presence of three or more criteria supports a diagnosis of polyarteritis nodosa with a sensitivity of 82 percent and a specificity of 87 percent.

B. Allergic Angiitis and Granulomatosis (Churg-Strauss Disease) This disorder is a form of necrotizing vasculitis with eosinophilia, pulmonary infiltrates, and severe asthma. Many findings seen in polyarteritis nodosa occur (e.g., fever, hypertension, skin nodules and purpura, neuropathy, and myocardial ischemia). Biopsy of affected tissues (e.g., skin nodules and tender muscles) reveals tissue infiltration by eosinophils and granulomatous vasculitis. Arthritis or arthralgia may occur in 21 percent of cases. Renal involvement is less severe than in classic polyarteritis nodosa. Asthma and pulmonary infiltrates usually precede systemic symptoms and signs by a mean of 2 years.

C. Polyangiitis Overlap Syndrome This disorder may have features of polyarteritis nodosa, Churg-Strauss disease, and hypersensitivity vasculitis. Because of this, classification is difficult, and such cases are placed in this diagnostic category. A patient with severe renal disease, mononeuropathy multiplex, aneurysms of small and medium-sized renal arteries, asthma, eosinophilia, polyarthritis or polyarthralgia, and cutaneous vasculitis involving small venules (i.e., palpable purpura) might be classified as having the polyangiitis overlap syndrome.

D. Wegener's Granulomatosis Polyarthralgia or polyarthritis occurs in up to 44 percent of cases. Upper airway disease is a prominent feature and includes purulent sinusitis (67 percent of cases), nasal ulceration, chronic rhinitis (22 percent), otitis media (25 percent), and hearing loss. Cough occurs in 25 percent and hemoptysis in 18 percent. Fever (34 percent), weight loss (16 percent), and anorexia may occur. Chest radiographs show bilateral pulmonary infiltrates (71 percent), which may be diffuse, nodular, or tumorlike. Cavitation of pulmonary lesions is common, while pleural effusions occur in 20 percent of cases. Renal involvement causes proteinuria, microhematuria, cellular casts, and an elevated creatinine level (11 percent of cases). Anemia, leukocytosis, and an elevated erythrocyte sedimentation rate are frequent findings. Rheumatoid factor may be present in up to 50 percent of severe cases. Antineutrophil cytoplasmic antibody (ANCA) levels are frequently elevated in the serum. Renal biopsy findings include a mild focal or segmental glomerulonephritis or focal necrotizing glomerulonephritis with crescents and extravascular granulomas. Results of immunofluorescent staining of glomeruli for immunoglobulins or complement are usually negative. Biopsy of involved nasal or sinus mucosa or lung tissue will allow a specific tissue diagnosis. Symptoms respond to combined therapy with prednisone and cyclophosphamide.

11. SUBACUTE BACTERIAL ENDOCARDITIS

This disorder causes fever, anorexia, weakness, weight loss, malaise, and delirium. The latter may be subtle but is often noticed by family members as mild confusion and memory loss. Low back pain, polyarthralgias, or polyarthritis may occur in up to 35 percent of cases. The peripheral joints affected are usually the larger proximal ones (e.g., knees, elbows, ankles, wrists, and shoulders). A mitral or aortic insufficiency murmur is usually present in patients without a history of drug addiction.

A tricuspid systolic murmur may be audible, a pulsating enlarged liver palpable, and a systolic V wave in the external jugular veins visible in an intravenous drug abuser with endocarditis-related tricuspid regurgitation. Patients with left-sided endocarditis may have cutaneous and conjunctival petechiae, reddish-brown to black splinter hemorrhages, cotton-wool perivascular exudates, and sometimes hemorrhages in the retina. Two-dimensional echocardiography may detect vegetations as small as 2 mm. The sensitivity for detection of vegetations varies between 60 and 90 percent. Blood cultures are usually positive (86 percent of cases). Joint symptoms, fever, anorexia, and delirium resolve within 2 to 3 days of initiation of intravenous antibiotic therapy. A therapeutic trial of parenteral antibiotic therapy in a blood culture-negative, clinically likely case is a useful test.

12. LYME DISEASE

This disease follows a tick bite received in an endemic area for the causative agent, *Borrelia burgdorferi*. Within 3 to 30 days, an annular, spreading skin lesion occurs at the bite site and achieves a diameter of 5 to 68 cm (mean, 15 cm). In 50 percent of untreated patients, a flulike illness accompanies the appearance and progression of the rash. Symptoms include fever, chills, myalgia, arthralgia, headache, neck pain and stiffness, fatigue, weakness, and malaise. If the diagnosis is not made and treatment initiated, up to 60 percent of patients may develop a recurrent oligoarthritis involving the knees, ankles, wrists, and small finger and toe joints or, less commonly, a symmetrical polyarthritis. Joint symptoms may wax and wane over a period of months or years.

Up to 15 percent of untreated patients may develop an acute aseptic meningitis or meningoencephalitis with mental changes (decreased memory, attention span, and mild confusion). Unilateral or bilateral facial palsy, diplopia due to abducens paralysis, and painful plexopathies, radiculopathies, or radiculoneuropathies may also occur. These radiculoneuropathies and plexopathies may cause extremity and truncal pain, paresthesias, and unpleasant dysesthesias.

The diagnosis is established by clinical criteria and confirmed by use of serologic tests for *B. burgdorferi* antibodies (ELISA and Western blot, or an indirect immunofluorescence assay). Treatment with parenteral ceftriaxone usually leads to improvement or resolution of rheumatologic and neurologic symptoms.

13. CRYSTAL-INDUCED ARTHRITIS

A. Polyarticular Gout The initial attack in acute gout is usually monoarticular (85–90 percent) and involves the

first metatarsophalangeal joint in 50 percent of cases. Initial episodes may also be polyarticular, as may subsequent attacks. Polyarticular gout begins with severe, aching pain, which is intensified by weight bearing or use, in the knees, ankles, and feet (83 percent of involved joints are in the lower extremities), wrists, elbows, and hands. A symmetrical or asymmetrical distribution of joint involvement may be present. The patient may be totally incapacitated and bedridden during the attack. Systemic symptoms, such as fever, myalgia, and weakness, are common. The knees, ankles, and other large joints may contain joint effusions, and the overlying skin may be warm, erythematous, swollen, and tender.

Severe skin hyperesthesia may be present in the periarticular area. Bursitis at the shoulder and elbow and Achilles tendinitis may accompany a polyarticular episode. The diagnosis can be confirmed by analysis of synovial fluid. There is an increased concentration of polymorphonuclear leukocytes in the synovial fluid as well as intracellular and extracellular monosodium urate crystals (84 percent of cases). Symptoms respond to colchicine and/or indomethacin therapy within 2 to 7 days.

The first attack of gout in a woman may be polyarticular in 26 to 35 percent of cases, while the initial episode in a man is polyarticular in only 3 to 10 percent. The uric acid level is elevated above 7 mg/dl in 97 to 98 percent of cases of acute gout. Precipitating causes of an attack of acute gout include trauma, dietary excess, exercise, alcohol, medical illness, surgery, and drugs (e.g., thiazide diuretics; vitamin B12 for pernicious anemia; administration of allopurinol or probenecid shortly after an attack; administration of radioactive phosphorous [^{32}P] for polycythemia vera; use of cytotoxic drugs for the leukemias; low doses of aspirin, high doses of nicotinic acid; and administration of the antituberculous drug pyrazinamide). Only 3 to 7 percent of cases of primary gout occur in women, most of whom are postmenopausal. Only 10 percent of patients with gouty arthritis have demonstrable tophi. Bony tophaceous lesions may be observed as "punched-out" round or oval, lytic, juxtaarticular lesions on plain radiographs of the hands, wrists, and feet.

B. Calcium Pyrophosphate Dihydrate Deposition Disease The average age of onset is 72, and the male/female ratio is 1.5:1. Up to 40 percent of attacks may be polyarticular. Two or more joints (e.g., knees, wrists, hips, ankles, elbows, shoulders, calcaneocuboid joints, and small joints of the fingers and toes) may become involved simultaneously, or a single joint may be affected, followed by a cluster attack involving one or more joints situated near the initially affected joint(s). A cluster attack begins 1 day or more after the initial attack.

The involved joints are swollen, warm, red, immobile, and painful. Fever, dizziness, headache, and mental confusion may occur. Synovial fluid contains an increased concentration of polymorphonuclear leukocytes and calcium pyrophosphate dihydrate crystals. Plain radiographs of the knees, shoulders, wrists, and/or ankles may demonstrate chondrocalcinosis. Attacks may be provoked by parathyroidectomy, other operative procedures (9.4 percent of cases), a severe medical illness (e.g., stroke or myocardial infarction; 24 percent of cases), or trauma.

Attacks of polyarthritis respond within 48 h to colchicine or indomethacin. Acute episodes are usually less severe than in gouty arthritis.

14. POLYARTHRITIS AND BOWEL DISEASE

A. Polyarthritis Associated with Inflammatory Bowel Disease   The onset of arthritis is usually abrupt, and in 80 percent of cases joint involvement coincides with the first symptoms of inflammatory bowel disease or occurs within the first year. In the remainder of cases, the arthritis may precede the bowel disease by 1 to 3 years. The knees, hips, and ankles are most frequently involved, but the interphalangeal, metacarpophalangeal, and metatarsophalangeal joints may also be affected. The arthritis is often migratory or additive. It may remain oligoarticular and asymmetrical or develop into a symmetrical polyarthritis.

The course of the arthritis is affected by the activity of the bowel disease in up to 74 percent of patients. Spontaneous resolution of each attack of arthritis occurs in 4 to 12 weeks. Episodes may recur at variable intervals.

Skin manifestations include erythema nodosum, pyoderma gangrenosum, and, less commonly, erythema multiforme. Painful oral ulcers may occur. Anemia, mild leukocytosis, and an elevated erythrocyte sedimentation rate may be present. Most patients are seronegative for rheumatoid factor and antinuclear antibody. Synovial fluids have cell counts in the inflammatory range, and there is a polymorphonuclear predominance. Radiographs show periarticular edema and juxtaarticular osteopenia.

The diagnosis of inflammatory bowel disease can be confirmed by colonoscopy and/or enteroclysis. Nonsteroidal anti-inflammatory drugs control joint pain and allow function. Bowel resection often leads to remission of the arthritis.

B. Bowel-Associated Dermatosis-Arthritis Syndrome   This disorder occurs in 20 percent of patients who have had a jejunoileal bypass procedure to treat obesity. Fever, chills, myalgias, polyarthralgia, and malaise are accompanied by an eruption of 2- to 4-mm erythematous, tender papules and pustules on the upper trunk and extremities. This disorder resolves spontaneously in 2 to 6 days and recurs every 1 to 6 weeks. Results of cultures of the blood and the pustules are negative. Similar episodes have also been reported after gastric surgery for ulcer disease and after colectomy or proctectomy for inflammatory bowel disease. Reversal of the bypass procedure or treatment of the inflammatory bowel disease results in cessation of attacks.

C. Whipple's Disease   This disease may present with an acute episode of symmetrical or asymmetrical polyarthralgia or polyarthritis. The knees, ankles, fingers, wrists, shoulders, elbows, hips, and temporomandibular joints may be involved. Examination may reveal normal joints or swelling, redness, warmth, and tenderness. Acute attacks may last 3 to 14 days and recur once or twice a month. Fever, chills, diaphoresis, fatigue, and malaise may accompany the joint symptoms. Weight loss and abdominal pain (95 percent of cases), diarrhea (78 percent of cases), and fatty stools may not develop for up to 10 years after joint symptoms begin. This disorder occurs with a male/female ratio of 9:1. The diagnosis may be confirmed by finding numerous macrophages containing PAS-positive, diastase-resistant bacilliform structures on a peroral jejunal biopsy or a synovial or lymph node biopsy. The causative bacillus of this disease has been identified as an actinomycete (i.e., *Tropheryma whippelii*) using a molecular genetic approach, but it has not been cultured on artificial media. Joint and intestinal symptoms respond to 4 weeks of tetracycline therapy.

15. SARCOID ARTHRITIS

Acute sarcoidosis may cause joint pain in 89 percent of patients, and arthralgia is associated with periarticular swelling in 63 to 69 percent of patients. The ankles and knees are most commonly involved, but any joint can be affected. Bilateral heel pain is a common presentation. Erythema nodosum and hilar adenopathy are frequent associated findings (Lofgren's syndrome). The joints are often tender, and the overlying skin warm, erythematous, and edematous. In some patients, joint pain is minimal and range-of-motion pain absent. Joint symptoms resolve within 1 to 4 months. Synovial biopsy usually reveals a nonspecific synovitis and, less commonly, granulomas. Muscle pain may occur, and biopsy of tender areas may reveal granulomata. Noninvasive evidence supporting a diagnosis of sarcoid arthritis includes detection of an elevated level of serum angiotensin-converting enzyme (75-percent sensitive) and a gallium citrate (^{67}Ga) radionuclide scan showing increased uptake over the salivary and lacrimal glands. A lymph node, skin, muscle, or lung biopsy that demonstrates noncaseating granulomas in the absence of other causes confirms the diagnosis. Symptoms improve or resolve with prednisone therapy.

16. POLYCHONDRITIS

The initial attack may cause erythema and painful swelling of the auricles, with sparing of the ear lobes; a symmetrical or asymmetrical polyarthritis, involving large and small joints and the parasternal articulations; costochondritis; arthritis of the spine; ocular inflammation (episcleritis, scleritis, conjunctivitis, or iritis); and laryngotracheal-bronchial inflammation. The polyarthritis is non-erosive and resolves spontaneously or with prednisone therapy. The diagnosis can usually be made on the basis of the unique auricular findings on examination and can be confirmed, if necessary, by auricular cartilage biopsy.

17. BEHÇET'S SYNDROME

The diagnosis of complete Behçet's syndrome requires the presence of oral, cutaneous, eye, and genital lesions. The presence of disease at less than four of these sites requires a diagnosis of incomplete Behçet's syndrome.

Painful oral ulcers, skin lesions (erythema nodosum, superficial thrombophlebitis, folliculitis, acnelike lesions, and pathergy), eye lesions (iridocyclitis, hypopyon, posterior uveitis, and chorioretinitis), and genital ulcers are major criteria for diagnosis and occur in the majority of patients. Polyarthralgia or polyarthritis (e.g., rheumatoid or Reiter's-like) affects large and small joints in up to 60 percent of cases. The knees and ankles are commonly involved. Synovial fluid reveals inflammatory-range cell counts, with a polymorphonuclear leukocyte predominance. Less frequent manifestations include colon ulcerations, epididymitis, arterial occlusions and aneurysms, and neurologic or neuropsychiatric disorders. Symptoms may respond to chlorambucil therapy.

18. POLYARTHRITIS ASSOCIATED WITH MALIGNANT DISEASE

A. Leukemia   Symmetrical and/or migratory polyarthritis and polyarthralgias may be associated with acute leukemia. Articular symptoms are more common in children. Joint pain may be disproportionately severe when compared to the appearance of the involved joints. The diagnosis may be confirmed by a peripheral blood smear or bone marrow examination. Rheumatoid factor and nodules have been reported in patients with leukemia. Chemotherapy of the leukemia may result in remission of the articular symptoms.

B. Carcinoma Polyarthritis   This disorder produces a seronegative symmetrical or asymmetrical polyarthritis that may be confused with rheumatoid arthritis. If associated with fever, it may be mistaken for adult-onset Still's disease. Eighty percent of women with this syndrome have carcinoma of the breast. The lower extremity joints are most frequently affected, and the wrists and hands are usually spared. Joint symptoms may have an abrupt onset. Treatment of the tumor may result in improvement or relief of joint symptoms. Polyarthralgia or polyarthritis may return if the neoplasm recurs.

C. Lymphoma   Arthritic manifestations may occur but are rare. Mono- or polyarthritis may develop. The diagnosis is dependent on the clinical findings and lymph node or bone marrow biopsy. Cutaneous T-cell lymphoma with polyarthralgia or polyarthritis (e.g., involving the metacarpophalangeal joints, wrists, elbows, shoulders, and feet) and erythroderma has been reported. Infiltration of synovial tissue with malignant cells or a reactive arthritis may be the cause of arthritic symptoms.

19. POLYARTHRITIS ASSOCIATED WITH FAMILIAL HYPERCHOLESTEROLEMIA (TYPE II HYPERLIPOPROTEINEMIA)

An acute migratory polyarthritis that may be mistaken for acute rheumatic fever occurs in 4 percent of patients with the heterozygous and in 56 percent of patients with the homozygous form of familial hypercholesterolemia. Atheromatous involvement of the aortic valve may cause aortic stenosis.

The joints most commonly involved include the knees, proximal interphalangeal joints, ankles, wrists, elbows, shoulders, and hips. The Achilles tendon may become inflamed. Polyarthralgia or polyarthritis, with joint swelling, tenderness, heat, and redness, may occur. Radiographs reveal no evidence of erosions unless they are related to xanthomas. Tendinous xanthomas on the hands and tuberous xanthomas of the knees, xanthelasma, arcus senilis, and hypercholesterolemia are associated findings. There is no bacteriologic or serologic evidence of a recent streptococcal infection. Joint symptoms usually resolve spontaneously in a few days but may recur. Attacks usually begin in childhood or adolescence and may antedate the appearance of xanthomas.

20. RARE CAUSES OF INFECTIOUS POLYARTHRALGIA OR POLYARTHRITIS

A. Secondary Syphilis   Systemic symptoms, such as fever (70 percent of cases), malaise, anorexia, weight loss, and polyarthralgias, begin 2 to 8 weeks after appearance of the primary lesion (i.e., chancre). Sore throat and hoarseness may also occur. Up to 90 percent of patients develop macular, maculopapular, papular, and/or pustular lesions on the trunk and proximal extremities. Macular and maculopapular lesions are most frequent, while pustular lesions occur in only a small percentage of cases. All of the listed types of rashes may be present simultaneously in a single patient. The presence of lesions on the palms and soles is suggestive of the diagnosis.

Condylomata lata (gray-white to erythematous, moist plaques) occur in the intertriginous areas, perianal region, vulva, scrotum, nasolabial folds, and interdigital webs. Mucous patches (gray erosions surrounded by erythema) appear in the mouth and pharynx or on the vulva, vagina, cervix, and glans penis. Erosions and aphthous ulcers may also occur in the mouth and throat. Polyarthritis, periostitis, and osteitis occur but are rare. Hepatitis, glomerulonephritis, or the nephrotic syndrome occur in a small number of cases. Central nervous system involvement may occur in up to 40 percent, with headache and a painful stiff neck the most common symptoms. The diagnosis can be supported by an RPR or a VDRL test (98–100-percent sensitive, except in AIDS) and confirmed by a fluorescent treponema antibody absorption test. Polyarthralgias and other symptoms and signs resolve rapidly with penicillin therapy.

B. Brucellosis Arthritis may occur in 22 to 34 percent of patients. It may be monoarticular or polyarticular and migratory or additive. The knees (52 percent of cases) and hips (52 percent) are most frequently involved. Ankles, shoulders, elbows, wrists, and finger joints may be affected. The lumbar spine and sacroiliac joints (47 percent) may also be involved. Fever (88 percent), headache, diaphoresis, chills, anorexia, weight loss, and myalgias accompany the joint symptoms. The liver may be enlarged in 17 percent and the spleen in 24 percent of cases. This disorder is usually acquired by drinking unpasteurized milk, eating cheese made from such milk, or inhaling aerosolized bacteria (e.g., abattoir workers).

The diagnosis may be confirmed by serologic methods (i.e., standard tube agglutination) or by positive blood, bone marrow, or synovial fluid culture results. The sensitivity of cultures is low in subacute or chronic cases. Symptoms respond to combined therapy with streptomycin and tetracycline or doxycycline and rifampin.

C. Rat-Bite Fever Fever, chills, headache, vomiting, and severe migratory polyarthralgias and myalgias begin 1 to 22 days after a rat bite. Those at risk include laboratory workers, farmers, and people living in rat-infested houses or rural areas. In many cases, there is no recollection of a rat bite.

After 2 to 4 days, a generalized maculopapular rash (93 percent of cases) develops and may become petechial. The extensor surfaces of the extremities, palms, and soles may be involved. Up to 50 percent of patients develop an asymmetrical migratory polyarthritis. The knees, ankles, elbows, wrists, shoulders, hips, proximal interphalangeal joints, and metacarpophalangeal joints may become warm, swollen, painful, and tender. Fever subsides spontaneously in 3 to 5 days, and the joint symptoms in 2 to 6 weeks, or recurrent fevers may occur. The presence of palmoplantar macules may lead to confusion with Rocky Mountain spotted fever and secondary syphilis.

The diagnosis can be established by synovial fluid culture on trypticase soy agar with 5% sheep blood at 35°C under microaerophilic conditions or on chocolate agar. Results of blood cultures in tryptic soy broth with resins may be positive. Three to 5 days of culture may be required. Since sodium polyanethol sulfonate may inhibit growth of some strains, use of culture medium not containing it is required. A biological false-positive test for syphilis occurs in 25 percent of cases.

Streptobacillus moniliformis is present in the mouths of 50 percent of wild and laboratory rats. Close contact with dogs, cats, pigs, squirrels, and dead rats may transmit the disease without a bite. Treatment with penicillin is rapidly effective.

D. Viral Arthritis: Rare Causes in the United States Polyarticular arthritis has been reported in rare cases of adenovirus (types 1 and 7), mumps virus, echovirus (types 6, 9, and 11), and coxsackievirus (B_2, B_3, B_4, and B_6). Herpes virus (Epstein-Barr virus, cytomegalovirus, varicella-zoster, and herpes simplex) tend to cause an oligoarthritis or monarthritis involving the larger joints.

Endemic and sometimes epidemic viral arthritis with fever, a maculopapular rash, and polyarthralgia or polyarthritis occur in Australia (Ross River virus), Africa, and Asia (chikungunya virus and Sindbis virus), South America (Mayaro virus), and Sweden (Ockelbo virus and Pogosta virus).

E. Poncet's Disease (Tuberculous Rheumatism) This rare manifestation of primary tuberculous infection causes a painful polyarthritis in association with fever and positive skin test results for tuberculosis (i.e., purified protein derivative). Joint radiographs are usually normal. The chest radiograph may be negative or show unilateral or bilateral apical or other infiltrates and hilar adenopathy. Sputum culture results may be positive for *Mycobacterium tuberculosis*. Symptoms usually respond to antituberculous drugs. The existence of this disorder has been questioned by some authors.

21. ALLERGIC SYNOVITIS

A. Food-Induced Polyarthralgia or Polyarthritis Polyarthralgia or pain limited to two or three joints may be associated with urticaria. Joint pain may be precipitated by ingestion of certain foods and prevented by an elimination diet. Many patients with food-related arthralgia are atopic and have a history of hay fever, asthma, eczema, and/or urticaria. Rarely, joint swelling may accompany the pain.

Common foods causing allergic arthralgia include eggs, wheat, milk, cheese, and other dairy products. Some patients with established arthritis (e.g., rheumatoid arthritis) may note worsening of joint symptoms after ingestion of specific foods. Skin testing, the radioallergosorbent (RAST) test, and an elimination diet may help identify the responsible food. Confirmation can be obtained in patients with equivocal findings by a double-blind food challenge using encapsulated lyophilized food and placebo (D-xylose). Symptoms may respond to elimination of the offending food and antihistamines.

B. Serum Sickness   Fever and chills begin 3 to 10 days after drug or serum administration. Polyarthralgia and/or polyarthritis occurs in the knees, ankles, wrists, hands, and feet. Pain at rest or only with joint use or movement occurs. The joints may be tender, warm, and swollen. Generalized lymphadenopathy and a maculopapular or urticarial rash and/or edema of the legs may occur in severe cases. Microhematuria and albuminuria and a rise in the serum creatinine level reflect immune complex-induced glomerulitis. Symptoms resolve within a few days of withdrawal of the offending drug. Penicillin and other antimicrobial drugs are frequently responsible (31 percent of cases in one series). Serum sickness, with fever and polyarthritis, has been reported after administration of streptokinase for the treatment of myocardial infarction and antivenin for snake bites that is prepared from equine serum.

C. Drug-Associated Polyarthralgia or Polyarthritis
Polyarthralgia or polyarthritis has been reported after therapeutic administration of quinidine, amphotericin B, cimetidine (600–1000 mg/day), levamisole, beta blockers (metoprolol and practalol), oral contraceptives, and barbiturates. Joint symptoms improve and resolve after discontinuance of the responsible drug.

D. Schönlein-Henoch Purpura   Patients may present with polyarthralgia or polyarthritis and a maculopapular rash on the legs and buttocks that may become purpuric (i.e., palpable purpura). Less commonly, skin nodules, vesicles, bullae, and ulceration may occur. Immune deposition occurs in postcapillary venules, resulting in a leukocytoclastic venulitis. Renal involvement causes proteinuria, microhematuria, and cylindruria and may result in creatinine elevation. Serum IgA levels may be elevated. Histopathologic and immunofluorescence studies of the kidneys reveal only mild mesangial proliferation or crescents and mesangial deposits of IgA, C3, and properdin. This disorder is uncommon after adolescence and is more frequent in males (male/female ratio, 2:1).

Infection, drugs (e.g., sulfonamides and penicillin), and exposure to exogenous antigens (e.g., possibly food antigens) have been considered to be precipitating events. Palpable purpura (vasculitic purpura) may also occur in systemic lupus erythematosus, rheumatoid arthritis, and essential mixed cryoglobulinemia. Prednisone may improve symptoms in some cases.

22. SUBCORNEAL PUSTULAR DERMATOSIS WITH POLYARTHRITIS

This disorder causes an erythematous rash with vesicles and pustules. A low-grade fever may be associated. Polyarthralgia or polyarthritis occurs, with swelling and tenderness of shoulder, wrist, knee, ankle, finger, and toe joints.

This disease has been treated symptomatically with nonsteroidal anti-inflammatory drugs with good results in some cases.

GENERALIZED JOINT PAIN REFERENCES

Acute Rheumatic Fever

Chun LT, Reddy DV, Yamamoto LG: Rheumatic fever in children and adolescents in Hawaii. *Pediatrics* 79:549–552, 1987.

Congeni B, Rizzo C, Congeni J, et al: Outbreak of acute rheumatic fever in northeast Ohio. *J Pediatr* 111:176–179, 1987.

Farrell AJ, Zaphiropoulos GC: First attack of rheumatic fever in an adult: The case for greater awareness. *Ann Rheum Dis* 49:1008–1009, 1990.

Griffiths SP, Gersony WM: Acute rheumatic fever in New York City (1969 to 1988): A comparative study of two decades. *J Pediatr* 116:882–887, 1990.

Livneh A, Sharma K, Sewell KL, et al: Multisystem disease in poststreptococcal arthritis. *Ann Rheum Dis* 50:328–329, 1991.

Ruttenberg HD: Acute rheumatic fever in the 1980s. *Pediatrician* 13:180–188, 1986.

Stollerman GH: Rheumatic fever, in Wilson JD, Braunwald E, Isselbacher KJ, et al (eds): *Harrison's Principles of Internal Medicine,* 12th ed. New York, McGraw-Hill, 1991, vol 1, pp 933–938.

Taranta A: Rheumatic fever, in McCarty DJ (ed): *Arthritis and Allied Conditions,* 11th ed. Philadelphia, Lea & Febiger, 1989, pp 1214–1226.

Tatengco MV, Weinhouse E, Jarenwattananon M, et al: Acute rheumatic fever in Wisconsin. *Wis Med J* 88:11–15, 1989.

Westlake RM, Graham TP, Edwards KM: An outbreak of acute rheumatic fever in Tennessee. *Pediatr Infect Dis J* 9:97–100, 1990.

Allergic (Food-Induced) Synovitis

Carini C, Fratazzi C, Aiuti F: Immune complexes in food-induced arthralgia. *Ann Allergy* 59:422–428, 1987.

Golding DN: Is there an allergic synovitis? *J R Soc Med* 83:312–314, 1990.

Polyarthritis—Adult-Onset Still's Disease

Arber N, Weinberger A, Fadila R, et al: Adult onset Still's disease. *Clin Rheumatol* 8:339–344, 1989.

Cassidy JT: Juvenile rheumatoid arthritis, in Kelley WN, Harris ED Jr, Ruddy S, et al (eds): *Textbook of Rheumatology.* Philadelphia, Saunders, 1981, vol 2, pp 1279–1305.

Cush JJ, Medsger TA Jr, Christy WC, et al: Adult-onset Still's disease: Clinical course and outcome. *Arthritis Rheum* 30:186–194, 1987.

Ohta A, Yamaguchi M, Tsunematsu T, et al: Adult Still's disease: A multicenter survey of Japanese patients. *J Rheumatol* 17:1058–1063, 1990.

Roberts-Thomson PJ, Ahern MJ, Southwood TR, et al: Adult onset Still's disease or coxsackie polyarthritis? *Aust N Z J Med* 16: 509–511, 1986.

Polyarthritis — Behçet's Syndrome
Ehrlich GE: Intermittent and periodic arthritis syndromes, in McCarty DJ (ed): *Arthritis and Allied Conditions,* 11th ed. Philadelphia, Lea & Febiger, 1989, pp 991–1009.
Moutsopoulos HM: Behçet's syndrome, in Wilson JD, Braunwald E, Isselbacher KJ, et al (eds): *Harrison's Principles of Internal Medicine,* 12th ed. New York, McGraw-Hill, 1991, vol 2, pp 1455–1456.

Polyarthritis — Bowel-Associated
Aldo-Benson MA: Enteropathic arthritis, in McCarty DJ (ed): *Arthritis and Allied Conditions,* 11th ed. Philadelphia, Lea & Febiger, 1989, pp 972–979.
Relman DA, Schmidt TM, MacDermott RP: Identification of the uncultured bacillus of Whipple's disease. *N Engl J Med* 327:293–301, 1992.
Scheib JS, Quinet RJ: Whipple's disease with axial and peripheral joint destruction. *South Med J* 83:684–687, 1990.
Schur PH: Psoriatic arthritis and arthritis associated with gastrointestinal diseases, in Wilson JD, Braunwald E, Isselbacher KJ, et al (eds): *Harrison's Principles of Internal Medicine,* 12th ed. New York, McGraw-Hill, 1991, vol 2, pp 1482–1484.

Polyarthritis — Bowel-Associated Dermatosis-Arthritis Syndrome
Dicken CH: Bowel-associated dermatosis-arthritis syndrome: Bowel bypass syndrome without bowel bypass. *J Am Acad Dermatol* 14:792–796, 1986.

Polyarthritis — Brucellosis
Al-Rawi ZS, Al-Khateeb N, Khalifa SJ: Brucella arthritis among Iraqi patients. *Br J Rheumatol* 26:24–27, 1987.
Khateeb MI, Araj GF, Majeed SA, et al: Brucella arthritis: A study of 96 cases in Kuwait. *Ann Rheum Dis* 49:994–998, 1990.
Lubani M, Sharda D, Helin I: Brucella arthritis in children. *Infection* 14:233–236, 1986.
Mousa ARM, Muhtaseb SA, Almudallal DS, et al: Osteoarticular complications of brucellosis: A study of 169 cases. *Rev Infect Dis* 9: 531–543, 1987.

Polyarthritis — Crystal-Induced
Alarcón GS, Reveille JD: Gouty arthritis of the axial skeleton including the sacroiliac joints. *Arch Intern Med* 147:2018–2019, 1987.
Howell DS: Diseases due to the deposition of calcium pyrophosphate and hydroxyapatite, in Kelley WN, Harris ED Jr, Ruddy S, et al (eds): *Textbook of Rheumatology.* Philadelphia, Saunders, 1981, vol 2, pp 1438–1454.
Kelley WN: Gout and related disorders of purine metabolism, in Kelley WN, Harris ED Jr, Ruddy S, et al (eds): *Textbook of Rheumatology.* Philadelphia, Saunders, 1981, vol 2, pp 1397–1437.
Levinson DJ: Clinical gout and the pathogenesis of hyperuricemia, in McCarty DJ (ed): *Arthritis and Allied Conditions,* 11th ed. Philadelphia, Lea & Febiger, 1989, pp 1645–1676.
Masuda I, Ishikawa K: Clinical features of pseudogout attack: A survey of 50 cases. *Clin Orthop* 229:173–181, 1988.
Ryan LM, McCarty DJ: Calcium pyrophosphate crystal deposition disease; pseudogout; articular chondrocalcinosis, in McCarty DJ (ed): *Arthritis and Allied Conditions,* 11th ed. Philadelphia, Lea & Febiger, 1989, pp 1711–1736.

Polyarthritis — Drug-Related
Hart FD: Drug-induced arthritis and arthralgia. *Drugs* 28:347–354, 1984.
Jones PB, Clague R, Freemont T: Acute inflammatory polyarthritis following streptokinase (letter to editor). *Br J Rheumatol* 29:402–403, 1990.
Khanna R, Chatterjee S: Polyarthritis: An unusual side effect of lithium. *J Clin Psychiatry* 52:43–44, 1991.
Sukenik S, Horowitz J, Katz A, et al: Quinidine-induced lupus ery-

thematosus-like syndrome: Three case reports and a review of the literature. *Isr J Med Sci* 23:1232–1234, 1987.

Polyarthritis — Familial Hypercholesterolemia
Bole GG: Arthritis associated with hyperlipidemia and hypercholesterolemia, in Kelley WN, Harris ED Jr, Ruddy S, et al (eds): *Textbook of Rheumatology.* Philadelphia, Saunders, 1981, vol 2, pp 1638–1646.
Rimon D, Cohen L: Hypercholesterolemic (type II hyperlipoproteinemic) arthritis. *J Rheumatol* 16:703–705, 1989.

Polyarthritis — Gonococcal
Goldenberg DL: Gonococcal arthritis, in McCarty DJ (ed): *Arthritis and Allied Conditions,* 11th ed. Philadelphia, Lea & Febiger, 1989, pp 1915–1924.
Handsfield HH: *Neisseria gonorrhoeae,* in Mandell GL, Douglas RG Jr, Bennett JE (eds): *Principles and Practice of Infectious Diseases,* 3d ed. New York, Churchill Livingstone, 1990, pp 1613–1631.
Kerle KK, Mascola JR, Miller TA: Disseminated gonococcal infection. *Am Fam Physician* 45:209–214, 1992.
Myers AR, Lane JM: Septic arthritis caused by bacteria, in Kelley WN, Harris ED Jr, Ruddy S, et al (eds): *Textbook of Rheumatology.* Philadelphia, Saunders, 1981, vol 2, pp 1551–1572.
O'Brien JP, Goldenberg DL, Rice PA: Disseminated gonococcal infection: A prospective analysis of 49 patients and a review of pathophysiology and immune mechanisms. *Medicine* 62:395–406, 1983.
Stein CM, Hanly MG: Acute tropical polyarthritis in Zimbabwe: A prospective search for a gonococcal aetiology. *Ann Rheum Dis* 46:912–914, 1987.
Zahari DT, Bakst S: Disseminated gonococcal infection involving the foot. *J Foot Surg* 28:405–409, 1989.

Polyarthritis — HIV-Associated
Bentin J, Feremans W, Pasteels J-L, et al: Chronic acquired immunodeficiency syndrome-associated arthritis: A synovial ultrastructural study. *Arthritis Rheum* 33:268–273, 1990.
Rosenberg ZS, Norman A, Solomon G: Arthritis associated with HIV infection: Radiographic manifestations. *Radiology* 173:171–176, 1989.

Polyarthritis — Idiopathic Hypereosinophilic Syndrome
Martín-Santos JM, Mulero J, Andréu JL, et al: Arthritis in idiopathic hypereosinophilic syndrome. *Arthritis Rheum* 31:120–125, 1988.

Polyarthritis and Infection
Tramont EC: *Treponema pallidum* (syphilis), in Mandell GL, Douglas RG Jr, Bennett JE (eds): *Principles and Practice of Infectious Diseases,* 3d ed. New York, Churchill Livingstone, 1990, pp 1794–1808.
Washburn RG: *Streptobacillus moniliformis* (rat bite fever), in Mandell GL, Douglas RG Jr, Bennett JE (eds): *Principles and Practice of Infectious Diseases,* 3d ed. New York, Churchill Livingstone, 1990, pp 1762–1764.

Polyarthritis and Lyme Disease
Duffy J: Lyme disease. *Infect Dis Clin North Am* 1:511–527, 1987.
Hoycke MM, D'Alessio DD, Marx JJ: Prevalence of antibody to *Borrelia burgdorferi* by indirect fluorescent antibody assay, ELISA, and Western immunoblot in healthy adults in Wisconsin and Arizona. *J Infect Dis* 165:1133–1137, 1992.
Lange WR, Schwan TG, Frame JD: Can protracted relapsing fever resemble Lyme disease? *Med Hypotheses* 35:77–79, 1991.
Malawista SE: Lyme disease, in McCarty DJ (ed): *Arthritis and Allied Conditions,* 11th ed. Philadelphia, Lea & Febiger, 1989, pp 1955–1965.
Steere AC: *Borrelia burgdorferi:* Lyme disease, Lyme borreliosis, in Mandell GL, Douglas RG Jr, Bennett JE (eds): *Principles and Practice of Infectious Diseases,* 3d ed. New York, Churchill Livingstone, 1990, pp 1819–1827.

Polyarthritis and Malignancy
Caldwell DS: Musculoskeletal syndromes associated with malignancy, in Kelley WN, Harris ED Jr, Ruddy S, et al (eds): *Textbook of Rheumatology.* Philadelphia, Saunders, 1981, vol 2, pp 1658–1671.

Seleznick MJ, Aguilar JL, Rayhack J, et al: Polyarthritis associated with cutaneous T cell lymphoma. *J Rheumatol* 16:1379–1382, 1989.

Polyarthritis and Polyarthralgia — Review

Anderson RJ: Polyarticular arthritis, in Kelley WN, Harris ED Jr, Ruddy S, et al (eds): *Textbook of Rheumatology.* Philadelphia, Saunders, 1981, vol 2, pp 393–402.

Case 27-1989, Case records of the Massachusetts General Hospital. *N Engl J Med* 321:34–43, 1989.

Hannonen P, Möttönen T, Oka M: Palindromic rheumatism: A clinical survey of sixty patients. *Scand J Rheumatol* 16:413–420, 1987.

Murtagh J: Arthralgia: A diagnostic strategy. *Aust Fam Phys* 19:1530–1532, 1990.

Pinals RS: Persistent fever and arthralgia in adults. *Hosp Pract (Off Ed)* 21(11A):35–43, 1986.

Rosenthall L: Nuclear medicine techniques in arthritis. *Rheum Dis Clin North Am* 17:585–597, 1991.

Polyarthritis — Polychondritis

Gilliland BC: Relapsing polychondritis and miscellaneous arthritides, in Wilson JD, Braunwald E, Isselbacher KJ, et al (eds): *Harrison's Principles of Internal Medicine,* 12th ed. New York, McGraw-Hill, 1991, vol 2, pp 1484–1490.

Herman JH: Polychondritis, in Kelley WN, Harris ED Jr, Ruddy S, et al (eds): *Textbook of Rheumatology.* Philadelphia, Saunders, 1981, vol 2, pp 1500–1508.

Trentham DE: Relapsing polychondritis, in McCarty DJ (ed): *Arthritis and Allied Conditions,* 11th ed. Philadelphia, Lea & Febiger, 1989, pp 1227–1233.

Polyarthritis and Poncet's Disease

Dall L, Long L, Stanford J: Poncet's disease: Tuberculous rheumatism. *Rev Infect Dis* 11:105–107, 1989.

Polyarthritis — Rat-Bite Fever

Holroyd KJ, Reiner AP, Dick JD: *Streptobacillus moniliformis* polyarthritis mimicking rheumatoid arthritis: An urban case of rat bite fever. *Am J Med* 85:711–714, 1988.

Polyarthritis — Reactive

Aho K, Leirisalo-Repo M, Repo H: Reactive arthritis. *Clin Rheum Dis* 11:25–40, 1985.

Calin A: Reiter's syndrome, in Kelley WN, Harris ED Jr, Ruddy S, et al (eds): *Textbook of Rheumatology.* Philadelphia, Saunders, 1981, vol 2, pp 1033–1046.

Cooper SM, Ferriss JA: Reactive arthritis and psittacosis. *Am J Med* 81:555–557, 1986.

Ford DK: Reactive arthritis: A viewpoint rather than a review. *Clin Rheum Dis* 12:389–401, 1986.

———: Reiter's syndrome: Reactive arthritis, in McCarty DJ (ed): *Arthritis and Allied Conditions,* 11th ed. Philadelphia, Lea & Febiger, 1989, pp 944–953.

Hannu TJ, Leirisalo-Repo M: Clinical picture of reactive salmonella arthritis. *J Rheumatol* 15:1668–1671, 1988.

Inman RD, Johnston MEA, Hodge M, et al: Postdysenteric reactive arthritis: A clinical and immunogenetic study following an outbreak of salmonellosis. *Arthritis Rheum* 31:1377–1383, 1988.

Keat A: Reiter's syndrome and reactive arthritis in perspective. *N Engl J Med* 309:1606–1615, 1983.

Keat A, Thomas B, Dixey J, et al: *Chlamydia trachomatis* and reactive arthritis: The missing link. *Lancet* 1:72–74, 1987.

Leirisalo-Repo M, Suoranta H: Ten-year followup study of patients with *Yersinia* arthritis. *Arthritis Rheum* 31:533–537, 1988.

Mermel LA, Osborn TG: *Clostridium difficile*-associated reactive arthritis in an HLA-B27 positive female: Report and literature review. *J Rheumatol* 16:133–135, 1989.

Rosenthal L, Olhagen B, Ek S: Aseptic arthritis after gonorrhoea. *Ann Rheum Dis* 39:141–146, 1980.

Taurog JD, Lipsky PE: Ankylosing spondylitis and reactive arthritis, in Wilson JD, Braunwald E, Isselbacher KJ, et al (eds): *Harrison's Principles of Internal Medicine,* 12th ed. New York, McGraw-Hill, 1991, vol 2, pp 1451–1455.

van den Broek MF, van de Putte LBA, van den Berg WB: Crohn's disease associated with arthritis: A possible role for cross-reactivity between gut bacteria and cartilage in the pathogenesis of arthritis. *Arthritis Rheum* 31:1077–1079, 1988.

Polyarthritis — Rheumatoid

Baum J, Ziff M: Laboratory findings in rheumatoid arthritis, in McCarty DJ (ed): *Arthritis and Allied Conditions,* 11th ed. Philadelphia, Lea & Febiger, 1989, pp 743–761.

Harris ED Jr: Rheumatoid arthritis: The clinical spectrum, in Kelley WN, Harris ED Jr, Ruddy S, et al (eds): *Textbook of Rheumatology.* Philadelphia, Saunders, 1981, vol 2, pp 928–963.

Lipsky PE: Rheumatoid arthritis, in Wilson JD, Braunwald E, Isselbacher KJ, et al (eds): *Harrison's Principles of Internal Medicine,* 12th ed. New York, McGraw-Hill, 1991, vol 2, pp 1437–1443.

McCarty DJ: Clinical picture of rheumatoid arthritis, in McCarty DJ (ed): *Arthritis and Allied Conditions,* 11th ed. Philadelphia, Lea & Febiger, 1989, pp 715–742.

Polyarthritis — Sarcoidosis

Schumacher HR Jr: Sarcoidosis, in McCarty DJ (ed): *Arthritis and Allied Conditions,* 11th ed. Philadelphia, Lea & Febiger, 1989, pp 1294–1300.

Sequeira W, Stinar D: Serum angiotensin-converting enzyme levels in sarcoid arthritis. *Arch Intern Med* 146:125–127, 1986.

Polyarthritis — Septic

Baker GL, Oddis CV, Medsger TA Jr: *Pasteurella multocida* polyarticular septic arthritis. *J Rheumatol* 14:355–357, 1987.

Epstein JH, Zimmermann B III, Ho G Jr: Polyarticular septic arthritis. *J Rheumatol* 13:1105–1107, 1986.

Moeser PJ, Costello PB, Gillikin S, et al: *Haemophilus influenzae* polyarthritis in an adult: An analysis of serotype b strains. *Rev Infect Dis* 13:61–63, 1991.

Salmeron C, Marty M, Richet H, et al: Primary meningococcal polyarthritis. *J Infect* 13:281–283, 1986.

Serushan M, Varghai M: Emphysematous septic arthritis in multiple joints due to *Streptococcus milleri. J Rheumatol* 15:517–519, 1988.

Vorne M, Salo S, Anttolainen I, et al: Septic *Haemophilus influenzae* polyarthritis demonstrated best with Tc-99m HMPAO labeled leukocytes. *Clin Nucl Med* 15:883–886, 1990.

Polyarthritis — Seronegative Rheumatoid Arthritis

Husby G, Gran JT: The differentiation between seronegative rheumatoid arthritis and other forms of seronegative polyarthritis: A review with suggested criteria. *Clin Exp Rheumatol* 5(suppl 1):97–100, 1987.

Kaarela K, Alekberova Z, Lehtinen K, et al: Seronegative rheumatoid arthritis: A clinical study with HLA typing. *J Rheumatol* 17:1125–1129, 1990.

Polyarthritis — Subcorneal Pustular Dermatosis

Lin RY, Schwartz RA, Lambert WC: Subcorneal pustular dermatosis with polyarthritis. *Cutis* 37:123–124,1986.

Ündar L, Göze, F, Hah MM: Subcorneal pustular dermatosis with seronegative polyarthritis. *Cutis* 42:229–232, 1988.

Polyarthritis — Systemic Lupus Erythematosus

Hahn BH: Systemic lupus erythematosus, in Wilson JD, Braunwald E, Isselbacher KJ, et al (eds): *Harrison's Principles of Internal Medicine,* 12th ed. New York, McGraw-Hill, 1991, vol 2, pp 1432–1437.

Rothfield N: Clinical features of systemic lupus erythematosus, in Kelley WN, Harris ED Jr, Ruddy S, et al (eds): *Textbook of Rheumatology.* Philadelphia, Saunders, 1981, vol 2, pp 1106–1132.

———: Systemic lupus erythematosus: Clinical aspects and treatment, in McCarty DJ (ed): *Arthritis and Allied Conditions,* 11th ed. Philadelphia, Lea & Febiger, 1989, pp 1022–1048.

Polyarthritis and Vasculitis

Davies DJ, Niall JF, Moran JE, et al: Migratory polyarthralgia and haemoptysis. *Med J. Aust* 151:302, 1989.

Fauci, AS: The vasculitis syndromes, in Wilson JD, Braunwald E, Isselbacher, KJ, et al (eds): *Harrison's Principles of Internal Med-*

icine, 12th ed. New York, McGraw-Hill, 1991, vol 2, pp 1456–1463.

Fauci AS, Leavitt RY: Vasculitis, in McCarty DJ (ed): *Arthritis and Allied Conditions*, 11th ed. Philadelphia, Lea & Febiger, 1989, pp 1166–1188.

Hunder GG, Conn DL: Necrotizing vasculitis, in Kelley WN, Harris ED Jr, Ruddy S, et al (eds): *Textbook of Rheumatology*. Philadelphia, Saunders, 1981, vol 2, pp 1165–1188.

Lightfoot RW Jr, Michel BA, Block DA, et al: The American College of Rheumatology 1990 criteria for the classification of polyarteritis nodosa. *Arthritis Rheum* 33:1088–1093, 1990.

Ralston SH, McVicar R, Finlay AY, et al: Lymphomatoid granulomatosis presenting with polyarthritis. *Scott Med J* 33:373–374, 1988.

Shenstone B, Schrieber L, Yong JLC, et al: Migratory polyarthralgia and hacmoptysis. *Med J Aust* 150:387–390, 1989.

Siegel DM, Siegel SF: An unusual presentation of periarteritis nodosa. *Ann Emerg Med* 17:365–367, 1988.

Polyarthritis — Viral

Fraser JRE: Epidemic polyarthritis and Ross River virus disease. *Clin Rheum Dis* 12:369–388, 1986.

Haile CA: Parvovirus and epidemic arthritis. *Md Med J* 39:939–944, 1990.

Malawista SE, Steere AC: Viral arthritis, in Kelley WN, Harris ED Jr, Ruddy S, et al (eds): *Textbook of Rheumatology*. Philadelphia, Saunders, 1981, vol 2, pp 1586–1601.

Naides SJ, Scharosch LL, Foto F, et al: Rheumatologic manifestations of human parvovirus B19 infections in adults: Initial two-year clinical experience. *Arthritis Rheum* 33:1297–1309, 1990.

Smith MA, Ryan ME: Parvovirus infections: From benign to life-threatening. *Postgrad Med* 84:127–128, 131–134, 1988.

Steere AC: Viral arthritis, in McCarty DJ (ed): *Arthritis and Allied Conditions*, 11th ed. Philadelphia, Lea & Febiger, 1989, pp 1938–1954.

Spondyloarthropathies

Bennett RM: Nonarticular rheumatism and spondyloarthropathies: Similarities and differences. *Postgrad Med* 87:97–99, 102–104, 1990.

Jacobs JC: Spondyloarthritis and enthesopathy: Current concepts in rheumatology. *Arch Intern Med* 143:103–107, 1983.

Khan MA, van der Linden SM: A wider spectrum of spondyloarthropathies. *Semin Arthritis Rheum* 20:107–113, 1990.

Thomson GTD, Johnston JL, Baragar FD, et al: Psoriatic arthritis and myopathy. *J Rheumatol* 17:395–398, 1990.

51

Acute Generalized Skin Pain

☐ DIAGNOSTIC LIST

1. Sun-induced skin injury
   A. Sunburn
   B. Phototoxicity
   C. Photoallergic dermatitis
2. Thermal burns
3. Acute bullous disorders
   A. Toxic epidermal necrolysis
   B. Mimics of toxic epidermal necrolysis
      1. Staphylococcal scalded skin syndrome
      2. Acute graft-versus-host disease
      3. Generalized fixed drug eruption
      4. Stevens-Johnson syndrome (erythema multiforme bullosum)
      5. Vesiculobullous systemic lupus erythematosus
      6. Bullous pemphigoid
      7. Pemphigus vulgaris
      8. Epidermolysis bullosa acquisita
4. Acute pustular lesions

   A. Generalized pustular psoriasis
   B. Impetigo herpetiformis
   C. Subcorneal pustular dermatosis

5. Panniculitis
   A. Erythema nodosum (septal panniculitis)
   B. Systemic nodular panniculitis (lobular panniculitis)
   C. Panniculitis of pancreatic origin (lobular panniculitis)
   D. Cytophagic histiocytic panniculitis
6. Sweet's syndrome
7. Glucagonoma syndrome
8. Erythroderma
9. Eosinophilic fasciitis
10. Generalized cellulitis
    A. Cellulitis in a lymphedematous limb
    B. Rapidly spreading clostridial cellulitis
11. Purpura fulminans
12. Acute urticaria
13. Psychogenic pain

☐ SUMMARY

Generalized *sunburn* results from excessive sun exposure during sunbathing. The skin on exposed areas is erythematous, warm, painful, and tender; cutaneous edema and blistering

often occur. Systemic symptoms such as fever, chills, malaise, nausea, weakness, and dizziness may occur in severe cases. Aspirin or indomethacin relieves some of the severe systemic manifestations, burning pain, and tenderness.

A severe sunburn reaction occurs after mild sun exposure in

a patient who has been ingesting a *phototoxic drug* (e.g., doxy-cycline or griseofulvin) or applying it to the skin (e.g., crude coal tar). *Photoallergic dermatitis* occurs after ingestion or topical application of a substance to which the patient is allergic. Sunlight, combined with the presence of the allergenic substance in the skin, results in a generalized papulovesicular, eczematous, and/or weeping dermatitis or blistering in sun-exposed regions. Chlorothiazides and phenothiazines are commonly used drugs that may be responsible for photoallergic reactions. Some sunscreening lotions contain para-aminobenzoic acid (PABA) esters or cinnamates that may cause generalized photoallergic dermatitis after sunbathing in patients sensitized to these substances by prior exposure.

Thermal burns may result from flames, hot steam, or scalding by hot water. First-degree burns cause skin erythema and edema (e.g., sunburn), while superficial partial-thickness (i.e., second-degree) burns cause vesiculation and blistering, and severe pain and skin tenderness. Deep partial thickness (i.e., second-degree) and full-thickness (i.e., third-degree) burns may appear pearly white or parchmentlike and translucent, or the skin may be charred (e.g., full-thickness flame burns). Pain is less or absent with deep partial-thickness or full-thickness burns, and tenderness is minimal. Adjacent areas with more superficial burns may cause pain and tenderness.

Toxic epidermal necrolysis (TEN) is usually caused by ingestion of a drug. Fever and large patches and plaques of painful, tender erythema develop on the trunk and extremities. The erythematous regions may coalesce to produce generalized erythroderma in up to 14 percent of cases. Large, flaccid blisters develop on the erythematous patches, and Nikolsky's sign is present over erythematous areas but not on normal-appearing skin. Sulfonamides, anticonvulsants, long-acting nonsteroidal anti-inflammatory drugs, antigout drugs (allopurinol and colchicine), and amoxicillin are the drugs most frequently responsible for TEN. Blistering and erosions involving the mouth, genitals, and/or conjunctivae occur in 85 to 95 percent of cases. Histopathologic studies reveal subepidermal blister formation, full-thickness epidermal necrosis, and damage to the basal cell layer. Results of immunofluorescence studies are usually negative. TEN has also been associated with systemic lupus erythematosus, leukemias, lymphomas, inflammatory bowel disease, and, rarely, vaccinations.

A number of blistering disorders may have an abrupt onset and may be mistaken for TEN. The *staphylococcal scalded skin syndrome* (SSSS) is one such disorder. SSSS is primarily a disease of infants and young children, but it may occur in adults who are being treated with immunosuppressive drugs or who have a chronic underlying systemic disease, such as a leukemia, lymphoma, or renal failure. Systemic symptoms (e.g., fever and malaise), skin pain, tenderness, erythema, and bullae formation occur. Mucous membrane involvement is usually limited to conjunctivitis, and the lesions beneath the ruptured bullae skin are less granular and wet-appearing than in TEN, since a portion of the epidermis remains on the surface in SSSS. Lesions may dry and crust rapidly with SSSS. Microscopic examination of a fragment of exfoliated skin reveals an intraepidermal cleavage plane at the level of the stratum granulosum. A biopsy of an early bulla reveals intraepidermal bulla formation with the split at or just below the stratum granulosum. Children usually have an upper respiratory, skin, or ear infection with a phage group II strain of *Staphylococcus aureus*. The site of the responsible staphylococcal infection in adults is less clearly defined. Circulating staphylococcal epidermolytic toxin is responsible for the epidermal damage.

An *acute graft-versus-host reaction* resembling TEN may follow bone marrow transplantation in 6 percent of cases. Diarrhea and abnormal liver function suggest that the cause is a graft-versus-host reaction. Some cases occurring after bone marrow transplantation are drug-related.

A *generalized fixed drug reaction* may mimic TEN. There is usually a history of a similar erythematous and/or blistering response of the skin to ingestion or parenteral administration of the same drug. Skin biopsy reveals epidermal necrosis, subepidermal bulla formation, and a superficial and deep dermal infiltrate of neutrophils, eosinophils, and lymphocytes. In patients with TEN or erythema multiforme bullosum, only the superficial dermal vessels are infiltrated with lymphocytes and histiocytes. Recurrent episodes of increasing severity and involvement of the same skin locations (verified by photography) suggest a diagnosis of generalized fixed drug eruption. Some cases initially diagnosed as TEN have been shown to be a generalized fixed drug eruption on the basis of the subsequent clinical course and histopathologic findings (i.e., deep dermal inflammatory cell infiltration).

The *Stevens-Johnson syndrome* is a severe form of erythema multiforme with mucous membrane and cutaneous bullae formation, resulting in extensive, painful erosion of epithelial surfaces. The rash consists of erythematous macules, papules, plaques, and target (iris) lesions. Flaccid bullae form on erythematous areas. The eyes (conjunctivitis), mouth (bullae and erosions), and the genitals are involved. The vermillion border of the lips may fissure and form hemorrhagic crusts that present a characteristic appearance. Many authors place the Stevens-Johnson syndrome on a severity continuum between erythema multiforme and TEN. Histopathologic findings in TEN and the Stevens-Johnson syndrome are very similar and cannot be used for diagnostic differentiation. *Vesiculobullous lesions may occur in patients with systemic lupus erythematosus*. Other criteria for the diagnosis of systemic lupus erythematosus are usually present. A skin biopsy demonstrates subepidermal blister formation and a dermal leukocytoclastic vasculitis. Granular deposits of IgG and IgM may be present in the basement membrane zone of involved and adjacent lesion-free skin.

Bullous pemphigoid results in the production of large tense bullae on apparently normal or erythematous skin. Eroded areas resulting from blister rupture are painful and tender and do not increase in size, in contrast to the enlarging coalescing erosions resulting from blister rupture in patients with pemphigus. An acute onset of bullous pemphigoid may occur, with fever and malaise, after administration of one of the penicillin drugs. This reaction may mimic erythema multiforme bullosum. Bullous pemphigoid causes subepidermal blisters, and there is IgG and C3 deposition in a linear pattern along the basement membrane zone. In cases simulating erythema multiforme bullosum, target lesions are usually present on the palms, soles, and other skin regions, and circulating antibody to basement membrane antigens may be demonstrable by indirect immunofluorescence studies. Oral bullae and erosions occur in 8 to 39 percent of cases and eosinophilia in up to 61 percent of cases.

Pemphigus vulgaris may have an acute onset and mimic TEN. Oral bullae and erosions may precede the skin eruption in 30 to 60 percent of cases. Crusted fissures may occur on the lips. Flaccid intraepidermal bullae are characteristic, and Nikolsky's and Asboe-Hansen signs are present, but target (iris) lesions are not. Histopathologic studies reveal intraepidermal blister formation and acantholysis. Direct immunofluorescence studies demonstrate intercellular deposition of IgG through the entire epidermis and oral epithelium. C3 may be present in intercellular areas in early acantholytic skin. Indirect immunofluorescence studies using patient sera are less reliable for definitive diagnosis.

Acute pemphigus may be precipitated by penicillamine, captopril, penicillin, rifampin, and possibly other drugs. *Epidermolysis bullosa acquisita* (EBA) is characterized by the presence of severe skin fragility and trauma-provoked blisters that rupture and heal with scarring and milia formation. In some cases, these clinical findings are absent, and the disease process is indistinguishable from that of bullous pemphigoid. In such cases, immunoelectron microscopy of perilesional skin for IgG deposits will reveal an upper dermal location just beneath the lamina densa in EBA patients and a lamina lucida deposition of IgG in patients with bullous pemphigoid. The sera of patients with EBA can be used in an indirect immunofluorescence assay with 1M NaCl-treated human skin to demonstrate dermal localization of circulating IgG antibody in EBA. Bullous pemphigoid circulating IgG antibody is localized in the epidermis or epidermis and dermis. EBA may be associated with systemic lupus erythematosus, inflammatory bowel disease, and other systemic disorders.

Generalized pustular psoriasis begins with severe skin pain, hyperalgesia, and fever. Skin erythema occurs in normal skin, and existing psoriatic plaques may become intensely red and edematous. Multiple pinpoint (1–2-mm) sterile pustules develop on erythematous patches and plaques. This disorder may occur in patients with psoriasis or in those with no prior evidence of psoriatic lesions (15 percent of cases). Toxicity, fever, and leukocytosis occur, and the skin burns and itches. Arthralgia or arthritis and ocular involvement (e.g., conjunctivitis, iridocyclitis, and corneal ulceration) may occur. Histopathologic study of pustule-bearing skin reveals a dermal perivascular infiltrate by mononuclear cells and neutrophil accumulation in the epidermis in spongiform pustules. Characteristic changes of psoriatic skin (e.g., elongated rete ridges) may be absent or difficult to find. *Impetigo herpetiformis* is a severe form of generalized pustular psoriasis usually occurring in pregnancy. It has a predilection for flexural areas, and healing is characterized by hyperpigmentation. *Subcorneal pustu-*

lar dermatosis may be mildly painful, tender, and pruritic or asymptomatic. Erythematous patches and plaques appear, and flaccid neutrophil-containing blisters (3–10 mm) form on their surface. Blister content is sterile. Erosions replace blisters and may form superficial crusts. Histopathologic examination reveals subcorneal pustules filled with neutrophils and a moderate dermal perivascular inflammatory infiltrate. This disorder has been associated with elevated serum IgA levels, IgA or IgG myeloma, IgA gammopathy, collagen vascular diseases, and generalized pustular processes.

Erythema nodosum (septal panniculitis) causes painful or painless, tender, red subcutaneous nodules on the lower legs, the thighs, and sometimes the upper extremities. Severe cases are associated with fever and ankle and/or knee pain. Joint swelling may occur. Biopsy of a subcutaneous nodule reveals vascular and perivascular septal inflammation and panniculitis of the adjacent fat. Septal hemorrhage and polymorphonuclear leukocyte and/or lymphocyte infiltration of the septal areas may be present. The causes of erythema nodosum include infections such as streptococcal pharyngitis, Epstein-Barr virus, coccidioidomycosis, histoplasmosis, blastomycosis, leprosy, primary tuberculosis, psittacosis, cat-scratch fever, lymphogranuloma venereum, leptospirosis, yersiniosis, and tularemia. Other conditions associated with erythema nodosum include acute and chronic leukemia, sarcoidosis, inflammatory bowel disease, sulfonamide or oral contraceptive administration, pregnancy, and Behçet's syndrome. Some cases are idiopathic.

Systemic nodular panniculitis (lobular panniculitis) causes painful, tender, erythematous subcutaneous plaques and nodules over a limited or large area of the body surface. Some erythematous plaques or nodules soften and discharge on oily white fluid resembling pus through the overlying skin. The fluid is liquified fat, and this can be demonstrated by examining a drop of this liquid under light microscopy using a Sudan stain for fat. Fever, chills, malaise, cutaneous pain, and prostration may be severe. Edema of the involved lower extremities may be extensive. Disorders associated with systemic nodular panniculitis include connective tissue diseases, lymphoproliferative diseases, α-$_1$-antitrypsin deficiency, and paraproteinemia associated with C1 esterase inhibitor deficiency.

A similar clinical picture of *generalized panniculitis* of the lobular type (i.e., biopsy of an acute lesion reveals necrotic lipocytes ["ghostlike" fat cells], interstitial infiltration of fat lobules by neutrophils and eosinophils, and basophilic deposits in the intercellular spaces, while chronic lesions demonstrate dead lipocytes surrounded by histiocytes and foam cells) may be caused by *pancreatitis* or by an *acinous carcinoma of the pancreas*. Serum amylase and lipase levels may be elevated, and abdominal, joint, and bone pain may occur. Accurate diagnosis of pancreatic disease can be made by a CT scan, endoscopic retrograde cholangiopancreatography, and/or needle biopsy of the pancreas. In some cases, exploratory laparotomy is required to obtain representative pancreatic tissue for histopathologic analysis.

Cytophagic histiocytic panniculitis presents with widespread, painful, tender, erythematous, and sometimes ecchymotic subcutaneous nodules and fever. Pancytopenia and hepatic and splenic enlargement may be associated. Biopsy reveals histiocytes containing red blood cells, leukocytes, and platelets (''beanbag cells'').

Sweet's syndrome (acute febrile neutrophilic dermatosis) may have an acute onset, with fever and the appearance of 2- to 10-cm oval or round, painful, tender, erythematous plaques and nodules. The nodules may be distributed over the face, neck, trunk, and extremities. Blisters and pustules may form on the surface of the erythematous plaques. A skin biopsy reveals infiltration of the upper and mid-dermis by neutrophils without an associated leukocytoclastic vasculitis. Conjunctivitis and an asymmetrical arthritis usually involving large joints may occur. Sweet's syndrome may follow an upper respiratory infection, or it may occur in a setting of inflammatory bowel disease. In up to one-third of cases, there is an underlying malignancy. An association of Sweet's syndrome with acute myeloid and acute myelomonocytic leukemia is commonly reported. Less frequently, it has been associated with myeloma and lymphoproliferative disorders. Sweet's syndrome is commonly associated with fever, leukocytosis, a dramatic response to prednisone, and no response to antibiotics.

The *glucagonoma syndrome* results in the formation of migratory erythematous plaques on the face, abdomen, perineum, and extremities. Flaccid bullae and vesicles may occur, resulting in painful erosions, crusted plaques, and skin necrosis. Lesions may form annular patterns. Hyperglycemia, an elevated serum glucagon, weight loss, stomatitis, and anemia occur. The cause is an alpha-cell tumor of the pancreas. Tumor excision results in resolution of all symptoms.

Acute *erythroderma* may cause burning pain and/or itching. There are generalized erythema and, commonly, edema of the entire body and face. The most likely cause of acute erythroderma is administration of a drug. Exacerbation of a chronic preexisting skin disease, such as contact dermatitis, atopic dermatitis, or psoriasis, is another major cause of acute erythroderma.

Eosinophilic fasciitis begins with painful swelling and redness of the skin of the extremities and trunk. A peau d'orange surface appearance may be present, and the skin feels firm, indurated, and thickened. Flexion and extension of the limbs may be impaired. The hands and face may be spared. Biopsy reveals a greatly thickened fascia. Eosinophilia of 10 to 40 percent is commonly present. Many patients respond to corticosteroid therapy.

Rapidly spreading painful and tender skin redness, swelling (*cellulitis*), and lymphangitic streaking may begin in an *edematous limb* and extend over the entire body in 12 to 24 h. Fever and chills are associated. The usual cause is a *group A streptococcus* or *S. aureus*.

Rarely, *Clostridium perfringens* may spread from an extremity or trunk wound and produce an extensive crepitant *cellulitis* involving large areas of subcutaneous tissue. Severe prostration, high fever, jaundice, and renal failure are associated, and the mortality rate is high. *Purpura fulminans* occurs as a complication of meningococcal septicemia and other fulminant infections. In patients with meningococcemia, extensive areas of skin, especially on the distal lower extremities, may become purpuric and necrotic, requiring extensive debridement if the patient survives. Shock, high fever, prostration, delirium, and coma are commonly associated. Symmetrical peripheral gangrene of digits, feet, and/or hands may occur, necessitating amputation during the convalescent period. Pain is associated with necrosis, adjacent inflammation, and secondary infection in necrotic areas.

Acute urticarial lesions may be pruritic or cause stinging or burning pain localized to the hive. Urticaria is associated with allergy to foods, food additives, drugs, insect bites, infections, and inhalants and also occurs with immune complex vasculitis (e.g., serum sickness).

Psychogenic pain and tenderness may occur over the entire body in the absence of any apparent abnormality of the skin. Stress intensifies the symptoms, and diazepam and similar drugs may lessen them.

☐ DESCRIPTION OF LISTED DISEASES

1. SUN-INDUCED INJURY

A. Sunburn Exposure of normal skin to sunlight will cause erythema after a latent period of 4 to 8 h. Prolonged

TABLE OF INCIDENCE

INCIDENCE PER 100,000 (APPROXIMATE)

Common (>100)	Uncommon (>5–100)	Rare (>0–5)
Sunburn	Phototoxicity	Toxic epidermal necrolysis
Thermal burns	Photoallergic dermatitis	Staphylococcal scalded skin syndrome
Erythema nodosum	Bullous pemphigoid	Acute graft-versus-host disease
Acute urticaria	Pemphigus vulgaris	Generalized fixed drug eruption
	Subcorneal pustular dermatosis	Stevens-Johnson syndrome
	Sweet's syndrome	Vesiculobullous systemic lupus erythematosus
	Erythroderma	Epidermolysis bullosa acquisita
		Generalized pustular psoriasis
		Impetigo herpetiformis
		Systemic nodular panniculitis
		Panniculitis of pancreatic origin
		Cytophagic histiocytic panniculitis
		Glucagonoma syndrome
		Eosinophilic fasciitis
		Generalized cellulitis
		Purpura fulminans
		Psychogenic pain

exposure to sunlight may cause severe erythema, pain, tenderness, and edema of the skin. Movement of the involved parts and pressure against the surface of a bed or chair intensify the discomfort. Blistering may occur in severely burned areas. Systemic symptoms such as chills, fever, nausea, weakness, and dizziness may occur. Sunburn is caused by ultraviolet B (UVB) radiation (wavelength, 290–340 nm), although the amount of UVB radiation is only 1 percent of the amount of ultraviolet A (UVA) radiation (wavelength, 340–390 nm). UVB radiation penetrates the dermis and has 1000 times the sunburn potency of UVA radiation. UVB radiation is also responsible for delayed melanogenesis (tanning), but UVA radiation can contribute to this cosmetically desirable effect when UVB radiation is blocked by use of a sunscreen lotion.

Sunburn may provoke an attack of the cutaneous manifestations of systemic lupus erythematosus, porphyria cutanea tarda, solar urticaria, and erythema multiforme.

Erythema after UVB radiation exposure is mediated by prostaglandins PGE_2 and PGF_2, and their effect can be inhibited by the administration of aspirin or indomethacin. Sunscreens prevent sunburn by absorbing UVB radiation before it reaches the skin.

B. Phototoxicity This nonimmunologic reaction results in a severe sunburn when the skin has been exposed to a photosensitizing compound and sunlight. Marked erythema, edema, blistering, and pain may occur after a brief exposure. Oral and topical phototoxicity inducers are listed in Table 51-1. Coal tar derivatives are found in cosmetics, drugs, dyes, disinfectants, and insecticides. Local phototoxic reactions are more common than generalized reactions, since these substances are used on a limited area of skin. Ingestion of a phototoxic drug followed by sunbathing can result in a severe, painful, generalized burn after a brief exposure to sunlight. Contact of moist skin with photosensitizing plants containing furocoumarins results in a phytophotodermatitis. This is usually restricted to the area of contact with the photosensitizing compound. Painful erythema, vesicles, and bullae develop in the contact area.

Table 51-1
PHOTOTOXICITY INDUCERS

Oral	Topical
Antimicrobial drugs	Coal tar derivatives
Doxycycline	Acridine
Griseofulvin	Anthracene
Sulfonamides	Pyridine
Nalidixic acid	Crude coal tar
Furocoumarins	Furocoumarins (psoralens)
Methoxsalen	Methoxsalen in lime, orange, celery, and
Trimethylpsoralen	dill

C. Photoallergic Dermatitis This dermatitis is produced by ingestion of a small amount of a photosensitizing substance that the patient is allergic to, followed by sunbathing. The result is a generalized papulovesicular, eczematous, and/or exudative dermatitis in the sun-exposed areas. The cutaneous reaction may extend to unexposed regions. Previous sensitization to the responsible drug is required. Drugs that may be responsible for photoallergic skin reactions include the chlorothiazides, quinethazone, chlorpropamide, phenothiazines, quinidine, and nalidixic acid. Sunscreening agents containing PABA esters, cinnamates, and digalloyl trioleate applied topically may cause a generalized photoallergic skin reaction after sunbathing. Photopatch testing can be used to identify substances causing contact dermatitis and photocontact sensitivity. Photoallergic reactions require the ingestion or topical application of a much smaller amount of photosensitizing substance than is required for a phototoxicity effect.

2. THERMAL BURNS

These injuries to the skin are described as first-, second-, or third-degree or as partial- or full-thickness burns.

First-degree burns cause skin redness, edema, pain, tenderness, and warmth (e.g., sunburn). Second-degree burns (partial-thickness burns) may be superficial or extend into the deep dermal region. Superficial partial-thickness burns are red, painful, tender, and moist. Blisters form and rupture, leaving large, painful denuded areas.

Deep partial-thickness burns are covered with necrotic epidermis. The underlying dermis may appear pearly or waxy white and does not bleed when abraded. The burn wound surface is dry and may be soft. Pinprick sensation may be decreased, but deep pressure sensation remains intact. Pain is mild to moderate.

Full-thickness, or third-degree, burns are usually pearly white or charred. The surface eschar is inelastic. It may be translucent or parchmentlike, and thrombosed, superficial veins may be seen beneath the eschar. This type of burn is usually painless and anesthetic. Pain may arise from adjacent partial-thickness burns.

Generalized partial- or full-thickness burns may be caused by hot steam, scalding in hot water, or flames.

3. ACUTE BULLOUS DISORDERS

A. Toxic Epidermal Necrolysis TEN begins with a brief prodrome of fever, myalgia, and arthralgia, sometimes associated with agitation and confusion (i.e., delirium). Severe burning pain involving the skin is associated with the appearance of small and large erythematous, tender patches. Flaccid blisters form in many of the erythematous areas, collapse, and slough, leaving a glistening, denuded, dermal surface that weeps a protein-rich exudate. Nikolsky's sign (i.e., shearing of the outer layer of the epidermis from the basal layer with sloughing of the epidermis produced by rubbing the skin surface firmly with a fingertip) is present only in erythematous regions. Some erythematous macules develop a darkened center but never form blisters or slough. These lesions have some resemblance to the target lesions of erythema multiforme. A painful, erythematous edema may develop on the palms and soles. Maximal extension and progression of lesions is complete in 12 to 72 h. In up to 14 percent of cases, the entire skin may become involved. The extent of skin blistering and sloughing, and not the amount of erythema, is the main determinant of prognosis and fluid requirements.

The frequency of mucous membrane involvement is estimated at 85 to 95 percent and may precede skin blistering by 24 to 72 h in 33 percent of cases. In one report of 87 cases, erosive mucosal lesions involved the conjunctivae in 78 percent, mouth in 93 percent, and genitalia in 63 percent. All sites were involved in over half the cases. The conjunctivae were never the only sites affected. Esophageal involvement may cause dysphagia and odynophagia. Endoscopy may reveal diffuse erosion of the esophagus in such cases. Esophageal stricture may occur as a complication of mucosal ulceration. Less commonly, bloody diarrhea may result from pseudomembranous or ulcerative lesions of the colon.

Respiratory symptoms are frequent and are due to tracheobronchial erosions and interstitial or alveolar pulmonary edema. The latter may result from overcorrection of hypovolemia when alveolar capillaries are leaky. Up to 20 percent of patients may require mechanical ventilation. Anemia (100 percent of cases), lymphopenia (90 percent), neutropenia (30 percent), and thrombocytopenia (15 percent) are the main hematologic abnormalities associated with TEN. Creatinine levels rise because of fluid losses from and into the skin and sometimes the gastrointestinal tract. Fluid replacement usually results in reduction of the elevated serum creatinine concentration. Extensive fluid losses require replacement of 4 liters/day or more.

Denuded skin with a protein-rich exudate is an excellent growth medium for bacteria. The commonest isolates from the skin are *S. aureus* and *Pseudomonas aeruginosa*. These organisms may cause local wound sepsis and invade the circulation, resulting in fatal septicemia. Histopathologic examination of blistered skin reveals subepidermal bullae. Changes occur in the basal cell layer as intercellular edema and then spread to involve the entire malpighian (i.e., prickle) layer. Necrosis may involve the entire epidermis as the lesion progresses. A superficial dermal infiltrate of lymphocytes and histiocytes is usually present. Results of direct immunofluorescence studies of biopsied skin are usually negative. Electron microscopy

shows areas of disruption of the lamina densa on the blister floor and necrotic basal cells with packed keratin.

TEN is usually associated with drug hypersensitivity. Table 51-2 lists the drugs that most frequently cause this disorder. Table 51-3 provides a measure of the relative risk involved by expressing the number of cases of TEN resulting from a specific drug in relationship to the total sales of that drug.

Mortality rates for TEN vary from 10 to 70 percent (mean, 29 percent). Diseases occasionally associated with the development of TEN include systemic lupus erythematosus, leukemias, lymphomas, and inflammatory

Table 51-2
DRUGS ASSOCIATED WITH TOXIC EPIDERMAL NECROLYSIS

Drugs	% of Cases
Sulfonamides	34
Co-trimoxazole	
Sulfamethoxazole/trimethoprim	
Anticonvulsants	18
Phenytoin	
Phenobarbital	
Carbamazepine	
Pyrazolones and other long half-life nonsteroidal anti-inflammatory drugs	18
Oxicams	
Fenbufen	
Sulindac	
Allopurinol	4

Note: Ampicillin, amoxicillin, and almost all other antibiotics, aspirin, and acetaminophen have been implicated.

Table 51-3
CAUSES OF TOXIC EPIDERMAL NECROLYSIS

Drug	Cases/Sales ($\times 10^{-8}$)
Nonsteroidal anti-inflammatory drugs	
Isoxicam	41
Oxyphenbutazone	18
Fenbufen	13
Piroxicam	4
Antimicrobial drugs	
Sulfadiazine	230
Co-trimoxazole	12
Ampicillin	9
Amoxicillin	5
Anticonvulsants	
Phenytoin	14
Carbamazepine	8
Phenobarbital	4
Analgesics and antigout drugs	
Colchicine	9
Diflunisal	4
Allopurinol	1.3

bowel disease. In addition to drug hypersensitivity, vaccination against measles, tetanus, diphtheria, or poliomyelitis may rarely cause TEN. Infection with herpes simplex virus or Mycoplasma pneumoniae is commonly associated with the Stevens-Johnson syndrome, but these agents have no apparent role in the causation of TEN.

Criteria for the diagnosis of TEN include (1) bullae and/or erosions over 20 percent or more of the body surface area; (2) bullae development on an erythematous base; (3) lesions occurring on non-sun-exposed skin; (4) skin sloughing off in sheets larger than 3 cm; (5) frequent mucous membrane lesions; (6) skin tender within 48 h of onset of rash; (7) fever; and (8) biopsy compatible with drug-induced TEN (basal layer necrosis).

B. Mimics of Toxic Epidermal Necrolysis

1. Staphylococcal Scalded Skin Syndrome SSSS occurs predominantly in infants and children and rarely in adults. Adult-type SSSS is usually limited to patients treated with immunosuppressive drugs or occurs in association with a severe underlying disease such as leukemia, Hodgkin's disease, or renal failure. Rarely, it has occurred in seemingly normal adults. Mucous membranes, with the exception of those in the eyes (e.g., conjunctivitis), are usually not affected.

The disease begins with fever, malaise, pain, tenderness, and diffuse redness of the skin (sunburned or scalded appearance). Within hours, large, flaccid bullae appear; and the upper layers of the epidermis wrinkle and slough after light finger pressure is applied (Nikolsky's sign), exposing a hyperemic, glistening surface. These erosions may be less granular and moist than those occurring in TEN, since a portion of the epidermis remains on the surface in SSSS. New bullae form for up to 48 h on tender, erythematous patches.

Perioral erythema, with crusts and fissures of the nasolabial folds and oral commissures, may develop. Areas of exfoliated skin usually dry within 48 h, and large, thick, seborrhea-like flakes appear at these sites. The diagnosis of SSSS can be confirmed by examination of a fragment of exfoliated skin to determine the cleavage level in the epidermis. In SSSS, the cleavage plane is intraepidermal within or just beneath the stratum granulosum. Histopathologic examination of a fixed or frozen skin biopsy reveals intraepidermal bulla formation at the level of the stratum granulosum and an absence of inflammatory cells in the upper dermis. In children, this toxin-mediated process is associated with a cutaneous, ear, or nasopharyngeal infection usually caused by *S. aureus* phage group II, types 55 or 71, and, rarely, by phage group I or III. Adults and older children usually do not get SSSS because they have circulating antibody to epidermolytic toxin.

2. Acute Graft-Versus-Host Disease Toxic epidermal necrolysis may follow bone marrow transplantation in 6 percent of cases. Some cases are caused by drugs, while other posttransplant cases associated with diarrhea and abnormal liver function tests are caused by graft-versus-host disease. The overall prognosis is very poor and, in one series of 9 bone marrow transplant patients, all died.

3. Generalized Fixed Drug Eruption Multiple oval or circular, painful, tender, red plaques and patches appear and may coalesce into a diffuse erythroderma. Bullae form during the first 48 h, collapse, and slough, leaving painful erosions. Biopsies of the involved skin reveal full-thickness skin necrosis, subepidermal bullae formation, and a superficial and deep dermal infiltrate of neutrophils, eosinophils, and lymphocytes. TEN and erythema multiforme cause full-thickness epidermal necrosis, but only the superficial dermal plexus is infiltrated with lymphocytes or histiocytes.

Patients with a widespread bullous fixed drug eruption usually give a history of similar previous attacks after ingestion of the same drug. The number and severity of lesions may increase with each administration of the drug, and there is a tendency of lesions to recur at the same sites with each attack. Such recurrences may be documented by photographic records or diagrams. The onset of symptoms within a few hours of drug ingestion is a helpful diagnostic clue. Symptoms resolve with withdrawal of the drug. The drugs that most frequently cause a fixed drug eruption include phenolphthalein, phenytoin, barbiturates, dapsone, quinine, quinidine, sulfonamides, tetracycline, and chlordiazepoxide.

4. Stevens-Johnson Syndrome (Erythema Multiforme Bullosum) This disorder is a severe form of erythema multiforme and has features of TEN (e.g., bullous lesions and epidermal necrosis). Erythema multiforme may appear as irregular round or oval, erythematous macules, papules, or plaques on the extensor surfaces of the extremities, the trunk, the dorsal surface of the hands and feet, and the palms and soles. Lesions may coalesce into large, extensive plaques. Target or iris lesions with an erythematous margin and a central bull's-eye of erythema or two concentric red or pink rings are abundant. On the lower extremity, lesions may be localized over the trochanteric region and knees. Other lesions include urticarial plaques, vesicles, and large bullae. A central bulla may form on a plaque or patch of erythema. This blister may be surrounded by a ring of vesicles (i.e., herpes iris lesion of Bateman).

The Stevens-Johnson syndrome usually begins with a high fever up to 40°C (104°F), sore throat and/or mouth, and headache. Vesicles and bullae form on the lips, tongue, and buccal mucosa. Ulceration rapidly occurs, with severe pain, crusting, and bleeding. Bilateral conjunctivitis, corneal ulceration, rhinitis, and epistaxis may occur. Hemorrhagic crusts are associated with fissures and erosions on the vermillion of the lips. Erosions on the genitalia are usually present. Bullae may form on erythematous cutaneous plaques, rupture, and collapse, resulting in local pain and tenderness. Pulmonary infiltrates, with cough and dyspnea, may occur, and renal failure may develop in severe cases. Possible causes of the Stevens-Johnson syndrome are listed in Table 51-4. The Stevens-Johnson syndrome is more likely to occur secondary to a viral or fungal infection or as a result of drug administration, but it may occur with the other causes of erythema multiforme, or it may be idiopathic.

Criteria for the diagnosis of Stevens-Johnson syndrome include (1) individual lesions less than 3 cm in diameter, with existing lesions that may coalesce; (2) target (iris) lesions; (3) mucous membrane involvement of at least two of three possible sites (i.e., mouth,

Table 51-4
CAUSES OF ERYTHEMA MULTIFORME AND THE STEVENS-JOHNSON SYNDROME

Infections	Doxycycline
Herpes simplex virus	Allopurinol
Epstein-Barr virus	Digitalis
Adenovirus	Hydralazine
Vaccinia	Penicillamine
Yersinia species	Salicylates
Tularemia	Nifedipine
Tuberculosis	Verapamil
Mycoplasma pneumoniae	Diltiazem
Dermatophytosis	Dapsone
Histoplasmosis	Gold
Coccidioidomycosis	Trimethoprim-sulfamethoxazole
Hepatitis B	Vaccines
Viral pneumonia	BCG
Influenza A	Diphtheria-tetanus toxoid
Coxsackievirus (B5)	Hepatitis B vaccine
Echovirus	Measles-mumps-rubella vaccine
Malaria	Poliomyelitis
Trichomoniasis	Malignant diseases
Chlamydia trachomatis	Hodgkin's and non-Hodgkin's
Chlamydia psittaci	lymphoma
Gonorrhea	Myeloma
Leprosy	Leukemia
Pseudomonas aeruginosa	Polycythemia vera
Syphilis	Internal carcinoma
Salmonella sepsis	Myeloid metaplasia
Staphylococcus	Collagen vascular diseases
Group A streptococcus	Dermatomyositis
Drugs	Polyarteritis nodosa
Sulfonamides	Rheumatoid arthritis
Tetracycline	Systemic lupus erythematosus
Penicillin	Discoid lupus erythematosus
Phenytoin	Deep radiation therapy
Carbamazepine	Pregnancy and menstruation
Barbiturates	Wegener's granulomatosis
Nonsteroidal anti-	Idiopathic ($\leq$50 percent of cases)
inflammatory drugs	

eyes, or genitalia); (4) fever; (5) biopsy compatible with erythema multiforme (i.e., full-thickness or scattered epidermal necrosis, perivascular lymphocytic or histiocytic infiltration of the upper third of the dermis, and subepidermal bulla formation); and (6) less than 20 percent of the body surface involved during the first 48 h and greater than 10 percent of body surface involvement present. Erythema multiforme is not painful, but erosive, bullous lesions are.

5. Vesiculobullous Systemic Lupus Erythematosus Patients with systemic lupus erythematosus may develop a generalized painful and tender vesiculobullous rash on sun-exposed or nonexposed skin. Vesicles may be single or grouped. Patients usually have a positive antinuclear antibody test and three or more other American Rheumatism Association criteria for the diagnosis of systemic lupus erythematosus. Biopsy of these lesions may reveal subepidermal vesicles containing polymorphonuclear leukocytes and fibrin at the tips of the dermal papillae. A leukocytoclastic vasculitis may be present in the superficial and middle dermis. Granular IgG and/or IgM deposition is present at the basement membrane zone in 100 percent of cases and IgA deposition in 64 percent. Lesions respond to prednisone or dapsone therapy.

6. Bullous Pemphigoid Large, tense bullae form on normal or erythematous, edematous skin areas. Rapid progression can lead to widespread cutaneous involvement. Bullae rupture and collapse, leaving eroded areas that tend to remain the same size, in contrast to the expanding erosions seen in pemphigus. These denuded areas are usually painful and tender. Oral bullae and erosions occur in 8 to 39 percent of cases, and eosinophilia may be present in 50 to 61 percent of cases.

Histopathologic study of early bullae reveals that they are subepidermal. Some bullae are infiltrate-poor (i.e., arise on normal appearing skin) or infiltrate-rich (i.e., arise in an erythematous area). The superficial dermal capillaries may show evidence of vasculitis produced by polymorphonuclear leukocytes, eosinophils, and lymphocytes. Eosinophilic spongiosis occurs in 51 percent of cases and an elevated serum IgE in 70 percent of cases. Direct immunofluorescence of involved or uninvolved skin reveals IgG or C3 deposits in a linear pattern along the basement membrane zone. C3 is present in 100 percent and IgG in 80 percent of cases. Immunoelectron microscopy has demonstrated that IgG is bound to an antigen in the lamina lucida with accentuation near hemidesmosomes. Most patients respond to corticosteroid therapy. Bullous pemphigoid has been induced by drug therapy (e.g., furosemide) and has been associated statistically with psoriasis, diabetes mellitus, rheumatoid arthritis, ulcerative colitis, and systemic lupus erythematosus.

Three to 10 percent of patients with bullous pemphigoid may have carcinoma. An increased incidence of neoplasm may occur in bullous pemphigoid patients without circulating antibasement membrane antibody by indirect immunofluorescence. Otherwise, no increased incidence of malignancy is associated with bullous pemphigoid.

An acute onset of bullous pemphigoid with fever, mimicking bullous erythema multiforme, has been reported in three patients as a result of sensitivity to penicillin G, amoxicillin, and phenoxymethyl penicillin. Other drugs reported to induce bullous pemphigoid include sulfasalazine, phenacetin, and topical fluorouracil. In the penicillin-induced cases, target lesions occurred on the palms and soles; direct immunofluorescence demonstrated linear deposition of IgG and C3 in the basement membrane zone; indirect immunofluorescence was positive in titers of 1:4 to 1:320; and prednisone therapy led to complete clearing of the bullous eruption without relapse.

7. Pemphigus Vulgaris   Thin-walled, flaccid bullae form, rupture, and leave large, painful, and tender erosions that ooze a protein-rich exudate and bleed easily. The unroofed area becomes crusted, enlarges, and coalesces with adjacent lesions. Nikolsky's sign is present, as is the Asboe-Hansen sign (pressure on the dome of an intact bulla with a fingertip forces fluid to spread under the apparently normal skin surrounding the bulla). Oral bullae and erosions occur and may precede skin lesions in up to 60 percent of cases. Crusted fissures may involve the vermillion of the lip. Throat and laryngeal lesions cause pain on swallowing and hoarseness. The conjunctivae, nasal mucosa, vagina, penis, and anus may also be involved.

Histopathologic studies reveal intraepidermal blister formation and acantholysis with detached epidermal cells lining or floating free in the blister cavity. A small, intact bulla should be biopsied for optimum diagnostic accuracy. Direct immunofluorescence reveals intercellular IgG through the entire epidermis and oral epithelium. C3 is also present in intercellular areas in early acantholytic skin. IgG also occurs in clinically normal skin.

Drug-induced pemphigus may occur with administration of penicillamine, captopril, penicillin, and rifampin. Myasthenia gravis, thymoma, epidermal carcinomas, and lymphomas have been associated with pemphigus-like rashes. Only 2 to 3 percent of patients with pemphigus have an associated malignancy. Rarely, ionizing radiation may induce pemphigus.

8. Epidermolysis Bullosa Acquisita   EBA is a rare disorder that is associated clinically with severe skin fragility, trauma-induced blisters, erosions on extensor areas of the limbs, and healing with scars and milia. These clinical findings can be used to differentiate this disorder from bullous pemphigoid. However, some cases of epidermolysis bullosa acquisita may mimic bullous pemphigoid by clinical, histologic, and immunohistologic criteria. A bullous pemphigoid-like clinical presentation of EBA may occur in 50 percent of cases, and 10 to 15 percent of patients diagnosed as having bullous pemphigoid may have EBA. EBA can be differentiated from bullous pemphigoid by immunoelectron microscopy of the skin. In bullous pemphigoid, IgG deposits are seen in the higher lamina lucida layer. In EBA, deposits occur in the upper dermis just beneath or associated with the dermal side of the lamina densa.

If immunoelectron microscopy is not available, indirect IgG immunofluorescence can be performed on 1M NaCl-treated human skin. Bullous pemphigoid anti-lamina lucida antibodies produce an epidermal or epidermal and dermal staining pattern on such skin, while EBA anti-sublamina densa antibodies cause only dermal staining. EBA is more resistant to corticosteroid therapy than is bullous pemphigoid. EBA may precede the onset of systemic lupus erythematosus or occur after its onset. There is a strong association of EBA with inflammatory bowel disease (30 percent of reported cases) and with other systemic diseases.

4. ACUTE PUSTULAR LESIONS

A. Generalized Pustular Psoriasis   Fever and malaise may precede skin symptoms by 1 to 2 days. Then, generalized skin pain and hyperalgesia may develop, followed by skin redness and edema. Previous psoriatic plaques may become very red and develop multiple pinpoint-sized (1- to 2-mm) pustules on their surfaces. In patients without existing psoriatic plaques (15 percent of cases), tiny superficial pustules develop in erythematous patches of skin. These painful and tender lesions spread to areas of uninvolved skin. Pustule formation occurs in herpetiform, polycyclic, arciform, or annular patterns, and pustules may coalesce into larger purulent blisters. Generalized erythroderma may develop. The lesions may spread and increase in severity or remit, only to flare again after a few days.

Severe toxicity, fever to 40°C (104°F), and leukocytosis to 32,000 cells/mm^3 may occur during periods of pustule formation. Generalized lymphadenopathy may occur. Patients complain of severe burning pain and itching of the skin.

Arthritis involving the distal interphalangeal joints or an asymmetrical polyarthritis and/or sacroiliitis may occur during an episode of generalized pustular psoriasis. Eye involvement may be severe, with a spectrum of disorders ranging from benign, purulent conjunctivitis to vision-threatening corneal ulceration or iridocyclitis. Bronchitis and pneumonia may occur in some cases. Secondary skin infection (e.g., cellulitis with group A streptococci) may occur. Laboratory abnormalities include hypoalbuminemia, a rise in liver enzyme and bilirubin levels, and a decrease in creatinine clearance and an elevation of the blood urea nitrogen and serum creatinine levels.

Histopathologic examination of the pustular lesions reveals dilated dermal vessels, a perivascular mononuclear cell infiltrate, and polymorphonuclear leukocyte accumulation in the epidermis as spongiform pustules (i.e., polymorphonuclear leukocytes are separated by narrowed keratinocytes). The pustules are found in a subcorneal location. Results of all Gram stains and cultures of pustule content are negative. During the acute phase, characteristics of psoriatic skin (elongated rete ridges) may be absent or difficult to find. Conservative management should be used for all cases that are not life-threatening. Systemic therapy (e.g., methotrexate, hydroxyurea, or a retinoid) should be used for fulminating, potentially lethal disease. Precipitants of generalized pustular psoriasis are listed in Table 51-5.

B. Impetigo Herpetiformis This pregnancy-initiated form of generalized pustular psoriasis arises most frequently in the third trimester. There is early and severe flexural involvement, and healing is characterized by hyperpigmentation. Ionized calcium depression may occur. This disorder may be life-threatening and may recur in a subsequent pregnancy or after administration of an oral contraceptive.

C. Subcorneal Pustular Dermatosis of Sneddon-Wilkinson This disorder causes a rash consisting of erythematous patches and plaques. Flaccid, 2- to 10-mm blisters,

Table 51-5
PRECIPITANTS OF GENERALIZED PUSTULAR PSORIASIS

Drugs
  Withdrawal of oral or topical corticosteroids in a patient with
    psoriasis vulgaris
  Nonsteroidal anti-inflammatory drugs
  Salicylates
  Penicillin
  Sulfonamides
  Lithium
  Morphine
  Alcohol
  Topical coal tar
  Pyrogallol
  Topical chrysarobin
  Potassium iodide
  Progesterone
  Antimalarials
  Oral contraceptive drugs
Infections
  Group A streptococci
  S. aureus bacteremia
Pregnancy
Sun exposure with or without sunburning

crusts, and erosions are superimposed on these erythematous areas. The blisters contain polymorphonuclear leukocytes, and results of Gram stains and cultures of blister fluid are negative. The erythematous lesions often form annular and serpiginous patterns.

Burning pain, tenderness, and/or pruritus may be associated with this eruption. It may be localized to flexural and intertriginous regions, or it may be extensive and generalized. Many patients are asymptomatic except for the presence of the cutaneous lesions. Histopathologic examination reveals subcorneal pustules containing polymorphonuclear leukocytes and a moderate perivascular dermal inflammatory infiltrate. IgG and C3 are absent in the epidermis and dermis on immunofluorescent study. This disorder may be associated with IgA or IgG myeloma, benign IgA monoclonal gammopathy, elevated IgA levels, seronegative spondyloarthropathy, rheumatoid arthritis, systemic lupus erythematosus, and generalized pustular psoriasis. Therapy with dapsone may be effective. One study has suggested that this disorder is an early form of generalized pustular psoriasis.

5. PANNICULITIS

A. Erythema Nodosum (Septal Type of Panniculitis) Fever, arthralgias, and extremity pain are early symptoms. Tender reddish nodules appear over the pretibial areas, knees, thighs, and in some cases the forearms. The lesions may cause spontaneous pain, or they may be painful only when touched. They vary in size from 1 cm to several centimeters and have indistinct, irregular margins. Lesion color may change from dark red to yellow-green in much the same way an ecchymosis evolves. The ankles and in some cases the knees may be painful on weight bearing and use. These joints may be swollen, warm, and tender. The leukocyte count may be normal or increased, and the erythrocyte sedimentation rate is elevated. Biopsy reveals vascular and perivascular septal inflammation and/or panniculitis in the adjacent fat. Septal hemorrhage with polymorphonuclear leukocyte or lymphocyte infiltration may be present. Immunofluorescence studies reveal deposition of IgG and/or IgM and complement in the walls of septal vessels. The causes of erythema nodosum are listed in Table 51-6.

B. Systemic Nodular Panniculitis (Lobular Type of Panniculitis) Painful, red, firm, and exquisitely tender nodules occur on the lower legs, ankles, thighs, trunk, and upper extremities, accompanied by high fever and diaphoresis. Edema of the lower extremities may accompany the presence of extensive plaques and nodules. Some large nodules may soften and rupture, discharging a yellow-white, creamy fluid that may be mistaken for pus. Examination of a drop of this exudate with a Sudan stain will reveal small and large fat globules without polymorphonuclear leukocytes. Large plaques and/or nodules may

Table 51-6
DISORDERS ASSOCIATED WITH ERYTHEMA NODOSUM

Cause	History	Examination	Laboratory/Imaging	Resolution May be Accelerated by Therapy with
Group A streptococcus infection	"Cold," sore throat, scarlet fever, or erysipelas	Normal throat or an exudative or nonexudative pharyngotonsillitis, desquamating rash, erysipelas	Positive throat culture for group A streptococcus, an elevated titer for anti-streptolysin O, anti-hyaluronidase, or anti-DNase B, elevated Streptozyme titer	Penicillin
Epstein-Barr virus	Sore throat, "swollen glands," fever, fatigue	Exudative tonsillitis, posterior cervical adenopathy, splenomegaly, hepatomegaly	Atypical lymphocytes on the peripheral blood smear in excess of 10%, positive Monospot test, IgM viral capsid antigen antibody positive	No therapy recommended
Sarcoidosis	Cough, dyspnea, wheezing, fever, polyarthralgia, myalgia, fatigue	Fever, uveitis, scattered rhonchi	Bilateral hilar adenopathy and/or parenchymal infiltrates on chest radiograph, ^{67}Ga scan uptake in salivary and lacrimal glands, elevated serum ACE level	Prednisone
Yersiniosis or *Campylobacter* infection	Diarrhea; abdominal pain (especially right lower abdomen), sore throat, fever, rigors	Abdominal tenderness in right lower abdomen Generalized abdominal tenderness	Positive stool cultures, rise in serum agglutinins to *Yersinia* species	Aminoglycosides or doxycycline
Coccidioidomycosis	Fever, cough, or no symptoms	Scattered rales, rhonchi, or negative chest examination	Pulmonary infiltrates, paratracheal adenopathy, positive skin test, positive tube precipitins, latex agglutination, or immuno-diffusion for IgM antibody; complement fixation less than 1:32 unless dissemination occurs	No therapy recommended
Histoplasmosis	Fever, cough, or no symptoms	Scattered rales; rhonchi; or negative chest examination	Pulmonary infiltrates and/or hilar adenopathy, positive complement fixation, positive skin test, positive agar gel precipitins, positive sputum culture	No therapy recommended
Blastomycosis	Fever, cough, or no symptoms	Scattered rales, rhonchi, or negative chest examination	Pulmonary nodules and cavitation or infiltrates and mediastinal adenopathy, positive skin test, positive immunodiffusion test to A antigen, histopathologic examination of tissue and use of special stains for fungi (Gomori methenamine-silver stain), positive smear and culture of sputum, tissue, or pus	No therapy recommended
Cat-scratch fever	History of cat scratch or cat contact, fever, localized or generalized lymph node enlargement	Fever, lymphadenopathy	Positive lymph node biopsy	No therapy available
Psittacosis	Fever, cough, mental obtundation	Rales, rhonchi, dullness, spleno-megaly, rash	Pneumonic infiltrate(s) in one or more lung fields, positive or rising titer on complement fixation or micro-IF tests for IgM or IgG antibody to *Chlamydia psittaci*	Tetracycline or erythromycin
Lymphogranuloma venereum	Sexual exposure; unilateral or bilateral femoral and/or inguinal pain, swelling, and tenderness	Fever, femoral and/or inguinal lymphade-nopathy, anorectal pain and discharge	Isolation of specific *Chlamydia trachomatis* serovars, complement fixation or micro-IF test for type-specific antibody	Doxycycline

(continued on page 777)

Table 51-6 *(continued)*
DISORDERS ASSOCIATED WITH ERYTHEMA NODOSUM

Cause	History	Examination	Laboratory/Imaging	Resolution May be Accelerated by Therapy with
Leptospirosis	Fever, malaise, headache, meningismus, dark urine	Fever, icterus, conjunctival suffusion	Leptospiral agglutinins elevated and/or increase over time, ELISA or dot-ELISA for leptospiral IgM antibodies highly sensitive and specific, abnormal liver function tests, abnormal urinalysis, elevated creatinine	Penicillin
Francisella tularensis	Contact with wild rabbits or muskrats, tick or deerfly bite	Conjunctivitis in one eye, ulcer or eschar on limb and regional adenopathy, high fever	Pneumonia (15–30% of cases) on chest radiograph, hilar adenopathy, positive culture of sputum or blood, rise in serum agglutinins (tube agglutination or microagglutination tests)	Streptomycin or tetracycline
Acute leukemia	Fever, fatigue, pallor, weakness, ecchymoses, splenomegaly and/or adenopathy in some patients	Fever, pallor, ecchymoses, lymphadenopathy, splenomegaly	Leukemia on peripheral smear and/or bone marrow	Antileukemic chemotherapy
Chronic leukemia	Fatigue, frequent infections, skin and mucosal bleeding, anemia	Generalized lymphadenopathy, hepatosplenomegaly, pallor	Leukemia on peripheral smear and/or bone marrow	Antileukemic chemotherapy
Crohn's disease or ulcerative colitis	Diarrhea, fever, abdominal pain, hematochezia	Abdominal tenderness, weight loss	Evidence of inflammatory bowel disease by colonoscopy, barium enema, and/or enteroclysis	Sulfasalazine, corticosteroids, surgical resection of diseased bowel
Erythema nodosum leprosum (leprosy)	Anesthetic skin lesions	Skin thickening with nodules, nerve thickening, anesthetic skin lesions, leonine facies	Detection of *Mycobacterium leprae* on skin biopsies and smears using acid-fast stains	Antimicrobial therapy with dapsone, clofazimine, and rifampin
Behçet's syndrome	Sore mouth with ulcers, genital ulcers, red eyes and blurred vision, and skin lesions (thrombophlebitis, acne, pustules, pathergy)	Oral ulcers, genital ulcers, anterior uveitis, hypyon, superficial thrombophlebitis, skin pustules, acneform rash, pathergy	None	Chlorambucil
Primary tuberculosis	Fever or no symptoms	Negative	Unilateral hilar node and unilateral or bilateral pulmonary infiltrates, positive tuberculin skin test	Isoniazid
Idiopathic	No symptoms	No signs, except erythema nodosum	No specific laboratory abnormalities	No therapy recommended
Pregnancy	Nausea, vomiting, hyperosmia, urinary urgency and frequency	Uterine enlargement, Hegar's sign, Cullen's sign	Positive pregnancy test	No therapy recommended
Sulfonamide	History of sulfonamide ingestion, pain in limbs; fever may occur	Erythema nodosum and sometimes fever	None	Discontinuance of drug
Oral contraceptives	History of oral contraceptive use, pain in limbs; fever may occur	Erythema nodosum and sometimes fever	None	Discontinuance of drug

coalesce. Lesions may occur all over the body in any subcutaneous area. Fever, arthralgia, and malaise may precede or begin with the appearance of the skin lesions. This disorder may present initially as an acute process, but it has a tendency to recur. Corticosteroids may be effective. Many cases are idiopathic, while others are associated with connective tissue disorders (systemic lupus erythematosus [lupus profundus] and systemic sclerosis), lymphoproliferative diseases (lymphoma and histiocytosis), α_1-antitrypsin deficiency, and paraproteinemia with C1 esterase inhibitor deficiency.

Biopsy of a nodule reveals lobular panniculitis. Early lesions may demonstrate foci of fat necrosis with other areas containing normal-appearing fat lobules. The cytoplasm of some fat cells may appear basophilic and granular, and nuclear staining is poor or absent (''ghostlike'' fat cells). Infiltration by polymorphonuclear leukocytes and eosinophils may be prominent in the intercellular spaces. Deposits of basophilic material around dead fat cells are related to calcium soap formation in the interstitium. More chronic lesions contain dead lipocytes surrounded by infiltrating histiocytes and associated sheets of foam cells. Biopsy is useful in diagnosis. Clinical examination and tests for pancreatic disease and the other disorders listed are required before a case of lobular panniculitis can be labeled idiopathic.

C. Panniculitis of Pancreatic Origin (Lobular Type of Panniculitis)

Painful, red, tender, and sometimes fluctuant subcutaneous nodules and placques appear on the legs, arms, and trunk. Edema of the legs may be prominent. Fever, chills, prostration, profound weakness, and diaphoresis are associated symptoms. Joint symptoms occur in 60 percent of cases and may result in erosive joint changes. Fat necrosis in a periarticular area may drain into a joint, causing severe synovitis. Bone marrow fat necrosis may result in lytic bone lesions. Serum amylase and lipase levels may be elevated, and eosinophilia occurs in 25 percent of cases. Abdominal pain may result from the primary pancreatic lesion or from intraabdominal fat necrosis. The causes of pancreatic panniculitis include alcoholic pancreatitis (50 percent), posttraumatic pancreatitis (5 percent), and acinous carcinoma of the pancreas (30 percent). A CT scan or endoscopic retrograde cholangiopancreatography can image a carcinoma, and the diagnosis can be confirmed by a needle or open biopsy (i.e., exploratory laparotomy) of the tumor. The course of this disorder is dependent on the nature of the pancreatic disease.

D. Cytophagic Histiocytic Panniculitis

This systemic disease may present with fever and widespread painful, 1- to 5-cm, tender, red, and/or ecchymotic subcutaneous nodules. Hepatosplenomegaly, pancytopenia, and abnormal liver function may be associated. Fat lobules are infiltrated by histiocytes and granulocytes, and fat necrosis and hemorrhage are prominent findings. Histiocytes are filled with phagocytized red blood cells, lymphocytes, platelets, and neutrophils (''beanbag cells''). This disorder follows a malignant and lethal course, with eventual death from hemorrhage.

6. SWEET'S SYNDROME (ACUTE FEBRILE NEUTROPHILIC DERMATOSIS)

This disorder begins with fever (72 percent of cases); 2- to 10-cm erythematous, painful, tender, and oval or circular nodules and plaques that appear on the face, neck, trunk, arms, and sometimes the legs (100 percent of cases); and neutrophilic leukocytosis (61 percent of cases). Pustular and vesicular lesions may appear on the surface of some of the erythematous plaques, giving the appearance in some cases of a multilocular blister. Skin biopsy reveals dense infiltration of the upper and middermis by polymorphonuclear leukocytes without an associated leukocytoclastic vasculitis. Conjunctivitis and an asymmetrical arthritis usually involving large joints (25 percent of cases) may also occur. Sweet's syndrome may follow an upper respiratory infection (67 percent of cases in one series), or it may be associated with inflammatory bowel disease. An association with malignancy occurs in up to one-third of reported cases. Acute myeloid and myelomonocytic leukemia are the malignant diseases most commonly associated with Sweet's syndrome. Patients with Sweet's syndrome and multiple myeloma or a lymphoproliferative disorder have also been reported.

Polyarthralgia or polyarthritis and conjunctivitis are uncommon in cases associated with acute leukemia, while anemia in the absence of malignancy is infrequent. Some authors have considered the vesiculopustular dermatosis associated with the bowel-bypass syndrome and bullous pyoderma gangrenosum to be variants of Sweet's syndrome. Su and Liu have proposed diagnostic criteria for the diagnosis of Sweet's syndrome. The two major criteria are (1) an abrupt onset of painful and/or tender erythematous or violaceous plaques or nodules and (2) neutrophilic infiltration of the dermis without leukocytoclastic vasculitis. Minor criteria include (1) an antecedent fever or infection; (2) accompanying fever, joint pain, conjunctivitis or a malignancy; (3) leukocytosis; and (4) a good response to corticosteroids and not antibiotics. The presence of both major criteria and two minor criteria are required for a definite diagnosis of Sweet's syndrome.

Sweet's syndrome responds rapidly to prednisone (40–60 mg/day). Colchicine or indomethacin may also be effective.

7. GLUCAGONOMA SYNDROME (NECROLYTIC MIGRATORY ERYTHEMA)

Migratory erythematous plaques occur on the face, abdomen, perineum, and extremities. Flaccid bullae and vesicles develop and rupture, producing large erosions and exudative crusting plaques and areas of skin necrosis. Lesions are often annular (circinate or gyrate patterns) plaques. Perioral lesions (erosions with crusting), stomatitis, and weight loss occur. Hyperglycemia, hypoaminoacidemia, an elevated serum glucagon level, and anemia are usually present. Skin biopsy of an early skin lesion reveals epidermal necrosis and intraepidermal separation with neutrophils in the spaces between epithelial cell layers. Results of immunofluorescence studies are negative.

Up to 80 percent of tumors responsible for the glucagonoma syndrome are malignant, and 50 percent have metastases when they are explored. The glucagonoma syndrome may mimic TEN, erythema multiforme, or pemphigus foliaceous. Complete removal of the tumor may result in resolution of all symptoms.

8. ERYTHRODERMA

Erythroderma is characterized by diffuse erythema and mild-to-moderate edema of the skin of the entire body associated with mild burning discomfort and/or severe pruritus. Malaise (34 percent of cases) and subjective chilliness (34 percent) may accompany the rash, and fever may occur in 33 percent of cases. Generalized lymphadenopathy may be present in 26 percent. Acute erythroderma is most commonly caused by a drug reaction. There is no history of skin disorder. Drugs commonly associated with erythroderma include phenytoin, penicillins, allopurinol, thiazides, sulfonamides, gold, isoniazid, phenobarbital, iodides, terbutaline, and quinacrine. Failure to discontinue drug therapy once skin erythema begins may increase the probability of progression to exfoliative dermatitis. Preexisting dermatoses are another major cause of erythroderma. Contact dermatitis, atopic dermatitis, psoriasis, pityriasis rubra pilaris, lichen planus, pemphigus foliaceous, and erythema multiforme may become more severe and present with generalized skin erythema and edema.

Erythroderma with a more insidious onset and chronic course may be associated with cutaneous T-cell lymphoma, Hodgkin's disease, or leukemia. Idiopathic erythroderma constitutes 16 to 50 percent of cases. Skin biopsy may be diagnostically helpful in up to 50 percent of patients. Corticosteroids are effective in the management of acute erythroderma caused by drug hypersensitivity.

9. EOSINOPHILIC FASCIITIS

There is an abrupt onset of painful swelling and erythema of the skin of the extremities and trunk. Flexion and extension of the limbs may be limited by the overlying edematous, painful, thickened skin. A peau d'orange appearance of the skin surface may be present. The hands and face are not affected in most cases. Biopsy reveals a mild lymphocytic and plasma-cell infiltrate of muscle and marked thickening of the fascia. Eosinophilia of 10 to 40 percent is commonly present. Hematologic abnormalities may include pancytopenia, anemia, and/or thrombocytopenia. A good response to corticosteroids is usual, but some patients are resistant to steroid therapy.

10. GENERALIZED CELLULITIS

A. Cellulitis in a Lymphedematous Limb Patients with chronic lymphedema of an extremity (e.g., postmastectomy lymphedema) may develop an acute painful cellulitis with erythema, heat, and tenderness that spreads rapidly up the limb and then over the trunk and into the other extremities. Fever, rigors, and generalized pain accompany the diffuse subcutaneous inflammatory process. The usual cause is a streptococcal species or *S. aureus* that enters the lymphedematous limb by way of a break in the skin. There is a prompt response to antibiotic therapy. Recurrent attacks of extensive cellulitis may occur in susceptible individuals.

B. Rapidly Spreading Clostridial Cellulitis This infection occurs as a complication of a contaminated wound. The local wound may appear infected, and it may drain a brown, watery, malodorous fluid. Subcutaneous crepitus may be palpable near the wound, and *Clostridium perfringens* can be observed on a Gram stain and/or grown in culture. Up to 5 percent of cases of clostridial cellulitis are fulminant, with rapid spread of clostridial infection through the subcutaneous tissues of the initially involved limb to the trunk and other extremities. Mild pain, skin edema, erythema, and crepitus occur. Fever, prostration, jaundice, and renal failure may develop due to the toxicity of the infectious agent. Patients with severe rapidly spreading cellulitis have a high mortality rate.

11. PURPURA FULMINANS (PURPURA GANGRENOSUM)

Severe and extensive ecchymoses of the skin occurs during the course of a febrile toxic illness. This disorder has been most frequently reported in association with *Neisseria meningitidis* bacteremia in children and young adults.

Other infections reported with purpura fulminans include *Streptococcus pneumoniae* bacteremia (especially in patients with functional or anatomic asplenia), scarlet fever, and varicella. Fever, rigors, prostration, delirium, coma, a diffuse maculopapular or petechial rash, headache, nausea, vomiting, nuchal rigidity, hypotension, and shock are common components of the clinical presentation of meningococcal septicemia. Transient depression of plasma levels of protein C and protein S occur during disseminated intravascular coagulation and may contribute to the tendency of patients with meningococcal sepsis to develop cutaneous thromboses and hemorrhagic gangrene of the skin. Purpura fulminans may occur in the absence of disseminated intravascular coagulation, and there is no correlation between the severity of the disseminated intravascular coagulation and the extent of the purpura.

Purpuric lesions often contain large numbers of bacteria, as demonstrated on biopsies and smears of excised skin. Meningococci are visible in endothelial cells and neutrophils. The purpuric lesions may represent a local Schwartzman reaction. Gangrene of one or more extremities, sometimes requiring amputation, may occur.

Purpura is usually most extensive in areas with reduced blood flow. Purpuric gangrene may result in necrosis of the underlying skin, subcutaneous fat, and muscle. Sharp demarcation of necrotic tissue from adjacent viable tissue occurs in a "cookie cutter" fashion. The purpuric areas require excision, as does a full-thickness burn, since the epidermis, dermis, and subcutaneous tissue are necrotic. Such lesions may be painless and anesthetic, but an inflammatory reaction in the surrounding viable skin, sloughing of necrotic tissue and secondary infection, and surgical excision of necrotic tissue may give rise to moderately severe pain. In some cases, single or multiple limb amputations are required. This disorder usually occurs in small children, but it may also occur in young adults. Treatment has included heparin, intravenous penicillin, administration of antithrombin III, and plasmapheresis.

A poor prognosis (40–100 percent mortality) in meningococcal sepsis is predicted by the presence of two or more of the following findings on admission: (1) petechiae for less than 12 h, (2) shock, (3) coma, (4) high fever, (5) a low or normal peripheral leukocyte count, (6) thrombocytopenia, (7) absence of meningitis (<20 white blood cells/mm^3 of spinal fluid), and (8) disseminated intravascular coagulation.

12. ACUTE URTICARIA

Whitish or reddish evanescent papules or plaques surrounded by erythema occur at multiple sites on the face, neck, trunk, and extremities. Individual lesions may sting, burn, tingle, or itch.

Urticarial lesions remain for 1 to 3 h and then gradually resolve. Antihistamine and/or corticosteroid therapy may relieve symptoms and prevent the occurrence of new le-

Table 51-7
CAUSES OF ACUTE URTICARIA

Insect bites and stings	Promethazine
Food	Propylthiouracil
Cheese	Quinidine
Chocolate	Quinine
Garlic	Saccharin
Melons	Sulfonamides
Onions	Others
Peanut butter	Food additives
Pork	Azo dyes (e.g., tartrazine)
Shellfish	Benzoic acid derivatives
Spices	Citric acid
Strawberries	Egg and fish albumin
Tomatoes	Penicillin
Others	Salicylates
Drugs	Yeasts
Alcohol	Infections
Allopurinol	*Chlamydia psittaci*
Aspirin	Epstein-Barr virus
Aminoglycosides	Group A streptococcal throat
Barbiturates	and skin infections
Chlorpromazine	Hepatitis B virus
Contrast dyes used in	*Treponoma pallidum*
radiographic studies	Serum sickness following
Gold	parenteral administration of
Griseofulvin	serum or a drug
Hydantoins	Inhalants
Hydralazine	Aerosols
Insulin	Animal dander
Iodides	Cosmetics
Menthol	Cottonseed
Mercury	Feathers
Morphine	Formaldehyde
Nonsteroidal anti-inflammatory	Grass
drugs	Molds
Penicillin	Pollens
Phenobarbital	Blood products
Pilocarpine	Emotional stress (e.g., cholinergic
Polio vaccine	urticaria)
Procaine	

sions. Possible causes of acute generalized urticaria are listed in Table 51-7.

13. PSYCHOGENIC PAIN

Some patients may complain of generalized skin burning or stinging pain and tenderness in the absence of an eruption. Scalp tenderness and pain associated with gentle traction of scalp hair may be present. The mechanism is unknown, and symptoms may be intensified by stress and reduced by diazepam and similar drugs.

GENERALIZED SKIN PAIN REFERENCES

Bullous Disorders — Review

Woolridge WE: Three blistering diseases: Why proper management is critical. *Postgrad Med* 88:103–104, 106, 1990.

Cutaneous Disorders — Review

Schaefer DG, Wolf JE: Common dermatologic disorders. *Clin Plast Surg* 14:209–222, 1987.

Sternbach G, Callen JP: Dermatitis. *Emerg Med Clin North Am* 3: 677–692, 1985.

Dermatitis — Atopic

Atherton DJ: Diagnosis and management of skin disorders caused by food allergy. *Ann Allergy* 53:623–628, 1984.

Oakes RC, Cox AD, Burgdorf WHC: Atopic dermatitis: A review of diagnosis, pathogenesis, and management. *Clin Pediatr (Phila)* 22: 467–475, 1983.

Dermatitis — Contact

Baer RL: Poison ivy dermatitis. *Cutis* 37:434–436, 1986.

Dahl MV, Pass F, Trancik RJ: Sodium lauryl sulfate irritant patch tests: 2. Variations of test responses among subjects and comparison to variations of allergic responses elicited by *Toxicodendron* extract. *J Am Acad Dermatol* 11:474–477, 1984.

Gayer KD, Burnett JW: *Toxicodendron* dermatitis. *Cutis* 42:99–100, 1988.

Marks JG Jr, DeMelfi T, McCarthy MA, et al: Dermatitis from cashew nuts. *J Am Acad Dermatol* 10:627–631, 1984.

Mitchell JC, Guin JD, Maibach HI, et al: Allergenicity of *Toxicodendron sylvestre* (Anacardiaceae): *Contact Dermatitis* 12:113–114, 1985.

Oltman J, Hensler R: Poison oak/ivy and forestry workers. *Clin Dermatol* 4:213–216, 1986.

Resnick SD: Poison-ivy and poison-oak dermatitis. *Clin Dermatol* 4:208–212, 1986.

Woolridge WE: Acute allergic contact dermatitis: How to manage severe cases. *Postgrad Med* 87:221–224, 1990.

Dermatitis — Herpetiformis

Accetta P, Kumar V, Beutner EH, et al: Anti-endomysial antibodies: A serologic market of dermatitis herpetiformis. *Arch Dermatol* 122: 459–462, 1986.

Economopoulou P, Laskaris G: Dermatitis herpetiformis: Oral lesions as an early manifestation. *Oral Surg Oral Med Oral Pathol* 62:77–80, 1986.

Ingber A, Feuerman EJ: Pemphigus with characteristics of dermatitis herpetiformis: A long-term follow-up of five patients. *Int J Dermatol* 25:575–579, 1986.

Jawitz J, Kumar V, Nigra TP, et al: Vesicular pemphigoid vs. dermatitis herpetiformis. *J Am Acad Dermatol* 10:892–896, 1984.

Karpati S, Torok E, Kosnai I: Discrete palmar and plantar symptoms in children with dermatitis herpetiformis Duhring. *Cutis* 37:184–187, 1986.

Kumar V, Beutner EH, Chorzelski TP: Antiendomysial antibody: Useful serological indicator of dermatitis herpetiformis. *Arch Dermatol Res* 279:454–458, 1987.

Sander HM, Utz MMP, Peters MS: Bullous pemphigoid and dermatitis herpetiformis: Mixed bullous disease or coexistence of two separate entities? *J. Cutan Pathol* 16:370–374, 1989.

Volta U, Cassani F, DeFranchis R, et al: Antibodies to gliadin in adult coeliac disease and dermatitis herpetiformis. *Digestion* 30:263–270, 1984.

Drug Reactions — Review

Arnold HL Jr, Odom RB, James WD: Contact dermatitis: Drug eruptions, in Arnold HL Jr, Odom RB, James WS (eds): *Andrews' Diseases of the Skin*, 8th ed. Philadelphia, Saunders, 1990, pp 89–130.

Bigby M, Stern RS, Arndt KA: Allergic cutaneous reactions to drugs. *Prim Care* 16:713–727, 1989.

Kaplan AP: Drug-induced skin disease. *J Allergy Clin Immunol* 74:573–579, 1984.

Eosinophilic Fasciitis

Arnold HL Jr, Odom RB, James WD: Connective tissue diseases (eosinophilic fasciitis), in Arnold HL Jr, Odom RB, James WD (eds): *Andrews' Diseases of the Skin*, 8th ed. Philadelphia, Saunders, 1990, pp 159–185.

Gilliland BC. Systemic sclerosis (scleroderma) (eosinophilic fasciitis), in Wilson JD, Braunwald E, Isselbacher KJ, et al (eds): *Harrison's Principles of Internal Medicine*, 12th ed. New York, McGraw-Hill, 1991, vol 2. pp 1443–1448.

Epidermolysis Bullosa Acquisita

Boh, E, Roberts LJ, Lieu T-S, et al: Epidermolysis bullosa acquisita preceding the development of systemic lupus erythematosus. *J Am Acad Dermatol* 22:587–593, 1990.

Gammon WR, Briggaman RA, Woodley DT, et al: Epidermolysis bullosa acquisita: a pemphigoid-like disease. *J Am Acad Dermatol* 11:820–832, 1984.

Kero M, Niemi K-M, Kanerva L: Pregnancy as a trigger of epidermolysis bullosa acquisita. *Acta Derm Venereol (Stockh)* 63:353–356, 1983.

Kurzhals G, Stolz W, Meurer M, et al: Acquired epidermolysis bullosa with the clinical feature of Brunsting-Perry cicatricial bullous pemphigoid. *Arch Dermatol* 127:391–395, 1991.

Labeille B, Gineston J-L, Denoeux J-P, et al: Epidermolysis bullosa acquisita and Crohn's disease: A case report with immunological and electron microscopic studies. *Arch Intern Med* 148:1457–1459, 1988.

Lacour J-P, Juhlin L, El Baze P, et al: Epidermolysis bullosa acquisita with negative direct immunofluorescence. *Arch Dermatol* 121: 1183–1185, 1985.

McCuaig CC, Chan LS, Woodley DT, et al: Epidermolysis bullosa acquisita in childhood: Differentiation from hereditary epidermolysis bullosa. *Arch Dermatol* 125:944–949, 1989.

Woodley DT: Immunofluorescence on salt-split skin for the diagnosis of epidermolysis bullosa acquisita (editorial). *Arch Dermatol* 126:229–231, 1990.

Woodley DT, Gammon WR: Epidermolysis bullosa acquisita: An autoimmune disease with distinctive immunoultrastructural features. *Cutis* 32:521–527, 1983.

Wuepper KD: Repeat direct immunofluorescence to discriminate pemphigoid from epidermolysis bullosa acquisita (comment). *Arch Dermatol* 126:1365, 1990.

Epidermolysis Bullosa — Heriditary

Eady RAJ: Diagnosing epidermolysis bullosa. *Br J Dermatol* 108:621–626, 1983.

Fine J-D: Epidermolysis bullosa: Clinical aspects, pathology, and recent advances in research. *Int J Dermatol* 25:143–157, 1986.

Fine J-D, Bauer EA, Briggaman RA, et al: Revised clinical and laboratory criteria for subtypes of inherited epidermolysis bullosa: A consensus report by the Subcommittee on Diagnosis and Classification of the National Epidermolysis Bullosa Registry. *J Am Acad Dermatol* 24:119–135, 1991.

Haber RM, Hanna W, Ramsay CA, et al: Hereditary epidermolysis bullosa. *J Am Acad Dermatol* 13:252–278, 1985.

Schofield OMV, Fine J-D, Verando P, et al: GB3 monoclonal antibody for the diagnosis of junctional epidermolysis bullosa: Results of a multicenter study. *J Am Acad Dermatol* 23:1078–1083, 1990.

Skerrow CJ: The electron microscope and the antibody: Trends in the diagnosis of epidermolysis bullosa. *Br J Dermatol* 115:123–124, 1986.

Tabas M, Gibbons S, Bauer EA: The mechanobullous diseases. *Dermatol Clin* 5:123–136, 1987.

Winship IM, Winship WS: Epidermolysis bullosa misdiagnosed as child abuse: A report of 3 cases. *S Afr Med J* 73:369–370, 1988.

Erythema Multiforme

Beacham BE, Schuldenfrei J, Julka SS: Sarcoidosis presenting with erythema multiforme-like cutaneous lesions. *Cutis* 33:461–463, 1984.

Brown FH, Houston GD, Phillips M, et al: Erythema multiforme following Cardizem therapy: Report of a case. *Ann Dent* 48:39–40, 1989.

Edmond BJ, Huff JC, Weston WL: Erythema multiforme. *Pediatr Clin North Am* 30:631–640, 1983.

Elias PM, Fritsch PO: Erythema multiforme, in Fitzpatrick TB, Eisen AZ, Wolff K, et al (eds): *Dermatology in General Medicine*, 2d ed. New York, McGraw-Hill, 1979, pp 295–303.

Fisher AA: Erythema multiforme-like eruptions due to topical miscellaneous compounds: 3. *Cutis* 37:262–264, 1986.

———: Unusual reactions associated with allergic reactions to nickel. *Cutis* 47:86, 88, 1991.

Goldberg GN: Erythema multiforme controversies and recent advances. *Adv Dermatol* 2:73–90, 1987.

Huff JC: Erythema multiforme. *Dermatol Clin* 3:141–152, 1985.

Irvine C, Reynolds A, Finlay AY: Erythema multiforme-like reaction to "rosewood." *Contact Dermatitis* 19:224–225, 1988.

Ledesma GN, McCormack PC: Erythema multiforme. *Clin Dermatol* 4:70–80, 1986.

Lewis MAO, Lamey P-J, Forsyth A, et al: Recurrent erythema multiforme: A possible role of foodstuffs. *Br Dent J* 166:371–373, 1989.

Erythroderma

Arnold HL Jr, Odom RB, James WD: Seborrheic dermatitis, psoriasis, recalcitrant palmoplantar eruptions, and erythroderma, in Arnold HL Jr, Odom RB, James WD (eds): *Andrews' Diseases of the Skin*, 8th ed. Philadelphia, Saunders, 1990, pp 194–226.

Dahl MV, Swanson DL, Jacobs HS: A dermatitis-eosinophilia syndrome: Treatment with methylprednisolone pulse therapy. *Arch Dermatol* 120:1595–1597, 1984.

Danno K, Kume M, Ohta M, et al: Erythroderma with generalized lymphadenopathy induced by phenytoin. *J Dermatol* 16:392–396, 1989.

Gaspari AA, Lotze MT, Rosenberg SA, et al: Dermatologic changes associated with interleukin 2 administration. *JAMA* 258:1624–1629, 1987.

Hidano A, Yamashita N, Mizuguchi M, et al: Clinical, histological, and immunohistological studies of postoperative erythroderma. *J Dermatol* 16:20–30, 1989.

King LE Jr, Dufresne RG Jr, Lovett GL, et al: Erythroderma: Review of 82 cases. *South Med J* 79:1210–1215, 1986.

Ray-Chaudhuri K, Boggild M: Hypersensitivity to carbamazepine presenting with a leukemoid reaction, eosinophilia, erythroderma, and renal failure. *Neurology* 39:436–438, 1989.

Wengrower D, Tzfoni EE, Drenger B, et al: Erythroderma and pneumonitis induced by penicillin? *Respiration* 50:301–303, 1986.

White WB, Shornick JK, Grant-Kels JM, et al: Erythroderma with spongiotic dermatitis: Association with common variable hypogammaglobulinemia. *Am J Med* 78:523–528, 1985.

Wiesenthal AM, Ressman M, Caston SA, et al: Toxic shock syndrome: 1. Clinical exclusion of other syndromes by strict and screening definitions. *Am J Epidemiol* 122:847–856, 1985.

Fixed Drug Eruption — Generalized

Baird BJ, DeVillez RL: Widespread bullous fixed drug eruption mimicking toxic epidermal necrolysis. *Int J Dermatol* 27:170–174, 1988.

Duhra P, Porter DI: Paracetamol-induced fixed drug eruption with positive immunofluorescence findings. *Clin Exp Dermatol* 15:293–295, 1990.

Sowden JM, Smith AG: Multifocal fixed drug eruption mimicking erythema multiforme. *Clin Exp Dermatol* 15:387–388, 1990.

Glucagonoma

Arnold HL Jr, Odom RB, James WD: Erythema and urticaria, in Arnold HL Jr, Odom RB, James WD (eds): *Andrews' Diseases of the Skin*, 8th ed. Philadelphia, Saunders, 1990, pp 131–158.

Goltz RW, Burgdorf WHC: Figurate erythemas (necrolytic migratory erythema), in Fitzpatrick TB, Eisen AZ, Wolff K, et al (eds): *Dermatology in General Medicine*, 2d ed. New York, McGraw-Hill, 1979, pp 669–674.

Immunodermatology — Review

Ahmed AR: Diagnosis of bullous disease and studies in the pathogenesis of blister formation using immunopathological techniques. *J Cutan Pathol* 11:237–248: 1984.

Black MM, Bhogal BS, Willsteed E: Immunopathological techniques in the diagnosis of bullous disorders. *Acta Derm Venereol (Stockh)* 69(suppl 151):96–105, 1989.

Gammon WR, Kowalewski C, Chorzelski TP, et al: Direct immunofluorescence studies of sodium chloride-separated skin in the differential diagnosis of bullous pemphigoid and epidermolysis bullosa acquisita. *J Am Acad Dermatol* 22:664–670, 1990.

Cockerell CJ: Reevaluation of routine histology in the diagnosis of blistering diseases. *Semin Dermatol* 7:171–177, 1988.

Helm KF, Peters MS: Immunodermatology update: The immunologically mediated vesiculobullous diseases. *Mayo Clin Proc* 66:187–202, 1991.

Leonard JN, Haffenden GP, Unsworth DJ, et al: Evidence that the IgA in patients with linear IgA disease is qualitatively different from that of patients with dermatitis herpetiformis. *Br J Dermatol* 110:315–321, 1984.

Pardo RJ, Penneys NS: Location of basement membrane type IV collagen beneath subepidermal bullous diseases. *J Cutan Pathol* 17:336–341, 1990.

Panniculitis

Arnold HL Jr, Odom RB, James WD: Diseases of subcutaneous fat, in Arnold HL Jr, Odom RB, James WD (eds): *Andrews' Diseases of the Skin*, 8th ed. Philadelphia, Saunders, 1990, pp 570–578.

Bullock WE: *Mycobacterium leprae*: Leprosy, erythema nodosum leprosum, in Mandell GL, Douglas RG Jr, Bennett JE (eds): *Principles and Practice of Infectious Diseases*, 3d ed. New York, Churchill Livingstone, 1990, pp 1906–1914.

deMoragas JM: Panniculitis, in Fitzpatrick TB, Eisen AZ, Wolff K, et al (eds): *Dermatology in General Medicine*, 2d ed. New York, McGraw-Hill, 1979, pp 784–794.

Foster DW: The lipodystrophies and other rare disorders of adipose tissue, in Wilson JD, Braunwald E, Isselbacher KJ, et al (eds): *Harrison's Principles of Internal Medicine*, 12th ed. New York, McGraw-Hill, 1991, vol 2, pp 1883–1887.

Pemphigoid — Bullous

Ahmed AR, Newcomer VD: Bullous pemphigoid: 2. Clinical features. *Clin Dermatol* 5:6–12, 1987.

Alcalay J, David M, Ingber A, et al: Bullous pemphigoid mimicking bullous erythema multiforme: An untoward side effect of penicillins. *J Am Acad Dermatol* 18:345–349, 1988.

Bhawan J, Milstone E, Malhotra R, et al: Scabies presenting as bullous pemphigoid-like eruption. *J Am Acad Dermatol* 24:179–181, 1991.

Bushkell LL, Jordon RE: Bullous pemphigoid: A cause of peripheral blood eosinophilia. *J Am Acad Dermatol* 8:648–651, 1983.

Camisa C, Neff JC, Rossana C, et al: Bullous lichen planus: Diagnosis by indirect immunofluorescence and treatment with dapsone. *J Am Acad Dermatol* 14:464–469, 1986.

Crotty C, Pittelkow M, Muller SA: Eosinophilic spongiosis: A clinicopathologic review of seventy-one cases. *J Am Acad Dermatol* 8:337–343, 1983.

Flotte TJ: Pathology of pemphigoid. *Clin Dermatol* 5:71–80, 1987.

Jordon RE: Bullous pemphigoid, cicatricial pemphigoid, and chronic bullous dermatosis of childhood, in Fitzpatrick TB, Eisen AZ, Wolff K, et al (eds): *Dermatology in General Medicine*, 2d ed. New York, McGraw-Hill, 1979, pp 318–323.

Korman N: Bullous pemphigoid. *J Am Acad Dermatol* 16:907–924, 1987.

Logan RA, Bhogal B, Das AK, et al: Localization of bullous pemphigoid antibody: An indirect immunofluorescence study of 228 cases using a split-skin technique. *Br J Dermatol* 117:471–478, 1987.

MacFarlane AW, Verbov JL: Trauma-induced bullous pemphigoid. *Clin Exp Dermatol* 14:245–249, 1989.

Mayou SC, Black MM, Holmes RC: Pemphigoid "herpes" gestationis. *Semin Dermatol* 7:104–110, 1988.

Muramatsu T, Shirai T, Iida T, et al: Antigen specificities of antibasement membrane zone antibodies: Immunofluorescence and Western immunoblotting studies. *Arch Dermatol Res* 280:411–415, 1988.

Roenigk RK, Dahl MV: Bullous pemphigoid and prurigo nodularis. *J Am Acad Dermatol* 14:944–947, 1986.

Rongioletti F, Parodi A, Rebora A: Dyshidrosiform pemphigoid: Report of an additional case. *Dermatologica* 170:84–85, 1985.

Thivolet J, Barthelemy H: Bullous pemphigoid. *Semin Dermatol* 7:91–103, 1988.

Urano-Suehisa S, Tagami H, Yamada M, et al: Bullous pemphigoid, figurate erythema and generalized pigmentation with skin thickening in a patient with adenocarcinoma of the stomach. *Dermatologica* 171:117–121, 1985.

Pemphigoid—Cicatricial

Mondino BJ: Cicatricial pemphigoid and erythema multiforme. *Ophthalmology* 97:939–952, 1990.

Roenigk R, Vance JC: Cicatricial pemphigoid: A rare but important bullous skin disease with mucosal involvement. *Minn Med* 66:557–561, 1983.

Pemphigus

Arnold HL Jr, Odom RB, James WD: Chronic blistering or pustular dermatoses, in Arnold HL Jr, Odom RB, James WD (eds): *Andrews' Diseases of the Skin,* 8th ed. Philadelphia, Saunders, 1990, pp 534–559.

Galimberti RL, Kowalczuk AM, Bianchi O, et al: Chronic benign familial pemphigus. *Int J Dermatol* 27:495–500, 1988.

Gibson LE, Muller SA: Dermatologic disorders in patients with thymoma. *Acta Derm Venereol (Stockh)* 67:351–356, 1987.

Hodak E, David M, Ingber A, et al: The clinical and histopathological spectrum of IgA-pemphigus: Report of two cases. *Clin Exp Dermatol* 15:433–437, 1990.

Jordan RE: Pemphigus, in Fitzpatrick TB, Eisen AZ, Wolff K, et al (eds): *Dermatology in General Medicine,* 2d ed. New York, McGraw-Hill, 1979, pp 310–317.

Kouskoukis CE, Ackerman AB: What histologic finding distinguishes superficial pemphigus and bullous impetigo? *Am J Dermatopathol* 6:179–181, 1984.

Low GJ, Keeling JH: Ionizing radiation-induced pemphigus. *Arch Dermatol* 126:1319–1323, 1990.

Maciejowska E, Jablonska S, Chorzelski T: Is pemphigus herpetiformis an entity? *Int J Dermatol* 26:571–577, 1987.

Phototoxicity and Photoallergic Dermatitis

Arnold HL Jr, Odom RB, James WD: Dermatoses due to physical factors, in Arnold HL Jr, Odom RB, James WD (eds): *Andrews' Diseases of the Skin,* 8th ed. Philadelphia, Saunders, 1990, pp 22–50.

Parrish JA, White HAD, Madhu AP: Photomedicine, in Fitzpatrick TB, Eisen AZ, Wolff K, et al (eds): *Dermatology in General Medicine,* 2d ed. New York, McGraw-Hill, 1979, pp 942–994.

Phytophotodermatitis

Henderson JAM, DesGroseilliers J-P: Gas plant (*Dictamnus albus*) phytophotodermatitis simulating poison ivy. *Can Med Assoc J* 130:889–891, 1984.

Porphyria

Murphy GM, Wright J, Nicholls DSH, et al: Sunbed-induced pseudoporphyria. *Br J Dermatol* 120:555–562, 1989.

Psoriasis—Pustular

Barth JH, Baker H: Generalized pustular psoriasis precipitated by trazodone in the treatment of depression. *Br J Dermatol* 115:629–630, 1986.

Cimitan A, Fantini F, Giannetti A: Clinical trial with Cyclosporin A. *Acta Derm Venereol Suppl (Stockh)* 146:159–163, 1989.

Farber EM, Van Scott EJ: Psoriasis, in Fitzpatrick TB, Eisen AZ, Wolff K, et al (eds): *Dermatology in General Medicine,* 2d ed. New York, McGraw-Hill, 1979, pp 233–247.

Hu G-H, O'Connell BM, Farber EM: When does psoriasis become pustular? *Cutis* 35:527–528, 1985.

Katz M, Seidenbaum M, Weinrauch L: Penicillin-induced generalized pustular psoriasis. *J Am Acad Dermatol* 17:918–920, 1987.

Lotem M, Ingber A, Segal R, et al: Generalized pustular drug rash induced by hydroxychloroquine. *Acta Derm Venereol (Stockholm)* 70:250–251, 1990.

Lotem M, Katzenelson V, Rotem A, et al: Impetigo herpetiformis: A variant of pustular psoriasis or a separate entity? *J Am Acad Dermatol* 20:338–341, 1989.

Lyons JH III: Generalized pustular psoriasis. *Int J Dermatol* 26:409–418, 1987.

Matsubara M, Komori M, Koishi K, et al: Generalized pustular psoriasis and bacteremia. *J Dermatol* 10:525–529, 1983.

Sanchez NP, Perry HO, Muller SA, et al: Subcorneal pustular dermatosis and pustular psoriasis. *Arch Dermatol* 119:715–721, 1983.

Shelley WB, Shelley ED: Pustular psoriasis: From the wheelchair to the dance floor. *Cutis* 38:150, 1986.

Purpura Fulminans

Arnold HL Jr, Odom RB, James WD: Cutaneous vascular diseases (purpura fulminans), in Arnold HL Jr, Odom RB, James WD (eds): *Andrews' Diseases of the Skin,* 8th ed. Philadelphia, Saunders, 1990, pp 944–990.

Densen P, Weiler JM, Griffiss JM, et al: Familial properdin deficiency and fatal meningococcemia: Correction of the bactericidal defect by vaccination. *N Engl J Med* 316:922–926, 1987.

Drapkin MS, Wisch JS, Gelfand JA, et al: Plasmapheresis for fulminant meningococcemia. *Pediatr Infect Dis J* 8:399–400, 1989.

Emparanza JI, Aldamiz-Echevarria L, Perez-Yarza G, et al: Prognostic score in acute meningococcemia. *Crit Care Med* 16:168–169, 1988.

Fourrier F, Lestavel P, Chopin C, et al: Meningococcemia and purpura fulminans in adults: Acute deficiencies of proteins C and S and early treatment with antithrombin III concentrates. *Intensive Care Med* 16:121–124, 1990.

Ikeda C, Capozzi A: Management of skin loss in meningococcal infection. *Ann Plast Surg* 19:375–377, 1987.

Jacobsen ST, Crawford AH: Amputation following meningococcemia: A sequela to purpura fulminans. *Clin Orthop* 185:214–219, 1984.

Kingston ME, Mackey D: Skin clues in the diagnosis of life-threatening infections. *Rev Infect Dis* 8:1–11, 1986.

Powars DR, Rogers ZR, Patch MJ, et al: Purpura fulminans in meningococcemia: Association with acquired deficiencies of proteins C and S. *N Engl J Med* 317:571–572, 1987. Letter to the editor.

Ramilo AC, Jackson MR, Wise RD, et al: *Mycoplasma* infection simulating acute meningococcemia. *Arch Dermatol* 119:786–788, 1983.

Rimar JM, Fox L, Goschke B: Fulminant meningococcemia in children. *Heart Lung* 14:385–391, 1985.

Schaller RT Jr, Schaller JF: Surgical management of life-threatening and disfiguring sequelae of fulminant meningococcemia. *Am J Surg* 151:553–556, 1986.

Weinmann A: Meningococcemia. *Aust Fam Phys* 19:757–759, 1990.

Pyoderma Gangrenosum

Baskin LS, Dixon C, Stoller ML, et al: Pyoderma gangrenosum presenting as Fournier's gangrene. *J Urol* 144:984–986, 1990.

Green LK, Hebert AA, Jorizzo JL, et al: Pyoderma gangrenosum and chronic persistent hepatitis. *J Am Acad Dermatol* 13:892–897, 1985.

Hay CRM, Messenger AG, Cotton DWK, et al: Atypical bullous pyoderma gangrenosum associated with myeloid malignancies. *J Clin Pathol* 40:387–392, 1987.

Holmlund DEW, Wåhlby L: Pyoderma gangrenosum after colectomy for inflammatory bowel disease: Case report. *Acta Chir Scand* 153: 73–74, 1987.

Klein JD, Biller JA, Leape LL, et al: Pyoderma gangrenosum occurring at multiple surgical incision sites. *Gastroenterology* 92:810–813, 1987.

Malkinson FD: Pyoderma gangrenosum vs. malignant pyoderma (editorial). *Arch Dermatol* 123:333–337, 1987.

Mir-Madjlessi SH, Taylor JS, Farmer RG: Clinical course and evolution of erythema nodosum and pyoderma gangrenosum in chronic ulcerative colitis: A study of 42 patients. *Am J Gastroenterol* 80: 615–620, 1985.

Rand RP, Brown GL, Bostwick J III: Pyoderma gangrenosum and progressive cutaneous ulceration. *Ann Plast Surg* 20:280–284, 1988.

Schwaegerle SM, Bergfeld WF, Senitzer D, et al: Pyoderma gangrenosum: A review. *J Am Acad Dermatol* 18:559–568, 1988.

Spiers EM, Hendrick SJ, Jorizzo JL, et al: Sporotrichosis masquerading as pyoderma gangrenosum. *Arch Dermatol* 122:691–694, 1986.

Vose JM, Armitage JO, Duggan M, et al: Pyoderma gangrenosum or cutaneous lymphoma: A difficult clinical diagnosis. *Cutis* 42:335–337, 1988.

Walling AD, Sweet D: Pyoderma gangrenosum. *AFP* 35:159–164, 1987.

Wernikoff S, Merritt C, Briggaman RA, et al: Malignant pyoderma or pyoderma gangrenosum of the head and neck? *Arch Dermatol* 123:371–375, 1987.

Staphylococcal Scalded-Skin Syndrome

Elias PM, Fritsch PO: Staphylococcal scalded-skin syndrome, in Fitzpatrick TB, Eisen AZ, Wolff K, et al (eds): *Dermatology in General Medicine,* 2d ed. New York, McGraw-Hill, 1979, pp 306–310.

Mirabile R, Weiser M, Barot LR, et al: Staphylococcal scalded-skin syndrome. *Plast Reconstr Surg* 77:752–756, 1986.

Swartz MN, Weinberg AN: Infections due to gram-positive Bacteria, in Fitzpatrick TB, Eisen AZ, Wolff K, et al (eds): *Dermatology in General Medicine,* 2d ed. New York, McGraw-Hill, 1979, pp 1426–1445.

Takiuchi I, Sasaki H, Takagi H, et al: Staphylococcal scalded-skin syndrome in an adult. *J Dermatol* 13:372–376, 1986.

Todd JK: Staphylococcal toxin syndromes. *Annu Rev Med* 36:337–347, 1985.

Stevens-Johnson Syndrome

Adunsky A, Steiner ZP, Eframian A, et al: Stevens-Johnson syndrome associated with *Mycoplasma pneumoniae* infection. *Cutis* 40:123–124, 1987.

Nunn P, Kibuga D, Gathua S, et al: Cutaneous hypersensitivity reactions due to thiacetazone in HIV-1 seropositive patients treated for tuberculosis. *Lancet* 337:627–630, 1991.

Patterson R, Dykewicz MS, Gonzales A, et al: Erythema multiforme and Stevens-Johnson syndrome: Descriptive and therapeutic controversy. *Chest* 98:331–336, 1990.

Shear NH: Diagnosing cutaneous adverse reactions to drugs. *Arch Dermatol* 126:94–97, 1990. Editorial.

Subcorneal Pustular Dermatosis

Dal Tio R, DiVito F, Salvi F: Subcorneal pustular dermatosis and IgA myeloma. *Dermatologica* 170:240–243, 1985.

Dallot A, Decazes JM, Drouault Y, et al: Subcorneal pustular dermatosis (Sneddon-Wilkinson disease) with amicrobial lymph node suppuration and aseptic spleen abscesses. *Br J Dermatol* 119:803–807, 1988.

Hashimoto T, Inamoto N, Nakamura K, et al: Intercellular IgA dermatosis with clinical features of subcorneal pustular dermatosis. *Arch Dermatol* 123:1062–1065, 1987.

Kasha EE Jr, Epinette WW: Subcorneal pustular dermatosis (Sneddon-Wilkinson disease) in association with a monoclonal IgA gammopathy: A report and review of the literature. *J Am Acad Dermatol* 19:854–858, 1988.

Kohl PK, Hartschuh W, Tilgen W, et al: Pyoderma gangrenosum followed by subcorneal pustular dermatosis in a patient with IgA paraproteinemia. *J Am Acad Dermatol* 24;325–328, 1991.

Marsden JR, Millard LG: Pyoderma gangrenosum, subcorneal pustular dermatosis and IgA paraproteinaemia. *Br J Dermatol* 114:125–129, 1986.

Murphy GM, Griffiths WAD: Subcorneal pustular dermatosis. *Clin Exp Dermatol* 14:165–167, 1989.

Roger H, Thevenet JP, Souteyrand P, et al: Subcorneal pustular dermatosis associated with rheumatoid arthritis and raised IgA: Simultaneous remission of skin and joint involvements with dapsone treatment. *Ann Rheum Dis* 49:190–191, 1990.

Saulsbury FT, Kesler RW: Subcorneal pustular dermatosis and systemic lupus erythematosus. *Int J Dermatol* 23:63–64, 1984.

Schieferstein G, Brattig N, Berg PA, et al: Subcorneal pustular dermatosis of Sneddon-Wilkinson: A long-term immunologic case study. *Arch Dermatol Res* 276:65–68, 1984.

Ündar L. Göze F, Hah MM: Subcorneal pustular dermatosis with seronegative polyarthritis. *Cutis* 42:229–232, 1988.

Venning VA, Ryan TJ: Subcorneal pustular dermatosis followed by pyoderma gangrenosum. *Br J Dermatol* 115:117–118, 1986.

Sweet's Syndrome

Callen JP: Acute febrile neutrophilic dermatosis (Sweet's syndrome) and the related conditions of "bowel bypass" syndrome and bullous pyoderma gangrenosum. *Dermatol Clin* 3:153–163, 1985.

Clemmensen OJ, Menné T, Brandrup F, et al: Acute febrile neutrophilic dermatosis: A marker of malignancy? *Acta Derm Venereol (Stockh)* 69:52–58, 1989.

Sherertz EF: Pyoderma gangrenosum versus acute febrile neutrophilic dermatosis (Sweet's syndrome) (letter to editor). *Am J Med* 83:1011–1012, 1987.

Su WPD, Liu H-NH: Diagnostic criteria for Sweet's syndrome. *Cutis* 37:167–174, 1986.

T-Cell Lymphomas — Mycosis Fungoides

Barnhill RL, Braverman IM: Progression of pigmented purpura-like eruptions to mycosis fungoides: Report of three cases. *J Am Acad Dermatol* 19:25–31, 1988.

Fisher AA: Allergic contact dermatitis mimicking mycosis fungoides. *Cutis* 40:19–21, 1987.

Fox PA: Mycosis fungoides. *Br J Clin Pract* 43:458–460, 1989.

Furness PN, Goodfield MJ, Maclennan KA, et al: Severe cutaneous reactions to captopril and enalalpril: Histological study and comparison with early mycosis fungoides. *J Clin Pathol* 39:902–907, 1986.

Hawkins KA, Schinella R, Schwartz M, et al: Simultaneous occurrence of mycosis fungoides and Hodgkin disease: Clinical and histologic correlations in three cases with ultrastructural studies in two. *Am J Hematol* 14:355–362, 1983.

Klapman MH: Cutaneous diseases preceding diagnoses of lymphoreticular malignancies. *J Am Acad Dermatol* 20:583–586, 1989.

Lawrence CM, Marks JM, Burridge A, et al: The nature of mycosis fungoides. *Q J Med* 58:281–293, 1986.

Lazar AP, Caro WA, Roenigk HH Jr, et al: Parapsoriasis and mycosis fungoides: The Northwestern University experience, 1970 to 1985. *J Am Acad Dermatol* 21:919–923, 1989.

McFadden NC: Mycosis fungoides: Unsolved problems of diagnosis and choice of therapy. *Int J Dermatol* 23:523–530, 1984.

Neill SM, DuVivier A: A case of mycosis fungoides mimicking actinic reticuloid. *Br J Dermatol* 113:497–500, 1985.

Neuman K: Blue polka dots: An unusual presentation of mycosis fungoides. *Cutis* 33:373–374, 1984.

Patel SP, Holtermann OA: Mycosis fungoides: An overview. *J. Surg Oncol* 22:221–227, 1983.

Payne CM, Nagle RB, Lynch PJ: Quantitative electron microscopy in the diagnosis of mycosis fungoides: A simple analysis of lymphocytic nuclear convolutions. *Arch Dermatol* 120:63–75, 1984.

Rosen ST, Gore R, Brennan J, et al: Evaluation of computed tomography and radionuclide scanning in the staging of cutaneous T-cell lymphoma. *Arch Dermatol* 122:884–886, 1986.

Sarnoff DS, DeFeo CP: Coexistence of pemphigus foliaceus and mycosis fungoides. *Arch Dermatol* 121:669–672, 1985.

Sausville EA, Eddy JL, Makuch RW, et al: Histopathologic staging at initial diagnosis of mycosis fungoides and the Sézary syndrome: Definition of three distinctive prognostic groups. *Ann Intern Med* 109:372–382, 1988.

Simon GT: The value of morphometry in the ultrastructural diagnosis of mycosis fungoides. *Ultrastruct Pathol* 11:687–691, 1987.

Slevin NJ, Blair V, Todd IDH: Mycosis fungoides: Response to therapy and survival patterns in 85 cases. *Br J Dermatol* 116:47–53, 1987.

Tosca AD, Varelzidis AG, Economidou J, et al: Mycosis fungoides: Evaluation of immunohistochemical criteria for the early diagnosis of the disease and differentiation between stages. *J Am Acad Dermatol* 15:237–245, 1986.

Ward PE: Podiatric considerations in mycosis fungoides. *J Am Podiatr Med Assoc* 78:572–576, 1988.

Welykyj S, Gradini R, Nakao J, et al: Carbamazepine-induced eruption histologically mimicking mycosis fungoides. *J Cutan Pathol* 17:111–116, 1990.

Yamamura T, Aozasa K, Sano S: The cutaneous lymphomas with convoluted nucleus: Analysis of thirty-nine cases. *J Am Acad Dermatol* 10:796-803, 1984.

T-Cell Lymphomas—Sézary Type

Buechner SA, Winkelmann RK: Sézary syndrome: A clinicopathologic study of 39 cases. *Arch Dermatol* 119:979–986, 1983.

Burg G, Kaudewitz P: Where are we today in the diagnosis of cutaneous lymphoma? *Curr Prob Dermatol* 19:90–114, 1990.

Duangurai K, Piamphongsant T, Himmungnan T: Sézary cell count in exfoliative dermatitis. *Int J Dermatol* 27:248–252, 1988.

Ikai K, Uchiyama T, Maeda M, et al: Sézary-like syndrome in a 10-year-old girl with serologic evidence of human T-cell lymphotrophic virus type I infection. *Arch Dermatol* 123:1351–1355, 1987.

Scheman AJ, Steinberg I, Taddeini L: Abatement of Sézary syndrome lesions following treatment with acyclovir. *Am J Med* 80:1199–1202, 1986.

Sheehan-Dare RA, Goodfield MJD, Williamson DM, et al: Ulceration of the palms and soles: An unusual feature of cutaneous T-cell lymphoma. *Acta Derma Venereol (Stockh)* 70:523–525, 1990.

Sentis HJ, Willemze R, Scheffer E: Histopathologic studies in Sézary syndrome and erythrodermic mycosis fungoides: A comparison with benign forms of erythroderma. *J Am Acad Dermatol* 15:1217–1226, 1986.

Yamada M, Takigawa M, Iwatsuki K, et al: Adult T-cell leukemia/lymphoma and cutaneous T-cell lymphoma: Are they related? *Int J Dermatol* 28:107–113, 1989.

Toxic Epidermal Necrolysis

Carmichael AJ, Tan CY: Fatal toxic epidermal necrolysis associated with cotrimoxazole (letter to editor). *Lancet* 2:808 809, 1989.

Chan H-L, Stern RS, Arndt KA, et al: The incidence of erythema multiforme, Stevens-Johnson syndrome, and toxic epidermal necrolysis. *Arch Dermatol* 126:43–47, 1990.

Dan M, Jedwab M, Peled M, et al: Allopurinol-induced toxic epidermal necrolysis. *Int J Dermatol* 23:142–144, 1984.

Dolan PA, Flowers FP, Araujo OE, et al: Toxic epidermal necrolysis. *J Emerg Med* 7:65–69, 1989.

Fritsch PO, Elias PM: Toxic epidermal necrolysis, in Fitzpatrick TB, Eisen AZ, Wolff K, et al (eds): *Dermatology in General Medicine*, 2d ed. New York, McGraw-Hill, 1979, pp 303–306.

Goldstein SM, Wintroub BW, Elias PM, et al: Toxic epidermal necrolysis: Unmuddying the waters (editorial). *Arch Dermatol* 123:1153–1156, 1987.

Halebian PH, Shires GT: Burn unit treatment of acute, severe exfoliating disorders. *Annu Rev Med* 40:137–147, 1989.

Hannah Ba, Kimmel PL, Dosa S, et al: Vancomycin-induced toxic epidermal necrolysis. *South Med J* 83:720–722, 1990.

Kelly DF, Hope DG: Fatal phenytoin-related toxic epidermal necrolysis: Case report. *Neurosurgery* 25:976–978, 1989.

Lyell A: Requiem for toxic epidermal necrolysis (letter to editor). *Br J Dermatol* 122:837–838, 1990.

Nadna A, Kaur S: Drug-induced toxic epidermal necrolysis in developing countries (letter to editor). *Arch Dermatol* 126:125, 1990.

Pietrantonio F, Moriconi L, Torino F, et al: Unusual reaction to chlorambucil: A case report. *Cancer Lett* 54:109–111, 1990.

Rasmussen JE: Causes, diagnosis, and management of toxic epidermal necrolysis. *Compr Ther* 16:3–6, 1990.

Revuz J, Penso D, Roujeau J-C, et al: Toxic epidermal necrolysis: Clinical findings and prognosis factors in 87 patients. *Arch Dermatol* 123:1160–1165, 1987.

Roujeau J-C, Chosidow O, Saiag P, et al: Toxic epidermal necrolysis (Lyell syndrome). *J Am Acad Dermatol* 23:1039–1058, 1990.

Roujeau J-C, Guillaume J-C, Fabre J-P, et al: Toxic epidermal necrolysis (Lyell syndrome): Incidence and drug etiology in France, 1981–1985. *Arch Dermatol* 126:37–42, 1990.

Small RE, Garnett WR: Sulindac-induced toxic epidermal necrolysis. *Clin Pharm* 7:766–771, 1988.

Solinas A, Cottoni F, Tanda F, et al: Toxic epidermal necrolysis in a patient affected by mixed essential cryoglobulinemia. *J Am Acad Dermatol* 18:1165–1169, 1988.

Stern RS, Chan H-L: Usefulness of case report literature in determining drugs responsible for toxic epidermal necrolysis. *J Am Acad Dermatol* 21:317–322, 1989.

Tuggle DD, Smith SH: Toxic epidermal necrolysis: Recognition and treatment. *J Enterostomal Ther* 17:208–211, 1990.

Whittington RM: Toxic epidermal necrolysis and co-trimoxazole (letter to editor). *Lancet* 2:574, 1989.

Urticaria

Burdick AE, Mathias CGT: The contact urticaria syndrome. *Dermatol Clin* 3:71–84, 1985.

Geller M: Cold-induced cholinergic urticaria: Case report. *Ann Allergy* 63:29–30, 1989.

Kivity S, Schwartz Y, Wolf R, et al: Systemic cold-induced urticaria: Clinical and laboratory characterization. *J Allergy Clin Immunol* 85:52–54, 1990.

Shaw DW, Hocking W, Ahmed AR: Generalized cutaneous mastocytosis and acute myelogenous leukemia. *Int J Dermatol* 22:109–112, 1983.

Smith ML, Orton PW, Chu H, et al: Photochemotherapy of dominant, diffuse, cutaneous mastocytosis. *Pediatr Dermatol* 7:251–255, 1990.

Tarvainen K, Salonen J-P, Kanerva L, et al: Allergy and toxicodermia from shiitake mushrooms. *J Am Acad Dermatol* 24:64–66, 1991.

Witkowski JA, Parish LC: Scabies: A cause of generalized urticaria. *Cutis* 33:277–279, 1984.

Vasculitis

Francès C, Boisnic S, Blétry O, et al: Cutaneous manifestations of Takayasu arteritis: A retrospective study of 80 cases. *Dermatologica* 181:266–272, 1990.

Pun YLW, Barraclough DRE, Muirden KD: Leg ulcers in rheumatoid arthritis. *Med J Aust* 153:585–587, 1990.

Viral Exanthems

Cherry JD: Viral exanthems. *Curr Probl Pediatr* 13:1–44, 1983.

Rouchouse B, Bonnefoy M, Pallot B, et al: Acute generalized exanthematous pustular dermatitis and viral infection. *Dermatologica* 173:180–184, 1986.

Schwartz RA, Jordan MC, Rubenstein DJ: Bullous chickenpox. *J Am Acad Dermatol* 9:209–212, 1983.

I|N|D|E|X

Page numbers in boldface refer to the major discussion of description of diseases; *t* indicates tables.